HOSPITAL MEDICINE
Just the Facts

Editors

Sylvia C. McKean, MD, FACP

Medical Director, Brigham and Women's Academic Hospitalist Service
Associate Professor of Medicine
Harvard Medical School
Boston, Massachusetts

Adrienne L. Bennett, MD, PhD

Director, Division of Hospital Medicine
Associate Professor of Clinical Medicine
The Ohio State University College of Medicine
Columbus, Ohio

Lakshmi K. Halasyamani, MD

Vice President, Quality and Systems Improvement
Saint Joseph Mercy Health System
Ann Arbor, Michigan

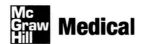

New York   Chicago   San Francisco   Lisbon   London   Madrid
Mexico City   Milan   New Delhi   San Juan   Seoul
Singapore   Sydney   Toronto

1 2 3 4 5 6 7 8 9 0   QPDQPD   12 11 10 9 8

ISBN 978-0-07-146395-9
MHID 0-07-146395-X

This book was set in Times Roman by International Typesetting and Composition.
The editor was James F. Shanahan.
The production supervisor was Phil Galea.
Project management was provided by Sam RC, International Typesetting and Composition.
Quebecor World Dubuque was printer and binder.

This book is printed on acid-free paper.

NOTICE

Cataloging-in-Publication data for this title is on file at the Library of Congress.

Science can never be a closed book. It is like a tree, ever growing, ever reaching new heights. Occasionally the lower branches, no longer giving nourishment to the tree, slough off. We should not be ashamed to change our methods; rather we should be ashamed never to do so.
— Charles V. Chapin (1856–1941)

This book is dedicated to the multidisciplinary teams of professionals who work every day to transform the hospital setting for our patients and families.

CONTENTS

Contributors   xi
Foreword   xix
Acknowledgments   xxiii

Section 1
THE HOSPITALIST MOVEMENT

1 Hospital Medicine in the United States: Growth,
       Prevalence, and Challenges
       Winthrop F. Whitcomb   1
2 The Role of the Hospitalist as Defined in the Core
       Competencies in Hospital Medicine
       Daniel D. Dressler   3
3 Innovative New Roles in the Hospital
       Lance Rachelefsky and Sylvia C. McKean   7

Section 2
SYSTEMS—HOSPITALISTS AS LEADERS
IN PATIENT SAFETY

4 General Overview of Patient Safety
       Sylvia C. McKean and Allan Frankel   13
5 Adverse Drug Events   *Frank Federico*   21
6 Medication Discrepancies and Medication
       Reconciliation   *Jeffrey L. Schnipper*   24
7 Polypharmacy   *Jatin K. Dave and
       Juergen Bludau*   30
8 Patient Safety: Preventing and Responding
       to Adverse Events   *Allen Kachalia and
       Tejal K. Gandhi*   36

Section 3
QUALITY IMPROVEMENT

9   Quality Improvement for the Hospitalist
Lakshmi K. Halasyamani and Erin R. Stucky   41

Section 4
HOSPITALIST AS MANAGER

10   Management for Hospitalists
Michael Friedlander and Mohammad Salameh   47

Section 5
HOSPITALISTS AND CARE TRANSITIONS AND TEAMWORK

11   Principles of Good Teamwork   *Janet Nagamine*   53
12   Strategies to Optimize Length of Stay
Kathleen M. Finn   57
13   Handoffs   *Vineet Arora and Julie Johnson*   62
14   Discharge Summaries   *Marcy G. Carty and Namita S. Mohta*   68
15   Patient Education in the Hospital   *Marie Neaton*   72
16   Managing Test Results at Hospital Discharge
Christopher L. Roy   76

Section 6
EVIDENCE-BASED MEDICINE

17   An Introduction to Evidence-Based Medicine
Eduardo Ortiz   81
18   Evidence-Based Medicine—Testing
Sylvia C. McKean and Eduardo Ortiz   91
19   The Growing Importance of Cost-Effectiveness
Analysis in Managing Hospitalized Patients
Jerome Lewis Avorn   96
20   Hospitalist As Researcher   *LeRoi Hicks*   99

Section 7
HOSPITALIST CLINICAL CORE COMPETENCIES
Cardiovascular Illness

21   Chest Pain   *Timothy D. Brennan*   105
22   Suspected Angina   *Aaron S. Wenger*   112
23   Acute Coronary Syndromes   *Hacho Bohossian*   120
24   Advanced Cardiac Life Support   *Apoor Patel*   127
25   Atrial Fibrillation and Atrial Flutter
Robert D. Winslow   129

26 Supraventricular Tachycardia   *Mara Giattina*   137

27 Sinus Bradycardia and Atrioventricular Blocks
Apoor Patel   147

28 Ventricular Arrhythmias   *Beth Liston*   152

29 Heart Failure due to Diastolic Dysfunction
Colleen M. Crumlish and James C. Fang   156

30 Heart Failure due to Systolic Dysfunction
Colleen M. Crumlish and James C. Fang   159

31 Syncope   *Daniel W. Mudrick*   168

32 Hypertensive Urgencies/Emergencies
Renee Y. Meadows   174

33 Secondary Hypertension   *Renee Y. Meadows*   182

Endocrine Disorders

34 Diabetic Ketoacidosis and Hyperosmolar
Hyperglycemia   *Mohammad Salameh*   188

35 Hyperglycemia in the Critical Care Unit
A. Rebecca Daniel   194

36 Hyperglycemia in Noncritically-Ill
Hospitalized Patients   *Aditi R. Saxena
and Merri L. Pendergrass*   198

37 Hypothyroidism and Hyperthyroidism
Rachael Fawcett and Erik K. Alexander   205

Gastrointestinal Illness

38 Abdominal Pain   *Norton J. Greenberger*   211

39 Abnormal Liver Enzymes and Acute Hepatitis
Mary Ann H. Sherbondy   217

40 Cirrhosis   *Thomas M. Shehab*   220

41 Colitis and Diarrhea, Including *Clostridium
difficile*   *Marvin Ryou*   223

42 Crohn's Disease   *Jonathan Levine
and Robert Burakoff*   231

43 Ulcerative Colitis   *Scott Hande
and Robert Burakoff*   235

44 Diverticular Disease and Diverticulitis
Norton J. Greenberger   240

45 Pancreatitis   *Eric R. Schumacher*   242

46 Small Bowel Obstruction   *Lynn Wilkinson*   247

47 Upper Gastrointestinal Bleeding
Naresh T. Gunaratnam   251

48 Lower Gastrointestinal Tract Bleeding
Naresh T. Gunaratnam   256

Hematological Derangements

49 Anemia in the Hospitalized Patient
*Eric Kupersmith, Susan Coutinho McAllister,
and Alpesh Amin*   260

50 Sickle Cell Disease *Andrew D. Campbell* 263
51 Thrombocytopenia *Rovie Mesola* 268
52 Transfusion Medicine *Susan Coutinho McAllister, Eric Kupersmith, and Alpesh Amin* 272

Infectious Diseases

53 Fever of Unknown Origin
David Oxman and Harry Schrager 278
54 Bacterial Endocarditis *John J. Ross* 282
55 Community- and Hospital-Acquired UTI
John J. Ross 289
56 Hospital-Acquired Bacteremia
Danielle Scheurer 294
57 Influenza *John J. Ross* 296
58 Skin and Soft Tissue Infections
Ranjan Chowdhry and Harry M. Schrager 300
59 Viral Gastroenteritis *Harry Schrager* 308
60 Antibiotic Resistance *John J. Ross* 310

Neurologic Illness

61 Confusion: Examination and Differential
Diagnosis *Zeina Chemali* 316
62 Delirium *Jatin K. Dave, Colleen M. Crumlish, and James Rudolph* 323
63 Ischemic Stroke/Transient Ischemic Attacks
Susan L. Hickenbottom 328
64 Cerebral Hemorrhage *Galen V. Henderson* 335
65 Meningitis/Encephalitis *Susan L. Hickenbottom* 339
66 Seizure *Susan L. Hickenbottom.* 344

Psychiatric Illness

67 Assessing Capacity for Medical Decision Making
David F. Gitlin and Ajita Mathur 350
68 Behavioral Disturbances That Interfere
with Medical Care *Michelle Nichols,
Bernard Vaccaro, and David F. Gitlin* 355
69 Drug Overdose *A. Rebecca Daniel* 360
70 Management of Patients with Alcohol Abuse
Sylvia C. McKean 373
71 Management of Patients with Drug Abuse
Mohammad Salameh 379
72 Management of Suicidal Patients
*Christine K. Kim, Meghan Kolodziej,
and David F. Gitlin* 383

Pulmonary Illness/Critical Care Medicine

73 Shortness of Breath *Andrew S. Karson
and Sylvia C. McKean* 388

74 Asthma *Andrew S. Karson* 395

75 Chronic Obstructive Pulmonary Disease
Andrew S. Karson 402

76 Acute Respiratory Failure *Abigail R. Lara*
and William J. Janssen 407

77 Community-Acquired Pneumonia
Adrienne L. Bennett 412

78 Hospital-Acquired, Ventilator-Associated
and Healthcare-Acquired Pneumonia
Nathan J. O'Dorisio 422

79 Complications of Pneumonia *Karen Catignani* 426

80 Sepsis and Septic Shock *William J. Janssen* 432

81 Ventilatory Support *Joshua J. Solomon,*
Ryan McGhan, and William J. Janssen 438

Renal Illness

82 Prevention of Acute Renal Failure in the Hospital
Glen M. Kim 446

83 Acute Renal Failure *Prabhdeep Sandhu*
and Adam C. Schaffer 452

84 Chronic Kidney Disease *Li-Li Hsiao*
and Valerie Luyckx 458

85 Care of the Hospitalized Dialysis Patient
J. Kevin Tucker 464

86 Acid-Base Disorders *David V. Gugliotti* 469

87A Disorders of Sodium and Water
Kambiz Zandi-Nejad and Chin C. Tang 477

87B Disorders of Potassium
Kambiz Zandi-Nejad and Chin C. Tang 484

Venous Thromboembolism

88 Prevention of Venous Thromboembolism
in Medical and Surgical Patients
Sylvia C. McKean 494

89 Venous Thromboembolism *Amir Jaffer*
and Franklin Michota 501

90 Anticoagulant Therapies *Rosalyn M. Nazaria*
and Michael Laposata 506

Section 8
HOSPITALISTS AS EXPERTS

91 Deconditioning *Joanne Borg-Stein*
and Claudia Wheeler 515

92 Nutrition and the Hospitalized Patient
Vihas Patel and Malcolm K. Robinson 520

93 Pain Management *Darin J. Correll* 527

94   Palliative Care: Overview and Symptom Management
         Jane deLima Thomas and David F. Giansiracusa   539
95   Palliative Care: Caring for the Dying Patient
         David F. Giansiracusa and Jane deLima Thomas   545
96   Palliative Care: Communication
         David F. Giansiracusa and Jane deLima Thomas   549

Section 9
HOSPITALISTS CARING FOR SPECIAL POPULATIONS

97   Care of Vulnerable Populations   *Cheryl Clark*   557
98   Inpatient Care of the Frail Older Adult
          Anne Fabiny   563
99   Oncologic Emergencies for the Hospitalist
          Rundsarah Tahboub   569
100   Skilled Nursing Facility Care   *Darrell W. Craig*   579

Section 10
HOSPITALIST AS MEDICAL CONSULTANT

101   Preoperative Evaluation of the Patient Undergoing
          Noncardiac Surgery   *Satyen S. Nichani*
          and Steven L. Cohn   585
102   Perioperative Medication Management
          Vibhu Sharma and Steven L. Cohn   592
103   Preoperative Screening Tests
          Ali Azarm and Steven L. Cohn   599
104   Postoperative Complications
          Danielle Scheurer and Cregg Ashcraft   604
105   Surgical Comanagement   *Shaun Frost*   611

Section 11
HOSPITALIST AS TEACHER

106   Adult Learning Principles and Hospitalist
          Medicine   *Grace Huang*   615
107   Teaching Venues for the Hospitalist
          Bradley A. Sharpe   617
108   Teaching on a Team   *Cindy Lai*   621
109   Feedback and the Hospitalist   *Anjala Tess*   625
110   Scholarship and Career Development for the
          Hospitalist Clinician Educator
          Preetha Basaviah and Subha Ramani   627

Index   635

CONTRIBUTORS

Erik K. Alexander, MD, Assistant Professor of Medicine, Division of Endocrinology, Director, Medical Student Education, Harvard Medical School, Boston, Massachusetts

Alpesh Amin, MD, MBA, FACP, Professor and Chief, Division of General Internal Medicine, Executive Director, Hospitalist Program, Vice Chair for Clinical Affairs and Quality, Department of Medicine, Associate Program Director, Internal Medicine Residency, University of California, Irvine Medical School, Irvine, California

Vineet Arora, MD, MA, Assistant Professor, Department of Medicine, Assistant Dean, Pritzker School of Medicine, Associate Program Director, Internal Medicine Residency, University of Chicago, Chicago, Illinois

Cregg Ashcraft, MD, Assistant Professor of Clinical Medicine, Division of Hospital Medicine, Department of Internal Medicine, The Ohio State University Medical Center, Columbus, Ohio

Jerome Lewis Avorn, MD, Professor of Medicine, Chief, Division of Pharmacoepidemiology and Pharmacoeconomics, Brigham and Women's Hospital, Harvard Medical School, Boston, Massachusetts

Ali Azarm, MD, Clinical Assistant Professor of Medicine, Department of Medicine, Kings County Hospital Center, SUNY Downstate, Brooklyn, New York

Preetha Basaviah, MD, Clinical Associate Professor, Department of Medicine, Stanford University School of Medicine, Stanford, California

Adrienne L. Bennett, MD, PhD, Director, Division of Hospital Medicine, Associate Professor of Clinical Medicine, The Ohio State University College of Medicine, Columbus, Ohio

Juergan Bludau, MD, Clinical Instructor, Chief, Division of Aging, Brigham and Women's Hospital, Harvard Medical School, Boston, Massachusetts

Hacho Bohossian, MD, Assistant Professor of Medicine, Hospital Medicine, Department of Medicine, Newton-Wellesley Hospital, Tufts Medical School, Boston, Massachusetts

Joanne Borg-Stein, MD, Assistant Professor, Chief of Physical Medicine and Rehabilitation (PMR), Medical Director, NWH Spine Center, Spaulding-Wellesley, Harvard Medical School, Boston, Massachusetts

Timothy Brennan, MD, Clinical Assistant Professor, Division of Hospital Medicine, Department of Internal Medicine, The Ohio State University Medical Center, Columbus, Ohio

Robert Burakoff, MD, PhD, Professor of Medicine, Clinical Chief, GI Division, Brigham and Women's Hospital, Harvard Medical School, Boston, Massachusetts

Andrew Campbell, MD, Clinical Assistant Professor, Division of Pediatric Hematology/Oncology, Department of Pediatrics and Communicable Diseases, Women's Hospital, University of Michigan Medical Center, Ann Arbor, Michigan

Marcy Carty, MD, MPH, Clinical Instructor, Senior Consultant, Center for Clinical Excellence, Brigham and Women's Academic Hospitalist Service, Division of General Internal Medicine, Harvard Medical School, Boston, Massachusetts

Karen Catignani, MD, Clinical Assistant Professor, Division of Hospital Medicine, Department of Internal Medicine, The Ohio State University Medical Center, Columbus, Ohio

Zeina Chemali, MD, Director, Neuropsychiatry Group, Director, Neuropsychiatry Fellowship Department Medical Director, Division of Cognitive and Behavioral Neurology, Brigham and Women's Hospital, Harvard Medical School, Boston, Massachusetts

Ranjan Chowdhry, MD, Fellow, Department of Infectious Diseases and Immunology, UMass Memorial Medical Center, University of Massachusetts Medical School, Worcester, Massachusetts

Cheryl Clark, MD, PhD, Clinical Instructor of Medicine, Brigham and Women's Academic Hospitalist Service, Division of General Internal Medicine, Harvard Medical School, Boston, Massachusetts

Steven L. Cohn, MD, FACP, Chief, Division of General Internal Medicine, Director. Medical Consultation Service, Clinical Professor of Medicine, SUNY Downstate, Brooklyn, NY

Darin J. Correl, MD, Clinical Instructor in Anesthesia, Director, Postoperative Care Pain Service, Department of Anesthesiology, Brigham and Women's Hospital, Harvard Medical School, Boston, Massachusetts

Darrell W. Craig, MD, Director of Palliative Care, Department of Internal Medicine, Saint Joseph Mercy Health System, Ann Arbor, Michigan

Colleen Crumlish, MD, Clinical Instructor, Brigham and Women's Academic Hospitalist Service, Division of General Internal Medicine, Harvard Medical School, Boston, Massachusetts

A. Rebecca Daniel, MD, Hospitalist, Department of Internal Medicine, Saint Joseph Mercy Hospital, Ann Arbor, Michigan

Jatin Dave, MD, Clinical Instructor in Medicine, Division of Aging, Brigham and Women's Hospital, Harvard Medical School, Boston, Massachusetts

Daniel D. Dressler, MD, MSc, Assistant Professor of Medicine, Hospitalist Medical Director, Emory University Hospital, Emory Medical School, Atlanta, Georgia

Anne Fabiny, MD, Assistant Professor, Chief of Geriatrics, Cambridge Health Alliance, Harvard Medical School, Boston, Massachusetts

James Fang, MD, Associate Professor of Medicine, Associate Director for Clinical Affairs, Medical Director of Heart Failure, Transplant, and Circulatory Assistance, University Hospitals, Case Western Reserve School of Medicine, Cleveland, Ohio

Rachel Fawcett, MD, Clinical and Research Fellow, Division of Endocrinology, Brigham and Women's Hospital, Harvard Medical School, Boston, Massachusetts

Frank Federico, Content Director, Institute for Healthcare Improvement, Cambridge, Massachusetts

Kathleen M. Finn, MD, Clinical Instructor, Associate Director, Clinician Educator Service, Massachusetts General Hospital, Harvard Medical School, Boston, Massachusetts

Allan Frankel, MD, Faculty, Institute of Health Improvement, Principal, Lotus Forum, Division of General Internal Medicine, Brigham and Women's Hospital, Harvard Medical School, Boston, Massachusetts

Michael Friedlander, MD, Hospitalist, Department Chair, Internal Medicine, Saline Hospital, Saline, Michigan

Shaun D. Frost, MD, Regional Medical Director, Cogent Healthcare, Nashville, Tennessee

Tejal K. Gandhi, MD, Assistant Professor of Medicine, Executive Director, Quality and Safety, Brigham and Women's Hospital, Harvard Medical School, Boston, Massachusetts

Maria Giattina, MD, Fellow, Division of Cardiology, Brigham and Women's Hospital, Harvard Medical School, Boston, Massachusetts

David F. Giansiracusa, MD, FACP, Co-Director, Center for Pain and Palliative Care, Maine Medical Center, Portland, Maine

David Gitlin, MD, Assistant Professor of Psychiatry, Department of Psychiatry, Director, Division of Medical Psychiatry, Brigham and Women's and Faulkner Hospitals, Harvard Medical School, Boston, Massachusetts

Norman Greenberger, MD, Clinical Professor of Medicine, Senior Physician, GI Division, Brigham and Women's Hospital, Harvard Medical School, Boston, Massachusetts

David Gugliotti, MD, Clinical Assistant Professor of Medicine, Department of Hospital Medicine, Cleveland Clinic, Cleveland Clinic Lerner College of Medicine of Case Western University, Cleveland, Ohio

Naresh T. Gunaratnam, MD, Staff Physician, Section of Gastroenterology, Saint Joseph Mercy Hospital, Ann Arbor, Michigan

Lakshmi K. Halasyamani, MD, Vice President, Quality and Systems Improvement, Saint Joseph Mercy Health System, Ann Arbor, Michigan

Scott Hande, MD, Fellow, Division of Gastroenterology, Brigham and Women's Hospital, Harvard Medical School, Boston, Massachusetts

Galen V. Henderson, MD, Assistant Professor of Neurology, Director of Critical Care and Emergency Neurology, Department of Neurology, Brigham and Women's Hospital, Harvard Medical School, Boston, Massachusetts

LeRoi Hicks, MD, MPH, Assistant Professor of Medicine, Director, Brigham and Women's Academic Hospitalist Fellowship, Division of General Internal Medicine, Harvard Medical School, Boston, Massachusetts

Susan L. Hickenbottom, MD, MPH, Staff Physician, Section of Neurology, Director, Stroke Program, Saint Joseph Mercy Health System, Ann Arbor, Michigan

Li-Li Hsiao, MD, PhD, Instructor in Medicine, Renal Division, Brigham and Women's Hospital, Harvard Medical School, Boston, Massachusetts

Grace Huang, MD, Instructor in Medicine, BIDMC Hospitalist Service, Division of General Internal Medicine, Harvard Medical School, Boston, Massachusetts

Amir Jaffer, MD, Associate Professor of Medicine, Chief, Division of Hospital Medicine, Department of Medicine, Leonard M. Miller School of Medicine, University of Miami, Miami, Florida

William J. Janssen, MD, Instructor of Medicine, Division of Pulmonary Sciences and Critical Care Medicine, University of Colorado Health Sciences Center, Denver, Colorado

Julie Johnson, MSPH, PhD, Assistant Professor, Department of Medicine, University of Chicago, Chicago, Illinois

Allen Kachalia, MD, JD, Assistant Professor of Medicine, Brigham and Women's Academic Hospitalist Service, Director of Quality, Department of Medicine, Brigham and Women's Hospital, Harvard Medical School, Boston, Massachusetts

Andrew Karson, MD, MPH, Clinical Instructor of Medicine, Director, Clinical Decision Support Unit, Center for Quality and Safety, Massachusetts General Hospital, Harvard Medical School, Boston, Massachusetts

Christine K. Kim, MD, Fellow, Department of Psychiatry, Brigham and Women's Hospital, Harvard Medical School, Boston, Massachusetts

Glenn M. Kim, MD, Clinical Instructor of Medicine, Brigham and Women's Academic Hospitalist Service, Division of General Internal Medicine, Harvard Medical School, Boston, Massachusetts

Meghan Kolodziej, MD, Fellow, Department of Psychiatry, Brigham and Women's Hospital, Harvard Medical School, Boston, Massachusetts

Eric Kupersmith, MD, Assistant Professor of Medicine, Director, Hospitalist Medicine, Cooper University Hospital, Camden, New Jersey

Cindy Lai, MD, Assistant Clinical Professor, Department of Medicine, University of California, San Francisco Medical Center, University of California, San Francisco Medical School, San Francisco, California

Michael Laposata, MD, PhD, Professor of Pathology and Medicine, Pathologist-in-chief, Department of Pathology, Vanderbilt Medical Center, Vanderbilt University School of Medicine, Nashville, Tennessee

Abigail Lara, MD, Fellow, Division of Pulmonary Sciences and Critical Care Medicine, University of Colorado Health Sciences Center, Denver, Colorado

Jonathan Levine, MD, Clinical Research Fellow, Division of Gastroenterology, Brigham and Women's Hospital, Harvard Medical School, Boston, Massachusetts

Beth Liston, MD, Assistant Professor of Medicine, Division of Hospital Medicine, Department of Internal Medicine, The Ohio State University Medical Center, Columbus, Ohio

Valerie Luyckx, MD, Assistant Professor of Medicine, Renal Division, Brigham and Women's Hospital, Harvard Medical School, Boston, Massachusetts

Ajita Mathur, MD, Fellow, Department of Psychiatry, Brigham and Women's Hospital, Harvard Medical School, Boston, Massachusetts

Susan Coutinho McAllister, MD, Assistant Professor of Medicine, Cooper University Hospital, Camden, New Jersey

Ryan McGhan, MD, Fellow, Division of Pulmonary Sciences and Critical Care Medicine, University of Colorado Health Sciences Center, Denver, Colorado

Sylvia C. McKean, MD, FACP, Associate Professor of Medicine, Medical Director, Brigham and Women's Academic Hospitalist Service, Division of General Internal Medicine, Brigham and Women's Hospital, Harvard Medical School, Boston, Massachusetts

Renee Y. Meadows, MD, FACP, Department of Hospital Medicine, Ochsner Medical Center, New Orleans, Louisiana

Rovie Mesola, MD, Clinical Assistant Professor, SUNY Downstate, University Hospital of Brooklyn, Brooklyn, New York

Franklin A. Michota, MD, Department of Hospital Medicine, Cleveland Clinic, Cleveland, Ohio

Namita S. Mohta, MD, Clinical Instructor, Clinical Consultant, Partners Health Care Business Planning, Brigham and Women's Academic Hospitalist Service, Division of General Internal Medicine, Harvard Medical School, Boston, Massachusetts

Daniel Mudrick, MD, Fellow, Division of Cardiology, Duke University Health Systems, Duke University School of Medicine, Durham, North Carolina

Janet Nagamine, MD, Hospitalist, Kaiser Permanente, Santa Clara, California

Rosalynn M. Nazarian, MD, Clinical Fellow in Pathology, Resident in Anatomic and Clinical Pathology, Massachusetts General Hospital, Harvard Medical School, Boston, Massachusetts

Marie Neaton, RN, APN, Heart Failure Program, Saint Joseph Mercy Hospital, Ann Arbor, Michigan

Satyen S. Nichani, MD, Staff Physician, Department of Internal Medicine, University of Michigan Health System, Ann Arbor, Michigan

Michelle Nichols, MD, Fellow, Department of Psychiatry, Brigham and Women's Hospital, Harvard Medical School, Boston, Massachusetts

Nathan O'Dorisio, MD, Assistant Professor of Clinical Medicine, Division of Hospital Medicine, Department of Internal Medicine, The Ohio State University Medical Center, Columbus, Ohio

Eduardo Ortiz, MD, MPH, Senior Medical Officer, Division for the Application of Research Discoveries, National Heart, Lung, and Blood Institute, National Institutes of Health, Bethesda, Maryland

David Oxman, MD, Fellow, Critical Care, Brigham and Women's Hospital, Boston, Massachusetts

Apoor Patel, MD, Fellow, Division of Cardiology, Cornell Medical Center, Cornell Medical School, New York

Vihas Patel, MD, Instructor in Surgery, Department of Surgery, Brigham and Women's Hospital, Harvard Medical School, Boston, Massachusetts

Marie Pendergrass, MD, Associate Professor of Medicine, Division of Endocrinology, Brigham and Women's Hospital, Boston, Massachusetts

Lance Rachelefsky, Administrator, Brigham and Women's Academic Hospitalist Service, Brigham and Women's Hospital, Boston, Massachusetts

Subha Ramani, MBBS, MMEd, MPH, Associate Professor of Medicine, Boston University School of Medicine, Boston, Massachusetts

Malcolm Robinson, MD, Assistant Professor of Surgery, Director, Metabolic Support, General and GI Surgery, Brigham and Women's Hospital, Harvard Medical School, Boston, Massachusetts

John Ross, MD, Clinical Instructor of Medicine, Brigham and Women's Academic Hospitalist Service, Division of General Internal Medicine, Brigham and Women's Hospital, Harvard Medical School, Boston, Massachusetts

Christopher L. Roy, MD, Assistant Professor, Associate Director, Brigham and Women's Academic Hospitalist Service, Division of General Internal Medicine, Harvard Medical School, Boston, Massachusetts

James L. Rudolph, MD, SM, Clinical Instructor, Geriatric Research Education and Clinical Center, VA Boston Healthcare System, Associate Physician, Division of Aging, Brigham and Women's Hospital, Harvard Medical School, Boston, Massachusetts

Marvin Ryou, MD, Fellow, Division of Gastroenterology, Brigham and Women's Hospital, Harvard Medical School, Boston, Massachusetts

Mohammad Salameh, MD, Associate Program Director, Internal Medicine Residency Program, Saint Joseph Mercy Hospital, Ann Arbor, Michigan

Prabhdeep Sandhu, MD, Clinical Assistant Professor of Medicine, Department of Medicine, Kings County Hospital Center, SUNY Downstate, Brooklyn, New York

Aditi R. Saxena, MD, Clinical and Research Fellow, Division of Endocrinology, Brigham and Women's Hospital, Harvard Medical School, Boston, Massachusetts

Adam Schaffer, MD, Clinical Instructor of Medicine, Director, Brigham and Women's Academic Hospitalist Medicine Consultation Service, Division of General Internal Medicine, Brigham and Women's Hospital, Harvard Medical School, Boston, Massachusetts

Danielle Scheurer, MD, MSc, Clinical Instructor of Medicine, Director, Brigham and Women's Hospital General Medical Service, Brigham and Women's Academic Hospitalist Service, Division of General Internal Medicine, Harvard Medical School, Boston, Massachusetts

Jeffrey L. Schnipper, MD, MPH, Assistant Professor of Medicine, Research Director of Brigham and Women's Academic Hospitalist Service, Division of General Internal Medicine, Harvard Medical School, Boston, Massachusetts

Eric L. Schumacher, DO, Assistant Professor of Clinical Medicine, Division of Hospital Medicine, The Ohio State University Medical Center, Columbus, Ohio

Harry Schrager, MD, Clinical Instructor in Medicine, Newton-Wellesley Hospitalist Service, Department of Medicine, Harvard Medical School, Boston, Massachusetts

Vibhu Sharma, MD, Clinical Assistant Professor, Division of Hospital Medicine, Department of Medicine, SUNY Downstate, Brooklyn, New York

Bradley A. Sharpe, MD, Assistant Clinical Professor, Assistant Chief of the Medical Service, University of California, San Francisco Department of Medicine, San Francisco, California

Mary Ann H. Sherbondy, MD, MS, Staff Physician, Division of Gastroenterology, Henry Ford Health System, Detroit, Michigan

Thomas M. Shehab, MD, Director of Research, Department of Internal Medicine, Saint Joseph Mercy Hospital, Ann Arbor, Michigan

Joshua Solomon, MD, Fellow, Division of Pulmonary Sciences and Critical Care Medicine, University of Colorado Health Sciences Center, Denver, Colorado

Erin R. Stucky, MD, Clinical Professor of Pediatrics, Rady Children's Hospital and Health Center San Diego (RCHSD), University of California San Diego, San Diego, California

Rundsarah Tahboub, MD, Medical Director, Hospital Medicine Service, Adjunct Faculty of the Grant, Family Medicine Residency Program, Grant Medical Center, Columbus, Ohio

Chin C. Tang, MD, Assistant Professor of Medicine, Division of Hospital Medicine, UMass Memorial Medical Center, University of Massachusetts Medical School, Worcester, Massachusetts

Anjala Tess, MD, Assistant Professor, Beth Israel Deaconess Medical Center Hospitalist Program, Associate Residency Program Director in Internal Medicine, Department of Medicine, Beth Israel Deaconess Medical Center, Harvard Medical School, Boston, Massachusetts

Jane Delima Thomas, MD, Clinical Instructor, Associate Director for the Harvard Palliative Medicine Fellowship Program, Division for Psycho-Oncology and Palliative Care at Dana Farber Clinical Institute, Harvard Medical School, Boston, Massachusetts

J. Kevin Tucker, MD, Assistant Professor of Medicine, Renal Division, Brigham and Women's Hospital, Harvard Medical School, Boston, Massachusetts

Bernard Vaccaro, MD, Fellow, Department of Psychiatry, Brigham and Women's Hospital, Harvard Medical School, Boston, Massachusetts

Lawrence D. Wellikson, MD, FACP, CEO, Society of Hospital Medicine, Philadelphia, Pennsylvania

Aaron S. Wenger, MD, Clinical Assistant Professor, Division of Hospital Medicine, Department of Internal Medicine, The Ohio State University Medical Center, Columbus, Ohio

Claudia Wheeler, DO, Resident Physician, Department of Physical Medicine and Rehabilitation, Spaulding Rehabilitation Hospital, Harvard Medical School, Boston, Massachusetts

Lynn Wilkinson, MD, Staff Physician, Fletcher Allen Health Care, Burlington, Vermont

Robert Winslow, MD, Staff Cardiologist, Cardiac Specialists, Fairfield, Connecticut.

Winthrop F. Whitcomb, MD, Assistant Professor of Medicine, Director, Performance Improvement, University of Massachusetts Medical School, Mercy Medical Center, Springfield, Massachusetts

Kambiz Zandi-Nejad, MD, FASN, Instructor in Medicine, Renal Division, Brigham and Women's Hospital, Harvard Medical School, Boston, Massachusetts

FOREWORD

Hospital Medicine has now become an established part of the medical landscape. Right now hospital medicine is more about promise and potential than delivering on the high expectations as our nation's hospitalists seek to define themselves and prepare for the future that is almost here. As the professional medical society for hospitalists, the Society of Hospital Medicine has been involved in defining hospital medicine. This practical book is another step in this long and important journey.

The hospital of the future will be patient centered, built on defined measurable quality, and delivered by engaged teams of health professionals, including nurses, pharmacists, case managers, and, of course, physicians. Hospitalists will need to be at the center of the reinvention of acute care, using their clinical skills, but just as importantly obtaining training in leadership, management, and systems thinking.

Hospitalists have been portrayed by some as simply replacing internists, family practitioners, and pediatricians in the inpatient setting. While this is true on the face of it, hospitalists bring so much more to the table. Certainly, hospitalists need to be the inpatient experts in the common medical conditions that acutely ill patients bring to the hospital. These clinical conditions (e.g. heart failure, pneumonia, stroke, DVT) have been defined in SHM's Core Competences for Hospital Medicine (Supplement to the Journal of Hospital Medicine, February 2006) and form the substance for this text.

Because of their focus on only inpatient care and the volume of clinical cases, hospitalists will become the inpatient experts. Already hospitalists see more admissions for CHF than cardiologists, manage more inpatient diabetics than endocrinologists, and have become the de facto experts in DVT and pulmonary embolism. As neurologists have more and more tilted their practices to outpatients, hospitalists have become the inpatient experts in stroke, dementia, delirium, and many acute neurologic syndromes. Practice does make perfect, but more to the point, hospitalists can and must be the experts in the nuances of acute care.

In my medical career as a busy internist in the "old days", it was enough to make the right diagnosis and order the correct therapy. Today's hospitalists must be aware of disease specific performance standards and participate in implementation strategies to define what will be measured. Once measured hospitalists are critical team members that will work with nurses, pharmacists, case managers, other physicians, and the hospital administration to develop and implement changes in health care work flow to improve on performance.

Hospitalists will also need to be part of the re-engineering of their hospitals. We are moving into an era of accountability where hospitals will need to be both efficient and effective and hospitalists must do their part. This will take the form of working with the hospital team to make sure all patients who need parenteral antibiotics receive them within 4 hours of coming to the hospital. Hospitalists will need to work with the Emergency Department (ED) professionals and the intensivists to make both the ED and the ICU work better and to make the flow throughout the hospital seamless and efficient.

Working with pharmacists, hospitalists need to be well versed in pharmacoeconomics, using not necessarily the least expensive therapeutic agent, but the one that has the best chance of getting the patient better quicker and keeping them out of the hospital. Working with the nurses and the case managers, hospitalists need to fashion the route to the ideal hospitalization for each inpatient they see. Where does diagnosis and therapy intersect with patient education and the important transition from inpatient to outpatient, especially in today's health care world where patients are often discharged not fully cured, but well enough to leave the hospital and the expense of inpatient care?

Hospital medicine is not limited to just replacing the traditional internist and family practitioners in the care of general medical patients. Surgeons and medical subspecialists now routinely rely on hospitalists to co-manage their patients, freeing them up to concentrate on their specialty expertise. Hospitalists need to be the experts in perioperative care, palliative and end of life care as well as certain aspects of critical care.

The time has come for a new vision of the role of the physician. We have moved from the lone ranger physician, operating as a unique individual to cure his patients. We are evolving to healthcare delivered by teams of health professionals. To assume a formative role in creating these teams, hospitalists need information and training to manage groups of hospitalists and provide leadership for other heath health professionals. Unfortunately, most of these skills are not taught in medical schools or residency programs. Yet they are essential if hospital medicine is to achieve the promise of this new specialty.

Practical books such as this one take a giant step to bringing together the current body of usable knowledge to help hospitalists succeed in this challenging environment. SHM has developed a set of Core Competencies that comprehensively defines the body of knowledge needed to be a complete hospitalist. To support this, SHM is developing web-based tools for education and to give hospitalists the resources to improve quality. SHM has also seen the need for courses on practice management and leadership to train the next generation physician leaders. We must all work together to close the knowledge gap.

There are now increased expectations for better quality outcomes, delivered in an efficient hospital setting. Those that pay for health care, the government and America's businesses, want more for their health dollar-better, predictable outcomes and accountability. Hospitalists are being asked to do things no physicians have been charged with before- saving their hospitals and insurance companies money, while making the hospital a safer and more efficient enterprise. In our roles in patient communication and palliative care and with our 24/7 presence, hospitalist work to make the hospital a kinder and gentler patient centered enterprise.

So many stakeholders- physicians, hospital executives, nurses, pharmacists, insurance companies, and patients- have grasped the potential of hospitalists to be a force of improvement at their hospitals and this ahs fueled the growth of hospital medicine, which has been nothing short of remarkable. Today more than half of the nation's hospitals have hospitalists working to improve health care. Soon there will be hospitalists at most if not all hospitals. They will be called upon to play a significant role in improving the health of their patients and leading their institutions into the future.

Hospitalists bring the enthusiasm and energy to take this on. Hospitalists need to rely on books like this one for up to date information designed to help them succeed. SHM will do our part to provide additional resources specific to hospitalists. Together we will supply our nation's hospitalists with the tools and resources to do the difficult, but necessary and rewarding job ahead.

Laurence D. Wellikson, MD, FACP
Chief Executive Officer
Society of Hospital Medicine

ACKNOWLEDGMENTS

Our special thanks to all the expert reviewers listed here.

Rebecca Barron, MD
Brigham and Women's Hospital
Division of Pulmonary and Critical Care
Boston, MA
Chapter 74, *Asthma*
Chapter 75, *Chronic Obstructive Lung Disease*

David C. Brooks, MD
Director of Minimally Invasive Surgery
Brigham and Women's Hospital
Boston, MA
Chapter 46, *Small Bowel Obstruction*

David F Giansiracusa, MD, FACP
Co-Director, Center for Pain and Palliative
  Care
Maine Medical Center
Portland, ME
Chapter 93, *Pain Management*

J. Roessner
Senior Writer
Institute for Healthcare Improvement
Cambridge, MA
Chapter 4, *General Overview of Patient Safety*

John Ross, MD
Hospitalist, infectious disease specialist
Brigham and Women's Academic Hospitalist
  Service
Brigham and Women's Hospital
Boston, MA
Chapter 41, *Colitis and Diarrhea, including
  Clostridium difficle*
Chapter 53, *Fever of Unknown Origin*
Chapter 56, *Hospital-acquired Bacteremia*
Chapter 58, *Skin and Soft Tissue Infections*
Chapter 59, *Viral Gastroenteritis*
Chapter 65, *Meningits/encephalitis*
Chapter 78, *Hospital-Acquired, Ventilator-
  Associated and Healthcare-Acquired
  Pneumonia*

Section 1
THE HOSPITALIST MOVEMENT

1 HOSPITAL MEDICINE IN THE UNITED STATES: GROWTH, PREVALENCE, AND CHALLENGES

Winthrop F. Whitcomb

KEY FACTORS IN THE GROWTH OF HOSPITALISTS—1990s

- The US hospitalist movement began in earnest in 1996.
- In 1999, the Society of Hospital Medicine defined hospitalists as "physicians whose primary professional focus is the general medical care of hospitalized patients. The position may involve patient care, teaching, research, or administration."[1]
- For many years prior to 1996, there were small numbers of hospitalists—though the name was not in widespread use—practicing in various parts of the country.
- Two major events ignited the growth of hospitalists and can be identified as the beginning of the US "Hospitalist Movement":
  - The appearance of "The Emerging Role of 'Hospitalists' in the American Healthcare System" in August of 1996[2]
  - The formation of the Society of Hospital Medicine in January of 1997[3]
- Drivers of the US hospitalist movement in the mid to late 1990s included[4]
  - Increased efficiency gained by dedicated inpatient physicians/providers (hospitalists)
  - Reduced length of stay (LOS) and cost per case under hospitalist care
  - Shortage of primary care physicians to care for emergency department unassigned patients requiring hospitalization
  - Surgeons' declining interest in general perioperative and nonoperative care
  - Increasing acuity of patient illness in the hospital and outpatient settings
  - Increasing challenges for physicians in mastering both inpatient and outpatient knowledge
  - Payers' demands for careful utilization of hospital resources
  - Primary physicians' departure from the hospital because of lifestyle concerns
  - Poor physician reimbursement for hospital care

GROWTH OF HOSPITALISTS—2000–PRESENT

- As of 2007, there are an estimated 20,000 hospitalists in the United States. The growth rate remains explosive, with hospitalists prevalent at both academic and community hospitals, regardless of size. The American Hospital Association 2005 Survey of US hospitals indicates that:
  - Forty percent of 4936 US hospitals have hospitalists on staff (20% growth since 2004).
  - For hospitals with 200 or more beds, 70% have hospitalists on staff.
  - On average, there are 8.3 physician hospitalists per hospital.
- The major causes of the growth of hospital medicine in the 1990s remain in effect today; however, a number of factors have emerged or intensified. Drivers of hospitalist growth from 2000–present include
  - Mounting pressures on primary care physicians are driving them to focus solely on office care (recruitment challenges, practice overhead [including malpractice costs], stagnant reimbursement, growing regulatory burdens, career dissatisfaction, the demand for sustainable work-life balance, explosion of medical information)

- Patient throughput challenges in hospitals
- Reduction in resident work hours causing the growth of hospitalist-managed "uncovered" services in academic medical centers
- The need for physician engagement in hospital quality, patient safety, and system improvement
- The legitimization of hospital medicine as a bona fide specialty
- The attractiveness of the hospital medicine career to physicians in training and those practicing traditional primary care
- The growing number of underinsured

- Hospital medicine remains a young field, with hospitalists practicing for a relatively short tenure, and trained predominantly as generalists. Key attributes of hospitalists are
  - Median age: 37 (40% 35 years old or younger, <10% more than 50 years old)
  - US medical graduates: 75%
  - Years as a hospitalist: 3
  - Generalists (internal medicine/pediatrics/family practice): 96% (in 1997 only 51%)
- The majority of hospitalists are internists; however, an important element of hospital medicine is derived from pediatricians. Training background of hospitalists:[5]
  - General internal medicine: 79%
  - Subspecialty internal medicine: 3%
    - Total internal medicine: 82%
  - Pediatrics: 12%
  - Medicine pediatrics: 3%
  - Family practice: 3%

EFFICACY OF HOSPITALIST SYSTEMS: EFFECTS ON COST, PATIENT SATISFACTION, AND QUALITY

- As of 2002
  - Fifteen of nineteen published studies[6] found significant decreases in hospital costs (avg. 13.4%) and LOS (avg. 16.6%)
  - Two of nineteen studies showed decreases in LOS but not cost; two showed no decrease in cost or LOS
  - Five studies showed satisfaction preserved under hospitalists vs. traditional pneumocystis carinii pneumonias (PCPs) (no reports of lower satisfaction)
- A number of studies since then have confirmed the effect on cost savings and LOS reduction under hospitalist versus traditional hospital care.[7,8]
- Based on these data, it can be concluded that hospitalist care results in cost savings and LOS reduction when compared to traditional hospital care.
- The data on patient satisfaction are not robust enough to draw definitive conclusions. However, patient

TABLE 1-1 Peer-Reviewed Publications Demonstrating a Mortality Benefit to Hospitalist Care

- Meltzer D et al. *Ann Intern Med.* 2002;137:866–874.
  - 6511 patients studied prospectively between 1997 and 1999
  - Year 2, mortality 4.2% for hospitalist vs. 6.0% nonhospitalists ($P = 0.04$)
  - Year 2 (LOS) ($P = 0.01$) and cost ($P = 0.01$) reduced for hospitalists vs. nonhospitalists, 0.49 day shorter and $782 less
- Auerbach A et al. *Ann Intern Med.* 2002;137:859–865.
  - 5308 patients studied retrospectively more than 2 years
  - Over study period, risk of death lower for patients under hospitalist care (adjusted relative hazard 0.71) and at 30 and 60 days
  - Year 2 cost ($P = 0.002$) and LOS ($P = 0.002$) decreased for hospitalists
- Tenner PA et al. *Crit Care Med.* Mar 2003;31(3):986–987.
  - Compared survival in a pediatric ICU under 24-hour hospitalist vs. traditional attending-resident coverage
  - Odds ratio of survival of 2.8 for the hospitalist vs. traditional attending-resident coverage ($P = .013$)
  - Retrospective cohort design

LOS, length of stay.

satisfaction with hospitalist care has not been shown to suffer when compared to traditional hospital care.
- There is insufficient evidence to determine whether quality of care is enhanced, unchanged, or diminished under hospitalist care when compared to traditional care.
- Table 1-1 lists three of the most prominent published studies examining mortality, each demonstrating a benefit.[9,10,11] Despite these trials, there is insufficient evidence to conclude that hospitalist care offers a definitive mortality benefit.

CHALLENGES FACING HOSPITAL MEDICINE

- Two major factors account for most of hospital medicine's important challenges:
  - The fledgling nature of the field
  - The explosive growth in number of and demand for hospitalists
- Top challenges for hospitalist programs: survey of 396 lead hospitalists (each respondent chose 3 categories)[5]:
  - Work hours/work life balance: 42%
  - Recruitment: 35%
  - Daily workload: 29%
  - Expectations/demand from hospital: 23%
  - Reimbursement and collections: 17%
  - Professional respect and job satisfaction: 17%
  - Career sustainability: 15%
  - Retention: 15%
  - Quality of care/quality indicators: 13%
  - Specialist availability for consultation: 11%
  - Bed capacity/throughput: 11%
- A number of threats to hospital medicine exist (see Table 1-2). Most of these relate to the following elements of hospitalist career satisfaction:

TABLE 1-2   Threats to Hospital Medicine

- Lack of practice management information
- Unclear professional boundaries (Should hospitalists admit patients who traditionally were on medical subspecialty or surgical services? Should hospitalists function as nighttime "house doctors?" To what extent should hospitalists be responsible for systemic hospital problems, such as patient flow or safety?)
- Limited/outdated systems for professional reward and recognition
- Shortage of hospitalists, making recruiting hospitalists difficult
- Archaic (encounter-based) payment paradigm doesn't recognize the need hospitalized patients have for round-the-clock care
- Workloads not well-defined

○ Inadequate reward and recognition
○ Poorly defined workloads and ill-defined schedules
○ Problems with professional autonomy

LOOKING AHEAD

Hospitalists, by the very nature of their professional practice, are uniquely positioned to achieve the six specific aims for improving healthcare quality in the inpatient setting,[12] that healthcare should be:

- *Safe:* avoiding injuries to patients from the care that is intended to help them
- *Effective:* providing services based on scientific knowledge to all who could benefit and refraining from providing services to those not likely to benefit (avoiding underuse and overuse)
- *Patient centered:* providing care that is respectful of and responsive to individual patient preferences, needs, and values and ensuring that patient values guide all clinical decisions
- *Timely:* reducing waits and sometimes harmful delays for both those who receive and those who give care
- *Efficient:* avoiding waste, in particular, waste of equipment, supplies, ideas, and energy
- *Equitable:* providing care that does not vary in quality because of personal characteristics such as gender, ethnicity, geographic location, and socioeconomic status

As hospitalists strive to meet the challenges faced presented by a rapidly emerging field, these aims can provide a paradigm from which to build the inpatient care models of the future, as well as rewarding and sustainable careers as experts in the practice of hospital-based medicine.

REFERENCES

1. Society of Hospital Medicine Board of Directors. 1999 from www.hospitalmedicine.org. Accessed January 10, 2008.
2. Wachter RM, Goldman L. The emerging role of "hospitalists" in the American healthcare system. *N Engl J Med.* 1996 15;335(7):514–517.
3. Press release. February 22, 2007. Society of Hospital Medicine. Philadelphia, PA.
4. *The Prevalence and Size of The Hospitalist Workforce in 2004 American Hospital Association Survey 2004.* American Hospital Association. Chicago, IL. 2004.
5. Society of Hospital Medicine 2005–2006. *Productivity Survey.* Society of Hospital Medicine; Philadelphia, PA: 2006.
6. Wachter RM, Goldman L. The hospitalist movement 5 years later. *JAMA.* 2002 Jan 23–30;287(4):487–494.
7. Everett GD, Anton MP, Jackson BK, et al. Comparison of hospital costs and length of stay associated with general internists and hospitalist physicians at a community hospital. *Am J Manag Care.* 2004 Sep;10(9):626–630.
8. Lindenauer PK, Rothberg MB, Pekow PS, et al. Outcomes of patients treated by hospitalists, general internists, and family physicians. Abstract. Presented at the Society of Hospital Medicine Annual Meeting. Dallas, TX. May 25, 2007.
9. Meltzer D, Manning WG, Morrison J, et al. Effects of physician experience on costs and outcomes on an academic general medicine service: results of a trial of hospitalists. *Ann Intern Med.* 2002;137:866–874.
10. Auerbach AD, Wachter RM, Katz P, et al. Implementation of a voluntary hospitalist service at a community teaching hospital: improved clinical efficiency and patient outcomes. *Ann Intern Med.* 2002 Dec 31;37(11):859–865.
11. Tenner PA, Dibrell H, Taylor, RP, et al. Improved survival with hospitalists in a pediatric intensive care unit. *Crit Care Med.* 2003 Mar;31(3):986–987.
12. The Institute of Medicine. *Crossing the Quality Chasm.* Washington, DC: The National Academies Press; 2001.

2 THE ROLE OF THE HOSPITALIST AS DEFINED IN THE CORE COMPETENCIES IN HOSPITAL MEDICINE

Daniel D. Dressler

OVERVIEW

HOSPITALIST

- Hospital medicine is the fastest growing group of specialized physicians in the United States today. It is estimated that there are currently more than 15,000 practicing hospitalists in the United States, with projected workforce needs in the United States estimated to be at least 30,000 hospitalists.

- Similar to specialties of emergency medicine and critical care medicine, hospital medicine is the next "site-based" specialty.
- In 2006, the American Board of Internal Medicine (ABIM) announced the decision to develop "focused recognition for hospital medicine" as a part of ABIM's maintenance of certification process.
- According to Robert Wachter, MD, professor of medicine at the University of California, San Francisco, a board member of ABIM, and a former president of the Society of Hospital Medicine, the board's decision to pursue recognition of hospital medicine is an acknowledgment of the unique focus of hospitalists.
- Hospitalists are defined as physicians whose primary professional focus is the general medical care of hospitalized patients. Their activities include patient care, teaching, research, and leadership related to hospital medicine (www.hospitalmedicine.org).
- Hospital medicine is a specialty of physicians leading, directing, and improving inpatient care.
- Hospital medicine offers opportunities for leadership, hospital administration, education and scholarship, and even clinical concentration.
- The core competencies of any medical specialty provide the necessary framework for that specialty to develop, refine, and evolve.

CORE COMPETENCIES

- The Society of Hospital Medicine published *The Core Competencies in Hospital Medicine: A Framework for Curriculum Development* (TCC) in 2006 to help define the field, set expectations for practice, and to spur curriculum development.
- Transitional care council (TCC) provides a framework for educators at all levels of medical education to develop curricula, train, and evaluate students, clinicians-in-training, and practicing hospitalists.
- TCC intentionally does not focus on content; rather specific competencies describe unambiguous, measurable learning objectives.
- TCC standardizes the expected outcomes of train and allows curriculum developers to create timely instruction appropriate for each specific training environment.
- TCC helps define the role of hospitalists, and suggests how knowledge, skill, and attitude acquisition might be evaluated.
- TCC provides developers of curricula and content with a standardized set of measurable learning objectives, while allowing them the flexibility needed to address specific contexts and incorporate advances in medicine.

- The intended audience includes educators of students, clinicians-in-training, and practicing hospitalists.
- TCC includes the most common and fundamental elements of inpatient care without an exhaustive listing of every clinical entity that may be encountered by a hospitalist.
- TCC clarifies the role of hospitalists as teachers and innovators for directors of continuing medical education, hospitalist fellowship directors, directors of hospitalist programs, residency program directors, medical school internal medicine clerkship directors, and hospital administrators and leaders.
- TCC also clarifies the role of hospitalists for health educators, potential employers, policy makers, and agencies funding quality improvement (QI) initiatives in the hospital setting.
- TCC should guide:
  - Teaching (what and how much)
  - Assessment (how to assess trainees and practicing hospitalists)
  - Design of systems to improve care quality and assure patient safety
  - Establishment of priorities for research in hospital medicine
- TCC can also be used to facilitate career choices post training.
- TCC topics (or chapters) are divided into three sections—clinical conditions, procedures, and healthcare systems (Table 2-1)—all integral components to the practice of hospital medicine.

EDUCATIONAL OBJECTIVES

CLINICAL CONDITION COMPETENCIES

- The core clinical topics include
  - Clinical areas which hospitalists encounter on a frequent basis and for which hospitalists can affect systems and processes of care
  - Those on which hospitalists focus in the design of institutional or global quality initiatives
- The core clinical topic list (see Table 2-1) reflects
  - The top nonsurgical discharge diagnoses
  - Conditions that are encountered with significant frequency in the hospital setting (eg, urinary tract infection [UTI], pneumonia, acute coronary syndrome)
  - Conditions that may be significantly life threatening in the hospital setting (eg, cardiac arrhythmias, sepsis)
  - Topics which hospitalists are likely to have significant involvement and impact to alter or refine processes of care, leading to improvement of care quality and/or efficiency (eg, perioperative care, venous thromboembolism)

TABLE 2-1   The Core Competencies in Hospital Medicine List of Chapters

CLINICAL CONDITIONS*	PROCEDURES	HEALTHCARE SYSTEMS
Acute coronary syndrome	Arthrocentesis	Business practices
Acute renal failure	Chest radiograph interpretation	Care of the elderly patient
Alcohol and drug withdrawal	Electrocardiogram interpretation	Care of vulnerable populations
Asthma	Emergency procedures	Communication
Cardiac arrhythmia	Lumbar puncture	Diagnostic decision making
Cellulitis	Paracentesis	Equitable allocation of resources
Chronic obstructive pulmonary disease	Thoracentesis	Evidence-based medicine
Community-acquired pneumonia	Vascular access	Hospitalist as consultant
Congestive heart failure		Hospitalist as teacher
Delirium and dementia		Information management
Diabetes mellitus		Leadership
Gastrointestinal bleed		Nutrition and the hospitalized patient
Hospital-acquired pneumonia		Palliative care
Pain management		Patient education
Perioperative medicine		Patient handoff
Sepsis syndrome		Patient safety
Stroke		Pharmacoeconomics, pharmacoepidemiology, and drug safety
Urinary tract infection		Practice-based learning and improvement
Venous thromboembolism		Prevention of healthcare-associated infections and antimicrobial resistance
		Professionalism and medical ethics
		Quality improvement
		Risk management
		Team approach and multidisciplinary care
		Transitions of care

*Clinical chapter list is not a complete compilation of all inpatient clinical conditions that hospitalists may care for in the inpatient setting (www.hospitalmedicine.org)

PROCEDURE COMPETENCIES

• Procedures competencies include those inpatient procedures that hospitalists are most likely to perform or supervise in their day-to-day care of hospitalized patients.
• The individual hospital setting, including local and regional variations, determines who might perform certain procedures depending on many factors, which may include the presence of trainees, specialty support including radiology, and procedure teams.
• The procedures included are those frequently performed during the course of routine practice of hospital medicine.
• Relevant procedure competencies are expected to afford proper performance, patient education and involvement, prevention of complications, and QI with respect to each inpatient procedure.

HEALTHCARE SYSTEMS COMPETENCIES

• These competency topics delineate themes integral to the successful practice of hospital medicine in diverse hospital settings.
• Many of the system topics focus on processes and systems of care that typically span multiple disease entities, and frequently require multidisciplinary input to create a coordinated effort of care quality and efficiency.
• The healthcare systems section chapters and core competencies direct hospitalists to lead and innovate within their own hospital practices, and to convey the principles of evidence-based inpatient medical care and systems-based practice to medical students, physicians in training, other medical staff, colleagues, and patients.
• In some healthcare systems chapters, the clinical approach spans multiple clinical entities and requires an organizational approach crossing several disciplines within medicine to optimize the hospital care (eg, care of the elderly patient, infection control, and antibiotic resistance).
• Other healthcare systems topics focus on educational themes that drive the practice of hospital medicine and lifelong learning and teaching required of hospitalists (eg, evidence-based medicine, patient education).
• Other healthcare systems topics identify much of the organizational approach that must be adopted by hospitalists in order to provide high quality of care while maintaining a functional and sound practice (eg, QI, transitions of care, risk management).
• Diagnostic decision-making:

- Chapter focused on symptom evaluation and management.
- Relevant part of triage, subsequent testing, and hospital care; the ability to develop a differential diagnosis and proceed with indicated testing and its interpretation.
- Therefore no symptom chapters are found in the clinical conditions section.
- Healthcare systems chapters help characterize and delineate the practice and scope of hospital medicine, especially with topics not taught in detail during most residency training programs.

ROLES OF THE HOSPITALIST

- Hospitalists are physicians who specialize in the care of hospitalized patients.
- Hospitalists are invested in helping hospitals function as effectively and efficiently as possible.
- The practice of hospital medicine requires proficiency of inter-related aspects of practice—clinical, procedural, and system-based competencies.
- Hospitalists subscribe to a systems organizational approach to clinical management and processes of care within the hospital.
- This systems approach, more than any level of knowledge or skill, is required to effectively and efficiently practice in the hospital setting.
- Hospitalists support and adhere to a multidisciplinary approach for the patients under their care (*lead, coordinate,* or *participate*).
  - They have interaction and integration with other hospital medical staff (eg, nursing, rehabilitation therapies, social services) and specialty medical or surgical services when indicated.
  - At minimum, hospitalists should *participate* in multidisciplinary teams for the care and process improvement with respect to clinical conditions within their organization.
  - However, they may also *lead* and/or *coordinate* teams in such efforts.
- Hospitalists should participate to various degrees in QI initiatives, focusing on measuring and improving processes or systems of care within the local institution or organization.
  - The level of involvement and role in QI initiatives may vary based on the system, resources, and hospitalist experience.
- Hospitalists must have a dedicated focus on care transitions that occur with their patients.
  - Such transitions may occur as patients enter the hospital, move from one location to another within the hospital, or leave the hospital.
  - Transition from one care setting or provider to another is a vulnerable time for patients, and requires thorough communication efforts, with patients, medical staff, and outpatient clinicians.
- Educators should utilize TCC (when applicable) as a foundation as they develop curricula in hospital medicine.
  - Hospitalists who create curricula should integrate educational learning domains, cognitive domain (knowledge), the psychomotor domain (skills), and the affective domain (attitudes), into their educational model.
  - Hospitalists remain dedicated to *system organization and improvement*, an added domain that requires integration of knowledge, skills, and attitudes and involvement of other medical services and disciplines for optimal patient care.
  - Medical educators should examine the outcomes of current training practices and assess what modifications of objectives, content, and instructional strategies should be made to better prepare the current and next generation of physicians to practice hospital medicine and improve the hospital setting.
  - Educators should consider a six-step approach (described in *Curriculum Development in Medical Education*) when developing curricula:
    - A problem and a need for improvement (the actual case and quality gap)
    - Needs assessment of targeted learners (hospitalists, clinicians-in-training)
    - Goals and specific measurable objectives (with competencies bridging the gap between traditional roles and setting expectations about the hospitalist role)
    - Educational strategies (with competencies providing structure and guidance to educational efforts)
    - Implementation (applying competencies to a variety of training opportunities and curricula)
    - Evaluation and feedback (ongoing nationally, regionally, locally)
- Hospitalists should strive to improve care processes, hospital work life, and the setting in which they practice.
- Hospitalists can develop and implement systems for best practices from admission through discharge and promote a culture of safety and quality within the hospital environment.

BIBLIOGRAPHY

Dressler DD, Pistoria MJ, Budnitz TL, et al. Core competencies in hospital medicine: development and methodology. *J Hosp Med.* 2006;1:48–56.

Kern DE, et al. *Curriculum Development for Medical Education: A Six-Step Approach.* Johns Hopkins University Press; 1998.

McKean SCW, Budnitz TL, Dressler DD, et al. "How to Use *The Core Competencies in Hospital Medicine: A Framework for Curriculum Development.*" *J Hosp Med.* 2006;1:57–67.

Pistoria MJ, Amin AN, Dressler DD, et al. Core competencies in hospital medicine. *J Hosp Med.* 2006;1(supplement 1):1–95.

Wachter RM, Goldman L. The emerging role of "hospitalists" in the American healthcare system. *N Eng J Med.* 1996; 335:514–517.

Wachter RM, Goldman L. The hospitalist movement 5 years later. *JAMA.* 2002;287:487–494.

3 INNOVATIVE NEW ROLES IN THE HOSPITAL

Lance Rachelefsky and Sylvia C. McKean

BACKGROUND

- The quality and safety movement in healthcare has led to the development of increased public awareness about factors to consider when choosing their healthcare providers.
- Third-party payers and employers have already started to use a variety of quality measures and criteria to establish reimbursement schedules and incentive programs for hospitals.
- For some hospitals, their scores on externally reported performance measures may translate into significant revenue lost or gained.
- At the same time that there is increased scrutiny on healthcare quality, there is also increasing healthcare disparity.
- Individuals in minority groups comprise approximately 80% of the 46.7 million uninsured people, or roughly 18% of the entire US population.
- The increasing cost of healthcare also takes a personal toll, with roughly 50% of all bankruptcy claims reportedly stemming from medical expenditures.
- The rise in healthcare costs has also been accompanied by increased attention to resident physician work hours and fatigue, with the implementation and strict monitoring of the 80-hour workweek for trainees.
- These challenges in healthcare delivery have allowed the hospitalist to not only focus on the medical care of the hospitalized patient, but to also assume a variety of other roles in the hospital. These roles include

  ○ Hospital administrator
  ○ Teacher
  ○ Physician advisor (PA) for utilization review
  ○ Procedure service leader and/or participant
  ○ Rapid response team (RRT) leader and/or participant
  ○ Partner with the emergency department (ED)
- There are significant opportunities for studying the impact of these innovative roles on healthcare delivery. The roles of hospitalists are evolving and the increasing presence of hospitalists is the first step in changing how we provide inpatient care.
- In light of these emerging new roles, it is vitally important for hospitalist programs and hospitals to set clear goals and expectations from the outset (Table 3-1).
- Hospitalist leaders need to work with their colleagues in order to ensure that current responsibilities and future initiatives are aligned with the mission of both the program and hospital (Fig. 3-1 and Table 3-2).

HOSPITALIST AS LEADER

- Hospitalists play a key role in ensuring that the inpatient system of care flows smoothly and effectively, allowing for the safe and efficient care of hospitalized patients (see Chap. 12).
- The hospitalist may also lead volume management during times of high patient census.
- Being on the front lines of inpatient care ideally positions the hospitalist as a leader of change in the healthcare system. In addition to the management of day-to-day logistics, they may be asked to oversee redesign of hospital care delivery. Hospital administration is now a defined career path for hospitalists.
- The presence of hospitalists has changed the healthcare system. The hospitalist can help promote:
  ○ Multidisciplinary collaboration among the entire inpatient care team, with the goal of delivering safer, more efficient, and higher quality patient care (see Chap. 11).
  ○ Dissemination of evidence-based medicine to cultivate multidisciplinary teaching and lifelong learning habits for all involved, including the hospitalist (see Sec. VI).
  ○ Quality improvement through the development of protocols and standards of care and the implementation of best practices. Examples of hospitalists as drivers of quality initiatives within the hospital include
    ▪ Protocols for the prevention and management of delirium
    ▪ Venous thromboembolism prophylaxis
    ▪ Glycemic control for diabetic patients
    ▪ Initiatives focused on improving patient handoffs and medication safety

TABLE 3-1 Alignment of Priorities with Goals and Core Values

EXPECTATIONS OF HOSPITAL MANAGEMENT THAT THE HOSPITALIST SERVICES

- Care for unassigned/uncompensated patients
- Reduce ALOS for medical and possibly surgical patients
- Supply 24/7 service (beeper and/or on-site)
- Standardize care and help implement hospital-wide guidelines and protocols
- Provide attending of record coverage for palliative care, other medical specialties, selected surgical patients
- Develop additional services (comanagement consultation, preoperative testing center, anticoagulation, palliative care, RRT, procedure service)
- Improve efficiency and quality of care at the ED-hospital interface (↓ patient ED to floor times, on-site direct patient care of admitted patients in the ED, management of chest pain unit, triage of patients to appropriate services)
- Triage of patients within network to most appropriate facility
- Increase chart documentation for core quality measures (such as smoking cessation counseling)
- Optimize billing for services provided (% submitted, level of coding)

EXPECTATIONS OF EXTERNAL INTERESTS

- Reaching network performance targets
- High satisfaction of outside primary care physician and other groups referring into the network
- Compliance with JCAHO regulations
- Meeting ACGME work hour requirements for residents and fellows
- Obtaining ≥90% core measure scores on publicly reported performance measures

WORK ENVIRONMENT

- Six different quality domains: safety, effectiveness, timeliness, patient centered, efficiency, and equity (Institute of Medicine)
- Hospitalist and healthcare team career satisfaction which integrates core values
  - Service excellence and patient safety
  - Continuous quality improvement and innovation
  - Professional growth, leadership, and scholarship

THE HOSPITALIST "REPORT CARD"—A STRATEGIC FRAMEWORK FOR ACTION: AT A GLANCE

- Articulates a shared vision of what is important for strategic planning
- Aligns goals with the strategic initiatives of the hospital and hospital network
- Reflects a consensus of what will be measured and reported as well as "stretch targets"
- After the data become available over a period of time, reassessment and feedback provided, group and individual targets can be set and compensation linked to goals
- Demonstrates the value added of a hospitalist service for hospital administrators
- Identifies areas which might be targeted for improvement by hospitalist leaders
- Creates a meaningful, motivating, and achievable blueprint for clinical enterprise

ACGME, Accreditation Council for Graduate Medical Education; ALOS, average length of stay; ED, emergency department; JCAHO, Joint Commission on Accreditation of Healthcare Facilities; RRT, rapid response team.

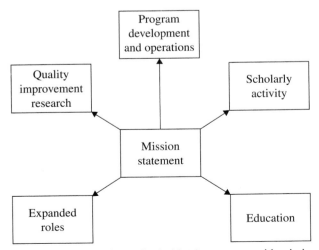

FIG. 3-1 The planning and prioritization process, with mission statement at the core.

- Hospitalists have become a crucial link in connecting the many providers a patient may have, and in this role ensure that no gaps exist across the continuum of care as a patient moves from inpatient to outpatient and extended care facilities and vice versa.

HOSPITALIST AS TEACHER

- One of the traditional teaching roles of a hospitalist is that of training the next generation of physicians, medical students and residents.
- This role has expanded to include physician assistants, nurse practitioners, and other physician extenders who have increasingly become key members of inpatient medical teams at many hospitals.
- The Accreditation Council for Graduate Medical Education (ACGME) has mandated work hour restrictions that have affected the hospitalist's role as a teacher and also the structure of clinical services,

Table 3-2   The Planning and Prioritization Process of Innovative New Roles Working Example

COMANAGEMENT WITH OTHER SERVICES

Problem	• Patient safety, satisfaction, quality issues related to traditional medical consultation service • Increasingly frail patients on other services with active medical comorbidities • Concern regarding hospitalist medical legal liability in the role of traditional medical consultant
Process of change	**Aim** • To improve patient care by leveraging a new infrastructure for success • To improve efficiency ($\downarrow$ALOS), eliminate redundancy, thereby improving resident work hours • To improve hospitalist, nursing, and patient satisfaction • To better meet ACGME educational reform (multidisciplinary teamwork) **Operations** • Explicitly state rules of "engagement" relating to multidisciplinary teamwork and respective roles • Establish treatment protocols • Delineate patient flow through the service and corresponding provider-to-provider communication at each step of the process **Finances** • Conduct regular meetings to revise "contract" as problems surface • Ensure adequate staffing, funding, and other resources • Outline procedure for billing • Build in recognition for success and incentives **Measurement** • Develop key metrics to measure the service with the goal to publish the results • PDSA throughout pilot for rapid cycle improvements • Hospitalist report card data pre- and post implementation • Daily multidisciplinary team meetings and ad hoc "huddles"
Options	• Pilot orthopedic-hospitalist surgical comanagement model • Develop other pilots involving selected surgical services • Create a new geographically organized comanagement service independent of surgical specialty • Collaborate with medical subspecialists, psychiatrists, and others to implement innovative new programs • Maintain status quo

ACGME, Accreditation Council for Graduate Medical Education; ALOS, average length of stay; PDSA, plan, do, study, act.

which some teams run without any resident physicians (see Sec. 6).

HOSPITALIST AS PHYSICIAN ADVISOR FOR UTILIZATION MANAGEMENT

• The physician advisor (PA) for utilization management role was developed to provide oversight of patients who did not meet established criteria for continued hospitalization. Typically, health plans employed PAs who would be contacted by nurse reviewers as a means to control costs (see Chap. 12).
• The PA serves as a consultant to the discharge planners and communicates with the attending physician to help resolve complex cases. The PA may also be the responsible party to determine medical necessity for care or make decisions regarding medical overrides.
• Physician override functions may include
  ○ Initial chart review by care coordinator/liaison nurse
  ○ Chart review by hospitalist PA, including review of data and communication with attending
  ○ Communication with the physician reviewer at the insurance company and review of the patient's medical issues and care plan. This communication results

in either an override of the initial denial, or delineates a plan for further information gathering which can include communication with
  ▪ The attending physician about the patient's need for on going hospitalization
  ▪ The patient about the status of his/her hospitalization
  ▪ The primary care physician about the ultimate disposition for the patient
• An effective PA role requires a structure and process as follows:
  ○ Regular utilization review meetings with case management
  ○ Availability to answer questions and as a resource when there are problems on the service relating to discharge planning
  ○ Collection of utilization review data relating to delay days as a tool to improve efficiency of care, identify waste within the system, and educate staff about alternative testing and sites of care.

RAPID RESPONSE TEAMS (RRTs)

• Hospitalists may be asked to participate in or lead RRTs to improve patient outcomes for individuals who develop a sudden change in clinical status.

- Failure to recognize or respond to a patient who has become clinically unstable outside of the intensive care unit setting may lead to greater than expected mortality.
- Resident work hour restrictions may also negatively impact on the ability of covering house staff to respond quickly and effectively to a changing clinical situation.
- University HealthSystem Consortium (UHC) benchmarking project, based on the Agency for Healthcare Research and Quality's (AHRQ's) failure to rescue metric, found wide performance variation among their members, namely, academic health centers in the United States.
  ○ UHC created an RRT database so that member healthcare centers could track key performance measures and outcomes through an online data collection tool.
- The Institute for Healthcare Improvement also posts information on its Web site including improvement stories and tools to measure changes.
  ○ Additional information: http://www.ihi.org/IHI/ Topics/CriticalCare/IntensiveCare/Tools, click "Rapid Response Teams."
- Studies are ongoing to determine if an effective RRT saves lives by bringing critical care expertise to the bedside of hemodynamically unstable patients on medical and surgical floors in a variety of settings.

PROCEDURE SERVICES

- Hospitalist services are increasingly developing procedure services as a means to improve access to important procedures.
- *TCC in Hospital Medicine* was published by the Society of Hospital Medicine to standardize the expectations for training and professional development for hospitalists and trainees. One section focuses on procedures commonly performed or supervised by hospitalists.
- *The Core Competencies in Hospital Medicine: A Framework for Curriculum Development* articulates the role of hospitalists to
  ○ Lead, coordinate, or participate in efforts to standardize how procedures are performed
  ○ Develop strategies to minimize institutional complication rates
  ○ Monitor hospitalists' and trainees' performance
- Traditional medical education was based on the motto: "See one, do one, teach one."
  ○ Trainees with variable backgrounds and expertise arrive at academic medical centers, perhaps using unfamiliar equipment to perform a procedure in

the middle of the night without attending level supervision.
  ○ Interventional radiology support and ultrasound imaging may also be unavailable during off-hours.
- The ACGME educational objectives now require outcomes measurement. It is no longer adequate that a trainee document that a given procedure has been performed "X" number of times. Trainees are now expected to document complication rates.
- Hospitalists have emerged as supervising attendings during off-hours when many procedures are performed.
- As their jobs increasingly interface with the intensive care units and EDs, hospitalists need to collaborate in establishing uniform goals, educational standards, and methods of evaluation for house staff procedural training.
  ○ The program should be comprehensive, but flexible in allowing services to determine their own mechanism of supervision.
  ○ Hospitalists developing procedure services need to establish measurable outcome targets.

HOSPITALISTS AS ED PARTNERS

- Hospitalists are now partnering with the ED staff to develop criteria for admission and help to facilitate care plans that do not include hospitalization.
- Operational challenges of providing care in the ED include the following:
  ○ The application of diagnostic or treatment protocols when patients have nonspecific symptoms or multiple comorbidities.
  ○ Implementation of guidelines which might be publicly reported.
  ○ Lack of outside supports in place for indigent patients and the impact of the medical legal environment on patient care.
  ○ Different or even conflicting priorities, as for example, admitting a patient to reduce ED length of stay versus preventing an unnecessary admission or facilitating appropriate triage through additional testing.
  ○ Different systems in place for the ED which is more protocol-driven than the medical and surgical inpatient service. Unfortunately, these systems may not "talk" to each other with resulting inefficiencies of care (requiring new orders for admissions to the hospital) and delays in medication administration.
  ○ Patient safety issues especially for those patients who must spend extended time in the ED because of no bed availability.
  ○ Venous thromboembolism prophylaxis, for example, should begin immediately but may not be on the radar screen of the busy ED physician.

- Hospitalists bring to the table expertise in the complexities of how the hospital works.
  - In order to get the proper plan set in motion as efficiently and safely as possible, especially during off-hours, communication at the ED–hospital interface is crucial.
  - One of the core competencies of hospital medicine relates to multidisciplinary teamwork and communication between specialties, rather than each working totally separate of the other, in the care of increasingly frail and vulnerable patients.
- Hospitalists and emergency medicine physicians are collaborating to develop improved systems of care at the ED–hospital interface (Fig. 3-2).
  - Hospitalist facilitator programs have been developed to promote appropriate transitions to the outpatient setting through timely follow-up plans.
  - The goal is to transition to home or to extended care facilities those patients who do not meet hospital criteria for admission, for whom the ED physician does not have access to resources or time to arrange.
  - On-site availability of hospitalists results in earlier response time to address medical issues that might arise in the ED, reconcile inpatient medications with outpatient medications, and to provide medical consultation for patients admitted to surgery.
  - Hospitalist availability and knowledge of the different services may also help expedite timely patient triage into the hospital to the appropriate medical subspecialty service with the potential of reducing diversion time during high census conditions.
- The role of the hospitalist is shifting from mostly a clinical consultative role for ED physicians to leading changes in the admission process, which may include:
  - Setting key process targets
  - Developing protocols for patients with selected clinical diagnoses at the ED hospital interface with the ED staff
  - Championing alignment of national performance targets such as venous thromboembolism prophylaxis and smoking cessation so that the network can reach target goals (eg, 90% or higher)
  - Providing attending availability 24/7, in some instances, as a rapid response admission service
- Using pay-for-performance incentives for improvements in efficiency:
  - Managing patients who do not yet have a bed available in the hospital
  - Leading RRTs/systems
  - Expediting safe transfers from the ED to other sites within the hospital network

SUMMARY

- The role of the hospitalist is evolving and may include broader roles in managing patients with specific problems relating to other specialties that may

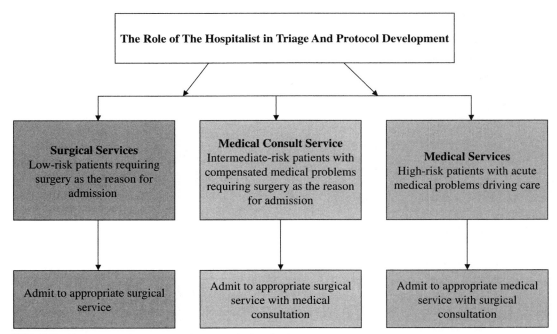

FIG. 3-2   Emergency department triage, surgical patients.

include psychiatry, oncology, and obstetrics. In addition, hospitalists comanage patients who have either undergone procedures or who are presenting with acute illness in the ED.

- As their work in quality improvement and education spans divisions and departments, interdisciplinary collaboration and communication have become central to the role of the hospitalist.
- Hospital medicine offers different career paths in administration, leadership, research, and clinician education and may further subspecialize as the field matures.
- Hospitalist leaders should actively align their goals with the strategic vision of their hospitals and actively engage in processes that improve the way we care for patients.
- Hospitalists need to measure their performance in order to target areas for improvement and to meet national performance standards and patient safety goals.

BIBLIOGRAPHY

Austin MT, Diaz JJ Jr, Feurer ID, et al. Creating an emergency general surgery service enhances the productivity of trauma surgeons, general surgeons, and the hospital. *J Trauma.* 2005:58(5):906–910.

Bodenheimer T, May JH, Berenson A, et al. Can money buy quality? Physician response to pay for performance. *Issue Brief Cent Stud Health Syst Change.* 2005;(102):1–4.

Halasyamani L, Kripalani S, Coleman E, et al. Transition of care for hospitalized elderly patients—development of a discharge checklist for hospitalists. *J Hosp Med.* 2006;1(6):354–360.

Kahn DN III, Ault T, Isenstein H, et al. Snapshot of hospital quality reporting and pay-for-performance under Medicare. *Health Aff.* 2006;25(1):148–162.

Pistoria M, Amin A, Dressler D, et al. Core competencies in hospital medicine: a framework for curriculum development. *J Hosp Med.* 2006;1(suppl 1):1.

Poon EG, Blumenfeld B, Hamann C, et al. Design and implementation of an application and associated services to support interdisciplinary medication reconciliation efforts at an integrated healthcare delivery network. *J Amer Med Inform Assoc.* 2006;13:581–592.

Ranji SR et al. Effects of rapid response systems on clinical outcomes: systematic review and meta-analysis. *J Hosp Med.* 2007;2:422–432.

Schnipper JL, Barsky EE, Shaykevich S, et al. Inpatient management of diabetes and hyperglycemia among general medicine patients at a large teaching hospital. *J Hosp Med.* 2006;1:145–150.

Vidyarthi AR, Arora V, Schnipper JL, et al. Managing discontinuity in academic medical centers: strategies for a safe and effective resident sign-out. *J Hosp Med.* 2006;1:257–266.

SYSTEMS—HOSPITALISTS AS LEADERS IN PATIENT SAFETY

4 GENERAL OVERVIEW OF PATIENT SAFETY

Sylvia C. McKean and Allan Frankel

THE ROLE OF THE HOSPITALIST IN PATIENT SAFETY

- From a clinical perspective a hospitalist today might be labeled a renaissance physician in that a requisite for success is a wide breadth of clinical knowledge to address complicated, acutely ill, and vulnerable hospitalized patients.
- Hospitalists see every aspect of care across many specialties and are more familiar with the overall hospital "domain" than their peers.
- As healthcare industrializes, meaning that cost and outcome become quantifiable and pathways that optimize these become clearer, hospitalists will require another set of skills pertaining to complex hospital environments that could be perhaps titled "Systems Specialists." These skills will extend beyond clinical care to the evaluation and management of systems of care. Few other physicians are better suited to this role.
- The sciences and concepts that now comprise *patient safety* are in many respects those that would support a system specialist.
- Ultimately, the truly skillful hospitalist will be as versed in patient safety and hospital-based systems re-engineering as in hospital-based clinical care, and a portion of their work time will be spent on change management and improvement.

THE PATIENT SAFETY MOVEMENT: A BRIEF HISTORY

- There are significant events in the past four decades that changed the relationship between patient, physician, government, and hospital and set the stage in the 1990s for an honest evaluation of healthcare errors.
- In the 1960s, Beecher's articles about the ethics of research brought clarity to the concept of informed consent and began a process of empowering patients. In so doing, the voice of patients and their reasonable expectations to receive reliable care began to surface.
- In the 1970s, the national mandate to make healthcare affordable brought Medicare and Medicaid and the categorization and coding of medical conditions. This brought a third party into the previously inviolable physician-patient relationship that had been so much a part of healthcare history, and afforded greater oversight and standardization of care.
- In the 1980s, patient activists brought to healthcare the concept of the "patient bill of rights," and further empowered patients.
- In all three decades, information technology kept apace supplying more and better information about healthcare in general, highlighting the need for standardization and simplification of care processes.
- Patient safety in the 1990s began with the publication in 1991 of *The Harvard Medical Practice Study*, a retrospective chart review of over 30,000 admissions in 1984 to New York state hospitals that showed that 3.7% of patients were affected by adverse drug events (ADEs) and 1% of patients were harmed because of negligence. Initially, and up to 1995, the findings were debated primarily within the healthcare literature.

- While the media has continuously published reports about individual patients' debacles in healthcare, few created the furor of Betsy Lehman's death when, in late 1994, she received a chemotherapy overdose at the Dana Farber Cancer Institute in Boston, Massachusetts. The resultant media discussion brought to public attention the *Harvard Practice Study* and findings from similar other research.
- The combination of increasing data similar to the Harvard study and individual stories like Betsy's led the US Congress to commission the Institute of Medicine (IOM), an academic group formally available to Congress to inform on medical issues, to evaluate and report on error in healthcare.
- In 1999, the IOM published *To Err Is Human* and in 2001 *Crossing the Quality Chasm: A New Health System for the 21st Century*[1] in which they reported on a large gap between what medical care can and should provide through advances in clinical knowledge and healthcare technology and the error-prone reality of current practice in the United States.
- While the exact numbers of "lives lost" from hospitalization was debated, the reports made clear that US healthcare systems failed to reliably deliver evidence-based therapies, that many medical services were not needed nor patient-centered, and some caused unnecessary harm or loss of life.
- These systemic failures—more than a few individual "bad apples"—wasted billions of dollars at a cost that threatened the health of the US economy and its citizens.
- These findings, viewed through a lens of 46 million Americans with no health insurance and a country that spent more on healthcare than any other, catalyzed efforts to evaluate and improve the American healthcare industry. National and state regulatory and quality groups weighed in with a wide variety of quality mandates and suggestions.
- Initially discordant and at times conflicting, the efforts beginning in the mid 1990s began to harmonize in the 2000s.
- The Agency for Healthcare Research and Quality (AHRQ) identified 25 patient safety practices and ranked the top five with "the greatest strength of evidence regarding their impact and effectiveness."[1] These included
  - Appropriate prophylaxis to prevent venous thromboembolism
  - Use of maximum sterile barriers during insertion of central lines to prevent central-line infections
  - Appropriate use of antibiotic prophylaxis to prevent surgical site infections
  - Semi recumbent positioning to prevent ventilator-associated pneumonia

- Information transfer between inpatient and outpatient pharmacy to prevent ADEs

AHRQ acquired national funding to support quality and safety-based research, making available 50–250 million dollars annually to health-based research and contracts.

- The Joint Commission on Accreditation of Healthcare Organizations (JCAHO) articulated national patient safety goals for hospitals which included
  - Reducing the risk of healthcare-associated infections
  - Accurately and completely reconciling medications across the continuum of care
  - Improving the effectiveness of communication among caregivers
  - Improving the safety of using medications

JCAHO accreditation standards and national patient safety goals also require communication of critical results, accurate patient identification, medication reconciliation, and standardized communication, including the opportunity to ask and respond to questions at the time of patient handoffs. JCAHO also requires hospitals to report "sentinel events."

- In an effort to limit fatigue-related error, the American College of Graduate Medical Education (ACGME) has gone beyond mandating work hour restrictions.
  - Applying scientific advances requires changing how we educate trainees, the ACGME Outcome Project has identified six areas for outcome-based education that will ensure competency, namely, medical knowledge, patient care, interpersonal and communication skills, professionalism, practice-based learning and improvement, and systems-based practice.
  - Education about error prevention and analysis is now mandated as part of residency curriculum.
- The National Quality Forum (NQF), a not-for-profit consensus-driven membership organization created to develop and implement a national strategy for healthcare quality measurement and reporting, released in 2003 a list of *30 best practices* following which The Leapfrog Group—Fortune 500 corporations organized through the Business Roundtable—endorsed the list as their *fourth* leap and then used the practices to engage other national and regulatory agencies to participate in an effort to harmonize metrics and goals.
- The result, in 2007, is a revision of the 30 practices that comprise a coordinated agenda for comprehensive patient safety that is endorsed by the major governmental payers—The Centers for Medicare and Medicaid Services and the Surgical Care Improvement, the primary hospital regulatory agency (JCAHO), major business roundtable (Leapfrog), primary quality group in the Unites States (the Institute for Healthcare Improvement [IHI]) and the national consensus group, NQF.

- The IHI, beginning early in the 1990s, used a highly successful collaborative teaching model in which many healthcare organizations would work together on projects, incorporating into their process industrial quality techniques like rapid cycle improvement.[2]
- In late 2004, the IHI initiated the *100,000 Lives Campaign* (http://www.ihi.org/IHI/Programs/Campaign/) asking hospitals to participate by implementing specific practices into their hospitals and measuring mortality. The national campaign interventions included the following:
  - Deploy rapid response teams (RRTs)
  - Deliver reliable evidence-based care for acute myocardial infarction
  - Prevent central-line infections
  - Prevent surgical site infections
  - Prevent ADEs
  - Prevent ventilator-associated pneumonia

The IHI reported 2 years later that hospitals participating in the *100,000 Lives Campaign* prevented an estimated 122,000 avoidable deaths.[2]

- In late 2006, IHI launched the *5 Million Lives Campaign*, asking participating hospitals to adopt 12 interventions—the six interventions in the *100,000 Lives Campaign,* plus six new interventions over a 24-month period through December, 2008. IHI estimates that 15 million incidents of harm occur annually—between 40 and 50 incidents of harm for every 100 hospital admissions.
  - To participate in IHI's *5 Million Lives Campaign,* hospitals must regularly report hospital profile and mortality data over the 2-year period.
  - Blue Cross Blue Shield Association contributed 5 million dollars to the campaign, which is expected to enlist more than 4000 US hospitals.
- Increasingly, hospitals will be required to publicly report on performance and adopt health plan "pay-for-performance" targets in order to receive predetermined at-risk reimbursement as part of their contracts with third-party payers. Between 2000 and 2007 the number of required publicly reported hospital measures increased from about 7 to 120, partly promoted by state and federal agencies, but also heavily endorsed by health plan and health insurance payers.
- In 2006, The Society of Hospital Medicine (SHM), the professional society of hospitalists, published *The Core Competencies in Hospital Medicine: A Framework for Curriculum Development.*
  - The goals of this publication are to improve patient care, guide educational reform, lead systems changes, and advance the field of hospital medicine in recognition of a quality and training gap.
  - For example, the healthcare systems chapters include patient safety, care transitions, care of vulnerable patients, and sign-outs.

SEEING HEALTHCARE THROUGH A DIFFERENT LENS—THE ANATOMY OF ERRORS

- A hospitalist primarily involved in clinical care is likely to view daily experience through a lens shaped by intensive clinical training.
  - In this venue, joy in work might be defined as the orchestration of data, interaction, and technique to achieve a patient's excellent clinical outcome.
  - The manifestation of success might be enhanced patient satisfaction, or seeing a patient's increased functional capacity or quality of life.
- A physician who is solely a patient safety systems specialist views the clinical world through a different lens, shaped by specific aspects of engineering, psychology, ethics and accountability, change management, and process improvement. Joy in work will vary based on the primary focus.
  - If engineering is the primary focus, success might be a simpler or more standardized mechanism for delivering care in which fewer errors occur or where the end result is achieved with greater reliability.
  - If quality metrics is the focus, success might be measured when a specific outcome goal is reached.
  - If culture is the focus, success might be measured by the degree of employee and physician mutual respect, the degree of trust that appears to be present in a clinical environment, how effectively teams work and communicate together, or patient satisfaction scores determined by care they are provided.
- With minimal reflection, the relationship between joy in clinical work and joy in patient safety work is obvious. The likelihood of seeing a patient's satisfaction with care or increased quality of life is dependent on an environment, molded by patient safety thinking, in which granular clinical care is most effectively delivered. The two bodies of knowledge must be woven together to achieve safe and reliable care.

THE COMPONENTS OF A SAFETY LENS—ENGINEERING AND RELIABLE DESIGN

- Reliability, the capacity of a process to deliver its intended result in a defined time, may be applied to healthcare as "defect free delivery of care for a patient." The phrase is purposively specific and presumes that "care" is almost always comprised of a series of actions or steps, and that "defect free" presumes that each step is performed flawlessly. A "patient" identifies that the unit of interest is each individual patient and the presumption is that a system can be made reliable for one patient, that the process can be replicated for the next and the next, and so forth.[3] Reliability, or its converse, defect rate, is measurable in a variety of ways. Patient safety experts are beginning to talk about reliability as defect rates of 10^{-1} ("ten to the minus one power") to 10^{-6} ("ten to the minus six power") where:

- 10^{-1} = One failure out of ten opportunities consistent with no articulated common processes such as medication management upon discharge.
- 10^{-2} = Up to 9 failures out of 100 opportunities consistent with processes with medium to high variation such as warfarin clinics.
- 10^{-3} = Up to 9 failures out of 1000 opportunities consistent with a well-designed system with low variation and cooperative relationships such as blood banking procedure and anesthesia intraoperative management.
- 10^{-4} = Up to 9 failures out of 10,000 opportunities consistent with a well-designed or redesigned process.
- Systems in healthcare with failure rates of 10^{-5} or 10^{-6} are rare.
- Model 10^{-1} reliability, predominantly the current status quo, is achievable through commonly understood and implemented basic failure prevention (intent, vigilance, and hard work).
  - Examples include common equipment, standard orders sheets, personal check lists, working harder next time, feedback of information on compliance and awareness, and training.
- Model 10^{-2} reliability requires basic failure prevention and mitigation.
  - Examples include decision aids and reminders built into the system, desired action the default based on evidence, standardization of process, redundancy, and scheduling. These take advantage of habits and patterns and rely on human factors and reliability science.
- Model 10^{-3} reliability requires determination of risk of critical failures and redesign of systems to address these areas.
  - Examples including adverse event surveillance systems, architectural redesign, failure modes and effects analysis, and application of Toyota Lean to entire processes.
- Reliable three-tier design is an improvement process in which sequential steps are taken to improve reliability.
  - For example, warfarin can be made safer through a standardized warfarin ordering algorithm to achieve a 10^{-1} defect rate in each step in the process.
  - Once successfully produced, these algorithms may achieve a 10^{-2} implementation rate if incorporated into a computerized physician order entry system.

However, there are likely to be patients who, for a variety of reasons, should be, but are not, placed into the algorithm.
  - Greater reliability (10^{-3}) might be gained if a pharmacist is assigned to identify and/or mitigate failure by finding patients not using the algorithm.
- Critical failure mode analysis is used to identify critical failures and then redesign.

CHANGING CULTURE

- Changing the standard of hospital care on a national scale requires coordinated improvements in more than information technology and physical architecture; it requires changing culture.
- Outstanding reliability requires cultural change to impact behaviors such as how we communicate and function on teams.
- Healthcare's current safety record results from the combination of a complex system that has taken shape less by forethought and design than by amorphous growth and historical precedent, and the limitations of human vigilance and behavior, shaped by intrinsic human error rates and a predisposition to deviate from standards and rules.
  - In the final analysis, "health care has safety and quality problems because it relies on outmoded systems of work."[1] Fortunately, "although we cannot change the aspects of human cognition that cause us to err, we can design systems that reduce error and make them safer for patients."[2]
- Culture might be best defined as "the way we do things around here" and is the composite of each individual's attitude toward their work, peers and the environment they work in, their patients, and their perceptions of themselves. In general, most healthcare providers have little formal understanding of hospital complexity and poor insight into their own limitations.
- In reality, there are about 40–80 steps for even the simplest of medication delivery processes—a much more complex process that originally suspected.
- The patient safety momentum has created public awareness, a call for educational reform to improve understanding, and a mandate to change how healthcare providers practice.

HUMAN ERROR

- While technological improvement is essential, it has not, to date, been able to fully mitigate the effect of human error.

- ○ Proficiency errors require technical training.
- ○ Communication and decision errors require team training.
- ○ Lack of compliance with standard procedure requires internal reviews of policies, procedures, and organization culture.
- If asked whether fatigue increases the likelihood of error, many physicians in the recent past, and even a few today, suggest that they personally are immune to this deleterious effect. Few understand the extraordinary catalysis that occurs when human limitations are combined with intense complexity.
- Active failures are those that occur at the point of a service delivery by medical and surgical personnel. Latent conditions—weaknesses in the organization—increase the likelihood of an active failure, which may be an error that is caught prior to reaching the patient, or may reach the patient and cause harm.
  - ○ A classic example of a latent condition is an organizational decision to cut back on nursing personnel with plans to rely on greater use of double shifts when workload requires it. The nurses are four times more likely to commit an active failure such as a medication error at hour 12 of a workday than at hour 1.
  - ○ For hospitalists, interruptions such as frequent beeper calls, RRT obligations, fatigue, handoffs, and lack of autonomy or control when specialty patients outside of their area of expertise are admitted to their service may predispose to error especially if consultants are not available.
  - ○ Each of these increased risks is likely to be associated with a "latent condition" predisposing the "active failure." Whether simply an error or a cause of patient harm is often determined by serendipity.
  - ○ Preplanning and vigilance have little beneficial effect in changing the likelihood of occurrence of an active failure if the latent condition persists that will continuously generate an environment that supports the failure.
- Human beings inherently deviate from norms.
  - ○ We regularly break rules. A glaringly obvious example is the normative speed of highway traffic, which is invariably above the speed limit. Each individual chooses their car speed based on personal satisfaction and a desire for a particular level of productivity that together are weighed against level of risk. The two factors determine the car's speed. We can apply the same criteria to every decision we make in healthcare. Upon personal reflection, it's likely that the reader will recognize that at any specific moment, a different mood will affect the way they combine the two aforementioned factors and alter the degree of risk they are willing to take.

- Human error is measurable and can be categorized.
  - ○ Humans have inherent limitations to short-term memory capacity (5–7 pieces of information) and limited multitasking ability (increased car accident rates when simultaneously driving and speaking on a cell phone).
  - ○ Our limitations are known to increase secondary to the effects of fatigue or stress.
  - ○ Humans err frequently and reproducibly. For example, we know from the human factors literature that errors of omission, such as forgetting to perform a certain task, are approximately 1 in 100. Errors of commission, such as misreading a label, occur at a rate of about 3 in 1000. These error rates increase under severe stress; an extreme example is the 1 in 4 error rate by new military recruits in a trench when live ammunition is being fired overhead.
- Application of behavioral and biological sciences will need to be further applied to the design of healthcare systems. Behavioral sciences include cognitive, experimental, organizational, and social psychology.
  - ○ Causes of error include cognitive overload, poor communication, flawed information processing, fatigue, workload, fear, and incorrect clinical decision-making.
  - ○ Team error is defined as failure to respond or failure to adhere to team or organizational standards.
  - ○ Failure to identify errors or "near misses" results from failure to recognize personal vulnerability under stressful conditions such as fatigue or personal problems, a culture of blame, and insufficient data such as observation of proficiency.
- Increasingly, simulation is used to facilitate dealing with situations prone to error without jeopardy.
  - ○ Industries such as aviation, manufacturing, and nuclear power provide lessons for US healthcare. Identifying types of errors and the processes uncovers latent factors that can induce error.
  - ○ Aviation's methodologies can be used to obtain essential data and develop interventions to mitigate error (Table 4-1). The US Veterans Health Administration implemented a "near-miss" reporting system based on the NASA aviation safety reporting system.
- Reliable three-tier design can be applied to improve aspects of culture, although the measurement is much more difficult. For example, if the goal is to improve teamwork
  - ○ Prevent initial failures (10^{-1}) by using intent and standardization to hire intelligently seeking individuals most likely to work well in teams, and developing "citizenship" criteria for behavior.
  - ○ Identify and/or mitigate failure (10^{-2}) through teamwork and communication training and feedback,

TABLE 4-1   Lessons from the Aviation Industry

THE AVIATION INDUSTRY	US HEALTHCARE SYSTEM
Infrequent aircraft accidents	Each year as many as 98,000 people die as a result of medical errors and many more suffer harm
Highly visible, massive loss of life	ADEs affect individuals; invisible
Exhaustive investigation into causal factors, public reports, remedial actions	No standardized method of investigation, documentation, dissemination
When error suspected, litigation and new regulations	When error suspected, litigation and new regulations
Errors result from physiological and psychological limitations of humans	Errors result from physiological and psychological limitations of humans
Team errors result from failure to act or deviation from established standards	Inaccurate self-perceptions relating to ability to perform under stress, fatigue leads to error
Error management based on understanding the nature and extent of error, changing conditions that induce error, determining behaviors that prevent or mitigate error, and personnel training	Punitive or fear of punitive incident reporting systems (litigation, interference with career advancement) and professional tolerance of misbehavior leads to underreporting of errors
Observation of flights in operation has identified failures of compliance, communication, procedures, proficiency, and decision making contributing to errors	Surveys in operating rooms have confirmed physicians and pilots have common interpersonal problem areas and similarities in professional culture
Systematic efforts to reduce frequency of error based on recognition that humans will inevitably make errors and the importance of reliable data on error	Inadequate error management programs to reduce the frequency and severity of adverse events. There are lessons that can be applied from the aviation industry

Adapted from Helmreich R.[9] ADEs, adverse drug events.

leadership engagement through walk rounds supported by effective use of the information discussed, and coordinated safety, quality, and risk functions in institutions.
○ Use multidisciplinary root cause analyses for learning and system design in conjunction with critical failure mode analysis of teamwork and communication issues that arise through adverse events reports and other data sources.

CONTINUOUSLY IMPROVING CARE

• A healthcare culture and physical environment can achieve reliable care delivery only if it manifests one essential characteristic, that of willingness to continuously learn. Learning requires that the system:
○ Monitors itself objectively for strengths and weaknesses.
○ Tests small changes, always seeking a safer or more efficient or more reliable mechanism.
○ Is willing and able to incorporate the positive results of small tests into everyday activities.
○ Is willing and able to spread the changes to other areas as needed.
This, in essence, is process improvement.
• All healthcare environments, even those deemed reliable, must continuously improve. There is no human produced system that doesn't need constant monitoring and improvement.
• Every healthcare provider must understand how to develop and participate in learning systems because of

the complexity of the care process, the changing personnel and personalities who come and go in healthcare institutions, and the constant likelihood that a care system will at any point in time need to incorporate new information, a new patient mix, or new technical devices.
• Many industries have developed process improvement and change management methodologies. Two common names attached to industry are Toyota Lean and Motorola's Six Sigma. Within healthcare the IHI has used "rapid cycle improvement." Each, in its own way, seeks to improve learning and facilitate change.
○ Toyota Lean may possibly be the most effective—and focuses primarily on the elimination of unnecessary steps in a process.
○ Six Sigma is a program designed to eliminate defects in a production process and healthcare may be viewed as the process of delivering care to a patient.
○ Rapid cycle improvement is a way of thinking about and applying small tests of change where the results are objectively viewed, applied to the next small test, and after a series of tests a viable permanent change process is delineated and implemented.
• Process improvement and clinical research have different goals:
○ The aim of classic research is the production of new knowledge.
○ In research, usually the test is blinded, there is an attempt to eliminate bias, there is a fixed hypothesis, extra data are usually obtained just in case they might be useful, and there is one large test. There may or may not be application of the results.

○ The goal of process improvement is the application of known knowledge to a system, and the improvement of that system through the application of human factors.

○ In tests of improvement, the tests are observable, bias is at best stable, just enough data are obtained (and no more usually because doing so requires unnecessary resources), rapid adaptation of changes occurs based on the results, and sequential tests are performed.

○ Rapid cycle improvement begins with hunches, theories, and ideas. Improvement results from a *series* of testing cycles where data are obtained that lead to changes that are incorporated if they appear to result in improvement.

• Rapid cycle improvement is at the heart of most improvement methods and its components should be known and understood by every healthcare provider. There is a step-by-step process that increases the likelihood of success, encapsulated in asking three questions:

○ What are we trying to accomplish?

○ What changes will we make?

○ How will we know that a change is an improvement?

• An overall aim should be established based on a perceived, and then measured, problem. Almost any type of problem can be addressed.

○ For example, if there is a general perception that employees do not believe the area they work in is safe, a survey might be given to test the hypothesis.

○ If the results of the survey corroborate the hunch, an "Aim Statement" might be that "at least 70% of staff surveyed will report a positive safety climate within 1 year."

• The aim should be unambiguous, clear, specific, numerical, and measurable. The aim should send a strong message in a stretch goal. Examples of aim statements include:

○ *Culture*—have at least 70% of staff surveyed reporting a positive safety climate within 1 year.

○ *High-hazard medications*—reduce ADEs involving anticoagulants by 75% within 9 months.

○ *Surgical*—achieve 100% compliance with appropriate selection and timing of prophylactic antibiotic administration.

○ *ICU*—reduce ADEs by 75% within 11 months.

○ *Reconciliation*—decrease errors from unreconciled medications by 50% within 6 months.

• Measurement is critical. Measures clarify the aim.

○ *Aim*—decrease the number of errors related to unreconciled medications by 75% in 1 year.

○ *Measure*—number of errors from unreconciled medications per 100 admissions.

○ *Formula*—the total number of errors related to unreconciled medications found in a sample of patient records, divided by the total number of patient records reviewed. Multiply the result by 100 to express a percentage.

○ *Process*—measures track whether a change has been made rather than the outcome. For example, percent of pneumonia patients receiving antibiotics before leaving the emergency department (ED) is a process measure.

• What changes will we make?

○ The cycle for learning and improvement involves:

▪ *Planning*—objectives, questions, and predictions of what will happen and why

▪ *Doing*—what modifications are to be made

▪ *Studying*—evaluating the results of what has been done

▪ *Acting*—utilizing what has been learned to incorporate in the next small test of change

• How will we know that a change is an improvement?

○ Measurement! Unlike measurement for research, however, the goal of rapid cycle improvement is to use small and rapid measurements that are just adequate to reasonably evaluate the change.

○ The purpose of measuring is to:

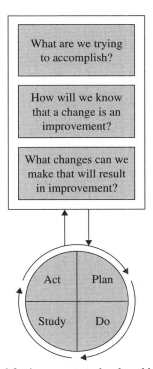

FIG. 4-1 Model for improvement developed by Tom Nolan. Used with permission from The Improvement Guide, Langley, Nolan et al. (*http://www.ihi.org/IHI/Topics/Improvement/ ImprovementMethods/HowToImprove/*)

- ▪ Increase the belief that the change will result in improvement
- ▪ Predict how much improvement can be expected from the change
- ▪ Learn how to adapt the change to local conditions
- ▪ Minimize resistance to implementation
- Changes made in the testing cycles tend to focus on the application of error reducing strategies. The goal is to design and prepare to implement changes to improve performance in your organization by setting aims, considering teams, establishing measures, and selecting changes. Error reduction strategies include:
  - ○ Avoid reliance on memory.
  - ○ Simplify and standardize the process.
  - ○ Use cultural, physical, and procedural constraints and forcing functions.
  - ○ Use protocols, checklists, and other reminders.
  - ○ Improve information access.
  - ○ Reduce handoffs and increase feedback.
  - ○ Decrease look-alikes.
  - ○ Automate carefully so that new types of errors are not introduced.
  - ○ Make errors visible so that harm can be minimized when they occur.

SUMMARY

- Hospitalists are in a position to teach what it actually means to care for patients and serve as role models as leaders of patient safety on the multidisciplinary team.
- Hospitalists have a responsibility to reduce patient harm by anticipating and treating predictable complications of hospitalization.
- Hospitalists have a responsibility to measure performance, establish patient safety goals, standardize care, critically review performance, and provide hospital-specific data to clinicians.
- Hospitalists should identify and lower barriers to patient safety standards, devise strategies to bridge the gap between knowledge and practice, develop automated reminder systems, and participate in quality improvement research.
- The hospitalist can play a central role in teaching about error and how teamwork and communication reduce error.
  - ○ The hospitalist can lead initiatives that promote teamwork and effective communication.
  - ○ The hospitalist must incorporate effective team behavior into their daily activities by observing team behavior, briefing teams on expectations, debriefing after activities, and measuring teamwork through observation.
  - ○ The hospitalist can commit to addressing problems in the context of how systems fail.
  - ○ The hospitalist can develop observation tools and structured communication to measure team performance and provide feedback over time.
- "The quality of care and the quality of caring are inseparable. We can hope for a day when medicine is practiced by knowledgeable, competent, and compassionate physicians who create high-quality therapeutic and healing relationships with patients and their families in the setting of safe, effective, and efficient healthcare systems."[4]

WEB RESOURCES

http://www.ihi.org/ihi
http://www.jointcommission.org/
http://www.leapfroggroup.org/
http://www.hospitalmedicine.org/
http://www.fda.gov/
http://www.acgme.org/acWebsite/home/home.asp

REFERENCES

1. IHI. *Crossing the Quality Chasm: A New Health System for the 21st Century*. Executive Summary. National Academy Press: 1999, Page 4.
2. *The Breakthrough Series: IHI's Collaborative Model for Achieving Breakthrough Improvement*. Boston, MA: Institute for Healthcare Improvement; 2003. http://www.ihi.org/IHI/Results/WhitePapers/TheBreakthroughSeriesIHIsCollaborativeModelforAchieving+BreakthroughImprovement.htm
3. *Improving the Reliability of Health Care*. Boston, MA: Institute for Healthcare Improvement; 2004. http://www.ihi.org/IHI/Results/WhitePapers/ImprovingtheReliabilityofHealthCare.htm
4. Nolan T. System changes to improve patient safety. *BMJ*. March 2000;320:771–777.
5. Berwick D. A primer on leading the improvement of systems. *BMJ*. 1996;312:619–662.
6. Brock W, Nolan K, Nolan T. Pragmatic science: accelerating the improvement of critical care. *New Horiz*. 1998;6:61–68.
7. James TC, Li MD. The quality of caring. *Mayo Clin Proc*. 2006 Mar;81(3):345–352.
8. Cohen HJ, Goodell B. Lessons on repairing distressed academic health centers. *Acad Clin Prac*. 2000;13(1):1–14.
9. Helmreich R. On error management: lessons from aviation. *BMJ*. 2000 Mar;320:781–785.

5   ADVERSE DRUG EVENTS

Frank Federico

OVERVIEW

- Medications are the most common intervention in healthcare.
- Medication errors are frequent, but not all errors result in harm or an adverse event.
- Several studies have identified adverse drug events (ADEs) as the single most frequent source of healthcare mishaps, continually placing patients at risk of injury.
- In 1991, Leape et al published one of the first studies that brought attention to the number and frequency of medical errors and injury.
- The medication system includes ordering/prescribing, preparation/dispensing, administration, and monitoring. The following rates of preventable inpatient ADEs were reported in a study by Bates[1]:
  - 56% at the stage of ordering
  - 34% at administration
  - 6% at transcribing
  - 4% at dispensing
- In order to minimize errors one must consider the system as a whole, as changes in one part of the system impact another part of the system.

DEFINITIONS

- An ADE is defined as an injury or harm resulting from medical intervention relating to a drug.
- An adverse drug reaction (ADR) is defined by WHO as "noxious and unintended, and which occurs at doses used in man for prophylaxis, diagnosis, or therapy." An ADR is an ADE.
- "A medication error is any preventable event that may cause or lead to inappropriate medication use or patient harm while the medication is in the control of the healthcare professional, patient, or consumer." National Coordinating Council Medication Error Reporting Program (NCCMERP) www.usp.org
- Potential ADEs may or may not be intercepted before reaching the patient.
  - An example of an intercepted potential ADE would be an order written for an acetaminophen overdose that is intercepted and corrected by a nurse before reaching the patient.
  - An example of a nonintercepted potential ADE would be an administered overdose of acetaminophen to a patient who did not suffer any sequelae.

- Any ADE that results from an error is considered preventable.

EPIDEMIOLOGY

- The types of ADEs experienced by patients range from allergic reaction to death.
- The Institute of Medicine (IOM) Committee that developed the Preventing Medication Errors 2006 report estimates that on average a hospitalized patient is subject to at least one medication error per day, with considerable variation in rate across facilities.
- In the report *To Err is Human*, the committee reported that 7000 deaths occur yearly because of medication errors.[2]
- Incidence rates of ADEs vary from 2 per 100 admissions[3] to 7 per 100 admissions among the hospitals that have conducted ADE studies. A precise national incidence rate is difficult to calculate because various researchers use different criteria to detect and identify ADEs. Kaushal et al reviewed 10,778 medication orders in a pediatric hospital and reported 115 potential ADEs (1.1%), and 26 ADEs (0.24%).
- One study estimated that 9.7% of ADEs caused permanent disability.
- Although ADEs cannot be predicted by patient characteristics or drug type, they are more likely to result in life-threatening consequences in intensive care unit (ICU) patients than in others. Classen at al estimated that the increased risk of death for a patient who experiences an ADE is nearly twice that of a patient who does not.

COST OF ADEs

- ADEs contribute to increased costs owing to the need for additional treatment, testing, and increased length of stay (LOS).
  - Researchers conducting an Agency for Healthcare Research and Quality (AHRQ)–funded study at Brigham and Women's Hospital and Massachusetts General Hospital found that, on average, ADEs increased the LOS by as much as 4.6 days and increased costs up to $4685.
  - Based on a rate of 400,000 ADEs per year in hospitalized patients, the IOM Committee (Preventing Medication Errors, July 2006) estimated that ADEs accounted for $3.5 billion (in 2006 dollars) of additional costs incurred by hospitals.
  - National hospital expenses to treat patients who suffer ADEs during hospitalization are estimated at between $1.56 and $5.6 billion annually.

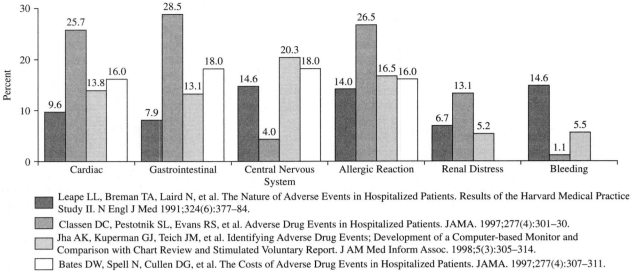

Leape LL, Breman TA, Laird N, et al. The Nature of Adverse Events in Hospitalized Patients. Results of the Harvard Medical Practice Study II. N Engl J Med 1991;324(6):377–84.

Classen DC, Pestotnik SL, Evans RS, et al. Adverse Drug Events in Hospitalized Patients. JAMA. 1997;277(4):301–30.

Jha AK, Kuperman GJ, Teich JM, et al. Identifying Adverse Drug Events; Development of a Computer-based Monitor and Comparison with Chart Review and Stimulated Voluntary Report. J AM Med Inform Assoc. 1998;5(3):305–314.

Bates DW, Spell N, Cullen DG, et al. The Costs of Adverse Drug Events in Hospitalized Patients. JAMA. 1997;277(4):307–311.

FIG. 5-1   Percent patients suffering selected injuries commonly studied among patients who experienced adverse drug events.
SOURCE: http://www.ahrq.gov/qual/aderia/figure1.htm

FACTORS THAT CONTRIBUTE TO ADVERSE DRUG EVENTS

• ADEs can result from errors, suboptimal delivery of care and as yet unknown ways to prevent them.
• Contributors to ADEs include:
  ○ Errors in prescribing, preparation, administration, and/or monitoring of medications.
  ○ Poor selection and management of medication regimen.
  ○ Poor or lack of monitoring for toxicities and side effects.
  ○ Drug interactions and therapeutic duplication.
  ○ Look-alike/sound-alike drug names and packaging.
  ○ Not having allergy information available.
  ○ Not having lab information available.
  ○ Equipment failures.
• Lack of standardization contributes to errors.
  ○ Rozich et al reported a reduction in hypoglycemic episodes when using a standardized insulin protocol.
  ○ The researchers report that standardization efforts to increase uniformity of practice are worth considering in other practice areas to increase safety and possibly reduce costs.

IDENTIFYING ADES

• Most hospital systems do not capture the majority of errors.[4]
• Studies of medical services suggest that only 1.5% of all ADEs result in an incident report and only 6% of ADEs are identified through traditional incident reporting or a telephone hotline.

• Incident reports or event reporting systems are voluntary reporting systems that are more likely to capture errors than ADEs.
• Chart reviews have been the foundation for research into medication errors and ADEs. This is an expensive process requiring time and dedicated personnel. There are limitations such as the reliability of reviewers to judge the presence of ADEs, and incomplete or poor documentation in the charts.
• The use of "triggers," or clues, to identify ADEs is an effective method developed by the Institute for Healthcare Improvement (IHI) for measuring the overall level of harm from medications in a healthcare organization (www.ihi.org).
  ○ Tracking ADEs over time is a useful way to tell if changes the team is making are improving the safety of the medication system.
• Direct observation is more effective in detecting errors during preparation and administration of medications. Disadvantages include:
  ○ The time needed for training and conducting the observation.
  ○ Confidentiality of data and how it may be used against an individual practitioner.
  ○ The focus on the individual performance rather than on the system as a whole.

STRATEGIES TO REDUCE ADES

• Standardize and simplify core medication processes in known high-risk areas (eg, protocols and templates, standard doses).
• Redesign delivery systems using proven human factors principles.

- Do not use unapproved abbreviations.
- Integrate clinical pharmacists into patient care.
- Make information available at the point of care (eg, laboratory data, allergy information).
- Implement technology wisely.
- Partner with patients.
- Create safety cultures that minimize blame and maximize communication.
- Perform medication reconciliation (see Chap. 30).
- Incorporate redundancy checks for high-alert medications that, even when used as intended, may cause harm or injury to the patient. Medications listed in this category include anticoagulants, insulin, narcotic/opiates, and concentrated electrolytes. A more extensive list can be found on www.ismp.org
- Add a second or double check at various stages of the medication process.
  - This check can be in the form of another individual from the same discipline or may include a different discipline.
  - The second check must be independent and should not be used instead of developing a reliable process that prevents errors from happening in the initial step.
- Formulary control and failure mode and effect analysis (FMEA) (www.patientsafety.gov) for new additions should be evaluated from the perspective of safety as well as efficacy and cost.
  - As new drugs are added to the formulary, hospitals should take a proactive approach to addressing potential errors.
  - Using a simplified FMEA, ask questions such as how likely is it that a prescriber will make an error in ordering this medication; how likely is it that the pharmacy will make an error in preparing or distributing this medication; and how likely is it that a nurse will make an error when administering this medication.
  - Does the drug name look like or sound like any other drug name? Does the packaging look like any other drug package?
  - Are any special monitoring parameters required when this drug is used?
  - Is any special equipment needed to prepare or administer this medication?
- Hospitalists can play an active role on pharmacy and therapeutic committees to ensure that the right questions are asked when drugs are added to the hospital formulary.

INFORMATION TECHNOLOGY

- Information technology (IT) holds the promise of improving hospital efficiency, reducing medical errors, and consolidating clinical information at the bedside where decisions are made.

- Although IT has great potential to improve patient safety and reduce medical errors including ADEs, it can also introduce new types of errors while addressing prior safety concerns.
- Computerized physician order entry (CPOE) is a term used to refer to a computer-based system used to order medications and other patient treatments. Use of CPOE provides for complete and legible orders.
- Optimal systems include clinical decision support that prompts the user as to appropriate drug, dose, frequency, and monitoring parameters.
- Systems with clinical decision support will also complete drug allergy checks, drug-laboratory value checks, and drug-drug interaction checks, as long as the clinician enters the correct information.
- IT also provides resources for ongoing research and many institutions have an IT infrastructure group.

THE ROLE OF THE HOSPITALIST

- The role of the hospitalist has evolved from improving hospital efficiency as the coordinator of inpatient care to leading innovative initiatives to promote patient safety.
- Many hospitalists are already implementing CPOE at their institutions. Some are working as physician-liaisons to their institution's patient safety and informatics officers and IT staff.
- Hospitalists work at the intersection of clinical medicine and applied informatics and are in a unique position to continually evaluate these complex information systems, how individuals interact with them, and how they affect workflow and patient care.
- Hospitalists can lead in researching and improving the information exchange at transitions of care; under standing and applying informatics solutions to workflow disruption caused by information systems, CPOE implementation, and clinical decision support; developing ways of standardizing aspects of hospital care that can improve quality, efficiency, and safety; and finally, educating house staff and medical students on the importance of information management as a fundamental aspect of our careers as physicians.

REFERENCES

1. Bates DW, Cullen DJ, Laird N, et al. Incidence of adverse drug events and potential adverse drug events: implications for prevention. *JAMA.* 1995;274:29–34.
2. Kohn L, Corrigan J, Donaldson M. *To Err is Human, Building a Safer Health System.* Washington, DC: Institute of Medicine, The National Academies Press, 2000.

3. Bates DW, Spell N, Cullen DJ, et al. The costs of adverse drug events in hospitalized patients. *JAMA*. 1997;277(4): 307–311.
4. Cullen D, Bates D, Small S, et al. The incident reporting system does not detect adverse events: a problem for quality improvement. *Jt Comm J Qual Improv*. 1995;21: 541–548.

6 MEDICATION DISCREPANCIES AND MEDICATION RECONCILIATION

Jeffrey L. Schnipper

SCOPE OF THE PROBLEM

- Drug therapies are the most common treatments in medical practice; their potential for both alleviating and causing illness is amply illustrated.
- Suboptimal drug therapy can result in avoidable patient suffering and even mortality because of drug side effects or inadequate control of disease or its symptoms.
  - One type of medication-related problem, adverse drug events (ADEs, broadly defined as any injury caused by medication) are particularly worrisome, preventable, and prevalent, especially during and following hospitalization (see Chap. 5).
- One newly appreciated cause of ADEs, especially at transition points such as hospital admission and discharge, is medication discrepancies.
- Medication discrepancies—that is unexplained differences between regimens, patients think they should be taking and those ordered by their physicians, or between documented regimens across different sites of care—are very common, especially after hospital discharge.
  - In one randomized controlled trial of a pharmacist intervention during and after hospital discharge, medication discrepancies were found to be the cause of slightly over half of all preventable ADEs that occurred within 30 days of discharge.[2]
- Discrepancies differ from problems of medication adherence (ie, differences between regimens patients think they should be taking and what they actually take) because the problem is one of communication and documentation more than patient motivation.
- Discrepancies can have serious consequences, including prolonged periods of over- or under treatment.

- The extent of the problem has been demonstrated in several recent studies, including three among general medical inpatients showing unexplained discrepancies on hospital admission or discharge in 49% to 54.4% of patients,[2–4] with approximately half these discrepancies having potential for patient harm.

CAUSES OF MEDICATION DISCREPANCIES

- Medication discrepancies occur for a variety of reasons:
  - Physicians may not obtain a comprehensive and accurate medication history at the time of admission.
  - Patients may be unaware of the medication regimens they were taking prior to admission, in part owing to receipt of medications from multiple providers, inadequate health literacy, and lack of patient involvement in their own care.
  - The medication history elicited from the patient at hospital admission is further affected by language barriers, the patient's current health status, the physician's medication history interviewing skills, and time constraints.
  - Physicians may not consult other important sources of medication information, including family members, prescription lists or bottles, outpatient medical records, and community pharmacy records.
  - These corroborating sources of medication information, including outpatient medical records, are often incomplete or inaccurate.
  - Additionally, multiple inpatient providers may independently take medication histories for the same patient, including a physician, nurse, or inpatient pharmacist, without recognizing or correcting differences among the various lists.
  - The most common error in the admission medication history involves omitting a medication taken at home.
- To complicate matters, significant alterations in a patient's medication regimen can occur several times during the hospitalization.
  - The acute illness may cause physicians to hold certain medications, discontinue others, or change prescribed doses during hospitalization.
  - At most hospitals, closed drug formularies necessitate substitution of one medication for another drug in the same class during the patient's hospital stay.
  - Changes from long-acting to short-acting medications are also routinely made in the name of tighter control (eg, of blood pressure).
  - In one study of hospitalized elders, 40% of all admission medications were discontinued by discharge and 45% of all discharge medications were newly started during the hospitalization.[5]

- At the time of discharge, the current medication regimen is not always reconciled with the preadmission medication regimen in a thoughtful manner.
  - Errors of reconciliation include failure to resume medications held or modified at admission for clinical reasons, failure to resume medications that were substituted in the hospital for formulary or pharmacokinetic reasons, and failure to stop newly started medications that were only required during the hospitalization (eg, for prevention of venous thromboembolism or stress ulcers).[6]
  - It is difficult even in hospitals with advanced electronic health information systems to prompt physicians to make these necessary changes.
- Finally, hospital discharge is often an extremely rushed event, making effective patient-provider communication difficult.
  - In one report, hospitalized elderly patients received an average of 5.3 minutes of medication education, and half of patients received no education at all.[7]
- In addition, hospital admission and discharge are often associated with discontinuity of care and miscommunication among providers. This may be particularly true with the use of hospitalists.
- Patients, especially the elderly, may become confused by how to reconcile their new and old regimens upon returning home.
  - Even 3 days after discharge, 29% of patients have unexplained medication discrepancies.[2]
  - One month after hospital discharge, regimen errors, including adding or deleting a drug or errors in dosing, can be found in 50% to 90% of patients.[8–10]
- Medication discrepancies can be *intentional* or *unintentional*.
  - If intentional, then there is no error. In the inpatient setting, the *timing* of an unintentional medication discrepancy can be at hospital admission (ie, between the preadmission medication regimen and the admission orders), at intra hospital transfer (ie, between preadmission medications and posttransfer orders, taking into account the patient's clinical status and their pretransfer medication regimen), and/or at hospital discharge (ie, between preadmission medications and discharge orders, again taking into account the patient's clinical status and their predischarge medications).
  - An unintentional discrepancy can be one of several *types.*
    - Omission of a medication; a change in dose, route, or frequency; a medication substitution; or an additional medication
- Finally, the *reason* for an unexplained discrepancy can be either a "history error" (eg, not including aspirin on the preadmission medication list (PAML),

thus explaining why it is not ordered at discharge), or a "reconciliation error" (eg, aspirin not restarted at discharge despite being present on the PAML and clinically indicated at discharge).

RISK FACTORS

- Studies have shown several risk factors for ADEs, in general and during and after hospitalization.
  - Patient age
  - Number of prescribed medications
  - Use of several classes of medications, including cardiac medications (including beta-blockers and angiotensin-converting enzyme [ACE] inhibitors), analgesics (including opiates and nonsteroidal anti-inflammatory drugs [NSAIDs]), antibiotics, antidepressants (including selective serotonin reuptake inhibitors [SSRIs]), diabetic medications, anticoagulants, and corticosteroids.
- Risk factors for medication discrepancies are less well defined, but may include the following:
  - Greater number of medications prescribed
  - High-risk medication classes
  - Number of changes made to medications during the hospitalization
  - Lack of patient familiarity with their preadmission medication regimen
  - Inadequate health literacy

EVIDENCE

- The prevalence of medication discrepancies and their potential for harm is only beginning to be appreciated and to receive attention from healthcare agencies.
  - The Joint Commission on Accreditation of Healthcare Organizations (JCAHO) now mandates medication reconciliation at the time of hospital admission and discharge in an effort to reduce discrepancies.
  - Reconciliation is "a process of identifying the most accurate list of all medications a patient is taking, including name, dosage, frequency, and route, and using this list to provide correct medications for patients anywhere within the healthcare system."[15]
  - Expectations for implementation include the resolution of any discrepancies and the communication of a complete list of the patient's medications to the next provider of service (within or outside the organization) and to the patient at the time of hospital discharge.[14]
- The evidence to support medication reconciliation is limited, but convincing.
  - In one investigation, when nursing staff obtained and pharmacists verified orders for home medications, the accuracy of admission medication orders increased from 40% to 95%.[16]

○ In other works, according to pharmacist-led medication reconciliation, significant discrepancies were found in approximately 25% of patients' medication histories and admission orders.[17]

○ In the absence of pharmacist intervention, the authors predicted that 22% of the discrepancies could have caused some form of patient harm during hospitalization, and 59% may have contributed to an adverse event if the error continued after discharge.[17]

○ Others report that orders were changed as a result of reconciliation for 94% of patients being transferred out of the intensive care unit.[18]

○ Finally, in a randomized controlled trial of a pharmacist intervention at discharge in which medication reconciliation was the most common action performed, preventable ADEs at 30 days were detected in 11% of control patients and 1% of intervention patients. Medication discrepancies were the cause of half the preventable ADEs in the control group.[2]

SYSTEMS IMPROVEMENT—THE PROCESS OF MEDICATION RECONCILIATION[19]

• An overview of the complete medication reconciliation process is shown in Fig. 6-1.

○ The process begins with taking an accurate and complete medication history and documenting it in a prominent place. This history should be confirmed by a second clinician and any discrepancies resolved.

○ The PAML should then be reconciled with the hospital admission orders; ideally, one clinician explicitly documents the planned action on admission of each preadmission medication, while a second clinician confirms that the reconciliation has been performed as planned.

○ At any time during the hospitalization, any uncertainties about the PAML should be clarified and updates to it should be made based on the most complete and accurate data.

○ If there is an intra hospital transfer, the preadmission and pretransfer medication lists should be explicitly used to create the post-transfer medication list, and this reconciliation process should be confirmed.

○ Similarly, at hospital discharge, the preadmission and predischarge medication lists should be used to create the hospital discharge orders and this reconciliation process confirmed by a second clinician.

○ The discharge medication orders and all changes from the PAML should be explicitly communicated to the patient and the receiving postdischarge provider.

○ Each of these processes is described in detail below. Note that the primary and secondary clinicians in Fig. 6-1 may be different personnel at different times, for example, a pharmacist may take the medication history while a physician writes the admission orders; a nurse may confirm the PAML while a pharmacist may confirm reconciliation. These designations are used to connote cross-checking of various stages of the process.

TAKING THE PREADMISSION MEDICATION HISTORY

• Optimal strategies for obtaining a complete medication history are shown in Table 6-1.

• These include asking patients about the following:

○ A typical day and what medications they take at different times of the day

○ Whether they get prescriptions from more than one doctor

  ▪ Nonoral medications (eg, inhalers, patches, etc.)

○ Dosage and indication for all medications

○ Length of therapy and timing of last dose

○ Over-the-counter products, herbals, vitamins, and supplements

○ Allergies

○ How many doses they have missed in the last week to assess adherence

• Forms are also available to help patients maintain a medication history (eg, from the American Association of Retired Persons Web site).

• Ideally, the process of obtaining medication history will involve the integration of several sources of information.

○ Patient and caregiver recollection

○ Lists of medications from the patient or caregiver

○ Prescription bottles

○ Outpatient medical records

○ Prescription refill information from community pharmacies

• Any discrepancies in the information obtained from these various sources should be explicitly resolved with the patient and/or caregiver. Assistance from a pharmacist or the patient's outpatient physician(s) may also be required.

CONFIRMATION AND UPDATING OF THE PREADMISSION MEDICATION LIST

• Ideally, the accuracy of the PAML should be confirmed by a second clinician (for example, at Brigham and Women's Hospital, the list is first built by the medical resident, after which the nurse confirms it with the patient).

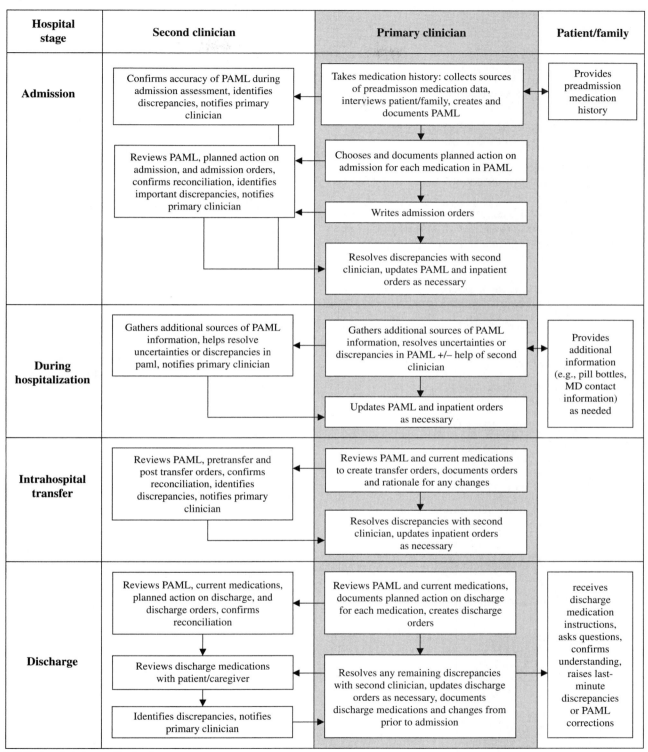

PAML: Preadmission medication list.

FIG. 6-1 Process of medication reconciliation.
SOURCE: Adapted with permission from: Poon EG, Blumenfeld B, Hamann C, et al. Design and implementation of a application and associated services to support interdisciplinary medication reconciliation efforts at an integrated healthcare delivery network. *J Am Med Inform Assoc.* 2006;13:581–592.[20]

TABLE 6-1 Tips for Taking a Complete and Accurate Medication History

- Ask about
  - Medication allergies and reactions
  - A typical day and what medications the patient takes at different times of the day
  - If the patient receives medication prescriptions from more than one provider, obtain the contact information for each prescribing provider
  - The patient's community pharmacy(ies) and phone number or town
  - How sure the patient is of their medications; who knows their medications the best
  - Various types of medications: tablets, oral liquids, eye drops, ear drops, nasal sprays, inhalers, patches, creams, lotions, injections, suppositories
  - Over-the-counter products, herbals, vitamins, and supplements
  - The indication for each medication
  - The strength, dose, and frequency of all medications (eg, one 20 mg tablet twice a day; 440 mcg inhaler, 2 puffs twice a day)
  - As needed medications and how often the patient uses them typically and recently
  - How long the patient has been taking the medication
  - The last time the patient took the medication
  - How many doses the patient has missed in the last week; explore reasons for nonadherence: cost, access to a pharmacy, lack of appreciation of need for medication, side effect, etc.
  - Potential side effects: type, duration, severity, actions taken by patient and prescriber
- Compare patient/caregiver information to objective sources of information: prescription pill bottles, outpatient medication lists, recent discharge or transfer orders, pharmacy refill information
- Explore discrepancies among the various sources of information
- Obtain additional objective information if patient unsure of medications or any discrepancies among sources

---

- Any uncertainties, discrepancies, or additional sources of medication information should prompt a conversation between the two clinicians and a plan to resolve the issue (eg, calling the family to have them bring in pill bottles from home, or contacting the patient's primary care physician or community pharmacy).
- This process may need to continue well after admission in order to obtain the most accurate and complete preadmission medication history possible.
- Note that while this process of confirmation is somewhat redundant, it replaces useless redundancy (ie, multiple clinicians taking separate medication histories without any communication or attempt to resolve differences) with purposeful cross-checking (ie, clinicians working together off a single PAML to iteratively refine it over time).

RECONCILING MEDICATIONS AT ADMISSION

- Once the preadmission medication regimen is confirmed, it should be entered on a standardized form and placed in a prominent place in the chart.
- This list should then be compared against the patient's medication orders at hospital admission. The planned

action for each of these medications at admission (eg, continue at same dose/route/frequency, continue at a different dose/route/frequency, substitute with a different medication in the same class, or discontinue) should be made explicit by the ordering clinician (usually the admitting physician).
- A second clinician (eg, a hospital pharmacist) should review the PAML, the planned action on admission for each medication, and the actual admission orders to make sure that reconciliation has indeed taken place.
- Clinically important discrepancies should prompt communication among clinicians and a plan to resolve the issue, including correction of unintentional discrepancies and appropriate documentation of intentional changes.

RECONCILING MEDICATIONS AT TRANSFER

- During intrahospital transfer, the preadmission medications and current (pretransfer) hospital medication list should be used to create coherent transfer orders based on the patient's clinical status. Ideally, the planned action on transfer for each medication from both these lists should be made explicit and clearly documented.
- A second clinician (eg, the accepting physician) should review these three lists (preadmission, pretransfer, and post-transfer) and the planned actions on transfer to confirm that reconciliation has taken place properly.
- Transfers from the intensive care unit to a hospital floor are especially prone to medication errors, as this is often the time when many preadmission medications need to be restarted.

RECONCILING MEDICATIONS AT DISCHARGE

- At hospital discharge, the preadmission list needs to be compared with the current hospital medications in order to create a coherent set of discharge orders. The planned action on discharge should be made explicit.
- A second clinician (eg, the nurse or pharmacist who provides discharge medication instructions to the patient) should review all three lists (preadmission, predischarge, and discharge) and the planned actions on discharge to confirm that reconciliation has indeed taken place properly.
- The discharge summary and written patient instructions should contain a clear list of the discharge medications and an explicit explanation of how this regimen is different from the one taken prior to admission (eg, which medications are new, which involve a change in dose or frequency, and which old medications should no longer be taken).

- Avoiding overarching orders such as "continue home medications" and "resume all medications" is crucial to patient safety at discharge.
- During patient discharge counseling, the provider should emphasize these changes, as well as the indications, directions and potential side effects of all new medications.

STAFFING ISSUES

- Staff responsibilities for obtaining and documenting an accurate list of preadmission medications and reconciling medications at admission, transfer, and discharge should be well defined and based on the resources available at each institution.
- Ultimately, it becomes the physician's duty to ensure provision of correct and complete medication information.
- If possible, partnering with clinical pharmacists seems to provide optimal results, as pharmacists have received formal education and have experience taking medication histories, which may make them the ideal interviewer for all patients admitted to the hospital.
- Unfortunately, pharmacists are responsible for only about 5% of medication history interviews taken in US hospitals, and they only participate in about 33% of discharge counseling.
- Patients who are at high risk for medication discrepancies, as noted above under risk factors, may require additional counseling or pharmacist involvement for effective reconciliation.

ROLE OF INFORMATION TECHNOLOGY

- To date, most medication reconciliation systems have relied on paper. This may be adequate when inpatient medication orders are also done using paper.
- However, in hospitals that use computer physician order entry (CPOE), a paper process creates additional steps and inefficiencies that may impede adoption. In those hospitals, it may be preferable to use a computerized system. Besides better integration with CPOE, such a system may have several advantages:
  - The ability to automatically pull various electronic sources of medication information with which to build the PAML, such as outpatient medication lists, pharmacy prescription fill information, and medication regimens from skilled nursing facilities. Such advantages depend, of course, on the availability and interoperability of these sources.
  - The ability to remind and prompt clinicians to perform medication reconciliation.
  - Facilitation of documentation of medication lists across transitions in care, the changes made to these lists, and the reasons for changes made.
  - Increased portability and legibility of medication information from various locations within a hospital.
  - The ability to "line up" various medication lists by medication class, allowing for easier comparison of regimens across transitions in care.
  - The generation of reports that, for example, explicitly document differences between preadmission and discharge medication regimens and automatically paste the report into a discharge summary.
- Partners Healthcare, Inc., has created an application with many of these features.[20] Its effects on patient outcomes are currently being evaluated.

CONCLUSION

- Medication discrepancies are very common at transitions in care and are a major source of ADEs during and after hospitalization.
- Medication reconciliation is the process of taking a complete and accurate preadmission medication history, explicitly comparing that regimen to admission, transfer, and discharge orders, and communicating the current regimen to the next provider of care at all transitions.
  - This process is designed to prevent medication discrepancies and improve patient safety and is now mandated by the JCAHO.
  - Each hospital should have a system in place for ensuring that each step of medication reconciliation is performed as accurately as possible.
  - This process likely involves the collaboration of physicians, nurses, and pharmacists, and might include the use of information technology.
- Hospitalists will likely have a major role in designing and implementing medication reconciliation protocols at their hospitals.

REFERENCES

1. Coleman EA, Smith JD, Raha D, et al. Posthospital medication discrepancies: prevalence and contributing factors. *Arch Intern Med.* 2005;165:1842–1847.
2. Schnipper JL, Kirwin JL, Cotugno MC, et al. Role of pharmacist counseling in preventing adverse drug events after hospitalization. *Arch Intern Med.* 2006;166:565–571.
3. Cornish PL, Knowles SR, Marchesano R, et al. Unintended medication discrepancies at the time of hospital admission. *Arch Intern Med.* 2005;165:424–429.

4. Gleason KM, Groszek JM, Sullivan C, et al. Reconcilation of discrepancies in medication histories and admission orders of newly hospitalized patients. *Am J Health Syst Pharm.* 2004;61:1689–1695.

5. Beers MH, Dang J, Hasegawa J, et al. Influence of hospitalization on drug therapy in the elderly. *J Am Geriatr Soc.* 1989;37:679–683.

6. Holzmueller CG, Hobson D, Berenholtz SM. Medication reconciliation: are we meeting the requirements? *J Clin Outcomes Mgmt.* 2006;13:441–444.

7. Alibhai SM, Han RK, Naglie G. Medication education of acutely hospitalized older patients. *J Gen Intern Med.* 1999;14:610–616.

8. Bedell SE, Jabbour S, Goldberg R, et al. Discrepancies in the use of medications: their extent and predictors in an outpatient practice. *Arch Intern Med.* 2000;160:2129–2134.

9. Cochrane RA, Mandal AR, Ledger-Scott M, et al. Changes in drug treatment after discharge from hospital in geriatric patients. *BMJ.* 1992;305:694–696.

10. Omori DM, Potyk RP, Kroenke K. The adverse effects of hospitalization on drug regimens. *Arch Intern Med.* 1991;151:1562–1564.

11. Forster AJ, Murff HJ, Peterson JF, et al. Adverse drug events occurring following hospital discharge. *J Gen Intern Med.* 2005;20:317–23.

12. Gandhi TK, Weingart SN, Borus J, et al. Adverse drug events in ambulatory care. *N Engl J Med.* 2003;348:1556–1564.

13. Gandhi TK, Weingart SN, Seger AC, et al. Outpatient prescribing errors and the impact of computerized prescribing. *J Gen Intern Med.* 2005;20:837–841.

14. Joint Commission on Accreditation of Healthcare Organizations. 2006 Critical Access Hospital and Hospital National Patient Safety Goals. http://www.jcaho.org/accredited+organizations/patient+safety/06_npsg/06_npsg_cah_hap.htm.

15. Institute for Healthcare Improvement. Medication Reconciliation Review: Luther Midelfort—Mayo Health System. http://www.ihi.org/IHI/Topics/PatientSafety/Medication Systems/Tools/Medication+Reconciliation+Review.htm. Accessed November 27, 2006.

16. Whittington J, Cohen H. OSF healthcare's journey in patient safety. *Qual Manag Health Care.* 2004;13:53–59.

17. Gleason KM, Groszek JM, Sullivan C, et al. Reconciliation of discrepancies in medication histories and admission orders of newly hospitalized patients. *Am J Health Syst Pharm.* 2004;61:1689–1695.

18. Pronovost P, Weast B, Schwarz M, et al. Medication reconciliation: a practical tool to reduce the risk of medication errors. *J Crit Care.* 2003;18:201–205.

19. Kripalani S, Jackson AT, Schnipper JL, et al. Promoting effective transitions in care at hospital discharge: a review of key issues for hospitalists. *J Hosp Med.* 2007; In press.

20. Poon EG, Blumenfeld B, Hamann C, et al. Design and implementation of a application and associated services to support interdisciplinary medication reconciliation efforts at an integrated healthcare delivery network. *J Am Med Inform Assoc.* 2006;13:581–592.

7 POLYPHARMACY

Jatin K. Dave and Juergen Bludau

OVERVIEW

- Polypharmacy is defined as the use of more medication than is clinically justified. In addition to inappropriate prescribing, it can also include incorrect dispensing and dosing.
- A higher number of appropriate medications is a common scenario, especially for older adults. The reasons for this include:
  - The addition of new drug treatments.
  - New indications for older drug treatments.
  - Lower thresholds for treating risk factors in preventative medicine.
  - The changing staging system for conditions like heart failure when earlier staging incorporates high-risk asymptomatic stages.
  - Combination therapy in selected situations to decrease the incidence and/or severity of adverse drug reactions, prevent the development of resistance, and increase the efficacy.
  - An aging population often with multiple pathologies.
- Appropriate use of a larger number of medications is called *rational polypharmacy*. This is especially common in older patients with multiple chronic conditions such as diabetes, heart failure, or coronary artery disease.
  - The need for multiple medications should be weighed against the risk of increased side effects/medication errors, reduced compliance, and increased cost of combination therapy.
  - Carefully balanced prescribing with risk/benefit analysis for an individual patient to achieve the desirable outcome and if possible reduce the number of medications is often necessary to prevent polypharmacy.
- Underuse of effective medications is also common. Therefore in addition to reducing prescribing of inappropriate medications, efforts should be targeted toward optimally prescribing effective medications.

EPIDEMIOLOGY

- Risk of polypharmacy is especially high in older adults because of higher prevalence of comorbidities, multiple providers, and sensory/cognitive impairment. Older adults are also vulnerable owing to a lack of physiologic reserve associated with aging called homeostenosis.

- The risk of polypharmacy is an important problem for hospitalized patients because of:
  ○ Association between hospitalization and polypharmacy.
  ○ Harms of polypharmacy.
  ○ Opportunities for medications modification during hospitalization.
  ○ Inadequate reconciliation of medications at the time of discharge.
- Hospitalizations present high-risk events during which significant medication changes are made and may lead to polypharmacy and inappropriate prescribing.
- Studies on prevalence of polypharmacy and interventions to prevent and manage polypharmacy in hospitalized patients are limited.
  ○ Changes in medication regimen are common in hospitalized patients. In a study of 197 older adults admitted to one hospital, 40% of all admission medications were discontinued by discharge and 45% of all discharge medications were newly started during the hospitalization.[1]
  ○ In another study, patients were discharged on an average of 8 medications, emphasizing both the importance of rational polypharmacy as well as the need for interventions to prevent/manage polypharmacy.[2]
- Polypharmacy is associated with adverse outcomes (including adverse drug events; hospitalizations; noncompliance; higher costs; and poor health outcomes such as falls, incontinence, cognitive impairment, and functional decline).
- Polypharmacy was associated with increased risk (5% to 10% increase in risk with each drug) of adverse drug reactions, noncompliance, and increased cost.[3,4,5]
  ○ In a study of 315 consecutive elderly patients admitted to an acute care hospital, 11.4% of admissions were because of noncompliance and 16.8% were caused by adverse drug reactions.
  ○ The patients admitted for adverse drug reactions took on average 6.3 medications compared to 3.8 medications in patients admitted for other reasons unrelated to adverse drug reactions, emphasizing the importance of avoiding polypharmacy.
- Polypharmacy is associated with increased risk of falls, incontinence, cognitive impairment, and functional decline.[6]
- Polypharmacy is also a predictor of post discharge mortality in older adults.[7]
- In a recent study, inappropriate medication use was directly associated with the number of medications, suggesting that polypharmacy may serve as a marker of quality of care.[8]
  ○ The number of drugs can be used to trigger a medication review.
  ○ However, the traditional number-based definitions (>5 or >7 drugs) are not realistic or useful because many patients require multiple drugs.

ETIOLOGY

- Since the development of polypharmacy is often multifactorial, including provider factors, patient factors, and system-related factors, multidimensional strategies are often required for prevention of polypharmacy (Table 7-1).
- Factors contributing to polypharmacy include (1) overuse of inappropriate prophylactic medications (especially proton pump inhibitors), (2) overuse of as-needed medications, and (3) prescription cascade.
  ○ The number of drugs increases with the number of clinician visits and hospitalizations.

TABLE 7-1 Etiology and Strategies for Preventing Polypharmacy

	ETIOLOGY	STRATEGIES
Provider factors	Multiple providers	Clear communication with specialists and primary care providers
	Prescription cascade	Suspect drugs as etiology of any new symptoms and use nonpharmacological treatment when possible
	Duplication	A careful and frequent review of medication list and bottles, therapeutic debridement
Patient factors	Lack of education concerning medications	Education at appropriate level
	A tendency toward self-treatment	A careful review of all medications including OTC and herbal medication
	Multiple disease states	A pill is not needed for every ill, careful prescribing with medication trial with measurable goals, when possible consult a pharmacist
System factors	Lack of sophisticated decision support systems	Development and implementation of evidence-based decision support systems
	Lack of access to pharmacy data	National electronic medical records system with access to pharmacy data
	Formulary differences across care settings	Medication reconciliation and careful communication

OTC, over-the-counter.

- Clinicians often inappropriately prescribe a new medication to treat the side effects of another drug frequently leading to a prescribing cascade.[9]
  - Also, the extent of repeat/duplicate prescribing is alarming, according to earlier studies, which show >70% prevalence. This number can increase with inappropriate medication reconciliation, especially in older adults.
- The limited time available for discussion for any sort and the time required at times to explain the rationale for not prescribing a medication compared to the time required for just prescribing it contributes to polypharmacy.
  - Careful patient education to demystify the myth of a "pill for every ill" is often necessary.
- Older age, female sex, multiple disease, recent hospitalization, and depression are known patient factors for polypharmacy.[10,11]
- System-related factors are the most challenging yet important contributors to polypharmacy.
  - A default dosing without the proper decision support system incorporating patient-related factors in early computerized physician order entry (CPOE) systems can lead to inappropriate doses in high-risk populations.
  - Limited knowledge of geriatric pharmacology and a tendency to click on a default option in routine CPOE systems as well as the power of inertia lead to polypharmacy and inappropriate dosing.
  - Inappropriate use of reminders and audits could also lead to polypharmacy, especially in frail older patients, in which some of the quality indicators have limited applicability.
- Because of the increasing number of efficacious drugs, it is important to differentiate preventable/manageable polypharmacy from rational/legitimate polypharmacy.
- Common conditions that may occur as a result of polypharmacy and common drug offenders causing these conditions are highlighted in Table 7-2.

STRATEGIES FOR PREVENTION AND MANAGEMENT

- Reduction of polypharmacy is one of the principal health protection goals in Healthy People 2000 (Table 7-3).
- We recommend a stepwise method, using an interdisciplinary approach including clinician, pharmacist, and information systems on admission, during hospitalization and on discharge focusing on risk stratification (Fig. 7-1).
  1. Risk stratification: Any patient with high-risk drug indicators or patient indicators is considered at high

TABLE 7-2   Common Conditions Caused by Polypharmacy and Drugs Likely to Cause These Conditions

Delirium	Antihistamines (diphenhydramine)
	Anticholinergics
	Older antihypertensives (reserpine, methyldopa, propranolol, clonidine)
	Antipsychotics
	Benzodiazepines
	Narcotics (at higher doses)
	H2 blockers (cimetidine)
	NSAIDs (especially indomethacin)
Constipation	Narcotics
	Calcium channel blockers
	Anticholinergics
	Tricyclic antidepressants
Diarrhea	Colchicine
	Donepezil
	Erythromycin
	Laxatives
	Levothyroxine
	Metformin
	Misoprostol
Liver dysfunction	NSAIDs
	Statins
	Antiepileptic drugs
	Antituberculosis drugs
Renal dysfunction	Diuretics
	Cyclosporine
	Methotrexate
	Amphotericin B
	Aminoglycosides
	Phenytoin
	Ciprofloxacin
Leg edema	Calcium channel blockers
	NSAIDs
	Prednisone
Hypertension	NSAIDs
	Prednisone
	Pseudoephedrine
Hypotension/falls/ dizziness/balance disturbances	Antihypertensives (especially diuretics, nitrates, calcium channel blockers)
	Antipsychotics
	Tricyclic antidepressants
	Antiparkinsonian agents
Anemia/ thrombocytopenia/ leucopenia	Chloramphenicol
	Cytotoxics
	NSAIDs
	Colchicine
	Sulfonamides
	Thiazides
	Antiepileptics
Hypoglycemia	Beta-blockers
	H2 receptor blockers
	Acetaminophen
	Alcohol
Hyponatremia	Thiazide diuretics
	Antidepressants (especially SSRIs)
	ACE inhibitors
	Antineoplastic agents
	Sulfonylurea
	Antipsychotics
	Anticonvulsants (especially carbamazepine

ACE, angiotensin-converting enzyme; NSAIDS, nonsteroidal anti-inflammatory drugs; SSRIs, selective serotonin reuptake inhibitors.

TABLE 7-2 Common Conditions Caused by Polypharmacy and Drugs Likely to Cause These Conditions (*Continued*)

Incontinence	Diuretics
	Antihistamines (diphenhydramine)
	Anticholinergics (disopyramide)
	Antispasmodics (dicyclomine)
	Antiparkinsonian agents
	Tricyclic antidepressants
	Antipsychotics
	Benzodiazepines
	Narcotics
	Alpha-blockers (prazosin, terazosin)
	Alpha-agonists (OTC nasal decongestants)
	Calcium channel blockers
Depression	Beta-blockers
	Calcium channel blockers
	Neuroleptics
Dyspepsia	NSAIDs
	Erythromycin
	Bisphophonates

NSAIDs, nonsteroidal anti-inflammatory drugs; OTC, over-the-counter.

risk for polypharmacy. High-risk drug indicators include:

- >12 doses of medications per day or >9 active medications.
- Specific medications: digoxin, warfarin.
- Anticonvulsants, antipsychotics, sedatives/hypnotics, benzodiazepines, narcotics, anticholinergics.
- High-risk drug combinations and high-risk disease-durg interactions (Table 7-4).

High-risk patient indicators include:

- Six or more active chronic medical diagnoses.
- Prior adverse drug reaction.
- Body mass index (BMI)<20 kg/m^2.
- Age >75 years.

- Impaired renal or liver function.
- Cognitive impairment.

2. Careful review and adjustments.

In high-risk patients, a thorough medication history, including over-the-counter/herbal medications, a consultation with a pharmacist, and assessment of adherence may help in managing polypharmacy.

- Assessment of indication/need, adherence, magnitude of prioritization (based on the risk assessment), potential for simplification, and feasibility of discontinuation trial will help determine the intensity of *therapeutic debridement*.
- Learning what patients should versus what they can actually take is the most important and at times challenging step in preventing polypharmacy especially in high-risk patients.
- Individualized adjustment with the goal of simplifying a medical regimen based on patient capabilities, once-a-day dosing, availability of combinations, and alternate routes (eg, per rectal route if patient is nauseous because of medications) is often necessary.
- Whether the inpatient setting is an ideal setting for medications change or not is debatable. If the patient is admitted for a medical problem for which drug regimen adjustment is necessary, then the hospital setting is likely the appropriate setting for a change. Hospitals provide a unique opportunity to discontinue certain medications owing to the feasibility of close monitoring if required.
- Awareness of common contributors and strategies to overcome those factors are critical to prevent and manage polypharmacy (Table 7-5).

3. Monitoring, follow-up, and communication to other providers are critical and include:
- A constant review of the need, compliance, and monitoring for common side effects.

TABLE 7-3 Role of Each Member of the Team During Each Phase of Hospitalization to Prevent Polypharmacy

	ON ADMISSION	DURING HOSPITALIZATION	ON DISCHARGE
Patient	Bring up-to-date medication list and all medication bottles when possible	Keep patients informed of any changes	Recheck/reconcile the home medications to prevent duplications and stockpiling
Clinician	• Assess the patient's risk for polypharmacy • Adjust medical regimen, eg, tapering of unnecessary high-risk medications • Communicate to all involved providers about the adjustments	Make necessary adjustments (therapeutic debridement) and monitor for any side effects	• Discontinue unnecessary as-needed and prophylactic medications • Update the primary care provider about the discharge medications • Schedule an f/u for high-risk medications and medication changes
Pharmacist/Nursing	• Review and update list • Recommend adjustment especially for high-risk interactions	Help patient and team simplify the regimen Educate about the common side effects	• Educate patient on medication changes • Provide up-to-date list with indication, duration, and doses
Information systems	• Decision support based on patient-related factors such as age, renal function • Provide an up-to-date list for medication reconciliation	Reminders for high-risk medications and recommendations for efficacious medications	• Facilitate the transfer of information to primary care provider and medication reconciliation

f/u, follow-up.

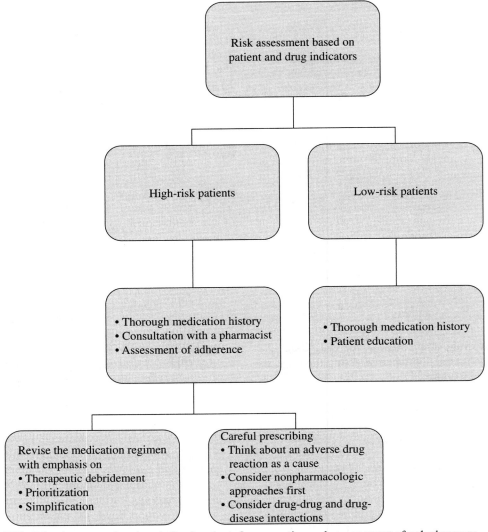

FIG. 7-1 An approach to hospitalized patients for prevention and management of polypharmacy.

TABLE 7-4 Common Drug-Drug and Disease-Drug Interactions

DRUG-DRUG	DISEASE-DRUG
Warfarin-NSAIDs (or sulfa drugs or macrolides or quinolones or phenytoin)	Cognitive impairment, anticholinergics
Digoxin, amiodarone (or verapamil)	Arrhythmia, tricyclic antidepressants
ACE inhibitors: potassium supplements and spironolactone	Falls/dizziness, diuretics
	Hyponatremia, SSRI
	Seizure disorder, bupropion
	Obesity, olanzapine
	Constipation, calcium channel blockers
	Insomnia, decongestants
	Parkinson disease, metochlorpropamide
	Gastric ulcer, NSAIDs

ACE, angiotensin-converting enzyme; NSAIDs, nonsteroidal anti-inflammatory drugs; SSRI, selective serotonin reuptake inhibitor.

○ Succinct and timely communication (including a query to subspecialists if needed) to all providers.
○ Reassessment of the necessity based on patient-centered goals of care and clinical condition. For example, the need for statins should be reconsidered in a patient with advanced dementia, anorexia, or weight loss of 10 lb over the last 6 months.
4. Careful prescribing includes:
   ○ Consideration of risk of adverse drug reactions, drug-drug interactions, and drug-disease interactions for any new medication.
   ○ Identification of high-risk medications based on age, organ dysfunction (renal failure, liver failure, or heart failure), and drug interactions.
   ○ Prescriptions for conditions only when indicated with specific goals in mind using a time-limited trial.

TABLE 7-5 Contributors to Polypharmacy and Strategies to Overcome Them

CONTRIBUTORS	STRATEGIES
Overuse of prophylactic medications	• Standardized protocols • Timely discontinuation of prophylactic
Overuse of as-needed medications	• Standardized protocols • Timely discontinuation of as-needed medications
Inappropriate medication reconciliation	Careful review of medication with the patient and PCP on admission and discharge
Prescription cascade	• Consider medication side effect as the cause of all new symptoms until proven otherwise • Use of effective nonpharmacological strategies first when possible
Duplication caused by formulary change	Review home medication on discharge
Nonadherence	• Simplification with least frequent dosing needed • Tie doses to scheduled daily activities, meals, sleep/wake cycle • Cognitive assessment • Education • Support • Medication flow sheet • Medication organization equipment
Stockpiling	Brown bag test and discard all unnecessary medications
Duplication	• Communication among prescribers with specific clarification of who will monitor what • Periodic review
Inertia	Drugs without indications (or proven benefits) should be carefully stopped!

PCP, primary care physician.

○ Consideration of patient's age, adherence, renal function, hepatic function, allergies, side effects, cost of the drug, and potential for drug-drug and drug-disease interaction when selecting the drug, its duration, and its dose.
○ Patient education regarding goals for medication, common side effects, and guidance on management of these side effects.

CARE TRANSITIONS

• Care transitions increase risk of polypharmacy.
• A clear communication among providers about indication, dose duration of each medication, recent relevant laboratory results, and a plan for managing high-risk medications is essential to reduce the risk and harm of polypharmacy at each transition.

SUMMARY

• Polypharmacy, defined as the use of more medications than is clinically justified, is an important target to improve quality of care provided to hospitalized patients.
• Hospitalists are in a unique position to make certain medication adjustments otherwise not feasible at home.
• The etiology of polypharmacy is often multifactorial, involving provider, patient, and system factors; requiring an interdisciplinary approach on admission, during hospitalization, and on discharge from the hospital to prevent/manage polypharmacy. Individualized interventions based on risk assessment may reduce the risk and prevent harm from polypharmacy.

• Care transitions increase the risk of polypharmacy.
• A clear communication of indication, dose, duration of each medication, recent relevant laboratory results, and plan for managing high-risk medication is essential to reduce the risk and harm of polypharmacy.

BIBLIOGRAPHY

Beers MH, Dang J, Hasegawa J, et al. Influence of hospitalization on drug therapy in the elderly. *J Am Geriatr Soc.* 1989;37:679–683.

Benner JS, Glynn RJ, Mogun H, et al. Long-term persistence in use of statin therapy in elderly patients. *JAMA.* 2002;288:455–461.

Bjerrum L, SÃ¸gaard J, Hallas J, et al. Polypharmacy: correlations with sex, age, and drug regimen. *Eur J Clin Pharmacol.* 1998;V54:197–202.

Col N, Fanale JE, Kronholm P. The role of medication noncompliance and adverse drug reactions in hospitalizations of the elderly. *Arch Intern Med.* 1990;150:841–845.

Hanlon JT, Pieper CF, Hajjar ER, et al. Incidence and predictors of all and preventable adverse drug reactions in frail elderly persons after hospital stay. *J Gerontol A Biol Sci Med Sci.* 2006;61:511–515.

Iwata M, Kuzuya M, Kitagawa Y, et al. Underappreciated predictors for postdischarge mortality in acute hospitalized oldest-old patients. *Gerontology.* 2006;52:92–98.

McMillan DA, Harrison PM, Rogers LJ, et al. Polypharmacy in an Australian teaching hospital. Preliminary analysis of prevalence, types of drugs, and associations. *Med J Aust.* 1986;145:339–342.

Rochon PA, Gurwitz JH. Optimising drug treatment for elderly people: the prescribing cascade. *BMJ.* 1997;315:1096–1099.

Schnipper JL, Kirwin JL, Cotugno MC, et al. Role of pharmacist counseling in preventing adverse drug events after hospitalization. *Arch Intern Med.* 2006;166:565–571.

Steinman MA, Seth Landefeld C, Rosenthal GE, et al. Polypharmacy and prescribing quality in older people. *J Am Geriatr Soc.* 2006;54:1516–1523.

Ziere G, Dieleman JP, Hofman A, et al. Polypharmacy and falls in the middle age and elderly population. *Br J Clin Pharmacol.* 2006;61:218–223.

8 PATIENT SAFETY: PREVENTING AND RESPONDING TO ADVERSE EVENTS

Allen Kachalia and Tejal K. Gandhi

OVERVIEW

- Adverse events are inevitable in clinical practice. Many are expected consequences of treatment, and some are foreseeable risks or complications of treatment. However, some adverse events—those that result from errors—are regarded as preventable.
- Patient safety principles seek to reduce the occurrence of preventable adverse events by eradicating errors in medical care.
- Errors and adverse events frequently trigger a broad range of legal, regulatory, and ethical obligations.
- When an error in medical care occurs, issues surrounding apology and disclosure can be very challenging.

BACKGROUND

- The burden of medical error and injury has captured significant attention since the Institute of Medicine (IOM) published its landmark report, *To Err Is Human: Building a Safer Health System* (2000), and followed with *Crossing the Quality Chasm: A New Health System for the 21st Century* (2001). These reports heightened not only the medical profession's interest in addressing the problem of errors in medicine, but also that of the public.
- Based largely on studies of injury in the inpatient setting, the IOM has estimated that approximately 44,000–98,000 patients annually die because of medical error in US hospitals. At the time of the *To Err is Human: Building a Safer System* report, the lower estimate placed medical error as the eighth leading cause of death in the United States.
- A significant amount of patient safety research today focuses on the inpatient environment because high patient acuity, frequent patient turnover, and multiple personnel changes are thought to raise the risks of serious and preventable injuries.
- Many hospital medicine programs strive, as one of their primary goals, to improve patient safety during hospitalization and related transitions in care.

PRINCIPLES IN PATIENT SAFETY

- The science of patient safety improvement is based on a systems approach to error. Aviation and engineering industries pioneered the approach, providing the basis for many principles in the healthcare arena.
  - Definitions in the field of patient safety often vary. The variation in taxonomy is largely attributable to the relative youth of the field. Table 8-1 provides a list of commonly employed definitions.
- Improvement is realized by building better systems of care delivery, as opposed to focusing on a given individual's behaviors. Goals include identifying where human error is likely to occur and then designing, and redesigning, processes to prevent or intercept errors (Table 8-2).
- A fundamental premise to a systems approach is that all clinicians try to exercise appropriate care and skill at all times; however, providers will still make mistakes regardless of how carefully they act.
- The recognition that error is inevitable heralds the notion that, when a mistake happens, blame should not be placed on individuals. Instead, the emphasis should remain on determining where and how the system could have prevented the error from reaching the patient.
- Systems are often analyzed through a framework of systems or contributing factors, that is, the reasons that "contributed" to the adverse event. Categories of such factors include:
  - Organizational context (eg, Were adequate resources dedicated to the provider?)
  - Work environment (eg, Was the lighting sufficient?)
  - Team and communication (eg, Was enough information transmitted during a handoff?)
  - Individual (eg, Was the provider adequately rested?)
  - Device design (eg, Was the equipment designed so that it could be used without unnecessary confusion?)
- Hospitals often charge quality improvement and risk management offices with improving patient safety. A

TABLE 8-1   Some Commonly Used Terms and Definitions in Patient Safety

Adverse outcome	Any harm to a patient. The cause of the harm can be the patient's underlying disease or because of medical treatment or management.
Adverse event	An adverse outcome that results from medical treatment (or management).
Error (IOM definition)	Either the use of a wrong plan to achieve a goal (error of plan) or the failure of a plan to be completed as intended (error of execution). An error can be an act of commission or omission.
Preventable adverse event	An adverse event resulting from an error.
Near miss	An error that, for some fortuitous reason, does not result in an adverse outcome. A near miss can be an error that was intercepted or one that reached a patient but did not yield injury.
Negligence	In general, the failure of a caregiver to provide the amount of care and skill that a reasonably prudent practitioner in the same specialty practicing in similar circumstances would provide. This level of care and skill is often referred to as the "standard of care." The definition of negligence can vary slightly from state to state based on judicial precedent and statutes.
Sentinel event (JCAHO definition)	An unexpected occurrence involving death or serious physical or psychological injury, or the risk thereof.
Disclosure	The notifying of a patient or family member about an error or adverse event that has occurred in the course of medical care.
Reporting	The notifying of an internal, regulatory, or state entity about an error or adverse event that has occurred in the course of medical care.
RCA and FMEA	A multidisciplinary investigation conducted to elucidate the root cause(s) of an adverse event. A proactive investigation to uncover latent errors. The analysis of a process in each of its parts (or steps). Each part is evaluated and scored for: the probability that a breakdown could occur, the likelihood that the breakdown would go undetected by other parts of the process, and the severity of the potential harm. Processes with higher scores are prioritized for intervention first.

FMEA, failure mode and effects analysis; RCA, root cause analysis.

number of tools for a systems focused analysis are available for this task.

○ To evaluate why an adverse event occurred, a root cause analysis (RCA) may be performed. An RCA is conducted by assembling a multidisciplinary group to discuss and investigate the event, and then reviewing relevant aggregate data. Based on the findings, steps to prevent similar events from happening in the future may be implemented.

○ Institutions do not have to wait for an error to determine where and how make care safer. New processes (or changes in current ones) should be evaluated to identify and prevent failures before they happen. One method to achieve this goal is a failure mode and effects analysis (FMEA), which is described in Table 8-1.

TABLE 8-2   Selected Examples of High-Priority Patient Safety Strategies for the Inpatient Setting

Ensure deep venous thrombosis prophylaxis in all appropriate patients
Use two patient identifiers when giving blood, medication, or providing a procedure
Read back verbal orders
Conduct clear and timely handoffs that, when appropriate, include medication lists
Ask patients to recount informed consent discussions
Chart patient preferences for life-saving treatments
Ensure active participation of a pharmacist in medication use
Utilize dedicated anticoagulation clinics
Evaluate all patients undergoing elective surgery for cardiac risk and provide beta-blockers when appropriate
Reconcile medications at admission and discharge
Use antibiotic prophylaxis for surgery
Utilize protocols to avoid contrast-related nephropathy
Utilize methods to prevent catheter-related infections (including sterile barriers and antibiotic-coated catheters)
Use real-time ultrasound guidance during central venous catheter placement
Ensure appropriate hand-washing
Vaccinate health workers for influenza
Continuously aspirate subglottic secretions for ventilated patients
Utilize strategies to prevent malnourishment in the hospital
Use computerized physician order entry
Staff intensive care units with intensivists

Data from Shojania et al. (2001).

HOSPITAL-SPECIFIC SAFETY INTERVENTIONS

• Patient safety research and improvement efforts have begun to demonstrate where harm often occurs and what clinical areas should receive priority.
• Important sources of preventable inpatient injury include:
  ○ Medication use (particularly during ordering)
  ○ Wound infections
  ○ Poor handoffs and transitions in care (including discharge)
  ○ Technical complications from surgery
• Patient safety organizations have identified priority areas of intervention. Their selection was based on a host of factors: the amount and severity of harm occurring, the ability of an intervention to prevent the harm and the strength of the evidence supporting it, and feasibility of implementing the intervention. Table 8-3 provides a list of interventions highly pertinent to hospital medicine.

TABLE 8-3 Key Principles in Patient Safety

Errors in medical care are common and many adverse events preventable

Embrace a system approach

Blame should not be the focus when errors occur. Rather, the system of care should be improved when errors occur

Numerous valuable strategies to reduce harm have already been identified

Developing a culture of safety is a high-priority need

Reporting of adverse events is critically important to improving safety

A large barrier to reporting and disclosure remains the fear of a lawsuit and liability. Evidence of the effect disclosure exerts on malpractice liability remains inconclusive. However, ethical obligations and patient preference support disclosure. Legal and regulatory mandates for disclosure may also exist

Disclosure should be conducted with honesty and sincerity, and not lay blame on any caregiver. Disclosure should include an assurance that an investigation will be conducted and that potential steps to prevent future harm will be taken

- Voluntary reporting has been identified as an on going and critical need to better target and design safety interventions. Improved data collection would permit valuable analyses of where and how errors are occurring. Many institutions have an internal voluntary safety reporting process that should be utilized when an error, near miss, or adverse event occurs.

LAWS AND REGULATIONS

- The occurrence of an error or adverse event (whether preventable or not) can trigger legal and regulatory requirements. The mandated obligations vary, and are based on a multitude of factors that include the type of error, cause of the event, type of harm, severity of harm, and state (jurisdiction) in which the event occurred.
  - Regulatory requirements
    - Joint Commission on the Accreditation of Healthcare Organization (JCAHO) standards contain an investigative and disclosure requirement.
      - JCAHO requires that institutions conduct an RCA for all sentinel events and if necessary, take steps to prevent events from repeating in the future. Hospitals are encouraged, but not required, to report to JCAHO any sentinel event.
      - JCAHO also requires that patients and, when appropriate, their families are informed about the outcomes of care, treatment, and services that have been provided, including unanticipated outcomes. "Unanticipated outcome" has not been specifically defined.
  - State law
    - Peer review:
      - To encourage internal quality and patient safety improvement efforts, most states provide some

level of statutory "peer-review protection" for members participating in, and information elicited and collected during, qualified endeavors. Protection for members can mean insulation from legal liability during these activities. Information that garners protection cannot be used in legal proceedings.

- The nature of the activities and information protected is very state specific. It is important to note that, even if a member or activity enjoys peer-review protection, that protection can be lost if all required conditions for protection are not met.
  - Reporting and disclosure:
    - At least 27 states have some type of reporting requirement for errors or adverse events. State laws continue to evolve and vary broadly on what must be reported, how reporting must occur, and who will have access to report information.
    - At least six states require, in certain circumstances, disclosure of an error or adverse event to a patient or family member.
    - A majority of, but not all, states have passed what are commonly known as "I'm sorry" laws. Varying by state, these laws may protect provider expressions of sorrow or apology after an adverse event from being used in a court of law as proof of liability.
  - Federal law
    - At present, a federal mandatory reporting requirement for errors or adverse events does not exist.

DISCLOSURE AND APOLOGY

- Ethical principles: Notwithstanding the legal or regulatory obligations described above, ethical obligations of physicians support disclosure. Three relevant ethical principles include respect of patient autonomy, fiduciary duty to patients, and equity (dealing fairly with patients). Medical societies and scholars have voiced support for disclosure with some advocating that ethical principles mandate disclosure.
- Patient and provider expectations: Beyond the legal, regulatory, and mandates, a key concern centers upon what patients and providers expect and want when an adverse event or medical error occurs.
  - Patients prefer to be informed of all errors in their care. This appears to be true for errors regardless of extent of the resultant harm, ranging from trivial to serious, and even for errors with no harm (near misses)
  - Patients may often expect some type of compensation or provider discipline when a medical error occurs.

- Physicians demonstrate mixed feelings regarding the disclosure of error. In one study, 77% of physicians reported that physicians should be required to tell patients when errors are made in their care.[5] However, in the same survey, 86% of physicians felt that hospital reports of serious medical errors should be confidential.
- Physicians tend to define error more narrowly than patients.
- In today's environment of increasing transparency, hospitals are increasingly adopting institution specific disclosure policies.
- **Malpractice fears:** An oft-cited barrier to error reporting and disclosure malpractice risk. Providers voice concern that an apology may lead to lawsuits and liability that would not otherwise have existed.
  - When an adverse event owing to negligence occurs, it is estimated that only 2% to 3% of the time does a malpractice claim result.
  - The association between disclosure and malpractice liability remains unknown. Multiple anecdotal reports, and some "before and after" analyses, have suggested that total liability may decrease, but these data are not controlled or adjusted. While most agree that the average payment per claim will decrease with disclosure, it remains unknown whether the absolute number of lawsuits will rise or fall.
  - The quality of patient relationship with their physician is thought be an important factor that leads patients to file a claim. Of patients and families that sue, many do so because of feeling ignored or neglected, sensing a cover-up, or wanting an explanation of the event.
  - The severity of a patient's injury or disability (and not underlying negligence in care) has been shown to be a driver of claims and payment.
- **Key principles for apology and disclosure:** The combination of (1) legal, regulatory, and ethical mandates; (2) difficulty in elucidating the relation between disclosure and malpractice; and (3) evidence on the importance of good physician-patient relationships has led some experts to offer the following considerations at the time of an error or adverse event:
  - Caregivers should request and secure the involvement of risk management upon discovery of the event. Risk management can provide not only expertise and advice on relevant regulatory requirements and next steps, but also support and sources of support.

- Caregivers should remember that an adverse event can be a difficult emotional time for all involved, including patients, families, and providers.
- Support, emotional or otherwise, should be provided as soon as possible for patients, families, and providers. Multiple resources exist and include patient and family relations services, chaplaincy services, risk management offices, patient safety offices, and employee assistance programs. Availability is institution dependent.
- Conversations with patients and families should, at all times, be conducted with honesty and sincerity. Communication techniques in Chap. 96, Palliative Care: Communication, may be helpful in this setting as well.
- During discussions with the patients and families at the time of the error of adverse event, the "entire story" will often not be known without an investigation. Blame should not be placed on any individuals, even if it seems that the error was blatant. However, it is permissible to say, "I am sorry, this happened."
- It is reasonable to assure patient and families that all necessary steps to prevent future harm will be taken.
- Discussions (and relevant details of) with patients and family members should be documented contemporaneously.

BIBLIOGRAPHY

Blendon RJ, DesRoches CM, Brodie M, et al. Views of practicing physicians and the public on medical errors. *N Engl J Med.* 2002;347(24):1933–1940.

Brennan TA, Leape LL, Laird NM, et al. Incidence of adverse events and negligence in hospitalized patients. Results of the Harvard Medical Practice Study I. *N Engl J Med.* 1991;324(6):370–376.

Institute of Medicine. *To Err is Human: Building a Safer System.* Washington, DC: National Academy Press; 2000.

Institute of Medicine. *Crossing the Quality Chasm: A New Health System for the 21st Century.* Washington, DC: National Academy Press; 2001.

Shojania KG, Duncan BW, McDonald KM, et al. *Making Health Care Safer: A Critical Analysis of Patient Safety Practices.* Rockville, MD: Agency for Health Care Research and Quality; 2001. Report no. 43.

Vincent C, Young M, Phillips A. Why do people sue doctors? A study of patients and relatives taking legal action. *Lancet.* 1994;343(8913):1609–1613.

QUALITY IMPROVEMENT

9   QUALITY IMPROVEMENT FOR THE HOSPITALIST

Lakshmi K. Halasyamani and
Erin R. Stucky

BACKGROUND

- Quality improvement (QI) efforts have historically been delegated to nonclinicians in healthcare settings.
- However, as the regulatory focus on quality and patient safety issues has evolved over the past few years, it is clear that meaningful improvements in clinical care delivery will occur only through successful engagement of those on the frontlines providing the care.
- Partnerships between regulatory agencies (Joint Commission [JC]) and payers (Centers for Medicare and Medicaid Services [CMS]) have led to public reporting of specific quality measures and the linkage of those measures to tiered reimbursement schedules.
- The Accreditation Council for Graduate Medical Education (ACGME) and many, if not all, American board organizations assessing qualifications of physicians have integrated quality improvement and systems-based practice expectations into residencies and certification processes.
- Useful definitions of quality include:
  - Meeting the needs and exceeding the expectations of those we serve
  - Delivering all and only the care that the patient needs
  - Healthcare value = high-quality patient outcomes ÷ cost
- There are traditionally two levels to improve quality and safety

  - Individual level
    - Education and training
    - Physician's awareness
  - Process and systems level
    - Multidisciplinary
    - Changing the practice environment
    - Eliminating barriers and unnecessary steps

A MODEL FOR IMPROVEMENT

- One frequently used model for improvement is shown in Fig. 9-1.
- This model relies on asking three critical questions.
  - What is it that we are trying to improve?
  - How will we know that a change is an improvement?
  - What changes can we make that will result in improvement?
- The answers to those questions are then used to test interventions through the plan, do, study, act (PDSA) cycle, also known as the Shewhart-Deming cycle.
- The model for improvement will be discussed further later in this section.

THE MULTIDISCIPLINARY TEAM

- There are myriad opportunities for improvement in the hospital and the hospitalist can help to identify those that are critical to patient safety and quality of care.
- However, the backbone of any improvement effort is the multidisciplinary team.
- Team composition should reflect all stakeholders.
  - Typically this includes a leader, facilitator, and members such as 1–2 hospitalists, 1–2 subspecialists (per area/issue), 1–3 residents/fellows, 1–2 bedside nurses, nurse practitioner, top five clinician "users" as obtained from hospital discharge data, pharmacist, nursing supervisor/unit nursing leader.

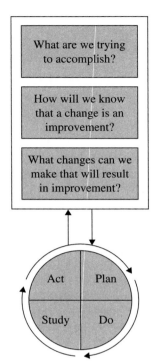

FIG. 9-1 A model for improvement developed by Tom Nolan. Used with permission from The Improvement Guide, Langley, Nolan et al.

○ Others should be added as appropriate, such as respiratory therapy, nutrition, social work, or discharge planning.
○ A data analyst may also be of value if available.
• Group dynamics suggest 7–10 individuals may be best to ensure engaged participation and reach consensus on issues.
• Hospitalists may serve in a variety of roles on a team including:
○ Team leader, often a member of an oversight steering group:
  ▪ Schedules and chairs team meetings
  ▪ Sets the agenda
  ▪ Records team activities
  ▪ Reports to management
○ Team facilitator:
  ▪ Owns the process
  ▪ Oversees the dynamics of the team and helps to ensure each team member's opinions are heard
  ▪ Clarifies decision-making processes
○ Team member:
  ▪ Brings fundamental knowledge about a topic
  ▪ Helps with implementation of proposed interventions
  ▪ Should evolve into future team leaders
  ▪ Represents all of the key process owners, stakeholders

TABLE 9-1   Team Ground Rules

• Members
  ○ Attend meetings regularly
  ○ Are equal and respected for their unique expertise
  ○ Speak freely and in turn
  ○ Attack problems, not people
• Meetings and timeline
  ○ Start and end on time
  ○ Perform work electronically between meetings
  ○ Adhere to a specific agenda for face-to-face meetings
  ○ Complete the project within 1–3 months from inception
• Consensus
  ○ Honesty before cohesion
  ○ All agreements kept unless renegotiated
  ○ Team speaks with "one voice" outside meeting setting
  ○ Silence equals agreement

• Each team should develop team ground rules that explicitly state team members' expectations (Table 9-1).
• Features of a good team include
  ○ *Safe*: no personal attacks
  ○ *Inclusive*: open to potential contributors and views
  ○ *Open*: considers all ideas fairly
  ○ *Consensus-seeking*: finds a solution all members can support

CHOOSING A PROJECT
• One of the first things a team will do is choose a specific area for improvement.
• Potential improvement projects are everywhere and it is important for the group to develop a collaborative process for project selection.
• When choosing a project, think about:
  ○ A process that requires redoing (new evidence or technology exists)
  ○ A process that is done differently by each of those who perform it (variability in practice)
  ○ A process that is a hassle (high risk for process error)
  ○ A process that has questionable value (evidence refuting clinical or system improvement)
• Factors involved in project selection include internal and external drivers. Internal drivers are factors related to interest in and effectiveness of implementation at your institution. External drivers include new evidence or external agency mandates. Examples of these include:
  ○ *Scope and importance of the problem*: high volume, high risk, high cost
  ○ *Level of evidence for potential solution*: national or societal guidelines
  ○ *Regulatory priorities*: Joint Commission on the Accreditation of Healthcare Organization (JCAHO) and Institute for Healthcare Improvement (IHI) reporting

° *Institutional priorities*: hospital board strategic plans
° *Implementation issues and challenges*: clinical pharmacist availability
° *Feasibility of potential solutions*: information technology barriers

IMPROVEMENT MODEL
- After the team chooses a project area, the next step is delineating a plan of improvement.
- One frequently used model for improvement is shown in Fig. 9-1.
- This model relies on asking three critical questions:
  ° What is it that we are trying to improve?
  ° How will we know that a change is an improvement?
  ° What changes can we make that will result in improvement?
- And then using the answers to those questions to test interventions through the PDSA cycle. The PDSA cycle recognizes that all improvement efforts are iterative and grounded in testing and evaluating changes over time.
- Linked to the first question—what is it that we are trying to improve—is the development of the *aim* statement.
- The aim statement is the most important step in defining the goals of the project.
- Good aim statements should have the following features (Table 9-2):
  ° Specific
  ° Measurable
  ° Aggressive yet achievable
  ° Relevant
  ° Time-bound

PLAN

CREATING MEASUREMENT SYSTEMS AND COLLECTING DATA
- One of the barriers that a team may face is developing a measurement system that includes strategies to collect data.

TABLE 9-2 Examples of Good Aim Statements

- In 6 months, we will improve our rates of venous thromboembolism (VTE) prophylaxis by 50%.
- In 1 year we will decrease the number of patients experiencing a catheter-associated blood stream infection by 50%.
- In 6 months, we will improve our rates of documenting smoking cessation for patients with community-acquired pneumonia to 100%.

- Important measurement principles include:
  ° Seek usefulness, not perfection
  ° Integrate measurement into daily routine
  ° Use qualitative and quantitative data
  ° Use sampling
  ° Plot data over time
- Specific measures can fall into one of the following categories:
  ° Outcome measures
    ▪ How is the system performing across a variety of outcomes such as clinical, resource, and financial?
    ▪ What is the clinical result?
    ▪ What safety measure is important?
  ° Process measures
    ▪ Are tools developed being used?
  ° Structure measures
    ▪ Are there differences between patient care settings?
    ▪ Are there differences among providers, specialties, and so forth?

Balancing measures are changes designed to improve one part of the system causing new problems in other parts of the system?

Critical to any data review is for the data to be relevant to the problem identified and the aim statement developed.

- Some reasons to collect data include:
  ° Understanding variation in a process
  ° Monitoring a process over time
  ° Assessing changes in processes
  ° Providing a common reference point
  ° Providing an accurate basis for predicting future performance
- Data collection sources may include systems already in place or may require the team to develop a novel strategy or submit a specific data request.
- Sources of data include:
  ° Administrative data
    ▪ Hospital claims data
    ▪ Pharmacy computer system
  ° Clinical data
    ▪ Chart review
    ▪ Electronic medical record review
  ° Evidence from published peer-reviewed literature
  ° Interviews, surveys
  ° Local and national expert opinion
  ° Direct observations of care
- Once data are collected, it should be summarized in a format that allows the team to understand it so the conclusions from the data review are meaningful and helpful in influencing the next test of change. The team may need to involve data analysis experts to help the group understand the data so the conclusions are valid.

• The specific method of displaying data is not as important as understanding the data presented and using the same methodology over time.

COMMON QUALITY IMPROVEMENT TOOLS
• There are several quality improvement tools that can be used in various stages of project development, implementation, and assessment.
• These tools help the team understand the issues, target interventions, and understand the implementation issues involved in choosing specific interventions.
• Common QI tools and their uses are listed in Table 9-3.

DO

EFFECTING CHANGE
• The steps above may require 1–3 face-to-face meetings, with electronic communication to all members highlighting remaining questions between meetings. The team leader and facilitator are responsible for ensuring that timelines are established and deadlines are met.
• After final agreement is reached, administrative steps such as posting order sets and real-time education of end users should occur. Typically these steps are institution-specific, most often performed by all team members in conjunction with hospital personnel.
• Key to successful implementation is to make it EASY: Evidence-based, Actionable, Standardized, and Yours.

STUDY AND ACT

MONITORING AND RAPID CYCLE IMPROVEMENT
• After a defined period, typically 3 months, data should be obtained and reviewed by the team. A summary of findings can be sent electronically, with key questions highlighted by the team leader and facilitator.
• Small tests of change result in the most rapid improvements. Results of the first data extraction can be acted upon within 1–2 weeks, with the most actionable modifications made to algorithms or order sets.
• Any questions which cannot be resolved electronically within 1–2 weeks should be tabled for a future face-to-face meeting.
• A face-to-face meeting should occur when the team determines an issue requires focused attention, or at a predetermined time interval such as 6 months post-initial implementation/revision.
• Successes should be shared across the institution by electronic updates or presentations at key department or hospital meetings.

TABLE 9-3 Common QI Tools

NAME OF TOOL	DESCRIPTION	PRIMARY USEFULNESS
Brainstorming	Method of generating list of ideas and encouraging team member creativity, team members give ideas in turn, can be done verbally or on note cards	Problem identification Solution/intervention planning yes it is a single point.
Process mapping/flow chart	Picture of all of the steps in a process; allows every step to be delineated and its relationship to the other steps understood	Problem identification Solution/intervention planning
Nominal group technique	Prioritize ideas (could be generated through brainstorming) and achieve consensus through written voting	Problem identification Solution/intervention planning
Affinity diagram	Organize and summarize ideas by theme to understand problem/solutions; done in conjunction with brainstorming	Problem identification Solution/intervention planning
Cause and effect diagram (also known as fishbone or Ishikawa diagram)	Used to identify and prioritize causes of a specific problem; organized display of factors resulting in specified outcome	Problem identification Data analysis
Pareto chart	Graphical display that compares relative weights of frequencies of specific variables; helps to identify area for largest impact	Problem identification Data analysis Result evaluation
Failure mode and effects analysis (FMEA)	Prospective risk analysis strategy by identifying potential or actual errors for each process step (delineated through process mapping); allows priority assessment through weighting system based on severity, occurrence, and detection of errors identified	Problem identification Data analysis Solution/intervention planning Result evaluation (can redo FMEA and see if errors have been eliminated)
2 × 2 tables	Can be used to prioritize data or interventions; table consists of yield vs. feasibility	Data analysis solution/intervention planning
Control chart	Consists of a run chart (data plotted over time) with statistically determined upper and lower control limits; helps to determine whether performance is stable (not necessarily ideal) or if there has been a shift.	Problem identification Data analysis Result evaluation

FMEA-Failure mode and effects analysis.

SUMMARY

- Hospitalists are well positioned to be leaders and member of multidisciplinary quality improvement teams and to perform quality improvement research.
- Critical to the success of any project is an effective team that has successfully focused its target for improvement.
- The model for improvement can serve as a useful guide for teams embarking on QI efforts.
- QI tools can help to clarify the issues and identify potential interventions to improve and measure performance.

BIBLIOGRAPHY

Boluyt N, Lincke CR. et al. Quality of evidence-based pediatric guidelines. *Pediatrics.* 2005;115(5):1378–1391.

Brown MS, Ohlinger J., et al. Implementing potentially better practices for multidisciplinary team building: creating a neonatal intensive care unit culture of collaboration. *Pediatrics.* 2003;111(4):e482–e488.

Bucuvalas JC, Ryckman FC, Arya G, et al. A novel approach to managing variation: outpatient therapeutic monitoring of calcineurin inhibitor blood levels in liver transplant recipients. *J Pediatr.* 2005;146(6):744–750.

Deming W. Edwards. *Out of the Crisis.* Cambridge, Massachusetts, MA: MIT Press; 1986. ISBN 0-911379–01-0.

Horbar JD, Plsek PE, et al. NIC/Q 2000: establishing habits for improvement in neonatal intensive care units. *Pediatrics.* 2003;111(4):e397–e410.

Institute of Medicine reports at http://www.iom.edu/CMS/2955.aspx

Jackson JK, Vellucci J, et al. Evidence-based approach to change in clinical practice: introduction of expanded nasal continuous positive airway pressure use in an intensive care nursery. *Pediatrics.* 2003;111(4):e542–e547.

Langley GJ, Nolan KM, Nolan TW, et al. *The Improvement Guide.* Jossey-Bass; 1996.

Onady GMR, Marc A. Evidence-based medicine: searching literature and databases for clinical evidence (search tools). *Ped Rev.* 2004;25(10):358–63.

Richardson PJ, Sobo EJ, Stucky ER. Child health services research: applications, innovations, and insights. In: *Standardized Approaches to Clinical Care, Pathways, and Disease Management.* San Francisco, CA: Jossey-Bass; 2003: 275–309.

Sharek PJ, Baker R, et al. Evaluation and development of potentially better practices to prevent chronic lung disease and reduce lung injury in neonates. *Pediatrics.* 2003; 111(4):e426–e431.

Solberg LI, Klevan DH, et al. Crossing the quality chasm for diabetes care: the power of one physician, his team, and systems thinking. *J Am Board Fam Med.* 2007;20(3):299–306.

WEB RESOURCES

http://www.hospitalmedicine.org/Content/NavigationMenu/HQPS/QualityImprovementTools/Quality_Improvement_.htm

http://www.IHI.org

Section 4
HOSPITALIST AS MANAGER

10 MANAGEMENT FOR HOSPITALISTS

Michael Friedlander and Mohammad Salameh

BACKGROUND

- The purpose of this chapter is to provide a framework that may be used to evaluate employment opportunities and resources for further professional development in nonclinical areas.
- For anyone starting a career in hospital medicine, it is important to evaluate a given locale and how it fits into one's professional and personal long-range plans.
- In order to select a hospital or group that will allow a given physician to explore and nurture their interests and allow for professional growth, the physician should reflect on their core values, and recognize that their needs will change over time depending upon their career and family obligations.
- The Society of Hospital Medicine (SHM) has developed a white paper on career satisfaction. This paper emphasizes "job fit," finding a match between the hospitalists and work and provides tools that employers and individual hospitalists can use to create a positive work environment.
  - The white paper is divided into the four pillars of career satisfaction: autonomy/control, workload/schedule, reward/recognition, and community/environment.
  - For each of the four pillars, the paper outlines recommendations and specifies tools that hospitalist employers can use to improve the work environment.
  - Also included within the paper is a questionnaire that individual hospitalists can use to identify what

factors are important to them in a job and how their current position is meeting their needs.
- Each practice setting faces unique challenges and more research is needed to better understand what makes for a long and satisfying career in hospital medicine.

COMMON HOSPITALIST GROUP MODELS

NATIONAL HOSPITALIST COMPANIES

- A number of these entities now exist. They operate off of a percentage of billing margin (typically 15%–20%) and provide the opportunity for an individual to receive a competitive salary with attached benefits.
- Usually the opportunity for bonus or incentive is somewhat limited in the range of 10%–15%, and usually the company has a contractual relationship with the health system that includes 24-hour coverage.
- Under this structure night coverage is usually included in the offered contract. This responsibility needs to be well clarified and well defined in the contract.
- Advantages of this system include:
  - Geographic flexibility as members can move from one site to another
  - Administrative structures that handle the billing issues
  - Lucrative stipends often available and shared by physician members for night and rapid response coverage
  - Electronic medical record (EMR) and malpractice coverage already in place
- Disadvantages of this system may include:
  - Possible loss of autonomy in decision-making.
  - Perception of national hospitalist companies as having too much "alliance" to the hospital.

○ Required signing of noncompete clauses that are often difficult to enforce and can at times result in financial burden when negated.
○ Contract negation with health systems with minimal physician input.

HOSPITAL EMPLOYMENT MODELS

• Hospitals may employ hospitalists directly and negotiate with each individual separately to provide both clinical and administrative services.
• Many of the hospitals that utilize this model have teaching programs and the core faculty of educators also provides clinical hospital services.
• Advantages of this system may include:
  ○ Competitive benefits package and malpractice coverage
  ○ Considerable opportunity for teaching residents and junior faculty
  ○ Higher job security
  ○ Career growth opportunities through committee work, research projects, and other administrative tasks
  ○ Easier recruitment of new hospitalists primarily from the residency program because of academic role
• Disadvantages of this system include:
  ○ Loss of autonomy when owing to decision-making by the hospital administrators instead of hospitalists
  ○ Hospital bureaucracy for contract negotiations, dismissal of unproductive members, and obtaining strong ancillary staff much less efficient and very challenging
  ○ Limited income growth because of considerable salary component to their contracts with less incentive provisions
  ○ Complex communication issues with referring doctors because of another layer of residents

PRIVATE HOSPITALIST PRACTICES

• While this concept may seem somewhat intimidating, there are an ever-increasing number of physicians who have realized that they prefer the autonomy and potential economic upside that comes with developing their own practice.
• Because this type of practice may require a very high initial financial risk, one must evaluate the practice climate and competition, and analyze the current local benchmarks for length of stay (LOS), cost per case, readmission rates, and quality initiatives information available through the hospital.
• This type of practice requires a considerable amount of financial and time commitment up front, but the potential for financial gain is much higher.

• There is a growing trend toward this type of hospitalist service that coincides with the growth of the hospitalist movement.
• Advantages of this system include:
  ○ Autonomy in decision-making.
  ○ Potential for greater financial gains and freedoms.
  ○ Greater flexibility in hiring practices that can focus on keeping productive physician members and terminating members who are less productive.
  ○ More investment in the success of the group which is a strong motivating factor in fostering high-quality, efficient care.
• Disadvantages of this system include:
  ○ Greater financial risk even though the potential gains are higher.
  ○ Recruiting may be challenging as benefits packages such as malpractice coverage, 401k, retirement, and health insurance may not be as competitive as those provided by a hospital or a hospitalist corporation.
  ○ Because of the typical small size of these groups, the loss of a member resulting career change or lack of productivity may place an undue burden on other member physicians.
  ○ In starting the group, a lag time of at minimum 12 weeks is typical before seeing any significant revenue and therefore initial losses are not unusual and this fact may result in members leaving the group.

STARTING A HOSPITALIST PROGRAM

• Strong negotiations with the hospital as all three models will require some financial support from the host hospital, especially in providing charity care to uninsured patients.
• More importantly for the two private models, a legal team can aid in negotiations and in tailoring a contract.
• Strong legal representation will also provide guidance for the selection of malpractice coverage.
  ○ For example, if the group members want to perform procedures, coverage for these procedures must be included in the malpractice policy.
  ○ Individual members will need to determine whether the policy selected has tail coverage that will cover members once and if they leave the group. Depending on the locale, this type of coverage may cost 2 years of premium payments ($6000–$25000 per year), an important financial consideration.
• Ensuring satisfaction of the referral base is essential to ensure that primary care physicians continue to use the hospitalist group to admit patients. Patients will communicate their experiences to their doctors and this can significantly affect a hospitalist program's success.

- Developing relationships with services such as orthopedic surgery, neurosurgery, and psychiatry are also essential as much of the revenue for hospitalist services comes from consults initiated by these services.
- Because hospitalists spend all of their clinical time in the hospital, it is natural that they will be called upon to sit on hospital committees, especially formulary and quality improvement committees and any committee that is collaboration between doctors and nursing.
- Hospitalists should also support their professional SHM through active participation that provides opportunities for networking and learning new strategies for success. The SHM has numerous committees and task forces working on issues central to the practice of hospital medicine.
- Available through the SHM Web site are resources relating to practice management.

FINANCIAL VIABILITY OF THE HOSPITALIST SERVICE AND QUALITY CONSIDERATIONS

- Once a facility decides to utilize hospitalists to cover all or some of their inpatients, it is imperative that parameters are put in place to ensure the financial and quality success of the service.
- The majority of hospitals already have a significant amount of data available that can be used to monitor this success. Therefore, whether a private group is in place or the hospitalist group is employed by the health system, there must be a system in place to utilize and organize these data and ultimately apply it to real practice.
- Further, the hospitalist group must provide quality patient care that can be measured and reproduced.

ELEMENTS OF A SUCCESSFUL PROGRAM

- The hospitalist director has day-to-day responsibilities of running the service, including scheduling, conflict resolution, ensuring communication with nursing staff and other services, ensuring standards of care are met, and creating protocols for handoffs and sign-outs.
  - This role entails the use of data provided by the hospital to determine staffing needs, ways to improve efficiency, and to give feedback to their doctors.
  - In addition, as an advocate of the physicians they are representing, the director must represent the group to hospital administration and serve as an effective

liaison between the hospitalist group and the hospital administration.
- Useful statistics and data can generate a quarterly hospitalist report card:
  - *LOS data*: national guidelines regarding LOS for specific DRGs are available and can be compared to institutional numbers. These data can be useful in monitoring consistency in workup, treatment, and clinical decision-making among members of the hospitalist group and between different hospitalist groups.
  - *Decreased LOS*: A decreased LOS translates to more resource availability, less nursing cost, and a more productive bottom line for the hospital. A decreased LOS must factor in readmission rates and the patient population being served.
  - *Readmission rates*: Routine evaluation of readmission rates may identify areas of variance. Members of the group with consistently higher readmission rates for the same DRG may also need to have their clinical work reviewed.
    - High readmission rates result in increased utilization of resources and lower reimbursements. Therefore, the group that can demonstrate a lower rate relative to peers may also have a better financial standing with the hospital.
  - *Core measure performance*: These are disease-specific, externally reported measures that may be used for pay-for-performance incentives. They are one measure of quality of care and the number of diseases that will have associated core measures will grow over the next few years. Hospitalist groups that demonstrate compliance with these measures may be able to advocate more effectively for resources
- All data collected should be used to constructively give feedback and to motivate the group to excel. Some groups have linked compensation to performance on some parameters and it is unclear how that linkage translates into improvements in patient care or improvements in group dynamics and overall performance.
  - Work relative value units (wRVU)/provider— according to SHM's survey of national hospitalist groups, a 0.93 clinical FTE translates to a median of 3213 wRVUs. This information may not apply to academic tertiary hospitalists groups who in fact may be on service an average of 23 weeks in the year, according to University Health System Consortium (UHC) benchmarking project of academic hospitalist groups within the participating hospitals.
  - Any provider falling below this number or other similar benchmark may need to have their work

audited by the hospitalist director. These data can be used to ensure that all members of the group are clinically productive.

- The director of the hospitalist service should set up an administrative structure that empowers other hospitalists to take the lead in innovation whether it is quality improvement, research, or education.
  ○ Titles such as director of the hospitalist quality improvement task force or educational scholarship provide recognition, encourage individuals to find niches within the organization, and may ultimately facilitate funding for nonclinical time for important activities.
  ○ Providing annual awards to recognize exemplary efforts relating to the core mission of the group can aid in professional recognition within the hospital and medical school.
- Often physician leaders are chosen because of their clinical skills with the assumption that they will become effective leaders that require a different skill set.
- Leadership academies through multiple organizations, including the SHM and the American College of Physicians, provide additional training for hospitalists so that they can be effective leaders and negotiators.

BILLING AND DOCUMENTATION

- Effective and appropriate billing is one of the most important means to maintain financial viability for the hospitalist group.
- It is imperative that members of the group review changes to documentation requirements and regulatory rules regarding billing in order to optimize payments for charges.
- Because of the complexities of inpatient procedure, and consult billing, the hospitalist director must ensure that all physicians in the group have some formal training regarding billing and documentation.
- It is important to have a system in place that ensures that all hospitalists bill for their encounters and measure billing activity so that lapses can be rectified. Especially when there are no incentives in place, billing may take a low priority relative to other obligations.
- This expectation not only ensures maximizing reimbursement, but also will help prevent audits from regulatory bodies. Further, appropriate documentation is vital to help reduce physician liability and is a key in preventing malpractice claims.
- There are a growing number of computer applications that have been developed to assist in both assigning

the correct level of service to be billed and in submitting the bills to the payers.
- There are resources through the SHM Web site on billing and coding.

COMMUNICATION

- Communication is critical to the patient's care. In addition to direct communication to the patient, the hospitalist must communicate effectively with nursing and other members of the patient's care team, the referring physician (and follow-up physician) and with the other members of the hospitalist group. (See Chapter 2).
- Physician-nurse communication is a mainstay of inpatient medicine. Nurses are the first responders regarding any urgent issues that develop and spend a majority of their time at the patient bedside. Therefore, it is critical for the hospitalist group to create a system where nurses can easily determine who to call in the event a patient issue may arise.
- Lack of a successful cross-coverage or rapid response system can lead to poor patient care and failure of the hospitalist group. Hospitalists that share call coverage or use a moonlighting service for admissions and cross-cover must have a means of communicating pertinent patient data with their colleagues.
- Physician communication with their referral base is also critical for success. A hospitalist group that maintains excellent communication with the primary or principal care physicians (PCPs) who refer patients for admission can increase their exposure and the number of PCPs that they cover. See the chapter on discharge summaries (Chapter 14) for strategies to improve the discharge transition. Systems can be created to facilitate timely communication such as "hospitalist lines" for messages for busy primary care physicians, computer, and ancillary support.
- Furthermore, good communication with noninternal medicine services will also lead to increased consults and more revenue. In addition, both of these practices greatly improve the quality of patient care. (See chapter on medical comanagement.)
- Physician hand offs or transfers of care are also vital for high-quality care. A hospitalist system that has standards for hand offs and sign-out would be expected to decrease medical errors and high-quality care will only increase the exposure and competitiveness of the group. (See the chapter on hand offs for additional information.)

BIBLIOGRAPHY

Burger A, Holmboe E, Rifkin WD, et al. Comparison of hospitalists and nonhospitalists regarding core measures of pneumonia care. *Am J Manag Care.* 2007;13:129–32.

Dichter J. (ed). Tools and strategies for an effective hospitalist program. HcPro, Inc. 2006.

Dressler DD, Pistoria MJ, Budnitz TL, et al. Amin AN. The core competencies in hospital medicine: a framework for curriculum development. *J Hosp Med.* 2006 Jan–Feb.

Huddleston JM, Long KH, Naessens JM, et al. Hospitalist–orthopedic comanagement reduced minor complication rates without increasing length of stay or cost. *Ann Intern Med.* 2004;141:28–38.

Kralovec PD, Miller JA, Wellikson L, et al. The status of hospital medicine groups in the United States. *J Hosp Med.* 2006 Mar;1(2):75–80.

Piturro M. Hospital Business Drivers. *The Hospitalist.* 2006 Mar;3:47–9.

Salerno SM, Hurst FP, Halvorson S, et al. Principles of effective consultation: an update for the 21st-century consultant. *Arch Intern Med.* 2007 Feb 12;167(3):271–5.

WEB RESOURCES

http://www.hospitalmedicine.org/AM/Template.cfm?Section=Careers

http://www.hospitalmedicine.org/Content/NavigationMenu/ResourceCenter/PracticeResources/Practice_Resources.htm

http://www.hospitalmedicine.org/AM/Template.cfm?Section=Search_Advanced_Search&section=SHM_Initiatives&template=/CM/ContentDisplay.cfm&ContentFileID=3084

HOSPITALISTS AND CARE TRANSITIONS AND TEAMWORK

11 PRINCIPLES OF GOOD TEAMWORK

Janet Nagamine

BACKGROUND

- Working successfully in teams is one of the most crucial skills in the practice of medicine.
- Many of these skills can be taught and incorporated systematically into patient care processes.
- Teamwork is increasingly being viewed as a competency and accrediting bodies such as Association of American Medical Colleges (AAMC) and Accreditation Council for Graduate Medical Education (ACGME) now include specific teamwork-related competencies for medical students and residents.
- The Society of Hospital Medicine (SHM) also includes a team approach and multidisciplinary care chapter in *The Core Competencies: A Framework for Curriculum Development* that defines specific knowledge, skills, and attitudes related to teamwork.
- The impetus behind these requirements in medical training is the increasing recognition that teamwork and communication failures in healthcare are common and can result in patient harm. The typology of errors that human beings make may be unintentional or violations.
  - Communication was determined to be the root cause in over 80% of sentinel events involving delays in treatment, and over 70% of cases involving wrong site surgery.
  - Many of these cases exemplify a group mindset of following the leader even when the leader of the team goes down the wrong path. In addition, stress,

fatigue, burnout, and multitasking can negatively impact on cognitive function and vigilance.
  - Highly reliable industries such as aviation require specific team training in crew resource management (CRM) in order to ensure that personnel function in a coordinated and effective manner. All staff is required to participate in training that emphasizes flattening of steep hierarchies and promoting clear, open communication that facilitates achievement of desired outcomes.
- Training of healthcare providers as teams is a pragmatic, effective strategy for enhancing patient safety and reducing medical errors. Using examples from other industries, leaders in healthcare can promote a culture of safety through effective teamwork building and systems improvement.
  - Systems can be put in place to address communication failures through effective teamwork, computer support, and multiple checks.
  - Errors of omission such as failure to turn on a machine, errors of commission such as misreading a label on a drug, and errors under severe stress can be avoided through standardization of procedures and policies.
  - Team members can play a critical role in cross-monitoring of colleagues—in essence, looking out for each other—and in communicating essential team information.
- Comprehensive, evidence-based approaches to medical team training require teaching, observing, and measuring teamwork and communication competency.

TEAMWORK IN HEALTHCARE

- Teamwork generally has not been regarded as an important facet of medical performance and there may be confusion relating to the identification of team members, role definition, and expectations for effective teamwork.

- During the twentieth century individual blame and physician autonomy in decision making were deeply embedded in the culture of medicine. Medical schools and residency programs did not educate physicians about the concepts of error, inherent limitations of human beings and complex systems, approaches of other industries to reduce error, and how teamwork and communication can reduce error rates in healthcare systems.
- Although physicians work with other professionals such as nurses, pharmacists, respiratory therapists, and physical therapists, interdisciplinary teams that function in a coordinated or integrated manner have not been operational in many settings.
  - Trained in distinctly different disciplines with varied educational focus and approach to patient care, team members may function independently and not interface directly with other healthcare providers directly involved in the care of a single patient.
  - Physicians and nurses are often referred only to colleagues in their respective disciplines when asked about teamwork.
  - Instead of team "sign-out", physicians sign out to physicians, nurses to nurses, residents to residents and likewise only provide feedback with their peers.
- Time constraints and different schedules limit face-to-face interaction in order to exchange thoughts, share observations, or communicate management plans directly.
  - Communication usually occurs via charts and computer, relying on notes and orders to "coordinate" care while team members function in parallel or independent of each other.
  - In fact, e-mail and other forms of communication by computer have increasingly replaced telephone or face-to-face dialogue.
- The hierarchical relationship that physicians have with other healthcare providers makes clarification of any uncertainty difficult and often leads to the communication failures seen in adverse events.
  - Another component of this hierarchical relationship is a culture of perfection that emphasizes individual agency rather than collective thinking and shared decision making.
  - Although physicians play a less dominant role than previously, there is continued adherence to traditional hierarchical behavior patterns which inhibit open communication and contribute to adverse events. Physicians and other team members may

fear that appropriate inquiry of actions taken by a superior may jeopardize a positive evaluation of their performance, or they may hesitate to assert themselves due to a concern about being wrong.
  - Members of the healthcare team have divergent views regarding role expectations and what constitutes effective teamwork. Studies on teamwork comparing survey responses of physicians with other health professionals consistently show that physicians rate levels of teamwork much higher than nonphysicians.
- Research in non-healthcare industries has identified many of the competencies necessary for effective teamwork and validated strategies exist in other domains.
  - Many of these principles and strategies are applicable to the environment of clinical medicine. The teamwork issues we currently face are quite similar to the issues faced by aviation prior to initiating CRM programs.
  - Strong hierarchy and power differential as well as lack of clarity regarding specific tasks and roles were two major challenges seen in aviation and similarly serve as major barriers to effective teamwork in healthcare.
- Teamwork is a complex and dynamic process in which members interact and collaborate to achieve desired outcomes.
  - A misguided emphasis on congenial working relationships as sufficient for successful teamwork may actually promote error.
  - The development of the specific skills and behaviors that are necessary for effective team performance and delivery of safe care requires training and evaluation.

PROMOTING EFFECTIVE TEAMWORK

- Effective teamwork requires the willingness of team members to cooperate toward a shared goal.
- Key features of a team include members with defined roles, defined tasks, and task interdependency.
- One model for medical teamwork is shown in Fig. 11-1. The model illustrates how the concepts of roles, tasks, and task interdependency can be implemented to accomplish shared goals.
- Formal teamwork training in high-risk industries such as aviation include techniques and specific

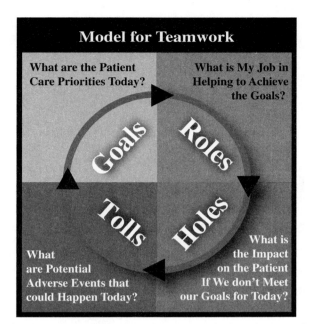

FIG. 11-1 One model of medical teamwork. Questions to ask include (1) What information do we need to make an accurate clinical assessment?
(2) What clinical outcomes are we trying to impact today?
(3) How will we know that we are progressing toward those outcomes?
(4) What interventions should we do that may lead to improved outcomes?

teamwork behaviors that ensure roles are clearly defined and plans are discussed and mutually agreed upon.
• Table 11-1 contrasts characteristics of effective versus ineffective teams.

TABLE 11-1   Contrasting Characteristics of Effective and Ineffective Teams

EFFECTIVE TEAMS	INEFFECTIVE TEAMS
Mutual goal setting	Lack of understanding of goals or plans
Sense of shared responsibility and interdependence recognized and addressed	Turf mentality Silo operations Interdependence not recognized or addressed
Clear understanding of roles, responsibilities, and tasks to be done	Ambiguity of roles, responsibilities, and tasks to be done
Inclusive, different perspectives welcome	Exclusive, other perspectives not sought
Open communication and safety in sharing ideas, observations, and making suggestions despite "rank"	Closed communication; not safe to share observations, ideas, or make suggestions: "know your place"
Members function in a coordinated manner	Lack of coordination

BUILDING TEAM-BASED CARE MODELS

• Successful teamwork requires strong leadership support, namely,
  1. Leadership by example—Mutual respect, explicit personal acknowledgement of error, recognition that all members of the team are capable of error, and evaluation of all errors or near misses through systems analysis rather than individual blame
  2. Daily clarification of specific team behaviors that all members of the team agree to
  3. Dedication of resources for team training
Goals of care include effective teamwork to get the job done correctly the first time. In order to accomplish this goal, there must be effective communication by the team leader. Effective communication strategies include:
  ○ Brief the team to set the plan for the day and establish expectations.
  ○ Verbalize the plan with explicit concise information.
  ○ Ask for feedback from *all* members of the team and modify plan accordingly.
  ○ Promote awareness for the potential of error and how team members can help monitor each other and safeguard against error.
• Examples where it is useful to set goals of care in advance of the encounter include:
  ○ Establishment of a contract with a noncompliant patient
  ○ Family meetings to discuss end-of-life issues
  ○ Any teaching session to establish ground rules for learning
  ○ Standardization of protocols for performing a procedure
• SBAR is a framework for communication that can be used in any practice situation, especially for instances that require modification of action, handoffs, and presentations to physicians.
  ○ *Situation*—Succinct description of the problem
  ○ *Background*—Synopsis of critical information
  ○ *Assessment*—Speaker's evaluation
  ○ *Recommendation*—Specific action plan for the listener
• Closed-loop communication requires the listener to repeat back the information. Not only does this ensure that the communication is heard and understood but this also promotes team awareness.
• Debriefing is a communication tool to review what went well and what did not so that corrective action can be taken by the team when a similar situation arises again.
  ○ Frequently used after cardiac codes, this exercise can be used effectively after procedures, difficult family meetings, adverse events, misdiagnosis, and routinely at the end of the day or week.

○ Specific action steps should be identified and referred to people responsible to improve the system of care. Usually, this requires standardization of procedures and processes that facilitate safe and high-quality care.

INPATIENT CARE DELIVERY

• Both interpersonal and organizational factors must be addressed in order to build effective teams.
• The presence of hospitalists has changed the system of healthcare delivery. Now hospitalists have an opportunity to demonstrate that they can improve patient safety by developing and building models of interdisciplinary teamwork and collaboration.
• Interpersonal and organizational factors that facilitate teamwork among physicians and nurses include:
  ○ Interdisciplinary rounds and meetings
  ○ Collaborative practice orders, critical pathways, and protocols
  ○ High-quality, competent people committed to effective teamwork
  ○ Culture in which concern for the patient is paramount
  ○ Continuity, longevity, and specialization of staff
  ○ Established mechanisms for constructive conflict resolution
  ○ Committed unit/service medical directors
  ○ Nurse manager support
• Creating specific workflow structures and partnerships that overcome the traditional logistical challenges of interdisciplinary teamwork shows promise.
• Some organizations have implemented documentation tools to facilitate team-based care and communication.
  ○ One example is the daily goals sheet developed and implemented in the ICU at Johns Hopkins hospital.
  ○ The daily goals sheet makes explicitly clear what the goals are and members of the team must initial the sheet on each shift. Demonstrated outcomes include improvement of resident and nurse understanding of plans from 10% to 95% and a decrease in LOS from 2.2 days to 1.1 days.
• Care transitions are also vulnerable times for patients and demand effective teamwork. (See Chap. 14 on discharge summaries and sign-out).

CONCLUSION

• Successful teamwork is a core competency that requires training, evaluation, and feedback.
• Hospitalists are responsible for creating medical management plans not only for patients but also for leading healthcare teams.

• Hospitalists can shape how the healthcare team functions by explicitly setting goals of open dialogue and collaboration to overcome logistical and social barriers that get in the way of optimal patient care.
• Hospitalists are in a unique position to change and improve the delivery of healthcare by facilitating team training.

BIBLIOGRAPHY

Baker DP, Gustafson S, Beaubien J, et al. *Medical Teamwork and Patient Safety: The Evidence-based Relation.* Rockville, MD: http://www.ahrq.gov/qual/medteam/; Literature Review. AHRQ Publication No. 05-0053, April 2005. Agency for Healthcare Research and Quality.

Cannon-Bowers JA et al. Defining competencies and establishing team training requirements. In: Guzzo RA, Salas E (eds). *Team Effectiveness and Decision Making in Organizations.* San Francisco, CA: Jossey-Bass; 1998:333–381.

Dunnington GL, Williams RG. Addressing the new competencies for residents' surgical training. *Acad Med.* 2003;78(1):14–21.

Franklin C et al. Developing strategies to prevent in-hospital cardiac arrest: analyzing responses of physicians and nurses in hours before the event. *Crit Care Med.* 1994;22(2):244–247.

Greenfields LJ. Doctors and nurses: a troubled partnership. *Ann Surg.* 1999;230(3): 279–288.

Groff H. Teamwork failures noted in malpractice claims. In: Forum 2003 July; 23(3). Risk Management Foundation of the Harvard Medical Instituions.

Helmreich RL, Merritt AC. *Culture at Work in Aviation and Medicine: National, Organizational and Professional Influences.* Brookfield, VT: Ashgate; 1998.

Joint Commission. *Root Causes of Sentinel Events: All Categories.* Oakbrook, IL: Joint Commission. http://www.jointcommission. org/NR/rdonlyres/FA465646-5F5F-4543-AC8F-E8AF6571E372/ 0/root_cause_se.jpg Accessed June 7, 2007.

Page A. (ed.) *Keeping Patients Safe: Transforming the Work Environment of Nurses.* Institute of Medicine. Washington, DC: National Academies Press; 2003.

Pistoria MJ, Dressler DD, Budnitz TL; Society of Hospital Medicine. The core competencies in hospital medicine: a framework for curriculum development. *J Hosp Med.* 2006; 1(suppl. 1):48–56.

Pronovost P, Berenholtz S, Dorman T, et al. Improving communication in the ICU using daily goals. *J Crit Care.* 2003;18(2):71–75.

Rogers SO, Gawande AA, Kwaan M, et al. Analysis of surgical errors in closed malpractice claims at 4 liability insurers. *Surgery.* 2006 Jul;140(1):25–33.

Schmalenberg C, Kramer M, King C, et al. Excellence through evidence: securing collegial/collaborative nurse-physician relationships. Part 1. *J Nurs Adm.* 2005;35(10):450–458.

Schmalenberg C, Kramer M, King C, et al. Excellence through evidence: securing collegial/collaborative nurse-physician relationships. Part 2. *J Nurs Adm.* 2005;35(11):507–514.

Sexton JB, Thomas EJ, Helmreich RL, et al. Error, stress and teamwork in aviation and medicine: cross-sectional surveys. *BMJ.* 2000;320:745–749.

Thomas EJ, Sexton JB, Helmreich RL. Discrepant attitudes about teamwork among critical care nurses and physicians. *Crit Care Med.* 2003 Mar;31(3):956–959.

Uhlig P, Brown J, Nason AK, et al. System innovation: Concord hospital. *Jt Comm J Qual Improv.* 2002 Dec;28(12):666–672.

WEB RESOURCES

Society of Hospital Medicine Quality Improvement Resource Rooms Care Transitions

Society of Hospital Medicine Quality Improvement Resource Room

http://www.hospitalmedicine.org/AM/Template.cfm?Section= Quality_Improvement_Resource_Rooms&Template=/CM/ HTMLDisplay.cfm&ContentID=6566

12 STRATEGIES TO OPTIMIZE LENGTH OF STAY

Kathleen M. Finn

BACKGROUND/OVERVIEW

- Up until 1982, US hospitals were reimbursed on a per diem basis. Given payment for each day of hospitalization, the longer the stay the more the hospitals and physicians were paid. As expected this encouraged relatively long average length of stay (LOS).
- In 1982, the federal government adopted the prospective payment system (PPS) for reimbursement on hospitalized Medicare patients. The system dictated a fixed amount for each patient hospitalized regardless of how many days they stayed in the hospital. The fixed reimbursement was based on 1 of 511 federal diagnosis related groups (DRGs) defined by the patient's diagnosis, surgical procedure, age, comorbidities, complications, and other factors.
  - After the PPS implementation by the federal government for Medicare, the system was rapidly adopted by the states for Medicaid programs and by many private insurance plans.
  - Suddenly LOS in the hospital mattered financially. Hospitals would lose money if patients stayed longer than the DRG allotted, and potentially save/make money if efficiency of care was optimized.

TABLE 12-1   Hazards of Hospitalization

Deconditioning
Nosocomial infections
Hospital-acquired delirium
Hospital-acquired renal failure
Deep vein thrombosis (DVT)
Line infections
Medication errors

- Hospitals and researchers began looking at ways to optimize LOS and to do this without adversely affecting patient care. Through the 1980s and 1990s, there were numerous studies published on optimizing LOS.
  - Hospitals did succeed in reducing LOS. Between 1985 and 2001, the average LOS declined 1.7 days from 6.6 to 4.9 days. Yet, studies indicated that LOS was still too long.
  - In the last 10 years, the hospitalist movement has contributed to further reductions in the LOS. Hospitalists enhance patient throughput by responding to changes in the patient's condition in real time, and are skilled in navigating hospital systems to maximize the efficiency of resource utilization.
  - Hospitalist programs have grown rapidly around the country as hospitals hope to optimize their LOS and save money.
- As inpatient physicians, hospitalists are aware there are other important reasons to optimize LOS besides individual hospital reimbursement.
  - Patient safety is a significant factor since the longer a patient stays in the hospital the more he or she is exposed to the potential, and not inconsiderable, hazards of hospitalization (Table 12-1).
    - The Institute of Medicine (IOM), in its landmark report *To Err is Human: Building a Safer Health System*, estimated that hospital admission is the eighth leading cause of unnecessary death in the United States, ahead of motor vehicle accidents and breast cancer.
  - Other reasons to optimize LOS include
    - Reducing national healthcare costs.
    - Alleviating high census conditions, allowing for more patients to be cared for with the same increasingly scarce hospital resources.

DEFINITION OF LOS

- LOS is defined as the time between a patient's admission to the hospital and his or her time of discharge from the hospital. LOS is influenced by many factors, including
  - Patients' responses to treatment, their clinical condition at time of hospitalization, as well as their comorbidities

- Patients' social situations and the availability of an outpatient support system, such as the availability of a family member to become a temporary caregiver
- Federal regulations (such as the Medicare 3-day rule, requiring a 3-day LOS for Medicare to reimburse skilled nursing facility care)
- Availability of insurance to cover medications and treatments in the outpatient setting (common examples: low-molecular-weight heparin and home intravenous antibiotic therapy)

- LOS is often reported as an observed to expected ratio where the expected LOS is based on benchmarking data from Medicare, similar hospitals (such as the University HealthSystem Consortium) or consensus statements.
  - Hospital administrators often use the LOS metric as a measure of efficiency.
  - One of the IOM-specific aims for improving healthcare quality is that healthcare should be efficient—avoiding waste, in particular waste of equipment, supplies, ideas, and energy (and by extension, the waste of hospital bed days).
- With the decline in LOS, there has been concern for increase in mortality and readmission as a possible consequence. However, the literature does not support the relationship of shortened LOS with increased mortality or readmission rates.
  - Baker et al looked at 83,445 Medicare patients in Ohio with five diagnoses from 1991 to 1997 and found that readmission rates remained stable for all except heart failure. Postdischarge mortality was unchanged except for those with do not resuscitate orders.
  - In a multicenter hospital study, Lindenauer and colleagues compared hospitalist care to general internists and family physicians for 7 common diagnoses. Compared with general internists and family physicians, hospitalists had a significantly shorter LOS but there was no difference in death rates and 14 day readmissions. An accompanying editorial comments this study has clearly demonstrated shortening LOS has no adverse events on patient outcomes.
- While discharges to other facilities will reduce LOS and cost of care for the acute-care hospital, it is unclear if it reduces overall health costs or merely shifts the costs to other providers.
  - Fitzgerald et al demonstrated keeping hip replacement patients in the acute hospital 2 days longer to prevent a 1-week stay in a rehabilitation facility.
  - Some studies have shown earlier discharges actually increased the number of outpatient visits to primary care physicians and specialists as well as increased home nursing needs.

FACTORS THAT INCREASE LOS

- Patient complexity and hospital complications are medical care-related factors that can increase LOS. However, there are other factors that can increase LOS that may be related to the efficiency of the systems of care rather than the medical care itself.
- "Unnecessary days" or "delay days" are the description for days patients spend in the hospital when they do not need that level of care.
  - Private companies, like InterQual and MCAP, have emerged and produced tools that could be used to evaluate whether patients met criteria to be in the hospital. These tools or utilization guidelines were based on outcome studies and physician consensus.
    - Insurers apply these utilization guidelines to determine if each day of hospitalization is appropriate, and may deny coverage for days they determine to be unnecessary.
    - Hospitals and healthcare organizations can utilize these tools to learn their total number of unnecessary inpatient days and search for the specific causes in their organization.
  - Applying InterQual to 858 medical and surgical admissions at 43 veterans administration hospitals, Weaver et al found an average LOS of 12.7 days of which 6.8 days did not meet acute care level.
- What are the causes of delay days? One study at an academic teaching hospital found that 30% of patients on the general internal medical and gastrointestinal services experienced delays in discharge of an average of 2.9 days and that overall 17% of hospital days were unnecessary. In addition, 41% of all delay days were due to the unavailability of a bed at a subacute-care facility. The most frequent reasons for delay in discharge were
  - Scheduling of tests (31%)
  - Unavailability of postdischarge facilities (18%)
  - Physician decision making (13%)
  - Discharge planning (12%)
  - Scheduling of surgery (12%)
- Delays waiting for a bed at a postdischarge facility remain an ongoing problem:
  - Closed rehabilitation facilities and nursing homes because of financial insolvency
  - Inadequate numbers of psychiatric facilities, making it difficult to place mentally ill patients
  - A shortage of drug treatment centers, making it difficult to place patients with substance abuse issues
  - A lack of adequate centers skilled at managing patients with dual diagnoses of psychiatric disorders and substance abuse
  - Inadequate support services and shelters for homeless (and typically uninsured) patients

WAYS TO OPTIMIZE LOS AND IMPROVE PATIENT OUTCOMES

- There are a variety of ways to improve efficiency and optimize LOS (Table 12-2).

HOW TO IMPROVE QUALITY OF CARE

- As outlined by the IOM, healthcare should be safe (avoiding injuries to patients from the care that is intended to help them) and effective (providing services based on scientific knowledge to all who could benefit and refraining from providing services to those not likely to benefit, avoiding under use and overuse).
- One major attempt in medicine to improve quality of care was the development of guidelines and pathways.
- The terms practice guidelines, clinical guidelines, clinical pathways, or critical pathways are often used interchangeably in the literature.
  - Guidelines (both practice and clinical) are consensus statements of best practices, some derived from evidence-based medicine (nearly 50% are not), that are developed to assist practitioners in making optimal patient management decisions.
  - Pathways are management plans that provide a sequence of actions necessary to achieve goals and optimize efficiency. Pathways are often based on guidelines but not always.

- While practice guidelines have existed in medicine for many years, the late 1980s saw a rapid growth in the development of both guidelines and clinical pathways. This was fueled not only by the change in reimbursement but also the rise of healthcare costs, reports of large variation in practice among physicians and growing evidence of inappropriate utilization.
  - These guidelines and pathways were viewed as a way to improve and standardize patient care as well as remove inefficiencies in the healthcare system and reduce LOS.
  - The push for clinical pathways and guidelines came at a national level. In 1988, the Physician Payment Review Commission, which advises Congress, and the US Department of Health and Human Services both recommended using practice guidelines.
  - In 1989, the IOM convened a group of national experts to discuss guidelines. They recommended clinical guidelines be based on patient outcomes research.
  - Medical organizations, health plans, researchers, and public officials all expressed increasing interest in the development and implementation of practice guidelines and pathways. Millions of dollars were spent on their development on a national and local level.
  - The Agency for Healthcare Policy and Research established a national clearinghouse Web site for evidence-based medicine guidelines (see references for Web address).

TABLE 12-2   Ways to Optimize LOS

Clinical pathways	Help to standardize practice, reducing inefficiency, and improving quality of care
Discharge planning	Start discharge planning at time of admission
	Anticipate patients' discharge needs and plan ahead
	Work closely with case management
	Participate in interdisciplinary rounds to improve communication and help identify problems early
	Identify patients who need extended care facilities early on and discuss with patient and family
Communication	Set expectations early on about LOS. This allows patients and families to plan ahead
	Caution people they may not feel fully back to their baseline health status at time of discharge.
	Describe a time line and trajectory for improvement
	Communicate daily with patients' and their families and PCPs
Minimize hazards of hospitalization	Monitor for medication errors and minimize polypharmacy
	Remove tethers like foleys, oxygen tubes, and intravenous lines to limit deconditioning and nosocomial infection
	Evaluate the patient for risk of DVT and prescribe appropriate prophylaxis
	Evaluate patients for mobility issues and limit in-hospital deconditioning
	Minimize polypharmacy and other risks that contribute to delirium
	Minimize risks that contribute to hospital-acquired renal failure
Risk factors that increase LOS	Age >85
	History of dementia or cognitive impairment
	Poor nutrition
	Incontinence
	History of falls
	History of stroke
	Diabetes

○ National organizations disseminated guidelines and pathways with the assumption that these would change practice. The new guidelines differed from older versions in that they focused on evidence-based medicine, quality of care, and appropriateness of practice.

• During the 1990s, there were many single-institution-based studies that confirmed the benefits of guidelines and pathways to patient care and LOS, and found no negative effects on patients such as increased mortality or readmission (surrogate markers for care quality).

○ Weingarten et al in 1994 evaluated a practice guideline for chest pain showing a decreased LOS (0.91 days) and a cost reduction of $1397 per patient. No difference was found in the hospital complication rate, mortality, or patient satisfaction.

○ In a 1993 meta-analysis, Grimshaw et al looked at 59 published studies of clinical pathways and found all but four studies showed improvement in the process of care. However, the size of improvement varied significantly. The authors found the most successful pathways were locally developed with specific educational interventions for the particular system that employed them. National guidelines that were published in journals or mailed to groups were not found to be effective.

○ Lomas and colleagues studied the national consensus guidelines for cesarean delivery and found most obstetricians were aware of the guidelines and said they were compliant. Yet 2 years after the guidelines' release, there was no change in cesarean section rates. The authors concluded guidelines should not be developed in isolation but at the local level with resources for implementation and education.

• Given that most studies were single-institution-based trials, are the results from these studies accurate and generalizable? There are very few randomized multi-centered studies on clinical pathways to answer that question.

○ Shaneyfelt et al evaluated 279 guidelines from 1985 to 1997, and found only 51% were developed using methodological standards and only 33.6% identified and summarized evidence.

○ One multicenter study found that the implementation of several surgical pathways resulted in a lower LOS, but at the same time overall LOS for those areas decreased even in hospitals without pathways.

○ Marrie et al in one of the few medical multihospital randomized trials found that a critical pneumonia pathway could maintain quality and decrease resource use in Canada.

• Physicians have not globally embraced pathways as a vehicle to improve patient care. There has been resistance on the basis of "cookbook medicine" or loss of professional autonomy. In addition, while pathways may work well for patients with a single illness or undergoing procedures, it is not clear they work as well for complex medical inpatients with multiple comorbidities and problems requiring balanced management.

• After nearly two decades of the development and use of guidelines and pathways, they are believed to improve quality of care, reduce LOS, and create efficiency, with no detrimental effects to patient care, but this has not been consistently shown in the literature.

• Should hospitalists use guidelines/pathways to improve patient care and reduce LOS? While pathways may not be the panacea that was hoped for in the late 1980s, "homegrown" single institution's pathways implemented with educational support have been shown to improve patient care and reduce LOS. Given hospitalists know their own hospital systems the best, they are well suited to develop and facilitate implementation of guidelines and pathways for their own institutions.

IMPROVING EFFICIENCY AND CARE TRANSITIONS

• The IOM noted that healthcare should be timely, reducing waits and sometimes harmful delays for both those who receive care and those who give care.

• Improving the transition of care at discharge can have a significant impact on optimizing LOS.

• In the study by Selker et al, physician's decision making and discharge planning accounted for a quarter of the reasons for delays.

• In addition to testing and decision making delays, the discharge transition itself can be slow and cumbersome.

• The discharge process should begin upon admission, and requires effective teamwork among physicians, nurses, therapists, case managers/social workers, and other members of the healthcare team to anticipate the discharge needs and proactively prepare to implement the discharge plan.

• Involvement of patients and families, and setting expectations for the goals of the hospitalization and the expected time course to accomplish them, is also crucial.

CASE MANAGEMENT

• The role of the case manager and expansion of case management departments has grown to promote a more coordinated discharge process.

- Typically made up of nurse case managers and social workers, and often combined with utilization review, case management focuses on anticipating and preparing for patients' needs after they leave the hospital and coordinating the discharge plan.
- Case managers know available resources in the community and what various insurers will cover, and can identify appropriate alternative sites of care.
- Case managers and social workers can make referrals to acute or subacute care facilities early in the hospital stay to minimize the delay in procuring an appropriate bed.
- Moher et al showed the benefit of case management with a reduction in LOS from 9.4 days to 7.3 days with a concomitant increase in patient satisfaction.

HOSPITALISTS

- Increasing communication between hospital-based physicians and outpatient physicians can allow for an earlier discharge. For example, a patient with chest pain who is deemed low risk and has ruled out may be able to be safely discharged over the weekend, rather than wait until Monday for a stress test, if the PCP is aware of the admission and can expeditiously arrange for an outpatient stress test.
- Varnava et al found that discharge days were not just based on clinical decisions but also determined by the day of the week, Fridays being the biggest day for discharges in hospitals. Increasing awareness of clinical indications for discharge may reduce this bias.
- Smith et al found there was an increase in LOS during physician's switch periods due to delays in decision making or planning as the new physician gets to know the patient's history.
- Strategies to improve this process include
  ◦ Standardized and thorough sign-out processes
  ◦ Expectations that physicians should "tie up lose ends" before going off service
  ◦ Schedules that maximize continuity of care (block or block-shift models)
  ◦ Preparing the discharge plans for patients that could go home on the transition day or during a weekend.
- Hospitalists can evaluate delay days on their services and identify the barriers to timely discharge, and participate in systems-based improvements to remove those barriers (such as lack of availability of diagnostic testing on the weekend).
- Hospitalists can collaborate with case managers and local rehabilitation and skilled nursing facilities to facilitate discharges. Some strategies that have been employed include:
  ◦ Creating "discharge appointments" both to improve LOS and increase patient flow. The appointments are given to patients and families with an expected date and time of discharge, so arrangements can be made for transportation home, and the physician, nurse, and/or case manager can be available to review discharge instructions (especially any changes in medications) and answer questions. While results on LOS have been mixed, discharge appointments do set expectations for patients and families and give them time to plan.
  ◦ Collaborating with the PCP and/or physicians who practice home care, and with visiting nurses, can allow patients (particularly frail elders) to be discharged early into a safe and familiar environment. Visiting nurses can monitor patients and ensure compliance with treatments.
  ◦ Hospitalists have started follow-up clinics for recently discharged patients. This allows patients to be discharged earlier and monitored frequently even if their primary care physician is not available to see them soon after discharge, or they do not have a PCP.
  ◦ This intervention may especially benefit homeless or uninsured patients with limited access to outpatient care.
  ◦ Disadvantaged and difficult to place patients can drive up LOS as many delay days accrue while trying to find a safe discharge plan. One Boston group is teaming up with the state's Medicaid program and the department of public health to designate a number of beds in an already existing rehabilitation facility for these difficult to place patients.
  ◦ Some hospitals with high volumes of discharges to skilled nursing facilities have partnered with such facilities to set aside a proportion of their beds for patients from that referral hospital. Such arrangements may include collaboration on post-acute care guidelines or pathways to enhance the care that can be provided in the facility for patients with particular discharge diagnoses, and/or the availability of appropriate subspecialists to do follow-up rounds or comanage patients at the facility.
  ◦ Some hospitalist groups also provide skilled nursing facility care to help achieve a more seamless transition from acute care to skilled care.

BIBLIOGRAPHY

Agency for Healthcare Research and Quality, US Department of Health and Human Service: National Guideline Clearinghouse www.guideline.gov.

Baker DW, Einstadter D, Husak SS, et al. Trends in postdischarge mortality and readmissions. Has LOS declined too far? *Arch Intern Med.* 2004;164:538–544.

Fitzgerald JF, Moore PS, Dittus RS. The care of elderly patients with hip fractures. Changes since implementation of the prospective payment system. *N Engl J Med.* 1988; 319: 1392–1397.

Grimshaw J, Russel IT. Effect of clinical guidelines on medical practice: a systematic review of rigorous evaluations. *Lancet.* 1993;342:1317–22.

Kohn LT, Corrigan JM, Donaldson MS, et al. *To Err is Human: Building a Safer Healty System. Committee on Quality of HealthCare in Mserica, IHI.* National Academy Press, Washington, DC: Nov 1999.

Kostis WJ, Demissie K, Marcella SW, et al. Weekend versus weekday admission and mortality from myocardial infarction. *N Engl J Med.* 2007;356:1099–1109.

Lindenauer PK, Rothberg MB, Pekow PS, et al. Outcomes of care by hospitalists, general internists, and family physicians. *N Engl J Med.* 2007;357:2589–2600.

Lomas J, Anderson GM, Domnick-Pierre K, et al: Do practice guidelines guide practice? The effect of a consensus statement on the practice of physicians. *N Engl J Med.* 1989;321:1306–1311.

Marrie TJ, Lau CY, Wheeler SL, et al. A controlled trial of a critical pathway for treatment of community-acquired pneumonia. *JAMA.* 2000;283:749–755.

Moher D, Weinberg A, Hanlon R, et al. Medical team coordinator and length of hospital stay. *Can Med Assoc J.* 1992;146: 511–5.

Selker HP, Beshansky JR, Pauker SG, et al. The epidemiology of delays in a teaching hospital. *Med Care.* 1989;27(2):112–130.

Shaneyfelt TM, Mayo-Smith MF, Rothwangl J. Are guidelines following guidelines? *JAMA.* 1999;281:1900–1905.

Smith JP, Mehta RH, Das SK, et al. Effects of end-of-month admission on LOS and quality of care among inpatients with myocardial infarction. *Am J Med.* 2002;112(4):288–293.

Varnava AM, Sedgwick JE, Deaner A, et al. Restricted weekend service inappropriately delays discharge after acute myocardial infarction. *Heart.* 2002;87:216–219.

Weaver FM, Guihan M, Hynes DM, et al. Prevalence of subacute patients in acute care: results of a study of VA hospitals. *J Med Sys.* 1998;22(3):161–172.

Weingarten SR, Riedinger MS, Conner L, et al. Practice guidelines and reminders to reduce duration of hospital stay for patients with chest pain: an interventional trial. *Ann Intern Med.* 1994;120(4):257–263.

13 HANDOFFS

Vineet Arora and Julie Johnson

SCOPE OF THE PROBLEM

- An increased focus on the vulnerability of transfers of patient care between providers (handoffs) has occurred for a variety of reasons.

○ The implementation of restricted resident duty hours by the Accreditation Council of Graduate Medical Education (ACGME), coupled with the demand for 24-hour shift coverage by various groups, such as Leapfrog, are two reasons for increased attention to handoffs.

○ The Joint Commission on the Accreditation of Healthcare Organizations (JCAHO) has made handoffs a national patient safety goal in 2006. The JCAHO mandate "requires hospitals to implement a standardized approach to handoff communications and provide an opportunity for staff to ask and respond to questions about a patient's care" (Table 13-1).[1]

- Poor communication at the time of handoffs has been implicated in near misses and adverse events in a variety of healthcare contexts, including nursing handoffs, physician sign-out of patients, and emergency medicine shift changes.

- Despite the increased focus on the vulnerability of the handoff, few medical trainees or hospitalists receive formal education on how to perform an effective handoff.

TERMINOLOGY ("PATHOPHYSIOLOGY")

- Other terms for the handoff include "sign-out," "sign-over" and "handover." These different terms refer to a difference in the approach to manage care over the 24-hour day. The distinction between handoff and sign-out has carried over into studies of information transfers under short call and cross-coverage schedules.

○ "Sign-out" and "sign-over" are used when a "day" provider or team transfers care to an evening or night shift, such as short-call or night float. Patients move from an active period of management to a "holding phase" until their regular provider returns. While the physician who accepts the sign-out will be dealing with emergencies, the planning and ongoing care of patients are often on hold.

  ▪ Sign-out can either refer to the written document or electronic file used to transfer patient information during "handoffs" or to the verbal communication that occurs during the "handoff."[7]

○ "Handoff" and "handover" are used to refer to the 24-hour, 7-day continuous management of the patient. The accepting physician is often fully empowered to manage all aspects of patient care (i.e., nursing, intensive care unit (ICU), emergency department (ED), and so forth).

  ▪ An effective handoff includes the transfer of critical patient information needed to continue care for that patient, and the acceptance of the professional responsibility of continued care for a patient.

TABLE 13-1   JCAHO Handoff National Patient Safety Goal: Improve the Effectiveness of Communication Among Caregivers[1]

Requirement 2E	Implementation Expectations
• Requires hospitals to implement a *standardized approach* to handoff communications and provide an opportunity for staff to ask and respond to questions about a patient's care.	1. The organization's process for effective handoff communication includes: interactive communications allowing for the opportunity for questioning between the giver and receiver of patient information.
Rationale for Requirement 2E	2. The organization's process for effective handoff communication includes: up-to-date information regarding the patient's care, treatment and services, condition, and any recent or anticipated changes.
• The primary objective of a handoff is to provide accurate information about a patient's care, treatment and services, current condition, and any recent or anticipated changes. The information communicated during a handoff must be accurate in order to meet patient safety goals.	3. The organization's process for effective handoff communication includes: a process for verification of the received information, including repeat-back or read-back, as appropriate.
• In healthcare there are numerous types of patient handoffs, including, but not limited to:	4. The organization's process for effective handoff communication includes an opportunity for the receiver of the handoff information to review relevant patient historical data, which may include previous care, treatment, and services.
○ Nursing shift changes, temporary responsibility for staff leaving the unit for a short time	5. Interruptions during handoffs are limited to minimize the possibility that information would fail to be conveyed or would be forgotten.
○ Physicians transferring complete responsibility for a patient; physicians transferring on-call responsibility	
○ Anesthsiologist report to post-anesthesia recovery room nurse	
○ Nursing and physician handoff from the ED to inpatient units, different hospitals, nursing homes and home healthcare	
○ Critical laboratory and radiology results to physicians	

EVIDENCE

Strategies from other industries and applications to healthcare

- Human factors researchers conducted direct observations of handoffs in other 24-hour high-risk industries such as aviation, transportation, and nuclear power.

- ○ They proposed a series of effective strategies that could be applied to healthcare, which included the following (Table 13-2):
- ○ The use of standardization and a face-to-face verbal update with interactive questioning emerged as two key strategies from these observations that resonate with the JCAHO goals.

TABLE 13-2   Handoff Coordination and Communication Objectives and Strategies

INFERRED OBJECTIVES	STRATEGY
1 Improve handoff update effectiveness	Face-to-face verbal update with interactive questioning
2 Improve handoff update effectiveness	Additional update from practitioners other than the one being replaced
3 Improve handoff update effectiveness	Limit interruptions during update
4 Improve handoff update effectiveness	Topics initiated by incoming* as well as outgoing†
5 Improve handoff update effectiveness	Limit initiation of operator actions during update
6 Improve handoff update effectiveness	Include outgoing team's stance toward changes to plans and contingency plans
7 Improve handoff update effectiveness	Read-back‡ to ensure that information was accurately received
8 Improve handoff update efficiency and effectiveness	Outgoing writes summary before handoff
9 Improve handoff update efficiency and effectiveness	Incoming assesses current status
10 Improve handoff update efficiency and effectiveness	Update information in the same order every time
11 Improve handoff update efficiency and effectiveness	Incoming scans historical data before update
12 Improve handoff update efficiency and effectiveness	Incoming reviews automatically captured changes to sensor-derived data before update
13 Improve handoff update efficiency and effectiveness	Intermittent monitoring of system status while "on call" §
14 Improve handoff update efficiency and effectiveness	Outgoing has knowledge of previous shift activities
15 Increase access to data	Incoming receives primary access to the most up-to-date information
16 Increase access to data	Incoming receives paperwork that includes handwritten annotations
17 Improve coordination with others	Unambiguous transfer of responsibility
18 Improve coordination with others	Make it clear to others at a glance which personnel are responsible for which duties at a particular time
19 Enable error detection and recovery	Overhear others' updates
20 Enable error detection and recovery	Outgoing oversees incoming's work following update
21 Delay transfer of responsibility during critical activities	Delay the transfer of responsibility when concerned about status/stability of process

*Incoming, personnel arriving to begin their shift
†Outgoing, personnel ending their shift.
‡Read-back, verbal repeat of information that was just heard to verify accuracy.
§On call, personnel who are assigned responsibility to be available to provide support on an "as needed" basis during a scheduled time.
Emily S. Patterson, et. al. Handoff strategies in settings with high consequences for failure: lessons for health care operations. *Int J Qual Health Care.* 2004;16(2):125–32, by permission of Oxford University Press.

- Use of structured language (i.e., "read-back" or "SBAR") can improve the comprehension of information transmitted at the time of a handoff.
  ○ "Read-backs" have been shown to reduce the number of errors during requested read-back of 822 lab results. All errors were detected and corrected. Furthermore, the use of a read-back was cost-effective.
  ○ "SBAR" or the situational briefing model is a technique used in aviation to communicate critical content (Table 13-3). This model has been

TABLE 13-3   Situation Debriefing Model "SBAR"

SBAR report to physician about a critical situation

S	**Situation**
	I am calling about <u><patient name and location></u>.
	The patient's code status is <u><code status></u>.
	The problem I am calling about is _____.
	      I am afraid the patient is going to arrest.
	I have just assessed the patient personally:
	Vital signs are: Blood pressure _____/_____, Pulse _____, Respiration _____and temperature ____.
	I am concerned about the:
	    Blood pressure because it is over 200 or less than 100 or 30 mm Hg below usual.
	    Pulse because it is over 140 or less than 50.
	    Respiration because it is less than 5 or over 40.
	    Temperature because it is less than 96 or over 104.

B	**Background**
	The patient's mental status is:
	    Alert and oriented to person place and time.
	    Confused and cooperative or noncooperative.
	    Agitated or combative.
	    Lethargic but conversant and able to swallow.
	    Stuporous and not talking clearly and possibly not able to swallow.
	    Comatose. Eyes closed. Not responding to stimulation.
	The skin is:
	    Warm and dry
	    Pale
	    Mottled
	    Diaphoretic
	    Extremities are cold
	    Extremities are warm
	The patient is not or is on oxygen.
	    The patient has been on _____ (l/min) or (%) oxygen for _____ minutes (hours).
	    The oximeter is reading _____%.
	    The oximeter does not detect a good pulse and is giving erratic readings.

A	**Assessment**
	    This is what I think the problem is: <u><say what you think is the problem></u>.
	    The problem seems to be cardiac infection neurologic respiratory _____
	    I am not sure what the problem is but the patient is deteriorating.
	    The patient seems to be unstable and may get worse, we need to do something.

R	**Recommendation**
	I suggest or request that you <u><say what you would like to see done></u>.
	    transfer the patient to critical care
	    come to see the patient at this time.
	    Talk to the patient or family about code status.
	    Ask the on-call family practice resident to see the patient now.
	    Ask for a consultant to see the patient now.
	Are any tests needed:
	    Do you need any tests like CXR, ABG, EKG, CBC, or BNP?
	    Others?
	If a change in treatment is ordered then ask:
	    How often do you want vital signs?
	    How long to you expect this problem will last?
	    If the patient does not get better, when would you want us to call again?

effective in improving communication between clinicians. The SBAR process is defined as follows:

- *Situation*: Briefly state the nature of the problem, how it started, and how severe it is. Clearly communicate the patient's name and room number.
- *Background*: Give pertinent background information for the situation such as vital signs or code status.
- *Assessment*: What is your assessment of the patient's situation?
- *Recommendation*: What is your recommendation? Do orders need to be changed? Does the patient need to be moved?

In hospital physician handoffs (Table 13-4)

- Although few studies of in-hospital physician handoffs exist to date, these studies describe barriers to effective handoffs and how these barriers may compromise patient care.
- One study of internal medicine residents developed a taxonomy to describe effective and poor communication (Table 13-5).
- At least two studies have demonstrated benefits with the implementation of a computerized sign-out system in academic teaching hospitals. However, it is important to note that these computerized sign-out systems cannot substitute for a successful communication act and human vigilance will still be required to ensure a proper verbal handoff.

TABLE 13-4 Taxonomy of Sign-Out Quality

POOR SIGN-OUT	EFFECTIVE SIGN-OUT
Content omissions	Written sign-out patient content
• Medications or therapies	• Code status
• Tests or consults	• Anticipated problems
• Medical problems	• Active problems
◦ Active	• Baseline examination
◦ Anticipated	• Pending test or consults
• Baseline status	Overall features
• Code status	• Legible
• Rationale of primary team	• Relevant
Failure-prone communication processes	• Up-to-date
• Lack of face-to-face communication	Verbal sign-out
• Double sign-out ("night float")	• Face to face
• Illegible or unclear handwriting	• Anticipate
	• Pertinent
	• Thorough

Arora V, Johnson J, Lovinger D, et al. Communication failures in patient signout and suggestions for improvement: a critical incident analysis. *Qual Saf Health Care.* 2005;14:401–407.

SYSTEMS IMPROVEMENT

- Developing a standardized handoff protocol can help to meet the JCAHO national patient safety goals and potentially improve communication and transfer of professional responsibility during handoffs.
  - ◦ The handoff protocol should be tailored for users. To do this, take into account the culture of the discipline (i.e., surgery, medicine, nursing, and so forth), the

TABLE 13-5 Studies of In-Hospital Physician Handoffs

AUTHOR	STUDY TYPE	METHODS OR INTERVENTION	FINDINGS	IMPLICATIONS
Arora V, et al. 2005.[2]	Qualitative	Interns interviewed after a call night using critical incident technique to report near misses and adverse events due to deficient sign-out.	Sign-out communication failures include omitted content (such as medications, active problems) or failure-prone communication processes (such as lack of face-to-face discussion). These failures lead to uncertainty during medical decisions, resulting in inefficient or poor care. Interns desire relevant face-to-face verbal sign-outs that anticipate issues; and legible, accurate, updated, standardized written sign-out sheets.	Suggestions can be used to design educational programs and build effective sign-out systems.
Solet DJ, et al. 2005.[13]	Descriptive, observational	Reviewed the literature on patient handoffs and evaluated the patient handoff process in their internal medicine residency program.	Considerable variation observed in the quality and content of handoffs. Barriers to effective handoffs include noisy, distracting physical settings that impede conversation; the hierarchal nature of medicine (which can discourage open discussion between health professionals); language barriers among doctors; lack of face-to-face communication; and time pressures.	Important need to develop standard educational practices that address these barriers.

(Continued)

TABLE 13-5 Studies of In-Hospital Physician Handoffs (*Continued*)

AUTHOR	STUDY TYPE	METHODS OR INTERVENTION	FINDINGS	IMPLICATIONS
Petersen LA, et al.[14]	Pre- and post-analysis to evaluate intervention	Pre- and post-analysis of preventable adverse events to evaluate the effect of implementation of computerized sign-outs.	Rate of preventable adverse events among the 3747 patients admitted to the medical service decreased from 1.7% to 1.2% ($p < .10$) with computerized sign-out. In the baseline period, the odds ratio (OR) for a patient suffering a preventable adverse event during cross coverage was 5.2 (95% confidence interval [CI], 1.5–18.2; $p = 0.01$), but was no longer significant after the intervention (OR, 1.5; 95% CI, 0.2–9.0).	Computerized sign-out may have reduced the risk for medical injury associated with discontinuity of inpatient care.
Van Eaton EG et al., 2005.[15]	Randomized cross-over study of intervention	Central, web-based system that stores sign-out information; downloads patient data (vital signs, laboratories); and prints them to rounding, sign-out, and progress note templates.	Improved efficiency through: (1) halved prerounding time spent copying data ($p < .0001$); shortened team rounds by 1.5 min/patient ($p = 0.0006$); and residents finishing work sooner (82.1% agree or strongly agree). Improved patient care by: (1) fewer patients missed on rounds (2.5 vs. 5 patients/team/month, $p = 0.0001$); (2) 40% more of resident prerounding time spent seeing patients ($p = 0.36$); (3) increased resident perceptions of sign-out quality (70% agree or strongly agree) and continuity of care (66% agree or strongly agree).	Information technology systems cannot only improve the quality of care but also address the importance of efficiency.

institution, and the local environment in which the handoff is occurring (i.e., busy ICU, ED, and so forth).
○ The goal of the handoff protocol is to standardize both process and content, within each discipline. While differences in the protocol across different disciplines are to be expected, deviations from the protocol within each discipline must be reduced.
• A process map can be very useful in getting buy-in and assessing the integrity of the handoff process.

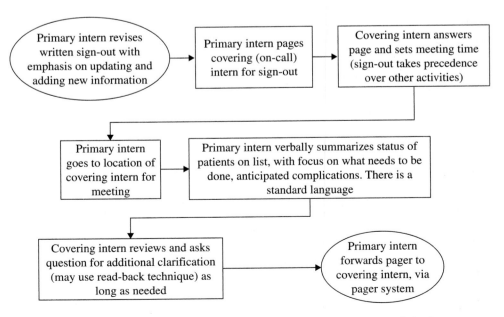

FIG. 13-1 Sample handoff process map for University of Chicago internal medicine interns.

Some important questions to ask about the process are the following:

○ Where does the process begin and end? Is there a clear transfer of content and professional responsibility? Are there any gaps in the process? Where are the redundancies or unnecessary steps that do not add value to the process (Fig. 13-1)?

• A checklist of critical content can help to standardize the information that is communicated in addition to improving the transmission of that information (Fig. 13-2).

○ An ideal checklist is customized to one's institution and practice and contains examples of jargon routinely used to transfer information.

• This handoff protocol (process map and checklist) can be used to train new personnel and also observe handoffs in real time to monitor the adherence to the protocol.

✓ **P**roblem List

☐ Any Pertinent Past Medical History (i.e. Cerebral Palsy, Seizure Disorder, etc.)
☐ Systems-based List of Current Problems
☐ Focus on Any Invasive Tubes/Devices (i.e. Patients has g-tube or trach)

✓ **E**xpected Tasks to be Done

☐ Any Labs to Check on and What to Do About Them
☐ Tests to Order or Follow-up on (CT scans, etc.)

✓ **D**iagnostic One-liner

☐ Includes Age, Sex, Relevant Past History Related to Current Problem and Current Chief Complaint/Reason for Hospitalization (4 yo F with History of Chronic Severe Asthma here with Status Asthmaticus)

✓ **I**f/Then

☐ Frequent Issues to be Expected with a Plan to Resolve Using IF/Then Format (i.e. "If HTN, Please Give Hydralazine," "CIS" etc.)

✓ **A**dministrative Data/Advanced Directives

☐ Patient Name, Medical Record Number
☐ Room Number
☐ Admission Date
☐ Primary Inpatient Team, Attending
☐ Family Contact Information
☐ Weight/BSA (Body Surface Area)
☐ Code Status

✓ **T**herapeutics

☐ Medications (Updated List of Medications with Doses (esp Dates that Any Antibiotics were Started and Duration)
☐ Diet with Any Weaning Orders—Is the Patient NPO?
☐ IVF
☐ Oxygen with Weaning Instructions

✓ **R**esults and Other Important Facts

☐ Labs (i.e. Recent Hgb/Hct, etc.)
☐ Cultures (esp Any Outside Hospital Cultures that were Obtained)
☐ Radiology Test Results
☐ Consults

✓ **IV** Access/Invasive Devices

☐ IV Access and What to Do If It Comes Out Overnight (i.e. "Has PIV, Must be Replaced If It Falls Out")
☐ Any Invasive Devices Listed in Problem List

✓ **C**ustody and Consent Issues

☐ Is the Patient DCFS (Division of Child and Family Services)—If yes, Need to Get Consents from Them
☐ Child Protective Services Involved?
☐ Parental Custody or Any Issues Related to Parental Custody

FIG. 13-2 Handoff checklist for pediatrics residents at the University of Chicago.

REFERENCES

1. Joint Commission on Accreditation of Healthcare Organizations. Joint Commission announces 2006 national patient safety goals for ambulatory care and office-based surgery organizations [Internet]. [cited 2005 September 1]. Available from: http://www.jcaho.org/news+room/news+ release+archives/06_npsg_amb_obs.htm

2. Arora V, Johnson J, Lovinger D, et al. Communication failures in patient signout and suggestions for improvement: a critical incident analysis. *Qual Saf Health Care.* 2005;14: 401–407.

3. Ebright PR, Urden L, Patterson E, et al. Themes surrounding novice nurse near miss and adverse-event situations. *J Nurs Adm.* 2004;34:531–538.

4. Beach C, Croskerry P, Shapiro M. Center for Safety in Emergency Care. Profiles in patient safety: emergency care transitions. *Acad Emerg Med.* 2003;10:364–367.

5. Horwitz LI, Krumholz HM, Green ML, et al. Transfers of patient care between house staff on internal medicine wards: a national survey. *Arch Intern Med.* 2006;166: 1173–1177.

6. Philibert I, Leach DC. Re-framing continuity of care for this century. *Qual Saf Health Care.* 2005;14(6):394–396.

7. Vidyarthi AR, Arora V, Schnipper JL, et al. Managing discontinuity in academic medical centers: Strategies for a safe and effective resident sign-out. *J Hosp Med.* 2006;1: 257–266.

8. Arora V, Johnson J. Meeting the JCAHO national patient safety goal: a model for building a standardized handoff protocol. *Jt Comm J Qual Saf.* 2006;32(11):646–655.

9. Patterson ES, Roth EM, Woods DD, et al. Handoff strategies in settings with high consequences for failure: lessons for healthcare operations. *Int J Qual Health Care.* 2004;16: 125–132.

10. Barenfanger J, Sautter RL, Lang DL, et al. Improving patient safety by repeating (read-back) telephone reports of critical information. *Am J Clin Pathol.* 2004;121:801–803.

11. Leonard M, Graham S, Bonacum D. The human factor: the critical importance of effective teamwork and communication in providing safe care. *Qual Saf Health Care.* 2004; 13(Suppl I):i85–90.

12. Haig KM, Sutton S, Whittington J. SBAR: a shared mental model for improving communication between clinicians. *Jt Comm J Qual Patient Saf.* 2006;32(3):167–175.

13. Solet DJ, Norvell JM, Rutan GH, et al. Lost in translation: challenges and opportunities in physician-to-physician communication during patient handoffs. *Acad Med.* 2005;80(12): 1094–1099.

14. Petersen LA, Orav EJ, Teich JM, et al. Using a computerized sign-out program to improve continuity of inpatient care and prevent adverse events. *Jt Comm J Qual Improv.* 1998;24:77–87.

15. Van Eaton EG, Horvath KD, Lober WB, et al. A randomized, controlled trial evaluating the impact of a computerized rounding and sign-out system on continuity of care and resident work hours. *J Am Coll Surg.* 2005;200: 538–545.

14 DISCHARGE SUMMARIES

Marcy G. Carty and Namita S. Mohta

BACKGROUND

The hospitalist plays an integral role in ensuring a safe transition for discharged patients. This role is made more difficult by the following trends:
- Decreasing length of stay (LOS) and increasing case mix index (CMI)
  ○ Hospitalized patients are admitted and discharged sicker than ever before.
  ○ At same time, inpatient LOS is steadily declining.
- Growing number of handoffs
  ○ With the Accreditation Council of Graduate Medical Education (ACGME) resident hours restrictions, patients admitted to academic medical centers with house staff are handed off, or transitioned, to other caregivers (night floats, covering teams) multiple times throughout their stay and even in nonteaching settings there may be multiple clinicians involved in the patient's care. Therefore, discharges are often performed by someone other than the admitting physician, thus important details may be lost.
  ○ The advent of hospitalist attendings often creates additional systematic discontinuities, with transition on admission and transition postdischarge back to the primary care physician (PCP)/subspecialist who will provide follow-up care.
- Rising number of medications per patient
  ○ As population ages, number of chronic problems increases and necessitates more complex medical regimens. The average number of prescriptions per person rose from 7.3 to 11.6 between 1992 and 2002.
  ○ Growth of new pharmaceuticals is projected to continue with over 1000 products in the development pipeline.
- Increasing number of discharges to extended care facilities
  ○ Intermediate steps involving long-term care facilities create more transitions of care, and more opportunity for adverse events. Between 1985 and 1999, the percentage of discharges from hospitals transferred to long-term care facilities doubled, from 4.3% to 9%.

GOALS OF AN EFFECTIVE DISCHARGE CARE TRANSITION

- The discharge planning process begins at admission (Fig. 14-1), and should

TABLE 14-1   Case Concerning Discharge Summary

Ms S is an 86-year-old female with a history of CAD, CHF, and DM who was admitted to a community hospital with sepsis from a urinary tract infection.

• She improved with treatment consisting of IV fluid and several broad spectrum antibiotics, which were quickly narrowed to a quinolone.
• She was deemed stable for hospital discharge on hospital day #4 to a local rehabilitation facility for continued antibiotics and physical therapy.
• After three days at the facility, she became febrile and hypotensive and was readmitted to the hospital.
• In the emergency department (ED), her blood sugar was noted to be 671.

What happened?

• On discharge, medication reconciliation was not performed and her PO diabetes medications were not restarted.
• Her discharge summary did not indicate that the accepting provider needed to follow-up on pending urine culture sensitivities. Upon review, the bacteria were resistant to quinolones.

How could this readmission have been avoided?

• Contain all key elements, including pending test results at discharge.
• The discharge summary should communicate the plan for unresolved medical problems at the time of discharge, including specific information about what the receiving physicians should do.

○ Prevent redundancy in diagnostic evaluations and avoid delays in future diagnosis and treatment.
○ Lay out a therapeutic/next step plan for the receiving physician for the patient's outstanding medical issues.
○ Ensure continuity during future hospitalizations.

The discharge summary should

○ *Contain all key elements:* Qualitative data suggest that many outpatient providers are dissatisfied with discharge summaries they receive because they are missing data regarding *discharge diagnosis*, *abnormal test results*, *medications,* and *follow-up plans*.
○ *Communicate the plan for unresolved medical problems at the time of discharge:* Several qualitative studies have shown that poor communication of the follow-up plan and outstanding issues at the time of discharge leads to adverse events; discharge summaries should contain specific information about

what the follow-up physicians need to do, when they should do it, and what they should watch for in the patient being passed off to them.
○ *Be brief:* van Walraven et al found that physicians felt quality of discharge summaries was substantially lower if length was greater than two pages.
○ *Follow a standardized format:* van Walraven et al found that outpatient physicians preferred discharge summaries in a standardized format that prompted inpatient providers to provide key elements that ensured information most relevant to ongoing care.

• The discharge process should
○ *Guarantee that the PCP/referring physician receives the discharge summary within a specific predefined number of days:* Recent studies have shown that between 25% and 40% of discharge summaries never reach the intended postdischarge clinician. Given most follow-up appointments are within 1–2 weeks, several best practice hospitals have a goal of all discharge summary reaching the outpatient providers within 5 business days.
○ *Ensure that the patient is educated regarding their medications and the discharge follow-up plan prior to discharge:* Schnipper et al identified drug-related problems during and after hospitalization and found unexplained discrepancies between discharge medication lists and postdischarge regimens in 29% of patients, and medication nonadherence in 23% of patients.
○ *Make certain that direct communication occurs between the discharging physician and follow-up clinician(s):* In a prospective cohort study of patients discharged from a general medical service, Forster et al found that almost 20% of patients had an adverse event postdischarge, 75% of which were preventable or ameliorable. The most common deficit was poor communication between the hospital caregivers and either the patient or the PCP.

ELEMENTS OF EFFECTIVE PATIENT INSTRUCTIONS

When a patient is discharged from the hospital, he/she is inundated with a variety of information and it is important to highlight the critical elements so that the patient has a safe care transition.

The delineation of patient instructions is frequently a multidisciplinary process and it is important that the hospitalist coordinates all of the various care management and follow-up instructions in a document that facilitates an effective care transition. When thinking about the elements of effective patient instructions, consider the following question: What does the patient absolutely need to do in the next 72 hours?

Admit

• Discuss code status
• Confirm home medications
• Ask about social situation
• Communicate with PCP and Referring MD (ask patient who should be contacted)

• Reconcile medications
• Educate patient on discharge meds and confirm understanding of changes
• Communicate directly with PCP on follow-up plan

Discharge

FIG. 14-1   Hospitalist Role in Planning for Patient Discharge.

ELEMENTS OF AN EFFECTIVE DISCHARGE SUMMARY

When thinking about the elements of an effective discharge summary, it is important to consider the following questions:

- Who will be reading the discharge summary?
  - Healthcare providers who have never met your discharged patient may be caring for him/her in a semi-acute setting (visiting nurses and doctors at skilled nursing facilities). This team's primary, and often only, source of information about the patient is the hospital discharge summary.
  - Patients receive care in a variety of settings from an ever-growing number of healthcare providers. In the case of hospitalized patients, for example, 70% of patients experience between two and three transfers in the first 3 months after discharge from acute care hospitals.
  - Different types of clinicians will need varying types/amount of information, and often the discharge summary will be shared by all of them. For example, the visiting nurse seeing a patient will need to be told in follow-up visits to check daily weights while the PCP will need to know the last creatinine and medication regimen at discharge.

- What information will healthcare providers need to take care of this patient after discharge?
  - The Society of Hospital Medicine (SHM) has recently published a discharge checklist for hospitalists, included in Table 14-2. This checklist includes the elements of an effective discharge summary, patient instructions, and critical information that need to be communicated to the follow-up clinician.
  - Each hospital has their own format for generating discharge summaries, whether they be dictated or electronically automated. Regardless of the template format, the framework outlined in the SHM checklist should form the basis of what is included in the summary and what is passed on during the transition handoff.

TABLE 14-2 Ideal Discharge of an Elderly Patient—A Hospitalist Checklist

DATA ELEMENTS	PROCESSES		
	DISCHARGE SUMMARY	PATIENT INSTRUCTIONS	COMMUNICATION TO FOLLOW-UP CLINICIAN ON DAY OF DISCHARGE
Presenting problem that precipitated hospitalization	x	x	x
Key findings and test results	x		x
Final primary and secondary diagnoses	x	x	x
Brief hospital course	x		x
Condition at discharge, including functional status and cognitive status if relevant	x—functional status o—cognitive status		
Discharge destination (and rationale if not obvious)	x		x
Discharge medications:			
Written schedule	x	x	x
Include purpose and cautions (if appropriate) for each	o	x	o
Comparison with preadmission medications (new, changes in dose/freq. unchanged, "meds should no longer take")	x	x	x
Follow-up appointments with name of provider, date, address, phone number, visit purpose, suggested management plan	x	x	x
All pending labs or tests, responsible person to whom results will be sent	x		x
Recommendations of any subspecialty consultants	x		o
Documentation of patient education and understanding	x		
Any anticipated problems and suggested interventions	x	x	x
24/7 call-back number	x	x	
Identify referring and receiving providers	x	x	
Resuscitation status	o		
And any other pertinent end-of-life issues			

*x = Required element.
†O = Optional element.
Adapted from: Halasyamani LK, Kripalani S, Coleman E, et al. Transition of care for hospitalized elderly patients—development of a discharge checklist for hospitalists. *J Hosp Med.* 2006;1:354–360.

- Discharge summary "pearls"
  - A general rule of thumb when writing the discharge summary is "What would I want to know if I was responsible for the care of this patient?"
    - Identification of new drug allergies, intolerances, any recommended drugs that did not work, any medication changes, specifics about high-risk drugs such as warfarin (dosages, follow-up check, and who is responsible), time course for administration of antibiotics
    - "New" information about the patient such as suspected substance abuse or dementia that would require outpatient follow-up, incidental findings on imaging that require follow-up with specified time intervals, identified healthcare proxy, end-of-life wishes, and family issues
    - Names of consultants, contact information, and synopsis of recommendations
    - Pending tests at discharge
  - It is also important to remember what not to include in a discharge summary. Often, the value of the information is diluted by superfluous data that is not helpful to receiving care providers or too long.

SYSTEMS IMPROVEMENT

- Based on the above discussion, the key to a good discharge summary, and more importantly a good postdischarge handoff, is communication in multiple venues and at multiple levels:
  - Communication with the patient predischarge
  - Communication with the outpatient providers (both via a written discharge summary and often a more direct communication such as a phone conversation)
  - Communication with future admitting hospitalists via the discharge summary (as part of the patient's longitudinal medical record)
- Based on research and personal experience initial systems improvement should focus on the following areas:
  - *Set communication standards and measure the implementation:* Select a physician champion and develop a short-term team with departmental leadership, referring physicians and hospitalists tasked with developing communication guidelines for the discharge summary between inpatient and outpatient physicians:
    - When (admission, discharge, change in status)
    - How (e-mail, phone, pager)

While setting guidelines also ensure that your group chooses specific goals and measures for each process and notes how they will be followed over time.

- *Weigh the pros and cons of automating and standardizing the production of the discharge summaries at your institution:* There are pros (more efficient, standardized sections, less dictation cost, forces summarization) and cons (often poorer quality content, rely on the provider typing rather than dictating) to automating the discharge summary.
- *Ensure that hospitalists and house staff are educated on what a proper discharge summary and an ideal discharge process are:* Frain et al found that physicians in training felt a lack of guidance regarding what to include in a discharge summary. Also, writing/dictating more than 20 discharge summaries per week conflicted with the need to attend to active inpatients, which caused an innate conflict on the part of the house staff. We support a highly structured educational curriculum starting in medical school on how to best communicate over transitions of care.
- *Develop an audit system:* We believe that discharge summaries should be routinely audited. This will ensure that problems with documentation are addressed and may improve completeness. It will also reinforce the importance of discharge summaries to hospitalists and physicians in training.

BIBLIOGRAPHY

Forster AJ, Murff HJ, Peterson JF, et al. The incidence and severity of adverse events affecting patients after discharge from the hospital. *Ann Intern Med.* 2003;138:161–167.

Frain JP, Frain AE, Carr PH. Experiences of medical senior house officers in preparing discharge summaries. *BMJ.* 1996; 312:350.

Halasyamani LK, Kripalani S, Coleman E, et al. Transition of care for hospitalized elderly patients—development of a discharge checklist for hospitalists. *J Hosp Med.* 2006;1: 354–360.

Schnipper JL, Kirwin JL, Cotugno MC, et al. Role of pharmacist counseling in preventing adverse drug events after hospitalization. *Arch Intern Med.* 2006;166:565–571.

Van Walraven C, Seth R, Austin PC, et al. Effect of discharge summary availability during the postdischarge visits on hospital readmission. *J Gen Intern Med.* 2002;17:186–192.

Van Walraven C, Mamdani M, Fang J, et al. Continuity of care and patient outcomes after hospital discharge. *J Gen Intern Med.* 2004;19:624–631.

15 PATIENT EDUCATION IN THE HOSPITAL

Marie Neaton

BACKGROUND

- The Institute of Medicine (IOM) has defined patient-centered care as one of the six aims for healthcare improvements in the twenty-first century.
- Patient-centered care requires that all members of the healthcare team effectively educate patients and families so that they can actively participate in decision making relating to their care plans. This goes beyond informed consent.
- *The Core Competencies: A Framework for Curriculum Development* by the Society of Hospital Medicine (SHM) has identified patient education as a fundamental core competency for hospitalists.
- The American Association of Family Practitioners (AAFP) core educational guidelines define patient education as "the process of influencing patient behavior and producing the changes in knowledge, attitudes, and skills necessary to maintain or improve health."
- Behavior change is a complex process that requires more than increased knowledge.
  ○ A longitudinal perspective acknowledges the difficulty that patients have in following medical regimens.
  ○ It is a process that occurs over time and requires the integration of knowledge into daily action through trial and error.
- The hospital stay provides an opportunity that goes beyond teaching patients and families about their diagnosis, tests, treatment plans, and ongoing care after discharge.
- Patient-centered care includes patient education that
  ○ Empowers patients to ask questions and take an active role in their care
  ○ Facilitates insight into behaviors that put patients at risk so that they can modify behavior accordingly
  ○ Teaches patients self-management skills for acute and chronic disease care
  ○ Provides specific contact information relating to community resources postdischarge

PATIENT EDUCATION AND PATIENT SAFETY

- Recognition that patient education is central to patient safety and a critical component to reduce hospitalizations and readmissions, regulatory agencies and professional organizations include patient education as part of their standards of care. For example, the Joint Commission of Accreditation of Hospital Organizations (JCAHO) has selected an educational intervention, the provision of written heart-failure–specific discharge instructions, as a core measure of quality for hospitalized heart-failure patients.
  ○ The impact of this intervention has been demonstrated in a randomized controlled trial comparing the effects of a structured 1-hour education session with a nurse educator to usual discharge education for heart failure patients (Koelling et al).
  ○ The combined endpoint of rehospitalization or death occurred in 47% of the education group vs. 65% of the control group.
  ○ Patient's reports of self-care practices such as doing daily weights were higher in the intervention group.
- Other examples of positive impact of patient education on health outcomes include
  ○ Improvements in diabetes control and fewer complications
  ○ Reduced emergency department (ED) visits and hospitalizations for asthmatics and improved self-management skills with lower morbidity (The National Asthma Education Program)
  ○ Positive impact on blood pressure control, mortality exercise, and diet for patients with cardiac disease
- The recommendations for patient education that may take different forms are to focus on survival skills and the behaviors needed for self-management, rather than on broader concepts such as disease pathophysiology or pharmacology.
- Despite a lack of clear outcomes for a particular type of educational intervention, all organizations dealing with chronic illness have identified patient education as a critical part of programs designed to improve clinical outcomes for chronic diseases.

PATIENT ADHERENCE TO PRESCRIBED THERAPIES

- Lack of compliance or failure to follow the treatment plan is a widespread problem.
  ○ For example, several studies of heart failure patients reported that they took only 70% of their medications and had high rates of nonadherence to the rest of their treatment plan, such as following a sodium-restricted diet.
  ○ It is estimated that nonadherence contributes to more than 60% of the hospital readmissions for heart failure.
- Even with patient education, some patients continue to not follow a treatment plan.

- Adherence is a complex behavioral process and not as simple as learning to follow specific directions. Adherence requires patients to internalize information about medical care plans and make choices.
- Poor adherence to the prescribed regimen or instructions can lead to
  ○ A poor understanding of complex instructions or complex medical regimens that involve multiple behavior changes
  ○ Low health literacy
  ○ Reduced cognition, hearing, vision, and concentration, especially common in hospitalized patients
  ○ Financial constraints
- Factors that facilitate adherence include
  ○ Simplified regimens
  ○ Integration of self-management behaviors into daily routines
  ○ Development of achievable goals
  ○ Feedback on adherence to recommended treatment plan

HEALTH LITERACY

- The IOM defines health literacy "as the degree to which individuals have the capacity to obtain, process, and understand basic health information and services needed to make appropriate health decisions."
- According to the IOM report on health literacy, nearly half of all American adults—90 million people—have difficulty understanding and acting upon health information. These difficulties include the ability to read, comprehend, and act on health information as well as perform basic numerical tasks such as "taking 2 tablets every 8 hours."
- The 1992 National Adult Literacy Survey found that 75% of respondents with a chronic disease also had low literacy skills. In the 2003 report, adults over age 65 continued to have the lowest literacy scores of any age group partly attributed to a decline in reading skills that appear to decline with advancing age. The elderly are also more likely to have other problems that may affect literacy including decreased vision, hearing loss, impaired cognition, and multiple chronic illnesses.
- The medium for health education also may be a factor in non-compliance with healthcare plans.
- For example, health related materials are commonly written at a 10th grade or higher level instead of the required fifth-sixth grade reading level.
- Low health literacy has been linked in many studies to poor health outcomes: the IOM report states that those with low literacy are more likely to make errors with their medication, less likely to complete medical treatments, and more likely to become hospitalized (see Chap. 97).

CHRONIC ILLNESS

- Approximately 120 million Americans have one or more chronic illnesses that account for 70% to 80% of healthcare costs.
- In the Medicare population, 25% of recipients have four or more chronic conditions accounting for two-thirds of Medicare expenditures. These numbers will only increase as the population continues to age.
- Chronic illnesses require patients to take extensive responsibility in the day-to-day management of their care.
- Key concepts of self-management include the ability to
  ○ Monitor illness
  ○ Manage symptoms and treatments
  ○ Cope with chronic physical and psychosocial changes
- The focus of the patient education of chronic disease is self-management, namely, how to
  ○ Develop problem-solving skills
  ○ Improve self-efficacy (the belief that the patient can positively impact their health)
  ○ Apply knowledge to individual circumstances
- Clinicians are advised to focus on goal setting, problem-solving strategies, and to link patients to self-management programs in the community.

STRATEGIES TO IMPROVE SELF-MANAGEMENT OF CHRONIC DISEASES

- Motivational interviewing techniques have been identified as an effective strategy to focus the patient interaction on problem solving, and identifying and reducing barriers to self-management. Motivational interviewing involves asking provocative questions and then discussing the responses.
- In the hospital setting asking focused questions can be helpful in assessing a patient's understanding about his/her illness and required self-management. For examples of questions, see Table 15-1.

TABLE 15-1 Questions that Patients Should be Asked

"Many people have some trouble taking their medications every day. What kind of trouble have you had taking your medication? What problems might happen at home?"

"These are the symptoms of heart failure. Did you have any of these symptoms before you came into the hospital? What do you think caused them? What do you do when you get these symptoms?"

"What are you afraid might happen because of your diabetes? Do you think you can have any impact on that?"

"Lots of people have trouble picking low-salt foods when they eat out. Have you had these problems?"

"It can be hard to follow the doctor's advice at home. What gives you the most difficulty?"

• Asking questions, and listening to and discussing responses help the patient in identifying barriers, beliefs, and priorities for action. This collaborative nonjudgmental approach can be an effective strategy to identify barriers and problem solve real-life situations.

INTERVENTIONS

ASSESS FOR LITERACY

• Low literacy is frequently hidden and not readily admitted to. Even if asked, the patient may deny problems with reading.
• *Observe:* Look for behavioral indicators, such as asking someone else to read or having difficulty completing forms.
• *Ask:* "Many people have trouble reading health information. Do you have any trouble with this?"
• *Assess:* "Can you read these instructions to me (Their question should be asked in private.)"
• *Evaluate comprehension:* Use open-ended questions. "Tell me what you understand about your disease." "When you go home, what will you do to control your diabetes?"

STRATEGIES FOR EFFECTIVE EDUCATION

• Education requires repetition; it is important to repeat the key points and to use more than one method. Remember that patient education is a team approach and a responsibility of all disciplines. It is most effective when the whole team delivers a consistent message.
• *Say it:* Patients do regard the physician as an authority and are influenced by medical recommendations. Verbal instructions are important. "The doctor said you should. . . ."
• *Repeat it:* Assume that only a small portion is actually retained and understood. Important information should be repeated. "It is very important that you take your warfarin each day and have your blood levels drawn." "You are going home on a medication called clopidogrel. Take it everyday to prevent blood clots from forming in your stent. It can prevent a heart attack."
• *Write it:* Written materials provide a reference for both: the patient, and caregivers and the next care provider. They also reinforce the education given. Reviewing written materials with the patient can be an effective strategy. Written instructions should include the diagnosis and a detailed treatment plan including changes in medication, other appointments, activity, diet, and when to seek further medical advice. Just providing a written piece of information without a verbal explanation is not a highly effective strategy, especially for people with lower health literacy.
• *Close the loop or teach back:* This is a simple, highly effective strategy to increase understanding and correct misunderstandings. Assess the patient's comprehension by having them tell you what they understand. "So tell me what you know about taking clopidogrel and why it is important." "Before you go home I want to be sure you have all the information that you need. Can you please explain to me what you will do to control your pain at home?"
• *Use multiple methods:* Using videos, pictures, diagrams, schedules, or tables can increase learning. Reviewing written materials with the patient also improves comprehension. Involve the family and caregivers in the educational process as well.

READING LEVEL

Whether it is preprinted material or personalized written discharge instructions, the "keep it simple" principle is facilitates compliance
• Use shorter words and sentences. Sentences should be no more than 8–15 words long. Express one idea per sentence. Use words that are one-two syllables as often as you can.
• Use common everyday language and avoid medical jargon if possible. "It's positional vertigo and quite benign" is not as meaningful as "You get dizzy when you change positions. While uncomfortable, it should go away and it does not cause other health problems."
• The simple measure of gobbledygook (SMOG) index is an easy method to use to assess reading level (Table 15-2) and a SMOG calculator is available online at http://webpages.charter.net/ghal/SMOG.html
• In general, physicians tend to overestimate the patients reading level and use recommended strategies infrequently.

SYSTEM CHANGES

• Provide written discharge instructions for common diagnoses, whether they are on a computer or preprinted.
• Standardize common, critical information such as how to take and monitor warfarin.
• Assess reading level of materials and work to reduce it. Use short sentences, small words, and larger fonts. Use dark ink on light paper, and use headers, subheadings, or a question and answer format to increase readability.

TABLE 15-2 SMOG Readability Formula

1. Select 30 sentences from the text to be assessed. Count 10 consecutive sentences near the beginning of the text, 10 in the middle, and 10 near the end. A sentence is any string of words ending with a period, question mark, or exclamation point.
2. In these 30 sentences, count every word containing three or more syllables. Include repetitions.
3. Estimate the square root of the number of polysyllabic words counted by taking the square root of the nearest perfect square.
4. Add 3 to the approximate square root. This gives the SMOG grade which is the reading grade that a person needs to fully understand the text.

Example

Total number of words with 3 or more syllables:	78
Nearest perfect square:	81
Square root:	9
Add 3:	12
The grade level would be grade 12.	

Adapted from: G. Harry McLaughlin. SMOG grading. *Journal of Reading* 1969;5:639–646; and Hoffman T, Worrall L. Designing effective written health education materials: consideration for health professionals. *Dis Rehab.* 2004;26(19):1166–1173.

- Supplement educational efforts with videos, DVDs, or closed-circuit TV programs available for common health problems or treatment plans.
- Use charts, models, pictures, and diagrams to clarify message.
- Develop standards for patient education and a multi-disciplinary team to implement them. Develop a "tool kit" with standardized content, outcomes, and materials and methods to support the plan.
- The bottom line is patient education remains a critical and necessary part of each hospital stay. Effective education requires repetition, clarity of message, simple language, and interaction with the patient.

BIBLIOGRAPHY

Behar-Horenstein LS, Guin P, et al Improving patient care through patient-family education programs. *Hosp Top.* 2005:83(1)21–27.

Billek-Sawney B, Reicherter EA. Literacy & the older adult. Educational considerations for health professionals. *Top in Ger Rehab.* 2005;21(4):275–281.

Coleman MT, Newton KS. Supporting self management in patients with chronic illness. *Am Fam Physician.* 2005;72: 1503–1510.

Hoffman T, Worrall L. Designing effective written health education materials: consideration for health professionals. *Dis & Rehab.* 2004;26(19):1166–1173.

Institute of Medicine of the National Academies. Report Brief: Health Literacy: A Prescription to End Confusion. April 2004; Available at: www.iom.edu

Koelling TM, Johnson ML. Discharge education improves clinical outcomes in patients with chronic heart failure. *Circulation.* 2005;111:179–185.

McLaughlin GH. SMOG grading: a new readability formula. *Read.* 1969;5:639–646.

National Network of Libraries of Medicine. Health literacy: Consumer Health Manual. Available at: http://nnlm.gov/outreach/consumer/hlthlit.html

Powell CK, Kripalani S. Brief report: resident recognition of low literacy as a risk factor in hospital readmission. *J Gen Intern Med.* 2005;20:1042–1044.

Rankin SH, Stallings KD. *Patient Education: Issues, Principles, Practices.* 3rd ed. Philadelphia, PA: Lippincott; 1996.

Redman BK. *The Practice of Patient Education.* 8th ed. St. Louis, MO: Mosby; 1997.

US Department of Education, Institute of Education Sciences, National Center for Statistics, 1992 National Adult Literacy Survey, and 2003 National Assessment of Adult Literacy. Available at: http://nces.ed.gov/NAAL

US Department of Health & Human Services. *Healthy People 2010: Understanding & Improving Health.* 2nd ed. Washington DC: US Government Printing Office; November 2000. Available at www.health.gov/healthypeople/

White H. Adherence and outcomes: it's more than just taking pills. *Lancet.* 2005;366:1989–1991.

Williams MV, Baker DW, Honig EG, et al. Inadequate literacy is a barrier to asthma knowledge and self care. *Chest.* 1998;114:1008–15.

WEB RESOURCES

Health literacy

1. Harvard School of Public Health, Health Literacy Studies. http://www.hsph.harvard.edu/healthliteracy/Comprehensive Web site with many links and literacy information, tools, and guides for writing patient education materials.
2. National Assessment of Health Literacy (NAAL) http://nces.ed.gov/naal
   Contains the 2003 NAAL report & statistics on literacy in the United States
3. Center for Health Care Strategies
   a. www.chcs.org
      Nine fact sheets available about health literacy, its impact on health outcomes, and strategies for designing patient education for patients with low literacy.
   b. Report on Literacy and Health Outcomes. Evidence Report/Technology Assessment No. 87. www.ahrq.gov
      Summarizes data related to health impacts of low literacy and interventions to improve health outcomes.

Writing guides

1. *Simply Put.* Developed by the Centers for Disease Control & Prevention (CDC).
   http://www.cdc.gov/od/oc/simpput.pdf Provides tips for writing simply and translating technical information into common language.

2. *Clear and to the Point. Guidelines for using plain language at NIH.*
   http//:execsec.od.nih.gov/plainlang/guidelines/index.html
   Gives more tips on writing simply and clearly.
3. *The SMOG Readability Calculator by G. Harry McLaughlin*
   http://webpages.charter.net/ghal/SMOG.html
   Contains a SMOG score calculator and other links.

Selected sites with patient education materials

1. American Diabetes Association www.diabetes.org
2. American Heart Association www.americanheart.org
3. American Lung Association www.lungusa.org
4. Arthritis Foundation www.arthritis.org
5. Heart Failure Society of America: Patient education modules www.abouthf.org
6. National Cancer Institute www.cancer.gov/cancerinfo/
7. National Diabetes Education Program www.ndep.nih.gov
8. National Digestive Diseases Information Clearinghouse http//:digestive.niddk.nih.gov
9. National Heart, Lung, & Blood Institute www.nhlbi.nih.gov
10. Vascular Disease Foundation www.vdf.org
11. Vascular Web www.vascularweb.org

Chronic illness

1. Improving chronic illness care www.improvingchroniccare.org
   Web site contains many tools & resources for providers to use in managing the care of those with a variety of chronic illnesses.

16 MANAGING TEST RESULTS AT HOSPITAL DISCHARGE

Christopher L. Roy

OVERVIEW

- The transition of care from hospital to home has been identified as a hazardous time for patients.
- Due in part to the rising prevalence of hospitalist services, discontinuity between inpatient and outpatient providers is increasingly the rule rather than the exception.
- Failures of communication between providers have been shown to account for more than half of all preventable adverse events in the postdischarge period.
- Although many physicians rely on the discharge summary for communication, it may not include key details about medications, pending test results, and follow-up plans and may not be available at all at the first postdischarge visit.

- Test results that are still pending at discharge may be particularly likely to fall through the cracks during this transition for the following reasons:
  - They may be considered relatively minor details after an eventful hospital admission.
  - They may be numerous.
  - Lines of responsibility for follow-up may not be clear.
  - It may not be obvious that they are not finalized or that they may change after discharge (e.g., in the case of a radiology report that has yet to be reviewed by an attending radiologist or a sensitivity panel returning on a positive culture).
- In recent years, national organizations have underscored the importance of test result follow-up in general:
  - As a national patient safety goal for 2005, the Joint Commission on Accreditation of Healthcare Organizations (JCAHO) challenged hospitals to "measure, assess, and, if appropriate, take action to improve the timeliness of reporting, and the timeliness of receipt by the responsible licensed caregiver, of critical test results and values." In *20 tips to help prevent medical errors* the Agency for Healthcare Research and Quality (AHRQ) tells patients that when it comes to test results, "If you have a test, don't assume that no news is good news."[6]
- In the outpatient setting, several authors have studied follow-up of test results and found major deficiencies, with the majority of physicians reporting delays in reviewing test results, dissatisfaction with their ability to manage results, and failures to notify patients of normal, and sometimes even abnormal, results.
- Inadequate management of test results has the potential to affect not only patient safety but also malpractice claims. One major malpractice insurer reports a failure to follow-up results as accounting for one-quarter of diagnosis-related claims.
- In the outpatient setting, the same physician ordering the test is generally the physician who will follow up on the result. However, in the transition from hospital to home, responsibility for result follow-up is not always clear. Multiple providers (including hospitalists, consultants, and house staff) are often involved in caring for the patient in hospital, and multiple individuals order tests. Several questions often arise in this situation:
  - If a result is pending for several days to weeks after a patient has left the hospital, does the responsibility for follow-up shift to the outpatient physician?
  - If so, when and how does this transfer of responsibility occur?
  - If the pending test and need for follow-up is documented in the discharge summary, does this absolve the inpatient physician of the responsibility?

EPIDEMIOLOGY AND PHYSICIAN AWARENESS OF TEST RESULTS PENDING AT DISCHARGE

- In a recent prospective study, we collected data on test results that were pending on the day of discharge at two academic medical centers, and surveyed hospitalists and primary care physicians about those that were potentially clinically actionable. This was the first and only study of the epidemiology and physician awareness of "postdischarge results."
- We hypothesized that these postdischarge results were common, were frequently overlooked in a patient's transition from inpatient to outpatient physicians, and that some might have important clinical consequences.
- Our objectives were to determine the prevalence and characteristics of postdischarge laboratory and radiology results and to determine physician awareness of those results that were important clinically
- Among 2644 patients discharged over 5 months, 1095 patients (41%) had pending results on the day of discharge.
- Of 2033 pending results, 877 (43%) were found to be abnormal when the results returned, and 191 (9%) were considered potentially actionable on the basis of a review of the discharge summary.
- When surveyed on these potentially actionable results, hospitalists and primary care physicians (PCP) stated they were unaware of 62%, and they were unaware the test had been ordered in 33%.
- Surveyed physicians agreed that 33% required clinical action and that 13% were urgent.
- Most of the urgent results were microbiology (blood, urine, and wound cultures) that necessitated starting or changing antibiotic therapy. One patient who had been admitted with new atrial fibrillation had an undetectable thyroid stimulating hormone level.
- Examples of actionable but nonurgent results included
  - Incidental findings of pulmonary nodule(s) or opacities on chest radiography or computed tomography (CT) that required follow-up
  - Positive serologic testing for *Helicobacter pylori* in setting of gastrointestinal bleeding
  - A new diagnosis of hepatitis C in a setting of presumed alcoholic hepatitis
  - Unexplained iron deficiency
- Our findings have important implications for patient safety on several fronts:
  - First, the volume of pending postdischarge results (both normal and abnormal) was high, averaging about one outstanding result for each discharged patient. About 9% of these were potentially actionable, and some were urgent. The sheer volume of

postdischarge results thus calls for a high-reliability results management system.
  - Second, inpatient and primary care physicians' awareness of potentially actionable results was low, with an overall awareness rate of only 38%. The standard of care at our organizations during the study period was essentially to rely on the vigilance of individual clinicians to track these postdischarge results, and clearly this is not sufficient.
  - Finally, there was also a low awareness that a test was ordered, suggesting that multiple team members were ordering the tests, that there was imperfect communication about these tests with the physician discharging the patient, and that lines of responsibility were not clear.

DESIGNING AN IDEAL POSTDISCHARGE RESULTS MANAGEMENT SYSTEM

- The high volume and low physician awareness of postdischarge results provides justification for a high-reliability system of follow-up for these results to avoid the catastrophic cases such as those presented in Table 16-2 and 16-3.
- The remainder of this chapter outlines key concepts in developing an ideal system for your hospitalist practice (Fig. 16-1).

ESTABLISH LINES OF RESPONSIBILITY AND IDENTIFY RESPONSIBLE PROVIDERS

- Clear lines of responsibility for test follow-up in addition to clear identification of responsible providers form the necessary foundation of a postdischarge result management system.
- Lines of responsibility should be established at the time of test ordering and reconfirmed at hospital discharge.
  - Avoid a system that creates a sense of diffused responsibility, when multiple providers care for the same patient.
  - Instead, create a system of planned redundancy in which one provider is held primarily responsible and a multilayered fail-safe mechanism is put into effect if the responsible provider fails to act on abnormal test results.
- In most cases, the ordering physician will have primary responsibility for test result follow-up.
  - Your practice should discuss exceptions to this rule, contingency plans if the ordering physician is unavailable, and whether this responsibility can be delegated.

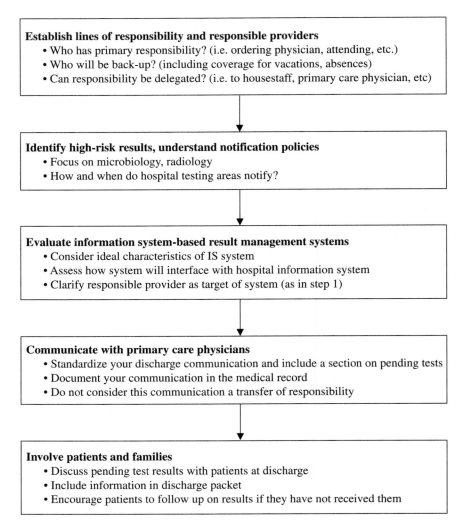

FIG. 16-1 Developing an ideal postdischarge results management system.

- Consider centralizing all test result follow-up with one position or individual, for example, having a physician assistant or nurse practitioner screen all postdischarge test results.
  - The main drawback of a centralized system is that this individual would not know the clinical context and thus the urgency of an abnormal result.

IDENTIFY HIGH-RISK RESULTS AND UNDERSTAND NOTIFICATION POLICIES OF YOUR HOSPITAL'S TESTING AREAS

- Consider which postdischarge results are more common and more likely to be actionable. In our study, most actionable results were from microbiology and radiology.
- Understand your laboratory and radiology department policies for notifying providers about abnormal results.

- Microbiology results, mainly culture data and sensitivities, frequently take several days to be finalized, increasing the likelihood that the patient will have been discharged when the result is finalized. Laboratory personnel may notify the responsible physician of some results but not others, for example, when a patient develops positive blood cultures, but not when the antibiotic sensitivity panel becomes available.
- Radiology results are first preliminarily dictated or discussed with the inpatient team. The final report is entered only when an attending physician reads the study, which may be several hours later, and may differ from the preliminary report. Unless these amendments to the preliminary report are directly communicated to the responsible inpatient physician, it may be assumed that the final report will be unchanged.
- Your practice should understand how each testing area within your hospital handles abnormal results,

noting specifically which results require active communication (i.e., page) and how changes to preliminary reports are communicated to providers.

EVALUATE INFORMATION-SYSTEM–BASED RESULTS MANAGEMENT SYSTEMS

- An ideal postdischarge results management system would leverage the power of modern information systems.
- Postdischarge results would be centralized in a results management system that is integrated into the hospital's clinical information system and that is able to alert users to severely abnormal results.
- The application would be seamlessly embedded within the inpatient electronic medical record and be able to cull pending and final results from the clinical data repository, prioritizing the results on the basis of the type of result and degree of abnormality, and placing them in a centralized queue for users to review.
- Additional features would include automatic notification of severely abnormal results by alphanumeric page or e-mail, and patient notification of results with automatically generated letters.
- Similar systems have been tested and successfully implemented to address results management in the outpatient setting and could serve as a model for inpatient systems.
- In organizations with computerized provider order entry (CPOE), responsibility for the result should be assigned when the test is ordered, confirmed, and, if necessary, modified, at discharge.
- The results management system could be integrated with the discharge order so that pending results must be reviewed at discharge and could allow the discharging physician to assign responsibility for the result and select their preferred mode of notification of the result when it is finalized.
- Information systems-based management of postdischarge results is attractive but also has limitations:
  - Most centers are limited by the cost and difficulty of integrating such a system into the hospital's information systems.
  - Any results management system will be unsuccessful without clear guidelines regarding roles and responsibility for follow-up.
  - The process of result management must be clear to all providers caring for a patient, and a back-up system must be in place if those assigned primary responsibility are not available.
  - If the system depends on administrative databases to identify the responsible providers, these must be exquisitely accurate.

TABLE 16-1   Summary Points

- Test results that return after hospital discharge are common and can be overlooked by hospitalists and PCPs, resulting in potential harm to patients
- Clarifying how your practice and your hospital currently handles postdischarge results is a key first step
- Designing an ideal system will involve identifying responsible providers, focusing on high-risk test results, considering information-systems–based solutions, improving communication with PCPs, and involving patients and families.

  - The system must not unduly burden busy clinicians with unnecessary alerts and warnings.
  - The rules by which results are prioritized must be robust enough to filter out less urgent results, and the user should be able to set their preference about how to be notified.

COMMUNICATE WITH THE PCP

- Your discharge communication with the PCP should highlight information about pending tests, and this communication should be documented in the medical record.
- Consider standardizing your communication at discharge with a template that includes pending tests and follow-up plan.
- Although this communication is extremely important, it should not be considered a transfer of the primary responsibility for postdischarge result follow-up, unless clearly stated and understood as so.

INVOLVE PATIENTS AND FAMILIES

- The patient and family members may be a largely untapped resource when it comes to postdischarge result follow-up.

TABLE 16-2   Case 1: Postdischarge Test Result Follow-up Failure

A 45-year-old man is admitted with headaches and a blood pressure of 230/120 mm Hg.
- He has no past medical history and is on no medications.
- He has no family history of hypertension.
He is managed successfully with antihypertensive medications.
- The intern orders a 24-hour urine collection for catecholamines as a workup for pheochromocytoma.
- These results are pending at hospital discharge, but they are not mentioned in the discharge summary.
During the subsequent 6 months, he is readmitted twice with hypertensive urgencies before his PCP notices that the previously ordered 24-hour urine catecholamines are elevated. He undergoes a magnetic resonance imaging (MRI) that reveals an adrenal mass consistent with pheochromocytoma.
- The mass is resected with resolution of his hypertensive crises.

TABLE 16-3   Case 2: Postdischarge Test Result Follow-up Failure

A 37-year-old woman with advanced AIDS is admitted with fever, mental status changes, and bilateral pulmonary nodules.
- Blood cultures grow *Staphylococcus aureus,* and she is successfully treated with nafcillin.
- The pulmonary nodules are thought to be septic emboli, but invasive fungal disease is also a possibility
- A serum beta glucan (a test predictive of early invasive fungal disease) is ordered and is still pending on the day of discharge.

She is readmitted to the intensive care unit 6 days later with obtundation and worsening pulmonary opacities.
- The beta glucan is noted to be positive, having been available 4 days before the readmission.
- Antifungal therapy is begun but she dies of respiratory failure within 24 hours.
- Autopsy confirms invasive aspergillosis of the lungs and central nervous system.

- Consider including pending test results with the discharge information packet and telling patients that they should not assume "no news is good news." If they do not obtain the results from their physician, they should be encouraged to seek them out.
- Several organizations are developing web-based "patient portals" where patients can not only book appointments and send messages to their physician but also review test results.

SUMMARY

- A failure to follow up on postdischarge results can result in adverse outcomes for patients, as illustrated in the cases presented in the sidebars above.
- We have documented important gaps in physician awareness of these results.
- Designing a system to address this problem poses challenges similar to those seen when designing a system for test result management for outpatients, but unique challenges are posed by the transition of care that frequently accompanies hospital discharge.
- An ideal postdischarge result management system should rest on a foundation characterized by unequivocal lines of responsibility for result follow-up and accurate identification of responsible providers.

Parts of this chapter are republished with kind permission from *Joint Commission Resources.*

BIBLIOGRAPHY

Agency for Healthcare Research and Quality: *Patient Fact Sheet: 20 Tips to Help Prevent Medical Error.* http://www.ahrq.gov/consumer/20tips.htm (Last accessed Mar 2, 2006).

Boohaker EA, Ward RE, Uman JE, et al. Patient notification and follow-up of abnormal test results: a physician survey. *Arch Intern Med.* Feb 12, 1996;156:327–31.

Coleman EA, Berenson RA. Lost in transition: challenges and opportunities for improving the quality of transitional care. *Ann Intern Med.* Oct 5, 2004;141:533–56.

Forster AJ, Murff HJ, Peterson JF, et al. The incidence and severity of adverse events affecting patients after discharge from the hospital. *Ann Intern Med.* Feb 4, 2003;138:161–7.

Harvard Risk Management Foundation. Reducing office practice risks. *Forum.* 20: p. 2, 2000.

Joint Commission on Accreditation of Healthcare Organizations: *National Patient Safety Goals for 2006.* http:// www.jcaho.org/accredited+organizations/patient+safety/ npsg.htm (Last accessed Mar 1, 2006).

Moore C, Wisnivesky J, Williams S, et al. Medical errors related to discontinuity of care from an inpatient to an outpatient setting. *J Gen Intern Med* Aug. 2003;18:646–51.

Poon EG, Gandhi TK, Sequist TD, et al. "I wish I had seen this test result earlier!": dissatisfaction with test result management systems in primary care. *Arch Intern Med.* Nov 8, 2004;164:2223–8.

Poon EG, Wang, SJ, Gandhi TK, et al. Design and implementation of a comprehensive outpatient results manager. *J Biomed Inform.* Feb–Apr 2003;36:80–91.

Roy CL, Poon EG, Karson AS, et al. Patients safety concerns arising from test results that return after hospital discharge. *Ann Intern Med.* Jul 19, 2005;143:121–8.

Roy CL, Poon EG, Gandhi TK, et al. Managing test results during the transition from hospital to home: the experience of two academic medical centers. In: Schiff GD (ed). *Getting Results: Reliably Communicating and Acting on Critical Test Results.* Oakbrook Terrace, IL: Joint Commission Resources; 2006:19–29.

Weingart SN, Rind D, Tofias Z, et al. Who uses the patient internet portal? The PatientSite experience. *J Am Med Inform Assoc.* Jan–Feb 2006;13:91–5. Epub 2005 Oct 12.

van Walraven C, Seth R, Laupacis A. Dissemination of discharge summaries: not reaching follow-up physicians. *Can Fam Physician.* Apr 2002;48:737–42.

EVIDENCE-BASED MEDICINE

17 AN INTRODUCTION TO EVIDENCE-BASED MEDICINE

Eduardo Ortiz

WHAT IS EVIDENCE-BASED MEDICINE?

- Evidence-based medicine (EBM) is the *thoughtful* and *judicious* use of the best available evidence for making decisions about healthcare.
- The EBM approach uses scientific evidence as the foundation for clinical decision-making based on whether a service or intervention improves health outcomes.
- EBM helps clinicians and patients work together to make more cost-effective decisions by maximizing the use of effective care and minimizing the use of ineffective care.
- Appropriate application of EBM principles means integrating scientific evidence with clinical experience and judgment, patient values and preferences, quality-of-life issues, costs, and other important factors that help inform and influence medical decisions (Fig. 17-1).
- The EBM process typically begins during an encounter between a clinician and patient that generates a clinical question about diagnosis, treatment, or prognosis.
- There are five steps in the EBM process as traditionally taught (the "five As"):
  1. Assessing the patient and/or situation
  2. Asking the right question
  3. Acquiring the evidence
  4. Appraising the evidence
  5. Applying the evidence
- Some EBM teachers add an additional step to this process:

6. Assessing its impact

- Asking the right clinical question is a key component of the EBM process and often determines the results and success of the subsequent steps. The EBM approach to asking a clinical question uses the PICO format, which involves developing a question that contains four distinct components that are structured as follows:
  - P = patient or problem
  - I = intervention (therapy, diagnostic test, service, and so forth) of interest
  - C = comparison to the intervention of interest
  - O = outcome of interest (Table 17-1 includes for examples of structured clinical questions using the PICO format)
- Unfortunately, the scope of this chapter does not allow us to cover all of the other steps in detail, so we have provided references later in this chapter (see EBM resources and EBM Internet sites that you can use to learn more about each of these steps).

OUTCOME MEASURES

- There are three important types of health-related outcome measures with which you should be familiar.
- A *process measure* is a measure of some process that occurs in healthcare. Healthcare processes refer to the way interventions and services are organized and carried out.
  - Examples of process measures include frequency of hemoglobin A1C testing in patients with diabetes, frequency of blood pressure measurements in patients with hypertension, frequency of hand washing by physicians before and after seeing patients, use of aspirin and beta-blockers in patients admitted to the hospital with a myocardial infarction (MI), and number of labs drawn or imaging tests performed during a hospital stay.
- An *intermediate outcome* (also known as a *surrogate measure* or *surrogate outcome*) is usually based on

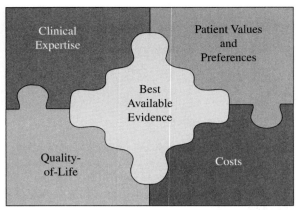

FIG. 17-1 Conceptual model of EBM. One way to think about EBM is to picture a jigsaw puzzle comprised of multiple pieces. Sitting at the center of this puzzle and forming its foundation is the "evidence piece." However, without all the other pieces in their proper places, you cannot complete the puzzle. The other pieces are made up of the other factors that must be considered when making clinical decisions—clinical experience and judgment, patient values and preferences, quality-of-life issues, costs, and so forth.

biochemical, physiologic, pharmacologic, or laboratory measures.
  ○ Examples of intermediate outcomes include laboratory values like serum hemoglobin A1C and low-density lipoprotein (LDL) cholesterol, individual blood pressure values, bone mineral density, and the number of premature ventricular contractions.
• The third and most important type of health measure is the *health outcome*. Health outcomes are important clinical endpoints that people actually experience and care about (both positive and negative).
  ○ Examples of health outcomes include mortality, MI, amputation, renal failure, blindness, impotence, and pain.
• The distinction between these three types of measures is important because changes in process measures or

TABLE 17-1 Examples of Structured Clinical Questions Using the PICO Format (P = Patient or Problem, I = Intervention, C = Comparison, O = Outcome)

1. In critically ill patients (P), does the use of a pulmonary artery catheter (I), compared to no catheter (C), reduce length of stay (O) or mortality (O)?
2. In patients with cancer and chemotherapy-induced neutropenia (P), does the routine use of prophylactic antibiotics (I), compared to no prophylaxis (C), reduce mortality (O)?
3. In patients with ST-elevation MI treated with aspirin and thrombolytics (P), is low molecular weight heparin (I) better than unfractionated heparin (C) or placebo (C) for preventing reinfarction (O) or reducing mortality (O)?

intermediate outcomes do not necessarily result in improvements in health outcomes.
  ○ There are many examples in the medical literature where improvements in process measures or intermediate outcomes did not result in improved health outcomes, including examples where intermediate outcomes improved while health outcomes worsened.
  ○ An example of this phenomenon is the Cardiac Arrhythmia Suppression Trial (CAST) by Pratt and Moye, 1990, where the treatment of patients hospitalized with acute MIs with antiarrhythmic medications resulted in decreased ventricular arrhythmias (an intermediate outcome), but it increased mortality (a more important health outcome) by 3.6 fold. Prior to this study, the standard of care for patients admitted with acute MIs included the routine use of antiarrhythmic medications because they decreased ventricular arrhythmias.
• *Reading tip*—In general, clinical decisions that affect patients should be based on evidence that a service or intervention improves important health outcomes. If process measures or intermediate outcomes are used to support clinical decisions, there should be evidence (whenever possible) of a causal link demonstrating that improvements in the process measure or intermediate outcome will result in meaningful improvements in important health outcomes. For example, there is good evidence that lowering blood pressure (an intermediate outcome) in hypertensive patients reduces their risk of stroke, MI, and heart failure.

LEVELS OF EVIDENCE

• The strength of the evidence is an important factor when making evidence-based medical decisions.
• US Preventive Services Task Force (USPSTF), a highly-respected national panel of experts in prevention and primary care, has developed the following grading scale for rating the quality of evidence and a grading scheme for recommendations about a given clinical practice (see http://www.ahrq.gov/clinic/3rduspstf/ratings.htm)
  ○ *Good evidence*—Includes consistent results from well-designed, well-conducted studies in representative populations that directly assess effects on health outcomes. High-quality RCTs and systematic reviews/meta-analyses of such trials provide the highest levels of evidence.
  ○ *Fair evidence*—Includes sufficient results to determine effects on health outcomes, but the strength of the evidence is limited because of problems with the number, quality, or consistency of the individual studies, generalizability to routine practice, or indirect nature of the evidence on health outcomes.

Nonrandomized controlled studies such as cohort studies, case-control studies, and observational studies provide fair levels of evidence.

○ *Poor evidence*—Includes insufficient results to assess the effects on health outcomes because of limited number or power of studies, important flaws in their design or conduct, gaps in the chain of evidence, or lack of information on important health outcomes. Poorly conducted studies with significant methodological flaws, opinions from "experts" in a field without explicit critical appraisal, case series, physiologic studies, and bench research represent the lowest levels of evidence.

• A number of organizations, such as the Oxford Centre for Evidence-Based Medicine's Levels of Evidence and Grades of Recommendation, the American Academy of Family Physicians' Strength of Recommendation Taxonomy (SORT), and the Grading Recommendations Assessment, Development, and Evaluation (GRADE) Working Group have developed their own evidence-rating scales.

• *Reading tip*—Well-developed, evidence-based guidelines should provide explicit ratings on the levels of evidence and strength of recommendations used to formulate the guideline. If they do not, you should be wary of the guideline. When reading the medical literature or listening to medical presentations, rate the quality of the evidence being presented and use this information to guide whether you should incorporate the evidence into your practice.

STUDY DESIGN

• Most study designs can be divided into *experimental studies* and *observational studies*. Experimental studies are those in which the investigator controls the conditions under which the study is conducted. *Clinical trials* (also known as *controlled trials, controlled clinical trials,* or *intervention trials*) are examples of experimental studies.

EXPERIMENTAL STUDIES

• *Randomized controlled trials (RCTs)* randomly assign patients into their respective study groups. Randomization helps ensure that the experimental and comparison groups are as similar as possible in all characteristics except for the intervention being studied. It is important to make sure that the experimental design truly lends itself to proper randomization.

• *Reading tip*—Look in the Study Methods section of the article to see if randomization occurred, and, if so,

how it was conducted. Determine whether the experimental and comparison groups are comparable in terms of numbers (eg, were the number of participants similar in each arm of the study?); important demographic and socioeconomic characteristics (eg, sex, race, education, income, geographic location); risk factors; comorbidities; or other variables that could influence the results.

• RCTs generate the highest level of evidence because well-designed and conducted RCTs are the best types of studies for minimizing the biases that can compromise the validity of research results.

• RCTs can either be *single-blinded, double-blinded,* or *triple-blinded.*

○ Single-blinded RCTs require that the subjects participating in a study are "blinded" as to which intervention they are receiving (eg, the experimental drug or placebo).

○ Double-blinded RCTs require both the subjects participating in a study and the investigators conducting the study are unaware of what intervention the study subjects are receiving.

○ Triple-blinded RCTs require that the persons analyzing the data are not aware of what intervention the study subjects are receiving (in addition to blinding the study subjects and the investigators). Triple-blinding is also sometimes used to describe studies where other outcome assessors not directly involved in the study (eg, radiologists reading chest x-rays in a study on the treatment of pneumonia) are unaware of whether the patients whose films they are reading are in the experimental group or the comparison group.

○ In medical studies, ensuring that the experimental drug and the placebo are made to look, smell, and taste alike is a common blinding technique. In surgical studies, the use of sham surgical procedures is another blinding technique.

• *Allocation concealment* is when measures are taken to keep investigators and study subjects from knowing into which study group the next enrolled subject will be assigned. Allocation concealment is important because manipulating the enrollment of subjects in a study can undermine the randomization process and bias the results.

○ One allocation concealment technique is to assign randomization (eg, which patients go into the active drug group and which ones go into the placebo group) from a central site for a large multicenter study, therefore preventing the investigators from an individual study site from knowing into which group the next patient entering the study will be assigned.

○ Another example of an allocation concealment technique is to randomly distribute sealed, opaque envelopes that assign the study subjects into their groups. This prevents an investigator or patient from looking through the envelope to figure out which group the next subject will be assigned to, thereby figuring out the randomization pattern and manipulating enrollment into study and comparison groups.

- *Reading tip*—When you read an article, look to see if allocation concealment was used and whether the methods employed were adequate.

OBSERVATIONAL STUDIES

- *Observational studies* are studies where the investigators do not control the conditions of the study; rather, the investigators are simply observers, collecting and analyzing data on subjects where events have occurred naturally over a prescribed time course. Observational studies come in many forms, but three common ones are *cohort, case-control, and cross-sectional studies*.
- In *cohort studies*, the investigators begin with a study cohort (eg, a group of patients) that have been exposed to some risk factor or intervention and then follow this cohort forward in time to see what outcomes occur. Along with this study cohort, the investigators simultaneously study a control group that have not been exposed to the risk factor or intervention and follow them forward in time to see what outcomes occur. Because cohort studies begin with an exposure and follow the cohort forward in time until an outcome occurs, cohort studies are prospective in nature (ie, forward-looking).
- In *case-control studies*, the investigators begin with a group that already has the outcome of interest and then look retrospectively (ie, back in time) to ascertain their exposures. Along with these *cases*, the investigators also identify a *control group* without the outcome of interest and look retrospectively to see ascertain their exposures. Because case-control studies always begin with a group that already has a specific outcome (eg, patients with heart failure, asthma, lung cancer, diabetes, and so forth), all case-control studies are retrospective in nature.
  - The most important issue in case-control studies is how the cases and controls are selected. Both groups should be as similar as possible in important characteristics that are known to influence the probability of the outcome.
  - As a general rule, case-control studies should have at least 1 control for every case. Increasing the number of controls up to a case-control ratio of 1:3 or 1:4 can improve the validity of the results even further. However, using more than 3 or 4 controls for every case offers no further advantage, as you reach a point of diminishing return.

  - *Reading tip*—Look to see if the investigators used at least one control for every case and that both cases and controls were well-matched on important characteristics that are known to affect the outcome of interest.
  - The methods used to collect retrospective data on past exposures, characteristics, etc. in case-control studies should be collected in a standardized, uniform manner in both the cases and controls in order to minimize the possibility of introducing bias, which can compromise the validity of the results.
  - *Reading tip*—Look to see if there are any differences in the methods used to collect this information. If so, these differences may have unduly biased the results.
  - Because of the limitations inherent in the nature of their design, *case-control studies cannot prove causation*. However, they can demonstrate potential associations that can later be tested in a more rigorous fashion through controlled clinical trials.
- *Cross-sectional studies*, also known as *prevalence surveys*, look at an entire population at a given point in time and simultaneously assess the prevalence of specific outcomes and exposures in that population. Cross-sectional studies can also be used to compare outcomes and exposures between two or more populations to see if differences in exposures might be associated with differences in outcomes between the different populations.
  - Because outcomes and exposure are assessed simultaneously in cross-sectional studies, there is no way of knowing whether the exposure preceded (and thereby caused) the outcome. Like case-control studies, cross-sectional studies therefore cannot prove causation.
  - Cross-sectional studies can identify possible associations between exposures and outcomes, thereby generating hypotheses for further testing using more rigorous methods like controlled clinical trials.
- *Systematic reviews* are studies that use a standardized, systematic approach to answer a specific clinical question by summarizing the best available evidence from all the appropriate existing studies. Systematic reviews should adhere to standard methodological principles, including use of a preplanned strategy to conduct a comprehensive search for all relevant studies in the subject area, application of evidence-based principles to appraise the validity of each study, and synthesis of the data to answer a specific clinical question. Systematic reviews can be qualitative or quantitative.
  - A qualitative systematic review summarizes the results of the primary studies but does not combine the results of each study into a single pooled estimate of effect.

○ A quantitative systematic review, or *meta-analysis*, takes things a step further by employing statistical techniques to mathematically combine the results of the different studies into a single pooled estimate of effect.

○ Systematic reviews are a good resource to help you keep up-to-date with the vast amounts of medical information published in the literature, especially when the individual studies are small or yield conflicting results.

○ By combining the results of multiple studies, they increase power and create more precise estimates of treatment effects.

○ Combining multiple studies that involve different study populations, providers, and treatment settings also provides evidence that is applicable to a broader population.

• Unlike systematic reviews, *narrative reviews* are traditionally written by an expert in the field as a summary or update of a particular topic in medicine and usually include information on disease pathophysiology, diagnosis, and treatment.

○ Although narrative reviews can provide a good overview of a topic, they do not apply the same standardized, rigorous approach to searching, appraising, and synthesizing the literature that is necessary for conducting a proper systematic review and helps ensure the validity of the results and recommendations.

○ Recommendations in a narrative review are often based on the author's expertise and opinion, which makes them prone to bias

• *Reading tip*—A high-quality systematic review or meta-analysis that includes all the appropriate RCTs is considered by many to represent the highest level of evidence.

STATISTICAL SIGNIFICANCE

• Tests of statistical significance are used in hypothesis testing and help us determine the degree to which sampling variability due to chance may account for the results observed in a study.

• When we test for statistical significance, we use the *null hypothesis*. By convention, the null hypothesis takes the default position that there is no difference between two or more interventions, groups, etc. Investigators must either accept the null hypothesis (eg, there is no real difference between drug A and drug B) or reject the null hypothesis (eg, there really is a difference—drug A is better than drug B).

• The *P* value is the probability that an effect as great (or greater) as that observed in a study (eg, when comparing two or more interventions) could have occurred by chance, if in fact there really was no difference between the two.

○ By convention, results are said to be statistically significant if the *P* value (also known as the *alpha level*) is < 0.05, which means there is less than a 5% (1 in 20) chance that the difference observed was due to chance.

○ A *Type I* or *alpha error* occurs if we claim there is a difference between two interventions (eg, drug A is better than drug B) when in fact there is no difference (drug A is equivalent to drug B).

○ A *Type II* or *beta error* occurs if we claim there is no difference between two interventions (eg, drug A is equivalent to drug B) when in fact there really is a difference (eg, drug A is better than drug B). By convention, *beta* is usually set at 0.20.

○ *Power* is determined by 1 − beta. By convention, the power of most studies is set at $1 - 0.20 = 0.80$ or 80%. This means that the study has an 80% chance of finding a difference between two interventions if one truly exists.

○ When designing studies, investigators can calculate in advance the risk they are willing to take of drawing erroneous conclusions in both directions. By convention, studies are usually conducted using a *P* value (alpha level) of 0.05 (ie, 5% risk of concluding the two interventions are different when in fact they are not—a false positive result) and beta of 0.20 (ie, 20% risk of concluding the two interventions are not different when in fact they are—a false negative result).

○ This purposefully places more of a burden on investigators to demonstrate that there really is a difference between two interventions than to demonstrate that there is no difference. In other words, it is more difficult to obtain a false positive result than a false negative result. The burden of proof is to show that the experimental therapy really is better than currently proven therapies or no therapy at all.

○ Results that are statistically significant ($P < 0.05$) may still be due to chance, although as the *P* value becomes smaller and smaller (eg, $P < 0.0001$), this becomes less likely.

○ Likewise, results that are not statistically significant ($P > 0.05$) may not be due to chance. For example, a difference in a study between two interventions with a *P* value of 0.06 means that the probability that this result was due to chance is 6% (if in fact there was no real difference between the two interventions). However, it also means you have a 94% probability that the difference is not due to chance.

• *Statistical significance has nothing to do with clinical significance*. Results can be statistically very significant ($P < 0.0001$) and yet be clinically insignificant.

○ The magnitude of the P value is related to two factors: (1) sample size of the study and (2) magnitude of the difference in effect size. The larger the sample size, the smaller the P value. The larger the effect size between two or more interventions (eg, 60% reduction in mortality between two groups in a study vs. a 20% reduction), the smaller the P value. If you have a large enough sample size in your study, any difference you find will be statistically significant (eg, not due to chance).

○ *Reading tip*—One of the most important questions you should ask after determining whether a finding is statistically significant is: Are the results *clinically significant*? In other words, "so what?"

○ Results that are not statistically significant may still be very important clinically (eg, 50% reduction in death, MI, stroke, renal failure, blindness, etc.). Imagine that you recently read about a study that demonstrated a mortality reduction of 50%, but the P value was 0.10. This means that there is a 10% probability that the results were due to chance and a 90% probability that the results were not due to chance.

○ *Reading tip*—Ask whether it is appropriate to automatically dismiss the results of a study simply because of an arbitrary cutoff at a P value of 0.05, especially if the findings have important clinical implications. Remember that statistical significance is just a tool that should be used to inform and guide your decisions.

• Statistical significance only has to do with the probability that the result obtained was due to chance. Statistical significance does not inform you as to whether a study was designed or conducted properly. A statistically significant finding can result from a study that was poorly designed and improperly conducted, leading to methodological problems and erroneous results.

• When well-conducted studies do not demonstrate a statistically significant difference between two interventions, there are two issues to consider. The first is that there really is no significant difference between the two interventions, that is, they are equivalent. The second is that there really is a difference, but the power was insufficient to demonstrate the difference. This means the study did not include enough patients to detect a difference between the two groups. If more patients had been studied, the difference would have been detected.

• Confidence intervals (CI) are another way of determining statistical significance. The 95% CI, which is most commonly used and analogous to a P value of 0.05, means that if you repeated a test 100 times, the true value would fall within this range 95 out of

100 times. But 5% of the time (analogous to $P = 0.05$), it would fall outside this range because of chance.

○ Like a P value, the CI lets you know whether an association is statistically significant at a given level (by convention, we usually use the 95% CI, which corresponds to a P value of 5%).

○ In a study looking at the relative risk (RR) between two interventions, if the CI crosses 1.0 (if the risk in one group relative to the risk in the other group is 1.0, then there is no difference between the two groups), then the result is not statistically significant and corresponds to a P value > 0.05. If the CI does not cross this threshold, then it is statistically significant, corresponding to a P value < 0.05. Sometimes the threshold value is set at 0.0 rather than 1.0, depending on the type of study and measures being used (Fig. 17-2 is an example of how point estimates and CIs are commonly represented in graphic form).

○ The width of the CI provides additional information that you cannot obtain from P values—the range in which the true result will fall 95% of the time.

○ For example, if an intervention reduced mortality by 25% (known as the *point estimate*) with a CI of 12% to 48%, it would be written as: relative risk reduction (RRR) 25%, 95% CI 12% to 48%; or it could be expressed as: RR 0.75, 95% CI 0.52–0.88. This means if you repeated the experiment 100 times, 95% of the time the RRR would fall within the range of 12% to 48%. Because there will be a range of responses among the population (ie, not everyone will have the same exact RRR), 25% (the *point estimate*) represents the average RRR over the entire population studied.

○ As the sample size in a study becomes larger, the CIs will become narrower (eg, less variability in the range of results), which gives you more confidence in the accuracy of your point estimate

RELATIVE RISK REDUCTION, ABSOLUTE RISK REDUCTION, AND NUMBER-NEEDED-TO-TREAT

• Risk is defined as the event rate for any outcome of interest. It is calculated as follows: number of persons having the event/number of persons receiving the intervention. For example, the number of women in a study taking tamoxifen who die from breast cancer/number of women in the study taking tamoxifen.

• RR is the risk in one group (eg, the intervention group)/the risk in another group (eg, the control group). For example, the risk of dying from breast cancer in the group taking tamoxifen/the risk of

Odds Ratio Meta-analysis Plot (Random Effects)

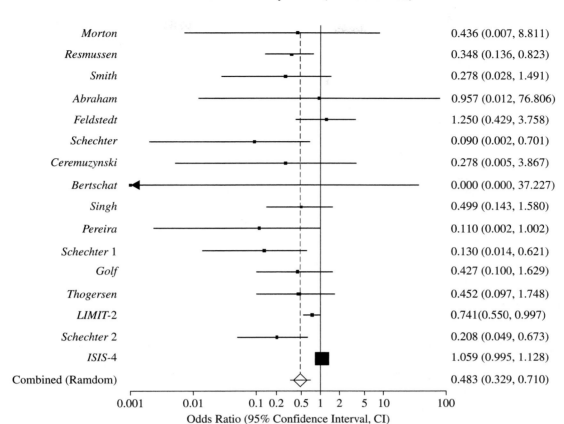

Morton	0.436 (0.007, 8.811)
Resmussen	0.348 (0.136, 0.823)
Smith	0.278 (0.028, 1.491)
Abraham	0.957 (0.012, 76.806)
Feldstedt	1.250 (0.429, 3.758)
Schechter	0.090 (0.002, 0.701)
Ceremuzynski	0.278 (0.005, 3.867)
Bertschat	0.000 (0.000, 37.227)
Singh	0.499 (0.143, 1.580)
Pereira	0.110 (0.002, 1.002)
Schechter 1	0.130 (0.014, 0.621)
Golf	0.427 (0.100, 1.629)
Thogersen	0.452 (0.097, 1.748)
LIMIT-2	0.741(0.550, 0.997)
Schechter 2	0.208 (0.049, 0.673)
ISIS-4	1.059 (0.995, 1.128)
Combined (Ramdom)	0.483 (0.329, 0.710)

Odds Ratio (95% Confidence Interval, CI)

FIG. 17-2 Example of 95% CIs of odds ratios in a meta-analysis plot. The black squares represent the point estimates for each study result while the horizontal lines represent the CIs. The diamond represents the cumulative point estimate from all the studies combined. Note that any horizontal line that crosses 1.0 is not statistically significant at a *P* value of 0.05. Six of the individual studies do not cross the 1.0 threshold; they are thus statistically significant. SOURCE: Available at: http://www.public-health.com/help/meta_analysis/cochrane_plot.htm. Accessed December 1, 2006.

dying from breast cancer in the group not taking tamoxifen.

- RRR is how much the risk is reduced in one group (eg, the intervention group) in proportion to (ie, relative to) how much it is reduced in another group (eg, the control group). It can be calculated in one of two ways.
  - |(experimental event rate − control event rate)/ control event rate|
    Note that the result is an absolute value, so it is always positive.
  - 1 − RR (if you know the RR)
- Absolute risk is the actual number of events that occur in each group (eg, number of deaths in the experimental group and number of deaths in the control group).
- Absolute risk reduction (ARR) is the absolute difference in risk between the experimental group and the control group. It is calculated as follows:

| experimental event rate − control event rate |

- Number-needed-to-treat (NNT) is the number of patients who need to be treated to achieve the outcome of interest over the studied time course. It is calculated as follows: 1/APR (Table 17-2 uses an example to show how to calculate and interpret RR, RRR, ARR, and NNT).
- The distinction between RRR and ARR is important because the ARR (and subsequently NNT) can vary substantially depending on the underlying baseline risk for a particular outcome.
  - For example, a treatment may reduce the risk of a bad outcome by 50%, which sounds impressive. However, if the baseline risk is very low (eg, the risk is only 1/1000), then a 50% RRR will only decrease the risk from 1/1000 to 0.5/1000, and 2000 patients (NNT) will have to be treated to achieve the benefit for 1 person. The other 1999 patients treated

TABLE 17-2 A Hypothetical Case to Illustrate how to Calculate and Interpret Relative Risk, Relative Risk Reduction, Absolute Risk Reduction, and Number-Needed-to-Treat

1. An oncology trial is testing a new treatment for colorectal cancer. The 4-year mortality for patients in the experimental treatment group is 30%. In the control group, mortality is 50%. What are the RR, RRR, ARR, and NNT?
2. RR = risk of death at 4 years for those receiving the new treatment ÷ risk of death at 4 years in the control group.

   $0.3 \div 0.5 = 0.6$ or 60%
3. RRR =
   1 − RR =
   1 − 0.6 = 0.4 or 40%.
   This means that patients in the new treatment group have a 40% relative reduction in the risk of death at 4 years compared to the control group.
4. The other way to calculate RRR and arrive at the same answer is:

$$\frac{|\text{Experimental event rate} - \text{control event rate}|}{\text{control event rate}}$$

$$\frac{|0.3 - 0.5|}{0.5}$$

   = 0.4 or 40% reduction.
5. ARR =
   | experimental event rate − control event rate | = | 0.3 − 0.5 |
   = 0.2 or 20%
   This means that patients in the new treatment group have a 20% absolute reduction in the risk of death at 4 years compared to the control group.
6. NNT = 1 / ARR = 1 / 0.2 = 5.
   This means that 5 patients would have to be treated in order to prevent one death at 4 years.

TABLE 17-3 The Effects of Varying Baseline Risks for a Particular Outcome (e.g., Risk of a Myocardial Infarction) on Relative Risk Reduction, Absolute Risk Reduction, and Number-Needed-to-Treat. As the Baseline Risk Decreases, Note how the RRR Remains Constant while the ARR Decreases and the NNT Increases

Baseline risk	10%	5%
RRR = 50%	ARR = 5%	NNT = 20
Baseline risk	1%	0.5%
RRR = 50%	ARR = 0.5%	NNT = 200
Baseline risk	0.1%	0.05%
RRR = 50%	ARR = 0.05%	NNT = 2000

EVIDENCE-BASED RESOURCES

- When searching for answers to clinical questions, the "5S" model has been proposed as a method for selecting evidence-based resources. The "5S" model uses a hierarchical strategy for finding the current best evidence to answer clinical questions. It is comprised of *studies, syntheses, synopses, summaries*, and *systems* (Fig.17-3).
  - As you move upward from the base of the triangle, less effort and expertise is required on the part of the user in terms of searching, retrieving, analyzing, and interpreting the evidence.
  - *Studies* refer to original studies.
  - *Syntheses* refer to systematic reviews, meta-analyses, and evidence reports.
  - *Synopses* refer to brief structured summaries of evidence from original studies or systematic reviews. Synopses provide information narrowly focused on a specific aspect of care (eg, effects of angiotensin-converting enzyme [ACE] inhibitors on mortality and hospitalization in patients with congestive heart failure [CHF]). *ACP Journal Club* is an example.
  - *Summaries* refer to resources that integrate evidence from original studies and systematic reviews to provide a more comprehensive summary of the evidence about the management of a particular condition (eg, CHF). Evidence-based guidelines that summarize the management of conditions are included in this category.
  - *Systems* refer to information systems that provide clinicians with evidence-based decision support about individual patients. An example would be an electronic medical record system with imbedded clinical decision support in the form of patient-specific rules and reminders.
  - *Reading tip*—In general, the most efficient search strategy to find answers to your clinical question is to

will not achieve the benefit, but they still incur the costs, side effects, and inconvenience of treatment. Table 17-3 for an example of how varying the baseline risk of a particular outcome affects the RRR, ARR, and NNT.
  - *Reading tip*—In addition to the RRR, always calculate the ARR and NNT before making decisions about whether an intervention should be implemented or recommended.
- If the experimental group ends up with worse outcomes than the control group (ie, the risk in the experimental group is higher than in the control group), then you use relative risk increase (RRI), absolute risk increase (ARI), and number-needed-to-harm (NNH) rather than RRR, ARR, and NNT, respectively. The calculations, however, are the same as described previously.
- For interventions that result in positive outcomes (as opposed to those that reduce bad outcomes), you can apply the same calculations as above and simply substitute the terms relative benefit increase (RBI) and absolute benefit increase (ABI) for RRR and ARR, respectively.

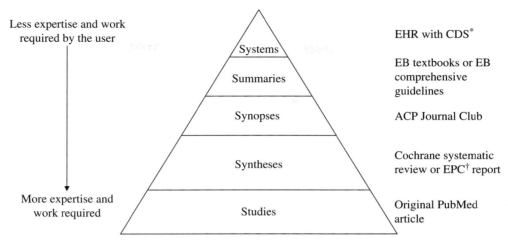

FIG. 17-3   The "5S Hierarchical Model" for organizing and using evidence-based health information resources.

*Electronic Health Record with Clinical Decision Support
†Evidence-Based Practice Center

SOURCE: Adapted from: Haynes RB. Of studies, syntheses, synopses, summaries, and systems: the "5S" evolution of information services for evidence-based healthcare decisions. *ACP J Club.* 2006; Nov–Dec(145):A8.

begin with the resource at the highest level of the triangle available to you and work your way down until you find the best answer to your clinical question.

EVIDENCE-BASED MEDICINE RESOURCES

- *Two excellent books for learning more about EBM*
  1. Straus SE, Richard WS, Glaziou P, et al. Evidence-Based Medicine: How to Practice and Teach EBM. 3rd ed. Edinburgh: Churchill Livingstone; 2005. ISBN 0443074445.
  2. Guyatt G, Rennie D. User's Guide to the Medical Literature: Essentials of Evidence-Based Clinical Practice. American Medical Association; 2001. ISBN 1579471919.
- *ACP Journal Club (ACPJC) (www.acpjc.org)*
  ACPJC is published bimonthly and summarizes articles from over 100 leading journals. The articles are chosen based on their clinical relevance in internal medicine core areas and must meet explicit EBM methodological criteria to be included. Each article is reviewed and presented in a structured abstract that allows for rapid review of the basic methods and results. Commentary by an expert in the relevant clinical field places the findings in the greater context of the existing literature.
- *BMJ Updates (http://bmjupdates.mcmaster.ca/ index.asp)*
  BMJ updates provides daily e-mail alerts and a searchable database of best evidence from the medical literature. Over 130 journals are regularly screened. Clinical articles are selected by experts according to explicit criteria, with high reproducibility and periodic quality assurance checks. Each article is also rated on its clinical relevance and newsworthiness on a scale of 1–7 by at least three practitioners in each discipline for which the article might be pertinent. The database is linked to PubMed so readers can see the abstract (if available) and can occasionally access the full-text article. Once you have registered (which is free), you can sign up for daily email alerts of articles that are likely to be of interest to you based on information you provide during registration.
- *Clinical evidence (http://clinicalevidence.bmj.com/ ceweb/index.jsp)*
  Clinical evidence is an international, peer-reviewed resource that summarizes the current state of knowledge and uncertainty about the prevention and treatment of clinical conditions, based on thorough searches and appraisal of the literature.
- *The Cochrane Library (http://www3.interscience. wiley.com/cgi-bin/mrwhome/106568753/HOME)*
  The Cochrane Library is a set of databases updated quarterly by the Cochrane Collaboration that contains high-quality, independent evidence to inform healthcare decision-making. The library's premier database contains over 3000 completed reviews prepared by members of the Collaboration. Each Cochrane review addresses an explicit clinical question related to therapy and prevention. The reviews bring together the relevant research findings on the

topic, synthesize the evidence, and then present it in a standard, structured way. Each review uses explicit methods to minimize bias and is peer-reviewed. Cochrane reviews have been shown to be of higher methodological quality than other systematic reviews and are considered by many to be the first-line resource when questions of therapeutic or preventive measures arise.

• *Database of Abstracts of Reviews of Effects (DARE) (http://www.york.ac.uk/inst/crd/crddatabases.htm)*
DARE is a public domain, full-text database containing summaries of systematic reviews which have met strict methodological quality criteria. DARE is produced by the expert reviewers at the National Health Services Centre for Reviews and Dissemination at the University of York in the United Kingdom. The database covers a broad range of health and social care topics and can be used for answering questions about the effects of interventions, as well as for developing guidelines and policy-making. DARE covers topics such as diagnosis, prevention, rehabilitation, screening, and treatment. It is updated monthly. Because DARE is one of the databases maintained in the Cochrane Library, a search of the Cochrane Library for systematic reviews will retrieve records from both DARE and the Cochrane Database of Systematic Reviews.

• *Evidence-Based Practice Centers (EPCs) (http://www.ahrq.gov/clinic/epc)*
The EPCs, supported by the Agency for Healthcare Research and Quality, develop evidence reports and technology assessments on topics relevant to clinical, social science/behavioral, economic, and other healthcare organization and delivery issues—specifically those that are common, expensive, and/or significant for the Medicare and Medicaid populations. These reports are used for informing and developing coverage decisions, quality measures, educational materials and tools, guidelines, and research agendas.
Reports are available at: http://www.ahrq.gov/clinic/epc/epcseries.htm.

• *US Preventive Services Task Force (USPSTF) (http://www.ahrq.gov/clinic/uspstfix.htm)*
The USPSTF, supported by the Agency for Healthcare Research and Quality (AHRQ), is an independent panel of experts in primary care and prevention that conducts rigorous, impartial assessments of the scientific evidence on the effectiveness of a broad range of clinical preventive services, including screening, counseling, and preventive medications.

• *National Guideline Clearinghouse (NGC) (http://www.guideline.gov)*
NGC, which is maintained by AHRQ, is a comprehensive database of evidence-based clinical practice guidelines and related documents. It provides free access to objective, detailed information on clinical practice guidelines to facilitate their dissemination, implementation, and use.

• *National Institute for Health and Clinical Excellence (NICE) (http://www.nice.org.uk)*
NICE, part of the UK National Health Service (NHS), is an independent organization responsible for providing national guidance on the promotion of good health and the prevention and treatment of ill health. NICE produces guidance in the following areas of health:
1. Clinical practice—guidance on the appropriate treatment and care of people with specific diseases and conditions
2. Health technologies—guidance on the.use of new and existing medicines, treatments, and procedures
3. Interventional procedures—guidance on whether interventional procedures used for diagnosis or treatment are safe enough and work well enough for routine use
4. Public health—guidance on the promotion of good health and the prevention of ill health for those working in the NHS, local authorities, and the wider public and voluntary sector.

• *Scottish Intercollegiate Guidelines Network (SIGN) (http://www.sign.ac.uk)*
SIGN was formed in 1993, and its objective is to improve the quality of healthcare for patients in Scotland by reducing variation in practice and outcome through the development and dissemination of national clinical guidelines containing recommendations for effective practice based on current evidence. Membership includes all the medical specialties, nursing, pharmacy, dentistry, allied health professions, patients, health service managers, social services, and researchers.

BIBLIOGRAPHY

Chobanian AV, Bakris GL, Black HR, et al. Seventh Report of the Joint National Committee on Prevention, Detection, Evaluation, and Treatment of High Blood Pressure. *Hypertension*. 2003;42: 1206–1252.

Ebell MH, Siwek J, Weiss BD, et al. Strength of Recommendation Taxonomy (SORT): a patient-centered approach to grading evidence in the medical literature. *Am Fam Physician*. 2004;69(3):548-556. Available at: http://www.aafp.org/afp/20040201/548.html. Accessed on October 31, 2006.

Haynes RB. Of studies, syntheses, synopses, summaries, and systems: the "5S" evolution of information services for evidence-based healthcare decisions. *ACP J Club*. 2006; Nov–Dec(145):A8.

Hennekins CH, Buring JE. *Epidemiology in Medicine.* Boston, MA: Little, Brown, and Company; 1987.

Levels of Evidence and Grades of Recommendations. Oxford Centre for Evidence-Based Medicine Levels of Evidence. Available at: http://www.cebm.net/levels_of_evidence.asp. Accessed October 31, 2006.

Pratt CM, Moye LA. The cardiac arrhythmia suppression trial: background, interim results, and implications. *Am J Cardiol.* 1990;65(4):20B–29B.

Sackett DL, Haynes RB, Guyatt GH, et al. *Clinical Epidemiology: A Basic Science for Clinical Medicine.* 2nd ed. Toronto: Little, Brown, and Company; 1991.

The Grading of Recommendations Assessment, Development, and Evaluation (GRADE) Working Group. Available at: http://www.gradeworkinggroup.org/index.htm. Accessed on January 29, 2008.

US Preventive Services Task Force. Available at: http://www.ahrq.gov/clinic/uspstfix.htm. Accessed October 30, 2006.

US Preventive Services Task Force Ratings: Strength of Recommendations and Quality of Evidence. *Guide to Clinical Preventive Services.* 3rd ed. Rockville, MD: Agency for Healthcare Research and Quality; 2000–2003. Periodic Updates. Available at: http://www.ahrq.gov/clinic/3rduspstf/ratings.htm. Accessed October 30, 2006.

WEB RESOURCES

The following internet sites provide information for learning more about EBM and also contain some useful EBM tools:

- A ScHARR introduction to evidence-based practice on the Internet (http://www.shef.ac.uk/scharr/ir/netting)
- Centre for Evidence-Based Medicine, Oxford (http://www.cebm.net/index.asp)
- Centre for Evidence-Based Medicine, University Health Network (http://www.cebm.utoronto.ca)
- Canadian Medical Association Journal Evidence-Based Medicine Series (http://www.cmaj.ca/cgi/collection/evidence_based_medicine_series)
- EBM Teaching Tips Online (www.ebmtips.net)
- Evidence-Based Medicine Resource Center, New York Academy of Medicine in partnership with the Evidence-Based Medicine Working Group of the American College of Physicians, New York Chapter (http://www.ebmny.org)
- Centre for Health Evidence (CHE), University of Alberta (http://www.cche.net). CHE contains the full-text prepublication version of the Users' Guides to Evidence-Based Practice, originally published as a series in the Journal of the American Medical Association, on behalf of the Evidence-Based Medicine Working Group.
- Introduction to Evidence-Based Medicine Tutorial, Duke University Medical Center Library and University of North Carolina at Chapel Hill Health Sciences Library (http://www.hsl.unc.edu/services/tutorials/EBM/index.htm)

18 EVIDENCE-BASED MEDICINE—TESTING

Sylvia C. McKean and Eduardo Ortiz

OVERVIEW

- Clinical expertise is the ability to use our clinical knowledge, skills, and experience to identify an individual patient's health state, address specific medical complaints, assess the individual risks and benefits of potential interventions, and incorporate personal preferences, values, and expectations into clinical decisions.
- Our diagnostic skills and clinical judgment often increase over time as we gain more experience, but our up-to-date knowledge and clinical performance may decline.
- The ability to quickly and accurately get to the bottom of a problem and make clinical decisions is one of the most highly regarded skills in the practice of medicine.
- There are many challenges in clinical decision-making including
  - Subjective assessments of events are often affected by factors unrelated to objective evidence.
  - Decisions are often unduly influenced by selective recall of previous events and personal biases.
  - Information used for decision-making is often incomplete, changing, and sometimes conflicting.
  - More information than is necessary is often collected before decisions are made.
  - Errors in assessing the diagnostic value of clinical evidence and errors in the revision of probability are common in medical practice. This may relate to technical considerations in testing.
    - For example, even the most recent multidetector-row spiral computed tomography (CT) scanner may miss an acute pulmonary embolism due to human factors in interpretation, technical limitations relating to body habitus and bolus of dye, and timing relating to onset of symptoms.
    - Another example is a radiologist overestimating the likelihood of cancer in a mass seen on imaging so as to not miss a malignancy.
    - In addition, some tests are more reproducible than others. For example, ultrasound examinations are more subjective and require more expertise than CT imaging. Lower extremity noninvasive studies performed by radiology fellows during off-hours may be less accurate than those performed by a certified vascular technician.

- In most teaching hospitals, the layers and status of staff, gamesmanship, and, more recently, work hour restrictions may promote the "shotgun approach" to workups.
- There are also forces at work that encourage clinicians to do more testing.
  - For example, fear of litigation or of patient complaints may lead to unnecessary testing.
  - There may also be other incentives such as financial reimbursement for testing or access to newer diagnostic technologies.
- Finally, what is considered a "normal" test may in fact be abnormal for a specific patient.
  - For example, a "normal" creatinine as a surrogate marker for the glomerular filtration rate (GFR) may in fact be consistent with an abnormal GFR in a frail elderly patient or in an African American.

- A diagnostic test should always be used to make a diagnosis or to establish a prognosis. Before ordering a test the clinician must ask the following questions:
  - Does the test distinguish between patients who have and those who do not have the disorder?
  - How good is the test? What is the probability that the test will provide the correct diagnosis?
  - Will the test change the management of the patient?
- Ideally the clinician should use the smallest number of tests, especially those tests that are expensive, invasive, or risky, to expeditiously identify the correct diagnosis.

MEASUREMENTS FOR EVALUATING A CLINICAL TEST (OR APPLIED BAYESIAN ANALYSIS)

- The simplest diagnostic test is one where the results of an investigation such as a physical examination finding, blood test, or radiographic study are used to classify patients into two groups according to the presence or absence of a symptom or sign. The terms positive and negative are used to refer to the presence or absence of the condition of interest.

SENSITIVITY/SPECIFICITY

- *Sensitivity or true negative rate*—Proportion of people with the target disorder who test positive (see Fig. 18-1). Sensitivity is also referred to as the *true positive rate (TPR)*. The formula for sensitivity is

$$\frac{\text{True positive (TP)}}{\text{True positives (TP)} + \text{False negatives (FN)}}$$

  - It is used to assist in assessing and selecting a diagnostic test.

		Condition		
		Present	**Absent**	
Test	+	TP	FP	PPV TP/TP + FP
	–	FN	TN	NPV TN/TN + FN
		Sensitivity TP/TP + FN	Specificity TN/TN + FP	

FIG. 18-1 2 × 2 table depicting sensitivity, specificity, positive predictive value, and negative predictive value.

  - When a symptom, sign, or test has a high sensitivity, a negative result rules out the diagnosis. A highly sensitive test with a low false-negative rate is good for screening.
  - A helpful reminder is *snout* (high *sensitivity* = better for ruling *out* a diagnosis).
- *Specificity*—Proportion of people without the target disorder who test negative. Specificity is also referred to as the *true negative rate (TNR)*. The formula for specificity is

$$\frac{\text{True negative (TN)}}{\text{True negatives (TN)} + \text{False positives (FP)}}$$

  - It is used in assessing and selecting a diagnostic test. When a symptom, sign, or test has a high specificity, a positive result rules in the diagnosis.
  - A highly specific test with a low false positive rate is good to confirm a disease.
  - A helpful reminder is *Spin* (high *specificity* = better for ruling *in* a diagnosis).
- Values of test sensitivity and specificity derived in one clinical population cannot necessarily be used to make accurate predictions about a different population.
- Test sensitivity increases with increasing severity of disease.
  - What this means is that there is a distribution of sensitivities and specificities across the spectrum of patients. The values of sensitivity and specificity are actually average values across the population.
  - Two institutions may have different averages when their mix of patients is different.
  - The predictive value of physical diagnosis signs will be higher when the disease is prevalent and lower when the disease is uncommon or unlikely.
  - For example, the predictive value of common physical signs for ascites depends on the prevalence of ascites in the patient population examined.
- *Reading tips*—Sensitivity and specificity are one approach for quantifying the diagnostic accuracy of a

test. In clinical practice, however, the test result is all that is known. We want to know how good the test is at predicting an abnormality. What proportion of the patients with abnormal test results is truly abnormal? The sensitivity and specificity do not answer this question. In addition to knowing the test's average sensitivity and specificity, the clinician must be aware of how the test performs in different segments of the population.

- The sensitivity and specificity alone do not give us the probability that the test will give the correct diagnosis. If the pretest probability of an underlying condition is sufficiently low, the physical examination looking for the underlying condition may not be worthwhile. For example, examiners do not routinely check for splenomegaly when a patient has a routine physical examination and feels well.
  - If the prior probability of splenic enlargement is less than 10%, the specificity of percussion or palpation for splenomegaly is not sufficiently high to rule in splenic enlargement even if both tests are positive.
- Evaluation of diagnostic tests performed only at the two ends of the disease spectrum (ie, only the sickest of the sick or the healthiest of the well) will seriously distort the apparent value of the tests.

PREDICTIVE VALUES

- The positive and negative predictive values (see Fig. 18-1) can be calculated for any disease prevalence.
- *Positive Predictive Value (PPV)*—Proportion of people with a positive test who truly have the target disorder.
  - The formula for PPV is

$$\frac{\text{True positive (TP)}}{\text{True positives (TP)} + \text{False positives (FP)}}$$

  - Unlike sensitivity and specificity, the PPV of a test improves as the prevalence of disease in a population increases.
- *Negative Predictive Value (NPV)*—Proportion of people with a negative test who truly are free of the target disorder.
  - The formula for NPV is

$$\frac{\text{True negative (TN)}}{\text{True negatives (TN)} + \text{False negatives (FN)}}$$

  - Unlike sensitivity and specificity, the NPV of a test improves as the prevalence of disease in a population decreases.
- *Reading tips*—As the prevalence of a condition in a population decreases, the PPV will decrease, while

the NPV will increase (ie, the test will be better for ruling out than ruling in a diagnosis). In general, you will obtain more value from a clinical symptom, sign, or diagnostic test when the likelihood of disease (eg, pretest probability) is in the range of 40% to 60%.
  - At this level the presence of the clinical finding or positive test result makes a strong case for the diagnosis, while a negative test result often eliminates the target disorder from your list of hypotheses.
  - For example, on the basis of only a patient's age, sex, location, and type of chest pain, the clinician can estimate a pretest probability—low, moderate, or high—that the causative factor accounting for chest pain is cardiac ischemia. This knowledge permits the appropriate ordering of exercise tolerance tests to rule in or rule out a diagnosis.
  - The predictive values of a test in clinical practice depend on the prevalence of the abnormality in the patients being tested. This may differ from the prevalence in a published study assessing the usefulness of the test.
  - If the prevalence of the disease in a population is very low, the predictive value of a positive test will not be very good even if the sensitivity and specificity are high. Thus in screening the general population for diseases with low prevalence, it is inevitable that many people with positive test results will end up having false positive results.
- Prevalence (pretest or prior probability of disease)— The proportion of people with the target disorder in the population at risk at a specific time (point prevalence) or time interval (period prevalence). Prevalence includes all new cases plus old cases that are still alive (eg, all women with breast cancer in the United States in 2006), whereas incidence is the proportion of new cases (eg, women newly diagnosed with breast cancer in the United States in 2006).
- Posttest probability of disease—The proportion of patients with that particular test result who have the target disorder. The PPVs and NPVs are the revised estimates of the same probability for those subjects who test positive and negative (posterior probabilities).

LIKELIHOOD RATIO

- Likelihood ratio (LR) represents the likelihood that a given test result would be expected in a patient with the target condition compared with the likelihood that the same result would be expected in a patient without the target condition. The LR indicates the value of the test for increasing certainty about a positive diagnosis.

- *LR positive*—Ability of positive test result to confirm the disease status.

  LR positive = (Sensitivity)/(1 − Specificity)

- A LR > 1 produces a post-test probability that is higher than the pre-test probability. Good tests for ruling in a target disorder have high LRs (eg, LR = 10) (low false positive rate).
- A high LR may show that the test is useful, but it does not necessarily follow that the test is a good indicator of the presence of disease.
- *LR negative*—Ability of negative test result to confirm nondiseased status.

  LR negative = (1 − Sensitivity)/(Specificity)

- A LR < 1 produces a post-test probability that is lower than the pre-test probability. Good tests for ruling out a disorder have small LRs (eg, LR = 0.1) (low false negative rate).
- The LR is more stable than sensitivity and specificity when the prevalence of disease changes.
- Unlike sensitivity and specificity, where the results are dichotomous and limit the test result options to either "positive" or "negative," LR can be generated for multiple levels of the diagnostic test result. The LR can be used to calculate the increase in the probability of disease with a positive test result (LR positive) or decrease in probability of disease with a negative test (LR negative) for any baseline level of disease prevalence.
  - The LR can be used to shorten a list of diagnostic hypotheses because the pretest "odds" of the target disorder (the ratio of the probabilities for and against a particular diagnosis) multiplied times the LR for the diagnostic test result = the post-test odds for the target disorder.
  - The LR strategy allows you to carry out sequences of diagnostic tests. The post test probability for the one test becomes the pre-test probability for a second, independent diagnostic test.
- *Reading tips*—Although the LR, PPV, and NPV are all known as posttest probabilities (ie, inform the clinician the probability that a patient has—or does not have—a disorder after the test results are known), the LR incorporates both the sensitivity and specificity of the diagnostic test. Unlike PPV and NPV, LRs are not affected by the underlying prevalence or incidence of the disorder.
  - When a LR = 1 for a diagnostic test, the test does not change the pretest probability.
  - A LR < 0.1 or > 10 results in significant changes from the pretest to post test probability.
  - The LR negative is the ability of the test to rule out a disorder—ability of the test to confirm nondisease status. The LR positive is the ability to rule in a disorder—ability of the test to confirm disease status.

- When there are multiple symptoms and signs, the LR for each symptom and sign may be incorporated into a prediction rule (with points for each symptom or sign). Using this information, the clinician can focus the history and physical examination on those symptoms and signs that most reliably make the diagnosis, for example in determining whether a preoperative patient with a systolic murmur requires screening for the presence of aortic stenosis.

THE NOMOGRAM

- A nomogram is a graphical calculating tool that makes it easy to determine the probability of a target disorder by converting pre-test probabilities into post-test probabilities for diagnostic test results when the pre-test probabilities and LR are known (Fig. 18-2).

RECEIVER OPERATING CURVE CHARACTERISTICS

- An ideal test would have a sensitivity and specificity of 100%. In the real world, however, trade-offs have to be made between sensitivity and specificity, which are determined by where one sets the cutoff point for a diagnosis using a particular test. As the cutoff point is changed, sensitivity and specificity move in opposite directions (eg, sensitivity increases while specificity decreases or vice versa).
- When screening the general population for target disorders, the optimal cutoff point depends on the circumstances.
  - When testing for a disorder that results in substantial morbidity and mortality if not detected and treated early (eg, screening a newborn for congenital hypothyroidism or phenylketonuria), the diagnostic cutoff point should be selected to ensure that no cases are missed (ie, low false negative rate or high sensitivity).
    - The trade-off is that the number of false positives will increase (ie, low specificity).
    - That is a risk worth taking because the consequences of missing the diagnosis could be disastrous, and further confirmatory testing could eliminate the false positives.
  - On the other hand, if you have a disorder where missing the diagnosis is not that crucial because the consequences of a missed diagnosis are minimal, especially if actions stemming from the positive test lead to invasive (and costly) testing or treatment, the diagnostic cutoff would be chosen to ensure that when a test was positive, the person really had the disorder (ie, low false positive rate or high specificity).
    - The trade-off is that the number of false negatives will increase (low sensitivity).

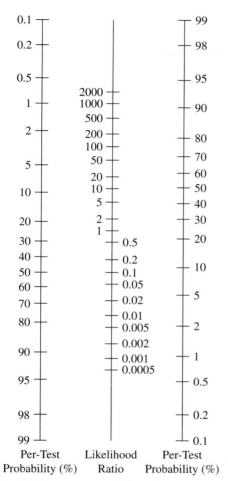

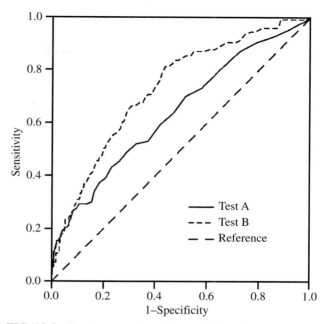

FIG. 18-3   Receiver operating characteristic (ROC) graph.

FIG. 18-2   A LR nomogram. Using the nomogram: Assume you have a patient with a 30% pretest probability of having coronary disease. Look at the left side of the nomogram, which represents the pretest probability, and locate 30 on the vertical line. Assume you apply a test with a LR of 2 (represented by the middle vertical line). Take your ruler and make sure the edge aligns with 30 on the left and 2 in the middle. The edge of the ruler crosses the ride vertical line at about 45%, which represents the posttest probability. This means that the probability of this patient having a disease increased from 30% to 45% based on the positive test result. If the LR is 5, the posttest probability increases to 66%. With a LR of 10, it increases to 82%.

- ROC curves allow clinicians to visualize the trade-offs of using different cutoff points in order to select an optimal test value that best distinguishes patients with the disorder from those without the disorder.
- The area under the ROC plot gives a global assessment of the test performance (ie, the diagnostic accuracy).
  - When comparing two or more tests, the test with the greatest area under the curve will be the better test for distinguishing patients with the disorder from those without the disorder.
  - The closer the ROC curve is to 1.0, the better the test.
  - A test that is completely nondiscriminatory results in a diagonal line from the bottom left corner to the top right corner and has an area under the curve of 0.5 (equivalent to tossing a coin) (Fig. 18-3).

THE RATIONAL USE OF DIAGNOSTIC TESTING: THE VALUE OF THE HISTORY AND PHYSICAL EXAMINATION

- The LRs of specific symptoms and signs during the patient encounter express the odds that a given finding on the history or physical examination would occur in a patient with, as opposed to a patient without, the target disorder.
- LRs are more powerful than sensitivity and specificity.
  - When a finding's LR is above 1.0, the probability of the disease goes up because the finding is more likely among patients with, than without, the disorder.

- ■ That is a risk worth taking because the consequences of missing the diagnosis are not severe, and the morbidity, costs, and so forth of a false positive diagnosis are substantial.
- When making healthcare decisions, the key is to find the appropriate balance. Receiver operating characteristic (ROC) curves can help.
- ROC curves are graphical displays that plot the TPR (sensitivity) of a test on the y axis and the false positive rate ($1 -$ specificity) of a test on the x axis for all possible cutoff points.

- ○ When the LR is below 1.0, the probability of disease goes down because the finding is less likely among patients with, than without, the disorder.
- ○ When the LR is close to 1.0, the probability of disease is unchanged because the finding is equally likely in patients with, and without, the disorder.
- Relative size of the LRs for the brief, immediate, and relatively inexpensive history taking usually dwarf LRs derived for the longer, delayed, and relatively expensive testing.
- Appropriate use of physical findings can reduce reliance on sophisticated and expensive tests, reduce the incidence of misdiagnoses, and reduce lengths of stay.
- The problem lies not so much in the test but in the way the clinician uses the results. The abnormal findings must be interpreted in the context of the patient's clinical presentation.
- Deciding whether or not to perform a diagnostic study involves balancing its risks and costs vs. the information it could provide. When we perform diagnostic studies on patients with low probabilities of disease, we must be concerned about false positive test results unless the tests are highly specific.

DIAGNOSTIC STRATEGY

- Learn the LRs for key symptoms and signs and several levels (rather than just positive and negative results) of diagnostic tests.
- Identify the logical sequence of diagnostic tests (whenever feasible).
- Estimate the pretest probability of disease for the patient, and using either a nomogram or conversion formulas, apply the LR that corresponds to the first diagnostic test result.
- While remembering that the resulting post-test probability or odds from the first test becomes the pretest probability or odds for the next diagnostic test, repeat the process for all the pertinent symptoms, signs, and laboratory studies that pertain to the target disorder. However, these combinations may not be independent, and convergent diagnostic tests, if treated independently, will combine to overestimate the final posttest probability of disease.

BIBLIOGRAPHY

Elstein A, et al. Evidence base of clinical diagnosis: clinical problem solving and diagnostic decision-making: selective review of the cognitive literature. *BMJ.* 202;321:729–732.

Etchells E, Bell C, Robb K. Does this patient have an abnormal systolic murmur. *JAMA.* 1997;277:564–561.
Kassirer JP. Teaching problem-solving—how are we doing? *N Engl J Med.* 1995;332(22):1507–1509.
Sackett DL, Richardson WS, Rosenberg W, et al. *Evidenced-Based Medicine: How to Practice and Teach EBM.* 2nd ed. Edinburg: Churchill Livingstone; 1997.
Sackett DL. The rational clinical examination: a primer on the precision and accuracy of the clinical examination. *JAMA.* 1992;267(19):2638–2644.
Sox HC, Blatt MA, Higghins MC, et al. *Medical Decision-Making.* Boston, MA: Butterworth-Heinemann; 1998.
Wachter R, Shojania K, Sane S, et al. The cognitive psychology of missed diagnoses. *Ann Intern Med* 2005;142:115–120.

WEB RESOURCES

- A collection of likelihood ratios for common tests, provided by the Cochrane Centre in Oxford, England (http:// cebm.jr2.ox.ac.uk/docs/likerats.html)
- Center for Evidence-Based Medicine (http://www.cebm.net/index.aspx?o=1043)
- Examples of how to interpret likelihood ratios (http://www.poems.msu.edu/InfoMastery/Diagnosis/likelihood_ratios.htm)
- This interactive nomogram takes the pain out of using likelihood ratios (LRs) to convert pretest probabilities into post-test probabilities for diagnostic test results with a known LR (http://www.cebm.net/index.aspx?o=1161)

19 THE GROWING IMPORTANCE OF COST-EFFECTIVENESS ANALYSIS IN MANAGING HOSPITALIZED PATIENTS

Jerome Lewis Avorn

EPIDEMIOLOGY/OVERVIEW

Increasingly, physicians who care for hospitalized patients are being asked to consider not just the efficacy and safety of the specific interventions they order, but also the relative cost-effectiveness, or clinical value of the intervention in relation to its expense. Rather than being seen as a kind of interference with the physician's role, this added responsibility is becoming an important component of appropriate care in the twenty-first century.

The costs of healthcare overall are rising beyond the point of affordability for many patients, and hospital-based care is a particularly fast-rising component of all healthcare expenditures. For those with private health insurance, this makes monthly premiums increasingly difficult to afford. In addition, many insurers and employers are increasing the amount of the deductibles or copayments which patients must shoulder themselves; some companies are dropping health insurance altogether. For patients who are covered by Medicare, the largest payor of hospital costs, increased hospital expenditures mean greater demands on the federal treasury: Medicare has been identified as the single most important economic crisis facing the US economy in the coming decades. The most important burden of all is borne by uninsured patients, who often must forego hospital care except in emergency situations, because of its expense.

COST-EFFECTIVENESS ANALYSIS

Because of these issues, it is vital for all hospital-based physicians to have a basic understanding of the principles of cost-effectiveness analysis—not to ration care, but for precisely the opposite reason. Responsible stewardship of our healthcare resources is needed to make sure that healthcare will remain affordable for as many patients as possible. Conversely, ignoring these issues will have the direct result of placing medical care beyond the reach of many of the most vulnerable patients who need it.

Cost-effectiveness analysis is simply the comparison of the clinical benefit which a patient derives from a given intervention (its effectiveness), compared with the cost of that intervention. Many expensive hospital-based interventions do not produce clinical benefit for the patient that is any greater than that produced by much less expensive strategies. This is most clear in the area of medication use, in which a costly brand-name product that is still under patent (eg, an angiotensin receptor blocker [ARB]) may be no better in controlling hypertension for most patients than a very inexpensive thiazide diuretic (despite a cost that can exceed $1000 per year for the ARB vs. under $50 per year for the diuretic).

Comparable examples have been carefully documented in relation to other hospital-based utilization, including:
• Cardiac catheterization and stent placement for patients with nonsevere angina whose symptoms (and longevity) could be equally well maintained with a medication regimen.
• The extensive use of costly imaging studies such as magnetic resonance imaging (MRI) which are often ordered nearly automatically, but which in many cases yield relatively small amounts of additional information to guide clinical decision-making.

The growing field of cost-effectiveness analysis is based on an increasingly sophisticated set of methodical approaches that are becoming more standardized. The effectiveness component can be defined at varying levels: the cost per MI treated, or hip fracture repaired, or appendix removed. However, it is preferable to consider effectiveness at a higher level that takes into account the clinical status of the patient beyond the period of hospitalization—and, whenever possible, throughout the remaining life span. Thus, a management strategy for MI that results in a higher survival rate should take into account all the additional life-years that a patient experiences after discharge. A treatment such as thrombolysis or angioplasty that is more successful in preventing longer term mortality would thus be considered more cost-effective than a less expensive intervention that did not confer this survival advantage. To measure this accurately requires considering the difference in outcome that was observed within the usually narrow confines of a clinical trial, and projecting it forward throughout the life expectancy of such patients to estimate the true value of the intervention.

It is also necessary to measure the *quality* of life following a given medical intervention. For example, a hospital-based treatment that carries a high risk of intracerebral hemorrhage, which could lead to many years spent in a persistent vegetative state, should be considered differently from an intervention which leads to a comparable number of years with excellent functional status. To accomplish this, the concept of the *quality-adjusted life-year (QALY)* was developed. This metric ranges from 100% for a year spent in perfect health to 0 for death. It is an attempt to describe the functional status of a patient with a given condition in a way that makes it possible to compare many different conditions with one another. A QALY analysis might, for example, determine that a patient with a severe hemiparesis would have a QALY that is worth only about 60% that of a patient in excellent health. The means by which these values are generated are understandably problematic, and quite approximate. Nonetheless, they begin to make it possible to compare interventions which yield results that are clinically quite different from one another.

The economic component of cost-effective analysis can be similarly arcane. One approach is to attempt to add up an institution's cost for providing a given service (eg, a 4-day admission for bacterial pneumonia, which would take into account the cost of nursing time, physician encounters, nonprofessional staff time, the expense of maintaining the hospital bed, the cost of all medications, intravenous fluids, and so forth). Alternatively, and far more simply, one can look up the amount which Medicare pays a hospital for a patient admitted with that particular diagnosis. This is both more straightforward and also quite accurate; whatever the actual expense incurred by the hospital in caring for such a patient, the cost to the Medicare program (and thus to the nation) of that hospitalization is equal to the amount paid by Medicare to the hospital.

Cost-effectiveness analyses are often based on RCTs of one intervention compared with another, suitably projected into the future life expectancy of the study subjects, often using computer models. For example, we can assume that a given intervention (eg, thrombolysis) for MI is much more costly initially, but results in a 1% reduction in mortality. (This was the case when tissue-type plasminogen activator [tPA] was first studied in comparison with its older and cheaper alternative, streptokinase.) The cost-effectiveness analysis would consider the additional up-front cost of using the more expensive agent, and then "spread out" that cost over the lifetime of a hypothetical cohort of 1000 patients who were given that drug vs. its less costly comparator. It could well turn out (as it did in the case of tPA) that the additional initial cost of the drug was "worth it" in relation to the additional number of QALYs that were gained in a population of patients who received it compared to streptokinase. This example also brings to light the very important issue of *perspective* in conducting (and reading) cost-effectiveness analyses. If payment by insurers were no different, irrespective of which thrombolytic agent was used, it would seem from the hospital's perspective that tPA would be a very cost-inefficient agent to use. However, it is universally accepted that the most appropriate perspective to take in such an analysis is that of society as a whole, for obvious reasons. When the well-being of patients viewed throughout their lifespan is taken into account, even a costly intervention that reduces mortality can be seen to be a "good buy" for society over the long term. The hospitalist can be uniquely qualified to take a leading role in balancing these issues. They play a central and continuing role in the life of the institution, and can be well situated to participate in formulary review, guideline development, and other allocation decisions. The hospitalist can bring to these discussions the perspective of a frontline physician engaged in direct patient care, while at the same time being able to consider the need for the institution to allocate its resources prudently.

ETHICAL CONSIDERATIONS

Prudent resource allocation on the institutional level is a particularly challenging role because in a marketplace-driven healthcare system, those who sell a particular product (whether it is a costly new medication, imaging equipment, or medical devices) generally invest considerable sums to promote it. This often raises conflict-of-interest issues for physicians who are drawn into such company-sponsored activities, whether as consultants, researchers, paid speakers, or just as recipients of free meals or gifts. (Physicians who act as "vendors" of their own expensive clinical consultative activities may also be in a conflict-laden role in relation to their services as well.) Manufacturers of new drugs, devices, and diagnostic or imaging equipment are very effective in making the case for their latest and most costly products. There is also a great deal of support available from industry to study and teach about such costly approaches. As a result, concern has grown that this abundance of industry support has made some research and educational activities resemble promotion more than science. By contrast, relatively little is spent promoting older interventions that are less profitable—even if they have the same efficacy and much greater cost-effectiveness than the "latest model." The perspective of rational cost-effective decisionmaking is often presented far less compellingly—and usually without the engaging promotion and free meals that often accompany such sales pitches. Hospitalists are key targets for such promotional activities, because their day-to-day decisions account for enormous sums of dollars of resource use.

Unfortunately, institutions sometimes ignore the societal view of cost-effectiveness and take a more narrow and self-serving perspective, in which the cost of caring for a particular kind of patient, or performing a given procedure, is compared with the reimbursement rate available for such care. This can result in the proliferation of services (and even whole institutions) devoted to maximizing that kind of care (such as whole-body scanning), even when the multiplication of such services is not in the interest of the healthcare system in its entirety.

Physicians sometimes worry that attention to cost-effectiveness might compromise their moral obligation to provide the best possible care to the individual patient for whom they are responsible. This can indeed be a problem, and one which has reached important proportions in the British National Health Service, where certain kinds of medical services which have been judged to be *not cost-effective* are simply not provided. In the United States, the crisis takes on a different form. Many physicians err on the side of providing all possible services to the patients for whom they are caring, for both ethical and remunerative reasons. But this approach, taken to excess, renders the healthcare system unaffordable for large groups of patients, even though the identities of the people who end up without affordable care may be unknown to a given physician.

EVIDENCE-BASED OUTREACH

There is one practical reconciliation to this apparent ethical paradox. It is based on the fact that a very large proportion of the interventions we provide to our patients, whether in the hospital or not, could well be replaced by clinical strategies that are far more cost effective, with absolutely no diminution in the benefit received by patients.

Several groups have successfully mounted programs to level the playing field in these informational wars. In the area of prescribing, a movement has developed known as "academic detailing" that uses the engaging, interactive manner of the pharmaceutical industry, but puts it in the service of evidence-based, cost-effective prescribing. Several programs in the United States, Canada, Australia, and Europe have reported good results in "de-marketing" overused drugs (including over-prescribed antibiotics in hospitalized patients) and replacing them with more appropriate choices. One large program has made its educational materials available for noncommercial use on the Internet. Economic analyses of this approach indicate that it can save the healthcare system far more than it costs to implement.

Other areas in which such evidence-based outreach can improve care and contain costs include more judicious use of imaging studies that do not meaningfully contribute to a patient's clinical management, restrained use of diagnostic studies such as endoscopies which are not likely to aid much in subsequent clinical decision-making, and wiser choices of medications, avoiding costly products which are no more effective than generic ones. In this way, physicians sensitive to the inevitably growing importance of cost-effectiveness considerations can continue to provide excellent care to their patients while playing a role in helping to contain the rapidly escalating costs of hospital care, which have begun to make health services unaffordable for many Americans.

BIBLIOGRAPHY

Avorn J. *Powerful Medicines: The Benefits, Risks, and Costs of Prescription Drugs.* New York, NY: Knopf; 2004.

Avorn J, Soumerai SB. Improving drug-therapy decisions through educational outreach. A randomized controlled trial of academically based "detailing." *N Engl J Med.* 1983; 308:1457–1463.

Brennan TA, Rothman DJ, Blank L, et al. Health industry practices that create conflicts of interest: a policy proposal for academic medical centers. *JAMA.* 2006;295:429–433.

Gold MR, Siegel JE, Russell LB, et al. *Cost-effectiveness in Health and Medicine.* New York, NY: Oxford University Press; 1996.

Kaslish SC, Gurwitz JH, Krumholz HM, et al. A cost-effectiveness model of thrombolytic therapy for acute myocardial infarction. *J Gen Intern Med.* 1995;10: 321–330.

Solomon DH, Glynn RJ, Baden L, et al. Academic detailing to improve use of broad-spectrum antibiotics at an academic medical center. *Arch Intern Med.* 2001;161:1897–1902.

WEB RESOURCES

- Independent Drug Information Service Web site. www.RxFacts.org
- National Institute for Clinical Excellence of the British National Health Service Web site. www.nice.org.uk

20 HOSPITALIST AS RESEARCHER

Leroi Hicks

OVERVIEW

- Developing research skills, although difficult, has the benefit of establishing expertise in the emerging field of hospital medicine that is critical in any new specialty. It also aids in academic and career promotion.
- Despite the opportunities and need for more research in hospital medicine, hospitalists are often hired by hospitals and other organizations to meet clinical demand. The time constraints of inpatient service can impede initiating and completing research projects.
- Many hospitalist services, especially new programs, hire physicians with little or no formal training in research, and provide little or no grant funding or protected time for scholarly activity.
- Most hospitalist programs, especially in the community, have very limited administrative support to facilitate quality improvement research in hospital medicine.
- Inexperienced researchers who are new to practicing as hospitalists may find it challenging to properly identify a dimension of research that can easily be coordinated with clinical work.
- This chapter will review how to protect time to conduct research, identify research areas and specific projects, develop a system to organize projects, seek out funding opportunities, and disseminate work through presentations and manuscripts.

NECESSARY STEPS

- A hospitalist-researcher should take the following essential steps to more easily initiate and develop research projects:
  - Identify research mentors and collaborators outside your clinical discipline.
  - Collaborate with other hospitalists and take advantage of resources within professional societies such as the Society of Hospital Medicine (SHM).
  - Find the proper agency/foundation from whom to obtain funding.
  - Disseminate work, through publication and conference presentations.
- Directors of hospitalist programs should advocate for administrative and financial support so that hospitalists can undertake projects that are aligned with the needs of their institutions.
  - Usually the time spent caring for patients during clinical rotations will preclude robust research activities, so protected time must be allocated for the research initiatives to be successful.
  - The time necessary to develop a research project, collect and analyze the data, and present research findings also requires dedicated time.
- Create a strategic plan.
  - Negotiate clinical schedule around grant/internal funding and conference deadlines.
  - Utilize clinical time to strictly focus on clinical work and multidisciplinary team teaching but merge research projects with clinical interests and activities in order to keep research initiatives moving forward.
  - Avoid added clinical and/or administrative responsibilities and focus on completing existing research and developing new projects during *nonclinical* time.
  - Use your environment as a "natural laboratory" (eg, pilot an intervention to improve patient satisfaction among a cohort of patients being cared for when you are on service to work out study logistics).
  - Block out time to write grants and do so repeatedly until you have obtained enough grant funding to pay for your nonclinical time.
- Select a research focus.
  - Identifying the type of research to conduct can be difficult, but should represent alignment of an individual's interests with the organization's need.

TABLE 20-1   Essential Steps to Establishing a Research Career

- Protect your time when you get it.
- Identify research dimension (e.g., quality improvement, clinical trials, and so forth).
- Develop a system to organize the work.
- Be ever vigilant for funding opportunities.
- Disseminate your work.

- Most research conducted by hospitalists can be divided into quality improvement research, outcomes research, and health services research.
- Identify a mentor.
  - Success as a hospitalist-researcher, at any level of development, is largely based on selecting the proper mentor to aid in selecting the right projects and identifying priority areas.
  - Although having a specified mentor is not essential to conducting research, mentors may be a significant help in navigating your career as a hospitalist researcher.
  - Strategies to look the best mentor include finding someone who is in or near your institution that either does similar work or whose work you respect and find innovative.
  - A mentor should be knowledgeable about how to conduct research, have experience working with others, be available, and be interested in your professional development.
- Select the right project. Work with your mentor to select a project that is
  - *Meaningful* by filling a knowledge gap or improving a significant problem by improving quality of care.
  - *Practical* with resources available to make this project successful. Important questions to ask are
    - Is this best studied through 1 or 2 data collection?
    - Is there available funding to support the project?
  - *Feasible* scope of work that can be accomplished in reasonable time frame.
    - Will this project be ready to turn over to research assistants (RAs) for data abstraction *before* you attend on your next ward rotation?
- Develop a study team.

TABLE 20-2   Examples of Common Research Dimensions for Hospitalists

- Quality improvement research
  1. Rapidly assess gaps in quality
  2. Develop short duration interventions
  3. Rapidly assess intervention and develop a new strategy to improve intervention
- Outcomes research
  1. Assess educational outcomes (e.g., resident proficiency in evaluating acid-base disturbances)
  2. Survey outcomes (e.g., evaluating patient satisfaction with hospitalist vs. primary care physician or surrogate)
  3. Conduct clinical trials (e.g., evaluating if introducing a pharmacist to nurses clinical rounds reduce medication errors)
- Health services
  1. Evaluate quality of continuing care (e.g., rates of meeting acceptable benchmarks for coronary disease care)
  2. Evaluate disparities in care (e.g., evaluate patients' racial or insurance-based differences in receipt of echocardiography in CHF)

○ A statistician, if available, to assist with developing study methodology and arranging plan for statistical tests to analyze the data.

○ A research coordinator, ideally someone hired to run daily operations of the project (eg, supervising assistants, monitoring data collection, handling Institutional Review Board [IRB] applications).

○ RAs, typically students trained to handle data collection

○ Computer programmer/analyst to store data electronically and perform data analyses using software.

• Write the research plan. The written research protocol is an essential part of documenting the proposed project for perusal by hospital administrators, IRB, and potential funding sources.

○ A very detailed written protocol will enable you to work out many logistics prior to beginning the study and will provide your collaborators and study staff with a clear roadmap for moving the study forward while the hospitalist is occupied with clinical responsibilities. Table 20-3 provides an example of how to structure the aims, background, and preliminary data sections of a written research protocol.

○ The remainder of the written research protocol should describe the study methods in detail. Research methods should include enough information to explain every aspect of the project from study subject selection to how data will be collected, stored, and analyzed (Table 20-4).

• Obtain funding. Another key facet of conducting research, as a hospitalist, is the ability to obtain funding for projects aimed at improving care.

○ While your hospital administration may be able to provide funding, typically in small amounts, it is helpful to consider external funding for projects.

○ External funding, often from foundations or the federal government, will typically provide higher amounts to support you and study staff, as well as indirect costs for your institution to support its infrastructure. Examples of funding sources and grant types are presented below.

■ Career development awards, typically sponsored by the National Institutes of Health (NIH) and foundations such as the Robert Wood Johnson Foundation, fund 4–5 years of work, mostly salary for investigator. The investigator is funded more than the specific project.

■ Small or pilot project funds provide funding for short range (1–2 years) projects without substantive preliminary data.

TABLE 20-3 Example Structure of Aims, Background, and Preliminary Data Sections of a Written Research Protocol

Study aims (1 page)	Briefly describe need for study and give a concise statement of hypotheses and study goals Example goal "To determine if rates of thrombosis prophylaxis can be improved using computerized decision support to hospitalists." Example hypothesis "Computerized reminders to hospitalists about use of low molecular weight heparin will reduce the incidence of venous thrombosis among hospitalized patients."
Background (1–2 pages)	Describe current relevant knowledge gap in the research literature. Describe why your proposed study may help fill the knowledge gap. Present reader with a conceptual model of why your study is important.
Preliminary data (2–3 pages)	Describe any relevant data obtained thus far and present enough data to assure the reader you are qualified to conduct the study. Example "Our examination of baseline rates of prophylaxis demonstrated that only 30% of hospitalized patients received low molecular weight heparin." Example "Each patient admitted to our hospitalist service has medication orders entered through a computerized order entry system."

TABLE 20-4 Example Structure of Methods Section of a Written Research Protocol

Overview	Explain in two or three paragraphs descriptions of overall study design and timeline for the project. Example "Controlled trial conducted over two years. The first 6 months will focus on examination of baseline use of low molecular weight heparin."
Study subjects	Describe who will be studied and how they are selected. Example "Hospitalists providing care to all patients admitted to general medical services and orthopedic surgical services will be randomized to either receive computerized reminders to start low molecular weight heparin or no reminders."
Data collection	Describe what information you will collect for the study outcome and how the data will be obtained. Describe each additional data element to be collected, the purpose for collecting the data, and how the data will be collected.
Data analyses	Describe how the data will be evaluated and what statistical methods will be used. Calculate the number of subjects you will need to study in order to adequately examine your aims.
Limitations	Describe limitations of study design and your attempts to address them.
Project management	Describe what key personnel are necessary for the study and their duties. Example personnel Statistician, research coordinator, RAs, and programmer
Human subjects	Describe what proportion of women, children, and minorities will be included. Describe security measures for storing data.

- External funding from NIH (known as R03s or R21s) and foundations (eg, Commonwealth Fund) sponsor pilot interventions or develop and test surveys.
- Internal funding from earmarked hospital research funds made available through department chairs, from healthcare system quality improvement or risk management funds, or from device or pharmaceutical companies may also be good sources.
  - Planning grants are typically NIH-sponsored grants (known as R24s or R34s) for up to 3 years for developing a new service or intervention and planning methods to adopt the service into usual practice.
  - Large project funding, sponsored by NIH (known as RO1s) or foundations, support projects for 3 to 5 years with costs > $250,000. Projects are typically funded as part of a call for proposals in particular area, or investigators have a good idea and solicit funding. Agency for Healthcare Research and Quality (AHRQ) is another potential source of funding.
- Disseminate the work. A critical aspect to success as a researcher is reporting findings from your work to others.
  - Establishing a track record of data presentations and publications is not only beneficial to career development, but also helps to inform administrators, policy makers, clinicians, and researchers about new knowledge gained as a result of your work.
  - In particular, adding information about how medical processes of care can be improved through data gained from research is a critically important role of the hospitalist researcher.
  - Dissemination of knowledge gained from projects usually takes place in three forms.
    1. Reports of findings for institutions/organizations (known as *white papers*)
    2. Journal publication (peer-reviewed full-length manuscripts or briefs)
    3. Meeting presentations (oral or poster presentation of abstract from project)
  - Of the methods listed above, disseminating data in the form of peer-reviewed manuscripts allows the largest audience an opportunity to learn from your work. Clinical research manuscripts require a specific format that varies slightly by the journal but consistently contains the following:
    - *Abstract*—Normally 150–250 words describing purpose for the study, a brief overview of the methods, key results, and one or two sentences in conclusion
    - *Introduction*—One page concisely describing scope of the problem (motivation for the study) and the study aims

- *Methods*—Describe methods in sufficient detail for the reader to replicate the study. Normally one or two paragraphs describing each of the following:
  - Study design
  - Study site(s) and participants (study subjects)
  - Data sources and variables collected
  - Data analyses
- *Results*
  - Describe findings from analyses outlined in methods
  - Use tables and figures to clearly present results.
  - Include results of comparisons (eg, odds ratio 2:3 [95% C.I. 1.2–4.8])
  - Do not repeat data from tables and figures in text
- *Discussion*
  - One paragraph summarizing key findings from paper
  - Details from prior literature and how study findings relate to prior published work
  - The limitations of the study and attempts to mitigate the limitations
  - One concluding paragraph stating the policy/clinical implications of the findings and new hypotheses developed

CONCLUSIONS

- The role of the hospitalist as researcher requires dedicated time and resources to be successful.
- It is difficult to protect research time; however it is easier if hospitalists facilitate combining research with clinical work.
- The pathway to independence in career and academic advancement depends largely on good working relationship with mentor and study collaborators.
- The more hospitalists attend to process and planning, the easier it will be to obtain funding and complete the project.
- Dissemination of findings from work through presentations and peer-reviewed manuscripts is critical to academic advancement and to promoting the field of hospital medicine.

BIBLIOGRAPHY

Docherty M, Smith R. The case for structuring the discussion of scientific papers. *Br Med J.* 1999;318:1224–1225.
Inouye SK, Fiellin DA. An evidence-based guide to writing grant proposals for clinical research. *Ann Intern Med.* 2005; 142:274–282.

Kaushansky K. ASCI presidential address: mentoring and teaching clinical investigation. *J Clin Invest.* 2004;114:1165–1168.

Lynn J, Nolan K, Kabcenell A, et al. Reforming care for persons near the end of life: the promise of quality improvement. *Ann Intern Med.* 2002;137:117–122.

Perneger TV, Hudelson PM. Writing a research article: advice to beginners. *Int J Qual Health Care.* 2004;16:191–192.

WEB RESOURCES

- For grant writing: National Institutes of Health, National Health, Lung, and Blood Institute Clinical Research Guide Web site. Available at: http://www.nhlbi.nih.gov/crg/index.php. Accessed April 3, 2007.

HOSPITALIST CLINICAL CORE COMPETENCIES

CARDIOVASCULAR ILLNESS

21 CHEST PAIN

Timothy D. Brennan

EPIDEMIOLOGY/OVERVIEW

- There are over six million visits for chest pain each year, making it the second most common presenting symptom, totaling 5.4% of all visits (The National Hospital Ambulatory Medical Care: 2004 Emergency Department Summary).
- Sixty percent to sixty-five percent of patients admitted for chest pain will be subsequently diagnosed with noncardiac chest pain. Billions of dollars are spent on the care of unnecessary admissions to rule out myocardial infarction (MI) for a heterogeneous group of patients, the majority of whom do not have ischemic chest pain.
- Despite coronary artery disease being the number one cause of death for both men and women, roughly 20,000 patients with coronary ischemia, 2% to 5% of acute myocardial infarction (AMI) are discharged annually from emergency departments (ED).
- Medical errors in the management of acute coronary syndromes (ACS) and missed diagnosis of AMI account for 20% of all malpractice settlements paid on behalf of emergency physicians.
- As the spectrum of disease causing chest pain ranges from acute/life threatening to relatively benign symptoms, the challenge for clinicians caring for a patient with chest pain is to rapidly rule out those diagnoses associated with a high morbidity and mortality, whether in the ED, office, or inpatient setting. While much of the focus on chest pain is in ruling out myocardial ischemia, the practicing physician must

always consider multiple possible causes before embarking on an ischemic chest pain pathway.

TRIAGE AND INITIAL MANAGEMENT

- Initial management of patients presenting with chest pain involves rapid initial assessment to identify or exclude life-threatening etiologies that require immediate therapeutic interventions.
- The initial evaluation and treatment, which should be completed within 10 minutes of presentation, includes:
  - A brief, focused history emphasizing risk factors for cardiac ischemia
  - Initial vital signs (including measurement of blood pressure [BP] in both arms)
  - An electrocardiogram (ECG)
  - Initiation of continuous cardiac monitoring
  - Supplemental oxygen therapy at 2 L of oxygen/min by nasal cannula, indicated regardless of pulse oximetry reading to help increase arterial oxygenation and improve coronary oxygen delivery
  - Peripheral intravenous (IV) access
  - Initial laboratory testing
    - Complete blood count (CBC) with differential
    - Chemistry profile with calcium and magnesium
    - Cardiac enzymes—at least an initial troponin as well as total CPK and CK-MB isoform
    - Portable chest x-ray (CXR)
  - Other laboratory tests to consider in the ED setting if clinical suspicion based on disease prevalence, risk factors, signs, and symptoms:
    - *Brain-type natriuretic peptide (BNP)*—volume overload
    - Thyroid-stimulating hormone (TSH)—*hyperthyroidism*
    - D-*Dimer*—pulmonary embolus
    - *Serum and urine toxicology screening*—cocaine and other stimulants

- In some urban centers, cocaine-associated chest pain continues to be a significant problem causing MI and cardiomyopathy.
  - Coronary vasospasm and infarction can occur in the setting of otherwise normal coronary arteries.
  - Beta-blockers should be used with caution in this population due to potential worsening of chest pain through unopposed alpha stimulation.
  - First-line treatment generally consists of nitrates, aspirin, and benzodiazepines.
  - Calcium channel blockers as an additive to nitrate therapy can be used if there is evidence of ST elevation or depression on the ECG.
- Most patients tolerate 325 mg of aspirin well as a one-time dose in light of the proven benefits of antiplatelet therapy early in MI.
  - AMI is one of the diagnoses for which the Joint Commission on Accreditation of Healthcare Organizations (JCAHO) and the Centers for Medicare and Medicaid (CMS) jointly collect and report quality measures. Two JCAHO/CMS AMI core measures are relevant to patients presenting with undifferentiated chest pain possibly due to AMI: *aspirin on arrival* and *beta-blockers on arrival.*
- By the time the above steps are completed, the physician should interpret the ECG and direct further therapies and diagnostic workup. If the ECG demonstrates evidence of AMI, management is as per Chap. 23 of this book.
- If the ECG is nondiagnostic for ischemic pain and initial cardiac enzymes are negative, the clinician still needs to initiate therapies allowing for the possibility of an unstable coronary syndrome as the cause of chest pain.
  - With the exception of profound bradycardia (heart Rate <50 beats/min) or suspected cocaine use, most patients tolerate a small dose of short-acting beta-blocker. Care should also be taken, however, in those patients with prolonged PR intervals or evidence of high-degree A-V block.
  - Patients should receive either sublingual or topical nitroglycerin.
    - Notable exceptions include hypotension (ie, systolic BP <95 mm Hg), ECG evidence of right ventricular infarct, recent use of phosphodiesterase inhibitors (sildenafil, vardenafil, tadalafil), or critical aortic stenosis.
    - Relief of chest pain with nitroglycerin is nondiagnostic, as gastrointestinal causes (ie, esophageal spasm and reflux disease) may also be relieved with nitroglycerin.
    - If chest pain responds to SL or topical nitrates, and the patient is still experiencing pain, and a high index of suspicion for ischemia exists, then the physician may want to consider a continuous nitroglycerin drip titrated until the patient is chest pain free (see Chap. 22).
- Many physicians will include a trial of a fast-acting gastrointestinal agent such as magnesium bromide for heartburn which may help in diagnosis.
- If chest pain persists after the administration of the above measures, pain relief should be attempted with IV morphine. Morphine is not only an analgesic agent but a vasodilator, particularly in the pulmonary vasculature, and an anxiolytic.
- Further initial management and evaluation is tailored based on the findings from the physician's focused history and physical examination, the response to these initial therapies, and the results of the initial ECG, laboratory, and CXR.
- At the present time, ~22% of EDs in the United States have chest pain centers (CPCs) as a part of their treatment strategy for chest pain (CP).
  - The ideal patient for an ED-based chest pain center is considered low risk for a cardiovascular event with negative initial supporting tests (ie, a normal or unchanged ECG and negative first set of cardiac enzymes). Most CPCs utilize stress testing as the definitive portion of the protocol after serial cardiac enzymes are negative.
  - CPCs have shown similar outcomes with regard to morbidity and mortality from cardiovascular events when compared to standard hospital admission.
  - The cost savings to the patient in terms of charges differs from study to study but ranges anywhere from as little as $1000 to over $4000.

CLINICAL PRESENTATION, DIFFERENTIAL, MAKING THE DIAGNOSIS

- Multiple etiologies exist for the development of chest pain: They can broadly categorized as thoracic, intrathoracic, or extrathoracic (Table 21-1).
  - Thoracic causes generally refer to injury to the integument such as muscles, tendons, bones, ligaments, and nerves.
  - Intrathoracic causes of chest pain can include vascular infarction, injury, or insufficiency. Additional causes can also include infection and mucosal injury.
  - Extrathoracic causes include systemic illnesses, referred pain, and psychiatric etiologies.
- Patients may offer or should be prompted to describe the chest pain by several different characteristics, which may provide clues to the differential diagnosis.

TABLE 21-1   Causes of Chest Pain

THORACIC ETIOLOGIES

Musculoskeletal (10%–15% of adults presenting to ED)	Costochondritis; Tietze syndrome; sternalis syndrome; xiphoidalgia; spontaneous sternoclavicular subluxation; rib pain with reproducible tender spot on the costal margin; posterior chest wall pain due to herniated thoracic disc; costovertebral joint dysfunction
	Thoracic joint involvement with rheumatologic diseases including: osteoarthritis; rheumatoid arthritis, and ankylosing spondylitis
	Chest wall trauma, including muscle strain, rib fractures, contusions, and many others
	Tumors
Skin	Herpes zoster including acute prior to appearance of the rash and postherpetic neuralgia; postradiation neuralgia

INTRATHORACIC ETIOLOGIES

Cardiac	Acute myocardial infarction
	Myocardial ischemia, including stable and unstable angina
	Angina syndromes associated with normal coronary arteries: variant (Prinzmetal's) angina; cardiac syndrome X
	Inflammation/infection: pericarditis, myocarditis
	Pericardial effusion from any underlying etiology
	Congestive heart failure; rare causes include stress-induced or takotsubo cardiomyopathy
	Valvular heart disease, including: mitral valve prolapse, aortic stenosis
	Arrhythmias, most frequently atrial fibrillation, premature ventricular contractions
Vascular	Aortic dissection
	Pulmonary thromboembolism
	Pulmonary hypertension; cor pulmonale
	Pulmonary infarction
Pulmonary	Pneumothorax, including tension pneumothorax
	Inflammation of the pleural space (with or without pleural effusion), including empyema and pleuritis from various underlying causes
	Infection: pneumonia, bronchitis
	Cancer
Gastrointestinal	Esophageal: gastroesophageal reflux; spasm (achalasia, nutcracker esophagus) esophagitis (infectious, medication-induced); rupture

EXTRATHORACIC AND SYSTEMIC DISEASES

Rheumatologic	Fibromyalgia
	Sarcoidosis
Psychiatric (20% of adults presenting to ED)	Anxiety disorders, including primary, hyperventilation, and panic disorder
	Affective disorders/depression
	Somatiform disorders such as delusions
Hematologic	Sickle cell acute chest syndrome
Neurologic	Neuropathic pain, cervical disc disease
Referred visceral pain	Biliary, including cholangitis, cholecystitis and choledocholithiasis, pancreatitis, peptic ulcer disease

- ○ Onset (acute or gradual)
- ○ Severity (usually on a pain scale of 0–10)
- ○ Quality (sharp, stabbing, dull, and so forth)
- ○ Radiation of pain (eg, neck, jaw, arm, or back)
- ○ Accompanying symptoms (shortness of breath, nausea, diaphoresis, abdominal pain, dizziness, and so forth)
- ○ Aggravating or relieving factors
- The clinician should also question about risk factors relating not just to ischemic cardiac disease but also venous thromboembolism, dissection, and other potentially life-threatening etiologies of chest pain.
- The process of investigating symptoms requires correlation of key information, namely, the clinical history including risk factors, physical examination, ECG, CXR, and laboratory tests.
- Although diagnosis is usually carried out during conditions of uncertainty, often with incomplete and sometimes inconsistent information, nevertheless, expeditious identification of the correct diagnosis using the smallest number of expensive and risky tests can be achieved by assigning patients to one of three groups:
  - ○ *Low pretest probability* (no risk factors, story sounds like something else, no supporting initial data)
  - ○ *Moderate pretest probability* (risk factors present, story could be something else or convincing story without risk factors)
  - ○ *High pretest probability* (risk factors and convincing story)
- The history and physical examinations are just like other diagnostic tests, in that expert opinion and disease prevalence can assign a pretest probability.
- The clinician then determines whether the patient needs additional testing, based on whether the test will actually change the pretest probability. The sensitivity,

specificity, and positive predictive value of the test combined with the pretest probability determine the post-test probability. The predictive accuracy of tests depends on test characteristics and disease prevalence.

- Although exercise tolerance testing has been the most extensively studied, in general, additional testing for patients with very low pretest probabilities is more likely to result in more false-positive results and/or incidental findings than reliably improving the likelihood that the patient actually has the disorder.
  - Useful test properties have the following characteristics:
    - Presence of signs = *rule in* the disorder (↑ specificity, ↑ positive predictive value, ↑ likelihood ratio (LR) +)
    - Absence of signs = *rule out* the disorder (↑ sensitivity, ↑ negative predictive value, ↓ LR −)

ACUTE MI

- For AMI, features that *rule in* MI (with cardiac enzymes the gold standard) are
  - Chest pain radiating to both left and right arms (LR 7.1)
  - New ST-segment elevation ≥1 mm (LR 5.7–53.9)
  - Any ST-segment elevation (LR 11.2)
  - New conduction defect (LR 6.3)
- Features that *rule out* MI include
  - Pleuritic chest pain (LR 0.2)
  - Chest pain sharp or stabbing (LR 0.3)
  - Positional chest pain (LR 0.3)
  - Chest pain reproduced by palpation (LR 0.2–0.4)
- Use of these criteria does not include unstable angina or other conditions that might require intervention (Panju et al).

UNSTABLE ANGINA

- For unstable angina, more than 20 years ago, the coronary artery surgery study (CASS) (Table 21-2) developed a simple scheme for the classification of angina that can discriminate between patients with coronary artery disease and those with negative stress tests and coronary angiograms. Pretest probability is estimated based on the age, gender, characterization of chest pain, and risk factors (diabetes, smoking, hyperlipidemia, and Q waves on ECG).
  - *Typical angina (all three factors)*—(1) chest heaviness, pressure, tightness, or burning; (2) provoked by exercise or emotional stress or cold; and (3) relieved with rest. Typically, these symptoms last longer than 2 minutes and less than 20 minutes in duration (unless the patient is having an AMI). Dyspnea, nausea, vomiting, diaphoresis, presyncope, and/or palpitations may be associated symptoms.
  - *Probable angina*—two factors
  - *Probably not angina*—one factor
  - *Nonanginal pain*—zero factors
- Then the clinician uses the pretest probability that reflects the prevalence of disease in a given population to determine whether performing an exercise tolerance test will benefit the patient. Do the test only if it will change the pretest probability significantly or for prognostic purposes. Intermediate pretest patients should have noninvasive testing. Noninvasive testing is not recommended for low- or high-risk patients except
  - For prognostic purposes in high-risk patients
  - For frequent chest pain in low-risk patients
- If the patient needs a stress test, then the clinician must ask the question whether the patient can *safely* undergo a stress test. This means that the patient should not have
  - An unstable coronary process such as ACS, prolonged QT, significant arrhythmia
  - An acute process such as deep venous thrombosis (DVT), pulmonary embolism (PE), and dissection
  - Coexisting severe illness such as anemia, bronchospasm, pulmonary edema, febrile illness, thyrotoxicosis, and pheochromocytoma
  - Critical aortic stenosis or severe hypertrophic cardiomyopathy
- The best test for the patient (standard exercise ECG test using a treadmill or bicycle; exercise imaging study using mibi, thallium, or echocardiography; pharmacologic stress imaging study using adenosine, persantine, or dobutamine; and cardiac catheterization) is based on the ability of the

TABLE 21-2 Pretest Probability that Chest Pain is Angina

	NONANGINAL PAIN		ATYPICAL ANGINA		TYPICAL ANGINA	
Age	Men	Women	Men	Women	Men	Women
30–39	4	2	34	12	76	26
40–49	13	3	51	22	87	55
50–59	20	7	65	31	93	73
60–69	27	14	72	51	94	86

With permission from: Diamond GA, Forrester JS: Analysis of probability as an aid in the clinical diagnosis of coronary artery disease. *N Engl J Med.* 1979;300:1350.

patient to exercise, the presence of baseline ECG abnormalities, prior digitalis therapy or revascularization, and the need to localize ischemia or assess viability.

∘ Although there are significant differences in cost, the differences in predictive accuracy of these

tests are modest, due to all of them being highly sensitive for severe disease.
∘ See Fig. 21-1. The diagnostic workup for cardiac etiologies of chest pain.
∘ For evaluation and management of ischemic cardiac chest pain, see Chaps. 22 and 23.

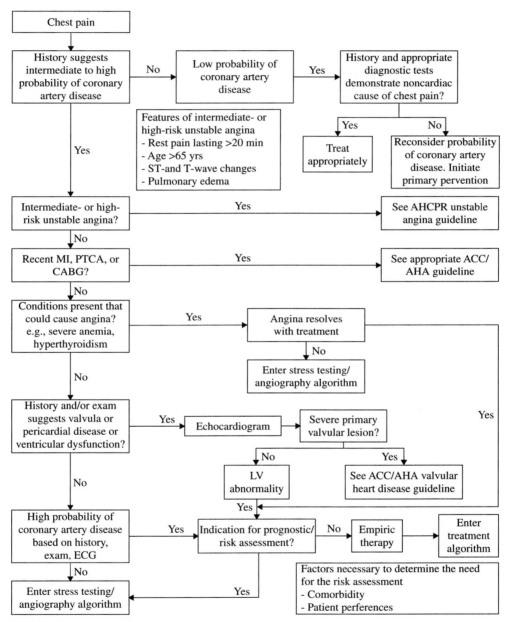

FIG. 21-1 Assessment of chest pain.
AHPCR, Agency for Healthcare Policy and Research; MI, myocardial infarction; PTCA, percutaneous transluminal coronary angioplasty; CABG, coronary artery bypass graft; ACC, American College of Cardiology; AHA, American Heart Association; LV; left ventricular; ECG, electrocardiogram.
Reproduced with permission from: Gibbons RJ, Chatterjee K, Daley J, et al. ACC/AHA/ACP-ASIM guidelines for the management of patients with chronic stable angina: a report of the American College of Cardiology/American Heart Association Task Force on Practice Guidelines (Committee on Management of Patients With Chronic Stable Angina) *J Am Coll Cardiol*. 1999;33:2092. (Copyright American College of Cardiology).

THORACIC AORTIC DISSECTION

- For thoracic aortic dissection, the studies are primarily retrospective reviews of nonindependently selected patients. A few physical findings may help *rule in* a thoracic dissection:
  - Focal neurologic deficit (LR + 6.6–33)
  - Pulse deficit (LR + 5.7)
- A prediction rule is based on (1) aortic pain characterized by severity, sudden onset, and tearing; (2) BP differential between two arms or pulse differential between arms; and (3) wide mediastinum.
  - *0 findings:* LR 0.1
  - *1 finding:* LR 0.5
  - *2 findings:* LR 5.3
  - *3 findings:* LR 66
- The patient who has suspected aortic dissection must urgently undergo a transesophageal echocardiogram, CT aortography, or direct aortic angiography to evaluate for dissection.
- Acute management includes admission to an intensive care unit (ICU), pain control and BP control with parenteral agents to achieve a systolic pressure of 100–120.
- Emergent vascular surgery and/or cardiothoracic surgery evaluation is necessary for any individual in whom the diagnosis of aortic dissection is being seriously entertained.

ACUTE PULMONARY EMBOLISM

- For acute PE, there are multiple clinical presentations and often nonspecific symptoms and signs.
  - Most patients have identifiable risk factors (PIOPED). For patients already hospitalized, hospitalization is a risk factor for acute PE.
  - When clinically suspected, the signs and symptoms depend on the size of the emboli.
    - Small to medium emboli are characteristically associated with dyspnea, chest pain, cough; tachypnea, and tachycardia in the majority. Mild fever <39°C is common and wheezing uncommon (<5%).
    - Massive emboli may cause syncope, chest pain, dyspnea, and signs of right ventricular dysfunction (right ventricular heave, RV S_3, increased jugular venous pressure [JVP], tricuspid regurgitation, accentuated P_2).
  - ECG is often abnormal but nonspecific. It is normal in 23% of patients with submassive acute PE and normal in 6% of patients with massive acute PE. $S_1Q_3T_3$ pattern was the first one described but there are many additional ECG findings in acute PE. It is clinically helpful chiefly in patients with no history of heart or lung disease.
  - Echocardiography will rarely visualize an acute PE and is usually normal despite PE. It is most useful for risk stratification and prognostication after the diagnosis of PE has been established.
  - CXR abnormalities occur in 84% of patients with acute PE even if no infarction is present. Elevation of hemi-diaphragm or atelectasis, effusion which is usually small and unilateral, and/or infiltrate, classically pleural based with a convex margin directed toward the hilum may be seen. Hampton's hump and oligemia are rarely seen.
  - D-Dimer has a high negative predictive value and a very low positive predictive value. It may be most useful for patients presenting to ED with no underlying comorbidities. An elevated D-Dimer is insufficient to diagnose PE in the inpatient setting.
  - The test reliability of ventilation/perfusion scans (V/Q) in patients with symptoms within the last 24 hours depends on the reading: high probability V/Q scans, LR + 18; intermediate, LR + 1.2; low, LR − 0.36; and normal or near normal LR − 0.10. V/Q scans are usually reserved for patients who cannot receive radiocontrast dye due to renal insufficiency. It is controversial whether V/Q scans are safer than chest PE protocol scans in pregnancy.

Chest PE protocol scans have emerged as the best screening test for PE. Chest PE protocol scans are superior to ventilation/perfusion imaging with a LR + 22, LR − 0.36. It is important to remember these studies have important limitations, which are as follows:
  - Detection of small isolated peripheral clots
  - Image quality decreased in patients with cardiovascular disease and morbid obesity
  - Sensitivity related to technical limitations (size, bolus), timing related to the onset of symptoms, and the human factor in interpretation
  - Pulmonary angiograms can identify peripheral or chronic emboli and emboli along the axial plane. Although the gold standard, pulmonary angiography is difficult to perform and expensive.

ACUTE PERICARDITIS

- For acute pericarditis, presentation depends on the etiology and whether a large effusion is present. Purulent pericarditis is characteristically an abrupt fulminant illness. Viral pericarditis may follow an upper respiratory infection, or may be associated with dyspnea or fever. Tuberculous pericarditis characteristically has an insidious onset and nonspecific symptoms. In addition to infectious disease, metastatic disease (lung, breast, melanoma), and autoimmune disease (systemic lupus erythematosus [SLE], rheumatoid arthritis) affect the presentation.

○ The history of chest pain is notably dull, stabbing, or aching and usually pleuritic. The pain may be brief, recurrent, waxing and waning in intensity usually over hours; aggravated by recumbency, cough, inspiration, or swallowing; and relieved by sitting up and leaning forward. The pain may radiate to the trapezius ridge but there may be a wide area of radiation. Sometimes the pain is felt at the cardiac apex synchronously with each heart beat.

○ The pericardial friction rub characteristically gets louder with inspiration and is best heard along the left sternal border but sometimes solely at the apex. A possible clue when the rub cannot be heard on examination is the association of fever with pain onset. Use the diaphragm of the stethoscope pressed firmly on the chest wall.

○ ECG findings may include
  ▪ A pattern of electrical alternans with beat-to-beat alternation of one or more components of the electrical tracing (usually the QRS complex);
  ▪ Low-voltage QRS, particularly in the setting of significant effusion;
  ▪ Evolution through four stages with acute pericarditis:
    • *Stage 1*—Diffuse ST elevation with reciprocal ST depression in leads aVR and V_1 and diffuse PR depression with reciprocal PR elevation in lead aVR
    • *Stage 2*—Normalization of ST and PR changes
    • *Stage 3*—Diffuse T-wave inversions
    • *Stage 4*—Normalization or persistence of diffuse T-wave inversions

○ Echocardiography (either transthoracic or transesophageal) remains the best method to visualize the pericardium.

○ Tamponade physiology must be ruled out by BP manometry during inspiration and expiration. The findings of a >10 mm Hg drop in BP recorded during inspiration in comparison to that recorded during exhalation is known as pulsus paradoxus and is diagnostic of tamponade physiology in the setting of a significant pericardial effusion.
  ▪ This is a medical emergency and must be referred immediately to a cardiologist for emergent pericardiocentesis.
  ▪ The internist caring for the patient should initiate intravenous fluids to increase right heart filling pressures and avoid the use of vasodilatory or negative chronotropic agents (beta-blockers, calcium channel blockers, etc).

ACUTE PNEUMOTHORAX

• Risk factors for acute pneumothorax include young tall individuals or those with connective tissue disorders, individuals with severe asthma or chronic obstructive pulmonary disease, or those who have had recent invasive procedures (such as central venous catheters).

• The presentation of sudden chest pain due to pneumothorax may have a Hammons crunch on physical examination and/or subcutaneous emphysema due to mediastinal air.

• The diagnosis of any clinically significant pneumothorax can most often be made from the CXR, preferably a posteroanterior (PA) and lateral also. In rare circumstances, a computed tomography (CT) scan of the chest may be needed to establish the diagnosis.

CONGESTIVE HEART FAILURE

• Congestive heart failure exacerbation primarily presents with dyspnea rather than chest pain unless there has been an antecedent MI.

• See Chaps. 29 and 30.

PULMONARY HYPERTENSION

• Patients with pulmonary hypertension experience chest pain related to exertion.

• The physical examination may reveal a giant "A" wave in the jugular venous pulsation, a loud pulmonary closure sound, and a right ventricular lift.

MITRAL VALVE PROLAPSE

• Although the chest pain in mitral valve prolapse (MVP) may mimic angina, the most common historical features are
  ○ Variable location and radiation with different episodes in the same patient
  ○ Spontaneous variation in symptom severity
  ○ Brief, fleeting chest pain, recurrent over a long time with inconsistent relationship to rest or exercise
  ○ Palpitations a prominent feature, often coexisting with the chest pain
  ○ Light-headedness, syncope, chronic fatigue, anxiety, and/or hyperventilation are more common with MVP than angina.

• Using the diaphragm of the stethoscope, the clinician should listen to the patient lying flat, turned to the left lateral position over the point of maximum impulse of

the left ventricle. In addition, the physician should listen with the patient sitting, standing, and squatting. At times the typical findings are only heard in one phase of respiration. The following may be suggestive of MVP:
  ○ No click or murmur
  ○ A single click, several clicks, usually in mid to late systole, but not always
  ○ A murmur, typically in mid to late systole, sometimes a "whoop" or "honk"

GASTROESOPHAGEAL REFLUX DISEASE

• One of the most common noncardiac causes of chest pain is gastroesophageal reflux disease (GERD), but this is a diagnosis of exclusion.
  ○ Clues to the diagnosis of GERD may include dyspepsia after eating a large meal, worsening symptoms while lying flat and excessive caffeine intake. Many patients with a final diagnosis of GERD will describe symptoms that worsened with exercise, usually after eating.
  ○ Remember that patients with gastrointestinal causes of chest pain may describe improvement in their symptoms after the administration of sublingual or topical nitroglycerin.
  ○ Patients with GERD can be initiated on a 4–6-week empiric therapeutic and diagnostic trial of a proton pump inhibitor and referred for follow-up with their primary care physician (PCP). Patients with ongoing symptoms of noncardiac chest pain of possible gastrointestinal etiology may need subsequent referral for a barium swallow/upper gastrointestinal series, esophagogastroduodenoscopy, or esophageal pH monitoring.

CARE TRANSITIONS

• There is no substitute for sound clinical intuition based on a thorough history and physical and review of the laboratory data, ECG, and CXR.
• If your institution does not possess a CPC for the evaluation of low-risk chest pain patients, you can refer to several risk assessment methods like the Goldman to identify those at moderate- to high risk for significant coronary artery disease. Those at low risk by risk factors and a low clinical suspicion for obstructive coronary artery disease (CAD) can be referred to their PCP for follow-up. PCP follow-up should focus on modifiable risk factors: cigarette smoking, control of hypertension, good control of blood sugar in diabetics, hyperlipidemia, and increasing exercise tolerance/weight loss.

BIBLIOGRAPHY

American Heart Association Heart and Stroke Statistics—2006 Update.
Brown KA. Prognostic value of thallium-201 myocardial perfusion imaging: a diagnostic tool comes of age. *Circulation.* 1991;83:363–381.
Diamond GA, Forrester JS. Analysis of probability as an aid in the clinical diagnosis of coronary artery disease. *N Engl J Med.* 1979;300:1350.
Gibler WB. Chest pain evaluation in the ED: beyond triage. *Am J Emerg Med.* 1994;12:121–122.
Goldman L, Cook EF, Brand DA, et al. A Computer protocol to predict myocardial infarction in emergency department patients with chest pain. *N Engl J Med.* 1988;318:797.
Goldman L, Weinberg M, Weisberg M, et al. A computer protocol to predict myocardial infarction in emergency department patients with chest pain. *N Engl J Med.* 988;318:797.
Hachamovich R, Berman DS, Shaw LJ, et al. Incremental prognostic value of myocardial perfusion SPECT for the prediction of cardiac death and myocardial infarction. *Circulation.* 1998;97:533–543. [published erratum *Circulation.* 1998;98:120.]
McCaig LF, Nawar EW. National Hospital Ambulatory Medical Care Survey: 2004 Emergency Department Summary. CDC Division of Health Care Statistics.
Panju AA, Hemmelgarn BR, Guyatt GH, et al. Is this patient having a myocardial infarction? *JAMA.* 1998;280:1256–1263.
PIOPED Investigators. Value of the ventilation/perfusion scan in acute pulmonary embolism. Results of the prospective investigation of pulmonary embolism diagnosis (PIOPED). *JAMA.* 1990;263:2753–2759.
Pope JH, Aufderheide TP, Ruthazer R, et al. Missed diagnosis of cardiac ischemia in the emergency department. *N Engl J Med.* 2000;342:1163.
Lettman NA, Sites FD, Shofer FS, et al. Congestive heart failure patients with chest pain: incidence and predictors of acute coronary syndrome. *Acad Emerg Med.* 2002;9:903.

22 SUSPECTED ANGINA
Aaron S. Wenger

EPIDEMIOLOGY/OVERVIEW

• Chest pain due to suspected coronary artery disease (CAD) is among the most common complaints addressed by hospitalists and constitutes one of the greatest challenges to healthcare systems worldwide.
  ○ CAD and its sequelae are the leading causes of death in developed countries. In the United States, heart disease accounted for ~700,000 deaths (28% of all deaths) in 2003.

○ Heart disease accounts for 8 cents of every dollar spent on healthcare in the United States, for a total annual cost estimated at 143 billion dollars.

○ Recent estimates put the prevalence of angina pectoris in the United States at 6.5 million persons affected, and the prevalence of acute myocardial infarction (MI) at 7.1 million persons affected.

○ Heart disease accounted for 4.4 million hospitalizations in 2004, 13% of all hospitalizations in the United States that year. Of these

- 17% (~750,00) were for acute MI
- 24% (~1.1 million or ~3.5% of all hospitalizations) were for suspected angina
- This chapter will discuss the approach to patients without acute coronary syndrome (see Chap. 23), but in whom after initial evaluation for chest pain (see Chap. 21), myocardial ischemia remains an important diagnostic consideration. These patients can be said to have suspected angina.

PATHOPHYSIOLOGY

- Angina pectoris denotes the subjective experience of chest pain secondary to myocardial ischemia, and is almost always secondary to CAD. It may, however, be due to nonatherosclerotic coronary vasospasm (Prinzmetal, or variant angina) or a complication of substance abuse (particularly cocaine).
- CAD (more precisely atherosclerotic coronary vascular disease) refers to the development of lipid-rich plaques in the walls of the coronary vessels. A significant role for inflammation (demonstrated by the infiltration of macrophages into atherosclerotic plaques with the formation of foam cells) is starting to be appreciated in this disease of dysregulated lipid metabolism exacerbated by unhealthy lifestyle choices (Table 22-1).
- The clinical presentation of CAD is characterized by two syndromes with distinct pathophysiologic underpinnings.
  ○ Chronic stable angina pectoris refers to classic anginal chest pain or its equivalents as a manifestation of myocardial ischemia secondary to an inability of stenotic coronary arteries to meet the oxygen demands of exercising heart muscle. It is typically relieved with

TABLE 22-1 Coronary Artery Disease Risk Factors

Age >55 in men or >65 in women
Current (or recent) cigarette smoking
Family history of MI or cardiac death at an early age
Hypertension
Hyperlipidemia
Chronic kidney disease
Diabetes mellitus is risk equivalent to a known prior history of coronary disease

MI, myocardial infarction.

the cessation of exertion, although a coronary vasodilator such as nitroglycerin may be required.
  ○ Acute coronary syndromes, on the other hand, are typically due to a rapid occlusion (or at least worsening of stenosis) secondary to plaque damage with resultant platelet plug and thrombus formation. The ischemic discomfort of an acute coronary syndrome is typically more severe than that of stable angina, and tends to be much more difficult to alleviate.

CLINICAL PRESENTATION/ DIFFERENTIAL/MAKING THE DIAGNOSIS

- Please refer to Chap. 21 for the differential diagnosis of chest pain.
- Anginal chest pain can be classified as typical angina, atypical angina, or noncardiac chest pain (Table 22-2).
- Only 60% to 70% of patients with myocardial ischemia present with chest discomfort. The remaining patients present with "silent" ischemia or with an "anginal equivalent," the most common being shortness of breath.
  ○ Other anginal equivalents may include nausea and vomiting, epigastric pain, syncope, palpitations, and occasionally ventricular arrhythmia and/or sudden cardiac death.
  ○ Supraventricular tachycardias including atrial fibrillation are rather rare as manifestations of coronary disease and myocardial ischemia.
  ○ Nonclassic presentations of myocardial ischemia are more likely among diabetics, women, and the elderly.
- The absence of chest pain in hospitalized patients later determined to have myocardial ischemia or infarction conveys significant prognostic information, including increased in-hospital mortality (23% vs. 9%), decreased likelihood of diagnosing MI, and decreased likelihood of receiving thrombolysis and/or percutaneous coronary intervention (PCI).
- Table 22-3 provides a rubric for CAD risk stratification on the basis of historic factors, which can then be utilized to assist the clinician in navigating the algorithm in Fig. 22-1.

TABLE 22-2 Characteristics of Typical Angina Pectoris

Substernal pressure-like discomfort
Brought on by exertion or distress
Alleviated by rest and/or nitroglycerin
Typical angina has all three of the above characteristics
Atypical angina has two of the above characteristics
Noncardiac chest pain has one or none of the above characteristics

SOURCE: Gibbons RJ, Chatterjee K, Daley J, et al. ACC/AHA/ACP-ASIM guidelines for the management of patients with chronic stable angina: a report of the American College of Cardiology/American Heart Association Task Force on Practice Guidelines (Committee on Management of Patients With Chronic Stable Angina) *J Am Coll Cardiol.* 1999;33:2092.

TABLE 22-3   Pretest Risk Stratification on the Basis of Chest Pain Character (see Tables 22-1 and 22-2)

	TYPICAL ANGINA	ATYPICAL ANGINA	NONCARDIAC CHEST PAIN
No risk factors	Intermediate risk	Low risk	Low risk
1–2 risk factors	Intermediate to high risk	Intermediate risk	Intermediate risk
>2 risk factors*	High risk	High risk	Intermediate to high risk

*Or a prior history of coronary artery disease or one of its risk equivalents (diabetes mellitus, peripheral vascular disease, and cerebrovascular disease).

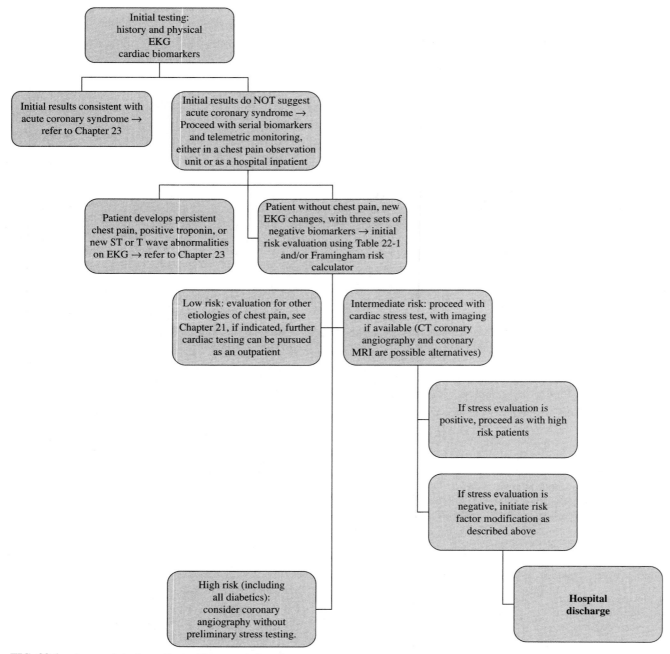

FIG. 22-1   Approach to the patient with suspected angina.

◦ In some cases, the initial workup may need to include assessment for some of the risk factors described in Table 22-1. Useful tests may include a fasting lipid panel, fasting blood glucose, serum creatinine, and hemoglobin A1C.

- The protocol in Fig. 22-1 may be recommended as a general approach to the patient with suspected angina, although obviously modifications may be required based on the multiple mitigating factors discussed above and the hospitalist's clinical judgment.

- All patients presenting with chest pain should immediately undergo electrocardiography (ECG). Unfortunately, while the initial ECG may reveal findings suggestive of an acute coronary syndrome (and thus has reasonable specificity, and, in the right patient population, positive predictive value), its sensitivity for the diagnosis of myocardial ischemia ranges from only 20% to 60%. The value of ECG findings alone for this purpose is substantially lower than biochemical diagnosis using troponin except in patients presenting with frank acute ST-segment elevation MI (STEMI).

- The main role of the ECG in the evaluation of suspected angina is to identify those patients with acute STEMI (who require immediate revascularization) and to suggest or support the role of myocardial ischemia as an etiology for the patient's chest discomfort. Thus, serial assays for serum markers of myocardial damage constitute the mainstay of contemporary diagnostic testing for myocardial ischemia in patients who do not meet initial criteria for an acute coronary syndrome.

- Contrary to frequently held opinion, there is very little difference between the kinetics of the initial rise in troponin and those of creatine kinase-MB (CK-MB) when newer assays for troponin are used. Troponin will be positive as early in the course of an acute coronary syndrome as CK-MB, but will remain positive for longer after the event.

- Given troponin's higher sensitivity and specificity, there is little clinical utility in routinely measuring CK and CK-MB. This is reflected in the American College of Cardiology/American Heart Association (ACC/AHA) guidelines for diagnosis of MI, which support the use of CK and CK-MB only when troponin testing is not available at a given facility. One additional use may be to clarify the timing of a coronary event in a patient with positive troponin and an unclear clinical history to differentiate between a recent and more temporally distant myocardial injury.

- The AHA/ACC definition of MI requires two measurements of troponin at least 6 hours apart. However, more recent studies suggest that greater than 80% of patients with MI will have a positive troponin measurement by 4 hours postpresentation. Therefore, a reasonable compromise would be to measure troponin at presentation, 4 hours post presentation, and 8 hours postpresentation. Obviously costeffectiveness would increase by omitting the third measurement if the first two show a pattern characteristic of MI.

- Although the specificity of troponin for MI in the clinical context of suspected angina is established, there are a number of other conditions which can cause elevations in this biomarker (Table 22-4).

TRIAGE AND INITIAL MANAGEMENT

- Except where absolutely contraindicated, all patients with suspected angina should be treated with aspirin and beta-blockers within 24 hours of presentation (see Chap. 21).

- Evaluation of cardiovascular risk factors and optimizing their management must be started during the hospital stay.
  ◦ There is substantial evidence linking cardiovascular prognosis in diabetic patients to the success of their glycemic control. All patients with diabetes and suspected angina should have their glycosylated hemoglobin A1c measured at the time of admission. This will facilitate optimization of the patient's home regimen for diabetes either during hospitalization or at the first postdischarge visit with the primary care physician (PCP).
    ▪ Given that there is a significant body of evidence supporting improved survival in diabetic CAD patients managed with insulin, this should be discussed with diabetic patients with suspected angina found to have CAD during their hospitalization. This does not necessarily need to be initiated prior to discharge, but an initial in-hospital discussion may facilitate such a therapeutic maneuver by the patient's PCP.
  ◦ Every patient evaluated for suspected angina should undergo fasting lipid testing (unless such results are available from within the 3 months preceding admission) and have therapy either initiated or titrated appropriately depending on comorbidities and the results of diagnostic testing for CAD.
  ◦ Hypertension must be managed aggressively in patients with CAD or significant risk thereof. Recent National Institutes of Health (NIH) (JNC-7, NHLBI) guidelines recommend control of blood pressure to less than 120/75 in patients with

TABLE 22-4 Elevated Troponin without Myocardial Infarction

There are a number of disease states which can lead to elevated troponin without the classic substrate of myocardial infarction secondary to atherosclerotic coronary stenosis or occlusion. Generally, the magnitude of troponin release in these confounding conditions is lower than that seen in acute coronary syndromes, but this is obviously more a tendency than a rule. Given that there is substantial epidemiologic and pathophysiologic overlap between some of the above conditions and coronary atherosclerosis, it is necessary to keep an open mind and open differential diagnosis when evaluating patients with mildly elevated troponin.

Chronic kidney disease
- Asymptomatic chronic elevations of serum troponin are not uncommon in patients with chronic kidney disease, particularly those with end-stage renal disease (ESRD).
- This elevation is much more common with troponin T than with troponin I, a potential advantage of the latter isoform for diagnosing MI in this patient population.
- Of note, the sensitivity and specificity of CK-MB for MI in patients with chronic kidney disease is confounded much more severely than troponin I.

Pulmonary disease
- Any pulmonary condition associated with right heart strain can cause these myocytes to release troponin. This has been observed with some frequency in patients with acute pulmonary embolism, and less commonly in patients with pulmonary hypertension or exacerbation of chronic obstructive pulmonary disease (COPD).

Catecholamine excess
- Autonomic nervous system dysfunction with abnormally elevated catecholamine release is posited as the explanation for the release of troponin from non-necrotic myocardium in conditions such as acute stroke and transient (stress-induced) cardiomyopathy.

Nonischemic myocardial injury
- Inflammatory
  ○ Myocarditis
  ○ Pericarditis
  ○ Sarcoidosis
  ○ Status postcardiac transplant
- Infiltrative
  ○ Amyloidosis
- Traumatic
  ○ Mechanical, as in myocardial contusion secondary to blunt trauma
  ○ Electrical; typically postdefibrillatory, but can also occur through accidental electrical trauma
- Chemical
  ○ Exposure to cardiotoxic agents such as anthracycline chemotherapy agents

Non-atherosclerotic myocardial ischemia ("demand ischemia")
- Critical illness, particularly sepsis and SIRS; frequently causes elevations in serum troponin. This may have prognostic significance, as at least one study has demonstrated substantially increased mortality in patients with sepsis and positive troponin.
- Tachycardia of any etiology has been rarely associated with elevated serum troponins in otherwise healthy patients with normal coronary arteriograms.
- Left ventricular hypertrophy may lead to demand ischemia and mild elevations in serum troponin through several mechanisms.
- Coronary vasospasm (Prinzmetal angina) can be severe and prolonged enough to lead to troponin release through the traditional mechanism of myocardial necrosis.

Chronic heart failure
- Patients with heart failure of nonischemic etiology may still have mildly elevated troponin due to myocardial strain and cardiac remodeling with myocyte apoptosis.

diabetes or any form of atherosclerotic vascular disease.
○ The inpatient hospitalization can be an excellent opportunity to initiate nicotine cessation efforts, possibly including nicotine replacement therapy (although this should be deferred until significant coronary stenosis is ruled out).

DISEASE MANAGEMENT STRATEGIES

- This section is devoted to the major modalities of diagnostic testing available for the identification of CAD in patients presenting with chest pain. Usually, this testing is performed in the inpatient/observation setting. However, at the discretion of the hospitalist, low-risk patients and intermediate-risk patients with atypical or noncardiac chest pain who rule out for MI with serial negative troponins may be considered for further testing as an outpatient.
- Most of the data on testing are from studies of men. Testing in women has a lower predictive value for the following reasons:
  ○ Lower disease prevalence
  ○ Suboptimal performance on stress tests, especially by elderly women
  ○ Higher false-positive ST depression
  ○ More false-negative pharmacologic studies (Echo, single-photon emission computed tomography [SPECT], positron emission tomography [PET])

• *Cardiac catheterization without preliminary noninvasive testing*—The negative predictive value of noninvasive testing in high-risk patients is too low to make these tests diagnostically useful. In patients with suspected angina and a high risk of CAD, noninvasive testing should be bypassed in favor of early catheterization, although exercise treadmill testing (ETT) may serve a prognostic purpose in such patients. The AHA/ACC guidelines recommend cardiac catheterization in high-risk patients if there is a high pretest probability of three vessel disease or left main disease.

 ◦ Diabetic patients should be treated with a very low threshold of suspicion for CAD, even if they present with atypical symptoms. The prevalence of significant CAD is very high in this population. Noninvasive testing has utility in prognosis and planning further therapy, although early cardiac catheterization for diagnosis and possible therapeutic intervention is reasonable in diabetic patients with angina.

 ◦ End-stage renal disease and peripheral vascular disease are considered CAD equivalents in the most recent recommendations of the NIH lipid management group. Noninvasive testing with ETT may provide prognostic information, but the high likelihood of a positive test often leads to additional invasive catheter-based studies. The chief drawback to cardiac catheterization in these patients is the risk of complications of the procedure itself, including the risk of contrast-induced nephropathy (CIN).

 ▪ CIN is particularly significant in that many of the patients at greatest risk for CAD, such as diabetics or patients with significant chronic kidney disease, are also at greatest risk of nephrotoxicity from iodinated contrast administration.

 ▪ In addition to the usual methods of preventing CIN (see Chap. 82), one modification which may be useful is to request that the cardiologist perform selective coronary angiography without ventriculography, thereby greatly reducing the total amount of contrast necessary to perform the procedure.

• *Cardiac stress testing* as a diagnostic modality initially consisted of electrocardiographic monitoring during exercise- or drug-induced elevations in heart rate and/or cardiac output. Exercise stress testing (EST) provides the following information:

 ◦ The presence of ischemia (in a standardized, validated, easy to perform, inexpensive protocol)

 ◦ Functional capacity (reproducible workload that induces ischemia)

 ◦ Prognosis (exercise capacity, hemodynamic response).

• Positive test results assess multiple data.

 ◦ ECG changes (ST depressions >2 mm are never falsely positive)

 ◦ Exertional hypotension (multivessel disease)

 ◦ Chest pain (angina or nonanginal)

 ◦ Slower than expected fall in heart rate at recovery

 ◦ Delay in fall of systolic blood pressure (SBP) at recovery

 ◦ Frequent ventricular ectopy

 ◦ The Duke treadmill score improves prognostic accuracy, especially in women.

 ▪ Duke treadmill score = Exercise time (minutes based on the Bruce protocol) – (5 × maximum ST-segment deviation in mm) – (4 × exercise angina).

 ▪ Exercise angina is scored as 0 = none, 1 = nonlimiting, and 2 = exercise limiting.

 ▪ Risk classification based on the Duke treadmill score—low-risk score ≥ +5; moderate-risk score –10 to +4; High-risk score ≤ –11.

• While the accuracy of stress testing has been significantly augmented by addition of imaging modalities, the basic stress ECG is the foundation for further understanding stress testing in general. The American College of Cardiology (ACC) has published a very thorough clinical practice guideline on stress testing, most recently updated in 2002. Briefly summarized, the ACC makes the following recommendations regarding the use of cardiac (ECG) stress testing (see also Table 22-5):

TABLE 22-5   American College of Cardiology Clinical Practice Guideline on Stress Testing

Class I (see footnote) Class I–Conditions for which there is evidence or general agreement that a given procedure or treatment is useful and effective. Class IIa–Weight of evidence/opinion is in favor of usefulness/efficacy. Class IIb–Usefulness/efficacy is less well established by evidence/opinion.	Patients at intermediate risk (see Table 22-3 for more information regarding determination of pretest risk) of having obstructive coronary artery disease as a cause of their chest pain Diagnosis of Prinzmetal (variant, vasospastic) angina Patients at low or high risk of having obstructive coronary artery disease as a cause of their chest pain; patients with LVH; and some patients with digoxin use (these conditions reduce the utility of stress testing as discussed below; stress ECG should *not* be used at all in patients on digoxin with >1 mm of ST depression at baseline)
Class III–Conditions for which there is evidence and/or general agreement that the procedure/treatment is not useful/effective and in some cases may be harmful.	Patients with pre-excitation syndromes (e.g. Wolff-Parkinson-White syndrome), ventricular pacing, >1 mm ST depression at baseline, and LBBB

ECG, electrocardiogram; LBBB, left bundle branch block; LVH, left ventricular hypertrophy.

○ Meta-analyses of studies evaluating the diagnostic utility of the stress ECG in populations without prior MI (the epidemiologically significant "diagnostic dilemma" group) yielded a mean sensitivity of 67% and a mean specificity of 72%, using one millimeter of horizontal or downward ST depression as the discriminant value. This equates to a diagnostic accuracy of 69%.

○ The sensitivity of any modality of cardiac stress testing is directly proportional to the severity of heart disease in the tested population.

○ The use of beta-blockers and antianginal medications can compromise the sensitivity of both standard ETT and ETT with imaging.

○ The following factors decrease specificity of cardiac stress testing: valvular heart disease; Wolff-Parkinson-White (WPW) syndrome, left ventricular hypertrophy, resting ST depression, and concurrent digoxin use.

○ Left bundle branch block (LBBB) or paced rhythms render the stress ECG nondiagnostic. Right bundle branch block (RBBB) renders ST depression in leads V_{1-3} uninterpretable, but the test should still have diagnostic utility in leads V_{5-6}, II, and aVF.

• *Cardiac stress testing with imaging:* In order to improve the yield of useful information, cardiac stress tests may include some sort of myocardial imaging, with the most common options being nuclear perfusion scanning and echocardiography. There are stress modalities utilizing cardiac magnetic resonance imaging (MRI), but these remain investigational and limited in their availability. Cardiac stress testing using PET is somewhat better established, but even less widely available than cardiac MRI. It is also quite time consuming and expensive compared to other modalities, without a significant advantage in diagnostic or prognostic accuracy.

○ A significant advantage of cardiac stress imaging over the basic stress ECG is that most of the confounding factors to stress ECG testing described above are negated by the ability to visualize myocardial wall motion and/or perfusion.

○ Myocardial perfusion imaging (MPI) uses tracers (SPECT mibi, PET rubidium 82) that are taken up by myocardial cells based on perfusion and viability.
  ▪ Initial distribution is based on myocardial blood flow.
  ▪ Images 3–4 hours later reflect viability not related to flow.
  ▪ An initial defect that resolves indicates viable myocardium and a perfusion defect.
  ▪ A defect on both initial and delayed images indicates myocardial scarring.

○ MPI using radionuclides include thallium and technetium.
  ▪ Both can have problems with image distortion or attenuation of images.

▪ Due to the shorter half-life of technetium, it is poorer at assessing functional viability.

○ Stress echocardiography produces images while the patient is at rest and during stress. A positive test detects the development or worsening of wall motion abnormalities. Function and viability can be assessed either with exercise or with pharmacologic agents (dobutamine).

○ Local availability influences preferred imaging study. In general, stress echocardiography has a higher specificity, better evaluates cardiac function, is shorter, and less expensive. Stress mibi or thallium has a higher sensitivity, better accuracy if there are multiple wall motion abnormalities, and a higher technical success rate.

○ Three pharmacologic agents can be used to provoke ischemia for patients unable to exercise.
  ▪ Dobutamine, a positive inotropic agent, through increased myocardial work
  ▪ Adenosine, a vasodilator, by increasing flow in coronaries without disease, thereby unmasking a coronary stenosis
  ▪ Dipyridamole, also a vasodilator

○ A normal stress MPI study portends a good prognosis even in those patients with known CAD, with a rate of cardiac death or MI as low as 0.9% per year.

○ Table 22-6 compares diagnostic performance of the various modalities of cardiac stress imaging. There are two significant caveats regarding the reported accuracy of these different modalities.
  ▪ They are studied in patients judged to have an intermediate pretest probability of CAD, the group of patients for whom cardiac stress tests were designed and may be expected to perform best. For various reasons, including medicolegal considerations and either incomplete clinical information or vagaries in the interpretation of that information, these tests are frequently used in a lower risk population. As discussed in the section on the stress ECG above, cardiac stress tests in such a population would be expected to have diminished accuracy, particularly in terms of their specificity. Using cardiac stress testing of any

TABLE 22-6 Sensitivity and Specificity of Various Modalities of Cardiac Stress Imaging

MODALITY	SENSITIVITY	SPECIFICITY
Stress ECG	68%	77%
Stress echocardiography	76%	88%
Stress SPECT MPI	88%	77%
Stress thallium MPI	79%	73%
Stress PET	91%	82%

ECG, electrocardiogram; MPI, myocardial perfusion imaging; PET, positron emission tomography; SPECT, single photon emission computed tomography.

TABLE 22-7   Verification Bias

- *Verification bias*, also known as workup bias, describes the confounding effect introduced when a diagnostic test under study is used to determine who will receive the "gold standard" test to which the studied test is being compared.
- The verification bias under discussion in this chapter occurs when only patients with positive stress tests receive coronary angiography. Thus, anyone with a false-negative stress test will not receive the gold standard test, and will not be included in the comparison group. This will artificially improve the sensitivity of the stress test. Conversely, anyone with a false-positive test *will* receive the gold standard test. This will by definition be negative, artificially worsening the specificity of the test under examination.
- The ethical and logistical dilemma introduced by verification bias in planning research studies is substantial, in that anyone enrolling must agree to undergo both the studied test *and* the gold standard test, regardless of the outcome of the initial test. This obviously increases considerably the expense of the study, and, when the gold standard test is invasive like coronary angiography, the risk to patients. This is why, to date, there have been very few studies of the diagnostic accuracy of stress testing designed in such a way as to eliminate verification bias.

modality in a low-risk population will increase the number of false-positives. This accounts for the class IIb recommendation stress testing received from the ACC in a low-risk population.

- The majority of meta-analyses of the diagnostic accuracy of cardiac stress testing do not eliminate primary studies confounded by verification bias (Table 22-7).
- See Table 22-8 for limitations of and contraindications to the various modalities of stress testing.
- *Alternatives to cardiac stress testing*—Cardiac catheterization is no longer the only diagnostic modality available for evaluating patients with suspected angina in whom all stress testing modalities were inadequate or contraindicated (see Table 22-8).
  - Computed tomography coronary angiography, in particular, has performed excellently as a diagnostic test, with sensitivity ranging approximately from 85% to 90% and a specificity typically greater than 90%.
  - Coronary MRA has a similar specificity, but its sensitivity is lower.
  - The advantages of PET and/or CT scans include

- Computed tomography scan corrects images created from emissions from the radionuclide tracer so no attenuation artifacts related to obesity, breast tissue
- Fast (approximately 40 minutes)
- Capable of assessing function and viability (low ejection fraction(EF), cardiomyopathy)
- Performed without requiring patients to put their hands over their head.
  - The disadvantages of CT, PET, and MRI cardiac imaging include
  - Expense
  - Inability to create exercise images
  - The risk of CIN (contrast-enhanced CT) and nephrogenic systemic fibrosis (gadolinium-enhanced MRA in patients with CKD)
  - The inability to perform PCI without subsequent cardiac catheterization and additional exposure to iodinated contrast
- Usually left ventricular function can be estimated by imaging stress tests. Patients with CAD and left ventricular systolic dysfunction (LVEF <40%) should be treated with either an angiotensin-converting enzyme (ACE) inhibitor or angiotensin receptor blocker (ARB),

TABLE 22-8   Limitations and Contraindications to Stress Testing

MODALITY	LIMITATIONS	CONTRAINDICATIONS
Exercise echocardiography	■ Decreased accuracy in patients with existing wall motion abnormalities ■ Moderate likelihood of inadequate images leading to increased numbers of nondiagnostic studies, particularly in obese or emphysematous patients	■ Inability to complete test ■ Severe COPD, while not an absolute contraindication, renders the likelihood of a technically inadequate study very high
Dobutamine echocardiography	In addition to limitations of exercise echo: ■ ECG less accurate than in patients with exercise stress	■ Aortic aneurysm ■ Recent MI ■ LV outflow tract obstruction ■ History of ventricular arrhythmia or severe cardiomyopathy ■ Systemic HBP
Exercise nuclear MPI	■ Diminished specificity in female patients due to "breast artifact" ■ Diminished specificity in patients with LBBB	■ Inability to complete test
Adenosine or dipyridamoleI nuclear MP	Limitations of exercise nuclear MPI plus: ■ Diminished specificity in patients with a ventricular pacemaker ■ Caffeine alters hemodynamic response	■ Hypotension ■ Sick sinus syndrome or high-grade AV nodal block ■ Severe COPD or asthma (bronchospasm may be reversible with aminophylline) ■ Concurrent oral dipyridamole therapy

except when contraindicated. It is important to document specific contraindications to both ACE inhibitor and ARB if the patient has an LVEF <40% and is not discharged on one of these medications.

CARE TRANSITIONS

- The results of any inpatient testing should be conveyed to the patient's PCP prior to the first posthospital visit.
- For all patients with CAD, close follow-up in the primary care environment is even more important, as the goals for management of hypertension (HTN), diabetes, and hyperlipidemia are more intensive in patients with coronary disease.

BIBLIOGRAPHY

Adams JE III, Bodor GS, Davila-Roman VG, et al. Cardiac troponin I: A marker with a high specificity for cardiac injury. *Circulation.* 1993:88;101–106.

American Heart Association. *Heart Disease and Stroke Statistics—2005 Update.* Dallas, TX: American Heart Association; 2005.

Braunwald E, Antman EM, Beasley JW, et al. ACC/AHA 2002 guideline update for the management of patients with unstable angina and non–ST-segment elevation myocardial infarction: a report of the American College of Cardiology/American Heart Association Task Force on Practice Guidelines (Committee on the Management of Patients With Unstable Angina). 2002. Available at: http://www.acc.org/qualityandscience/clinical/guidelines/unstable/incorporated/UA_incorporated.pdf

Canto JG, Frederick PD, Lambrew CT, et al. Prevalence, clinical characteristics, and mortality among patients with myocardial infarction presenting without chest pain. *JAMA.* 2000;283:3223–3229.

Cheitlin MD, Armstrong WF, Aurigemma GP, et al. ACC/AHA/ASE 2003 guideline update for the clinical application of echocardiography: a report of the American College of Cardiology/American Heart Association Task Force on Practice Guidelines (ACC/AHA/ASE Committee to Update the 1997 Guidelines for the Clinical Application of Echocardiography). 2003. American College of Cardiology Web Site. Available at: http://www.acc.org/qualityandscience/clinical/guidelines/echo/index_clean.pdf

Gibbons RJ, Abrams J, Chatterjee K, et al. ACC/AHA 2002 guideline update for the management of patients with chronic stable angina: a report of the American College of Cardiology/American Heart Association task force on practice guidelines (Committee to Update the 1999 Guidelines for the Management of Patients with Chronic Stable Angina). 2002. Available at http://www.acc.org/qualityandscience/clinical/guidelines/stable/stable_clean.pdf

Gibbons RJ, Balady GJ, Bricker T, et al. ACC/AHA 2002 guideline update for exercise testing: a report of the American College of Cardiology/American Heart Association Task Force on Practice Guidelines (Committee on Exercise Testing). 2002. American College of Cardiology Web site. Available at: http://www.acc.org/qualityandscience/clinical/guidelines/exercise/exercise_clean.pdf

Jaffe AS, Naslund U, Apple FS, et al. It's time for change to a troponin standard. *Circulation.* 2000;102:1216–1220.

Klocke FJ, Baird, MG, Lorell BH, et al. ACC/AHA/ASNC guidelines for the clinical use of cardiac radionuclide imaging: a report of the American College of Cardiology/American Heart Association Task Force on Practice Guidelines (ACC/AHA/ASNC Committee to Revise the 1995 Guidelines for the Clinical Use of Radionuclide Imaging). 2003. American College of Cardiology Web Site. Available at: http://www.acc.org/qualityandscience/clinical/guidelines/radio/index.pdf

Macrae AR, Kavsak PA, Lustig V, et al. Assessing the requirement for the 6-hour interval between specimens in the American Heart Association classification of myocardial infarction in epidemiology and clinical research studies. *Clin Chem.* 2006;52:812–818.

Schuijf DJ, Bax JJ, Shaw LJ, et al. Meta-analysis of comparative diagnostic performance of magnetic resonance imaging and multislice computed tomography for noninvasive coronary angiography. *Am Heart J.* 2006;151(2):404–411.

Swap CJ, Nagurney JT. Value and limitations of chest pain history in the evaluation of patients with suspected acute coronary syndromes. *JAMA.* 2005;294:2623–2629.

23 ACUTE CORONARY SYNDROMES

Hacho Bohossian

This chapter will focus on the management of acute coronary syndromes (ACS) once the diagnosis has been established (see Chaps. 21 and 22).

TRIAGE AND INITIAL MANAGEMENT

- ACS describes the presentation of a patient with unstable ischemic chest pain characterized by rest angina, new angina, and/or increasing angina that is more frequent and longer in duration than previously experienced.
- ACS itself can be furthermore divided into three entities based on the echocardiographic (ECG) findings.
  ○ ~30% are ST-elevation (Q-wave) myocardial infarction (STEMI)
  ○ ~25% are non-ST elevation (non–Q-wave) myocardial infarction (NSTEMI)
  ○ ~45% are unstable angina (UA)

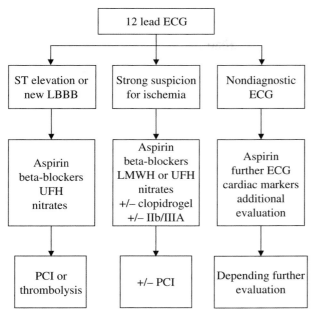

FIG. 23-1 Initial approach to suspected ACS.

- The difference between NSTEMI and UA is that the former has prolonged ischemia leading to elevation of cardiac marker; in the latter ischemia is transient and cardiac markers often remain normal. The two conditions are thus indistinguishable in the first 12–18 hours after presentation.
- Because the initial management of STEMI (patients benefit from reperfusion therapy) and NSTEMI are somewhat different, each will be discussed separately. Figure 23-1 outlines the initial approach to suspected ACS.
- Several best practices have been demonstrated to improve patient outcomes, and are embodied in the American College of Cardiology/American Heart Association (ACC/AHA) task force recommendations and the Joint Commission on Accreditation of Healthcare Organizations' (JCAHO's) core measures for the management of acute myocardial infarction (AMI) (*noted throughout the chapter in italics*) (Table 23-1).

TABLE 23-1 JCAHO Acute MI Core Measures

Aspirin on arrival
Aspirin prescribed on discharge
Beta-blockers on arrival
Beta-blocker on discharge
Angiotensin converting enzyme-I/angiotensin receptor blocker
  (ACE-I/ARB) for left ventricular systolic dysfunction (LVSD)
Adult smoking cessation advice/counseling
Mean time to thrombolysis—30 minutes or less
Mean time to PCI—120 minutes or less
Decrease in inpatient mortality

STEMI

- As it is obvious from its definition, the hallmark of STEMI is the presence of ST elevations of at least 1 mm in two contiguous leads. In addition, two other groups of patients are considered to have STEMI in the absence of true ST elevations.
  - Patients with a new left bundle branch block (LBBB)
  - Patients with acute true posterior myocardial infarction
    - The 12-lead ECG typically shows a tall R in V_1, and reciprocal ST depression and T elevation in V_{1-2}, often associated with concomitant inferior infarction. Acute true posterior myocardial infarction may be confirmed with obtaining additional V_{7-9} leads (or esophageal leads) showing ST elevation.
    - It is important to recognize right ventricular myocardial infarction that may be associated with inferior-posterior MI in 30% to 50% of patients. Despite clear lung fields, these patients may present with elevated jugular venous pressures, hypotension, and sometimes shock. All patients with inferior MI should have right-sided ECG precordial leads testing. The diagnosis of right ventricular MI using ECG criteria of ST-segment elevation of ≥ 1 mV in the right precordial leads V_4 can be confirmed by echocardiography. The initial proper management includes optimization of ventricular preload by volume loading, rate, and rhythm control, as well as avoidance of diuretics, nitrates, and vasodilators (which ordinarily would be prescribed for patients with left ventricular pump failure).
- Once the diagnosis is established, risk stratification may further identify patients at the highest risk and thus most likely to benefit from aggressive management. The thrombolysis in myocardial infarction (TIMI) risk score (Fig. 23-2) is a fairly widely used system to assess risk of in-hospital mortality.
- The major goal of initial therapy in STEMI is to relieve of ischemic pain and stabilization of hemodynamic status while assessment for thrombolysis or percutaneous coronary intervention (PCI) is being made. Hospitalists work with cardiologists and sometimes cardiac surgeons to determine the best strategy of care. Table 23-2 summarizes initial medical therapy for STEMI.
- The question of who benefits from reperfusion is complex and requires multidisciplinary teamwork. Multiple randomized trials have shown improved survival with PCI as compared to thrombolysis. The ACC/AHA task force has made the following recommendations regarding invasive therapy for STEMI:

Clinical Risk Indicators	Points
Historical	
Age	
>75	3
65–74	2
History of DM, HTN, or angina	1
Examination	
SBP <100 mm Hg	3
Heart rate >100/min	2
Killip class II–IV	2
Weight <67 kg	1
Presentation	
Anterior ST elevation or LBBB	1
Time to reperfusion therapy >4 hours	1
Total possible points	14

Prediction of In-Hospital Mortality With TIMI Risk Score for STEMI

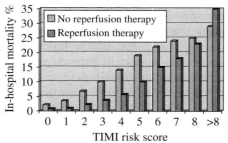

FIG. 23-2   Elements of TIMI risk score for STEMI. Modified with permission from: Morrow DA, Antman EM, Parsons L, et al. Application of the TIMI risk score for ST-elevation MI in the National Registry of Myocardial Infarction 3. *JAMA.* 2001;286:1356.

TABLE 23-2   Initial Medical Therapy for Patients with STEMI

Oxygen
If patient's Sao_2 <90% (but in practice given to all patients with STEMI)
Nitroglycerin
  SL nitroglycerin 0.4 mg tab every 5 minutes × 3
  IV nitroglycerin for relief of ongoing ischemic discomfort
  Nitroglycerin should not be administered to patients with hypotension, tachycardia, severe bradycardia, suspected RV infarction, or critical aortic stenosis
  Nitrates should not be administered to patients who have taken a phosphodiesterase inhibitor (sildenafil, vardenafil, tadalafil) within 24 hours
Morphine sulfate
  2–4 mg IV every 5–15 minutes
Aspirin
  160–325 mg chewed
Beta-blockers
  Oral or IV beta-blockers irrespective of fibrinolytic therapy or PCI

○ If PCI is available on-site or rapid transfer to a PCI facility can be arranged with a door-to-balloon time of 90 minutes, patients should undergo PCI (Table 23-3 lists the indications and risks of cardiac catheterization for STEMI).

○ If PCI is not available or it cannot be promptly arranged, patients should undergo thrombolysis (Table 23-4 lists the indications and contraindications of thrombolysis).

• The use of antiplatelet agents and thrombolytics in addition to aspirin is closely tied in to reperfusion strategies as follows:

○ Clopidogrel should be administered to all patients undergoing PCI with stenting (recommended loading dose varies between 300 mg and 600 mg with the latter being favored and a maintenance dose of 75 mg daily) and to all patients undergoing thrombolysis (loading dose 300 mg with a maintenance dose of 75 mg daily).

○ IIb/IIIa inhibitors should be given as early as possible in patients undergoing PCI. Patient scheduled to receive thrombolysis, however, should not receive IIb/IIIa inhibitors as these agents do not improve outcome in this set of patients and can lead to higher complication rates.

○ Despite its wide use, the evidence for heparin in STEMI is limited. The current recommendation from AHA/ACC includes the administration of unfractionated heparin or low-molecular heparin to all patients less than 75 years without renal dysfunction undergoing PCI and to the vast majority of patients undergoing thrombolysis.

• Multiple studies have revealed that both diabetic and nondiabetic patients with MI or a critical illness have improved outcomes from tight glycemic control. The ACC/AHA task force recommends insulin infusion (with the goal of normoglycemia) in patients with STEMI and a complicated course (Class I) as well as in patients with STEMI and hyperglycemia (Class II). Refer to Chaps. 35 and 36 for more information on management of diabetes in the hospitalized patient.

NSTEMI AND UA

• The initial medical regimen for patients with NSTEMI and UA is quite similar to the one used for STEMI (indeed all therapies listed in Table 23-2 should be given to patients with NSTEMI and UA as well). Tight glycemic control is just as important as in STEMI.

• There is, however, one very important difference in terms of reperfusion therapies: there is no

TABLE 23-3 Indications for PCI in STEMI and PCI Complications*

INDICATION	COMPLICATIONS (AND THEIR INCIDENCE)

Class I evidence
• *Patients with STEMI (including posterior MI and new LBBB) with onset of symptoms within 12 hours if performed in a timely fashion (balloon inflation within 90 minutes of presentation) by experienced personnel.*
• Additional considerations
  1. If symptoms duration less than 3 hours and door-to-balloon time is
    a. <1 hour, PCI is preferred
    b. >1 hour, thrombolytics is preferred
  2. If symptom duration is more than 3 hours, PCI is preferred
  3. PCI is also indicated for patients
    a. <75 years old and in cardiogenic shock within 36 hours following STEMI
    b. In severe congestive heart failure (CHF) within 12 hours following STEMI
Class IIa evidence
• PCI is reasonable in patients
    a. >75 years old and in cardiogenic shock within 36 hours following STEMI
    b. Whose symptoms started more than 12 hours prior but who have one of the following: severe CHF, persistent ischemia, hemodynamic instability, or electrical instability
	Cardiac complications
	• Dissection and abrupt closure of the target coronary artery (5% to 10%)
	• Intraluminal hematoma (7%)
	• Perforation of coronary artery (0.2% to 0.6%)
	• Occlusion of a branch vessel (14%)
	• STEMI as a result of PCI (0.4% to 1.0%)
	• NSTEMI as a result of PCI (5% to 30%)
	Noncardiac complications
	• Bleeding from puncture site (variable based on anticoagulation and antiplatelet agents used)
	• Bleeding from other sites, e.g., gastrointestine (GI) (variable based on anticoagulation and antiplatelet agents used)
	• ARF secondary to IV contrast (variable based on patient)
	• Stroke (0.1% to 0.4%)
	• Ventricular arrhythmias (4%)
	• Bacteremia/sepsis (0.5%)

*Class I—There is general consensus agreement that it is useful and effective.
Class II—There is conflicting evidence or divergence of opinion about the usefulness or efficacy.
Class IIa—Weight of evidence/opinion in favor of usefulness/efficacy.
Class IIb—Usefulness/efficacy is less well established by evidence/opinion.
Class III—General agreement that it is not useful/effective and is some cases may be harmful.

evidence to support the use of thrombolysis in NSTEMI.
• Additionally, there are some differences in the medical management particularly regarding the use of antiplatelet and anticoagulation therapy.
  ○ Several randomized trials have demonstrated improved survival in patients with UA or NSTEMI who received clopidrogel and underwent PCI. A separate issue remains about the timing of clopidrogel therapy as a small number of patients undergoing PCI may turn out to need coronary artery bypass graft (CABG).
  ○ All patients receiving PCI will benefit from IIb/IIIa inhibitors, while those not undergoing PCI should receive it only if they are high-risk patients.
  ○ The weight of evidence favors LMWH over UFH in NSTEMI/UA. Advantages include lower incidence

TABLE 23-4 Indications and Contraindications for Thrombolysis in STEMI

INDICATIONS	CONTRAINDICATIONS
Class I evidence • Patients with STEMI with onset of symptoms within 12 hours prior and ST elevation of at least 1mm in two contiguous leads • Patients with STEMI with onset of symptoms within 12 hours (even 24 hours) prior and new LBBB Class IIa evidence • Patients with STEMI with onset of symptoms within 12–24 hours prior and ST elevation of at least 1mm in two contiguous leads with continuing ischemic symptoms • Patients with STEMI with onset of symptoms within 12 hours (even 24 hours) prior and posterior MI	Absolute • Previous intracranial hemorrhage (ICH) • Known structural cerebral vascular lesion • Known malignant intracranial neoplasm • Ischemic stroke within three months • Suspected aortic dissection • Active bleeding or bleeding diathesis • Significant closed-head or facial trauma within 3 months Relative contraindication • Poorly controlled or chronic sustained hypertension (systolic blood pressure >180 mm Hg) • Ischemic stroke more than 3 months previously • Cardiopulmonary resuscitation (>10 minutes) or major surgery (within <3 weeks) • Recent internal bleeding • Noncompressible vascular puncture • Active peptic ulcer • Current use of anticoagulants: the higher the international normalized ratio (INR), the higher the risk of bleeding

of heparin-induced thrombocytopenia (HIT) and ease of administration.
• Finally, the most important decision in the management of NSTEMI is whether a patient should undergo early revascularization.
  ○ There are the occasional patients who will meet indication for urgent PCI. Patients with any of the following should proceed to PCI immediately:
    1. Cardiogenic shock
    2. Heart failure
    3. Recurrent chest pain
    4. Sustained ventricular tachycardia (VT)
  ○ The vast majority of patients will not have the above conditions: the question then is whether an early invasive, ie, PCI or conservative medical strategy is the better approach.
  ○ Patients with intermediate- or high-risk criteria will most likely benefit from early invasive strategy after the patient is stabilized on a medical regimen. The TIMI score for NSTEMI (Fig. 23-3) is the most commonly used model to estimate the benefits of an early invasive approach in this patient group.
  ○ Among other high-risk factors not addressed by TIMI are:
    1. Decreased left ventricular ejection fraction (LVEF)
    2. Prior PCI within 6 months or prior CABG

Clinical Risk Indicators	Points
Age >65	1
Presence of at least 3 risk factors for CAD	1
Prior coronary stenosis of >50%	1
ST-segment deviations on admission ECG	1
At least 2 anginal episodes in 24 hours	1
Elevated cardiac biomarkers	1
Aspirin use in last 7 days	1
Total possible points	7

Rate of Mortality, Recurrent MI, or Urgent PCI Based on TIMI Risk Socre in Non-ST Elevation ACS

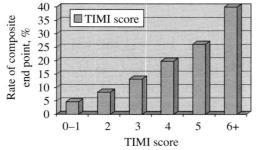

FIG. 23-3 Elements of TIMI risk score for NSTEMI. Modified with permission from: Antman EM, Cohen M, Bernink PJ, et al. The TIMI risk score for unstable angina/non-ST elevation MI: a method for prognostication and therapeutic decision making. *JAMA.* 2000;284:835.

  ○ Furthermore, there is evidence that if PCI is to be performed, it should be done within the first 4–48 hours. Some of the suspected reasons of improved outcome with PCI include antiplatelet therapy and coronary stenting, now commonly done with drug eluting stents.

DISEASE MANAGEMENT STRATEGIES

• Hospitalists are most likely to care for the ACS patient after the initial management has been performed in the emergency department (ED) or in a cardiac invasive laboratory by the cardiologist. Once the patient has stabilized from the ACS, an antiischemic regimen will be established within the first 24–48 hours. Table 23-5 summarizes this medical regimen.
• All patients with ACS should be on telemetry for at least 72 hours. Several arrhythmias may occur depending on the clinical setting.
  ○ Patients with STEMI could develop VT/VF (ventricular fibrillation)—Incidence is about 10% and the vast majority of these occur within the first 48 hours after infarction. Prophylactic administration of antiarrhythmic agents is not recommended; rather beta-blockers and the correction of hypokalemia and hypomagnesemia should be the main focus.
  ○ The incidence of VT/VF in patients with NSTEMI/UA is much smaller at around 2%.
• A common question raised by episodes of VT is about their prognostic significance. VT early in the course of an AMI (6–48 hours) does not portend a worse prognosis. VT later in the course (more than 48 hours), however, is associated with increased mortality. Such patients need additional outpatient cardiac evaluation; those patients with depressed LVEF may benefit from placement of an internal cardiac defibrillator (ICD).

CARE TRANSITIONS

• Risk stratification is an important part of the care transition in the evaluation of ACS. There are three main components of risk stratification: evaluation of LVEF, risk for arrhythmic death, and noninvasive stress testing.
  ○ All patients with ACS should have a cardiac echocardiogram to evaluate their LVEF because a depressed LVEF is associated with increased mortality. Initial measurements of LVEF can be misleading and should be generally repeated within 4–6 weeks for all patients found to have a reduced ejection fraction after MI.
  ○ Prevention of sudden cardiac death from an arrhythmic event is closely tied to the measurement of the EF.
    ▪ ICD indicated for patients with EF<30%

TABLE 23-5   Medications Commonly Used in Patient with ACS

MEDICATION	MECHANISM OF ACTION/BENEFIT	INDICATIONS	CONTRAINDICATIONS
Antiplatelet therapy			
—Aspirin	—Irreversible inhibition of thromboxane A2	*Should be administered immediately in any patient thought to have acute MI. Should be continued indefinitely at 81 mg daily*	—Allergy or intolerance (use clopidogrel instead) —Active bleeding —Severe untreated HTN
—Clopidogrel	—Inhibits binding of adenosine diphosphate (ADP) to its receptor thus inhibiting platelet aggregation	—All patients who undergo PCI with stenting (load 600 mg followed by 75 mg daily) —All patients undergoing thrombolysis (load 300 mg followed by 75 mg daily)	—Similar to aspirin —Do not give clopidogrel if patient going for CABG
IIb/IIIa Inhibitor	—Binds to the glycoprotein IIb/IIIa receptor preventing fibrinogen and von Willebrand factor from binding and activating platelet aggregation	—All patients undergoing PCI —Patients undergoing thrombolysis should not receive IIb/IIIa inhibitors	—Same as in aspirin —A IIb/IIIa inhibitor specific side effect is thrombocytopenia usually seen within 24 hours.
Beta-blockers	—Relief of ischemic pain by reducing HR, BP, and contractility —Decreased risk of VF/VT —Improved left diastolic function (by slowing HR) —Reduction in remodeling and thus improving LV hemodynamic function	*Initially beta-blockers should be given to all patients with ACS. Therapy in patients with documented MI should be continued indefinitely*	—Heart rate <60 —SBP<100 mm Hg —Severe LV failure —Shock —PR>.24 —Second- or third-degree AV block —Active asthma —MI caused by cocaine use
ACE-inhibitors (should be started within 24 hours after MI but not in the first 6 hours)	—Increases end-diastolic volume —Improves LVEF at 1 year post-MI	*All patients with MI (though data is strongest in those with STEMI and NSTEMI patient with LV dysfunction, hypertension, or diabetes)*	—Renal failure (not absolute contraindication) —Hypotension —Shock —History of bilateral renal artery stenosis
Nitrates	—Dilation of coronaries leading to increased perfusion of ischemic areas —Reduction of infarction size —Enhanced collateral flow	Should be continued for the first 24–48 hours in patients with recurrent ischemia, HTH, or CHF. Beyond that only continue if recurrent chest pain an issue and if patient already on beta-blocker/ACE-I	Use with caution or avoid if —Administration likely to cause hypotension —Patient has an RV infarction —Patient has significant aortic stenosis —Patient has taken a phosphodiesterase inhibitor for erectile dysfunction in last 24 hours
Statins	—Plaque stabilization —Atherosclerosis regression —Reduced inflammation —Reduced thrombogenicity	Start atorvastatin 80 mg daily in all patients. Titrate down to a dose achieving adequate LDL (current recommendation less than 100), will probably require statin therapy indefinitely	No absolute contraindications. Patients with liver disease will need absolute abstinence from alcohol and frequent monitoring
Aldosterone antagonists	—Significant reduction in blood pressure —Increase in serum K+ (possibly reducing cardiac arrhythmias) —Blocking the effects of aldosterone in the heart	Patients with MI and —LVEF<40% —On ACE-I —CHF or DM —Preserved renal function —Normal serum K+ Greatest benefit in first 30 days, optimal duration unknown	—Hyperkalemia —Acute or chronic renal failure (baseline creatinine >2.5 in men and >2.0 in women)
Calcium channel blockers	—No evidence for beneficial effect in ACS. —No mortality reduction in MI	Should be used only when beta-blockers not sufficient to control HTN. Short-acting dihydropyridines (e.g., nifedipine) should never be used in ACS because of increased mortality	—Heart rate <60 —SBP<100 mm Hg —Severe LV failure —Shock —PR>.24 —Second- or third-degree AV block

TABLE 23-6   Indications for Stress Testing for ACS*

ACC/AHA Guidelines for Exercise Testing Before or After Revascularization

Class I
1. Demonstration of ischemia before revascularization
2. Evaluation of patients with recurrent symptoms suggestive of ischemia after revascularization

Class IIa
1. After discharge for activity counseling and/or exercise training of cardiac rehabilitation of patients who have undergone coronary revascularization

Class IIb
1. Detection of restenosis in selected high-risk asymptomatic patients within the first 12 months after PCI
2. Periodic monitoring of selected, high-risk asymptomatic patients for restenosis, graft closure, incomplete coronary revascularization, or disease progression

Class III
1. Localization of ischemia for determining the site of intervention
2. Routine, periodic monitoring of asymptomatic patients after PCI or CABG without any specific indications

*Class I—There is general consensus agreement that it is useful and effective.
Class II—There is conflicting evidence or divergence of opinion about the usefulness or efficacy.
Class IIa—Weight of evidence/opinion in favor of usefulness/efficacy.
Class IIb—Usefulness/efficacy is less well established by evidence/opinion.
Class III—General agreement that it is not useful/effective and is some cases may be harmful.

- Holter monitoring and an electrophysiologic (EP) study for patients with ejection fraction (EF) of 31% to 40%
- No further evaluation for patients with EF>40%
  - Stress testing can be a fairly complicated issue during an admission for ACS. Table 23-6 summarizes the indications for stress testing in several common situations. A couple of points worth mentioning are
    - Stress testing prior to discharge is not indicated for patients who were fully revascularized, but rather for patients who have not undergone any PCI and or have not been fully revascularized even after PCI.
    - Because patients routinely have baseline ECG abnormalities, myocardial perfusion tests or echocardiography will be an essential part of the stress test regimen.
- It should be emphasized that early discharge (within 72 hours) after an uncomplicated ACS is considered safe and cost effective. The initiation of secondary prevention measures prior to discharge is an important priority. The medical therapy for secondary prevention is already addressed in detail in Table 23-5.

Additionally, lifestyle changes to be addressed prior to DC include
  - *Smoking-cessation counseling*
  - Dietary modification and weight reduction
  - Engagement in a routine exercise program (after undergoing noninvasive cardiac stress testing)
  - Referral to a cardiac rehabilitation program
- Communication with outpatient providers is crucial at the time of discharge. Patients with ACS will need close follow-up not only with their primary care physician for optimization of CAD risk factors, but they should also have a cardiology follow-up for any further necessary diagnostic/prognostic workup (such as repeat echocardiogram for LVEF assessment 4–6 weeks after acute MI) and for outpatient cardiac rehabilitation.
- Finally, patients with ACS have numerous questions about return to daily activities. While there is a paucity of data on this subject, a few points can be made.
  - Most people can return to work within 2 weeks.
  - Activities of daily living can be performed without concern and indeed should be encouraged.
  - Sexual activity may be resumed after 6 weeks with an uncomplicated post-MI course (no recurrence of angina, no arrhythmias, or congestive heart failure).
  - Driving can usually begin within a week of discharge.
  - Air travel should probably be avoided for the first 2 weeks.

BIBLIOGRAPHY

Antman EM, Anbe DT, Armstrong PW, et al. ACC/AHA guidelines for the management of patients with ST-elevation myocardial infarction—executive summary. A report of the American College of Cardiology/American Heart Association task force on practice guidelines (Writing Committee to Revise the 1999 Guidelines for the Management of Patients with Acute Myocardial Infarction). *Circulation.* 2004;110:588.

Antman EM, Cohen M, Bernink PJ, et al. The TIMI risk score for unstable angina/non-ST elevation MI: a method for prognostication and therapeutic decision making. *JAMA.* 2000;284:835.

Braunwald E, Antman E, Beasley J, et al. ACC/AHA 2002 guideline update for the management of patients with unstable angina and non-ST-segment elevation myocardial infarction—summary article. A report of the American College of Cardiology/American Heart Association task force on practice guidelines (Committee on the Management of Patients with Unstable Angina). *J Am Coll Cardiol.* 2002;40:1366.

Cannon CP, Braunwald E, McCabe CH, et al. Intensive versus moderate lipid lowering with statins after acute coronary syndromes. *N Engl J Med.* 2004;350:1495.

Cannon CP, Hand MH, Bahr R, et al. Critical pathways for management of patients with acute coronary syndromes: an assessment by the National Heart Attack Alert Program. *Am Heart J.* 2002;143:777.

Cannon CP, Weintraub WS, Demopoulos LA, et al. Comparison of early invasive and conservative strategies in patients with unstable coronary syndromes treated with the glycoprotein IIb/IIIa inhibitor tirofiban. *N Engl J Med.* 2001;344:1879.

Gibbons RJ, Balady GJ, Bricker JT, et al. ACC/AHA 2002 guideline update for exercise testing. A report of the American College of Cardiology/American Heart Association task force on practice guidelines (Committee on Exercise Testing). *Circulation.* 2002;106:1883.

Keeley EC, Boura JA, Grines CL. Primary angioplasty versus intravenous thrombolytic therapy for acute myocardial infarction: a quantitative review of 23 randomized trials. *Lancet.* 2003;361:13.

Morrow DA, Antman EM, Parsons L, et al. Application of the TIMI risk score for ST-elevation MI in the National Registry of Myocardial Infarction 3. *JAMA.* 2001;286:1356.

Popma JJ, Berger P, Ohman EM, et al. Antithrombotic therapy during percutaneous coronary intervention: the seventh ACCP conference on antithrombotic and thrombolytic therapy. *Chest.* 2004;126:576S.

Smith SC Jr, Feldman TE, Hirshfeld JW Jr, et al. ACC/AHA/SCAI 2005 guideline update for percutaneous coronary intervention—summary article. A report of the American College of Cardiology/American Heart Association task force on practice guidelines (ACC/AHA/SCAI Writing Committee to Update the 2001 Guidelines for Percutaneous Coronary Intervention). *J Am Coll Cardiol.* 2006;47:216.

24 ADVANCED CARDIAC LIFE SUPPORT

Apoor Patel

- Sudden cardiac arrest causes approximately 250,000 out-of-hospital deaths in the United States per year.
- The national and international survival rate of out-of-hospital sudden cardiac arrest remains <6%.
- The 2005 American Heart Association guidelines for cardiopulmonary resuscitation (CPR) and emergency cardiovascular care emphasize increasing the number of chest compressions per minute and *minimizing* interruptions in compressions.
- Until an advanced airway is in place, single rescuers should use a compression to ventilation ratio of 30:2, and 15:2 when at least two rescuers are present.

- Emergency medical services (EMS) personnel are no longer required to defibrillate patients with out-of-hospital cardiac arrest as soon as they arrive on the scene. If the call to arrival interval is greater than 5 minutes or EMS responders did not witness the arrest, EMS rescuers may give 5 cycles (about 2 minutes) of CPR before attempting defibrillation. There are insufficient data to recommend this strategy for in-hospital arrest at the current time.
- When an advanced airway (endotracheal tube, esophageal-tracheal combitube, laryngeal mask airway) is in place, continuous chest compressions should be provided at a rate of 100 compressions/min with complete recoil between compressions ("push hard, push fast"). Patients should be ventilated at 8–10 breaths/min.
- Instead of three stacked shocks for pulseless ventricular tachycardia/ventricular fibrillation (VT/VF), the new guidelines recommend only one shock followed by *immediate* CPR. Rhythm check and repeat shock should only occur after 2 minutes of continuous compressions. The rationale for this change is based on the high rate of first shock success with new biphasic defibrillators and rapidly declining efficacy of subsequent shocks.
- Know your defibrillator.
  - Biphasic defibrillators should be used
    - At a dose at which the specific defibrillator has been shown to terminate VF (usually 120–200J). If the effective dose of the device is unknown, 200J may be used for the first shock.
    - For synchronized cardioversion of atrial fibrillation at 100–120J (no official recommendations for atrial flutter or reentry synchronized ventricular tachycardia [SVT]).
  - Monophasic defibrillators should be used
    - At 360J for the initial and subsequent shocks
    - For synchronized cardioversion of atrial fibrillation (AF) at 100–200J, and for atrial flutter or reentry SVT at 50-100J
- All rescue interventions (intubation, medication administration) should be done in a manner which minimizes interruption of chest compressions.
- Vasopressors should be delivered while compressions are occurring to enhance drug delivery.
- Transcutaneous pacing is not recommended for asystole in the new guidelines.
- Full guidelines can be found at http://circ.ahajournals.org under the section Circulation Supplements.
- See advanced cardiac life support (ACLS) algorithms, and individual chapters on atrial fibrillation, supraventricular tachycardia, ventricular arrythmias and sinus bradycardia, and atrioventricular blocks.

VF AND PULSELESS VT

1. CPR until defibrillator ready
   30:2 ratio until intubated then 100 compressions/min with 8-10 breaths/min
2. Defibrillate
   Biphasic: Device-specific, usually 120–200J, if unknown, use 200J
   Monophasic: 360J
3. Resume Immediate CPR for 2 minutes (5 cycles)
4. Defibrillate
   Biphasic: Same as first dose or higher
   Monophasic: 360J
5. Epinephrine 1mg IV repeat q3-5
   Vasopressin 40U × 1 may replace first or second dose of epinephrine
6. Repeat steps 3–5
   Biphasic: Escalate dose
   Monophasic: 360J
7. Consider antiarrhythmics
   Amiodarone (*IIb*) 300 mg IV push (may repeat 150 mg push in 3–5 minutes)
   Lidocaine (*Indent.*) 1–1.5 mg/kg IV (may give additional 0.5–0.75 mg/kg IV push q5–10 to
   max dose 3 mg/kg)
   Magnesium (*IIb if hypomagnesemia*) 1–2 g IVq

DIFFERENTIAL DIAGNOSIS FOR PULSELESS ARREST (H6T5)

Hypovolemia
Hypoxia
Hydrogen ion (acidosis)
Hypo-/hyperkalemia
Hypoglycemia
Hypothermia
Toxins
Tamponade, cardiac
Tension pneumothorax
Thrombosis (coronary or pulmonary)
Trauma

WIDE COMPLEX IRREGULAR TACHYCARDIA

If atrial fibrillation with aberrancy, treat as irregular narrow complex tachycardia
If pre-excited atrial fibrillation (AF with Wolff-Parkinson-White [WPW]), avoid AV nodal blocking agents (adenosine, diltiazem, digoxin, verapamil)
   Consider amiodarone 150 mg IV over 10 minutes
If polymorphic VT, get expert consultation
If torsades de pointes, give magnesium (load with 1–2 g over 5–60 minutes, then infusion)

WIDE COMPLEX REGULAR TACHYCARDIA

If ventricular tachycardia or uncertain rhythm give
Amiodarone: 150 mg IV over 10 minutes (may repeat to max 2.2 g/24 h). See dosing in narrow complex regular tachycardia
Prepare for synchronized cardioversion
If SVT with aberrancy, give adenosine

NARROW COMPLEX IRREGULAR TACHYCARDIA

Differential diagnosis: Atrial fibrillation, atrial flutter with variable block, multi-focal atrial tachycardia (MAT)
1. *Unstable*: Synchronized cardioversion
2. *Stable*: Rate control. *Normal EF*: Beta-blocker or calcium channel blocker (CCB) such as diltiazem or verapamil. *Low EF*: Use beta-blockers and diltiazem with caution. Verapamil contraindicated

ATRIAL FIBRILLATION

Key Issues: Stable? Duration >48 hours? Reduced EF? WPW present?
1. *Unstable*: Cardioversion (start at 100J)
2. *Stable*: Rate control (with beta-blockade, diltiazem, verapamil). No chemical or electrical cardioversion if >48 hours duration without anticoagulation and documentation by TEE of no left atrial thrombus. If <48 hours can start heparin and cardiovert
Rate control agents include verapamil, diltiazem, beta-blocker, and digoxin. Rhythm control agents include amiodarone, ibutilide, propafenone, and flecainide. Expert consultation recommended

NARROW COMPLEX REGULAR TACHYCARDIA

Differential diagnosis: Sinus tachycardia, atrial flutter, reentry supraventricular tachycardia (SVT) such as AV nodal reentry and accessory pathway-mediated tachycardia, atrial tachycardia, junctional tachycardia
1. *Unstable*: Synchronized cardioversion
2. *Stable*: Vagal maneuvers or Adenosine 6 mg rapid IV, then 12 mg (may repeat × 1). Wait 1–2 minutes between doses
3. If rhythm converts was probably reentry SVT treat recurrence with adenosine, or can start long-acting nodal agent such as beta-blocker or diltiazem

(Continued)

NARROW COMPLEX REGULAR TACHYCARDIA (CONTINUED)

4. If rhythm does not convert consider persistence of reentry SVT, atrial flutter, or atrial or junctional tachycardia
    * *Normal EF*: Beta-blocker, calcium channel blocker (CCB) such as diltiazem or verapamil. Cardioversion only helpful if rhythm felt to be reentry SVT
    * *Low EF*: Use beta-blockers and diltiazem with caution. Verapamil contraindicated. Consider amiodarone. Cardioversion only helpful if rhythm felt to be reentry SVT

Drug Dosing
Verapamil: 2.5–5 mg IV over 2 minutes. Then repeat doses of 5–10 mg every 15–30 minutes, for total of 20 mg
Diltiazem: 0.25 mg/kg (10–20 mg) over 2 minutes, then can repeat at 0.35 mg/kg in 15 minutes
Lopressor: 5 mg IV slow over 5 minutes. May repeat × 2 q5 minutes
Amiodarone: 150 mg IV over 10 minutes, then 1 mg/mL infusion for 6 hours, then 0.5 mg/mL for 18 hours. Total daily dose <2.2 g

UNSTABLE BRADYCARDIA

Unstable bradycardia is defined as HR<60 and signs or symptoms of hypoperfusion such as altered mental status, ongoing chest pain, hypotension, or other signs of shock

1. Prepare transcutaneous pacing. Use without delay in type II second-degree- or third-degree block. Atropine likely ineffective in these patients
2. Atropine 0.5–1 mg IV q3-5 minutes for a total of 3 mg
3. Dopamine 2–10 μg/kg/min, or epinephrine 2–10 μg/kg/min while awaiting pacer or if pacing ineffective
4. Use transvenous pacing if needed

ASYSTOLE/PULSELESS ELECTRICAL ACTIVITY (PEA)

1. Immediate CPR for 5 cycles
2. Intubate and IV access
3. When IV/IO available give either
    * Epinephrine 1 mg IV/IO repeat q3-5 minutes
    * Vasopressin 40 U IV/IO to replace first or second dose of epinephrine
4. Consider atropine 1mg IV/IO for asystole or slow PEA. Repeat q3-5 minutes. Max three doses

ANAPHYLAXIS

1. High flow O_2
2. Epinephrine 0.3–0.5 mg (1:1000) IM q 15–20 minutes if no clinical improvement
3. If severe, epinephrine 0.1 mg (1:10,000) IV over 5 minutes
4. IVF, antihistamines, H2 blockers, inhaled beta-agonists (ipratropium in patients receiving beta-blockers), solumedrol, glucagons, 1.2 mg q5 minutes IM/IV for patients unresponsive to epinephrine
5. Consider early intubation

BIBLIOGRAPHY

Hazinski MF, Nadkarni VM, Hickey RW, et al. Major changes in the 2005 AHA guidelines for CPR and ECC: reaching the tipping point for change. *Circulation*. 2005;112:IV206–211.

Zheng ZJ, Croft JB, Giles WH, et al. Sudden cardiac death in the United States, 1989 to 1998. *Circulation*. 2001;104:2158-2163.

25 ATRIAL FIBRILLATION AND ATRIAL FLUTTER

Robert D. Winslow

EPIDEMIOLOGY/OVERVIEW

* Atrial fibrillation (AF) is the most common arrhythmia, accounting for approximately one-third of hospital admissions for arrhythmias.

* Over 2 million people in the United States are thought to have permanent or paroxysmal AF, with a prevalence of 0.4% in the general population.
    ○ The prevalence increases with age from <1% in those under 60 years old to >8% in those over 80 years old, and is higher in men than in women.
    ○ The prevalence increases as the severity of coexisting heart failure, ischemia, or valvular heart disease increases.
* AF is classified as
    ○ *Paroxysmal:* self-terminating, recurrent episodes of AF typically lasting less than 24 hours but sometimes up to 1 week
    ○ *Persistent:* lasting more than 1 week and requiring cardioversion for resumption of normal sinus rhythm (NSR)
    ○ *Chronic or permanent:* lasting more than 1 year, unresponsive to cardioversion
    ○ *"Lone" AF:* paroxysmal, persistent, or chronic AF, typically in patients less than 60 years old, without underlying cardiovascular disease and structurally normal hearts, who are deemed to be at lower risk of thromboembolism
* Atrial flutter (AFl) and AF may have identical presentation, workup, and management. Issues

specific to AFl are delineated as such throughout the chapter.

- Treatment of both rhythms is directed toward symptom relief and to the prevention of secondary complications, such as systemic embolism, syncope, myocardial ischemia, and heart failure.

PATHOPHYSIOLOGY

- AF is a disease process where there is disruption of normal atrial conduction of electrical impulses, replacing normal electrical activity with chaotic activity occurring throughout the atria.
- Electrical activity recorded from any one location will reveal irregular impulses, often occurring at a rate of 300–500 per minute.
- The ventricular rate in AF is related to conduction through the atrio ventricular (AV) node as well as sympathetic and parasympathetic influences on the AV node.
- Acute AF can be caused by a number of diseases, conditions, and exogenous or endogenous substances (Table 25-1).
- Chronic cardiac conditions can lead to the development of AF, such as valvular or coronary heart disease and hypertension, especially when accompanied by left ventricular hypertrophy (LVH) (Table 25-2).
- Any condition which would normally cause an increase in heart rate can cause a rapid ventricular response to AF such as pain, dehydration, fever, or the postoperative state.
- AFl is a regular atrial rhythm that results in fixed ration AV "block," that is, 2:1, 3:1, and so forth.
- Thromboembolism from thrombus formation in the left atrial appendage causes the major morbidity and

TABLE 25-2   Mechanisms of Atrial Fibrillation in Chronic Heart Disease

Valvular heart disease	Chronically elevated atrial pressures and atrial stretch
Ischemic heart disease	Atrial ischemia or infarction, as a consequence of chronic congestive heart failure
Hypertension	Diastolic dysfunction leading to increased atrial pressures (predominantly with LVH)
Chronic heart failure	Chronic elevation of filling pressures

mortality due to infarcts involving the brain, gastrointestinal (GI) tract, kidneys, and extremities.

CLINICAL PRESENTATION, DIFFERENTIAL, MAKING THE DIAGNOSIS

- AF can present with a wide range of symptoms, and should be in the differential of any patient who presents with symptoms possibly due to cardiovascular disease and of patients presenting with acute neurologic events.
- Symptoms can be caused by the irregularity of heart beats, the heart rate, or can be related to complex perturbations of cardiovascular function (Table 25-3).
- Typical cardiac symptoms include shortness of breath, palpitations, syncope, and angina.
  - AF with rapid ventricular response (RVR) commonly precipitates congestive heart failure in patients with diastolic dysfunction and myocardial ischemia in patients with coronary artery disease.
  - Patients with severe cardiac dysfunction or valvular disease are more likely to have significant reductions in cardiac output when in AF.

TABLE 25-1   Acute Causes of AF

Exogenous toxins/ stimulants	Alcohol, catecholaminergic drugs (pseudoephedrine, epinephrine, norepinephrine, dopamine, cocaine), prescription drugs (thyroid replacement hormones)
Endocrine	Thyrotoxicosis
Pericardial disease	Acute pericarditis (bacterial or viral), immune-mediated pericarditis (as in lupus or postinfarction pericarditis), postoperative pericarditis
Myocarditis	Acute myocardities affecting the atria
Pulmonary diseases	Any, but especially pneumonia, flares of chronic obstructive pulmonary disease, and pulmonary embolism
Postoperative state	
Infections	
Electrolyte disturbances	
Renal failure	

TABLE 25-3   Symptoms in AF and Physiologic Causes

Fast heart rate, palpitations	• Irregular and or rapid conduction through AV node to ventricles
Chest pain	• Rapid heart rate • Ischemia caused by increased demand and decreased diastolic coronary perfusion
Shortness of breath	• High left atrial filling pressures and resultant pulmonary edema • Reduced cardiac output from loss of atrial contribution to ventricular filling and reduced diastolic filling time
Ligh-theadedness, syncope	• Hypotension caused by reduced cardiac output
Fatigue, exertional intolerance	• Low cardiac output at rest and with exercise
Neurologic complaints, stroke	• Embolism from clot in left atrium
Polyuria	• Release of atrial natriuretic peptide
Cardiogenic shock	• Severe reduction in cardiac output

- Diagnosis and treatment should be directed toward the underlying condition that precipitated the rhythm disturbance and toward reducing thromboembolism risk.
- Some patients will have a past personal and/or a family history of AF or other cardiac diseases.
- The history does not reliably estimate the onset of AF because many episodes of AF do not produce symptoms.
- Physical examination findings of AF include an irregularly irregular heart rhythm, with or without tachycardia, and may include hypotension. Other findings, when present, typically relate to comorbidities (such as focal neurologic deficits in embolic stroke caused by AF or signs of heart failure exacerbation precipitated by AF with rapid ventricular response or signs of thyrotoxicosis).
  - The patient may be unaware of a rhythm disturbance, and the clinician may incidentally discover AF on physical examination.
- AF is diagnosed by electrocardiography (ECG) (Fig. 25-1) or through telemetry monitoring.
  - Hallmarks are an irregular rhythm with narrow QRS complexes and an absence of discreet P waves.
  - There can be coarse atrial activity seen in some leads, leading to the misdiagnosis of AFl.
  - Differential diagnosis of irregular narrow complex rhythms includes AF, AFl with variable block, and multifocal atrial tachycardia (MAT).
  - If there is any question about the atrial activity in a narrow complex irregular tachycardia, maneuvers to block conduction through the AV node (ie, carotid sinus massage) or administration of adenosine (which transiently blocks AV nodal conduction) can create a pause in ventricular activity which allows for more careful examination of atrial activity on a rhythm strip.
- The clinician should obtain the following laboratory studies:
  - TSH if AF is new, rates are more difficult to control, or thyroid disease is clinically suspected.
  - Creatinine kinase and cardiac troponins if suspected ischemic heart disease.
  - Baseline-activated partial thromboplastin time (PTT), prothrombin time (PT) and internationalized normal ratio (INR), hemoglobin, and platelet count.
  - Stool guaiac to look for occult gastrointestinal bleeding.
  - Electrolytes (including potassium and magnesium), blood urea nitrogen, creatinine, and liver function tests.

TRIAGE AND INITIAL MANGEMENT

- Place all admitted patients on continuous telemetry monitoring.
- Patients in AF should be assessed for severity of symptoms and hemodynamic compromise. Initial urgent/emergent therapies are dictated by the patient's heart rate and blood pressure.
  - If the patient is tachycardiac and hypotensive
    - Provide blood pressure support (intravenous fluids or pressors).
    - Use rate-slowing agents as the improved hemodynamics at slower heart rates can overcome deleterious effects of mediations on blood pressure.

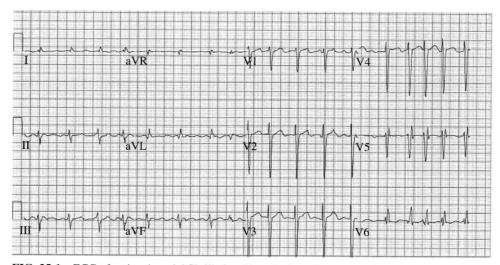

FIG. 25-1 ECG of patient in atrial fibrillation. Note the irregular, narrow QRS complexes. In some leads (e.g., V_1), there appears to be organized atrial activity, but inspection of all 12 leads (particularly the limb leads) reveals that there is no coordinated atrial activity.

- Proceed with urgent external cardioversion under conscious sedation if hypotension persists.
- Defibrillate to emergently cardiovert if unresponsive or in cardiogenic shock (see Chap. 24).
  ◦ If the patient is bradycardic and hypotensive
    - Attempt transcutaneous pacing.
    - Refer for urgent temporary transvenous pacemaker wire insertion.
  ◦ If the patient is tachycardic and has normal blood pressure
    - Use rate-slowing agents (Table 25-4).
  ◦ If the patient is normotensive with rate controlled AF, consider
    - Outpatient management with anticoagulation (or aspirin for low-risk patients)
    - AV nodal blocking agents
    - Close follow-up for consideration of cardioversion and other therapies
- Special considerations
The Wolff-Parkinson-White (WPW) Syndrome
  ◦ An irregular, wide complex rhythm should raise suspicion for "preexcited AF," which is caused by activation of the ventricles via accessory pathway rather than AV node.
    - Often there are narrow complex beats due to conduction down AV node.
    - Frequently there are variable degrees of fusion, with resultant variable QRS complex width.
  ◦ AV nodal agents, which can cause preferential conduction down accessory pathways and very rapid ventricular rates, should not be used alone. Treatment is directed at slowing conduction down accessory pathways, using antiarrhythmic medications such as IV propafenone (Table 25-5).
Postoperative patients with AF
  ◦ AF is extremely common after cardiac surgery, affecting as many as 50% of patients and occurring within 5 days of surgery. AF is also seen as a postoperative complication of noncardiac surgeries.
  ◦ Rate control can be difficult because of exogenous or endogenous sympathetic stimulation.
  ◦ Cardioversion may be necessary if there is hemodynamic instability or difficult to control rates.

TABLE 25-4   Medications Used for Rate Control in Atrial Fibrillation

CLASS	DRUG	DOSES	SIDE EFFECTS AND SPECIAL CONSIDERATIONS
Beta-blockers	Esmolol	500 mcg/kg IV load, then 60–200 mcg/kg/min	Not for preexcited atrial fibrillation (WPW) Side effects include
	Metoprolol	2.5–5 mg IV 25–100 mg bid po	• Hypotension • Bradycardia
	Atenolol	25–100 mg daily po	• Heart block • Exacerbations of heart failure • Exacerbations of reactive airway disease
Calcium channel blockers	Diltiazem	10–20 mg (0.25 mg/kg) IV bolus, then 5–15 mg/hr continuous IV gtt 120–360 mg po daily divided doses or sustained release	Not for preexcited atrial fibrillation (WPW) Side effects include • Hypotension • Bradycardia
	Verapamil	0.075–0.15 mg/kg IV 120–360 mg PO daily divided or sustained release	• Heart block • Exacerbations of heart failure
Digitalis glycosides	Digoxin	0.25 mg IV q2 hours, up to 1.0 g, or 0.5 mg IV followed by 0.25 mg IV × 2 doses q2-4 hours 0.125–0.375 mg po or IV daily	May use in combination with beta-blockers or calcium channel blockers, or as a single agent in patients with heart failure and no accessory pathway Side effects include • Bradycardia • Heart block • Digoxin toxicity, especially in patients with renal dysfunction
Antiarrhythmics	Amiodarone	150 mg IV bolus, then 0.5–1 mg/min for up to 12 hours	Should rarely be used Good for patients with preexcited atrial fibrillation (WPW) or heart failure. Suitable for use as a single agent. Helps maintain sinus rhythm Side effects include • Hypotension • Bradycardia • Phlebitis if given via peripheral IV

TABLE 25-5   Medications Used for Chemical Cardioversion in Atrial Fibrillation

DRUG	DOSES	SUCCESS RATES (CONVERSION TO NSR)	SIDE EFFECTS	SPECIAL CONSIDERATIONS
Propafenone Class IC	600 mg po × 1 1.5–2.0 mg/kg IV	56% to 83% within 2–6 hours	• Hypotension • Conversion to atrial flutter with rapid ventricular rate • Proarrhythmic	Excellent for preexcited atrial fibrillation (WPW) Need to observe for QRS and QT changes Poor choice if structural Heart disease present Can be used as a "pill-in-the-pocket"
Flecainide Class IC	300 mg po × 1	68% to 75% within 2–8 hours	• Dizziness • Visual disturbances • Dyspnea • Proarrhythmic	Can be used as a "pill-in-the-pocket"
Ibutilide Class III	1 mg IV over 10 minutes, may repeat × 1	60% to 70%	• 4% risk polymorphic ventricular tachycardia (higher in females) • Should be avoided in patients with heart failure or low ejection fractions because of higher proarrhythmic risk	Need to have normal serum concentrations of potassium (>4.0 mg/dL) and magnesium (>2.0 mg/dL) prior to administration Must monitor patients for QT prolongation and arrhythmias for 4 hours after administration
Dofetilide Class III	125–500 mcg daily po depending on renal function	60% to 70%	• QT prolongation	Many contraindications exist, must be a licensed hospital and practitioner to prescribe
Amiodarone Class III	IV: 150 mg bolus IV then 0.5–1 mg/min for up to 12 hours Oral: may load over several weeks	34% to 69% acutely; higher when combined with po maintenance therapy	• Hypotension • Bradycardia • Phlebitis if given via peripheral IV • Multiple side effects possible with chronic use (thyroid, pulmonary, dermatologic, and so forth)	Intravenous formulations are rarely indicated. Good for patients with preexcited atrial fibrillation (WPW) or heart failure Must monitor patients for QT prolongation, arrhythmias, and bradycardia Use with caution in patients with underlying severe pulmonary disease

○ Anticoagulation is appropriate if AF lasts more than 48 hours, or recurs. Patients should be considered for 30 days of anticoagulation and outpatient surveillance of AF.

○ Predictors of postoperative AF include:

  ▪ Increasing age
  ▪ Hypertension
  ▪ Preoperative history of AF
  ▪ Valvular heart disease
  ▪ Chronic obstructive pulmonary disease (COPD)
  ▪ Previous cardiac surgery
  ▪ Need for intra-aortic balloon pump or pressors postoperatively
  ▪ Mechanical ventilation >24 hours postoperatively
  ▪ Diabetes mellitus
  ▪ Postoperative withdrawal of beta-blockers if used preoperatively

○ Beta-blockers and amiodarone are the most common medications used to prevent and manage postoperative AF.

○ Frequently the management of postoperative AF is done in conjunction with a cardiologist.

• Once the patient is hemodynamically stabilized, the next steps are

  ○ To perform echocardiography to assess for a structurally normal heart (particularly left atrial size, ventricular size and function, and the presence of mitral valve disease) and the likelihood of successful conversion to/maintenance of normal sinus rhythm (NSR).

  ○ To quantify the duration of AF, if possible; however, this can be quite difficult as patients may have vague symptoms or may not be able to recall when symptoms started.

DISEASE MANAGEMENT STRATEGIES

- Management of AF can most effectively be accomplished with clinical care pathways that adhere to evidence-based practices and national guidelines (Fuster et al).
- There are three therapeutic goals in the long-term management of patients with AF.
  - Rate control
  - Rhythm control (which may not be necessary for many patients)
  - Prevention of systemic thromboembolism
- Rate control consists of medications to prevent tachycardia and anticoagulation. Avoidance of tachycardia in many patients will prevent hemodynamic instability, troublesome symptoms such as palpitations or poor exercise capacity, and the risk of developing cardiomyopathy, and the potential side effects of antiarrhythmic therapies. Target heart rates
  - Resting heart rate should be less than 80.
  - Recovery heart rate less than 110 after a 6 minutes walk.
  - No heart rate >110% of the age adjusted maximum (maximum heart rate is 220 minus age in years) by Holter monitoring.
- Medications used for rate control are agents that affect the AV node (Table 25-4).
  - Start with beta-blocking agents as first-line therapy to slow conduction and prolong refractoriness of the AV node.
  - Nondihydropyridine calcium channel blockers are second-line therapy if beta-blockers are contraindicated or not tolerated. These agents also slow conduction, prolong refractoriness, and depress myocardial contractility.
  - Digoxin generally should be used only as adjunctive therapy. Digoxin slows conduction, through parasympathomimetic and weak antiadrenergic mechanisms. The onset of action is slower than other agents and it is renally cleared. Digoxin does not cause hypotension or depress ventricular function. If digoxin is to be used in the treatment of AF, the following should be kept in mind:
    - If used alone, it will not control exercise-induced tachycardia. Hence, its use alone is in specific circumstances such as the sedentary elderly patient with heart failure. Target serum ranges for digoxin for patients with heart failure are 0.5–0.8 ng/mL
    - Systemic levels or effects can be increased in renal failure or by drug-drug interactions. Patients started on amiodarone should have their digoxin dose cut in half.
    - Serum concentrations of digoxin correlate poorly with symptoms and toxicity. Symptoms of

digoxin toxicity include nausea, visual disturbances, headache, and arrhythmias such as
  - *Slow, regularized AF:* AF with heart block
  - *Rapid regular rhythm:* accelerated junctional rhythm
  - Rarely accelerated ventricular rhythms
- Toxicity is associated with disturbances in serum electrolytes, especially potassium, magnesium, and calcium, which should be normalized.
- In addition to discontinuation of digoxin when toxicity is noted, antibodies against digoxin (Digibind) are rarely used (*only if* the arrhythmia is lifethreatening).
  - Amiodarone prolongs the action potential and refractory period, thereby slowing conduction. Although highly effective, amiodarone has significant adverse effects which include hypotension, bradycardia, nausea, constipation, and thyroid abnormalities. The long half-life of 60–90 days makes management of these complications difficult. (See the topic rhythm control in this chapter.
  - Surgical or catheter ablation may be considered in consultation with an electrophysiologist for patients who have frequent clinically significant recurrences despite antiarrhythmic drugs or cannot tolerate adequate doses of antiarrhythmic drugs.
    - Ablation of the AV node and insertion of a permanent pacemaker is highly effective in rate control.
    - Disadvantages include the need for anticoagulation due to persistent AF, loss of AV synchrony, and the need for permanent pacing.
- Rhythm control (with drug therapy or direct current reversion) is managed somewhat differently for patients with AF and AFI.

ATRIAL FIBRILLATION

- Patients with a shorter duration of AF and smaller left atrial size are more likely to revert to normal sinus rhythm.
- If AF is of less than 48 hours duration, and the patient has a structurally normal heart, it may be reasonable to proceed with chemical or electrical cardioversion. Exceptions include situations that are likely to be temporary such as AF following an alcoholic binge in young college student or in the stable postoperative patient with AF for whom anticoagulation would be a transient problem.
- If AF is of undetermined or more than 48 hours in duration or unstable, transesophageal echocardiography (if the initial study was transthoracic) can reliably exclude left atrial thrombus prior to cardioversion.

○ Alternatively, stable patients should be therapeutically anticoagulated for at least 4 weeks prior to elective direct current (DC) cardioversion.

○ Cardioversion can successfully convert AF to NSR in roughly 70% to 99% of the cases, and maintenance of normal sinus rhythm requires the addition of an antiarrhythmic regimen.

• Particularly with a new or first-time diagnosis of AF, patients should be considered for chemical or electrical cardioversion.

○ Rhythm control, consisting of antiarrhythmic medications to maintain sinus rhythm, are indicated when patients have persisted troublesome symptoms despite adequate rate control or when adequate rate control cannot be achieved.

○ The "pill-in-the-pocket" approach is an effective strategy for patients with structurally normal hearts and paroxysmal persistent AF that occurs without hemodynamic compromise, if an effective agent (single PO dose propafenone or flecainide) is identified for the patient in a supervised setting.

○ Rhythm control does not eliminate the need for anticoagulation. Recurrent episodes of AF are common and often asymptomatic.

• If patient is successfully converted to normal sinus rhythm, anticoagulation should be continued for at least 4 weeks to prevent systemic embolism.

• Medications used for conversion to sinus rhythm in the hospital setting are in Table 25-5.

○ Class Ic antiarrhythmics (propafenone, flecainide) which act primarily on sodium channels and slow conduction velocity of impulses within the atria.

■ Flecainide causes reduction in cardiac conduction, contractility, and is proarrhythmic. It is contraindicated in patients with systolic dysfunction or in patients with coronary artery disease. Because it may increase AV nodal conduction, it should be used with AV nodal blocking agents.

○ Class III antiarrhythmics (ibutilide, dofetilide, and amiodarone) which act primarily on potassium channels to prolong refractoriness of atrial tissue

■ Administration of oral amiodarone may result in 15% to 40% of patients reverting to NSR at 28 days

■ In the inpatient setting, patients often receive a loading bolus and infusion which may result in a reversion rate as high as 95%.

ATRIAL FLUTTER

• Rate control with AV nodal blocking drugs is often challenging.

○ Though 4:1 AV ratios (ventricular rates of approximately 70 bpm) might be able to be achieved temporarily with the patient at rest, increased patient activity can result in faster heart rates despite high doses of AV nodal agents.

○ For this reason, more expeditious cardioversion is often warranted for AFl even if it has been present for more than 48 hours.

○ AFl, in contrast to AF, can be pace terminated in many cases. This can be accomplished with some indwelling pacemakers or defibrillators with temporary pacemaker electrodes (eg, with the epicardial atrial wires sometimes present after open heart surgery)

○ Typical AFl is often approached with a high degree of success with percutaneous radiofrequency ablation.

• *Prevention of systemic thromboembolism*—All patients should be anticoagulated unless they have contraindications.

○ In the hospital setting, this may be accomplished initially with weight-based low-molecular-weight or unfractionated heparin (see Chap. 90).

○ For patients who have been in AF more than 48 hours, and are converted to sinus rhythm (either electrically or chemically), the patient should be maintained on therapeutic anticoagulation for at least the subsequent 4–6 weeks using warfarin with a target INR of 2:3.

CARE TRANSITIONS

• Patient education about their disease is important, as there are many factors which influence the treatment and outcome.

○ Patients should be made aware that even with appropriate therapy AF may be a lifelong problem.

○ Although they may still experience symptoms, they may also be asymptomatic (because of effective rate control), but are still at risk of complications of AF.

○ Avoidance of substances (alcohol, caffeine, stimulants, etc) that may trigger AF may improve prognosis.

• All patients without contraindication to anticoagulation should be sent out on an antithromboembolism regimen.

○ Approximately one in four strokes in the elderly are related to AF.

○ Patient characteristics associated with higher risk of thromboembolism include age >60, heart failure (particularly with left ventricular ejection fraction [LVEF] <35%), left atrial thrombus, rheumatic heart disease, coronary artery disease, diabetes mellitus, hypertension, or prior stroke. Such patients should be managed with long-term warfarin with a goal INR of 2:3.

■ Arrangements should be made for at least weekly prothrombin time (PT) and INR measurements to monitor warfarin therapy.

TABLE 25-6 CHADS2 Score and Thromboembolism Risk from AF

RISK FACTOR	CHADS2 SCORE
Heart failure	1
Hypertension	1
Age ≥75 years	1
Diabetes mellitus	1
Secondary prevention in patients with prior ischemic cerebrovascular attack/transient ischemic attack (CVA/TIA) or systemic embolism	2

CHADS2 SCORE	% PER YEAR OF THROMBOEMBOLIC EVENTS		NUMBER NEEDED TO TREAT
	NO WARFARIN	WARFARIN	
0	0.49	0.25	417
1	1.52	0.72	125
2	2.50	1.27	81
3	5.27	2.20	33
4	6.02	2.35	27
5–6	6.88	4.60	44

Data from: (for Score and Thromboembolism Risk from AF) Go AS, Hylek EM, Chang Y, et al. Anticoagulation therapy for stroke prevention in atrial fibrillation: how well do randomized trials translate into clinical practice *JAMA*. 2003;290:2685 and (for CHADS2 score) Gage BF, Waterman AD, Shannon W. Validation of clinical classification schemes for predicting stroke: results from the National Registry of Atrial Fibrillation *JAMA*. 2001;285:2864.

○ Patients at low risk for thromboembolism can be considered for therapy with aspirin instead of systemic anticoagulation. A CHADS2 score of zero is considered low risk, 1–2 intermediate risk, and ≥3 high risk (Table 25-6).
• All patients should be treated with beta-blockers or calcium channel blockers (as heart rate and blood pressure allow) to prevent rapid ventricular rates if AF is persistent or recurs.
  ○ Careful attention should be paid to outpatient medications, as many patients are on antihypertensive medications and the addition of rate controlling medications can have significant effects on blood pressure and significant drug-drug interactions.
• It is safe to discharge patients who are still in AF if they are adequately rate controlled (resting heart rate <80 and rate <110 after a 6-minute walk).
• Outpatient follow-up should be arranged for continued monitoring of symptoms and development of patient-specific treatment plans, including referral to a cardiologist or electrophysiologist when subsequent outpatient cardioversion is planned or other forms of rhythm control may be indicated.

BIBLIOGRAPHY

American Heart Association. Heart Disease and Stroke Statistics—2006 Update. American Heart Association; 2006.

Carlsson J, Miketic S, Windeler J, et al. Randomized trial of rate-control versus rhythm-control in persistent atrial fibrillation: the Strategies of Treatment of Atrial Fibrillation (STAF) study. *J Am Coll Cardiol*. 2003; 41:1690–1696.

Chevalier P, Durand-Dubief A, Burri H, et al. Amiodarone versus placebo and classic drugs for cardioversion of recent-onset atrial fibrillation: a meta-analysis. *J Am Coll Cardiol*. 2003;41:255–262.

Farshi R, Kistner D, Sarma JS, et al. Ventricular rate control in chronic atrial fibrillation during daily activity and programmed exercise: a crossover open-label study of five drug regimens. *J Am Coll Cardiol*. 1999;33:304–310.

Furberg CD, Psaty BM, Manolio TA, et al. Prevalence of atrial fibrillation in elderly subjects (the Cardiovascular Health Study). *Am J Cardiol*. 1994;74:236–241.

Fuster V, Rydén LE, Cannom DS, et al. ACC/AHA/ESC 2006 guidelines for the management of patients with atrial fibrillation: a report of the American College of Cardiology/ American Heart Association task force on practice guidelines and the European Society of Cardiology Committee for practice guidelines (Writing Committee to Revise the 2001 Guidelines for the Management of Patients With Atrial Fibrillation). *J Am Coll Cardiol*. 2006;48:e149–e246.

Naccarelli GV, Wolbrette DL, Khan M, et al. Old and new antiarrhythmic drugs for converting and maintaining sinus rhythm in atrial fibrillation: comparative efficacy and results of trials. *Am J Cardiol*. 2003;91:15D–26D.

Stroke Prevention in Atrial Fibrillation Investigators. Predictors of thromboembolism in atrial fibrillation: I. Clinical features of patients at risk. *Ann Intern Med*. 1992;116:1–5.

Tamariz LJ, Bass EB. Pharmacological rate control of atrial fibrillation. *Cardiol Clin*. 2004;22:35–45.

Wyse DG, Waldo AL, DiMarco JP, et al. A comparison of rate control and rhythm control in patients with atrial fibrillation. *N Engl J Med*. 2002;347:1825–1833.

26 SUPRAVENTRICULAR TACHYCARDIA

Mara Giattina

EPIDEMIOLOGY/OVERVIEW

- Supraventricular tachycardia (SVT) refers to paroxysmal tachyarrhythmias which involve the atria or atrioventricular (AV) junction or both. These arrhythmias are relatively common and a frequent cause of emergency department (ED) visits; and though infrequently the primary reason for hospital admission, commonly occur during inpatient admissions as a result of precipitating illness or drug interaction.
- This chapter provides
  - An overview of select SVTs
    - Atrial tachycardia (AT)
    - Atrioventricular reciprocating tachycardia (AVRT)
    - Atrioventricular nodal reciprocating tachycardia (AVNRT)
    - Multifocal atrial tachycardia (MAT)
    - Inappropriate sinus tachycardia
    - Junctional tachycardia
  - Acute diagnosis and management strategies
  - Long-term treatment strategies
  - Indications for referral to an electrophysiologist
- Aflutter and MAT, though not routinely classified as SVTs, are included as part of the differential diagnosis of SVT; for further discussion of atrial fibrillation (AF) and atrial flutter, please refer to Chap. 25.
- The failure to discriminate among AF, atrial flutter, and other SVTs in many studies complicates determination of the prevalence, associated risk factors, and responses to treatment for each of the specific arrhythmias.
  - SVT prevalence is approximately 2.25/1000.[1]
  - In a review of Medicare discharge cases from 1991 to 1998, SVT was diagnosed in 3.8% of discharges, atrial flutter in another 5.2%, with a case fatality rate around 1% and average length of stay (LOS) of 4.2–4.5 days.[2]
- Average age of onset is 57 with a wide age range. Occurrence is more frequent with advanced age and female gender.[1]
- Most forms of paroxysmal SVT (AVNRT, AVRT) are not associated with structural heart disease, though 48% to 90% of patients presenting with SVT report a history of cardiovascular disease. Those with "lone" SVT (no structural heart disease) tend to be younger and have faster heart rates.

PATHOPHYSIOLOGY

- All cardiac arrhythmias are produced by either abnormal impulse initiation (automaticity) or abnormal impulse conduction (reentrant circuits).[4] The SVT is then classified by the location of the ectopic focus or the reentrant circuit[5] (Fig. 26-1).
- *Abnormal automaticity:* In SVT, tissues with abnormal automaticity can reside in the atria, the AV node, or the nearby vessels. If the firing rate of the ectopic focus is greater than that of the sinus node, then the ectopic focus will become the predominant pacemaker of the heart.
  - *Atrial tachycardia:* Abnormal atrial automaticity is thought to cause focal atrial tachycardia. Of note, however, this rhythm can instead be from a very focal "micro reentrant" circuit.
  - *Junctional tachycardia:* Focal junctional tachycardia is characterized by abnormally rapid discharge from the AV node or bundle of His, is rare in the pediatric population, and even more uncommon in adults. More common in adults is nonparoxysmal junctional tachycardia, abnormal automaticity from high in the AV node, which shows a typical "warm-up" and "cool-down" pattern, and, though benign, may be a marker for more serious underlying condition, that is, digoxin toxicity.
- *Reentrant circuits:* Most types of SVT involve a reentrant mechanism. The requirements to initiate and sustain a reentrant circuit are (1) unidirectional block in one limb of the circuit, often because of the refractory period of the tissue and (2) slow conduction in another section of the circuit. Antiarrhythmic drugs work by increasing refractoriness (class III) or interfering with conduction (class I) thereby disrupting a reentrant circuit.
  - In atrial flutter the reentrant circuit occupies large areas of the atria, ("macro reentrant").
  - Atrioventricular reciprocating tachycardia depends on the presence of an accessory pathway, which is abnormal conduction tissue located between the atria and the ventricles.
    - The most common pathway ("orthodromic") begins with an atrial impulse blocked by the accessory pathway, but able to conduct slowly down the AV node.
    - This impulse excites the ventricles via the His-Purkinje system producing a narrow QRS complex, then travels by ventriculo-atrial (V-A) conduction via the accessory pathway, exciting the atria shortly after the ventricles ("short RP" tachycardia, where RP interval < PR interval on electrocardiogram [ECG]).

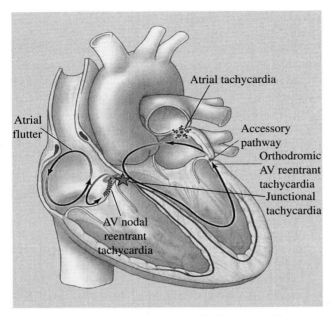

FIG. 26-1 Mechanisms of supraventricular tachycardia. Adapted from: Delacretaz E. Supraventricular tachycardia. *NEJM.* 2006;354:1039–1051.

- By the time the impulse reaches the AV node, it is again excitable thus propagating the circuit.
- AVRT is "antidromic" if the circuit is in the opposite direction, with A-V conduction down the accessory pathway, producing a wide QRS complex, then V-A conduction via the AV node.
  - AVNRT is similar to AVRT; however, there is no accessory pathway. Instead, both the A-V and V-A conduction travel through distinct pathways within the AV node, typically traveling antegrade down the slow pathway and retrograde via the fast pathway, activating the atria and ventricles almost simultaneously ("Short RP" or "no-RP" tachycardia).
    - In 5% to 10%, the circuit is in the reverse direction with fast A-V conduction and slow V-A conduction, producing a "long RP" tachycardia.
    - Regular paroxysmal SVT is most commonly due to AVRT or AVNRT.
  - Sinus node reentry is rare paroxysmal SVT with micro reentrant circuit within the sinus node and immediately surrounding atrial tissue.
- Sinus tachycardia (ST) can either be appropriate or inappropriate.
  - Physiologic ST is common during the inpatient setting in response to the underlying medical illness. Heart rate trends on telemetry monitoring may be helpful as ST is characterized by gradual changes in rate, whereas other SVTs are paroxysmal with abrupt changes in rate.

- Inappropriate sinus tachycardia is out of proportion or unrelated to underlying pathology. It is caused by abnormal automaticity or abnormal autonomic tone and is more common in females and healthcare workers.
  - Positional orthostatic tachycardia syndrome (POTS) manifests as severe orthostatic tachycardia without hypotension in patients with autonomic neuropathy. The mechanism is unknown, though splanchnic or peripheral blood pooling or reduced red cell mass are some of the proposed mechanisms.

CLINICAL PRESENTATION, DIFFERENTIAL, MAKING THE DIAGNOSIS

- SVT is most often asymptomatic though, when present, symptoms can include abrupt onset of palpitations, fatigue, polyuria, diaphoresis, chest discomfort, dyspnea, presyncope, or syncope.
  - Syncope occurs in approximately 15%, and is more common with associated structural heart disease or cerebrovascular disease.
  - If persistent, SVT may lead to tachycardia associated cardiomyopathy.
  - Symptoms may also manifest similarly to panic attacks.
  - Initial evaluation should focus on associated symptoms, whether palpitations are regular or irregular, frequency and duration of episodes, and possible triggers (Table 26-1).

TABLE 26-1 Palpitations—Precipitating or Predisposing Factors[4]

NONCARDIAC CAUSES	CARDIAC CAUSES
Caffeine, nicotine	CAD, old MI
Alcohol/withdrawal	CHF/cardiomyopathy
Certain drugs	Valvular disease
Antiarrhythmics	Congenital heart disease
Antidepressants	Primary electrical disorders (i.e., long
Antibiotics	QT syndrome, Brugada syndrome)
Antihistamines	Accessory pathways
Appetite suppressants	Other conditions that may cause
Stimulants	myocardial scarring (i.e.,
Hyperthyroidism	sarcoidosis, tuberculosis)
Anemia	
Hypovolemia	
Fever, infection	
Anxiety, lack of sleep	
Electrolyte disturbance	

Adapted from: Blomstrom-Lundqvist C., Scheinman MM, Aliot EM et al. ACC/AHA/ESC guidelines for the management of patients with supraventricular arrhythmias—executive summary: a report of the American College of Cardiology/American Heart Association Task Force on Practice Guidelines and the European Society of Cardiology Committee for Practice Guidelines (Writing Committee to Develop Guidelines for the Management of Patients With Supraventricular Arrhythmias) Circulation 2003;108(15):1871–909.

- The physical examination is usually not helpful in differentiating the diagnosis.
  - The physical examination should focus on signs of structural heart disease or acute underlying illness.
  - SVT can be associated with the "frog sign," the prominent jugular A waves from atrial contraction against a closed tricuspid valve.
- *The ECG:* Both resting ECG and telemetry/12-lead ECG analyses during the arrhythmia are pivotal in the differential and management of the arrhythmia. Whenever possible, a 12-lead ECG should always be taken during the SVT, though this should not delay immediate therapy if the patient is unstable. At a minimum, a monitor strip should be obtained from the defibrillator prior to direct current (DC) cardioversion.
  - A narrow complex tachycardia (QRS <120 ms) is almost always supraventricular in origin. Careful examination for P waves, and their relation to the QRS helps determine the specific diagnosis (Table 26-2 and Figs. 26-2 and 26-3). The P waves may be retrograde, and/or buried in the QRS, therefore difficult to discern. Telemetry monitoring can also be helpful to document sudden changes in rate suggesting SVT vs. a more gradual rate change characteristic of sinus tachycardia.
  - *Wide complex SVT:* A wide QRS may be a manifestation of a SVT, (as in SVT with preexisting or rate-related bundle branch block or SVT with conduction over an accessory pathway) though this occurs in <10%.[5] In unstable presentations, or where a preexisting diagnosis of SVT is not certain, these cases should be treated as ventricular tachycardia. The presence of a wide complex tachycardia warrants referral to an electrophysiologist.
  - *Accessory pathway:* A-V conduction over an accessory pathway may occur during any type of SVT: AF, atrial flutter, AT, AVNRT, or antidromic AVRT.
    - The baseline ECG should be carefully examined for evidence of pre-excitation (delta wave), and is generally sufficient to make the diagnosis of AVRT in a patient with paroxysmal regular palpitations.
    - However, the delta wave may be minimal or absent in approximately 30% of patients with an accessory pathway so its absence cannot exclude AVRT.
    - The presence of pre-excitation on resting ECG in a patient reporting paroxysmal irregular palpitations strongly suggests AF and Wolff-Parkinson-White (WPW) syndrome and should immediately trigger an EP referral. These patients are at risk for ventricular fibrillation (VF) and sudden death.[4]

- Additional diagnostics
  - Initial laboratory evaluation should include electrolytes and TSH.
  - An admission chest radiograph is helpful in evaluation of any exacerbating lung disease, congestive heart failure, or dilated cardiomyopathy.
  - Though uncommon, structural heart disease should be excluded with an echocardiogram.[4]
  - Exercise testing may be useful if the arrhythmia is clearly triggered by exertion.

TRIAGE AND INITIAL MANAGEMENT

- Refer to Fig. 26-4 for the acute management of SVT. Patients presenting with SVTs are rarely hemodynamically unstable, though in these cases, proceed directly to electrical cardioversion.
  - Electrical cardioversion can be used at any point in the algorithm with appropriate sedation and analgesia, if the following AV blocking agents fail, or if clinical condition worsens.
- *Vagal maneuvers:* Carotid sinus massage triggers increased vagal tone and sympathetic withdrawal, thus slowing conduction through the AV node.
  - After ascertaining the absence of a carotid bruit or the presence of carotid disease, 5–10 seconds of firm circular pressure is applied at the level of the cricoid cartilage.
  - Vagal tone can also be increased by having the patient Valsalva.
  - The response to these vagal maneuvers and to adenosine can be therapeutic and/or diagnostic, so should be performed with continuous ECG monitoring.
- *Adenosine:* The advantage of adenosine is its rapid onset and short half-life. The patient should have continuous ECG monitoring during the adenosine infusion, to aid in the diagnosis during the period of AV block (Table 26-3). Adenosine will terminate those SVTs depending on the AV node for propagation (AVRT, AVNRT).
  - Sixty percent to eighty percent of SVTs are successfully terminated after 6 mg of adenosine and 90% to 95% after 12 mg of adenosine.
  - If adenosine administration does not alter the rhythm, possibilities include inadequate dosing or the rare instance of narrow complex ventricular tachycardia of high septal or fascicular origin.
  - Bronchoconstriction and ventricular fibrillation are rare complications, so resuscitation equipment should be immediately available.
  - Adenosine is contraindicated in wide complex tachycardia and in heart transplant patients, and should be used with caution in patients with severe COPD or asthma.

TABLE 26-2 Differential Diagnosis of Regular Narrow Complex Tachycardia

ARRHYTHMIA	DISTINGUISHING ECG/TELEMETRY FEATURES	RESPONSE TO VAGAL MANEUVERS/ ADENOSINE	OTHER ASSOCIATED FEATURES	TREATMENT MODALITIES
Sinus tachycardia	Gradual increases and decreases in rate on telemetry monitor. P wave is upright in leads I, II, avF, and is negative in R	Transient rate slowing then reacceleration. Rare instance of sinus node reentry will terminate with adenosine	Associated with precipitating stressors, i.e., infection, hypovolemia, anemia, CHF	Treatment of underlying precipitant BB treatment in some cases where anxiety, MI, CHF, thyrotoxicosis, or inappropriate ST is the cause
Atrial tachycardia	Isoelectric horizontal baseline with distinct P waves. Heart rate 100–250. P wave often hidden in T wave. Can have gradual "warm up" and "cool down" in rate	Variable—Usually persistent atrial tachycardia with transient AV block. Infrequent sudden termination of arrhythmia	Commonly associated with underlying cardiac abnormalities, congenital heart disease, digitalis toxicity	Catheter ablation. Difficult to treat medically BB, CCB, disopyramide, flecainide, propafenone, sotalol, amiodarone
Atrial flutter	Undulating or "sawtooth" baseline. Atrial rate usually >260 beats/min	Persisting atrial flutter with transient AV block	Associated heart disease and age >60 common. Often occurs during acute underlying disease process	DCCV* Catheter ablation Rate control with BB, CCB. Chemical cardioversion* with dofetilide, amiodarone, sotalol, flecainide, quinidine, propafenone, procainamide, disopyramide
AVRT	Delta wave in 70% on resting ECG Rates 140–250	Sudden termination; arrhythmia ends with P wave following QRS	Structural heart disease uncommon	Catheter ablation preferred. Flecainide, propafenone, sotalol, amiodarone. BB or CCB if no pre-excitation on resting ECG
AVNRT	Pathognomic "no RP" tachycardia, or P wave partially hidden in QRS, producing a pseudo-R' in V1 and/or pseudo-S in inferior leads. Rates 140–250	Sudden termination; arrhythmia ends with P wave following QRS	Structural heart disease uncommon	Catheter ablation preferred therapy CCB, BB, flecainide, propafenone, sotalol, amiodarone, digoxin
Nonparoxysmal junctional tachycardia	Nonparoxysmal, with warm-up and cool-down periods. Heart rate 70–120	Gradual slowing then reacceleration of rate	Marker for more serious underlying disorder i.e., digitalis toxicity, postcardiac surgery, hypokalemia, myocardial ischemia, hypoxia	Treatment of underlying disorder or cessation of digoxin BB or CCB therapy if persistent
Multifocal atrial tachycardia	Irregular rhythm with 3 or more P wave morphologies. Rate usually not excessively rapid	Adenosine not indicated for irregular rhythm	Usually associated with underlying pulmonary disease, also seen with metabolic or electrolyte derangements	Treatment aimed at correction of underlying illness. Some reported success with CCB

*If present >48 hours, exclude presence of thrombus with transesophageal echocardiography before elective DCCV or chemical cardioversion. Long-term anticoagulation treatment for atrial flutter similar to that for AF.

• *Calcium channel blockers (CCBs) or beta-blockers:* Following vagal maneuvers and adenosine, if arrhythmia persists, proceed to trial of IV verapamil, IV diltiazem, or IV beta-blocker.

◦ Even in those patients with successful conversion with adenosine, over 50% of patients have recurrence of SVT; these patients should also be treated with an AV nodal blocking agent in order to maintain sinus rhythm.

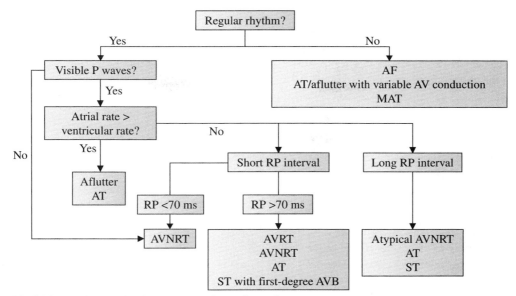

FIG. 26-2 ECG analysis of narrow complex tachycardia.
AF, atrial fibrillation; AT, atrial tachycardia; Aflutter, atrial flutter; MAT, multifocal atrial tachycardia;
AVNRT, atrioventricular nodal reciprocating tachycardia; AVRT, atrioventricular reciprocating tachycardia;
ST, sinus tachycardia; Short RP, RP interval<PR on ECG; Long RP, RP >PR.
Adopted from: Blomstrom-Lundqvist, Scheinman, et al. ACC/AHA/ESC Guidelines for the Management
of Patients with Supraventricular Arrhythmias. 2003.

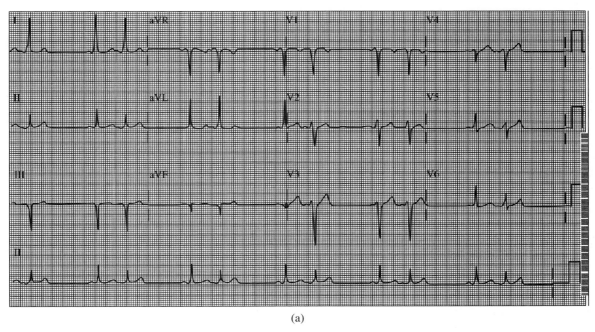

(a)

FIG. 26-3 ECG tracing in SVT.
a. Note the delta wave in this baseline resting ECG. ECG also notable for atrial bigeminy, with delta wave more evident
on the second beat, after a shorter R-R interval.
b. Transient atrial tachycardia. Not the P waves almost buried in the T wave. The termination of this long RP tachycardia
is notably without a P wave, therefore confirming AT in favor of atypical AVNRT.
c. Atrial flutter with 4:1 conduction. Note the sinusoidal baseline characteristic of typical atrial flutter.
d. AVNRT—Pathognomic pseudo R' in V1, which is actually the P wave buried in the terminal QRS complex. This
becomes evident when compared to this patient's baseline ECG (e).

STAT ECG

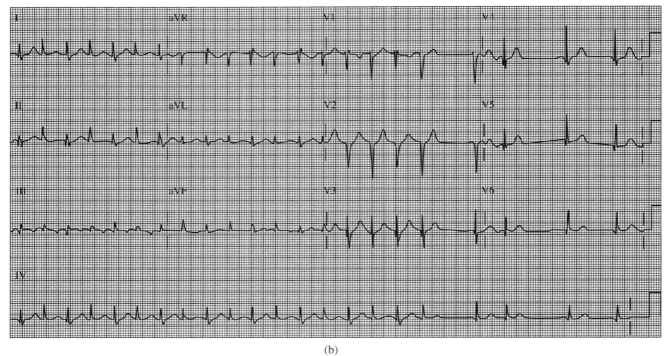

(b)

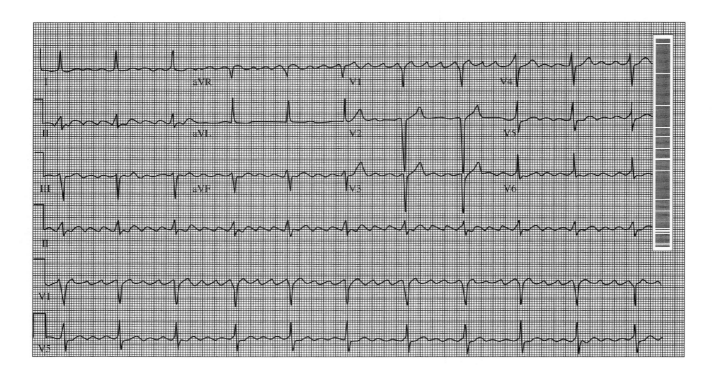

(c)

FIG. 26-3 *(Continued)*

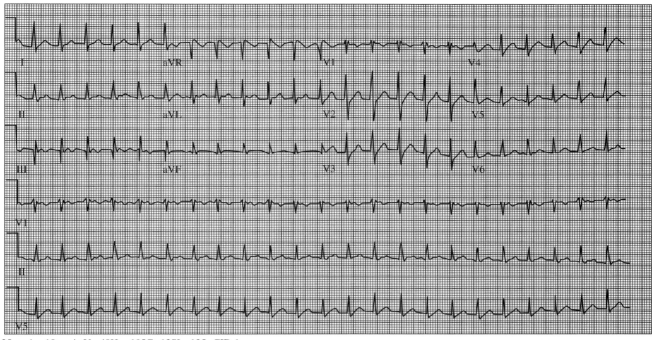

25mm/s   10mm/mV   40Hz   105C   12SL   135   CID:1

(d)

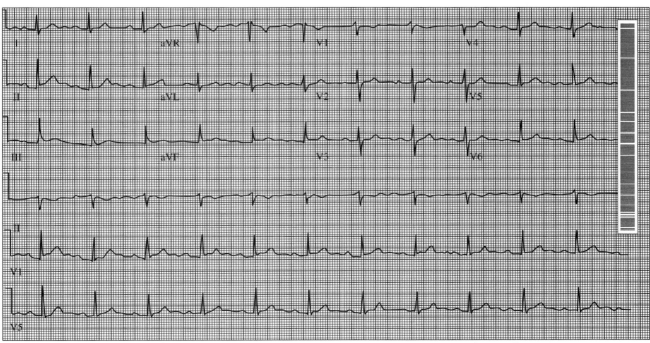

25mm/s   10mm/mV   150Hz   005C   12SL   229   CID:1

(e)

FIG. 26-3   *(Continued)*

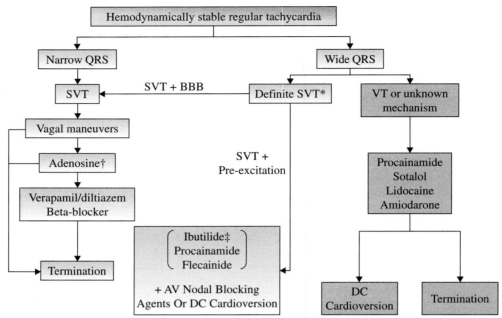

FIG. 26-4 Short-term management of narrow complex tachycardia.
*12-lead ECG during sinus rhythm must be available for diagnosis.
†Caution in patients with severe CAD, risk of AF and rapid ventricular rates in those with pre-excitation.
‡Should not be used in patients with LVEF<30% due to high risk of VT.

○ All these agents have side effects of hypotension, heart block, and negative inotropy, so the clinical condition of the patient should be reassessed before administration, and they should not be used in a patient with history of heart block, severe hypotension, or congestive heart failure.
○ These side effects are potentiated with the concomitant use of beta-blockers and CCBs.

• *Antiarrhythmic therapy:* If CCB and/or beta-blocker therapy is unsuccessful, consider the use of IV procainamide, propafenone, flecainide, or ibutilide.
○ These agents have major side effects of hypotension and bradycardia and can also be pro-arrhythmic.
○ Consider electrophysiologist (EP) consultation on the use of these antiarrhythmic agents.

TABLE 26-3   Pharmacologic Agents for Acute Treatment of SVT

DRUG	DOSE
Adenosine	6 mg rapid bolus followed by flush. If needed, repeat in 1–2 min with12 mg
Verapamil	5 mg IV every 3–5 min to maximum dose of 15 mg
Diltiazem	0.25 mg/kg over 2 min. If no response, additional dose of 0.35 mg/kg over 2 min. If needed, maintenance infusion of 5–15 mg/hr
Metoprolol	5 mg over 2 min, repeat every 5 min as needed to max dose of 15 mg
Esmolol	250–500 mcg/kg over 1 min. If needed, 4 min infusion of 50–200 mcg/kg/min
Propranolol	0.15 mg/kg over 2 min, dose not to exceed 1 mg/min
Procainamide	30 mg/min continuous infusion to a maximum dose of 17 mg/kg (maintenance infusion of 2–4 mg/min)
Flecainide	2 mg/kg over 10 min
Propafenone	2 mg/kg over 10 min
Ibutilide	If >60 kg: 1 mg over 10 min
If <60 mg: 0.01 mg/kg over 10 min
Repeat once if no response after 10 additional min

Adapted from: Delacretaz E. Supraventricular tachycardia. *NEJM*. 2006;354:1039–1051.

DISEASE MANAGEMENT STRATEGIES

- Not all patients with SVT require therapy, even if the arrhythmia is recurrent.
  - Generally the goal of treatment is improvement in quality of life.
  - The decision on whether to begin long-term therapy and/or to refer to an electrophysiologist is based on the severity of symptoms, presence of pre-excitation, the potential for successful catheter ablation, response to drug therapy, and patient preference (Fig. 26-5).
  - Consider EP referral for those started on chronic prophylactic therapy with class Ic or class III antiarrhythmic agents.
- *AV nodal blocking agents:* Calcium channel blockers, beta-blockers, and digoxin all decrease the number of events to a similar degree, with improvement in symptom frequency and severity in up to 60% of patients, but complete suppression is uncommon.[7] These agents
  - Provide rate control in atrial arrhythmias (aflutter, atrial tachycardia).
  - May abolish reentrant tachyarrhythmias dependent on AV nodal conduction (AVNRT, AVRT).

- Should not be used in patients with pre-excitation (Fig. 26-5).
- *Antiarrhythmic agents:* Class 1C (flecainide, propafenone) and class III (amiodarone, sotalol) drugs prevent recurrence of SVT in up to 80% of patients. No trials have directly compared these drugs to AV nodal agents.
  - These antiarrhythmic drugs should be used in combination with an AV nodal blocking agent because they can slow atrial arrhythmias sufficiently to allow 1:1 conduction through the AV node to the ventricles.
  - Though catheter ablation is preferred for patients with pre-excitation, both flecainide and propafenone are FDA approved to prevent SVT in this population.
  - Regardless, the side effects of class 1C drugs include proarrhythmia and merit caution before long-term use, especially in those with structural or ischemic heart disease.
  - Of note, amiodarone has been shown to be safe in structural heart disease;[4] however, catheter ablation should generally be recommended before committing a patient to long-term use.[5]
- *"Pill-in-the-pocket" approach:* This strategy, in which a patient takes one dose of a drug at the onset of symptoms, can be effective for those with prolonged (over

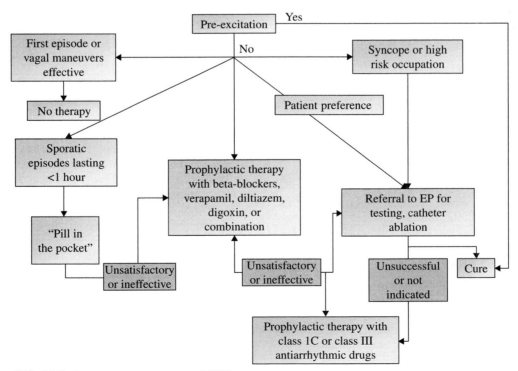

FIG. 26-5 Long-term management of SVT.
Adapted from: Delacretaz E. Supraventricular tachycardia. *NEJM.* 2006;354:1039–1051.

an hour) but infrequent episodes (only a few per year) that are well tolerated hemodynamically.

- ○ Drugs useful for this approach include verapamil (40–160 mg), various beta-blockers, flecainide (100–300 mg), and propafenone (150–450 mg).
- ○ The combination of diltiazem (120 mg) and propranolol (80 mg) has been shown to be superior to both placebo and flecainide, and is associated with reduced ED visits.[6]
- *Catheter ablation:* Although there have not been large randomized trials compared drug therapy to ablation, limited data suggests that catheter ablation improves quality of life and is more cost effective in the long term.
  - ○ It has been increasingly used for the treatment of AVRT by ablation of the accessory pathway, or treatment of AVNRT by ablation of the slow AV nodal pathway with success rates near 95%.[8]
  - ○ Though low, there is potential for the development of AF and sudden death in patients with WPW, supporting liberal indication for catheter ablation for those with accessory pathways.[4]
  - ○ Catheter ablation of focal atrial tachycardias has slightly lower success rates, around 85%.
  - ○ For reentrant atrial tachycardias, that is, atrial flutter, radiofrequency ablation is used with high success rates around 95%.
  - ○ Catheter ablation takes about 1–3 hours, can be performed as an outpatient procedure, or may require overnight hospitalization.
  - ○ Patients are recommended to take aspirin for a few weeks after a left-sided ablation to reduce the risk of embolization, but otherwise there is no special follow-up after the intervention.
  - ○ Complications occur in less than 2% to 3% of patients and include AV block and need for permanent pacemaker, structural damage to the heart, thrombosis, stroke, and rarely death.
- *Treatment in pregnancy:* Sustained arrhythmias are relatively rare in pregnancy. Of those women with preexisting SVT, symptomatic exacerbation occurs in about 20%. All antiarrhythmic drugs should be regarded as potentially toxic to the fetus, and should be avoided if possible, especially during the first trimester.
  - ○ All drugs used for the treatment of SVT are pregnancy class C, except sotalol (B), atenolol and amiodarone (D).
  - ○ There is considerable experience with adenosine, propranolol, metoprolol, digoxin, and flecainide in pregnancy.
  - ○ DC cardioversion can be used when necessary in all stages of pregnancy.

- ○ In women of reproductive age with symptomatic SVTs, catheter ablation should be recommended before contemplating pregnancy.
  - ▪ Although there is a risk of fetal exposure to radiation during the procedure, catheter ablation can be performed for drug refractory SVT, preferentially during the second trimester.

CARE TRANSITIONS

- For many patients with a normal resting ECG, the diagnosis remains unclear upon discharge.
- *Outpatient monitoring may be helpful:* Use an ambulatory 24-hour Holter monitor, or an event or loop recorder for less frequent episodes. An implantable loop recorder may be indicated in select cases with rare but hemodynamically significant episodes.
- Beta-blockers may be prescribed empirically. Patients should be taught vagal maneuvers, and should minimize common reversible predisposing factors (Table 26-1).
- Those with pre-excitation, wide complex tachycardia, those prescribed antiarrhythmic therapy or those who may be candidates for ablation warrant referral to an electrophysiologist.

REFERENCES

1. Orejarena LA, Vidaillet H Jr, DeStefano F, et al. Paroxysmal supraventricular tachycardia in the general population. *J Am Coll Cardiol.* 1998;31:150–157. (ACC10)
2. Baine WB, Yu W, Weis KA. Trends and outcomes in the hospitalization of older Americans for cardiac conduction disorders or arrhythmias , 1991–1998. *J Am Geriatr Soc.* 2001; 49:763–770. (ACC3)
3. Cairns CB, Neimann JT. Intravenous adenosine in the emergency department management of paroxysmal supraventricular tachycardia. *Ann Emerg Med.* 1991;20:717–721.
4. Blomstrom-Lundqvist C., Scheinman MM, Aliot EM et al. ACC/AHA/ESC guidelines for the management of patients with supraventricular arrhythmias—executive summary: a report of the American College of Cardiology/American Heart Association Task Force on Practice Guidelines and the European Society of Cardiology Committee for Practice Guidelines (Writing Committee to Develop Guidelines for the Management of Patients With Supraventricular Arrhythmias) Circulation 2003;108(15):1871–909.
5. Delacretaz E. Supraventricular tachycardia. *NEJM.* 2006;354: 1039–1051.
6. Alboni P, Tomasi C, Menozzi C et al. Efficacy and safety of out-of-hospital self-administered single-dose oral drug regimen in the management of infrequent, well-tolerated paroxysmal supraventricular tachycardia. *J Am Coll Cardiol.* 2001;37:548–553. (ACC211)

7. Winniford MD, Fulton KL, Hillis LD. Long-term therapy of paroxysmal supraventricular tachycardia: a randomized, double blind comparison of digoxin, propranolol, and verapamil. *Am J Cardiol.* 1984;54:1138–1139.
8. Kuck KH, Schluter M, Geiger M, et al. Radiofrequency current catheter ablation of accessory atrioventricular pathways. *Lancet.* 1991;337:1557–1561.

27   SINUS BRADYCARDIA AND ATRIOVENTRICULAR BLOCKS

Apoor Patel

EPIDEMIOLOGY/OVERVIEW

- Sinus bradycardia is defined as a heart rate (HR) <55–60 beats/min and is found commonly in both healthy and ill adults. The exact incidence of sinus bradycardia is unknown.
- In studies of normal adults, the mean afternoon HR was 70 beats/min in both men and women, but ranged from 46 to 93 in men and 51–95 in women. The average HR is the same regardless of age.
- In healthy adults, sinus bradycardia does not portend an adverse prognosis or effect longevity.

PATHOPHYSIOLOGY

- Normal cardiac conduction begins with impulse generation in the sinus node located in the right atrium. This impulse then travels electrically via the atria to the atrioventricular (AV) node and subsequently to the bundle of His. The bundle of His separates into the left and right bundle branches that in turn activate the left and right ventricles respectively.
- A balance between sympathetic and parasympathetic input on the conduction system determines the resting heart rate. Under resting conditions, parasympathetic input predominates.
- Bradycardia can be a normal finding in children and young adults. It can also be normal in well-conditioned athletes due to the presence of higher vagal tone in these patients.
- Bradycardia is more pronounced at night and at rest due to higher vagal tone during these periods.
  - In addition, sinus pauses (up to 2.5 seconds), sinoatrial block, junctional rhythms, and first and second-degree

AV block may all be normal variants occurring at night.
  - Young adults have an average decrease of 24 beats/min in their nocturnal heart rate.
- Sinus bradycardia is due to reduced impulse formation from the sinus node. AV blocks are due to conduction delays or impasses in the AV node or bundle of His.

CLINICAL PRESENTATION, DIFFERENTIAL, MAKING THE DIAGNOSIS

- Many patients with bradycardia are asymptomatic.
- However, patients may present with symptoms when their slow HR leads to a reduction in cardiac output. Light-headedness, dizziness, presyncope or syncope, shortness of breath, angina, heart failure, and fatigue all can be presenting symptoms of bradycardia.
- Etiologies of bradycardia that warrant immediate attention include patients with evidence of myocardial infarction, medication toxicity, sick sinus syndrome, neurologic symptoms suggestive of increased intracranial pressure, and electrolyte abnormalities.
- Once dangerous and potentially life-threatening etiologies have been assessed, a more detailed medical history should be obtained.
  - Carefully review medications to screen for nodal acting agents
  - Screen for symptoms of hypothyroidism
  - Screen for symptoms of obstructive sleep apnea
- The physical examination is generally nonspecific.
  - Physicians should look for stigmata of collagen vascular disease, infection, and hypothyroidism.
  - A careful cardiac examination should also be performed to assess for the presence of pathologic murmurs that may occur in the setting of endocarditis.
- While no specific guidelines exist for laboratory evaluation in patients with bradycardia, measurement of serum electrolytes and thyrotropin (TSH) is reasonable.
- All patients should have an electrocardiogram (ECG).
- The differential diagnosis of bradycardia is broad and can be approached by thinking in terms of causes intrinsic and extrinsic to the conduction system (Table 27-1).
- *Sick sinus syndrome:* The sick sinus syndrome is a disorder characterized by chronic sinus node dysfunction and is a common reason for pacemaker implantation. Sinus node dysfunction may be due to many of the intrinsic or extrinsic causes outlined above.
  - Idiopathic age-related fibrosis of the sinus node and conduction system is the most common etiology.
  - See Fig. 27-1 for illustrative examples. Patients may present with

TABLE 27-1   Causes of Bradycardia

INTRINSIC CAUSES	EXTRINSIC CAUSES
Idiopathic degeneration (aging)	Autonomically mediated
Infarction* or ischemia	syndromes
Infiltrative diseases	Neurocardiac syncope
Sarcoid	Carotid sinus
Amyloid	hypersensitivity
Hemochromatosis	Situational disturbances
Collagen vascular diseases	Coughing
Systemic lupus erythematosus	Micturition
Rheumatoid arthritis	Defecation
Scleroderma	Vomiting
Myotonic muscular dystrophy	Drugs
Surgical trauma	Beta-adrenergic blockers
Valve replacement	Calcium channel blockers
Correction of congenital	Clonidine
heart disease	Digoxin
Heart transplant	Antiarrhythmic agents
Familial diseases	Hypothyroidism
Infectious diseases*	Hypothermia
Chagas' disease	Neurologic disorders (elevated
Endocarditis	intracranial pressure)
	Electrolyte imbalances
	Hypokalemia
	Hyperkalemia

*These conditions cause atrioventricular conduction disturbances only.
Reproduced with permission from: Mangrum JM, DiMarco JP. The evaluation and management of bradycardia. *N Engl J Med.* 2000;342:703–709. (Copyright 2000 Massachusetts Medical Society).

- Inappropriate and severe bradycardia
- Alternating bradycardia and tachyarrhythmias such as atrial fibrillation or atrial flutter (known as the tachy-brady syndrome)
- Sinus arrest (failure of the sinus to node to generate an impulse)
- Sinus exit block (failure of impulse from sinus node to conduct to atria)
- Atrial fibrillation with a slow ventricular response (in the absence of AV nodal agents)

- *Myocardial infarction:* Sinus bradycardia and AV block may also occur with acute myocardial infarction (MI).
  - Patients with inferior MI are more likely to have transient bradyarrhythmias mediated by high vagal tone or local tissue edema around the SA or AV node. These patients often do not require permanent pacing, but may need a temporary pacer.
  - Patients with anterior MI are more likely to have necrosis of the conduction system and need permanent pacing.
- *Obstructive sleep apnea:* Patients with obstructive sleep apnea often have bradycardia that is more pronounced (<30 beats/min) during apneic episodes. Treatment of sleep apnea often leads to resolution of bradycardia.

Sinus bradycardia
  Normal P-wave axis with heart rate of
  <60 beats/min
  Every P wave followed by a QRS complex

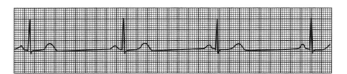

Sinus arrest
  Normal P-wave axis
  Every P wave followed by QRS complex
  Pauses of >3 seconds without atrial activity

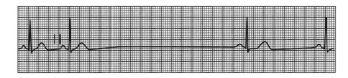

Sinoatrial exit block
  Normal P-wave axis
  Porgressive shortening of PP interval until one
  P wave fails to conduct (second degree, Type I)
  or sinus pause is an exact multiple of the base-
  line PP interval (second degree, Type II (shown))

Bradycardia—tachycardia syndrome
  Alternating periods of atrial tachyarrhythmias
  and bradycardia

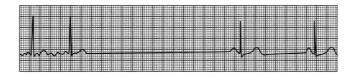

FIG. 27-1   Sinus abnormalities.
Reproduced with permission from: Mangrum JM, DiMarco JP. The evaluation and management of bradycardia. *N Engl J Med.* 2000;342:703–709. (Copyright 2000 Massachusetts Medical Society).

- *Atrioventricular blocks:* Atroventricular conduction may be delayed or fail to occur in the AV node or the bundle of His (Fig. 27-2). The various AV blocks may or may not be associated with bradycardia.
  - The causes of AV nodal blocks are similar to that of sinus bradycardia and are outlined in Table 27-2.
  - Endocarditis, Chagas disease, MI, and myocardial ischemia are usually only associated with AV nodal blocks and do not cause sinus bradycardia.
- Bifascicular block is either
  - A left bundle branch block (LBBB) or
  - The combination of right bundle branch block (RBBB) and either left anterior hemiblock (LAH) or left posterior hemiblock (LPH)
- Trifascicular block is
  - RBBB in association with LAH or LPH
  - Bifascicular block associated with first-degree AV block
  - Alternating RBBB and LBBB
- No formal triage and admission criteria exist for patients with hemodynamically stable bradycardia.
  - Patients with asymptomatic sinus bradycardia and first-degree AV block can be evaluated as outpatients.

Patients with second-degree type I AV block can also have an outpatient assessment if they have a narrow QRS complex and no evidence of a rapidly progressive process.
- Patients with symptoms that may be due to bradycardia should be admitted to the hospital.
  - Goals of admission include trying to definitively establish a connection between HR and symptoms, as this will guide whether to implant a pacemaker.
  - Patients with sinus bradycardia should be evaluated for their ability to increase their heart rate (HR) with exercise. They can be asked to walk or do straight leg raises with measurement of their HR before and after exercise. Inability to raise the HR suggests sinus node disease whereas an increase in HR suggests that the patient's resting bradycardia is physiologic (ie, athletes with high vagal tone).
  - Patients with second-degree type I AV block and a wide QRS suggesting concomitant bundle branch block should have urgent evaluation.
  - Patients with asymptomatic second-degree type II heart block and complete heart block should be

First-degree atrioventricular block
  PR interval of >.2 second
  Every P wave follwed by a QRS complex

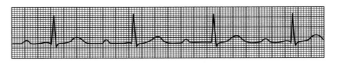

Second-degree atrioventricular block,
Mobitz type I (Wenckebach block)
  Progressive lengthening of PR interval and
  Shortening of RR interval until a P wave is blocked
  PR Interval after blocked beat is shorter than
  preceding PR interval

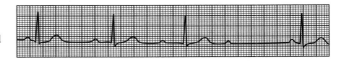

Second-degree atrioventricular block
Mobitz type II
  Intermittently blocked P waves
  PR inerval on conducted beats is constant

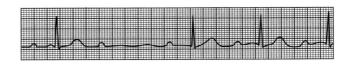

Second-degree, high-grade atrioventricular block
  Conduction ratio of 3:1 or more
  PR interval of conducted beats is constant

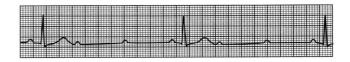

Third-degree atrioventricular block
  Dissociation of atrial and ventricular activity
  Atrial rate is faster than ventricular rate, which
  is of junctional or ventricular origin

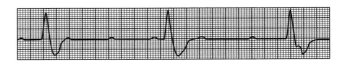

FIG. 27-2 Types of AV block.
Reproduced with permission from: Mangrum JM, DiMarco JP. The evaluation and management of bradycardia. *N Engl J Med.* 2000;342703-709. (Copyright 2000 Massachusetts Medical Society).

TABLE 27-2   Atrioventricular Blocks

TYPE OF BLOCK	ETIOLOGY	ECG FINDINGS
First-degree AV block	Conduction delay, usually through the AV node	• Prolonged PR interval (>.2 seconds) • PR interval constant
Second-degree AV block type I (Mobitz I or Wenckebach)	Progressive delay between atrial and ventricular conduction, leading to eventual failure of conduction. Conduction failure usually at the level of the AV node	• Gradually prolonging PR interval until get a dropped beat • Constant PP interval • PR interval after the dropped beat is the shortest • RR interval is progressively shorter leading up to dropped beat* • QRS complex usually narrow (suggesting block at level of AV node)
Second-degree AV block type II (Mobitz II)	Intermittent failure of conduction from the atria to ventricles. Conduction failure usually infranodal (His-Purkinje system)	• PR interval constant with intermittently dropped QRS • Constant PP interval • QRS complex usually wide (suggesting block is infranodal)
Advanced second-degree AV block	Intermittent failure of conduction from atria to ventricles. Block of two or more consecutive P waves	• Fixed ratio of P:QRS such as 2:1, 3:1, or higher • Since cannot analyze PR interval, difficult to discern if block is Mobitz type I or II • Narrow QRS suggests Mobitz type I while wide QRS suggests Mobitz type II
Third-degree or complete heart block	Complete failure of conduction from the atria to ventricles	• Constant PP and RR intervals with no consistent relationship between atrial and ventricular activity • Ventricular rate faster than atrial rate • Narrow QRS suggests junctional escape rhythm and presence of AV nodal block • Wide QRS suggests ventricular escape rhythm and presence of His-Purkinje block

*While the PR interval increases with each beat, the increment of increase actually decreases. Therefore, the RR interval shortens prior to the dropped beat.

admitted and evaluated by a cardiologist for possible permanent pacemaker placement. As these patients have a high rate of progression to unstable bradycardia, it is appropriate to have atropine and transcutaneous pacing pads near the patient in the event of a sudden decompensation.

TRIAGE AND INITIAL MANAGEMENT

• Any patient with unstable bradycardia (defined as bradycardia associated with altered mental status, ongoing severe ischemic chest pain, hypotension, seizures, or heart failure) should be admitted and managed according to advanced cardiac life support (ACLS) guidelines subsequently outlined in Chap. 24.
• Atropine functions as a vagolytic and is a common first-line agent for treatment of unstable bradycardia.
  ○ Atropine is helpful for sinus bradycardia, first-degree AV block, and second-degree type I AV block.
  ○ Atropine is generally ineffective for second-degree type II heart block since the level of block is below the AV node and thus atropine unresponsive.

  ○ Atropine should also be used with caution in patients with myocardial ischemia or infarction as it may increase the HR and thus worsen the ischemia or infarction zone.
  ○ Atropine is also ineffective in cardiac transplant patients as they lack vagal enervation.
• Dopamine and epinephrine are alternative agents to atropine for patients with unstable bradycardia.
• Unstable patients with type II second-degree or third-degree AV block usually require immediate pacing.

DISEASE MANAGEMENT STRATEGIES

• The American Heart Association (AHA), American College of Cardiology (ACC), and North American Society for Pacing and Electrophysiology (NASPE) have consensus guidelines for the implantation of pacemakers (Table 27-3). Indications for permanent pacing:
  ○ Class I indications are conditions in which there is general agreement that a given treatment is effective.

TABLE 27-3   Indications for Permanent Pacing

Indications for permanent pacing in sinus node dysfunction
Class I
    1. Documented symptomatic bradycardia including frequent sinus pauses that produce symptoms. This includes medication induced bradycardia for which there are no acceptable alternatives.
    2. Symptomatic chronotropic incompetence *

Indications for permanent pacing in acquired AV block in adults
Class I
    1. Third-degree and advanced second-degree AV block associated with†:
        a. Symptomatic bradycardia including heart failure
        b. Need to administer nodal agents that result in symptomatic bradycardia
        c. Asystole = 3 seconds or escape rate <40 beats/min in awake patients
        d. After catheter ablation of AV junction
        e. Postcardiac surgery AV block that is not expected to resolve
        f. Certain neuromuscular diseases with AV block
    2. Second-degree AV block regardless of type or site of block, with associated symptomatic bradycardia

Class IIa
    1. Asymptomatic third-degree AV block with ventricular rate >40 beats/min especially if cardiomegaly or left ventricular dysfunction is present
    2. Asymptomatic type II second-degree AV block with a narrow QRS. If QRS is wide, pacing becomes a class I indication (see next section regarding pacing for chronic bifascicular and trifascicular block)
    3. Asymptomatic type I second-degree AV block at intra- or infra-His levels found at electrophysiologic study performed for other indications
    4. First- or second-degree AV block with symptoms similar to those of pacemaker syndrome

Indications for pacing for chronic bifascicular and trifascicular block
    1. Intermittent third-degree AV block
    2. Type II second-degree AV block
    3. Alternating bundle-branch block

---

* Chronotropic incompetence defined as inability to achieve 85% of age predicted maximum heart rate (220-age) with exercise.
† Advanced second-degree AV block defined as 2:1 atrial to ventricular conduction ratio or higher (3:1, 4:1) such that one cannot discern between second-degree type I or second-degree type II AV block.
Adapted from: Gregaratos G, Abrams J, Epstein AE, et al. *Circulation.* 2002;106:2145.

○ Class II indications reflect conflicting evidence, with IIa indications having evidence in favor of a given treatment and IIb indications with less established evidence.

CARE TRANSITIONS

- Patients admitted with bradycardia should have close follow-up with their primary care physician (PCP) and/or cardiologist upon discharge.
  ○ Symptoms such as dizziness, light-headedness, extreme weakness, syncope, chest pain, and shortness of breath should lead to prompt medical evaluation.
- Medication reconciliation is important, especially if previous nodal agents were discontinued.
- Patients with pacemaker implantation should receive detailed instructions from the cardiology service regarding
  ○ Wound care and signs of pacemaker pocket infections
  ○ Driving and arm usage on the side of pacemaker implantation
  ○ Close monitoring of international normalized ratio (INR) for patients on coumadin to avoid pacemaker pocket hematoma formation

- The AHA has a helpful link for pacemaker care for patients: http://www.americanheart.org/presenter.jhtml?identifier=32

BIBLIOGRAPHY

Fuster V, Alexander RW, O'Rourke RA, et al. Hurst's the heart. 11th ed. In: Vijayaraman P, Ellenbogen K (eds). *Bradyarrhythmias and Pacemakers.* McGraw-Hill; 2004:893–926.

Gregoratos G, Abrams J, Epstein A, et al. ACC/AHA/NASPE Guideline Update for Implantation of Cardiac Pacemakers and Antiarrhythmias Devices: Summary Article. A report of the Americal College of Cardiology/American Heart Association task force on practice guidelines (ACC/AHA/NASPE Committee to Update the 1998 Pacemaker Guidelines). *Circulation.* 2002;106:2145–2161.

Haro LH, Hess EP. Arrhythmia in the Office. *Med Clin N Am.* 2006;90:431–438.

Mangrum JM, DiMarco JP. The evaluation and management of bradycardia. *N Engl J Med.* 2000;342:703–709.

Spodick DH. Normal sinus heart rate: sinus tachycardia and sinus bradycardia Redefined. *Am Heart J.* 1992;124:1119–1120.

Spodick DH, Raju P, Bishop R, et al. Operational definition of normal sinus heart rate. *Am J Cardiology.* 1992;69:1245–1246.

28 VENTRICULAR ARRHYTHMIAS

Beth Liston

EPIDEMIOLOGY/OVERVIEW

- Ventricular arrhythmias range from occasional ventricular premature complexes (VPCs) to ventricular fibrillation (VF) with cardiac arrest.
- VPCs are the most common arrhythmias and occur in both structurally normal and abnormal hearts.
  - More than 60% of healthy adult males will demonstrate VPCs on a 24-hour Holter monitor.
  - VPCs are more common in men than women, the elderly, and American people of African descent.
  - VPCs are also more common with structural heart disease, including ischemic heart disease postmyocardial infarction, dilated cardiomyopathy with heart failure, hypertrophic cardiomyopathy, congenital heart disease, valvular heart disease, specifically, aortic stenosis and mitral valve prolapse, and hypertensive heart disease with left ventricular hypertrophy.
  - Electrolyte disturbances (low potassium or magnesium) and faster sinus rates are also associated with VPCs.
  - The bizarre configuration of VPCs are typically but not invariably >120 msec with the T wave opposite the main QRS vector followed by a compensatory pause such that the interval from the proceeding beat to the following beat will be equal to two basic RR intervals. There is no preceding P wave.
- When there are multiple VPCs, they can be either monomorphic or polymorphic.
  - Monomorphic VPCs of similar morphology have not clearly been associated with increased mortality in patients with normal hearts.
  - Polymorphic VPCs or VPCs with different morphology associated with structural abnormalities or myocardial infarction (MI) do indicate an increased risk of mortality.
  - "R on T" refers to VPC landing at or near the apex of the T wave. These VPCs may increase the risk for sudden death by precipitating ventricular tachycardia (VT) or ventricular fibrillation (VF) in patients with ischemic events.
  - Late coupled VPCs may also precipitate VT or VF.
- The clinical significance of nonsustained VT (NSVT) is variable (Table 28-1).
  - In the documented absence of heart disease there is no associated increased mortality.
  - For patients with coronary artery disease and a left ventricular ejection fraction (LVEF) <40%, NSVT is a marker of poor prognosis.
- The prognosis of VT and VF is also determined by the clinical setting.
  - During the first 24–48 hours postmyocardial infarction is not associated with increased mortality.
  - If sustained VT develops within the first 6 weeks postmyocardial infarction the mortality is 75% in 1 year.
- VT or VF arrest cause more than two-thirds of the 450,000 sudden cardiac deaths that occur each year.

PATHOPHYSIOLOGY

- Arrhythmias result from abnormalities of depolarization, repolarization, or conduction.
- The three mechanisms underlying arrhythmias are reentry, automaticity, and triggered activity.
- Reentry is a disorder of impulse propagation requiring
  - A loop formed by two pathways with different conduction
  - Unidirectional block in one pathway
  - Slow conduction in the alternate pathway

  Reentry is the postulated mechanism of ventricular tachycardia in patients with a scar postmyocardial infarction. Bigeminy or trigeminy with constant coupling intervals between normal and VPC beats is a reentry arrhythmia.
- An arrhythmia caused by a disorder of automaticity occurs when latent pacemakers control the ventricular rate in response to catecholamines, electrolyte abnormalities, hypoxia, stretch, or drugs.
- Triggered activity is responsible for the majority of ventricular arrhythmias. Depolarization of cells after the absolute refractory period, termed afterdepolarization, can lead to another action potential that can be self-perpetuating. Catecholamine excess, hyperkalemia, hypokalemia, hypercalcemia, bradycardia, and digitalis toxicity cause after depolarizations.
- In a large proportion of cases, ventricular arrhythmias develop in the setting of structural heart disease. More severe coronary heart disease and polymorphism is associated with a worse prognosis.

CLINICAL PRESENTATION, DIFFERENTIAL, MAKING THE DIAGNOSIS

- Ventricular premature contractions are abnormal beats arising from the ventricular myocardium.
  - Ventricular premature complexes can be completely asymptomatic or manifest as palpitations. Rarely

TABLE 28-1   Clinical Significance of Nonsustained Ventricular Tachycardia

CLINICAL SETTING	SIGNIFICANCE
Normal heart	
Random finding	No adverse prognostic significance in the absence of occult pathology
During or post exercise	May predict IHD and increased cardiac mortality
Ischemic heart disease	
Acute MI<24 h	No adverse prognostic significance
Acute MI>24 h	Adverse prognostic significance
Chronic IHD with LVEF>40%	Prognostic significance unknown
Chronic IHD with LVEF<40%	Adverse prognostic significance
Dilated cardiomyopathy	Independent prognostic significance not established as opposed to LVEF
Hypertrophic obstructive cardiomyopathy	Probable adverse prognostic significance, especially in the young
Primary VF, congenital long QT, Brugada syndrome, ARVD, repaired congenital abnormalities, valvular disease, hypertension	Prognostic significance unknown

ARVD, arrhythmogenic right ventricular dysplasia; IHD, ischemic heart disease; LVEF, left ventricular ejection fraction; MI, myocardial infarction; VF, ventricular fibrillation.
With permission from: Katritsis DG, Cannon AJ. Nonsustained ventricular tachycardia: where do we stand? *Euro Heart J.* 2004;25:1093.

frequent VPCs or bigeminy can cause presyncope or syncope if the VPC does not have adequate stroke volume.

- The physical examination is often normal with an occasional irregular beat on cardiac auscultation although cannon a waves may be seen.
- In most cases, a VPC will be followed by a compensatory pause. Occasionally, they will travel retrogradely to the atrium or the AV node. In the atrium this will result in inverted P waves in leads II, III, and aVF and a shorter pause following the VPC. In the AV node this will cause prolongation of the next PR interval.

• NSVT is defined as three or more ventricular beats at a rate greater than 100 beats/min. NSVT terminates in less than 30 seconds without causing hemodynamic collapse.

- Examination and electrocardiographic (ECG) findings are similar to the signs and symptoms associated with VPCs although palpitations, lightheadedness, and syncope are more common.

• Sustained ventricular tachycardia is defined as beats at a rate of greater than 100 beats/min, lasting for more than 30 seconds or causing hemodynamic collapse.

- Ventricular tachycardia (VT) may also be monomorphic or polymorphic.
- Torsades de pointes is a specific type of polymorphic ventricular tachycardia with a QRS complex that changes in size and cycle length causing the beat to appear as if it is twisting around a baseline. It is associated with QT prolongation from several possible causes including electrolyte disturbances,

medication effects (Table 28-2), and congenital prolonged QT syndromes.

- If the rate is less than 100 but clearly a monomorphic ventricular arrhythmia then it is termed accelerated idioventricular rhythm (AIVR). This may commonly occur in the early phase postmyocardial infarction or after thrombolysis and is generally transient.

TABLE 28-2   Drugs that May Cause Torsades de Pointes

Drugs commonly involved
- Disopyramide
- Dofetilide
- Ibutilide
- Procainamide
- Quinidine
- Sotalol
- Bepridil

Other drugs
- Amiodarone
- Cisapride
- Calcium channel blockers: Lidoflazine (not marketed in the US)
- Antiinfective agents: Clarithromycin, erythromycin, halofantrine pentamidine, sparfloxacin
- Antiemetic agents: Domperidone, droperidol
- Antipsychotic agents: Chlorpromazine, heloperidol, mesoridazine, thioridazine, pimozide
- Methadone

*Further information on the strength of the evidence linking various drugs to torsades de pointes may be found at http://www.torsades.org
†The level of risk associated with these drugs depends on the dose and the population being treated; in general, the risk is probably less than 1%.
With permission from: Roden DM. Drug-induced prolongation of the QT interval. *NEJM.* 2004;350:1015.

○ Ventricular tachycardia is life threatening and must be recognized promptly. Although patients with VT may appear to be hemodynamically stable, VT frequently results in cardiovascular collapse and may further deteriorate to ventricular fibrillation. Supraventricular tachycardia (SVT) with aberrancy can be mistaken for VT and requires different therapy (Figs. 28-1 and 28-2 and Chap. 26).
  ▪ A wide complex tachycardia (WCT) should be managed presumptively in unstable patients as VT.
  ▪ If the patient is stable a thorough evaluation of the type and etiology of the arrhythmia should be done.
  ▪ Features of the history suggesting VT include older age, history of heart disease, presence of an implantable cardioverter defibrillator (ICD), and family history or patient history of ventricular arrhythmias. Historical features suggesting SVT are a young age and intermittent tachycardia occurring over several months in the absence of structural heart disease.

ECG Criteria That Favor Ventricular Tachycardia

1. AV Dissociation
2. QRS width: >0.14 s with RBBB Configuration
   >0.16 s with LBBB Configuration
3. QRS Axis: Left Axis Deviation with RBBB Morphology
   Extreme Left Axis Deviation (Northwest Axis) with LBBB Morphology
4. Concordance of QRS in Precordial Leads
5. Morphologic Patterns of the QRS Complex
   RBBB: Mono- or Biphasic Complex in V_1
   RS (*Only with Left Axis Deviation*) or QS in V_6

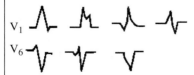

LBBB: Broad R Wave in V_1 or $V_2 \geq 0.04$ s
Onset of QRS to Nadir of S Wave in V_1 or V_2 of ≥ 0.07 s
Notched Downslope of S Wave in V_1 or V_2
Q Wave in V_6

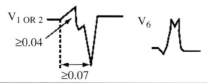

FIG. 28-1 ECG criteria that favor ventricular tachycardia. With permission from: Josephson ME, Zimetbaum P. The tachyarrhythmias. In: Kasper DL, Braunwald E, Fauci AS, et al, eds. *Harrison's Principles of Internal Medicine*. 16th ed. New York, NY: McGraw-Hill; 2005;1352.

Absence of an RS Complex in All Precordial Leads?

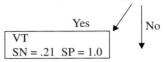

VT
SN = .21 SP = 1.0

R to S Interval > 100 ms in One Precordial Lead?

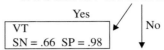

VT
SN = .66 SP = .98

Atrio-ventricular Dissociation:

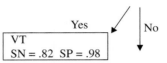

VT
SN = .82 SP = .98

Morphology Criteria for VT Present Both in Precordial Leads V_{1-2} and V_6?

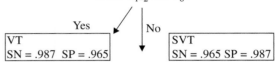

VT
SN = .987 SP = .965

SVT
SN = .965 SP = .987

SN: Sensitivity, SP: Specificity
With Permission from Brugada et al. 1991

FIG. 28-2 Algorithm for diagnosis of a wide complex tachycardia. With permission from: Brugada P, Brugada J, Mont L, et al. A new approach to the differential diagnosis of a regular tachycardia with a wide QRS complex. *Circulation.* 1991;83:5:1649.

  ▪ In VT signs of AV dissociation may be evident on clinical examination, including marked fluctuations of blood pressure and canon a waves.
  ▪ Carotid sinus pressure will slow or terminate SVT and rarely does also in VT.
  ▪ Electrocardiogram (ECG) criteria have been determined to differentiate between VT and SVT (Fig. 28-1). To apply these, the WCT must be classified as either right bundle branch block (RBBB) morphology with positive QRS complexes in leads V_1 and V_2 or left bundle branch block (LBBB) morphology with negative QRS complexes in V_1 and V_2.
  ▪ A diagnostic algorithm was created by Brugada et al to allow stepwise evaluation of the ECG in WCT (Fig. 28-2). If concordance is identified, an RS interval >.10 seconds is found in a precordial lead, AV dissociation is seen, or the above listed morphological patterns of the QRS complex suggest VT, then VT can be concluded with a sensitivity approaching 100%.

• Ventricular fibrillation is disorganized ventricular electrical activity most frequently associated with ischemia and precipitated by an early ventricular beat falling on the T wave.
• Ventricular fibrillation is always unstable and if not treated rapidly will result in death.

TRIAGE AND INITIAL MANAGEMENT

- In pulseless patients with VT or VF, advanced cardiac life support (ACLS) protocols should be followed (Chap. 24).
- Stable patients should be thoroughly evaluated for type and etiology of the arrhythmia. History taking, physical examination, and laboratory data should focus on common causes of ventricular arrhythmias including ischemic heart disease, hypoxia, and electrolyte disturbances.
  - ○ The 12-lead ECG should be evaluated to determine the type of arrhythmia as well as possible underlying etiologies including ischemia, conduction disturbances, and QT prolongation.
  - ○ Medication lists should be examined for drugs such as digitalis or agents that can prolong the QT interval (Table 28-2).
- Patients with VPCs and a structurally normal heart require no therapy other than reassurance. Beta-blockers can be used for those with bothersome symptoms.
- Similarly, a patient with NSVT and a structurally normal heart should be treated with beta-blockade alone.
- Ventricular ectopy in patients with ischemic heart disease is more concerning.
  - ○ Beta-blockers are clearly indicated in any patient who can tolerate them post-MI and are helpful in suppressing VPCs and NSVT.
  - ○ Amiodarone or sotalol can be considered in refractory symptomatic ventricular ectopy but have not been demonstrated to improve clinical outcome.
- In hemodynamically unstable patients with VT, synchronized cardioversion should be performed. Conscious patients should be sedated prior to therapy if possible. Monophasic cardioversion should begin with 100 J and successively increase to 360 J. Biphasic cardioversion should begin with shocks at 50–100 J. If synchronized cardioversion is not possible then unsynchronized cardioversion can be used.
- Stable monomorphic ventricular tachycardia can be treated by cardioversion (described above) or pharmacologically (use only one antiarrhythmic to decrease the potential for proarrhythmia).
  - ○ Procainamide is the drug of choice in patients with a normal LVEF and should be given at 30 mg/min until the arrhythmia terminates, QRS prolongation of greater than 50% occurs, a total of 17 mg/kg has been given, or until the patient becomes hypotensive.
  - ○ Amiodarone is the drug of choice in patients with impaired LVEF, and may be used in those with normal hearts. A bolus of 150 mg is given over 10 minutes followed by a drip of 1mg/min for the next 6 hours and then 0.5 mg/min until the rhythm is stabilized. Repeat boluses can be given every 10 minutes for a maximum dose of 2.2 g in 24 hours.
  - ○ Lidocaine is an alternative and may also be given in the setting of myocardial ischemia, starting with a bolus of 0.5–0.75 mg/kg and followed with a drip of 1–4 mg/min. Repeat boluses can be given with a maximum dose of 3 mg/kg/h.
- Polymorphic ventricular tachycardia without QT prolongation is frequently associated with ischemia and is usually unstable requiring cardioversion. However, IV beta-blockers and amiodarone may be helpful.
- Therapy for torsades de pointes should be directed toward the underlying cause for QT prolongation. Magnesium can be effective in terminating the rhythm if QT prolongation is present. Pacing may be necessary, particularly if the underlying etiology is due to heart block or symptomatic bradycardia.
- Sustained VT with a low elevation of cardiac enzymes should be treated similarly to sustained VT with no biomarker rise.

DISEASE MANAGEMENT STRATEGIES

- All individuals with ventricular ectopy should be evaluated and assessed for cardiac risk factors and ischemic and structural heart disease prior to hospital discharge.
  - ○ Pharmacologic or exercise stress testing should be done to detect undiagnosed coronary heart disease when the patients' cardiovascular risk is intermediate or greater.
  - ○ Coronary revascularization should be considered in patients with coronary heart disease. Cardiac catheterization may be conducted during the hospital stay if indicated by stress testing or known coronary heart disease.
  - ○ Echocardiography should be done in all patients with ventricular arrhythmias and suspected structural heart disease.
- Potassium and magnesium levels should be maintained within the normal range.
- Antiplatelet therapy and statins may decrease the risk of sudden cardiac death.
- Beta-blockers are the only antiarrhythmic medications indicated for primary prevention of sudden cardiac death, although amiodarone and sotalol may be considered for those with symptomatic ventricular ectopy refractory to beta-blockade.
- The previous practice of routine arrhythmia prophylaxis with lidocaine postmyocardial infarction is no longer recommended.

- Implantable cardioverter defibrillators (ICDs) are favored for secondary prevention of life-threatening ventricular arrhythmias as compared with antiarrhythmic drugs.
  - In patients with NSVT and an LVEF <40%, electrophysiology (EP) testing should be done with possible ICD placement. For those with a normal heart, the prognostic implications of NSVT are unclear and EP testing may be considered.
  - All individuals who have sustained ventricular tachycardia should undergo EP testing with possible ICD placement. Those with suspected ventricular tachycardia and coronary heart disease should also have EP evaluation.
  - Those who have survived cardiac arrest due to VT or VF should have an ICD placed prior to discharge.

BIBLIOGRAPHY

ACC/AHA/ESC 2006 guidelines for management of patients with ventricular arrhythmias and the prevention of sudden cardiac death. *Circulation.* 2006;114:385.

Brugada P, Brugada J, Mont L, et al. A new approach to the differential diagnosis of a regular tachycardia with a wide QRS complex. *Circulation.* 1991;83:5:1649.

Goldberger Z, Lampert R. Implantable cardioverter defibrillators: expanding indications and technologies. *JAMA.* 2006;295(7): 809.

Josephson ME, Zimetbaum P. The tachyarrhythmias. In: Kasper DL, Braunwald E, Fauci AS, et al, eds. *Harrison's Principles of Internal Medicine.* 16th ed. New York, NY: McGraw-Hill; 2005;342–1358.

Katritsis DG, Cannon AJ. Nonsustained ventricular tachycardia: where do we stand? *Euro Heart J.* 2004;25:1093.

Roden DM. Drug-induced prolongation of the QT interval. *NEJM.* 2004;350:1013.

29 HEART FAILURE DUE TO DIASTOLIC DYSFUNCTION

Colleen M. Crumlish and James C. Fang

EPIDEMIOLOGY/OVERVIEW

- The importance of heart failure with preserved left ventricular ejection fraction (LVEF), or diastolic heart failure, is increasingly being recognized.
- It is estimated that as many as 20% to 60% of patients with HF have a relatively normal LVEF. The prevalence of this patient population is increasing owing to the aging of the population, the increasing incidence of hypertension and diabetes mellitus, and a growing awareness and ability to make the diagnosis.
- The rate of hospitalizations for HF is similar in patients with preserved and reduced LVEF.
- Patients with HF with preserved EF have similar or only slightly better rates of survival than those with HF and depressed ejection fraction.
- Patients with HF with preserved LVEF are more likely to be older, to be female, and to have a history of hypertension and atrial fibrillation when compared with patients with reduced EF. Obesity, anemia, and diabetes are also commonly present.
- In contrast to HF with low LVEF, few clinical trials have been done in HF patients with preserved LVEF. No therapy has been shown to improve survival in diastolic HF.

PATHOPHYSIOLOGY

- Heart failure with preserved LVEF or diastolic heart failure is poorly understood and is likely a heterogeneous disorder. The definition of "preserved" LVEF is variable and can range from >40% to >50%.
- Heart failure with preserved LVEF has historically been attributed to reduced ventricular compliance and abnormal relaxation during diastole. Abnormal renal sodium and water handling, reduced vascular compliance, and anemia also play roles in diastolic HF.
- Diastolic function is often abnormal in patients with HF and reduced LVEF as well as those with preserved LVEF. The extent and type of diastolic dysfunction is variable in diastolic heart failure.
- Cardiac output, especially during exercise, may be limited by abnormal filling characteristics of the ventricles as well as chronotropic incompetence and lack of vasodilator reserve. In restrictive cardiomyopathies, for a given ventricular volume, the ventricular pressures may be inappropriately elevated, leading to pulmonary congestion, dyspnea, and edema.
- Chronic hypertension with resultant left ventricular hypertrophy is a major cause of diastolic HF.
- Several other recognized myocardial disorders are associated with HF and a normal LVEF, including restrictive cardiomyopathy, hypertrophic cardiomyopathy, and infiltrative cardiomyopathies.
- Patients with diastolic heart failure may have difficulty tolerating atrial fibrillation since the loss of atrial contraction can greatly reduce left atrial emptying, left ventricular (LV) filling, and LV stroke volume.

- Patients with diastolic HF may not tolerate tachycardia well since increases in heart rate shorten the duration of diastole and truncate the late phase of diastolic filling.
- Elevations in systemic blood pressure increase left ventricular wall stress and systolic load, which can impair myocardial relaxation in patients with diastolic HF.
- Ischemia can worsen diastolic dysfunction and symptoms of heart failure. Ischemia can result from coronary heart disease and/or left ventricular hypertrophy with subendocardial ischemia.

CLINICAL PRESENTATION, DIFFERENTIAL, MAKING THE DIAGNOSIS

- Diastolic dysfunction alone is insufficient to make the diagnosis of HF with preserved LVEF.
- The signs and symptoms of heart failure with preserved LVEF are similar to those in HF with low LVEF and cannot be used to distinguish between the two. Echocardiography remains the cornerstone of making the distinction between systolic and diastolic HF.
- See Table 29-1 for differential diagnosis in a patient with HF and normal LVEF:

TABLE 29-1   Differential Diagnosis in a Patient With Heart Failure and Normal Left Ventricular Ejection Fraction

Incorrect diagnosis of HF
Inaccurate measurement of LVEF
Primary valvular disease
Restrictive (infiltrative) cardiomyopathies
   Amyloidosis, sarcoidosis, hemochromatosis
Pericardial constriction
Episodic or reversible LV systolic dysfunction
Severe hypertension, myocardial ischemia
HF associated with high-metabolic demand (high-output states)
   Anemia, thyrotoxicosis, arteriovenous fistulae
Chronic pulmonary disease with right HF
Pulmonary hypertension associated with pulmonary vascular disorders
Atrial myxoma
Diastolic dysfunction of uncertain origin
Obesity

HF: Heart failure; LVEF: Left ventricular ejection fraction; LV: Left ventricular.
Reprinted with permission from: Hunt SA, Abraham WT, Marshall CH, et al. ACC/AHA 2005 guideline update for the diagnosis and management of congestive heart failure in the adult. a report of the American College of Cardiology/American Heart Association task force on practice guidelines (Writing Committee to Update the 2001 Guidelines for the Evaluation and Management of Heart Failure): developed in collaboration with the American College of Chest Physicians and the International Society for Heart and Lung Transplantation: endorsed by the Heart Rhythm Society. *Circulation.* 2005;112:e195.

- Heart failure, whatever the etiology, is a clinical diagnosis. The diagnosis is generally based upon the finding of typical signs or symptoms of congestive HF in a patient who has preserved systolic function, typically defined by LVEF. There may or may not be evidence of abnormal left ventricular relaxation, filling, diastolic distensibility, or diastolic stiffness. Evidence for diastolic dysfunction is often made by Doppler echocardiography but is load-dependent.
- Plasma concentrations of brain natriuretic peptide (BNP) and *N*-terminal pro-BNP may be increased in patients with diastolic HF and can improve diagnostic accuracy given the test's high negative predictive value.

TRIAGE AND INITIAL MANAGEMENT

- Regardless of the cause, acute heart failure is managed in the same manner. Initial treatment should focus on hemodynamic stabilization, oxygenation, and restoring filling pressure to optimal levels while searching for precipitating causes.
- No proven therapy for heart failure with preserved EF currently exists. Treatment should be directed toward symptoms, comorbid conditions, and physiologic factors known to contribute to impaired ventricular relaxation.
  - Control of systolic and diastolic hypertension
  - Control of ventricular rate in patients with atrial fibrillation
  - Control of pulmonary congestion and peripheral edema with diuretics
  - Coronary revascularization in patients with coronary heart disease in whom ischemia is thought to have an adverse effect on diastolic function
- See Table 29-2 for a summary of treatment recommendations.
- Occult coronary heart disease is a potentially reversible cause of diastolic heart failure and should be excluded.
- One randomized clinical trial (candesartan in heart failure assessment of reduction in mortality and morbidity [CHARM] study) showed a reduction in hospital admissions for HF in patients with New York Heart Association (NYHA) functional class II–IV and LVEF higher than 40% taking candesartan compared with placebo but no difference in cardiovascular mortality.

DISEASE MANAGEMENT STRATEGIES

- Studies suggest that hospital admission for HF can be prevented with multidisciplinary disease management programs. Functional status and quality of life can also be improved for HF patients. Appropriate

TABLE 29-2 Recommendations for Treatment of Patients With Heart Failure and Normal Left Ventricular Ejection Fraction

RECOMMENDATION	CLASS	LEVEL OF EVIDENCE
Physicians should control systolic and diastolic hypertension, in accordance with published guidelines	I	A
Physicians should control ventricular rate in patients with atrial fibrillation	I	C
Physicians should use diuretics to control pulmonary congestion and peripheral edema	I	C
Coronary revascularization is reasonable in patients with coronary artery disease in whom symptomatic or demonstrable myocardial ischemia is judged to be having an adverse effect on cardiac function	IIa	C
Restoration and maintenance of sinus rhythm in patients with atrial fibrillation might be useful to improve symptoms	IIb	C
The use of beta-adrenergic blocking agents, angiotensin-converting enzyme inhibitors, angiotensin II receptor blockers, or calcium antagonists in patients with controlled hypertension might be effective to minimize symptoms of heart failure	IIb	C
The use of digitalis to minimize symptoms of heart failure is not well established	IIb	C

Reprinted with permission from: Hunt SA, Abraham WT, Marshall CH, et al. ACC/AHA 2005 guideline update for the diagnosis and management of chronic heart failure in the adult: a report of the American College of Cardiology/American Heart Association task force on practice guidelines (Writing Committee to Update the 2001 Guidelines for the Evaluation and Management of Heart Failure): developed in collaboration with the American College of Chest Physicians and the International Society for Heart and Lung Transplantation: endorsed by the Heart Rhythm Society. *Circulation.* 2005;112:e194.

patients (multiple readmissions, high risk due to cognitive impairment or multiple comorbidities, persistent nonadherence) should be referred to heart failure management programs if available. A multidisciplinary team made up of physicians, HF nurses, dietitians, and pharmacists can provide

- Individualized education and counseling to the patient, family members, and caregivers that emphasize self-care
- Optimization of drug therapy
- Increased access to healthcare
- Early attention to signs and symptoms of fluid overload
- Close telephone follow-up after hospital discharge to assess symptoms and daily weights, adjust diuretic dosing, and answer questions regarding diet and medications

• As with patients with systolic HF, educating patients with diastolic HF and their families is critical and should start early in the hospitalization. Patient noncompliance with medications and diet is a common cause of clinical deterioration and readmission. *Discharge instructions* must address

- Medications (prescribed and what to avoid)
- Dietary restrictions (low-salt diet and possibly fluid restriction)
- Activity recommendations
- Signs and symptoms of worsening condition and what to do
- Close follow-up
- Weight monitoring (and what to do with weight gain)

• National guidelines strongly recommend *smoking cessation counseling* for smokers with cardiovascular disease, including HF.

• Immunization with influenza and pneumococcal vaccines is recommended.

CARE TRANSITIONS

• Clinically, HF patients can be discharged once optimal volume status is obtained, symptoms have resolved, and appropriate medications have controlled heart rate and blood pressure without hypotension or renal insufficiency.

• Patient and family should demonstrate an understanding of the discharge instructions regarding medications, diet, activity, daily weights, worsening symptoms, and follow-up.

• Close follow-up with a primary care physician or cardiologist within a week is mandatory to assess the patient's clinical status and tolerance of medications and to check for electrolyte abnormalities. Closer follow-up by telephone may be necessary to monitor weights and symptoms. Direct communication with the outpatient provider should be standard practice.

BIBLIOGRAPHY

Bhatia RS, Tu JV, Lee DS, et al. Outcome of heart failure with preserved ejection fraction in a population-based study. *N Engl J Med.* 2006;355:260–269.

Hunt SA, Abraham WT, Marshall CH, et al. ACC/AHA 2005 guideline update for the diagnosis and management of chronic heart failure in the adult: a report of the American College of Cardiology/American Heart Association task force on practice guidelines (Writing Committee to Update the 2001 Guidelines for the Evaluation and Management of Heart Failure): developed in collaboration with the American College of Chest Physicians and the International Society for Heart and Lung Transplantation: endorsed by the Heart Rhythm Society. *Circulation.* 2005;112:154–235.

Jessup M, Brozena S. Heart failure. *N Engl J Med.* 2003; 348:2007–2018.

Leite-Moreira AF. Current perspectives in diastolic dysfunction and diastolic heart failure. *Heart.* 2006;92:712–718.

Owan TE, Hodge DO, Herges RM, et al. Trends in prevalence and outcome of heart failure with preserved ejection fraction. *N Engl J Med.* 2006;355:251–259.

Yusuf S, Pfeffer MA, Swedberg K, et al. Effects of candesartan in patients with chronic heart failure and preserved left-ventricular ejection fraction: the CHARM-preserved trial. *Lancet.* 2003;362:777–781.

30 HEART FAILURE DUE TO SYSTOLIC DYSFUNCTION

Colleen M. Crumlish and James C. Fang

EPIDEMIOLOGY/OVERVIEW

- Approximately five million patients in the United States have heart failure (HF) with over 550,000 new cases diagnosed each year. The incidence of HF increases with age, approaching 10 per 1000 population after age 65.
- HF is the leading cause of hospital admissions in the Medicare population in the United States and is responsible for 6.5 million hospital days each year. Over the past decade, the rate of hospitalizations for HF has increased by 159%. About 45% of patients hospitalized with acute HF will be rehospitalized at least once (and 15% at least twice) within 12 months.
- Approximately 260,000 patients die of HF in the United States each year. The number of HF deaths has increased steadily despite advances in treatment, in part because of the aging of the population and improved survival after acute myocardial infarctions (MIs).
- More Medicare dollars are spent for the diagnosis and treatment of HF than for any other diagnosis. The estimated direct and indirect cost of HF in 2005 is $27.9 billion.
- The majority of HF patients in the hospital are managed by hospitalists.

- Heart failure has been identified by the Joint Commission on Accreditation of Healthcare Organizations (JCAHO) as a priority focus for hospital core measure development. The four HF core measures are
  - *HF-1:* Discharge instructions
  - *HF-2:* Evaluation of left ventricular systolic function
  - *HF-3:* Angiotensin-converting enzyme (ACE) inhibitor or angiotensin receptor blocker (ARB) for left ventricular systolic dysfunction
  - *HF-4:* Adult smoking cessation advice/counseling

PATHOPHYSIOLOGY

- HF is a complex clinical syndrome characterized by specific signs and symptoms, such as dyspnea and fatigue, that can result from any structural or functional cardiac disorder that impairs the ability of the ventricle to fill with or eject blood and meet the metabolic needs of the body.
- HF may result from disorders of the pericardium, heart valves, myocardium, or coronary circulation as well as rhythm disturbances. The majority of patients have symptoms due to an impairment of myocardial function, with or without a reduced ejection fraction.
- In developed countries, coronary artery disease is the leading underlying cause of left ventricle (LV) dysfunction. Other causes include
  - Hypertension
  - Cardiomyopathy
    - Idiopathic dilated cardiomyopathy
    - Familial cardiomyopathy
    - Hypertrophic cardiomyopathy
    - Toxins (eg, alcohol, cocaine)
    - Medications (eg, adriamycin)
    - Diabetes mellitus
    - Viral (coxsackie, echovirus, human immunodeficiency virus)
    - Infiltrative (amyloidosis, sarcoidosis, hemochromatosis)
    - Metabolic disorders (hypothyroidism)
    - Peripartum
  - Valvular heart disease (aortic stenosis, mitral regurgitation, or stenosis)
  - Tachyarrhythmias
  - High output states (hyperthyroidism, arteriovenous fistula, severe anemia, beriberi, Paget disease)
- HF is generally a progressive disorder that is a consequence of cardiac remodeling (eg, ventricular enlargement and hypertrophy), neurohormonal activation, and possibly genetic factors. Patients with HF have elevated circulating or tissue levels of norepinephrine, angiotensin II, aldosterone, endothelin, vasopressin,

and cytokines which act to adversely affect the structure and function of the heart. Neurohormonal activation increases the hemodynamic stresses on the ventricle by causing sodium retention and peripheral vasoconstriction.

- The 2005 ACC/AHA task force developed a new classification scheme outlining four stages in the evolution of the HF syndrome (Fig. 30-1), recognizing established risk factors, structural prerequisites, asymptomatic and symptomatic phases, and appropriate therapeutic interventions at each stage to reduce morbidity and mortality.
- Acute decompensated HF (cardiogenic pulmonary edema) is characterized by an elevation in left atrial and subsequently pulmonary venous and capillary

pressures. The net result may be transudation of excess fluid into the alveolar spaces, leading to decreased diffusing capacity, hypoxia, and shortness of breath.

CLINICAL PRESENTATION, DIFFERENTIAL, MAKING THE DIAGNOSIS

- The signs and symptoms of HF lack sensitivity and specificity. The clinical manifestations vary greatly depending upon the severity and chronicity of the presentation and degree of compensation.
- Reduced cardiac output causes fatigue and weakness and volume overload can lead to dyspnea at rest

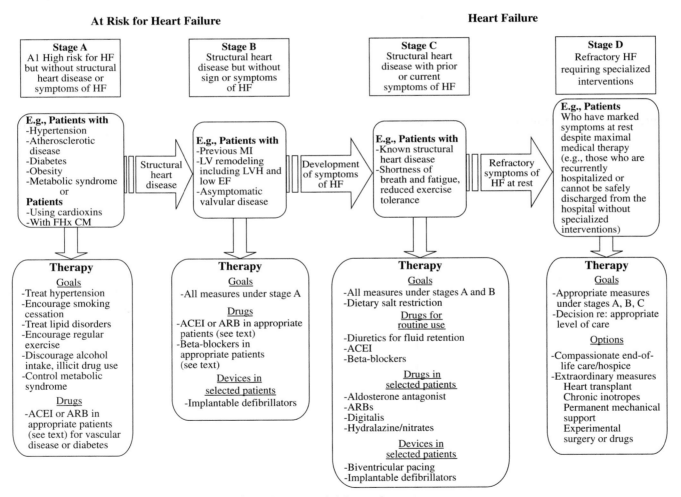

FIG. 30-1   Stages in the development of heart failure/recommended therapy by stage.
Reprinted with permission from: Hunt SA, Abraham WT, Marshall CH, et al. ACC/AHA 2005 guideline update for the diagnosis and management of chronic heart failure in the adult: a report of the American College of Cardiology/American Heart Association task force on practice guidelines (Writing Committee to Update the 2001 Guidelines for the Evaluation and Management of Heart Failure): developed in collaboration with the American College of Chest Physicians and the International Society for Heart and Lung Transplantation: endorsed by the Heart Rhythm Society. *Circulation.* 2005;112:e685.

and/or with exertion, orthopnea, paroxysmal nocturnal dyspnea, cough, edema, weight gain, and right upper quadrant discomfort from hepatic congestion. Chest pain may be present in both ischemic and nonischemic cardiomyopathy.

- Symptoms usually relate to impaired exercise tolerance, with or without symptoms related to fluid overload. Symptoms of exercise intolerance are assessed by the New York Heart Association (NYHA) functional classification and should be made in the ambulatory compensated state.
  - *I* = No symptoms
  - *II* = Symptoms with moderate or marked levels of activity
  - *III* = Symptoms with mild activity
  - *IV* = Symptoms at rest
- Physical examination findings consistent with elevated cardiac filling pressures and fluid overload include elevated jugular venous pressure, hepatojugular reflux, gallops (S_3 and S_4), pulmonary rales, hepatomegaly, ascites, and edema. A laterally displaced or prominent apical impulse and mitral regurgitation correlate with cardiac enlargement. Other murmurs can suggest valvular disease. Narrow pulse pressure, cool extremities, altered mentation, Cheyne-Stokes respiration, and a resting tachycardia suggest a marked reduction in cardiac output. Hypotension may indicate severe ventricular dysfunction and impending cardiogenic shock. The presence of peripheral edema and pulmonary rales, although relatively specific, are not sensitive and may be absent.
- The differential diagnosis for HF signs and symptoms includes
  - Myocardial ischemia
  - Pulmonary disease (pneumonia, asthma, chronic obstructive pulmonary disease, pulmonary embolus, pulmonary hypertension)
  - Sleep-disordered breathing
  - Obesity
  - Malnutrition
  - Hepatic failure
  - Renal failure
  - Hypoalbuminemia
  - Venous stasis
  - Depression
  - Deconditioning
  - Anxiety and hyperventilation syndromes
- There is no one diagnostic test for HF although ancillary testing (eg, brain natriuretic peptide [BNP], chest x-ray, echocardiography, and right heart catheterization) can be useful. It is largely a clinical diagnosis based upon a careful history and physical examination, supported by appropriate studies.

  - A low concentration of BNP has a high negative predictive value and may be useful in ruling out the diagnosis of HF in appropriate patients.
  - A BNP value >100 pg/mL diagnoses HF with a sensitivity, specificity, and predictive value of 90%, 76%, and 83%, respectively.
  - Brain natriuretic peptide is most useful in triage for patients presenting to the emergency department (ED) with dyspnea.
- Radiographic findings in acute pulmonary edema can range from minimal pulmonary vascular redistribution to marked cardiomegaly and extensive bilateral interstitial markings. Pleural effusions are seen in more chronic HF.

TRIAGE AND INITIAL MANAGEMENT

- Initial triage requires an assessment of resting pulmonary congestion (jugular venous distension, rales, abnormal chest radiograph) and hypoperfusion (cold clammy skin, hypotension, tachycardia, confusion, oliguria).
- Acute heart failure, whether in the context of new onset HF or in patients with established chronic HF, requires urgent treatment and should focus on hemodynamic stabilization, oxygenation/organ perfusion, and restoring filling pressure to optimal levels while searching for precipitating causes. See Fig 30-2.
- The causes and precipitating factors in acute HF include
  - Decompensation of preexisting chronic heart failure
  - Acute coronary syndromes
    - Myocardial infarction/unstable angina
    - Mechanical complication of acute myocardial infarction
  - Hypertensive crisis
  - Acute arrhythmia (ventricular tachycardia, ventricular fibrillation, atrial fibrillation or flutter, other supraventricular tachycardia)
  - Valvular regurgitation
  - Severe aortic stenosis
  - Acute severe myocarditis
  - Cardiac tamponade
  - Aortic dissection
  - Postpartum cardiomyopathy
  - High output syndromes
  - Noncardiovascular precipitating factors
    - Medical or dietary noncompliance
    - Infections (eg, pneumonia)
    - Severe brain insult
    - After major surgery
    - Reduction in renal function
    - Drug or alcohol abuse

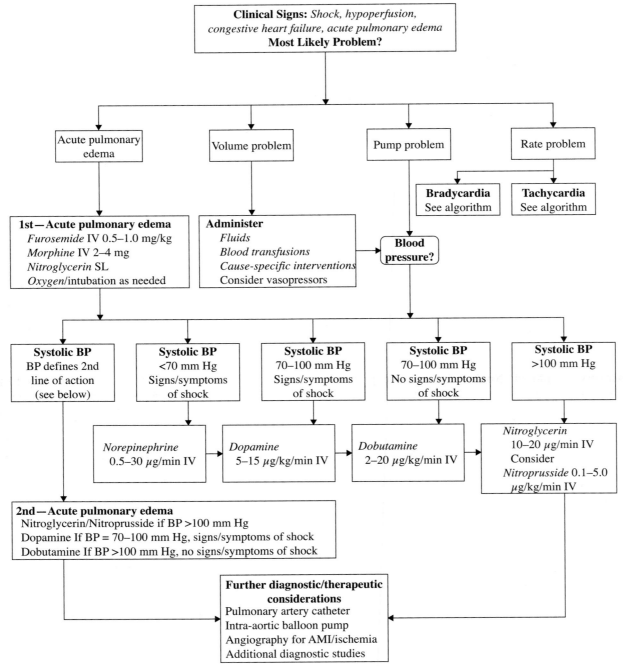

FIG. 30-2 The acute pulmonary edema, hypotension, and shock algorithm.
Reprinted with permission from: Guidelines 2000 for cardiopulmonary resuscitation and emergency cardiovascular care. Part 7: the era of reperfusion: section 1: acute coronary syndromes (acute myocardial infarction). The American Heart Association in collaboration with the International Liaison Committee on Resuscitation. *Circulation.* 2000:102(suppl 8):1–172.

- The following labs and studies should be obtained:
  - Complete blood count (CBC), urinalysis, serum electrolytes (including calcium and magnesium), blood urea nitrogen (BUN), serum creatinine, fasting blood glucose, cardiac biomarkers, lipid profile, liver function tests, and thyrotropin.
  - 12-lead electrocardiogram to identify rhythm, assess for acute coronary syndromes, detect conduction abnormalities and voltage, and assess loading conditions of the heart.
  - Chest radiograph to assess cardiac size and pulmonary congestion.

○ *Two-dimensional echocardiography with Doppler* is critical in the assessment of all patients with new onset HF. It provides information about left ventriclar ejection fraction (LVEF), LV size, wall thickness, valve function, right heart function, and pericardial disease. Repeat assessment of EF may be useful when the chronic HF patient has a major change in clinical status.

○ Brain natriuretic peptide or *N*-terminal pro-BNP (secreted by the cardiac ventricles in response to wall stress) can be useful in the urgent care setting when the diagnosis in patients presenting with dyspnea is uncertain. BNP has a good negative predictive value to exclude HF and can provide prognostic information if HF is confirmed.

○ In the workup of newly diagnosed HF, screening for hemochromatosis, sleep-disturbed breathing, or human immunodeficiency virus is reasonable in selected patients. Diagnostic tests for rheumatologic diseases, amyloidosis, or pheochromocytoma are reasonable if there is a clinical suspicion of these diseases (Class IIa recommendation/good supportive evidence).

- Supplemental oxygen should be initiated and pulse oximetry monitored. Noninvasive positive pressure ventilation, if necessary for respiratory failure, is associated with a significant reduction in the need for tracheal intubation and mechanical ventilation.

- In general, treatment begins with intravenous loop diuretics (furosemide is most commonly used), which in patients with adequate organ perfusion, will produce diuresis accompanied by a prompt drop in preload and relief of symptoms related to pulmonary edema. Intravenous loop diuretics may also exert a vasodilating effect. Peak diuresis typically occurs 30 minutes after administration and should be titrated to response. The administration of a thiazide diuretic such as metolazone 30 minutes prior to a dose of furosemide can potentiate its effect. Continuous infusions or hemofiltration can be considered when necessary. Overly rapid diuresis with an excessively rapid reduction in intravascular volume may result in symptomatic hypotension and/or worsening renal function.

○ Fluid balance must be measured closely along with daily weights to assess clinical efficacy of diuretic therapy.

○ Serum electrolytes and creatinine must be measured at least daily.

- A low-sodium diet (2 g daily) is recommended.

- Fluid restriction (<2 L/d) is recommended in patients with moderate hyponatremia (serum sodium <130 mEq/L) and should be considered to assist in treatment of fluid overload in other patients.

- In acute pulmonary edema, morphine may be useful because it induces venodilation and mild arterial dilatation and relieves breathlessness and anxiety.

- In the absence of symptomatic hypotension, intravenous vasodilator therapy may be considered as an addition to diuretic therapy for rapid improvement of congestive symptoms in patients with acute decompensated heart failure.

○ Nitrates decrease systemic and pulmonary vascular pressures and are coronary vasodilators.

○ Nitroprusside is indicated when there is a need for acute combined afterload and preload reduction (hypertensive emergency, acute aortic regurgitation, acute mitral regurgitation).

○ Nesiritide has venous, arterial, and modest coronary vasodilatory properties that reduce preload and afterload and has no direct inotropic effects. It is currently only approved for the acute relief of dyspnea in the patient with decompensated heart failure. Because of its hypotensive effects, it should be used only at recommended doses and with caution.

- Intravenous inotropic agents (dobutamine, milrinone, dopamine) are indicated in the presence of peripheral hypoperfusion (hypotension, decreased renal function) with or without pulmonary edema refractory to the above treatment modalities. The benefit of hemodynamic improvement may outweigh the risk of arrhythmias and increase in oxygen demand caused by these agents. These patients are most appropriately managed in cardiac care units. These agents should only be used for short-term circulatory support.

- The routine use of invasive hemodynamic monitoring in patients with acute decompensated heart failure is not recommended.

- Temporary mechanical circulatory assistance (intraaortic balloon counter-pulsation pump or ventricular assist device) may be indicated in patients not responding to pharmacologic therapy when there is reasonable potential for myocardial recovery with specific interventions (eg, bypass surgery). They can also be considered to help "bridge" appropriate patients to cardiac transplantation.

- Hemofiltration is a method of fluid removal that may benefit patients with acute decompensated HF accompanied by renal insufficiency or diuretic resistance. Advantages include adjustable fluid removal volumes and rates, no effect on serum electrolytes, and decreased neurohormonal activity.

- Emergent coronary angiography is indicated if an acute coronary syndrome is the cause of acute HF.

- Continuous electrocardiographic (ECG) monitoring is necessary during the acute decompensation phase. Arrhythmias may be a cause or complicating factor of HF.

- Patients with chronic HF are at increased risk of thromboembolic events. Appropriate prophylaxis should be initiated.
- A risk stratification tool developed from the Acute Decompensated Heart Failure National Registry (ADHERE) identified the following variables as predicting higher risk for in-hospital mortality:
  ○ BUN >43 mg/dL
  ○ Admission systolic blood pressure <115 mm Hg
  ○ Serum creatinine >2.75 mg/dL
- Other parameters that have been correlated with clinical outcomes in patients hospitalized with HF include age, heart failure etiology (ischemic cardiomyopathy has poorer prognosis), anemia, hyponatremia, B-type natriuretic peptide levels, and LVEF.

DISEASE MANAGEMENT STRATEGIES

- Studies suggest that hospital admission for HF can be prevented with multidisciplinary disease management programs. Functional status and quality of life can also be improved for HF patients. Appropriate patients (multiple readmissions, moderate to severe heart failure, high risk due to cognitive impairment or multiple comorbidities, persistent nonadherence) should be referred to heart failure management programs if available. A multidisciplinary team made up of physicians, HF nurses, dietitians, and pharmacists can provide
  ○ Individualized education and counseling to the patient, family members, and caregivers that emphasize self-care
  ○ Assistance with medication and dietary compliance
  ○ Optimization of drug therapy
  ○ Increased access to healthcare
  ○ Early attention to signs and symptoms of fluid overload
  ○ Close telephone follow-up after hospital discharge to assess symptoms and daily weights and to adjust diuretic dosing
- Hospitalists are in a key role to lead quality improvement initiatives to facilitate patient education and discharge planning, ensure adherence to evidence-based guidelines to improve patient outcomes, and to implement national quality measures. Initiatives include HF clinical pathways and preprinted HF discharge instructions and educational material. Discharge planning includes assuring that a scale is present in the home and arranging a visiting nurse or telephone follow-up soon after discharge and a clinic visit within 7–10 days.
- Educating patients with HF and their families is critical and should start early in the hospitalization. This can be achieved through discussions, videotapes, and reading materials.
- Patient noncompliance with medications and diet is a common cause of clinical deterioration and readmission. *Discharge instructions* must address
  ○ Medications (prescribed and what to avoid)
  ○ Dietary restrictions (low-salt diet and fluid restriction)
  ○ Activity recommendations
  ○ Signs and symptoms of heart failure and what to do
  ○ Close follow-up
  ○ Weight monitoring (and what to do with weight gain)
- National guidelines strongly recommend *smoking cessation counseling* for smokers with cardiovascular disease, including heart failure.
- Exercise training (aerobic) improves exercise capacity and quality of life in patients with mild to moderate heart failure in the short term. Optimal exercise protocols are not defined, but excessively strenuous physical exertion should be discouraged.
- Immunization with influenza and pneumococcal vaccines is recommended.
- Nutritional supplements and hormonal therapies should be avoided according to current guidelines.
- A crucial goal in the management of decompensated HF is optimizing the pharmacologic regimen in the chronic ambulatory state when the patient stabilizes. Goals shift to enhancing survival, minimizing symptoms and disability, improving functional capacity, and delaying disease progression.
- See Fig. 30-1 for recommended therapy by HF stage.
- Diuretics treat the sodium and fluid retention of HF. Their effects on morbidity and mortality are unknown. Once a decompensated HF patient achieves adequate IV diuresis, an oral regimen using the lowest diuretic doses to maintain euvolemia should be determined.
- *ACE inhibitors* have been shown to alleviate symptoms, improve clinical status, and reduce the risk of death and hospitalization and should be prescribed to *all patients with HF due to LV dysfunction with reduced LVEF* unless contraindicated (angioedema, pregnancy; caution with renal artery stenosis, or elevated levels of potassium).
  ○ Treatment with an ACE inhibitor should be initiated at low doses followed by gradual increments in dose if tolerated.
  ○ Adverse effects of ACE inhibitors include hypotension, worsening renal function, potassium retention, cough, and angioedema.
  ○ In patients who are hemodynamically or clinically unstable, it is recommended to interrupt treatment with the ACE inhibitors temporarily until the patient stabilizes.

- *Angiotensin II receptor blockers* should be used in patients who are ACE inhibitor-intolerant.
- Beta-blockers decrease the symptoms of HF, improve the clinical status of patients, enhance the patient's overall sense of well-being, and reduce the risk of death and the combined risk of death or hospitalization. Beta-blockers antagonize the sympathetic nervous system and thereby block the adverse consequences of adrenergic stimulation in HF. Three beta-blockers have been shown to be effective in reducing the risk of death in patients with chronic HF: bisoprolol, sustained-release metoprolol succinate, and carvedilol. Beta-blockers should be prescribed to all patients with stable HF due to reduced LVEF unless they have a contraindication to their use.
  - Acceptable patients for beta-blocker therapy should have no or minimal evidence of fluid overload or volume depletion and should not have required recent treatment with an intravenous positive inotropic agent.
  - Treatment with a beta-blocker should be initiated at very low doses followed by gradual increments to target doses used in the clinical trials.
  - Initiation of beta-blockers can cause fluid retention, fatigue, bradycardia and heart block, and hypotension, and therefore, requires very close monitoring and follow-up.
  - If patients develop fluid retention with or without symptoms on beta-blockers, the beta-blocker can be continued while the dose of diuretic is increased. If a patient deteriorates significantly demonstrating hypoperfusion or requiring IV inotropic drugs, it is recommended to stop or reduce treatment with beta-blockers temporarily until the patient stabilizes.
- Aldosterone antagonists (spironolactone and eplerenone) have been shown to reduce mortality and hospitalizations and improve functional class in patients with advanced heart failure as well as patients with HF after an acute MI. Addition of an aldosterone antagonist is recommended in selected patients with moderately severe to severe symptoms of HF and reduced LVEF who can be monitored for preserved renal function and normal potassium concentration. Creatinine should be less than or equal to 2.5 mg/dL in men or less than or equal to 2.0 mg/dL in women (to reduce the risk of hyperkalemia) and potassium should be less than 5.0 mEq/L.
- Digitalis can improve symptoms, quality of life, exercise tolerance, and hospitalization rates in patients with mild to moderate HF, but has no effect on mortality. It is currently considered second-line therapy for chronic heart failure (eg, Class II recommendation in ACC/AHA guidelines).

- The chronic HF guidelines suggest that the addition of a combination of hydralazine, an arterial vasodilator, and a nitrate, venodilators, is reasonable in patients with reduced LVEF who are already taking an ACE inhibitor and beta-blocker for symptomatic HF and who have persistent symptoms. The combination can also be considered in symptomatic patients who cannot be given an ACE inhibitor or ARB. A prospective, double-blind randomized trial conducted in African American patients with NYHA class III/IV HF demonstrated a mortality/morbidity benefit of isosorbide dinitrate plus hydralazine when added to a standard HF regimen. Time to first hospitalization and quality of life were also improved.
- Anticoagulation with warfarin is indicated in patients with HF who have experienced a previous thromboembolic event or who have paroxysmal or persistent atrial fibrillation. Anticoagulation should also be considered in patients with underlying disorders that may be associated with an increased thromboembolic risk (eg, amyloidosis, myocarditis). The evidence for benefit of chronic warfarin anticoagulation in patients with systolic heart failure in the absence of these previous indications is limited and is considered a class II indication.
- Certain drugs should be avoided or used with caution in HF patients.
  - Nonsteroidal anti-inflammatory drugs (NSAIDs) can cause sodium retention, peripheral vasoconstriction, and precipitate renal insufficiency and should be avoided in HF patients.
  - Thiazolidinediones have been associated with increased peripheral edema and symptomatic HF and should be avoided in patients with NYHA functional class III–IV symptoms of HF.
  - Most calcium channel blockers should be avoided because of their cardiodepressant effects.
  - Routine combined use of an ACE inhibitor, ARB, and aldosterone antagonist is not recommended given the risk for hyperkalemia.

CARE TRANSITIONS

- Clinically, HF patients can be discharged once near optimal volume status is obtained, symptoms have resolved, and appropriate medications are tolerated without hypotension or renal insufficiency.
- Patient and family should demonstrate an understanding of the discharge instructions regarding medications, diet, activity, daily weights, worsening symptoms, and follow-up.
- Follow-up with a primary care physician or cardiologist within a week is mandatory to assess the patient's clinical status and tolerance of medications and to

check for electrolyte abnormalities. Closer follow-up after discharge may be necessary by telephone to assure stable weights or continuing weight loss if needed and to adjust diuretic dosing. Direct communication with the outpatient provider or disease management team should be standard practice.

• The hospitalist should know indications for coronary angiography and revascularization, implantable cardioverter-defibrillator (ICD) placement, and cardiac resynchronization. Cardiology consultation should be sought to address these issues if not already reviewed with longitudinal care providers.

• The 2005 ACC/AHA guidelines on HF made the following recommendations for coronary angiography, unless the patient is not eligible for revascularization of any kind:

   ○ HF patients who have angina or significant ischemia (Class I).
      ■ In patients with both HF and angina, coronary revascularization can relieve symptoms of myocardial ischemia and coronary artery bypass surgery has been shown to lessen angina and reduce the risk of death in patients who have multivessel disease, reduced LVEF, and stable angina.

   ○ HF patients with chest pain that may or may not be of cardiac origin who have not had evaluation of their coronary anatomy (Class IIa).
      ■ Noninvasive testing may be misleading since inhomogeneous nuclear images and abnormal wall motion patterns are common in patients with a nonischemic cardiomyopathy.

   ○ HF patients who have known or suspected coronary artery disease but who do *not* have angina (Class IIa).
      ■ Observational data suggest that patients who have ischemic cardiomyopathy, HF, and no symptoms of angina, but have viable myocardium by noninvasive imaging demonstrate improved LV function and survival with revascularization compared with medical therapy (Fig. 30-3). Alternatively, patients without viable myocardium should not be revascularized.

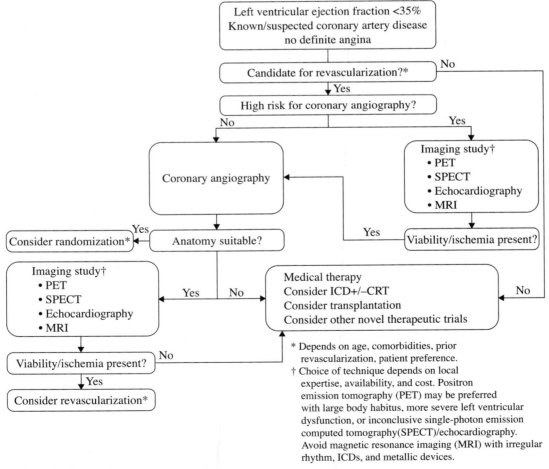

FIG. 30-3 Revascularization in ischemic cardiomyopathy.
Reprinted with permission from: Chareonthaitawee P, Gersh BJ, Araoz PA, et al. Revascularization in severe left ventricular dysfunction—the role of viability testing. *J Am Coll Cardiol.* 2005;46:572.

- Noninvasive imaging to detect myocardial ischemia and viability is reasonable in patients who have *known* coronary artery disease and *no* angina unless the patient is not eligible for revascularization (Class IIa).
- Less well supported by evidence, noninvasive imaging may be considered to define the likelihood of coronary artery disease in patients with HF and LV dysfunction (Class IIb).
- Recommendations for an ICD are
  - Secondary prevention to prolong survival in patients with current or prior symptoms of HF and reduced LVEF who have a history of cardiac arrest, ventricular fibrillation, or hemodynamically destabilizing ventricular tachycardia (Class I).
  - Primary prevention to reduce total mortality by a reduction in sudden cardiac death in patients with either ischemic heart disease (at least 40 days post-MI) or nonischemic cardiomyopathy (at least 9 months) who have an LVEF less than or equal to 30%, with NYHA functional class II or III symptoms while undergoing chronic optimal medical therapy, and have reasonable expectation of survival with a good functional status for more than 1 year (Class I).
  - ICDs are not warranted in patients with refractory symptoms of HF (stage D) or in patients with concomitant diseases that would shorten their life expectancy independent of HF.
- In addition to the mechanical disadvantages, ventricular dyssynchrony (as evidenced by a prolonged QRS duration) has been associated with increased mortality in HF patients. Dyssynchronous contraction can be alleviated by electrically activating the right and left ventricles in a synchronized manner with a biventricular pacemaker device (cardiac resynchronization therapy [CRT]). Evidence exists to support the use of CRT to improve symptoms, exercise capacity, quality of life, LVEF, and survival and to decrease hospitalization in patients with persistently symptomatic HF undergoing optimal medical therapy who have cardiac dyssynchrony.
- The Class I recommendation for cardiac resynchronization therapy is
  - Patients with LVEF less than or equal to 35%, sinus rhythm, and NYHA functional class III or ambulatory class IV symptoms despite recommended, optimal medical therapy and who have cardiac dyssynchrony, which is currently defined as a QRS duration greater than 120 msec.
- Patients with stage D HF, or refractory HF, have marked symptoms at rest despite maximal medical therapy and are best cared for by HF specialists. They may be eligible for specialized, advanced treatments, such as mechanical circulatory support, procedures to facilitate fluid removal (ultrafiltration or hemofiltration), invasive hemodynamic guided therapy, or cardiac transplantation. End of life and palliative care can also be reviewed and offered when appropriate.

BIBLIOGRAPHY

Anonymous. Guidelines 2000 for cardiopulmonary resuscitation and emergency cardiovascular care. Part 7: the era of reperfusion: section 1: acute coronary syndromes (acute myocardial infarction). The American Heart Association in collaboration with the International Liaison Committee on Resuscitation. *Circulation.* 2000:102(suppl 8):I172–I203.

Chareonthaitawee P, Gersh BJ, Araoz PA, et al. Revascularization in severe left ventricular dysfunction. *J Am Coll Cardiol.* 2005;46:567–574.

Cleland JGF, Daubert JC, Erdmann E, et al. The effect of cardiac resynchronization on morbidity and mortality in heart failure. *N Engl J Med.* 2005;352:1539–1549.

Fonarow GC, Adams KF, Abraham WT, et al. Risk stratification for in-hospital mortality in acutely decompensated heart failure. *JAMA.* 2005;293:572–580.

Forrester JS, Diamond GA, Swan HJ. Correlative classification of clinical and hemodynamic function after acute myocardial infarction. *Am J Cardiol.* 1977;39:137–145.

Heart Failure Society of America. Executive summary: HFSA 2006 comprehensive heart failure practice guideline. *J Card Fail.* 2006;12:10–38.

Hunt SA, Abraham WT, Marshall CH, et al. ACC/AHA 2005 guideline update for the diagnosis and management of chronic heart failure in the adult: a report of the American College of Cardiology/American Heart Association task force on practice guidelines (Writing Committee to Update the 2001 Guidelines for the Evaluation and Management of Heart Failure): developed in collaboration with the American College of Chest Physicians and the International Society for Heart and Lung Transplantation: endorsed by the Heart Rhythm Society. *Circulation.* 2005;112:154–235.

Jessup M, Brozena S. Heart failure. *N Engl J Med.* 2003;348:2007–2018.

Mueller C, Scholer A, Laule-Kilian K, et al. Use of B-type natriuretic peptide in the evaluation and management of acute dyspnea. *N Engl J Med.* 2004;350:647–654.

Nieminen MS, Bohm M, Cowie MR, et al. Guidelines on the diagnosis and treatment of acute heart failure. The task force on acute heart failure of the European society of Cardiology. *Eur Heart J.* 2005:1–36.

Pitt B, Zannad F, Remme WJ, et al. The effect of spironolactone on morbidity and mortality in patients with severe heart failure. *N Engl J Med.* 1999;341:709–717.

Rees K, Taylor RS, Sing S, et al. Exercise-based rehabilitation for heart failure. *Cochrane Database Syst Rev.* 2004, Issue 3. Art. No.: CD003331. DOI: 10.1002/14651858. CD003331.pub2.

Taylor AL, Ziesche S, Yancy C, et al. Combination of isosorbide dinitrate and hydralazine in blacks with heart failure. *N Engl J Med.* 2004;351:2049–2057.

Zipes DP, Libby P, Bonow RO, et al. *Braunwald's Heart Disease. A Textbook of Cardiovascular Medicine.* 7th ed. Philadelphia, PA: Elsevier Saunders; 2005:509–624.

31   SYNCOPE

Daniel W. Mudrick

EPIDEMIOLOGY/OVERVIEW

- Syncope is the abrupt loss of consciousness and postural tone due to cerebral hypoperfusion, with spontaneous recovery (without electrical or pharmacologic cardioversion).
- The diagnosis of syncope accounts for approximately 3% of emergency department (ED) visits, and 1% to 6% of hospital admissions in the United States. Many patients with a first episode of syncope or fainting never present for medical evaluation.
- Over an average of 17 years of follow-up in the Framingham heart study, Soteriades et al found that 11% of participants reported at least one syncopal episode. The overall incidence rate of a first report of syncope was 6.2 per 1000 person-years. Rising age, especially greater than 70, and cardiovascular disease were associated with higher incident rates of syncope.
- Sun et al estimated the direct medical costs of syncope-related hospitalizations in the United States in 2000 at $2.4 billion, with a mean cost of $5400 per hospitalization. The cost per diagnosis ranges widely, from $529 with an external loop recorder to $73,260 for electrophysiologic studies in patients without structural heart disease.
- Cardiac causes of syncope predict increased sudden death and all-cause mortality, while neurocardiogenic and orthostatic syncope have no increase in mortality compared to the general population (Fig. 31-1).
- Morbidity from syncope may be related to recurrent syncope, injury from falls or traffic accidents, and anxiety related to the condition.
  - In the Framingham heart study, only 28% of participants who had one syncopal event had a recurrent episode during the follow-up period. However, a person who has had an episode of syncope is much more likely to have a recurrence than a person with no such history is to have a first event (multivariable-adjusted hazard ratio 23.2).
  - Seventeen percent to thirty-five percent of patients with syncopal falls experience significant injury, and up to 7% may sustain fractures.

PATHOPHYSIOLOGY

- Syncope can be caused by any condition that transiently reduces cerebral blood flow by reducing cardiac output, decreasing peripheral vascular resistance, or obstructing blood flow in the central nervous system (CNS).
- A fall in mean arterial pressure below 40 mm Hg or a systolic blood pressure below 70 mm Hg generally results in loss of consciousness, though variations in cerebral perfusion, vascular reactivity, and baseline blood pressure may alter an individual's susceptibility to syncope.
- The classification of types of syncope is not consistent in the literature, but generally includes
  - Neurocardiogenic (or reflex-mediated) syncope (36%–62%)
  - Orthostatic syncope (2%–24%)
  - Cardiovascular syncope (10%–30%)
  - Other less-common causes of syncope including cerebrovascular (about 1%).
  - No clear cause of syncope is identified in many patients (18%–52%) (Table 31-1).

CLINICAL PRESENTATION, DIFFERENTIAL, MAKING THE DIAGNOSIS

- It is important to distinguish true syncope from other entities such as cardiac arrest (requiring cardiopulmonary resuscitation [CPR] or cardioversion), seizures, vertigo, transient ischemic attacks or cerebrovascular accidents, psychiatric disorders (eg, conversion disorder, malingering), coma, and drop attacks (loss of postural tone without loss of consciousness).
- The prevalence of syncope in a general population is much higher than the prevalence of epilepsy, 3% to 37% vs. 0.5%.
- A number of factors help distinguish syncope from seizure.
  - Syncope
    - Presence of coronary artery disease
    - Loss of consciousness with prolonged sitting or standing
    - Lightheadedness, nausea, diaphoresis, or dyspnea before loss of consciousness
    - Brief myoclonic jerks that last only a few seconds

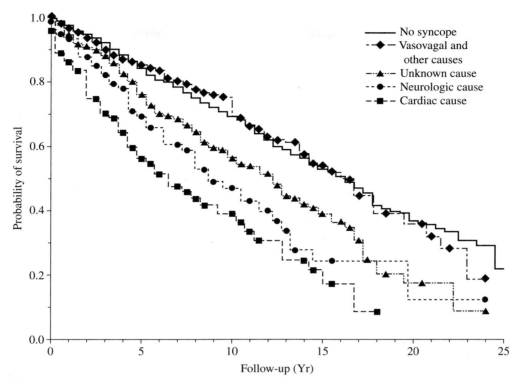

FIG. 31-1 Survival without syncope compared to survival with syncope, by cause of syncope.*
*P< .001 for the comparison between participants with and those without syncope. The category "Vasovagal and other causes" includes vasovagal, orthostatic, medication-induced, and other, infrequent causes of syncope.
From: Soteriades ES, Evans JC, Larson MG. Incidence and prognosis of syncope. _N Engl J Med._ 2002;347:882. (Copyright 2002 Massachusetts Medical Society. All rights reserved.)

TABLE 31-1   Causes of Syncope

- _Neurocardiogenic syncope_ is the result of a fall in peripheral vascular resistance due to autonomic hyperactivity, and has three closely related subgroups: vasovagal syncope, situational syncope, and carotid sinus syncope.
  - _Vasovagal syncope_ is thought to occur in susceptible individuals when cardiac hypercontractility (in the setting of noxious stimuli, prolonged standing, or underfilling) is misinterpreted by stretch receptors in the left ventricle, leading to a reflexive increase in parasympathetic tone and decreased sympathetic activity. This results in peripheral vasodilation and/or bradycardia, and may lead to loss of consciousness.
  - _Situational syncope_ is similar to vasovagal syncope, but occurs in specific settings such as during micturition, defecation, cough, or Valsalva (while playing an instrument, for example).
  - _Carotid sinus hypersensitivity_ results most often in a cardioinhibitory response with notable bradycardia and sinus pauses. Less commonly, there may be a vasodepressor response with hypotension, or a mixed response.
- _Orthostatic syncope_ is caused by a failure of the autonomic nervous system to prevent postural hypotension, and becomes more prevalent with advancing age.
  - Common causes include volume depletion, early sepsis from infections, medications (especially antidepressants), and alcohol.
  - Autonomic failure may be either primary, as in multisystem atrophy (Shy-Drager syndrome) or pure autonomic failure (Bradbury-Eggleston syndrome), or secondary, as in amyloidosis, diabetes, multiple sclerosis, or tabes dorsalis.
- _Cardiovascular causes of syncope_ include arrhythmias and mechanical causes.
  - The most common _electrical causes_ of syncope are atrioventricular block, sick sinus syndrome, and ventricular tachycardia. Other causes include supraventricular tachycardias, long QT syndrome with torsades de pointes, and Wolff-Parkinson-White syndrome.
  - _Mechanical causes_ include obstructive etiologies such as aortic stenosis, hypertrophic obstructive cardiomyopathy, mitral stenosis, pulmonary hypertension, pulmonary embolism, pulmonic stenosis, and atrial myxomas. Depressed cardiac output in cardiomyopathy, acute myocardial infarction, or tamponade can also lead to a transient global reduction in brain perfusion and cause syncope.
  - _Myocardial infarction_ can occasionally present as syncope, especially in older people, due to ischemia-induced ventricular tachycardia, depressed cardiac output secondary to myocardial dysfunction (especially in right-sided or posterior infarction), or reflex bradycardia (Bezold-Jarisch reflex).
- Other causes of syncope include _medication effects_ and polypharmacy, _anemia, metabolic derangements_ (e.g., hypoglycemia, hypokalemia, hypocapnea, or hypoxia), _cerebrovascular insults_ (e.g., posterior transient ischemic attack, subclavian steal syndrome, intermittent obstructive hydrocephalus, seizure-induced arrhythmogenic syncope, and migraine syncope), and _psychiatric conditions_ (e.g., panic with hyperventilation, and conversion disorders).

○ Seizure
  ▪ Tongue biting (especially lateral)
  ▪ Urinary incontinence
  ▪ Jerking movements lasting more than 30 seconds
  ▪ Prodromal déjà vu
  ▪ Head turning to one side during loss of consciousness
  ▪ Postictal confusion lasting more than a few minutes
• Neurocardiogenic syncope is extremely rare from a recumbent position; seizures and cardiac syncope may occur from any position.
• Cerebrovascular accidents may induce loss of consciousness, but will almost always be accompanied by focal neurologic deficits.
• In patients who present with injury and loss of consciousness, an attempt should be made to determine if any trauma preceded the fall or if the injuries resulted from loss of postural tone.

TRIAGE AND INITIAL MANAGEMENT

• Hospitalization is indicated for those with a significant likelihood of cardiac syncope, or those with debilitating symptoms (Table 31-2). Repeated hospitalizations for evaluation of recurrent syncope that has been worked up previously rarely result in a diagnosis.
• The most important goals of the initial workup of syncope are
  ○ To rule out acute processes such as myocardial infarction, pulmonary embolism, stroke, and so forth.
  ○ To identify patients with structural heart disease or underlying arrhythmias who are most likely to have cardiac syncope.
• Diagnosing the cause of syncope in a given patient can be very difficult, given the wide range of potential causes, the transient nature of the symptom, and the lack of gold-standard tests. Even so, a careful history, physical examination, and electrocardiogram (ECG) can suggest or confirm the cause of syncope in 40% to 70% of patients.
• Algorithms can be very useful in providing a systematic approach to the evaluation of syncope. The

TABLE 31-2   Indications for Hospitalization for Evaluation of Syncope

History or physical examination suggestive of coronary artery disease, congestive heart failure, ventricular tachycardia, valvular disease, or stroke
Abnormalities on the electrocardiogram suggestive of cardiac disease
Family history of sudden death
Severe injury or syncope while driving
Frequent episodes
Moderate to severe orthostatic hypotension
Advanced age, especially > 70

following algorithm (Fig. 31-2) established by Linzer et al provides a good framework for the workup of syncope.
• *History:* A detailed history including preceding symptoms, position at time of syncope, duration of loss of consciousness, and symptoms during recovery can be extremely important in determining the cause of syncope. When available, witnesses should be interviewed to corroborate or fill in details.
  ○ "Red flag symptoms" prior to the syncopal event, such as chest pain, shortness of breath, palpitations, low back pain, acute or severe headache, or focal neurologic changes, require further evaluation to rule out acute processes.
  ○ Underlying medical conditions and symptoms of concurrent illness (eg, pneumonia or urinary tract infection) may suggest an underlying etiology. Family history of sudden death should be determined.
  ○ A careful medication history is vital, with special attention to antihypertensives, diuretics, antiarrhythmics or nodal agents, medications that prolong the QT interval, sedatives, and potential drug-drug interactions.
  ○ Vasovagal syncope frequently occurs in the setting of pain, fear, or noxious stimuli, or with prolonged standing. It is often associated with a prodrome of lightheadedness, nausea, warmth, and/or diaphoresis, and a postsyncopal phase notable for severe fatigue and, possibly, a brief period of confusion.
  ○ Carotid sinus syncope should be suspected when syncope occurs with head turning, tight collars, shaving, choking, or other activities that could apply pressure to the carotid sinus.
  ○ Syncope during or immediately after micturition, defecation, cough, swallow, or Valsalva suggests situational syncope.
  ○ Loss of consciousness on standing or changing posture is often related to orthostatic hypotension.
  ○ Arrhythmia-induced syncope often occurs without prodrome, followed by sudden recovery.
  ○ Exertional syncope is worrisome for cardiac causes including aortic stenosis, hypertrophic obstructive cardiomyopathy, pulmonary hypertension, mitral stenosis, and coronary ischemia. Syncope in a well-trained athlete after exertion is often vasovagal.
• *Physical examination:* A comprehensive physical examination can provide evidence of cardiac or neurologic disease, and aid in the diagnosis of carotid sinus hypersensitivity and orthostatic hypotension.
  ○ Vital signs, including blood pressure in both arms and orthostatic signs, should be checked in all patients. Repeated postural testing is appropriate if there is a high level of clinical suspicion for orthostatic syncope. A decrease in systolic blood

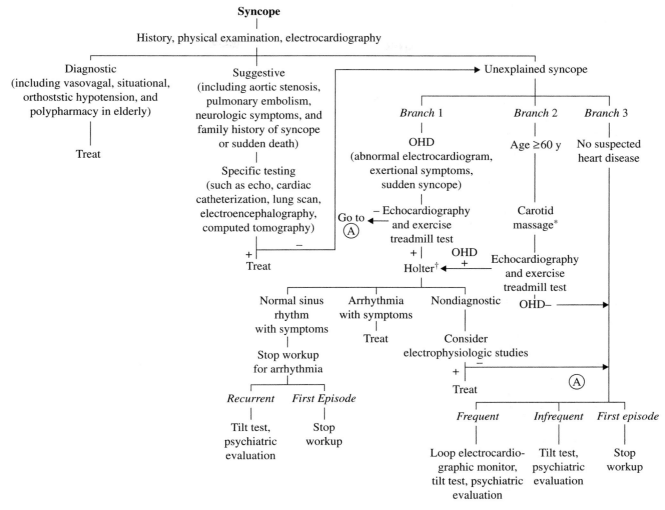

FIG. 31-2 Algorithm for diagnosing syncope.
From: Linzer M, Yang EH, Estes NA III. Diagnosing syncope. Part 1: value of history, physical examination, and electrocardiography. Clinical efficacy assessment project of the American College of Physicians. *Ann Intern Med.* 1997;126:989.

pressure ≥ 20 mm Hg or a decrease of systolic blood pressure to < 90 mm Hg with a change in position from lying to sitting or sitting to standing, is defined as orthostatic hypotension, regardless of symptoms.

○ Cardiovascular examination should focus on valvular findings, evidence of congestive heart failure or volume overload, extra heart sounds such as "tumor plops" or rubs, and peripheral pulses for signs of peripheral vascular disease or subclavian steal.

○ A detailed neurologic examination, including fundoscopy to identify embolic phenomena and search for carotid bruits, should be performed to evaluate for neurologic causes.

○ Carotid massage is indicated in patients with history suggestive of carotid sinus syncope, or age ≥ 60 years with syncope of unknown cause.

▪ Intravenous access and continuous ECG monitoring, blood pressure measurements, and pulse oximetry are required.

▪ Contraindications include myocardial infarction (MI), transient ischemic attack, or stroke within the past 3 months; or the presence of carotid bruits, ventricular fibrillation, or ventricular tachycardia.

▪ One side should be tested at a time. Longitudinal massage should be continued between 5 and 10 seconds per side.

▪ The test is considered positive with asystole of at least 3 seconds and/or a fall in systolic blood pressure of ≥ 50 mm Hg, without any symptoms; or ≥ 30 mm Hg with syncope or presyncope symptoms.

- All patients who present with syncope should have an ECG. ECG is a safe and relatively low-cost test that can suggest a specific diagnosis in 5% to 10% of patients, and can help rule out cardiac syncope.
  - Up to 90% of patients with cardiac syncope have abnormal ECG findings, while less than 10% of patients with neurocardiogenic syncope do.
  - Findings suggestive of specific etiologies of cardiac syncope are listed in Table 31-3.
- Laboratory tests are generally of little value in the evaluation of syncope. Peripheral blood glucose testing is reasonable in most patients. Tests that may be suggested by history and physical examination include hematocrit and stool guaiac, white blood count and cultures, urinalysis, chest radiograph, electrolyte levels, and drug/toxicology screening.
- All patients with pacemakers, defibrillators, or implantable loop recorders should have their devices interrogated.
- If heart disease is suspected, echocardiography and prolonged ECG monitoring should be performed.
  - In patients with evidence of heart disease, echocardiography is the test of choice to identify valvular or myocardial pathology. In patients with a negative cardiac history and a normal ECG, however, echocardiography is almost never helpful in determining the cause of syncope.
  - Continuous ECG monitoring, by telemetry as an inpatient or Holter monitor as an outpatient, for 24–48 hours (longer periods do not generally increase effectiveness) may be useful to diagnose or rule out arrhythmia as a cause of syncope if symptoms recur during monitoring.
  - Ambulatory monitoring is often more useful for ruling out arrhythmia as a cause of syncope than ruling in; in case series, approximately 2% of patients had documented arrhythmia with symptoms, while up to 15% had symptoms without evidence of arrhythmia.
  - In patients with evidence of structural heart disease who have nondiagnostic continuous ECG monitoring, referral for intracardiac electrophysiologic studies should be considered.
- If syncope occurs with exertion, or if chest pain precedes or follows syncope, myocardial infarction should be ruled out with serial enzymes, and an exercise stress test or myocardial perfusion study should be obtained. An echocardiogram should be obtained prior to stress testing to rule out aortic stenosis or hypertrophic cardiomyopathy.
- In patients with recurrent syncope without suspected heart disease, or in those with structural heart disease and negative ECG monitoring and electrophysiologic studies, outpatient head-up tilt table (HUTT) testing and prolonged electrocardiographic monitoring (with event recorders or implantable loop recorders) may be useful.
  - HUTT is used to further confirm or rule out neurocardiogenic syncope.
    - The test involves using a tilt table to place a patient in an upright position without active muscle flexion for up to 45 minutes. Various maneuvers can be used to increase the sensitivity of the test.
    - A test is considered positive if it reproduces symptoms in the setting of bradycardia or hypotension.
    - HUTT alone does not convincingly rule in or rule out neurocardiogenic syncope, but can be suggestive. If arrhythmia has been ruled out (ie, an event captured on ECG monitoring without arrhythmia, or a negative result on an electrophysiologic study), a positive HUTT is usually considered diagnostic for neurocardiogenic syncope.
    - In patients who experience loss of consciousness on HUTT without bradycardia or hypotension, a psychiatric disorder should be considered.

TABLE 31-3   Electrocardiographic Findings Suggestive of Syncopal Etiologies

FINDING ON ECG	UNDERLYING ETIOLOGY
Prolonged QT interval	Polymorphic ventricular tachycardia
Second- or third-degree heart block	Conduction system disease
Bundle branch or fascicular blocks	Conduction system disease
Other intraventricular conduction abnormalities (QRS ≥ .12 seconds)	Conduction system disease
Sinus bradycardia or sinoatrial block	Bradycardia and sinus pauses
Pre-excited QRS complexes (delta waves)	Supraventricular tachycardia with aberrancy (Wolff-Parkinson-White syndrome)
Negative T waves in right precordial leads, epsilon waves, and ventricular late potentials	Arrhythmogenic right ventricular dysplasia
Q waves suggesting prior myocardial infarction	Ventricular tachycardia
Right ventricular conduction delay (right bundle branch block pattern) with ST elevation in leads V_{1-3}	Congenital sodium channel abnormality (Brugada syndrome)
High QRS voltage, prominent septal Q waves in the lateral leads, and giant negative T waves in the precordial leads	Hypertrophic cardiomyopathy

- Event recorders and implantable loop recorders can be used for weeks to months; they increase the likelihood of capturing an event in patients with recurrent symptoms. Older event recorders that require activation by the patient to capture an event are often not as effective.
- Routine tests for neurologic causes of syncope (eg, electroencephalogram [EEG], magnetic resonance imaging [MRI] or computed tomography [CT] of the head and Doppler ultrasound of the carotids) are of low yield in true syncope unless there are focal neurologic findings or specific points of the history or examination to indicate evaluation.
- It is important to recognize the limitations of testing and to avoid initiating low-yield studies that may unnecessarily increase cost, patient discomfort, and length of stay (LOS).
- Hospitalists, in conjunction with cardiologists, electrophysiologists, and neurologists, are in a strong position to institute protocols for the appropriate workup of undifferentiated syncope.

DISEASE MANAGEMENT STRATEGIES

- Once a cause of syncope is identified, treatment should focus on the underlying process.
- If drug-induced syncope is diagnosed, the offending medication(s) should be reduced, administered at a different time of day, substituted, or discontinued.
- Syncope due to orthostatic hypotension is treated by expanding volume and increasing peripheral vascular resistance.
  - If possible, given concurrent health conditions, patients should be advised to avoid volume depletion and liberalize salt intake.
  - Medications that exacerbate orthostatic hypotension (antidepressants, diuretics, antihypertensives, sympathetic blockers) should be adjusted.
  - Patients can be taught techniques to minimize fluid shifts with change of position—slow transitions from lying to sitting or standing; flexing the legs or performing handgrip prior to standing; wearing fitted pressure stockings to decrease venous pooling in the lower extremities.
  - If the above techniques are ineffective, medications may be helpful.
    - Fludrocortisone (a mineralocorticoid) at 0.1–1.0 mg/d, titrated up slowly. Side effects include edema and hypertension, and it may be poorly tolerated in the elderly. Dose increases may be required over time as patients become desensitized.
    - Other pharmacologic options include alpha-1-adrenergic agonists including midodrine or phenylephrine, nonsteroidal anti-inflammatory drugs (NSAIDs), caffeine, and fluoxetine.
- Neurocardiogenic syncope can be difficult to treat. Interventions can be directed at many different points in the reflex cycle that leads to syncope.
  - Patients should be counseled to avoid or take precautions with recognized triggers, especially in situational or carotid sinus syncope, and to respond to prodromal symptoms by sitting down or, ideally, lying supine and raising legs.
  - Volume expansion and techniques to increase peripheral vascular resistance may be helpful, as described above, to treat orthostatics.
  - Beta-blockers are often used in an attempt to prevent the cardiac hypercontractility that initiates the reflex hypotension and bradycardia associated with syncope. Other medications that can sometimes be helpful include central acting agents such as selective serotonin reuptake inhibitors and vagolytics such as scopolamine.
  - If other strategies are ineffective or contraindicated, it is reasonable to consider pacemaker placement for recurrent neurocardiogenic syncope (including carotid sinus syncope), but only if bradycardia is demonstrated at the time of the event or on HUTT testing.
- Treatment of cardiac syncope usually requires consultation with a cardiologist or electrophysiologist for appropriate treatment of the underlying causes.
  - Syncope secondary to bradycardia from sinoatrial node dysfunction or high-grade atrioventricular blocks is an indication for pacemaker placement. Pacemakers are not indicated for empiric treatment in undiagnosed syncope if there is no documented bradycardia and an electrophysiologic study is negative.
  - Patients with documented ventricular tachycardia (VT) and syncope should be referred to an electrophysiologist for management of antiarrhythmic medications, and consideration of ablation and placement of a defibrillator. If VT is suspected but not documented in a patient with otherwise unexplained syncope, it is appropriate to refer to an electrophysiologist to test for inducible VT. If present, the patient should be treated as above.
  - Long QT with syncope should be referred to an electrophysiologist. Patients may respond to beta-blockers, and pacemaker and defibrillator placement should be considered. Medications with potential to prolong the QT interval should be avoided, and the patient should be told to notify all clinicians of the condition, especially when medications are prescribed.
  - Obstructive cardiac processes such as aortic stenosis and hypertrophic cardiomyopathy often require

surgical correction, though hypertrophic cardiomyopathy may be treated initially with negative inotropic agents such as beta-blockers and calcium channel blockers. In patients with outflow obstruction, vasodilators such as nitrates and inhibitors of the angiotensin system should be avoided, as should medications with positive inotropy, such as digoxin. Patients should be advised to consult with a cardiologist before engaging in athletics or heavy exertion.

○ Patients with cardiomyopathy and depressed ejection fraction who have syncope have a high risk of sudden cardiac death and death from other causes. They should be referred to cardiology for long-term management. There is a survival benefit from the placement of defibrillators; however, the decision to place a defibrillator needs to take into consideration the patient's other comorbidities and quality-of-life factors.

○ Patients with supraventricular tachycardias (SVTs) that result in syncope (especially those involving the atrioventricular node or an accessory pathway) should be seen by an electrophysiologist for possible initiation of antiarrhythmic medications and for consideration of ablation procedures.

CARE TRANSITIONS

• Appropriate length of hospitalization varies with the type of syncope. Discharge may be appropriate when a thorough workup has been completed, underlying causes have been treated, and follow-up treatments and tests have been arranged.

• Physicians should discuss activity or driving restrictions with patients prior to discharge.

○ If arrhythmia is suspected, driving should be proscribed until the workup is complete. Many states have specific driving restriction following any syncopal episode, often from 3 to 12 months. A physician's legal responsibility to notify the department of motor vehicles of a patient's history of syncope varies from state to state.

○ Small studies suggest that many patients do not heed driving instructions given by physicians. Nonetheless, it is important from a medicolegal standpoint to document that such instructions have been given to the patient.

• Reconcile admission and discharge medications and ensure the patient is aware of new or discontinued medications and changes in dosing, especially if specific drugs or polypharmacy are suspected in the syncopal episode.

• Contact the primary care physician (PCP) in a timely manner (ideally within 24 hours of discharge) regarding the patient's hospital course, diagnosis, treatment plan (particularly changes in medications), and any test that will need to be followed up, such as Holter monitors or tilt table testing.

BIBLIOGRAPHY

Goldschlager N, Epstein AE, Grubb BP, et al: Etiologic considerations in the patient with syncope and an apparently normal heart. *Arch Intern Med.* 2003;163:151.

Gould PA, Krahn AD, Klein GJ, et al: Investigating syncope: a review. *Curr Opin Cardiol.* 2006;21:34.

Grubb BP. Clinical practice. Neurocardiogenic syncope. *N Engl J Med.* 2005;352:1004.

Grubb BP. Neurocardiogenic syncope and related disorders of orthostatic intolerance. *Circulation.* 2005;111:2997.

Hadjikoutis S, O'Callaghan P, Smith PE. The investigation of syncope. *Seizure.* 2004;13:537.

Linzer M, Yang EH, Estes NA III. Diagnosing syncope. Part 1: value of history, physical examination, and electrocardiography. Clinical efficacy assessment project of the American College of Physicians. *Ann Intern Med.* 1997;126:989.

Miller TH, Kruse JE. Evaluation of syncope. Am Fam Physician. 2005;72:1492.

Sarasin FP, Junod AF, Carballo D, et al. Role of echocardiography in the evaluation of syncope: a prospective study. *Heart.* 2002;88:363.

Schnipper JJ, Kapoor WN., Diagnostic evaluation and management of patients with syncope. *Med Clin North Am.* March 2001;85(2):423-456.

Sheldon R. Tilt testing for syncope: a reappraisal. *Curr Opin Cardiol.* 2005;20:38.

Soteriades ES, Evans JC, Larson MG. Incidence and prognosis of syncope. *N Engl J Med.* 2002;347:878.

Sun BC, Emond JA, Camargo CA. Direct medical costs of syncope-related hospitalizations in the United States. *Am J Cardiol.* 2005;95:668.

32 HYPERTENSIVE URGENCIES/ EMERGENCIES

Renee Y. Meadows

EPIDEMIOLOGY/OVERVIEW

• Hypertension (HTN) affects approximately 50 million people in the United States and approximately one billion worldwide.

• Blood pressure classification is based on the average of two or more readings on at least three separate occasions over several weeks/months in a patient who is not on antihypertensive medication or acutely ill as follows:

○ *Normal blood pressure:* Systolic < 120 mm Hg and diastolic < 80 mm Hg

○ *Prehypertension:* Systolic 120–139 mm Hg or diastolic 80–89 mm Hg

○ Hypertension which requires pharmacologic treatment in those who do not respond to nonpharmacologic/lifestyle modifications
  - *Stage 1:* Systolic 140–159 mm Hg or diastolic 90–99 mm Hg (initial choice should be low-dose thiazide diuretic monotherapy per the recommendation of the seventh report of the Joint National Committee on Prevention, Detection,

Evaluation, and Treatment of High Blood Pressure [JNC7]).
  - *Stage 2:* Systolic ≥160 mm Hg or diastolic ≥100 mm Hg (typically requires at least two drugs to manage).
- Effective blood pressure control can be achieved in most hypertensive patients but the majority will require two or more antihypertensive medications in addition to lifestyle modification (Table 32-1).

TABLE 32-1 Pharmacologic Strategies for HTN Management

CATEGORY	ADVANTAGES AND SPECIFIC INDICATIONS FOR USE	DISADVANTAGES AND CONTRAINDICATIONS
INITIATION OF ANTIHYPERTENSIVE THERAPY		
Thiazide diuretic monotherapy at low dose	■ Cheap ■ Effective for most patients ■ Minimal side effects (hypokalemia, hyperuricemia, mild elevations in glucose) at low doses ■ Elderly ■ Black patients ■ Patients with edema or CHF ■ Osteoporosis	Absolute ■ Drug allergy ■ Rare cause of hypercalcemia Relative ■ History of gout ■ May cause sexual dysfunction in men
IF THIAZIDE ALONE INSUFFICIENT, ADD OR SUBSTITUTE ONE OF THE FOLLOWING (INDIVIDUALIZE TO PATIENT COMORBIDITIES WHERE APPROPRIATE)		
Angiotensin-converting enzyme (ACE) inhibitors	■ Mode of action synergistic with thiazide diuretics ■ CHF with low LVEF ■ Post-MI ■ LV hypertrophy ■ Diabetes ■ CKD with proteinuria	■ Angioedema ■ Hyperkalemia ■ Pregnancy Bothersome side effect ■ Dry cough (7% men and 15% to 20% women)
Angiotensin II receptor blockers (ARBs)	■ Same as ACE, but without the cough	■ Hyperkalemia ■ Pregnancy
Calcium channel blockers	■ No elevation of glucose or lipids, do not interfere with sympathetic system the way beta-blockers do ■ Preferred in patents who will not comply with sodium restriction and those on NSAIDs ■ First line in combination with thiazide diuretics in black or elderly patients ■ Also consider with angina, recurrent SVTs, Raynaud, migraine, diastolic dysfunction, esophageal spasm	■ Second- or third-degree heart block ■ Systolic dysfunction ■ Side effects include headache, dizziness, and peripheral edema
Beta-blockers	■ Resting tachycardia ■ CHF particularly due to diastolic dysfunction ■ Underlying CAD or angina ■ Migraine headache ■ Glaucoma ■ Essential tremor ■ Hyperthyroidism ■ Perioperative HTN	■ Asthma & COPD ■ Severe PVD ■ Raynaud phenomenon ■ Bradycardia ■ Second- or third-degree heart block ■ Diabetics prone to hypoglycemia ■ Less protective against stroke than other anti-HTN
SECOND-LINE OPTIONS		
Alpha-1 blockers	■ Lower LDL, raise HDL, decrease insulin resistance ■ BPH	■ Increased risk of CHF ■ Side effects include: HA, weakness, dizziness and syncope
Centrally acting sympatholytic agents	■ No adverse effects on glucose or lipids	■ High incidence of side effects including: dry mouth, sedation, sexual dysfunction ■ Rebound HTN with abrupt discontinuation
Aldosterone receptor blockers	■ Systolic heart failure	■ Hyperkalemia

Abbreviations: BPH, benign prostatic hyperplasia; CAD, coronary artery disease; CKD, chronic kidney disease; COPD, chronic obstructive pulmonary disease; HDL, high-density lipoprotein; LDL, low-density lipoprotein; LVEF, left ventricular ejection fraction; SVT, supraventricular tachycardia.

- Physician prescription of ineffective antihypertensive drug doses and inappropriate drug combinations, or patient nonadherence to antihypertensive therapy, may result in inadequate blood pressure control leading to hypertensive urgency or emergency.
  - Nearly 1% of hypertensive individuals will develop a hypertensive crisis.
  - Hypertensive crises account for over 25% of all medical emergencies presenting to the emergency department (ED) and 3% of all emergency room visits. Of these, over 75% are hypertensive urgencies while only 20% to 25% are hypertensive emergencies.
- Hypertensive crises include a variety of clinical situations that have in common elevated blood pressure (typically > 180/120 mm Hg) and progressive or impending target organ damage.
- Hypertensive emergency is severe hypertension with evidence of acute end-organ damage such as encephalopathy, unstable angina, stroke, dissecting aortic aneurysm, pulmonary edema, or eclampsia. The degree of blood pressure elevation is less important than the evidence of end-organ damage. These patients require aggressive reduction in blood pressure over minutes to hours.
- Hypertensive urgency is characterized by unexpected blood pressure elevation, possibly associated with headache, shortness of breath, epistaxis, or severe anxiety, but without evidence of end-organ damage. Blood pressure control for these patients may be achieved safely over one to several days.
- Resistant hypertension is the failure to reach goal blood pressure in asymptomatic patients who are adhering to full doses of an appropriate three-drug regimen that includes a diuretic. Drug interactions and secondary hypertension should be considered in these patients.
- *International Classification of Diseases, Ninth Revision, Clinical Modification (ICD-9-CM)* provides subcategories for systemic hypertension to designate the benign, malignant, or unspecified nature of hypertension. Historically, malignant hypertension is associated with papilledema. It is characterized by rapidly rising blood pressure, usually > 140 mm Hg diastolic, with findings of visual impairment and signs or symptoms of progressive heart failure, encephalopathy, or nephropathy.

PATHOPHYSIOLOGY

- Any disorder that causes HTN may cause a hypertensive emergency (Table 32-2).
- The necessary initiating step for acute hypertensive emergency with endothelial failure appears to be an initial abrupt rise in vascular resistance.

TABLE 32-2   Causes of Hypertensive Emergencies

Essential hypertension
Renal parenchymal disease
  Acute glomerulonephritis
  Vasculitis
  Hemolytic uremic syndrome
  Thrombotic thrombocytopenic purpura
Renovascular disease
  Renal-artery stenosis (atheromatous or fibromuscular dysplasia)
Pregnancy
  Eclampsia
Endocrine
  Pheochromocytoma
  Cushing syndrome
  Renin-secreting tumors
  Mineralocorticoid hypertension (rarely causes hypertensive emergencies)
Drugs
  Cocaine, sympathomimetics, erythropoietin, cyclosporin, antihypertensive withdrawal, interactions with monoamine-oxidase inhibitors (tyramine), amphetamines, lead intoxication
Autonomic hyperreactivity
  Guillain-Barré syndrome, acute intermittent porphyria
Central nervous system disorders
  Head injury, cerebral infarction/hemorrhage, brain tumors

SOURCE: Reprinted from Vaughan CJ, Delanty N. Hypertensive emergencies. *Lancet.* 2000;356(9227):411–417. (With permission from Elsevier).

- During an initial rise in blood pressure, the endothelium attempts to compensate for the change in vascular resistance through increased release of vasodilator molecules such as nitric oxide.
- When compensatory responses are overwhelmed, endothelial decompensation promotes further rises in blood pressure and endothelial damage.
- A cycle of homeostatic failure is initiated leading to progressive increases in vascular resistance and further endothelial dysfunction.
- Although the exact cellular mechanisms responsible for endothelial dysfunction are incompletely understood, disturbances of the renin-angiotensin-aldosterone system, loss of endogenous vasodilator mechanisms, proinflammatory responses induced by mechanical stretching and secretion of cytokines, upregulated expression of endothelial adhesion molecules, and release of local vasoconstrictors such as endothelin-1 are likely involved.
- Local inflammation leading to additive loss of endothelial function ultimately may trigger increases in endothelial permeability, inhibit local endothelial fibrinolytic activity, and activate the coagulation cascade.
- Platelet aggregation and degranulation on damaged endothelium may promote further inflammation, thrombosis, and vasoconstriction leading to end-organ damage of the renal, cardiovascular, and central nervous systems.

CLINICAL PRESENTATION, DIFFERENTIAL, MAKING THE DIAGNOSIS

- Severe asymptomatic HTN is defined as systolic blood pressure > 180 mm Hg or diastolic blood pressure > 110 mm Hg. These levels do not apply to pregnant patients. Severe HTN may be incidentally noted when patients are hospitalized for unrelated complaints.
- Patients presenting with hypertensive urgency have symptoms associated with severe HTN. Common signs and symptoms of hypertensive urgency include headache (22%), epistaxis (17%), and chest pain, dyspnea, dizziness, and psychomotor agitation (each ~10%). Previously unrecognized hypertension, monotherapy, noncompliance with prescribed regimens, or running out of antihypertensive medications may lead to hypertensive urgency.
- Patients with hypertensive emergency may have blood pressure that is extremely high (> 220/140 mm Hg), or < 180/110 mm Hg but with signs and symptoms of impending end-organ damage. The most common presenting symptoms are chest pain (27%), dyspnea (22%) and neurological deficits (21%).
  - Although the blood pressure level is not considered a criterion for the diagnosis of a hypertensive emergency, nonpregnant patients usually present with diastolic blood pressure exceeding 120 mm Hg.
  - The most prevalent associated complications include acute congestive heart failure (CHF) with pulmonary edema, cerebral infarction, hypertensive encephalopathy, acute myocardial infarction (MI) or unstable angina, intracerebral or subarachnoid hemorrhage, eclampsia, and aortic dissection.
- Initial assessment should address the duration as well as the severity of hypertension, adherence to current antihypertensive therapy, review of all current medications including prescription and nonprescription drugs such as sympathomimetic agents or the use of illicit drugs such as cocaine. Revealing a history of prior cerebrovascular, cardiovascular, or renal disease and direct questioning regarding current neurological, cardiovascular, or renal symptoms such as headache, blurred vision, seizures, chest pain, dyspnea, back pain, confusion, and edema are essential to the initial evaluation.
- The physical examination should begin with an assessment of blood pressure, with an appropriate-size cuff, in both upper extremities and in a lower extremity if peripheral pulses are markedly reduced. Brachial, femoral, and carotid pulses should be assessed. Aortic dissection may result in arterial compromise manifested by pulse deficits that may cause cerebral, limb, or gut ischemia. Blood pressure should be measured while the patient is both supine and standing to detect volume depletion due to pressure-induced natriuresis.
  - A cardiovascular examination should concentrate on evidence of heart failure (crackles, elevated jugular venous pressure, third heart sound or gallop). A new or increased regurgitant murmur may be heard as a result of an increase in left ventricular afterload.
  - A neurological examination should look for signs of hypertensive encephalopathy that include disorientation, a depressed level of consciousness, focal neurological deficits, and seizure activity. Because hypertensive encephalopathy is a diagnosis of exclusion, other causes of impending or ongoing neurologic compromise, such as stroke or subarachnoid hemorrhage, should be eliminated from the differential diagnosis by appropriate imaging.
  - The clinician should perform a funduscopic examination. The ophthalmoscopic classification of hypertension (Keith-Wagener-Barker) identifies four groups of changes graded according to the presence of sclerosis, general spasm, and focal spasm and whether hemorrhages, exudates, and papilledema are present. They are as follows:
    - *Group one:* Narrow arterioles compared to normal with minimal spasm
    - *Group two:* More pronounced spasm, arteriovenous nicking with bulging of some veins where arteries cross over and some sclerosis of the arteries referred to as a "copper wire" effect
    - *Group three:* Spasm, nicking, sclerosis, and evidence of hemorrhaging and exudates, with less definition of the optic disc
    - *Group four:* Group three findings plus the presence of papilledema
- Expeditious initial laboratory studies should include
  - A urinalysis with microscopic examination for proteinuria, hematuria, or red cell casts, suggesting renal parenchyma disease
  - A complete blood cell count with peripheral smear to detect schistocytes due to microangiopathic hemolytic anemia
  - A chemistry panel looking for electrolyte abnormalities and renal failure
  - An electrocardiogram (ECG) to look for myocardial ischemia and/or left ventricular hypertrophy
  - A chest radiograph for evidence of pulmonary edema or the presence of a widened mediastinum
  - Pregnancy test in females of child-bearing age
  - Toxicology screen in suspected cases of substance abuse

TABLE 32-3 Identifiable Causes of Hypertension

Sleep apnea
Drug-induced or drug-related
Chronic kidney disease
Primary aldosteronism
Renovascular disease
Chronic steroid therapy and Cushing syndrome
Pheochromocytoma
Coarctation of the aorta
Thyroid or parathyroid disease

SOURCE: From National Institutes of Health; National Heart, Lung, and Blood Institute; National High Blood Pressure Education Program. *The Seventh Report of the Joint National Committee on Prevention, Detection, Evaluation, and Treatment of High Blood Pressure.* Rockville, MD: National Institutes of Health; August 2004. NIH Publication No. 04-5230.

- Additional imaging looking for target end-organ damage may include
  - Chest computed tomography (CT) scan, transesophageal echo, or aortic angiogram—indicated for clinical suspicion of aortic dissection
  - Head CT scan when the clinical examination suggests altered mental status or focal findings suggesting cerebrovascular ischemia or hemorrhage.
- It is important to screen secondary causes of hypertension that may have precipitated the crisis. (See Chap. 33 and Table 32-3.)

TRIAGE AND INITIAL MANAGEMENT

- Asymptomatic patients with markedly elevated blood pressure but without acute target-organ damage may not require hospitalization, unless they are pregnant. They should receive immediate combination oral antihypertensive therapy, and close outpatient follow-up should be scheduled within a few days.
- Patients with severe hypertension or hypertensive urgency may be observed for several hours in ED during which time their antihypertensive therapy can be adjusted or resumed, if previously discontinued. Inability to comply with instructions or inability to obtain medication is an indication for hospitalization.
  - Some patients may benefit from treatment with an oral, short-acting agent such as captopril, labetalol, or clonidine followed by several hours of observation.
  - However, there is no evidence to suggest that failure to aggressively lower blood pressure in the emergency room is associated with any increased short-term risk to the patient who presents with severe hypertension.
  - If previously untreated, an oral regimen can be initiated.
  - Most importantly, patients should not leave the emergency room without a confirmed follow-up visit with their primary provider the next day.

- Patients with marked blood pressure elevations and acute target-organ damage require hospitalization. For example, indications for immediate hospitalization include grade III or IV fundoscopic findings, encephalopathy, MI, unstable angina, pulmonary edema, eclampsia, stroke, life-threatening arterial bleeding, aortic dissection, renal failure, or pregnancy.
- Patients with a hypertensive emergency should be admitted to an intensive care unit (ICU) or step-down/intermediate care unit for continuous monitoring of blood pressure and parenteral administration of an appropriate parenteral agent (Table 32-4).
- The initial goal of therapy in hypertensive emergencies is to reduce mean arterial blood pressure by no more than 25% (within minutes to 1 hour), then, if stable, to 160/100 to 110 mm Hg within the next 2–6 hours. If this level of blood pressure is well tolerated and the patient is clinically stable, further gradual reductions toward a normal blood pressure can be implemented in the next 24–48 hours.
  - Excessive reduction in blood pressure that may precipitate renal, cerebral, or coronary ischemia should be avoided. Short-acting agents administered intravenously are preferred.
- There are exceptions to the above recommendations.
  - Patients with an ischemic stroke in which there is no clear evidence from clinical trials to support the use of immediate antihypertensive treatment unless thrombolysis is required or hemorrhage is present. See Chap. 63.
  - The following drugs should be avoided in acute stroke:
    - Nifedipine which can cause the blood pressure to suddenly drop
    - Hydralazine and nitrates as potent, sometimes unpredictable, vasodilators which may also adversely affect cerebral autoregulation
    - Clonidine which may cause excessive sedation through a central mechanism
  - Patients with aortic dissection who should have their systolic blood pressure lowered to < 100 mm Hg if tolerated
- The therapeutic approach is dictated by the particular presentation and end-organ complications. Parenteral strategies include use of sodium nitroprusside, beta-blockers, labetalol, or calcium channel antagonists, magnesium for preeclampsia and eclampsia; and short-term parenteral anticonvulsants for seizures associated with encephalopathy. Novel therapies include the peripheral dopamine-receptor agonist, fenoldopam, and may include endothelin-1 antagonists.
- Clinical practices for the management of hypertensive urgencies and emergencies vary considerably in part because of the lack of evidence supporting the use of one therapeutic agent over another.

TABLE 32-4   Parenteral Drugs for Treatment of Hypertensive Emergencies

DRUG	DOSE*	ONSET OF ACTION	DURATION OF ACTION	ADVERSE EFFECTS†	SPECIAL INDICATIONS
VASODILATORS					
Sodium nitroprusside	0.25–10 μg/kg/min as IV infusion‡	Immediate	1–2 min	Nausea, vomiting, muscle twitching, sweating, thiocyanate and cyanide intoxication	Most hypertensive emergencies; caution with high intracranial pressure or azotemia
Nicardipine HCl	5–15 mg/h IV	5–10 min	15–30 min, may exceed 4 h	Tachycardia, headache, flushing, local phlebitis	Most hypertensive emergencies except acute heart failure; caution with coronary ischemia
Fenoldopam mesylate	0.1–0.3 μg/kg/min IV infusion	< 5 min	30 min	Tachycardia, headache, nausea, flushing	Most hypertensive emergencies; caution with glaucoma
Nitroglycerin	5–100 μg/min as IV infusion‡	2–5 min	5–10 min	Headache, vomiting, methemoglobinemia, tolerance with prolonged use	Coronary ischemia
Enalapril	1.25–5 mg every 6 h IV	15–30 min	6–12 h	Precipitous fall in pressure in high-renin states; variable response	Acute left ventricular failure; avoid in acute myocardial infarction
Hydralazine HCl	10–20 mg IV 10–40 mg IM	10–20 min IV 20–30 min IM	1–4 h IV 4–6 h IM	Tachycardia, flushing, headache, vomiting, aggravation of angina	Eclampsia
ADRENERGIC INHIBITORS					
Labetalol HCl	20–80 mg IV bolus every 10 min 0.5–2.0 mg/min IV infusion	5–10 min	3–6 h	Vomiting, scalp tingling, dizziness, nausea, heart block, orthostatic hypotension, bronchoconstriction	Most hypertensive emergencies except acute heart failure
Esmolol HCl	250–500 μg/kg/min IV bolus, then 50–100 μg/kg/min by infusion; may repeat bolus after 5 min or increase infusion to 300 μg/min	1–2 min	10–30 min	Hypotension, nausea, asthma, first-degree heart block, heart failure	Aortic dissection, perioperative
Phentolamine	5–15 mg IV bolus	1–2 min	10–30 min	Tachycardia, flushing, headache	Catecholamine excess

Abbreviations: IM, intramuscular; IV, intravenous.
*These doses may vary from those in the Physicians' Desk Reference (51st ed.).
†Hypotension may occur with all agents.
‡Require special delivery system.
Source: From National Institutes of Health; National Heart, Lung, and Blood Institute; National High Blood Pressure Education Program. *The Seventh Report of the Joint National Committee on Prevention, Detection, Evaluation, and Treatment of High Blood Pressure.* Rockville, MD: National Institutes of Health; August 2004. NIH Publication No. 04-5230.

- In *hypertensive urgencies and emergencies of pregnancy*, end-organ damage to both mother and fetus must be considered. Maternal risks are hypertensive encephalopathy and stroke, while the fetus may suffer acute fetal distress or placental abruption.
  - HTN in pregnancy is classified into one of five categories (Table 32-5).
  - For pregnant women with target-organ damage or significant preexisting chronic HTN, antihypertensive medication should be administered with a target of maintaining blood pressures below 150–160 mm Hg systolic or 100–110 mm Hg diastolic.
    - Treatment of chronic HTN in pregnancy reduces maternal risk but does not affect perinatal outcomes.
    - The selection of antihypertensive medication should be based on safety to the fetus. Oral methyldopa and labetalol are preferred.
    - Angiotensin-converting enzyme (ACE) inhibitors and angiotensin II receptor antagonists are contraindicated in pregnancy.

TABLE 32-5 Classification of Hypertension in Pregnancy

Chronic hypertension
- BP > 140 mm Hg systolic or 90 mm Hg diastolic prior to pregnancy or before 20 weeks gestation
- Persists >12 weeks postpartum

Preeclampsia
- BP > 140 mm Hg systolic or 90 mm Hg diastolic with proteinuria (> 300 mg/24 h) after 20 weeks gestation
- Can progress to eclampsia (seizures)
- More common in nulliparous women, multiple gestation, women with hypertension for > 4 years, family history of preeclampsia, hypertension in previous pregnancy, renal disease

Chronic hypertension with superimposed preeclampsia
- New-onset proteinuria after 20 weeks in a woman with hypertension
- In a woman with hypertension and proteinuria prior to 20 weeks gestation
  - Sudden two- to threefold increase in proteinuria
  - Sudden increase in BP
  - Thrombocytopenia
  - Elevated AST or ALT

Gestational hypertension
- Hypertension without proteinuria occurring after 20 weeks gestation
- Temporary diagnosis
- May represent preproteinuric phase of preeclampsia or recurrence of chronic hypertension abated in mid pregnancy
- May evolve to preeclampsia
- If severe, may result in higher rates of premature delivery and growth retardation than mild preeclampsia

Transient hypertension
- Retrospective diagnosis
- BP normal by 12 weeks postpartum
- May recur in subsequent pregnancies
- Predictive of future primary hypertension

Abbreviations: ALT, alanine aminotransferase; AST, aspartate aminotransaminase; BP, blood pressure.
SOURCE: From National Institutes of Health; National Heart, Lung, and Blood Institute; National High Blood Pressure Education Program. *The Seventh Report of the Joint National Committee on Prevention, Detection, Evaluation, and Treatment of High Blood Pressure.* Rockville, MD: National Institutes of Health; August 2004. NIH Publication No. 04-5230.

○ Treatment of preeclampsia (new onset of HTN and proteinuria at > 20 weeks gestation) includes hospitalization for bed rest, blood pressure control, seizure prophylaxis, and timely delivery. Preeclampsia may be mild or severe. Symptoms and signs include one or more of the following:
  ▪ Blurred vision, scotomata, headache, hypertensive encephalopathy, stroke
  ▪ Hepatic symptoms such as right upper quadrant (RUQ) pain, nausea/vomiting; transaminase elevations
  ▪ Severe HTN
  ▪ Thrombocytopenia
  ▪ Renal signs including nephrotic range proteinuria or oliguria
  ▪ Pulmonary edema
  ▪ Fetal growth restriction
○ Antihypertensive therapy does not prevent progression to eclampsia. Treatment is similar to that of hypertension in pregnancy. Magnesium sulfate is used to prevent progression from preeclampsia to eclampsia.
○ HELLP syndrome (hemolysis with a microangiopathic blood smear, elevated liver enzymes, and a low platelet count) may be a severe form of preeclampsia, although in 15% of cases there is no HTN or proteinuria.

▪ HELLP typically presents in the third trimester, but may occur postpartum or in the second trimester, with epigastric/RUQ pain, nausea, and vomiting being the most common symptoms.
▪ Diagnosis is based on the presence of laboratory abnormalities as follows: schistocytes on peripheral smear consistent with microangiopathic hemolytic anemia and a platelet count below 100,000; low serum haptoglobin; abnormal liver function tests including elevated indirect bilirubin and lactate dehydrogenase (LDH) (due to hemolysis) and mildly elevated aspartate aminotransferase (AST).
▪ Differential diagnosis includes fatty liver of pregnancy, hemolytic-uremic syndrome (HUS) and thrombotic thrombocytopenic purpura (TTP), viral hepatitis, gastroenteritis, and gallbladder disease.
▪ Clues to the diagnosis of fatty liver of pregnancy include an elevated prothrombin time (PT), partial thromboplastin time (PTT), creatinine, and low glucose.
▪ Acute renal failure, neurologic symptoms and fever suggest HUS and TTP.
▪ Treatment is delivery of the fetus, although in milder cases particularly at gestational ages < 34 weeks, supportive care similar to that in preeclampsia with

TABLE 32-6   Treatment of Acute Severe Hypertension in Preeclampsia

Hydralazine
- 5 mg IV bolus, then 10 mg every 20–30 min to a maximum of 25 mg, repeat in several hours as necessary

Labetalol (second-line)
- 20 mg IV bolus, then 40 mg 10 min later, 80 mg every 10 min for two additional doses to a maximum of 220 mg

Nifedipine (controversial)
- 10 mg po, repeat every 20 min to a maximum of 30 mg
- Caution when using nifedipine with magnesium sulfate, can see precipitous blood pressure drop
- Short-acting nifedipine is not approved by the Food and Drug Administration for managing hypertension

Sodium nitroprusside (rarely, when others fail)
- 0.25 ug/kg/min to a maximum of 5 ug/kg/min
- Fetal cyanide poisoning may occur if used for more than 4 h

SOURCE: From National Institutes of Health; National Heart, Lung, and Blood Institute; National High Blood Pressure Education Program. *The Seventh Report of the Joint National Committee on Prevention, Detection, Evaluation, and Treatment of High Blood Pressure*. Rockville, MD: National Institutes of Health; August 2004. NIH Publication No. 04-5230.

administration of corticosteroids to promote fetal lung maturation may be considered in consultation with a maternal–fetal medicine expert.
- Treatment for eclampsia (grand mal seizures) is the delivery of the fetus (Table 32-6).

DISEASE MANAGEMENT STRATEGIES

- Hospitalists are frequently asked to assist with ED throughput and critical care resource utilization and should be aware that most patients seen in the ED with severe hypertension do not meet the criteria for hypertensive emergency and do not require admission to the hospital for blood pressure control. However, true hypertensive emergencies require rapid intervention, diagnosis, and treatment in the intensive or intermediate care unit (depending on unit capabilities).
- Hospitalists may design algorithms for use in the ED to assist with initial triage and thus limit unnecessary admissions.
- Standardized order sets based on clinical guidelines are effective for the management of patients with hypertension associated with stroke, acute congestive heart failure (CHF), and acute MI. Care pathways may be developed to assist in compliance with Joint Commission for Accreditation of Healthcare Organization (JCAHO) core measures for these disease states.
- Hospitalists and pharmacists may play a key role in patient education prior to discharge from the hospital or ED. Patients presenting with uncontrolled hypertension in the ED may benefit most when education about their disease is reinforced.

- Hospitalists may recognize patients with refractory HTN or secondary HTN and make the appropriate referral to hypertensive specialists, endocrinologists, or surgeons.

CARE TRANSITIONS

- Patients presenting with uncontrolled HTN or hypertensive urgency, when clinically stable, may safely be sent home with oral agents and arrangements for close outpatient follow-up. Blood pressure may remain elevated at discharge as long as the patient is asymptomatic.
- Patients with hypertensive emergency generally require treatment for 24–48 hours in order to normalize blood pressure. Possible causes of the hypertensive emergency should be sought and complications treated prior to discharge.
- An appropriate antihypertensive medication regimen should be started and the patient should be educated about adherence and the signs and symptoms of related complications such as heart failure and stroke.
- Outpatient follow-up with the patient's primary care physician (PCP) should be arranged within 1–3 days. Communication with the patient's PCP should occur at the time of discharge if possible, and prior to the scheduled follow-up appointment. To ensure appropriate follow-up, the PCP must receive
  - A reconciled admission and discharge medication list, reflecting any changes in antihypertensive therapy
  - Results of any diagnostic testing

BIBLIOGRAPHY

Bales A. Hypertensive crisis: how to tell if it's an emergency or an urgency. *Postgrad Med.* 1999;105(5):119–126.

Bender SR, Fong MW, Heitz S, et al. Characteristics and management of patients presenting to the emergency department with hypertensive urgency. *J Clin Hypertens (Greenwich).* 2006 Jan;8(1):12–18.

Black HR, Elliott WJ, Neaton JD, et al. Baseline characteristics and elderly blood pressure control in the CONVINCE trial. *Hypertension.* 2001;37:12–18.

Cherney D, Straus S. Management of patients with hypertensive urgencies and emergencies: a systematic review of the literature. *J Gen Intern Med.* 2002;17:937–945.

Chobanian AV, Bakris GL, Black HR, et al. The seventh report of the Joint National Committee on Prevention, Detection, Evaluation, and Treatment of High Blood Pressure: The JNC 7 Report. *JAMA.* 2003;289:2560–2571.

Cushman WC, Ford CE, Cutler JA, et al. Success and predictors of blood pressure control in diverse North American settings: The antihypertensive and lipid-lowering treatment to prevent heart attack trial (ALLHAT). *J Clin Hypertens* (Greenwich). 2002;4:393–404.

National Institutes of Health; National Heart, Lung, and Blood Institute; National High Blood Pressure Education Program. *The Seventh Report of the Joint National Committee on Prevention, Detection, Evaluation, and Treatment of High Blood Pressure.* Rockville, MD: National Institutes of Health; August 2004. NIH Publication No. 04–5230.

Vaughan CJ, Delanty N. Hypertensive emergencies. *Lancet.* 2000;356(9227):411–417.

Vidt DG. Hypertensive crises: emergencies and urgencies. *J Clin Hypertens (Greenwich).* 2004 Sep;6(9):520–525.

Zampaglione B, Pascale C, Marchisio M, Cavallo-Perin P, et al. Hypertensive urgencies and emergencies. Prevalence and clinical presentation. *Hypertension.* 1996;27:144–147.

33 SECONDARY HYPERTENSION

Renee Y. Meadows

EPIDEMIOLOGY/OVERVIEW

- Secondary hypertension (HTN) is high blood pressure caused by an identifiable disorder. Treatment of the primary disorder may lead to partial or complete normalization of the blood pressure.
- Approximately 10% of hypertensive patients have secondary hypertension. The etiologies of secondary hypertension (Table 33-1) may be grouped into four broad categories: renal, renovascular, endocrine, and miscellaneous disorders.

- Secondary hypertension should be suspected in patients with refractory hypertension or if the history, clinical, and routine laboratory evaluations strongly suggest an identifiable secondary cause (early or late age of onset, vascular bruits, symptoms of catecholamine excess, unprovoked hypokalemia, or as a complication of pregnancy).
- Patients with secondary hypertension may present to the emergency department (ED) with hypertensive urgency or emergency or with other symptoms associated with their underlying condition (see Chap. 32). Secondary hypertension may be suspected by history or associated symptoms.
  - Patients with renovascular disease, pheochromocytoma, or drug-induced HTN are more likely to develop an unexpected hypertensive emergency.
  - Patients with renal parenchymal disease may develop acute on chronic kidney failure and volume overload requiring hemodialysis.
  - Patients with primary aldosteronism may present with weakness and hypokalemia rather than hypertensive crisis.
  - The symptoms associated with thyroid dysfunction or sleep apnea are more likely to prompt a patient to seek urgent medical attention than those of the HTN alone.
- Because the etiology of secondary HTN is diverse, routine screening of hypertensive patients for all causes is not economically feasible. Hospitalists should be aware of the diagnostic clues associated with the variety of causes of secondary HTN and cost-effective screening and treatment.

ETIOLOGIES OF SECONDARY HYPERTENSION

- Most patients with high blood pressure have essential HTN; however, in those with signs and symptoms suggestive of underlying conditions associated with HTN, an evaluation should be performed to rule out secondary HTN (Table 33-2).
- In general, secondary HTN may be suggested by
  - An acute rise in blood pressure over a previously stable baseline in a patient with preexisting essential hypertension
  - Negative family history for HTN
  - Severe, refractory/resistant, or malignant HTN
  - Age of onset prior to puberty or after age 55, or prior to age 30 in the absence of obesity or alcoholism or family history of HTN
- Because obesity and drugs (particularly alcohol abuse) are among the most common, potentially correctable

TABLE 33-1   Causes of Secondary Hypertension

Renovascular
 Renal artery atherosclerotic stenosis
 Fibromuscular dysplasia

Renal disease
 Chronic kidney disease
 Polycystic kidney disease
 Diabetic nephropathy
 Glomerulonephritis
 Tumors of the kidney

Endocrine
 Pheochromocytoma
 Primary hyperaldosteronism
 Cushing syndrome
 Hyperparathyroidism
 Acromegaly
 Thyroid dysfunction
 Hypercalcemia

Other
 Obesity
 Coarctation of the aorta
 Obstructive sleep apnea
 Pregnancy
 Increased intracranial pressure or intracranial hemorrhage
 Drugs (alcohol, oral contraceptives, cyclosporine, tacrolimus, decongestants, NSAIDs, erythropoietin)

causes of secondary HTN, they should be considered during the initial evaluation of patients with newly diagnosed HTN as well as patients with suspected secondary HTN.

- Renovascular HTN is the next most common, potentially correctable cause of secondary HTN.
  ○ Ten percent to forty-five percent of patients presenting with malignant hypertension have renovascular HTN.
- Once obesity, alcohol, and renovascular causes of secondary hypertension have been considered, the features of other causes of secondary HTN should be considered and appropriate screening tests performed (Table 33-2).
  ○ Renal causes of secondary HTN should be considered next.
  ○ Primary aldosteronism is the most common endocrine cause of secondary HTN. Once thought to be rare, the use of a simple and readily available screening test has increased the prevalence of primary aldosteronism to as high as 10% of hypertensive patients and as high as 40% in patients with resistant HTN.
  Obesity: Obesity is defined as a body mass index (BMI) over 30, although a BMI of 26–30 is considered to be significantly overweight.
- Body mass index charts are readily available.
- To calculate BMI

$$\text{(weight in pounds} \times 703) \div \text{(height in inches} \times \text{height in inches)}$$

- Weight loss and improved physical fitness that decreases the BMI by even a few points will help control obesity-related hypertension.
- The etiology of HTN in individuals with *obstructive sleep apnea (OSA)* is believed to involve both the obesity-HTN link and an independent role of OSA in HTN. Repeated periods of apnea-induced hypoxia and hypercapnea stimulate strong sympathetic nervous system discharges that directly elevate blood pressure. Stress from sleep deprivation alone may also raise blood pressure.
  ○ Patients are typically obese, snore, and may report excessive daytime fatigue.
  ○ HTN associated with obstructive sleep apnea improves with continuous positive airway pressure (CPAP), improvement of sleep quality, and weight loss.
  ○ No specific class of antihypertensive medication has been shown to be superior for blood pressure reduction in patients with OSA.
  Drugs: A number of drugs and substances may cause hypertension (see Table 33-3). Excessive ethanol consumption is of particular importance as one of the leading correctible causes of HTN.
- Alcohol abuse is covered in Chap. 70. Abstinence from alcohol will improve HTN in patients with alcohol-related HTN.

RENOVASCULAR HYPERTENSION

- Renovascular HTN is typically associated with
  ○ Fibromuscular dysplasia of the mid or distal portions of the renal arteries and branches in younger patients
  ○ Atherosclerotic stenosis of the proximal renal artery in patients over the age of 50
- Reduction of renal blood flow and perfusion pressure stimulates renin production giving rise to the actions of angiotensin and aldosterone causing sodium and water retention, increased blood volume, vasoconstriction, and increased cardiac output.
  ○ Unilateral renal artery stenosis leads to underperfusion of the juxtaglomerular cells, thereby producing renin-dependent hypertension. Unilateral renal artery stenosis may lead to nephrosclerosis in the nonischemic kidney.
  ○ HTN due to bilateral renal artery stenosis is a potentially reversible cause of progressive ischemic nephropathy that is mediated by multiple effector mechanisms, including the renin-angiotensin system, sympathetic nervous pathways, and alteration of the balance among nitric oxide, eicosanoids, and other vasoactive systems. If left untreated, bilateral renal

TABLE 33-2 Clinical Features and Recommended Testing in Secondary Hypertension

DISEASE	FEATURES	RECOMMENDED TEST/REFERRAL
Renovascular disease: atherosclerotic renal artery stenosis, renal fibromuscular disease	Systolic-diastolic abdominal bruits over the renal arteries Abrupt onset of severe hypertension Diastolic blood pressure ≥115 mm Hg Initial onset before age 30 or after age 50 Resistant hypertension Evidence of systemic atherosclerotic vascular disease or malignant hypertension Recurrent unexplained episodes of flash pulmonary edema Elevation of serum creatinine after initiation of ACE inhibitor or ARB	There are a variety of screening tests for renovascular hypertension, depending on equipment and expertise in institutions. Magnetic resonance angiography (MRA) and renal artery duplex ultrasonography are used. Spiral CT angiography or post-captopril renograms may be used if MRA is contraindicated and renal function is normal. However, there is no single best test for renovascular hypertension, and consultation with experts in your institution is recommended. Renal angiography is the gold standard but is not used for initial diagnosis due to risk of contrast nephropathy. Intravenous pyelogram is relatively contraindicated in diabetes and no longer recommended as screening test for renovascular disease.
Kidney disease: chronic glomerulonephritis, polycystic kidney disease, and hypertensive nephrosclerosis	Abnormal urine sediment Elevated serum creatinine Hematuria on two occasions or structural renal abnormality Proteinuria	Urinalysis; estimation of urinary protein excretion and creatinine clearance by using a single random urine test; renal ultrasound Consider referral to nephrology
Primary hyperaldosteronism	Unexplained hypokalemia Muscle cramps Polyuria Weakness	Plasma aldosterone and plasma renin activity 24-hour urinary aldosterone level on a high sodium diet or IV salt load test
Pheochromocytoma	Labile blood pressure Orthostatic hypotension Triad of headaches, palpitations, and sweating Tachycardia	Plasma free metanephrine and normetanephrine, 24-hour urine for metanephrines, catecholamines Consider referral to specialist
Cushing syndrome and other glucocorticoid excess states including chronic steroid therapy	Amenorrhea Increased dorsal fat Diabetes mellitus Edema Hirsutism Moon facies Purple striae Truncal obesity	History 24-hour urine for free cortisol Dexamethasone suppression test
Hyperparathyroidism	Hypercalcemia Polyuria/polydipsia Renal stones	Serum calcium and parathyroid hormone level
Hyperthyroidism	Anxiety Brisk reflexes Hyperdefecation Heat intolerance Tachycardia Tremor Weight loss Wide pulse pressure	Thyroid-stimulating hormone Free T4
Hypothyroidism	Fatigue Weight gain Hair loss Cold intolerance	Thyroid stimulating hormone Free T4
Sleep apnea	Daytime somnolence Fatigue Obesity Snoring or observed apneic episodes	Referral for sleep study
Aortic coarctation	Weak or delayed femoral pulses	Computerized tomography angiography
Drug or substance induced	Acute onset Hypertension with tachycardia	History Urine toxicology as indicated

SOURCE: Adapted from Veterans Administration, Dept of Defense. VA/DoD clinical practice guideline for diagnosis and management of hypertension in the primary care setting. Washington DC: Veterans Administration, Dept of Defense; August 2004: 99. and National Institutes of Health; National Heart, Lung, and Blood Institute; National High Blood Pressure Education Program. *The Seventh Report of the Joint National Committee on Prevention, Detection, Evaluation, and Treatment of High Blood Pressure.* Rockville, MD: National Institutes of Health; August 2004. NIH Publication No. 04-5230.

TABLE 33-3   Common Substances Associated with Hypertension in Humans

Prescription drugs
Cortisone and other steroids: mineralo- and gluco corticosteroids, adrenocorticotropic hormone
Estrogens: oral contraceptive agents with high estrogenic activity
Nonsteroidal anti-inflammatory drugs
Phenylpropanolamines and analogues
Cyclosporine and tacrolimus
Erythropoietin
Sibutramine
Ketamine
Desflurane
Carbamazepine
Bromocryptine
Metoclopramide
Antidepressants: especially venlafaxine
Buspirone
Clonidine and beta-blocker combination
Clozapine

Street drugs and "natural products"
Cocaine and cocaine withdrawal
Ma Huang, "herbal ecstasy," and other phenylpropanolamine analogues
Nicotine and nicotine withdrawal
Anabolic steroids
Narcotic withdrawal
Methylphenidate
Phencyclidine
Ketamine
Ergotamine and other ergot-containing herbal preparations
St. John's wort

Food substances
Sodium chloride
Ethanol
Licorice
Tyramine-containing foods (with monoamine oxidase inhibitor [MAOI])
Chemical elements and other industrial chemicals
Lead
Mercury
Thallium and other heavy metals
Lithium salts, especially the chloride salt

SOURCE: From National Institutes of Health; National Heart, Lung, and Blood Institute; National High Blood Pressure Education Program. *The Seventh Report of the Joint National Committee on Prevention, Detection, Evaluation, and Treatment of High Blood Pressure.* Rockville, MD: National Institutes of Health; August 2004. NIH Publication No. 04-5230.

artery stenosis can decrease renal perfusion which can progress to end-stage renal disease.
• Renovascular HTN is suggested by the following features:
  ○ Onset of hypertension before puberty or age 30, especially in white females, (fibromuscular dysplasia) or proven onset after age 50 (atherosclerotic stenosis)
  ○ Presence of symptoms associated with systemic atherosclerotic disease such as angina, claudication, or transient ischemic attacks
  ○ Moderate to severe HTN in patients with recurrent episodes of acute dyspnea, flash pulmonary edema, or otherwise unexplained congestive heart failure

  ○ Abdominal bruits or aortic aneurysm
  ○ Acute elevation in serum creatinine level that occurs after the initiation of therapy with an angiotensin-converting enzyme (ACE) inhibitor or angiotensin II receptor blocker (ARB) without significant reduction in blood pressure.
• Radiographic testing for renovascular disease is indicated only when the history is suggestive and a corrective procedure will be performed if significant renal artery stenosis is identified. The recommended tests will vary based upon renal function and clinical suspicion.
  ○ Captopril-enhanced radionuclide renal scan, duplex Doppler flow studies, and magnetic resonance angiography (MRA) may be used as noninvasive screening tests.
  ○ MRA may provide the best sensitivity and specificity.
  ○ Three-dimensional spiral computed tomography (CT) angiography may be as useful but carries the risk of contrast nephropathy.
  ○ Renal angiography is the gold standard for definitive diagnosis and permits concurrent revascularization.
• Management of renovascular hypertension includes medical, percutaneous interventional, and surgical therapies.
  ○ The current treatment of choice for eligible patients is percutaneous transluminal renal angioplasty (PTRA) with secondary stenting. There are ongoing randomized controlled trials comparing medical versus interventional therapy.
    ▪ Patients with atheromatous renal artery stenosis associated with aortic aneurysms and atheromatous disease require surgical revascularization and aortic reconstruction.
  ○ In patients with fibromuscular dysplasia, PTRA alone is the treatment of choice.
  ○ Anticipated outcomes following revascularization include improved blood pressure control and preservation of renal function.
  ○ Medical management is utilized for patients who are not candidates for interventional or surgical therapies due to the location of stenosis or presence of advanced loss of renal function, although medical therapy does not relieve the renal ischemia.
    ▪ Therapeutic options are the same as those for essential hypertension with the exception that ACE inhibitors and ARBs should be avoided when bilateral renal artery stenosis is present or suspected.

RENAL PARENCHYMAL DISEASE

• In secondary HTN due to renal disease, perfusion of renal tissue is decreased due to inflammatory and fibrotic changes in multiple small intrarenal vessels. There is usually increased intravascular volume and/or increased renin-angiotensin activity. Expanded plasma volume is associated with peripheral vasoconstriction caused by both activation of vasoconstrictor pathways (renin-angiotensin and sympathetic nervous systems) and inhibition of vasodilator pathways (prostaglandins, nitric oxide). Cardiac output is usually normal.

- Patients with glomerular diseases such as glomerulonephritis or polycystic kidney disease tend to have sodium retention and fluid overload.
- In diabetic nephropathy, this volume expansion may be accompanied by increased activity of the renin-angiotensin system due to regional ischemia or intraglomerular HTN.
- The most common are chronic glomerulonephritis, polycystic kidney disease, and hypertensive nephrosclerosis which are usually accompanied by a reduction in glomerular filtration rate and/or an active urine sediment.

• HTN due to renal disease is suggested by elevation in the serum creatinine and/or abnormal urinalysis.
- Random urine for microalbumin to creatinine ratio above 30 mg/g suggests underlying renal disease, often due to diabetes, and is associated with cardiovascular disease even in the absence of diabetes.

• Treatment for secondary HTN due to renal parenchymal disease includes dietary sodium and fluid restriction, diuretics, and ACE inhibitors.
- The blood pressure goal is less than 130/80 mm Hg.
- ACE inhibitors reduce protienuria and progression of renal failure, particularly in diabetics; however, they may cause hyperkalemia or acute renal failure in patients with chronic kidney disease.
- Angiotensin II receptor blockers are practical in ACE inhibitor–intolerant patients.
- Hydralazine and minoxidil are effective in resistant HTN.

PRIMARY ALDOSTERONISM

• In primary hyperaldosteronism, there is increased secretion of aldosterone from an adrenal adenoma or adrenal hyperplasia. Increased circulating aldosterone causes renal retention of sodium and water, increasing blood volume and arterial pressure. Plasma renin levels are generally decreased as the body attempts to suppress the renin-angiotensin system. Hypokalemia is associated with the high levels of aldosterone.

• Primary aldosteronism is the most common endocrine cause of secondary hypertension, but the clinical presentation may be nonspecific and frequently indistinguishable from that of essential hypertension.
- Hypokalemia, once considered a prerequisite for the diagnosis, is present in only about half of cases.
- Consider screening in patients with HTN and adrenal incidentalomas (adrenal mass found incidentally on CT or MRI imaging performed for other reasons).
- The plasma aldosterone (PA)/plasma renin activity (PRA) ratio is used as a screening test.
  - Prior to testing, all potentially interfering drugs such as diuretics, ACE inhibitors, ARBs, and beta-blockers must be discontinued. Spironolactone must be stopped at least 6 weeks prior to testing.
  - Elevated PA and PRA with PA/PRA of 10 suggests secondary hyperaldosteronism (causes include renovascular HTN, diuretics, renin-secreting tumors, coarctation, malignant HTN).
  - Decreased PA and PRA suggest congenital adrenal hyperplasia, exogenous mineralocorticoids (licorice), Cushing syndrome.
  - Decreased PRA and elevated PA with PA/PRA over 20 and PA over 15 suggest primary aldosteronism.
  - However, an elevated PA/PRA alone is not diagnostic because suppression of the plasma renin activity is not unique to primary aldosteronism. Some patients have low renin, essential HTN.
- Patients with positive screening test results should undergo aldosterone suppression testing: a salt load test with measurement of PRA and collection of a 24-hour urine specimen for potassium, sodium, creatinine, and aldosterone.
- Confirmatory testing and subtyping is frequently expensive and invasive. The cost of identifying and relieving one aldosterone-producing adenoma in every 100 hypertensive patients has been estimated to be $250,000 based on figures obtained from four major US medical centers.
- The subtype evaluation of primary aldosteronism is based on adrenal imaging (CT scan) and selective adrenal venous sampling.
  - Selective adrenal venous sampling is the gold standard for the diagnosis of a lateralized aldosterone secretion, as typically observed in aldosterone-producing adenomas.

• Adrenal hyperplasia or idiopathic hyperaldosteronism can produce hormonal abnormalities similar to those found with Conn adenalomas, but is rarely cured by adrenalectomy.

• Due to the detrimental cardiovascular effects of aldosterone, normalization of blood pressure is not the only goal in patients with primary aldosteronism. Reduction of circulating aldosterone or aldosterone receptor blockade may be accomplished surgically or with medical management.

○ Unilateral laparoscopic adrenalectomy is the preferred treatment option for patients with unilateral aldosterone-producing adenoma although normalization of blood pressure may not occur.

○ Hypertension due to bilateral adrenal hyperplasia or idiopathic hyperaldosteronism is not corrected by adrenalectomy and should be treated medically.[10,13] Medical management should include an aldosterone receptor antagonist such as spironolactone.

PHEOCHROMOCYTOMA

• Pheochromocytoma is a rare adrenal neoplasm although some may be extraadrenal and up to 10% are malignant. Catecholamine secretion by these tumors can result in catecholamine excess leading to alpha-receptor-mediated systemic vasoconstriction, which increases peripheral vascular resistance, and to beta-receptor-mediated increases in cardiac output.

• The classic triad of symptoms consists of episodic headache, sweating, and tachycardia; however, not all patients will have these three classic symptoms.

○ Some patients have paroxysmal hypertension but most present with what appears to be essential hypertension.

○ Because of the low prevalence, screening should be selective but would include patients with paroxysmal hypertension, an adrenal mass, orthostatic hypotension, or familial history of pheochromocytoma.

• The treatment for pheochromocytoma is adrenalectomy or removal of extraadrenal pheochromocytoma after localization of the functional tumor by CT or MRI. Laparoscopic adrenalectomy is preferred for small solitary intra adrenal pheochromocytomas.

○ Generally, preoperative alpha-blockade for blood pressure control is started 1–2 weeks prior to surgery.

○ Alpha-blockers may be followed by beta-blockers for control of tachycardia several days before surgery.

○ Patients may develop hypertensive emergencies before or during surgery which may be treated with nitroprusside.

MISCELLANEOUS CAUSES (TABLE 33-2)

• In *Cushing syndrome*, the adrenal gland generates excessive amounts of glucocorticoids due to an adrenal tumor or as the result of corticotropin (ACTH) production by pituitary hyperplasia or ACTH-like peptide production by an undifferentiated neoplasm.

The mechanism for the hypertension associated with Cushing syndrome is not fully understood but appears to be the result of increased vasoconstriction and increased peripheral resistance, though cardiac output may also rise.

○ Suspected in patients with cushingoid facies, central obesity/buffalo hump, easy bruising, proximal muscle weakness, typically with a history of steroid use.

○ 24-hour urine cortisol is usually the first screening test. Alternatives are serum or saliva late evening cortisol levels.

• It is unclear how *hyperparathyroidism* increases blood pressure, although secondary hyperparathyroidism may increase the intracellular calcium concentration *Hypercalcemia* can lead to vasoconstriction and hypertension. In general, it raises the intracellular calcium concentration, also leading to vasoconstriction and hypertension.

• *Thyroid disease* can lead to HTN, and patients with symptoms of thyroid disease (see Chap. 37) may be screened with a serum supersensitive thyrotropin (TSH) assay.

○ *Hypothyroidism* is associated with diastolic hypertension due to decreased cardiac output and increased systemic vascular resistance although the mechanism is not fully understood.

○ *Hyperthyroidism* is associated with systolic hypertension due to amplified cardiac output and peripheral vasoconstriction.

• *Coarctation of the aorta* is a congenital defect that obstructs aortic outflow leading to elevated arterial pressures proximal to the coarctation, for example, the head and arms. Distal pressures are not necessarily reduced as might be expected because reduced systemic blood flow, specifically reduced renal blood flow, leads to an increase in the release of renin and activation of the renin-angiotensin-aldosterone system. This in turn elevates blood volume and arterial pressure.

• *Preeclampsia*, a pregnancy-specific syndrome of exaggerated vasoconstriction and reduced organ perfusion, also causes hypertension due to increased blood volume and tachycardia increasing cardiac output.

BIBLIOGRAPHY

Kaplan NM. Resistant hypertension. *J Hypertens.* 2005; 23:1441–144-4.

Kaplan NM. The current epidemic of primary aldosteronism: causes and consequences. *J Hypertens.* 2004;22:863–869.

Khosla S. Renal artery stenosis: a review of therapeutic options. *Minerva Cardioangiol.* 2005;53:79–91.

Klabunde RE. *Cardiovascular Physiology Concepts.* Philadelphia, PA: Lippincott Williams & Wilkins; 2004.

Krakoff LR. Screening for primary aldosteronism: progress and frustration. *J Hypertens.* 2006;24:635–637.

Mulatero P, Stowasser M, Loh K-C, et al. Increased diagnosis of primary aldosteronism, including surgically correctable forms, in centers from five continents. *J Clin Endocrinol Metab.* 2004;89(3):1045–1050.

National Institutes of Health; National Heart, Lung, and Blood Institute; National High Blood Pressure Education Program. *The Seventh Report of the Joint National Committee on Prevention, Detection, Evaluation, and Treatment of High Blood Pressure.* Rockville, MD: National Institutes of Health; August 2004. NIH Publication No. 04-5230.

Omura M, Saito J, Yamaguchio K, et al. Prospective study on the prevalence of secondary hypertension among hypertensive patients visiting a general outpatient clinic in Japan. *Hypertens Res.* 2004;27:193–202.

Raine AE, Bedford L, Simpson AW, et al. Hyperparathyroidism, platelet intracellular free calcium and hypertension in chronic renal failure. *Kidney Int.* 1993;43(3):700–705.

Textor SC. Revascularization in atherosclerotic renal artery disease. *Kidney International.* 1998;53:799–811.

Veglio F, Morello F, Rabbia F, et al. Recent advances in diagnosis and treatment of primary aldosteronism. *Minerva Med.* 2003;94(4):259–265.

Veterans Administration, Department of Defense. VA/DoD clinical practice guideline for diagnosis and management of hypertension in the primary care setting. Washington (DC): Veterans Administration, Department of Defense; 2004:99.

Young WF Jr. Minireview: primary aldosteronism—changing concepts in diagnosis and treatment. *Endocrinology.* 2003;144:2208.

ENDOCRINE DISORDERS

34 DIABETIC KETOACIDOSIS AND HYPEROSMOLAR HYPERGLYCEMIA

Mohammad Salameh

EPIDEMIOLOGY/OVERVIEW

- Diabetic ketoacidosis (DKA) and hyperosmolar hyperglycemic state (HHS) are potentially life-threatening complications of both type 1 and type 2 diabetes.
- More than 100,000 patients with DKA are hospitalized annually in the United States.
- The mortality rate of DKA can be as low as 5% with optimal care but the mortality rate of HHS remains around 15%.
- The presence of coma, hypotension, and old or very young age has a significantly negative impact on prognosis.
- There is emerging evidence that intensive interventions by diabetes teams may diminish excess hospital mortality for patients with diabetes who undergo surgical procedures such as coronary artery bypass graft (CABG) and for those patients with acute stroke and myocardial infarction (MI). (See Chap. 35.) Whether this is also the case for DKA and HHS is unknown.
- The effect of physician specialty can influence outcomes. For DKA, endocrinologists have been shown to have better outcomes than generalists relating to length of stay (LOS) and readmission rates. More research is needed to determine the impact of hospitalists.
- Hospitalists should play a key role in implementing inpatient diabetes protocols, including a DKA standard order set, and ensuring that inpatient management is in line with recent research in the field.

PATHOPHYSIOLOGY

- DKA and HHS are likely not separate entities, but different manifestations of the same disease process. The following is known to occur:
  - Inadequate insulin for glucose metabolism and excess amounts of glucagon, a hormone normally suppressed by insulin presence, along with the other counter-regulatory hormones (catecholamines, cortisol, and growth hormone) causes uncontrolled hyperglycemia with or without ketoacidosis.

○ These hormonal changes in DKA and HHS lead to increased hepatic and renal glucose production and impaired glucose utilization in peripheral tissues.

○ As a stress response, catecholamine and cortisol production are increased, further stimulating increasing glucose levels (and ketoacid generation in DKA).

  ▪ In DKA, ketogenesis (beta-hydroxybutyrate and acetoacetate) is promoted both by insulin absence and glucagon overproduction through lipolysis, leading to release of free fatty acids into the bloodstream and hepatic fatty acid oxidation to ketone bodies.

▪ In HHS, lower ketogenesis is likely related to sufficient small amounts of circulating insulin to prevent lipolysis and subsequent ketogenesis.

  ○ Increasing glucose levels → osmotic diuresis with renal losses of sodium and fluid → hypovolemia and increased plasma osmolality → hypotension and neurologic deterioration.

• Infection most commonly causes DKA and HHS in susceptible individuals. Other common triggers include MI, stroke, pancreatitis, trauma, and drugs such as exogenous steroid use, thiazides, and sympathomimetic agents, alcohol and drug abuse.

  ○ New onset, inadequate, or discontinued insulin therapy in type 1 diabetics may present as DKA. In some instances noncompliance can be attributed to psychological problems, especially in young patients.

  ○ Diabetic patients who are unable to take fluids and elderly patients who do not know they have diabetes may develop HHS.

CLINICAL PRESENTATION, DIFFERENTIAL, MAKING THE DIAGNOSIS

• The development of DKA typically occurs within a day whereas HHS may take several days or weeks.

  ○ Early symptoms include polyuria, polydipsia, polyphagia, nausea, vomiting, weight loss, abdominal cramping (in DKA), and generalized weakness from dehydration.

  ○ Later symptoms include confusion, visual changes, seizures, obtundation, and coma (predominantly in HHS).

• It is important to inquire about other conditions or risk factors that may be associated with acidosis such as alcoholism, starvation, ingestion of toxins such as methanol, and chronic renal failure or drugs such as metformin and aspirin.

• Vital signs are consistent with hypovolemia and metabolic acidosis, including hypotension, tachycardia, and tachypnea. Temperature may vary depending on the triggering event.

  ○ Even in the presence of infection, patients can be afebrile.

  ○ Hypothermia is a poor prognostic sign and reflects peripheral vasodilation.

• Physical examination signs may reveal decreased skin turgor, dry mucosal membranes, mental status changes, shock, coma (more often in HHS), and breath with fruity odor or Kussmaul's respirations (in DKA).

• See Table 34-1 for the diagnostic criteria for DKA and HHS.

  ○ Type 1 diabetics may have mildly elevated or even normal blood sugars and still have DKA, identified by the presence of serum ketones.

  ○ Type 2 diabetics with HHS typically have blood sugars > 600 which causes a high serum osmolality > 320 with small amounts of urine and serum ketones and an anion gap < 12.

• The hospitalist should calculate the anion gap and effective plasma osmolality.

  ○ See Table 34-2 for calculation formulas.

• The hospitalist should order the following tests in addition to checking the blood glucose and confirming the presence of serum and urinary ketones: blood urea nitrogen (BUN)/creatinine (Cr), electrolytes, osmolality, complete blood count (CBC) with differential, blood cultures, urine cultures, electrocardiogram (ECG), and chest x-ray (CXR). Additional testing depends on the clinical setting.

  ○ Although pancreatitis can precipitate hyperglycemic crisis, the majority of patients with DKA have elevated amylase levels. The lipase level can also be elevated in patients with DKA.

  ○ A drug screen may be helpful. Some intoxicants can be measured directly such as methanol, ethylene glycol, and are associated with an elevated osmolar gap.

TRIAGE AND INITIAL MANAGEMENT

• All patients with a diagnosis of DKA or HHS must be admitted to the hospital to—at—minimum a monitored bed.

• Patients with a pH < 7.20 or patients presenting with end-organ damage such as MI, sepsis syndrome, stroke, or neurologic deterioration should be admitted to an intensive care unit (ICU).

• The goals for the first day include

  ○ Stabilization of the patient

  ○ Volume repletion

  ○ Correction of metabolic disturbances

  ○ Identification of triggers

TABLE 34-1   Differentiating DKA from HHS

| | DKA | | | |
	MILD	MODERATE	SEVERE	HHS
Diagnostic criteria and classification				
Plasma glucose (mg/dL)	> 250 mg/dL	> 250 mg/dL	> 250 mg/dL	> 600 mg/dL
Arterial pH	7.25–7.30	7.00 to < 7.25	< 7.00	> 7.30
Serum bicarbonate (mEq/L)	15–18	10 to < 15	< 10	> 15
Urine ketone*	Positive	Positive	Positive	Small
Serum ketone*	Positive	Positive	Positive	Small
Effective serum osmolality†	Variable	Variable	Variable	> 320 mOsm/kg
Anion gap‡	> 10	> 12	> 12	< 12
Mental status	Alert	Alert/drowsy	Stupor/coma	Stupor/coma
Typical deficits				
Total water (L)	6			9
Water (mL/kg)§	100			100–200
Na^+ (mEq/kg)	7–10			5–13
Cl^- (mEq/kg)	3–5			5–15
K^+ (mEq/kg)	3–5			4–6
PO_4 (mmol/kg)	5–7			3–7
Mg^{2++} (mEq/kg)	1–2			1–2
Ca^{2++} (mEq/kg)	1–2			1–2

*Nitroprusside reaction method.

†Calculation of effective serum osmolality: 2[measured Na^+ (mEq/L)] + [glucose (mg/dL)]/18.

‡Calculation of anion gap: $(Na^+) - [Cl^- + HCO_3^-$ (m/Eq/L)].

§Per kg body wt.

SOURCES: Data adapted from: American Diabetes Association. Hyperglycemic crises in patients with diabetes mellitus. *Diabetes care.* January 2001;24(suppl 1); Kitabchi AE, Umpierrez GE, Murphy MB, et al. Management of hyperglycemic crises in patients with diabetes mellitus (Technical Review). *Diabetes Care.* 2001;24:131–153; Matz R. Hyperosmolar nonacidotic diabetes (HNAD). In: Porte D Jr, Sherwin RS, eds. *Diabetes Mellitus: Theory and Practice.* 5th ed. Amsterdam: Elsevier; 1997:845–850.

• The goals for subsequent days include
  ○ Optimal insulin administration and adjustment so glucose levels < 180 mg/dL. Initiation of longer-acting insulin is important to avoid the following:
    ▪ Osmotic diuresis with consequent dehydration and metabolic derangements
    ▪ Impaired white blood cell (WBC) function
    ▪ Delayed gastric emptying
    ▪ Delayed hospital discharge
  ○ Feeding (if the patient is able)
  ○ Patient and family education

TABLE 34-2   Formulas to Calculate the Anion Gap and Effective Plasma Osmolality

Anion gap (AG)

  ○ AG = Na – (Cl + HCO_3)
  ○ Normal anion gap 3–12. In DKA, AG > 10 and usually > 12 Magnitude of AG corresponds with amount of keto acids and lower pH, thus more severe acidosis and illness.

Effective Plasma Osmolality (EPO)

  ○ EPO = [2 × Na (mEq/L)] + [glucose (mg/dL) ÷ 18]
  ○ *or* EPO = Measured osmolality – [BUN (mg/dL) ÷ 28]
  ○ Higher EPO (> 320–330 mOs/kg) → greater severity of neurologic compromise. This calculation is more important in HHS than in DKA.

  ○ Treatment of triggering condition(s)
  ○ Prevention of predictable complications of hospitalization
• Hydration should be based on the following principles:
  ○ The typical total water losses for DKA = 6 L and for HHS = 9 L.
  ○ There is no agreed upon "best" infusion rate so clinical judgment and repeated bedside assessments are required.
  ○ Replace estimated fluid deficits within the first 36–48 hours monitoring renal function, urine output, electrolytes, and the physical examination.
  ○ Avoid iatrogenic fluid overload by monitoring serum osmolality, especially in patients with renal or cardiac disease.
• Insulin management requires an insulin drip in most cases.

DISEASE MANAGEMENT STRATEGIES

SPECIAL CONSIDERATIONS IN DKA

• Keep in mind the following for DKA
  ○ Clearance of ketonemia takes longer than normalization of the blood sugar.

Complete initital evaluation. Check capillary glucose and serum/urine ketones to confirm hyperglycemia and ketonemia/ketonuria. Start IV fluids: 1.0 L of 0.9% NaCl per hour.[†]

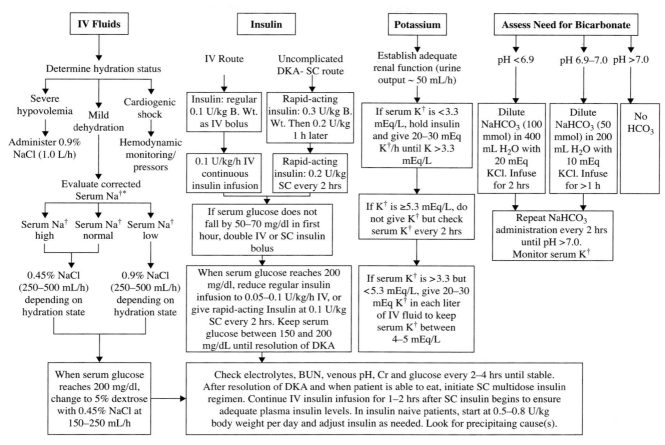

FIG. 34-1 Protocol for managing patients with DKA.

*DKA diagnostic criteria: blood glucose >250 mg/dl, arterial pH <7.3, bicarbonate <15 mEq/L, and moderate ketonuria or ketonemia.

†After history and physical examination, obtain arterial blood gases; CBC with differential, U/A, blood glucose, BUN, electrolytes, chemistry profile, and Cr levels STAT as well as an ECG. Obtain CXR and cultures as needed.

‡Serum Na should be corrected for hyperglycemia (for each 100 mg/dl glucose >100 mg/dl is one of , add 1.6 mEq to sodium value for corrected serum sodium value).

○ Criteria for resolution of DKA are glucose < 200 mg/dL, serum bicarbonate > 18 mEq/L, venous pH > 7.30, anion gap < 12 mEq/L.

○ If patients with type 1 diabetes do not receive insulin when their glucose normalizes, they will go back into DKA. Many patients assumed to have type 2 diabetes may actually have type 1 diabetes, so it is unwise to rely solely on an insulin sliding scale.

○ Generally, a bolus of 10–20 U is given at onset and patients are started on an insulin drip of 5–10 U/h initially.

  ▪ Regular insulin via intravenous infusion should be given until the ketoacidosis clears *and* the serum glucose concentration is < 250 g/dL.

▪ At that point, transition to subcutaneous (SC) insulin, given at least 1 hour prior to the cessation of the insulin infusion.

○ Newer longer-acting insulin formulations such as glargine provide more options. If a patient is ready for transition from an insulin drip to SC insulin at a time that glargine is normally given, one strategy may be to give an intermediate-acting formulation such as neutral protamine hagedorn (NPH) or novolin.

  ▪ Transition to a 24-hour formulation such as glargine once the patient is on a stable diet and blood sugars are < 200 g/dL

  ▪ Once a patient is transitioned to longer-acting SC insulin, adjustments to the regimen should be

Complete initial evaluation. Check capillary glucose to confirm hyperglycemia. IV fluids: 1.0 L of 0.9% NaCl per hour.[†]

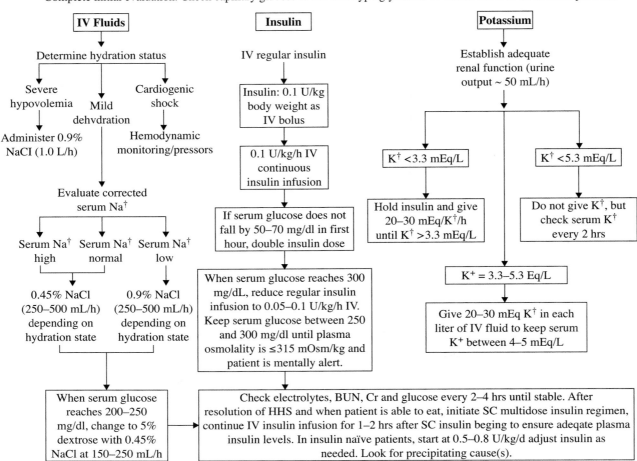

* Diagnostic criteria: blood glucose >600 mg/dl, arterial pH >7.3, bicarbonate >15 mEq/L, effective serum osmolality >320 mOsm/kg H$_2$O, and mild ketonuria or ketonemia. This protocol is for patients admitted with mental status change or severe dehydration who require admission to an ICU. For less severe cases, see text for management guidelines. Effective serum osmolality calculation: 2[measured Na (mEq/L)] + glucose (mg/dL)/18.

[†]After history and physical examination, obtain arterial blood gases, CBC with differential, U/A, plasma glucose, BUN, electrolytes, chemistry profile, and Cr levels STAT as well as an ECG. CXR and cultures as needed.

[‡]Serum Na should be corrected for hyperglycemia (for each 100 mg/dl glucose >100 mg/dl, add 1.6 mEq to sodium value for corrected serum value).

FIG. 34-2 Protocol for managing adult patients with HHS.

performed daily based on physiologic insulin replacement, eating, need for additional insulin, and recovery from coexisting illness. (See Chap. 36.)

• Electrolyte repletion is required because patients in DKA and HHS have total body deficits of water and electrolytes. Anticipate the following:
  ◦ Although patients are total body depleted, the potassium level is often elevated at presentation but will drop quickly with hydration and insulin infusion.
    ▪ Close monitoring of potassium levels, telemetry, and serial ECGs are generally used to ensure that

no cardiovascular sequelae occur from fluctuations of potassium.
    ▪ It is critical *not* to treat initial hyperkalemia with sodium polystyrene or other binding agents unless there are ECG changes or cardiovascular compromise from the elevated levels.
    ▪ The T waves on ECG will suggest serum potassium levels, often before the laboratory value returns.
    ▪ There is no reason to use potassium phosphate.
  ◦ Patients can present with either hyper- or hyponatremia; insulin and rehydration tend to drive the sodium upward as the blood sugar normalizes.

- Therefore, close monitoring of sodium is essential; normal saline may only need to be given for a short time.
- Switch to 5% dextrose when the serum glucose is < 200 mg/dL.
- Infusion of bicarbonate (HCO_3) to reverse acidosis and treat hyperkalemia in DKA is likely to be ineffective and may be harmful. Insulin administration blocks lipolysis, and ketoacidosis should resolve without bicarbonate.
  - If the pH is < 7.0 and the patient is hypotensive despite fluid resuscitation, intravenous bicarbonate drip may be administered to try to reverse the effect of severe chronic acidosis on left ventricular function.
  - Because bicarbonate will cause a decline in serum potassium, *never* give bicarbonate as a bolus.
- Magnesium levels may be high initially, but tend to be low.
  - Administer if < 1.8 mg/dL or if the patient has tetany.
  - Inability to correct hypokalemia may be secondary to low magnesium levels.
  - Lower levels are seen in patients with alcohol abuse or malnutrition.
- Like most of the other electrolytes, patients with DKA have total body phosphate depletion despite initially normal to elevated levels. Phosphate concentrations will decline with insulin therapy. However, phosphate repletion has not been shown to alter outcomes and may lead to severe hypocalcemia.
  - Supplement with sodium phosphate if < 1.0 mg/dL to avoid cardiac and skeletal muscle compromise.
  - Close monitoring is indicated to prevent respiratory compromise and musculoskeletal derangement.
- Once the acute phase of illness has resolved, usually within 24–48 hours, shift to oral diet.
- All patients should receive a nutritional assessment and education regarding diabetes and the importance of compliance.

SPECIAL CONSIDERATIONS IN HHS

- Unlike DKA, serum pH and serum ketones do not require monitoring.
- These patients tend to be older, more volume depleted and may have coexisting heart disease, hypertension, and kidney disease.
  - Serial bedside examinations to check for signs of fluid overload are critical and sometimes invasive monitoring is required to optimize therapy.
  - Patients are very sensitive to fluid hydration and sometimes insulin infusion is not necessary; however, blood sugar should be monitored very closely

(eg, at 1-hour interval for the first 24 hours or while on insulin infusion; check electrolytes at presentation and then at 4- to 6-hour intervals).
- These patients are at increased risk of arterial embolism and venous thrombosis.
  - Perform a baseline neurologic examination and frequent subsequent checks looking for new neurologic signs and symptoms.
  - Prescribe appropriate VTE pharmacologic prophylaxis for this high-risk population.

SPECIAL CONSIDERATIONS IN END-STAGE RENAL DISEASE

- These patients cannot clear electrolytes like potassium and phosphorus and medications (insulin) that are used to treat DKA and HHS.
- If potassium levels are very elevated, dialysis may be required to avoid cardiac complications.
- Aggressive fluid hydration is indicated in this population, but high rates for extended periods of time must be balanced with their inability to clear fluids; close monitoring for volume overload is necessary.

CARE TRANSITIONS

- Close outpatient follow-up is critical to ensure compliance and optimization of the diabetic regimen and to prevent readmission.
  - Nursing and support staff must teach patients about the importance of compliance with a diabetic diet, the use of insulin, and early signs of hyperglycemia to help prevent progression to DKA.
  - Patients must receive counseling on smoking cessation (as appropriate) and be informed about end-organ complications of diabetes.
  - A glycohemoglobin, although not a necessary test for workup and management of DKA, should be drawn at some point during hospitalization to determine adherence to, and effectiveness of, subsequent outpatient diabetes management.

BIBLIOGRAPHY

American Diabetes Association. Hyperglycemic crises in patients with diabetes mellitus. *Diabetes care.* January 2001;24:154–161.
Carroll P, Matz R. Uncontrolled diabetes mellitus in adults: experience in treating diabetic ketoacidosis and hyperosmolar coma with low-dose insulin and uniform treatment regimen. *Diabetes Care.* 1983;6:579–585.

Ilag LL, Kronick S, Ernst RD, et al. Impact of a critical pathway on inpatient management of diabetic ketoacidosis. *Diabetes Res Clin Pract.* 2003;62:23–32.

Kitabchi AE, Umpierrez GE, Murphy MB, et al. Management of hyperglycemic crises in patients with diabetes mellitus (Technical Review). *Diabetes Care.* 2001;24:131–153.

Kitabchi AE, Umpierrez GE, Murphy MB, et al. Hyperglycemic crises in adult patients with diabetes. *Diabetes Care.* 2006; 29(12):2739–2748.

Levetan CS, Passaro MD, Jablonski KA, et al. Effect of physician specialty on outcomes in DKA. *Diabetes Care.* 1999; 22:1790–1795.

Matz R. Hyperosmolar nonacidotic diabetes (HNAD). In: Porte D Jr, Sherwin RS, eds. *Diabetes Mellitus: Theory and Practice.* 5th ed. Amsterdam: Elsevier; 1997:845–850.

Morris LR, Murphy MB, Kitabchi AE. Bicarbonate therapy in severe diabetic ketoacidosis. *Ann Intern Med.* 1986;105:836–840.

Stoner GD. Hyperosmolar hyperglycemic state. *Am Fam Physician.* 2005;71:1723–1730.

Umpierrez GE, Casals MM, Gebhart SP, et al. Diabetic ketoacidosis in obese African Americans. *Diabetes.* 1995;44:790.

35 HYPERGLYCEMIA IN THE CRITICAL CARE UNIT

A. Rebecca Daniel

EPIDEMIOLOGY/OVERVIEW

- See Table 35-1 for risk factors associated with hyperglycemia in the critical care unit (CCU).
- Euglycemia was initially shown to be beneficial in the landmark study by Van den Berghe in 2001 who examined tight glycemic control in the surgical ICU setting. In that ICU setting, intensive insulin therapy was seen to be beneficial in reduction of many factors.
  - Overall hospital mortality in patients who stayed > 5 days (by 34%)
  - Bacteremia (by 46%)
  - Acute renal failure leading to dialysis (by 41%)
  - Polyneuropathy (by 44%)
- Subsequent studies by Van den Berghe in the medical ICU show less clear results.
  - Mortality was reduced in patients whose ICU stays were > 72 hours.
  - Mortality was increased in the patients whose ICU stays were < 72 hours.
  - Morbidity (newly acquired renal injury, time on the ventilator, LOS in the ICU) was reduced for all patients.
  - As a result of these and other studies, the American Diabetes Association (ADA) and the American College of Clinical Endocrinologists (AACE) have both recommended glucose targets.
  - The ADA currently recommends glucose targets "as close to 110 mg/dL as possible and generally < 180 mg/dL" for critically ill patients.
  - The AACE recommends the "upper limits for glycemic targets of 110 mg/dL in critically ill patients."
  - In addition, euglycemia or tight control (80–110 mg/dL) has shown to be beneficial in progression of the complications of diabetes (Table 35-2).
- A recent cost analysis of intensive glycemic control revealed substantial savings.
- Currently, there are no standardized protocols that are implemented nationally. Each institution should assess their system and the implementation of a feasible protocol with a team approach.

TABLE 35-1   Risk Factors Associated with Critical Illness-Induced Hyperglycemia

ETIOLOGY	MAJOR MECHANISM OF HYPERGLYCEMIA
Known diabetes mellitus	Relative or absolute insulin deficiency resistance or increased hepatic gluconeogenesis
Catecholamine infusion, particularly epinephrine and norepinephrine	Inhibition of insulin release
Elderly	Insulin deficiency
Obesity	Insulin resistance
Increased severity of illness	Excess counter-regulatory hormone concentration
Excess carbohydrate ingestion or infusion	Inadequate uptake of glucose
Acute or chronic pancreatitis	Insulin deficiency
Severe inflammation or infection	Insulin resistance
Hypothermia	Insulin deficiency
Uremia	Insulin resistance
Cirrhosis	Insulin resistance
Hypoxemia	Insulin deficiency

TABLE 35-2   Glycemic Goals for Critically Ill Patients

ADA	ACE
Blood glucose	< 110 mg/dL
Peak blood glucose	< 180 mg/dL

Abbreviations: ADA, American Diabetes Association; ACE, American College of Endocrinology.
Sources: Standards of Medical Care in Diabetes 2006. *Diabetes care.* 2006;s29 suppl S4–S42; American College of Endocrinology. American College of Endocrinology position statement on inpatient diabetes and metabolic control. *Endocr Pract.* 2004;10:77–82.

- The key point for success in management is a rigid protocol that can be nursing driven and physician supervised.
- See Chap. 34 for diagnostic criteria for DKA and HHS and management. Patients with severe DKA require admission to the ICU.

TRIAGE AND INITIAL MANAGEMENT

- The goal in management of hyperglycemia in the critical care setting is to improve blood glucose to at least below 180 mg/dL. While some patients may not require continuous infusions of insulin in the CCU, if blood sugars are not within the target range, the management should be reassessed.
- Tight control should be achieved by appropriately dosed insulin rather than the sliding scale technique.
- A complication of tight glucose control is hypoglycemia. For optimal outcomes, a protocol for identifying and managing hypoglycemia should be in place, especially in the critical care setting.
  - Usual symptoms may be difficult to elicit because of critical illness, concurrent drug therapy, and altered mental status. Hence, it is critical to frequently monitor the blood sugar and check if signs or symptoms of hypoglycemia develop.
  - Situations that precipitate hypoglycemia include
    - Liver disease
    - Decreasing fluids with glucose or lowering nutrition
    - Shock/sepsis
    - Renal disease that prevents clearance of insulin or oral antiglycemic drugs
    - Continuous venovenous hemofiltration (Vriesendorp et al. 2006)
    - Malnutrition
  - If blood glucose is < 50 mg/dL, recheck to be sure that the value is correct.
  - Recheck blood sugar every 15 minutes until blood glucose is > 70 mg/dL, treating with carbohydrates

or dextrose as deemed appropriate by the patient consciousness.
  - If patient can take in oral nutrition realize that 15 g of carbohydrates increase blood sugar 25–50 mg/dL.
  - Patients on ventilators or unconscious patients: give dextrose 25 g IV (1 amp D50) or glucagon 1 mg IV (SC or IM if no IV access). Recheck the blood glucose after 10 minutes, and repeat the D50 as needed. Glucagon can be repeated after 20 minutes.
  - If the patient is receiving an intravenous insulin drip, hold the insulin drip until the blood glucose is > 50 mg/dL. Recheck blood glucose every hour. Decrease and resume the insulin drip at half the previous dose once the blood glucose is 50–70 mg/dL.
  - Continue to follow blood sugars closely and initiate a dextrose drip as needed.
  - Etiology of the hypoglycemia should be evaluated.
- Indications for initiation of intravenous insulin therapy include:
  - Excess blood glucose above the target range in patients who are within 24 hours preoperative, intraoperative or 48 hours postoperative
  - Patient with acute MI/acute coronary syndrome with minimum of 24 hours post onset of event
  - Contraindication to oral or SC methods
  - Admitted with diagnosis of DKA or HHS
  - Poor control even with SC insulin
  - Persistent blood sugars in the range of 141–249 mg/dL. In patients with difficult to control hyperglycemia, additional considerations are given in Table 35-3
- Indications for transitioning from intravenous insulin drip to SC insulin are found in Table 35-4. The ability of the patient to take oral nutrition is an important aspect.
- Dietary management.
  - Often patients admitted to the CCU are too ill to have an oral intake and will require total parenteral nutrition or tube feedings.

TABLE 35-3   Persistent Insulin Management Issues

Consider sepsis
Lack of nutrition
Catecholamine effect from vasopressor use on the blood glucose levels
Concomitant steroid use or tapering
Administration of insulin through other sources such as TPN
Administration of additional glucose through other sources such as
   intravenous medications
Postoperative stress

Abbreviation: TPN, total parenteral nutrition.

TABLE 35-4   Indications for Transitioning to SC Insulin

Patient taking oral nutrition
Patients with DKA resolved
48 hours postsurgery and insulin dosing stable
24 hours after an MI with stable insulin requirements

○ Insulin management is often stable until the patient is able to intake oral supplements, which will cause fluctuations in the patient's glucose metabolism.
○ Physicians should also watch for the additional medications they may administer that would precipitate hyperglycemia such as glucocorticoids.
○ A nutrition consultation should be obtained for dietary education once the patient is able to communicate.
○ For additional information regarding dietary recommendations, refer to Chap. 88 for details.
• There are no specific clinical trials which provide a specific method of transitioning from insulin infusion to SC administration. A suggested method is provided in Table 35-5.
• Faster-acting insulin such as lispro or regular insulin requirements will need to be calculated once the patient is on enteral feedings or has oral intake (see the "1700" rule in Table 35-6).

DISEASE MANAGEMENT STRATEGIES

STROKE PATIENTS

• The diabetes position paper of 2006 stated that diabetics have a worse outcome after an ischemic stroke as witnessed in observational studies.
• The thirty-second international stroke conference presented a controversial outcome discovered in the

TABLE 35-5   Transitioning from Continuous Intravenous Insulin to SC Insulin

Review hourly dose of insulin required by the patient in the last 12–24 hours.
Multiply by 24 hours = daily insulin requirements.
Calculate basal insulin requirements: total daily insulin requirement × .5.

Problem
When reviewing your patient's insulin requirements over the past 24 hours, you note that the patient has required 2 units per hour. Patient is currently NPO, calculate the basal insulin requirement.

Answer
2 units × 24 hours = 48 units daily
48 units × .5 = 240 units
Option 1: Lantus 24 units in one daily dosing
Option 2: Lantus 12 units in AM and 12 units in PM
Option 3: Mixed products (NPH/70/30): 2/3 in AM and 1/3 in PM, so, 16 units in AM and 8 units in PM

TABLE 35-6   Using the "1700" Rule

Short- or rapid-acting insulin can be used to correct glucose values outside the target range.
Correction factor is defined by the effect of 1 unit of rapid- or short-acting insulin on the patient's blood glucose over 2–4 hours.
Correction factor = 1700/total daily insulin dose.
Problem: If patient used 100 units of insulin in 24 hours what is the correction factor and what does it imply?
Answer: Correction factor is 17 mg/dL, which means that 1 unit of insulin should reduce the blood glucose by 17 mg/dL within 2–4 hours.

SOURCE: Boucher J, Swift C, Franz M, et al. Inpatient management of diabetes and hyperglycemia: implications for nutrition practice and the food and nutrition professional. *J Am Diet Assoc.* 2007;107(1):105–111.

UK glucose insulin in stroke study (GIST-UK): decreased blood glucose levels in acute stroke was associated with a reduction in blood pressure, which could be harmful to acute stroke patients.
• The correlation between glucose and stroke is suspected to be attributable to the state of hyperglycemia causing intracellular acidosis and causing neuronal edema initially created by the ischemic insult.
• There are many benefits of tight glucose control in other populations, documented through clinical trials, yet we will need to await clinical rather than observational studies to adequately determine the effect of aggressive glucose management on acute stroke patients.

MYOCARDIAL INFARCTION

• Diabetes is a major cardiac risk factor for symptomatic or asymptomatic silent cardiac ischemia.
• Coronary vascular disease is the major cause of mortality in diabetics and is a major cause of morbidity.
• Eighty percent of fatalities associated with diabetes are caused by cardiovascular disease. The diabetes insulin-glucose acute myocardial infarction (DIGAMI) study showed that this mortality could be improved by insulin treatment of hyperglycemia in the setting of acute MI.
○ The American College of Cardiology and the American Heart Association guidelines recommend tight control with glucose < 110, with target HbA1C < 1% above normal, in addition to reduction of other major cardiac risk factors. See Chap. 23.

RENAL DISEASE

• An important aspect of management is avoiding progression of renal disease in diabetic patients leading to dialysis (Table 35-7).

TABLE 35-7 Nephrotoxic Precautions in Diabetics

Avoid:
Contrast dye (eg, excessive radiological studies/cardiac catheterization)
Overdiuresis
Nephrotoxic drugs (eg, antifungal medications)
Hypotension/hypovolemia

- The Hope (heart outcomes prevention evaluation) trial demonstrated the importance of angiotensin-converting enzyme inhibitor use in the management of diabetics with renal insufficiency and cardiovascular function, but in a critical care setting other factors such as blood pressure, electrolyte levels and acute renal failure may play a part in the initiation or continuation of such medications.

PERIOPERATIVE/POSTOPERATIVE MANAGEMENT OF HYPERGLYCEMIA

- Discontinue oral antiglycemics and patient insulin pumps.
- Society of Thoracic Surgeons (STS) stated that postoperative mortality is improved for CABG patients if blood glucose levels were kept below 200 mg/dL.
- Additional studies evaluated the importance of intraoperative glucose control and discovered that body mass index (BMI) and preinduction glycemia are predictors of perioperative insulin management.
- Always remember that the type 1 diabetic needs basal insulin the night prior to surgery.
- On morning of surgery do not administer oral antiglycemics or short-acting insulins, and discontinue operation of patient insulin pumps.
- Autonomic neuropathy puts diabetics at risk for aspiration and gastroparesis.
- Remember to keep head of bed at 45° angle, administer proton pump inhibitor, and give medications to increase gastric motility.
- Aggressive glycemic management is advocated to promote wound healing and optimize immune function.

CARE TRANSITIONS

- Start patient education in the CCU when the patient is able to communicate.
- Hemoglobin A1C is not an indicated test for inpatient diagnosis of diabetes but can be used to assess possible noncompliance or inadequacy of medical therapy within the past 120 days.
- Diagnostic testing includes a fasting blood glucose > 126 mg/dL or a random blood glucose > 200 mg/dL

with some symptoms of diabetes. These lab tests should be repeated in the outpatient setting in patients with stress-induced diabetes or those on steroid therapies.

- At the time of discharge if a new diagnosis of diabetes has been made patients should have referrals set up: eye examination, diabetic educator, family planning (fertile women), confirm that patient has an outpatient physician to continue management of their disease.
- When the patient is ready for transitioning insulin therapy from intravenous to SC forms, attempt to initiate or continue the insulin that will be continued as an outpatient. Financial stipulations may inhibit the patient from continuing the same insulin regimen as an outpatient.
- At the time of transfer of the patient out of the critical care setting remember to address the following issues:
  ○ Is the patient taking oral nutrition?
  ○ Does the patient's glucose remain in a range of 80–140? The patient should not have unexplained episodes of hypoglycemia.
  ○ Has the patient been on a stable dose of oral or SC insulin?

BIBLIOGRAPHY

American Diabetes Association Workgroup on Hypoglycemia. Defining and reporting hypoglycemia in diabetes: a report from the American Diabetes Association workgroup on hypoglycemia. *Diabetes Care.* 2005;28(5): 1245–1249.

American Diabetes Association. Standards of medical care in diabetes—2006. *Diabetes Care.* 2006;29(suppl 1): S4–S42.

American College of Endocrinology Task Force on Inpatient Diabetes and Metabolic Control: Metabolic Control: American College of Endocrinology position statement on inpatient diabetes and metabolic control. *Endocr Pract.* 2004;10:77–82.

Balkin M, Mascioli C, Smith V, et al. Achieving durable glucose control in the intensive care unit without hypoglycemia: a new practical IV insulin protocol. *Diabetes Metab Res Rev.* 2007 Jan;23(1):49–55.

Boucher J, Swift C, Franz M, et al. Inpatient management of diabetes and hyperglycemia: implications for nutrition practice and the food and nutrition professional. *J Am Diet Assoc.* 2007; 107(1):105–111.

Braithwaite SS, Edkins R, Macgregor LL, et al. Performance of a dose-defining insulin infusion protocol among trauma service intensive care unit admissions. *Diabetes Technol Ther.* 2006 Aug;8(4):476–488.

Brodows RG, Williams C, Amatruda JM. Treatment of insulin reactions in diabetics. *J Am Med Assoc.* 1984;252: 3378–3381.

Cammu G, Lecomte P, Casselman F, et al. Preinduction glycemia and body mass index are important predictors of perioperative insulin management in patients undergoing cardiac surgery. *J Clin Anesth.* 2007;19:37–43.

Coursin D, Connery L, Ketzler J. Perioperative diabetic and hyperglycemic management issues. *Crit Care Med.* 2004;32 (Suppl 4):S116–S125.

Cryer PE. Symptoms of hypoglycemia, thresholds for their occurrence, and hypoglycemia unawareness. *Endocrinol Metab Clin North Am.* 1999;28(3):495–500.

Desouza C, Salazar H, Cheong B, et al. Association of hypoglycemia and cardiac ischemia: a study based on continuous monitoring. *Diabetes Care.* 2003;26:1485–1489.

Furnary AP, Gao G, Grunkemeier GL, et al. Continuous insulin infusion reduces mortality in patients with diabetes undergoing coronary artery bypass grafting. *J Thorac Cardiovas Surg.* 2003;125:1007–1021.

Goldberg PA, Siegel MD, Sherwin RS, et al. Implementation of a safe and effective insulin infusion protocol in a medical intensive care unit. *Diabetes Care.* 2004 Feb;27(2): 461–467.

Kitabchi AE, Umpierrez GE, Murphy MB, et al. Hyperglycemic crises in diabetes. *Diabetes Care.* 2004;27(suppl 1): S94–S102.

Krinsley J, Jones R. Cost analysis of intensive glycemic control in critically ill adult patients. *Chest.* 2006;129(3): 644–650.

Levatan C. Controlling hyperglycemia in the hospital: a matter of life and death. *Clin Diabetes.* 2000;18:17–24.

Malmberg K, Ryden L, Efendic S, et al. Randomized trial of insulin-glucose infusion followed by subcutaneous insulin treatment in diabetic patients with acute myocardial infarction (DIGAMI Study): effects on mortality at 1 year. *J Am Coll Cardiol.* 1995;26:57–65.

Meijering S, Corstjens AM, Tulleken JE, et al. Towards a feasible algorithm for tight glycemic control in critically ill patients: a systematic review of the literature. *Crit Care.* 2006 Feb;10(1):R19.

Moghissi E, Hirsch Irl. Hospital management of diabetes. *Endocrinol Metab Clin North Am.* 2005;34:99–116.

Scott M Grundy, Ivor J Benjamin, Gregory L Burke, et al. Diabetes and cardiovascular disease: a statement for healthcare professionals from the American Heart Association Circulation. 1999;100:1134–1146.

American Diabetes Association standards of medical care in diabetes 2006. *Diabetes Care.* 2006;29(suppl 1):S4–S42.

The Heart Outcomes Prevention Evaluation Study Investigators. Effects of an angiotensin-converting enzyme inhibitor, ramipril, on cardiovascular events in high-risk patients. 2000;342(3): 145–153.

Van den Berghe G, Wouters P, Weekers F, et al. Intensive insulin therapy in critically ill patients. *N Engl J Med.* 2001;345:1359–1367.

Van den Berghe G, Wilmer A, Hermans G, et al. Intensive insulin therapy in the medical ICU. *N Engl J Med.* 2006 Feb 2;354(5): 449–461.

WEB RESOURCES

American College of Endocrinology. http://www.aace.com/college/
American Diabetes Association. http://www.diabetes.org/home.jsp
JCAHO diabetes certification. http://www.jointcommission.org

36 HYPERGLYCEMIA IN NONCRITICALLY ILL HOSPITALIZED PATIENTS

Aditi R. Saxena and Merri L. Pendergrass

EPIDEMIOLOGY/OVERVIEW

- Diabetes mellitus is a common comorbid condition among hospitalized patients.
  - In 2003, approximately 18% of all hospitalized adults had a secondary diagnosis of diabetes.
- Inpatient hyperglycemia has been associated with a number of adverse outcomes, including increased LOS, increased risk of infection, poor wound healing, decreased ability to live independently after discharge, and increased mortality.
- Randomized controlled trials have demonstrated that aggressive treatment of inpatient hyperglycemia improves outcomes in critically ill patients. However, no randomized controlled trials have been performed in noncritically ill patients.
- The ADA and American College of Endocrinology (ACE) advocate good glycemic control in hospitalized non-ICU patients. Goals for glycemic control in noncritically ill hospitalized patients are shown in Table 36-1.

TABLE 36-1 Glycemic Goals for Noncritically Ill Hospitalized Patients with Diabetes

PARAMETER	ADA	ACE
Premeal blood glucose (mg/dL)	90–130	< 110
Postprandial blood glucose	< 180	< 180

Abbreviations: ADA, American Diabetes Association; ACE, American College of Endocrinology.
SOURCES: From American Diabetes Association. Standards of medical care in diabetes–2006. *Diabetes Care.* 2006;29(suppl 1):S4–S42; American College of Endocrinology. American College of Endocrinology position statement on inpatient diabetes and metabolic control. *Endocr Pract.* 2004;10:77–82.

TABLE 36-2 Selected JCAHO Criteria for Inpatient Diabetes Certification

- All patients with a medical history of diabetes are identified as having a diagnosis of diabetes on admission and at discharge.
- An Hb_{A1C} is drawn at the time of admission, unless the Hb_{A1C} was drawn within 60 days prior to admission or the patient has received therapy that would confound the results.
- Blood glucose monitoring is ordered for all patients upon admission.
- Treatment plans for hypoglycemia and hyperglycemia are established for each patient.
- A plan for coordinating administration of insulin and delivery of meals is implemented.
- Hb_{A1C} results and any unresolved medical issues are communicated to the patient and the healthcare provider managing his or her diabetes care after discharge.

- In conjunction with the ADA, the Joint Committee on Accreditation of Healthcare Organizations (JCAHO) has developed an inpatient diabetes certification program. Highlights of the requirement for inpatient diabetes certification are outlined in Table 36-2.

PATHOPHYSIOLOGY

- Hyperglycemia occurs when there is a mismatch between insulin resistance, a condition of decreased insulin sensitivity, and insulin availability (from endogenous and/or exogenous sources).
  - Defects in *both* insulin sensitivity and insulin secretion are present in most patients with diabetes.
  - The major defect may be one of insulin deficiency (eg, type 1 diabetes).
    - It is crucial that these patients are recognized, as they require basal insulin at all times to prevent ketoacidosis.
    - Insulin should never be held, even when patients are NPO (Table 36-3).
  - The major defect may be insulin resistance (eg, type 2 diabetes).
    - These patients usually make some insulin, but not enough to balance the degree of insulin resistance.
    - Hyperglycemia potentially may be controlled without insulin, particularly if they are NPO or

TABLE 36-3 Clinical Characteristics of Patients with Insulin Deficiency

- Diagnosis of type 1 diabetes
- History of pancreatectomy or pancreatic dysfunction
- History of wide fluctuations in blood glucose levels
- History of DKA
- History of insulin use for > 5 years or history of diabetes for > 10 years

SOURCE: Adapted from Report of the Expert Committee on the Diagnosis and Classification of Diabetes Mellitus. *Diabetes Care.* 2002;25(suppl. 2): S5–S20.

have mild impairments in insulin secretion and/or insulin resistance.
  - If the patient has severe insulin resistance, because of illness and/or or underlying disease, they may require very high doses of insulin.
- The mismatch between insulin resistance and insulin availability frequently is augmented in hospitalized patients, even those without a preexisting diagnosis of diabetes.
  - Insulin resistance commonly increases during hospitalization because of several factors, including increases in stress hormones (eg, cortisol, catecholamines) and administration of certain medications such as corticosteroids and pressors.
- The mechanism by which hyperglycemia and relative hypoinsulinemia cause harm in inpatients remains unknown. Potential mechanisms for tissue and organ injury may be via the combined insults of infection, direct fuel-mediated injury, and oxidative stress and other downstream mediators.

CLINICAL PRESENTATION, DIFFERENTIAL, MAKING THE DIAGNOSIS

- Hospitalized patients with hyperglycemia fall into one of three categories:
  - Patients with a medical history of diabetes
  - Patients with previously unrecognized diabetes
  - Patients who exhibit hospital-related hyperglycemia ("stress hyperglycemia") that meets criteria of diabetes during hospitalization but who revert to having normal blood glucose levels before or soon after discharge
- Conceptualizing hospitalized patients with respect to these categories will aid in hospital management and anticipation of patient needs at the time of discharge.
  - Patients with a medical history of diabetes usually require insulin during the hospitalization.
  - Patients with previously unrecognized diabetes usually require insulin during the hospitalization and also may require diabetes medication (insulin and/or oral agents) at discharge.
  - Patients with stress hyperglycemia may require insulin during the hospitalization but usually do not require diabetes medication at discharge.
    - These patients are at a high risk for future type 2 diabetes and should be tested for diabetes 4–8 weeks after discharge.
- If a patient has no previous diagnosis of diabetes but has hyperglycemia in the hospital, it may be useful to obtain an Hb_{A1C} level.

○ If the Hb_{A1C} is above 6%, the patient likely has diabetes and may need treatment for this at the time of discharge.

○ Hyperglycemic inpatients with no prior history of diabetes and Hb_{A1C} below 6% usually will not require diabetes treatment when they are discharged.

DISEASE MANAGEMENT STRATEGIES

DIET

• Since 1994, the ADA has not endorsed any single meal plan or specified percentages of macronutrients.
• The use of terms such as "ADA diet," "no concentrated sweets," "no sugar added," or "liberal diabetic diet" is no longer appropriate. These diets unnecessarily restrict sucrose and do not reflect the current evidence-based nutrition recommendations.
• The "consistent carbohydrate" diabetes meal-planning system was developed to provide institutions with an up-to-date way of providing food service to hospitalized patients.
  ○ The system is not based on specific calorie levels, but rather on the amount of carbohydrate offered at each meal.
  ○ The amount of carbohydrate is consistent from meal to meal and day to day.
  ○ *Meals are based on heart-healthy diet principles—* Saturated fats and cholesterol are limited, and protein content falls within a usual diet's content of 15% to 20% of calories.
  ○ Instead of focusing on the type of carbohydrate foods served, the emphasis is on the total amount of

carbohydrate contained in the meal. The majority of carbohydrate foods should be whole grains, fruits, vegetables, and low-fat milk, but some sucrose-containing foods can be included as part of the total carbohydrate allowance.

○ These systems may ease difficulties in dosing prandial insulin, as the prandial dose can target the amount of carbohydrates provided in the meal.

○ They also reinforce the skill of carbohydrate counting, which is helpful to many diabetic patients in meal planning.

MEDICAL THERAPY

ORAL AGENTS
• Oral agents are usually ineffective in management of inpatient hyperglycemia and should be stopped on admission to the hospital.
  ○ Oral agents offer little flexibility or opportunity for titration.
  ○ In the inpatient setting, patients may develop contraindications, such as acute renal insufficiency and congestive heart failure, to common oral medications.
  ○ Adverse effects of oral agents, such as diarrhea, nausea, and fluid retention, may complicate the inpatient course (Table 36-4).

INTRAVENOUS INSULIN
• Medical literature provides strong evidence for benefit of intravenous (IV) insulin management in several inpatient settings, particularly when the following situations are applicable (Table 36-5).

TABLE 36-4 Inpatient Precautions for Commonly Prescribed Oral Agents

MEDICATION	PRECAUTION
Insulin secretagogues • Sulfonylureas (eg, glyburide, glipizide, glimepiride) • Meglitinides (repaglinide) • Phenylalanine derivatives (nateglinide)	• Risk for hypoglycemia, particularly in patients with poor nutritional intake and renal failure
Biguanides (metformin)	• Contraindicated in patients with active cardiac, liver, hepatic, or pulmonary disease • Following procedure, patients receiving iodinated intravenous contrast should have metformin held ~48 hours (until normal renal function is confirmed) • Adverse gastrointestinal side effects, eg, nausea and diarrhea, may interfere with assessment of other acute medical issues
Thiozolidinediones (rosiglitazone and pioglitazone)	• Contraindicated in Class 3 or 4 congestive heart failure • Fluid retention, the most common adverse effect, may complicate the assessment of other acute medical issues

TABLE 36-5 Reasons to Consider IV Insulin Therapy

PATHOPHYSIOLOGIC STATES	POSSIBLE DIAGNOSES
• Rapidly changing insulin requirements • Impaired perfusion of SC tissue (eg, severe, generalized edema) • Need for pressor support • Use of TPN	• DKA or HHS • Preoperative, intraoperative or postoperative care • Critical illness, including sepsis and cardiogenic shock • NPO status in type 1 diabetes • Exacerbated hyperglycemia in the setting of high-dose glucocorticoid therapy

Abbreviation: TPN, total parenteral nutrition.

SUBCUTANEOUS INSULIN

- Most patients with hyperglycemia, especially those who carry a diagnosis of diabetes mellitus, are most effectively managed with SC insulin during non-ICU hospitalization.
- Insulin may be safely administered even to patients without previously diagnosed diabetes.
  - As long as the prescribed doses do not exceed the total insulin requirements, the patient will not become hypoglycemic.
    - If the glucose level starts to fall too low, endogenous insulin secretion will reduce to compensate.
    - *Example*—If a person requires 40 U of insulin per day, and their own pancreas is making the equivalent of 30 U/d, they will "need" an extra 10 U/d. However, if 20 U of exogenous insulin are administered, the pancreas will decrease the endogenous secretion and only secrete 20 U.
- Profiles of available insulin formulations are listed below (Table 36-6).

SLIDING SCALE INSULIN

- Several studies have demonstrated that sliding scale insulin, *when used alone*, is ineffective. The ADA and other authorities strongly discourage the use of sliding scale insulin regimens *alone*, for the following reasons:
  - Sliding scales act retroactively and only treat hyperglycemia after it has already occurred.
  - These scales do not account for insulin sensitivity or amount of oral intake.
  - They may lead to widely fluctuating glucose levels and dangerous "stacking" of insulin doses, with resulting hypoglycemia.
    - In order to avoid insulin "stacking," short-acting insulin usually should *not* be given more frequently than every 4–6 hours.
  - Sliding scales give the illusion of glycemic control, instead of highlighting the need for daily proactive adjustment.

EFFECTIVE SUBCUTANEOUS REGIMENS

- Effective inpatient insulin regimens (see Tables 36-7, 36-8, and 36-9) typically include three components.
  - *Basal insulin*—Used to manage fasting and premeal hyperglycemia
    - This should comprise 50% of the total daily dose (TDD) of insulin.
  - *Nutritional or prandial insulin*—Controls hyperglycemia from nutritional sources (eg, discrete meals, total parenteral nutrition [TPN], IV dextrose)
    - This should comprise 50% of TDD of insulin.
  - *Supplemental or correctional insulin (AKA "sliding scale")*—Used in addition to scheduled insulin to control hyperglycemia that occurs despite the use of scheduled basal and nutritional insulin.
    - This should be proportional to the TDD of insulin.

TABLE 36-6 Duration of Action of Available Insulins

	TYPE OF INSULIN	ONSET OF ACTION	PEAK ACTION	EFFECTIVE DURATION
Rapid	Lispro	5–15 minutes	30–90 minutes	4–6 hours
Rapid	Aspart	5–15 minutes	30–90 minutes	4–6 hours
Rapid	Glulisine	10–15 minutes	30–90 minutes	3–5 hours
Short	Inhaled insulin*	10–20 minutes	30–90 minutes	4–6 hours
Short	Regular	30–60 minutes	2–3 hours	8–10 hours
Inter	NPH	2–4 hours	4–10 hours	12–18 hours
Long	Glargine	2–4 hours	None	20–24 hours
Long	Detemir	2 hours	None	12–20 hours

*Not recommended for inpatient use.

TABLE 36-7 Components of Effective Insulin Regimens

INSULIN COVERAGE	PHYSIOLOGIC BASIS	PREFERRED AGENTS
Basal	Controls fasting and premeal hyperglycemia	• Glargine • Detemir • NPH
Nutritional/prandial*	Controls hyperglycemia from nutritional sources (eg, dextrose infusion, TPN, enteral feedings, discrete meals, or nutritional supplements)	• Regular • Lispro • Aspart • Glulisine
Correctional/supplemental	Used *in addition to scheduled basal and nutritional insulin* to cover hyperglycemia that occurs despite scheduled insulin	• Regular • Lispro • Aspart • Glulisine

*In each patient, prandial and correctional insulin should be of same type, for example, if patient is receiving aspart insulin for prandial dosing, correction scale should be written for aspart insulin also.

TABLE 36-8 Insulin Regimen Based on Nutritional Status

NUTRITIONAL CATEGORY	BBG SCHEDULE	INSULIN REGIMEN
Eating discrete meals	qAC and qHS	• Basal insulin (~50% estimated TDD) ○ Eg, NPH, glargine, or detemir qd or divided bid • Nutritional insulin (~50% estimated TDD) ○ Eg, aspart, lispro, or glulisine divided tid ac • Supplemental insulin: aspart, lispro, or glulisine sliding scale tid ac
NPO	q6 hours	• Basal insulin (~50% estimated TDD) ○ Eg, NPH, glargine, or detemir qd or divided bid • Nutritional insulin: hold this component for NPO • Supplemental insulin: regular sliding scale q6 hours
Continuous tube feeds or continuous IV dextrose infusion	q6 hours	• Basal insulin (~50% estimated TDD) ○ Eg, NPH, glargine, or detemir qd or divided bid • Nutritional insulin (~50% estimated TDD) ○ Eg, regular q6 hours • Supplemental insulin: regular sliding scale q6 hours

Abbreviation: TDD, total daily dose.
*Initial TDD may be estimated as ~0.5–0.7 U/kg/d.

TABLE 36-9 Example Algorithm for Correction/Supplemental (AKA "Sliding Scale") Insulin

PREMEAL BLOOD GLUCOSE (mg/dL)	LOW-DOSE ALGORITHM (for patients requiring ≤ 40 U of insulin per day)	MEDIUM-DOSE ALGORITHM (for patients requiring 40–80 U of insulin per day)	HIGH-DOSE ALGORITHM (for patients requiring > 80 U of insulin per day)
150–200	1 unit additional insulin	1 unit	2 U
201–250	2 U	3 U	4 U
251–300	3 U	5 U	7 U
301–350	4 U	7 U	10 U
> 350	5 U	8 U	12 U

Source: Adapted from Clement S, Braithwaite SS, Magee MF, et al. Management of diabetes and hyperglycemia in hospitals. *Diabetes Care.* 2004;27:553–591.

Determining the Initial Inpatient Insulin Regimen

- If a patient has *not previously been treated with insulin*, a conservative estimate for initial insulin therapy in any patient is to start with a TDD that is typical for patients with type 1 diabetes mellitus (T1DM) (~0.5–0.7 U/kg/day).
- Half of the TDD should be given as basal insulin, and half as nutritional insulin.
  - *Example*—The initial TDD of a 70-kg person could be estimated as 70 kg × 0.6 U/kg/d = 42 U/d. This can be further divided into NPH insulin 10 qAM and 10 qHS + 7 Aspart tid qAC.
- This dose usually will underestimate the appropriate dose, especially in type 2 diabetes patients who have increased insulin resistance because of the stress of hospitalization.
  - If a patient has been *taking insulin as an outpatient*, the outpatient regimen usually should be continued on admission and adjusted to meet inpatient needs.
- The initial inpatient dose usually should be *increased* from the outpatient dose if the patient is very hyperglycemic on admission and/or has a history of poor outpatient glucose control (eg, high Hb_{A1C}).
- The initial inpatient dose usually should be *reduced* from the outpatient dose if the patient has a low current glucose value, a history of low values, worsening renal function, or is now NPO or at risk for poor nutritional intake while hospitalized.

Insulin Dose Adjustment

- After initial insulin orders are placed, bedside blood glucose (BBG) values should be monitored daily.
- Scheduled basal and nutritional insulin doses usually should be adjusted (increased or decreased) at least daily, based on the BBG results.
  - Basal and nutritional doses should be adjusted to maintain approximately a 50/50 ratio.
- In order to avoid hypoglycemia, insulin regimen should be changed if nutritional sources or content is changing.

PERIOPERATIVE/PROCEDURE CONSIDERATIONS

- On the day before procedure, administer usual doses of insulin.

TABLE 36-10   Factors Increasing Risk for Hypoglycemia

- Sudden decrease in oral intake or institution of NPO status
- Discontinuation of enteral or intravenous feeding
- Poor ingestion of food after premeal insulin administered
- Reduction in corticosteroid dose

TABLE 36-11   How to Titrate Insulin Regimen

Patient 1

Nutritional status: eating three discrete meals per day.
Current insulin regimen: glargine 30 U qHS and lispro 10 U qAC with meals. Patient 1 is also written to receive supplemental or correctional insulin according to medium-dose algorithm.

Blood glucoses on this regimen

Fasting (also prebreakfast): 260 mg/dL (receives 5 U supplemental lispro, in addition to 10 U scheduled lispro)
Prelunch: 277 mg/dL (receives 5 U supplemental lispro, in addition to 10 U scheduled lispro)
Predinner: 280 mg/dL (receives 5 U supplemental lispro, in addition to 10 U scheduled lispro)

1. To calculate new insulin doses for Patient 1, add all doses of insulin on this day to calculate TDD. *TDD* = 30 U (glargine) + 30 U (lispro scheduled with meals) + 15 U (supplemental insulin) = 75 U.
2. Divide new TDD into basal and nutritional doses: 50% of 75 (approximately 37 U) should be given as glargine and 50% (approximately 39 U) should be given as nutritional insulin. Further divide nutritional insulin to be given with each meal, 39 U over 3 meals is 13 U with each meal.
3. *New insulin regimen*: glargine 37 U qHS and lispro 13 U qAC with meals.

- On the day of procedure, a decision should be made to hold, reduce, or give full dose of basal insulin (eg, NPH, glargine, or detemir).
  - Basal insulin should never be held in patients with type 1 diabetes. For prolonged NPO status, the patient usually should be treated with an IV insulin infusion.
  - Basal doses may be reduced if BBG have been running low in patients with type 2 diabetes. If BBG values have been running high, it should not be reduced.
- Scheduled nutritional insulin should be held while nutrition is held (eg, the patient is NPO).
- The supplemental "sliding scale" insulin can be continued while nutrition is held.

DIABETES IN PREGNANCY

- Very good glycemic control during pregnancy improves perinatal outcomes.
- Glycemic goals for diabetes in pregnancy are lower than for nonpregnant patients—fasting < 95 mg/dL, preprandial < 100 mg/dL, 1-h postprandial < 140 mg/dL, and 2-h postprandial < 120 mg/dL.
- Oral agents are not recommended.
- Women with gestational diabetes may or may not require insulin.
- Most women with pregestational (type 1 or type 2) diabetes require insulin.
- The most commonly used insulins for diabetes in pregnancy are NPH, insulin lispro, and insulin aspart (all are category B).

- Pregnant patients' diabetes are best managed under the guidance of an endocrinologist, maternal-fetal medicine specialist, or other specialist with experience and expertise in this area.

CARE TRANSITIONS

- Effective discharge planning for patients with diabetes requires collaboration between several team members, including physicians (hospital attending, primary care physician [PCP] and endocrinologist), nurses, and diabetes educators.
- When creating a discharge plan for each patient, JCAHO suggests that the following issues should be addressed (Table 36-12):
  - Patients generally should be discharged to home on a medication regimen similar to the admission regimen (ie, the regimen prescribed by their PCP). Exceptions are listed below:
    - The patient has a contraindication to an admission medication.
    - There is evidence of severe hyperglycemia (eg, very high Hb_{A1C}) or hypoglycemia on admission regimen.
- For a patient who was not on insulin prior to admission but who requires insulin at time of discharge, the discharge insulin regimen usually should be as simple as possible (eg, a single injection of bedtime NPH, glargine, or detemir).
  - An exception for this is the newly diagnosed type 1 diabetic patient, who should be discharged to home on 3–4 injections per day.
- Patients generally should not be discharged to home on sliding scale insulin.
- Patients who require insulin injections and blood glucose monitoring after discharge should receive instruction how to perform these.
- If a medication has been changed or added, the patient should have prompt follow-up with their PCP.

TABLE 36-12   JCAHO Discharge Considerations (Inpatient Diabetes Certification)

- Hb_{A1C} results and any unresolved medical issues are communicated to the patient and the healthcare provider managing his or her diabetes care after discharge.
- Patients should be instructed on the use of a blood glucose meter and the importance of blood glucose monitoring.
- Prior to discharge, each patient who is newly diagnosed with diabetes should be educated on the signs, symptoms, and treatment of hypoglycemia and hyperglycemia.
- Patients should also receive instruction on sick day guidelines and how to dose medication in the setting of illness.

- For patients with no history of diabetes but who are diagnosed with stress hyperglycemia during the hospitalization, studies show that up to 60% of this population will meet diagnostic criteria for diabetes at follow-up testing.
  - Arrangements should be made for these patients to have follow-up testing for diabetes (eg, fasting plasma glucose) within 1–2 months following hospital discharge.

BIBLIOGRAPHY

ACOG Practice Bulletin. Clinical practice guidelines for obstetrician-gynecologists, number 60, March 2005: pregestational diabetes mellitus. *Obstet Gynecol.* 2005;105(3): 675–685.

American College of Endocrinology. American College of Endocrinology position statement on inpatient diabetes and metabolic control. *Endocr Pract.* 2004;10:77–82.

American Diabetes Association. Position statement: gestational diabetes. *Diabetes Care.* 2004;27(suppl 1):S88–S89.

American Diabetes Association. Standards of medical care in diabetes-2006. *Diabetes Care.* 2006;29(suppl 1):S4–S42.

Clement S, Braithwaite SS, Magee MF, et al. Management of diabetes and hyperglycemia in hospitals. *Diabetes Care.* 2004;27:553–591.

Hirsch IB. Insulin analogues. *N Engl J Med.* 2005;352: 174–183.

Mooradian AD, Bernbaum M, Albert SG. Narrative review: a rational approach to starting insulin therapy. *Ann Intern Med.* 2006;145:125–134.

Queale WS, Seidler AJ, Brancati FL. Glycemic control and sliding scale insulin use in medical inpatients with diabetes mellitus. *Arch Intern Med.* 1997;157:545–552.

Soran H, Younis N. Insulin detemir: a new basal insulin analogue. *Diabetes Obes Metab.* 2006;8:26–30.

Umpierrez GE, Isaacs SD, Bazargan N, et al. Hyperglycemia: an independent marker of in-hospital mortality in patients with undiagnosed diabetes. *J Clin Endocrinol Metab.* 2002;87:978–982.

WEB RESOURCES

American College of Physicians. http://diabetes.acponline.org/index.html

The glycemic control workbook on the SHM: http://www.hospitalmedicine.org/ResourceRoomRedesign/GlycemicControl.cfm

37 HYPOTHYROIDISM AND HYPERTHYROIDISM

Rachael Fawcett and Erik K. Alexander

EPIDEMIOLOGY/OVERVIEW

- The thyroid gland releases two forms of thyroid hormone: thyroxine (T4) and tri-iodothyronine (T3).
- All of the T4 in the body is made within the thyroid gland, whereas 80% of T3 is derived in the peripheral tissues.
- T3 affects the physiologic function of almost all bodily tissues through binding with a specific nuclear receptor and thereby regulating the transcription of thyroid-dependent genes.
- The peripheral conversion of T4 to T3 is decreased by various medications, including propranolol, corticosteroids, propylthiouracil (PTU), and amiodarone, and is down-regulated during the course of nonthyroidal illness.
- The synthesis and release of thyroid hormone are controlled by the pituitary-derived thyroid-stimulating hormone (also known as thyrotropin or TSH) under the influence of thyrotropin-releasing hormone (TRH) from the hypothalamus.
- TSH stimulates basic thyrocyte functions such as iodine uptake and organification and the synthesis and release of thyroid hormone.
- Both T3 and T4 are bound to proteins (primarily thyroxine-binding globulin) in the circulation that serve the dual purpose of preventing excessive tissue uptake and maintaining a readily accessible reserve of hormone. Several common medications affect levels of thyroxine-binding globulin without generally affecting the free thyroid hormone levels (estrogens, glucocorticoids, androgens).
- Hypothyroidism is more common than hyperthyroidism, though both have a disproportionate female predominance.
- While the risk of developing hyperthyroidism is similar throughout all decades of life, the risk of developing hypothyroidism substantially increases with age.
- Goiter (or enlargement of the thyroid) is common in patients with thyroid dysfunction. Effective examination of the thyroid is critical.
  - The neck should be palpated just below the cricoid cartilage.
  - The patient is asked to swallow, which raises the thyroid and improves the sensitivity of the examination.
  - In general, the left lobe, right lobe, and isthmus should all be examined separately for symmetry, overall size, and the presence of nodules via this mechanism.

HYPERTHYROIDISM

PATHOPHYSIOLOGY

- Hyperthyroidism is a disease of excess thyroid hormone production.
- Most thyrotoxicosis is because of Graves' disease or thyroiditis.
  - Graves' disease causes excess thyroid hormone production through an antibody that activates the TSH receptor on the thyroid gland.
  - Thyroiditis results in increased thyroid-hormone release from a damaged gland.
- Rarely, a toxic ("hot") adenoma, toxic multinodular goiter, factitious hyperthyroidism because of thyroid hormone consumption, or a struma ovarii may be causative.
- Iatrogenic hyperthyroidism is also common among patients taking levothyroxine (LT4) therapy. This can be purposeful (in the treatment of thyroid cancer), or incidentally caused by overprescribing LT4.
- Concurrent or recent amiodarone consumption can also induce thyrotoxicosis through multiple different mechanisms.

CLINICAL PRESENTATION, DIFFERENTIAL, MAKING THE DIAGNOSIS

- Consider the diagnosis of *hyperthyroidism* in patients with signs or symptoms of thyrotoxicosis (Table 37-1) or in those with diseases known to be caused or aggravated by thyrotoxicosis.
- There are several clinical presentations of hyperthyroidism.
  - Most patients will present with signs or symptoms typical of a hypermetabolic state and are classified as having *clinical hyperthyroidism.*
  - *Thyroid storm* is usually caused by rapid release of thyroid hormone (eg, large iodine load withdrawal of antithyroid drugs, treatment with radioactive iodine) in the setting of other illnesses such as surgery, infection, or trauma. Early recognition, prompt hospitalization (usually requires ICU), and consultation with endocrinology are the keys to a successful

TABLE 37-1 Signs and Symptoms of Hyperthyroidism and Hypothyroidism

HYPERTHYROIDISM	HYPOTHYROIDISM
Common symptoms	**Common symptoms**
• Nervousness or emotional lability	• Fatigue and excessive sleep
• Insomnia	• Weight gain
• Increased sweating	• Alopecia
• Heat intolerance	• Cold intolerance and constipation
• Palpitations	• Sluggish affect or depression
• Fatigue	• Bradycardia and fluid retention
• Weight loss	• Delayed deep tendon reflexes
• Hyperdefecation	• Loss of the lateral portion of the
• Menstrual irregularity	eyebrow
Common signs	**Common signs**
• Tremors	• Dry, coarse skin and hair
• Tachycardia or evidence of	• Periorbital puffiness
atrial fibrillation	• Bradycardia
• Proptosis of the eyes or extraocular	• Slow movements and speech
muscle palsy	• Hoarseness
• Stare, lid lag, or signs of Graves' orbitopathy	• Diastolic hypertension
• Goiter	• Goiter
• Pretibial myxedema	• Dementia or confusion

outcome (see section Disease Management Strategies). It is defined as a life-threatening condition manifested by an exaggeration of the clinical signs and symptoms of thyrotoxicosis:

■ Fever (> 38.5°C)
■ Cardiac dysfunction, often with marked tachycardia
■ Gastro hepatic dysfunction (diarrhea, emesis, hepatic failure)
■ Neurologic dysfunction, often with alteration of mental status (ranging from agitation to coma)
■ Systemic decompensation

○ "Apathetic thyrotoxicosis" develops in elderly patients with other disorders and patients describe nonspecific symptoms.

■ Apathetic hyperthyroidism is characterized by a lower frequency of goiter (found in 50%), fewer hyperadrenergic symptoms, and a predominance of cardiac findings including congestive heart failure and atrial fibrillation.
■ Biochemical tests demonstrate classic elevation of free T4 (FT4) with suppressed TSH.

○ Laboratory testing identifies *subclinical hyperthyroidism*.

■ Patients with subclinical hyperthyroidism have a low or undetectable TSH and a normal FT4.
■ Identification is important because subclinical hyperthyroidism can often be followed with periodic thyroid function tests in otherwise healthy patients younger than 60 years old.
■ Clinical assessment of concurrent or recent (within last 3 months) consumption of amiodarone should be queried.

• Patients with *acute nonthyroidal illness* may have TSH suppression that is part of the "euthyroid sick syndrome" and not because of underlying thyrotoxicosis.

○ TSH will be suppressed but the FT4 may be normal, elevated, or low. Most often TSH is not suppressed in acute nonthyroidal illness; rather values of 0.1–0.5 are common. The degree of suppression may correlate with the severity of the acute illness.
○ Additional testing over time is often required to make the diagnosis of euthyroid sick syndrome. Treatment is generally not indicated for euthyroid sick syndrome.

• Diagnostic testing

○ In hyperthyroidism, the TSH is low or undetectable and FT4 concentration is elevated.
○ If the TSH is suppressed and the FT4 normal, measure T3. T3 thyrotoxicosis (suppressed TSH, normal T4, elevated T3) is seen with increased frequency in patients with toxic multinodular goiters and autonomously functioning thyroid nodules.
○ If recent amiodarone consumption or delivery of intravenous iodinated contrast have been excluded as the etiology of hyperthyroidism, *radioactive iodine uptake (RAIU)* is the optimal test to *differentiate* between thyrotoxicosis owing to excess thyroid hormone production (*Graves' disease or a toxic adenoma*) and increased hormone release from a damaged thyroid (*thyroiditis*).

■ An elevated RAIU is consistent with excess thyroid hormone production (Graves' disease or toxic adenoma).

- A suppressed RAIU (usually < 5%) is consistent with hormone release from an inflamed thyroid gland (thyroiditis).
  - *Note—A radioactive iodine test cannot be performed if the patient has received iodinated contrast dye within the last 6 weeks.*
- *Amiodarone-induced hyperthyroidism* is a unique illness. Thyrotoxicosis in this setting can be caused by multiple mechanisms, and diagnostic radionuclide imaging is useless.

DISEASE MANAGEMENT STRATEGIES

- Treatment of hyperthyroidism is directed toward
  - Reducing synthesis and release of hormones from the thyroid
  - Antagonizing peripheral action of excess circulating thyroid hormone
  - Defining and treating the underlying cause
- The risks of hyperthyroidism are primarily related to cardiac function, arrhythmias, bone loss and osteoporosis, and a hypermetabolic state.
- Graves' ophthalmopathy is present in 10% to 25% of affected patients, though subclinical enlargement of extraocular muscles may be present in up to 70% of patients without overt eye disease. Smoking is the greatest modifiable risk factor for ophthalmopathy, and patients should be strongly counseled to avoid all tobacco products and secondhand smoke.
- Pretibial myxedema is a rare complication (< 5%) of Graves' disease.
- Once treated effectively, the overall risk associated with hyperthyroidism can be substantially diminished.
- Early in the treatment of thyrotoxicosis, iodine avoidance (such as contrast agent used in computed tomography [CT] scans) and exercise restriction are recommended.
- Thyroidectomy is a reasonable choice in rare thyrotoxic patients with concomitant suspicious (malignant) nodules and in patients who cannot tolerate or refuse radioactive iodine or antithyroid drugs. If pursued, however, the patient's thyroid status should be normalized prior to surgery.
- Thyrotoxicosis because of *thyroiditis* is managed conservatively because it is often self-limited.
  - Beta-blockers can be used for sympathomimetic symptoms (tachycardia, tremor, and anxiety).
  - Nonsteroidal anti-inflammatory drugs (NSAIDs) and, rarely, glucocorticoids are administered to reduce inflammation and discomfort.
- For patients with *Graves' disease* and *autonomously functioning thyroid nodules*, antithyroid drugs (see below) or radioiodine can be used, though patient preference, age, other comorbidities, severity of thyrotoxicosis, and the presence of Graves' ophthalmopathy must be taken into account.
- Antithyroid drugs are used for primary therapy of thyrotoxicosis, attainment of euthyroidism in preparation for thyroidectomy, and for use prior to radioiodine therapy in selected patients.
- Antithyroid drugs are also preferred to radioactive iodine in the presence of severe Graves' ophthalmopathy and thyroid storm.
- Most patients, however, ultimately select radioiodine as therapy for thyrotoxicosis caused by Graves' disease, toxic multinodular goiter, or autonomously functioning thyroid nodules. Radioiodine is also indicated in patients failing to achieve a remission after a course of antithyroid drugs.
- When antithyroid drugs are prescribed, *methimazole* is effective for most patients and is usually initiated at doses of 20 mg daily (Table 37-2). Individual requirements differ (ranging between 5 mg and 60 mg daily) and are based on periodic evaluation of thyroid function.
- Alternatively, PTU is preferred in pregnant patients and in those with an allergy to methimazole. PTU is frequently initiated at a dose of 100–200 mg three times daily, pending the severity of the illness.
- Pregnant women suffering from thyrotoxicosis should be managed in conjunction with endocrine and high-risk obstetrical consultation.
- With either drug, a baseline hepatic profile and CBC should be obtained. Patients should be counseled for the risk of hepatitis and agranulocytosis, both rare but potentially severe side effects. Patients should be instructed to discontinue the medication and seek medical advice if they develop a fever, sore throat, or other systemic illness after starting an antithyroid drug.
- If immediate control of severe thyrotoxicosis is required, inorganic iodine (*saturated solution of potassium iodine [SSKI]*) can be administered orally and is highly effective. This therapy, however, is self-limited in duration (3 weeks) and precludes further use of radioactive iodine for months thereafter.
- *Thyroid Storm* is managed similarly to other causes of thyrotoxicosis by targeting synthesis and release of thyroid hormone (PTU, methimazole, inorganic iodine), modifying peripheral action of thyroid hormone (beta-blockers, or more aggressive means are hemodialysis or plasmapheresis), and defining and treating precipitant causes. Equally as important is providing supportive care and preventing homeostatic decompensation.

TABLE 37-2 Initial Treatment Regimens for Hyperthyroidism

ETIOLOGY	INITIAL THERAPY
Unregulated production of excessive thyroid hormone	
Possible diagnosis: Graves' disease; functional ("hot") nodule or toxic adenoma; pregnancy (late 1st trimester); amiodarone-induced hyperthyroidism. *Biochemical and laboratory findings:* suppressed TSH; elevated T4 (or T3); **detectable** (or elevated) radioiodine uptake on thyroid scintigraphy. *Exception*: No radioiodine uptake will be detected in cases of amiodarone-induced hyperthyroidism, regardless of cause. **(Note: radionuclide imaging contraindicated in any pregnant individual)**	*If pregnant, involve endocrine and high-risk obstetric consultation.* *If recent amiodarone use within the last 3 months, involve endocrine consultation.* *All other cases, consider* a. Methimazole (starting dose: 20 mg daily; 5–60 mg daily titrated to normalization of FT4 concentration) *or* PTU (starting dose: 100–200 mg thrice daily; 100–900 mg TDD titrated to normalization of FT4 concentration) b. Beta-blocker (titrated to avoid hypotension, yet reduce heart rate modestly) c. SSKI; Inorganic iodine (**rarely needed only in severe cases;** starting dose: 3 drops in 8 oz. Liquid twice daily (7 days)
Release of preformed (stored) thyroid hormone	
Possible diagnosis: silent thyroiditis; postpartum thyroiditis; painful (de Quervain's) thyroiditis. Amiodarone-induced hyperthyroidism. *Biochemical and laboratory findings*: suppressed TSH; elevated T4 (or T3); **undetectable** (or elevated) iodine uptake on thyroid scintigraphy.	*Conservative therapy usually indicated unless patient severely symptomatic* *If recent amiodarone use within the last 3 months, involve endocrine consultation.* *As needed, consider* a. Beta-blocker (titrated to avoid hypotension, yet reduce heart rate modestly) b. Glucocorticoid (rarely needed for severe pain and thyroid inflammation; starting dose prednisone 20 mg twice daily × 7 days)

○ Aggressive treatment of fever with acetaminophen (preferred over salicylates which can displace thyroxine from serum binding proteins and increase free thyroid hormone levels), cooling blankets, or ice packs.

○ Careful monitoring of volume status because excess fluid loss can occur with fever, emesis, and diarrhea and may need to be replaced.

○ Monitoring for congestive heart failure that can be precipitated by atrial tachyarrhythmias, impairing myocardial activity.

○ Impaired adrenocortical reserve should also be contemplated, assessed diagnostically, and possibly treated with glucocorticoids (even if temporary until ruled out).

○ It is critically important to exclude underlying infection. Blood, urine, and possibly spinal fluid cultures in obtunded patients should be collected. In addition, implementing broad-spectrum antibiotics targeting the most likely source should be considered. The antibiotic regimen can be narrowed or discontinued after the culture data are known.

• *Amiodarone-induced hyperthyroidism* should also be managed in conjunction with endocrine consultation given the inability to obtain accurate radionuclide imaging, and the limited therapeutic options available in this unique setting.

CARE TRANSITIONS

• When thyrotoxicosis is caused by *thyroiditis*, repeat analysis of TSH and FT4 should be performed every 4–6 weeks until normalization. The typical pattern of thyrotoxicosis, followed by hypothyroidism, followed by normalization, usually spans 3–4 months.

• Following initiation of treatment for thyrotoxicosis, TSH and FT4 are monitored every 1–3 months for the first 3 months, and every 6–12 months thereafter once stable.

• Radioactive iodine is likely to cause permanent thyroid destruction requiring lifelong LT4 therapy.

HYPOTHYROIDISM

PATHOPHYSIOLOGY

Hypothyroidism is a disease of inadequate production of thyroid hormone.

• The most common causes of hypothyroidism are chronic, lymphocytic thyroiditis (Hashimoto disease), thyroidectomy, and radioactive iodine administration.

- Hashimoto disease is an autoimmune disease that may present at any age, but increases in prevalence with age. Onset is usually insidious and is usually associated with a goiter.
- The presence of thyroid peroxidase antibody (TPO antibody) is highly correlated with the presence of Hashimoto disease and can be useful in confirming the disease, or assessing the risk of developing hypothyroidism in the future.

CLINICAL PRESENTATION, DIFFERENTIAL, MAKING THE DIAGNOSIS

- There are several clinical presentations of hypothyroidism. Most patients will present with signs or symptoms typical of a hypometabolic state and are classified as having *clinical hypothyroidism.*
- In *subclinical hypothyroidism*, patients are asymptomatic, but biochemical testing reveals a mildly elevated TSH (5–10 µU/mL) and a normal FT4. Patients with subclinical hypothyroidism may not require treatment if asymptomatic and not desiring pregnancy (or not currently pregnant).
- *Myxedema coma* is a rare and extreme form of hypothyroidism manifested by features such as delayed reflexes; sparse hair; dry, scaly skin; and puffy facies. It is considered severe, life-threatening hypothyroidism. Frequently, hypothermia (eg, 80°F) or altered mental status is documented.
- In hypothyroidism, the serum TSH is elevated (> 10 µU/mL) in primary hypothyroidism (thyroid gland failure), but very rarely the TSH may be low or normal in conjunction with a low FT4-in secondary hypothyroidism.
- Patients with a mildly elevated TSH (5–10 µU/mL) and a normal FT4 have subclinical hypothyroidism.

DISEASE MANAGEMENT STRATEGIES

- The degree of hypothyroidism should be assessed in affected individuals. Biochemical and clinical parameters often correlate, though at times may be discordant.
- For patients with severe hypothyroidism (TSH > 100 µU/mL), several important facts must be considered in their care and instituting thyroid hormone replacement.
  - Morbidity and mortality in such patients are most often related to simultaneous (though often silent) infection, hypoventilation, or medication overdose.
  - Sedatives and narcotics should be avoided or their doses significantly reduced given reduced drug clearance caused by hypothyroidism.
  - Severely myxedematous patients should be considered for prophylactic antibiotic medication.
  - Additionally, the possibility of adrenal insufficiency should be considered in patients with severe hypothyroidism or myxedema. Until adrenal insufficiency is excluded, concomitant treatment of thyroid hormone and glucocorticoids should be considered.
- LT4 is the preferred treatment of hypothyroidism, and it safely, effectively, and reliably relieves symptoms and normalizes lab tests in hypothyroid patients (Table 37-3).
- LT4 is converted to T3 (the active hormone) primarily in peripheral tissues at an appropriate rate for overall metabolic needs.
- Treatment with a combination of LT4 and LT3 is not recommended, except in cases of life-threatening myxedema coma.
- While all patients with overt hypothyroidism (TSH > 10 µU/mL) should be treated, there is limited evidence that treatment of subclinical hypothyroidism is beneficial in nonpregnant patients.
- A full replacement dose of LT4 can be approximated by multiplying 1.7 µg/d by patient weight (kg).
- The severity of hypothyroidism should determine the urgency for replacement therapy.
- When possible, however, a modest dose of LT4 (50–75 µg daily) is preferred during the first week of therapy in those patients who are not in acute danger.
- An acute rise in thyroid hormone concentration can induce increased cardiac demand (and potential ischemia) or arrhythmias in predisposed patients. For this reason, caution should be exercised in those with known coronary artery disease or in patients over 80 years of age.
- *Mild-to-moderate hypothyroidism* can often be treated with 50–75 µg of LT4 daily.

TABLE 37-3   Therapy for Hypothyroidism

- LT4 is the preferred therapy for hypothyroidism. Combination T3/T4 therapy is not recommended except in cases of life-threatening, severe hypothyroidism.
- Full replacement of LT4 can be estimated: 1.7 µg/d × patient weight (kg).
- Most patients with Hashimoto's disease are normalized with LT4 doses 50–100 µg daily.
- Because LT4 replacement can worsen cardiac ischemia or induce arrhythmia, rapid replacement of LT4 should be avoided in the elderly unless the patient is severely ill. Clinical judgment must be used.

- At present, most patients can be safely monitored with TSH measurements every 4–6 months, evaluating for progression of disease. This recommendation excludes women seeking pregnancy or currently pregnant, who should be treated once TSH is outside the normal range because of greater maternal and fetal risk.

CARE TRANSITIONS

- Once LT4 treatment is initiated for hypothyroidism, therapy is usually lifelong.
- Serum TSH should be monitored 6–8 weeks after initiating therapy, and adjustments made to obtain a TSH value within the normal range.
- A full replacement dose of LT4 is approximately 1.7 μg/kg, though many patients require less because of remaining partial thyroid function.

THYROID NODULAR DISEASE

- Thyroid nodules are common, especially in women. The prevalence of thyroid nodules increases with age.
- Differentiating patients with malignant nodules from those with benign nodules is critical.
  - Typically, although important, does not require emergent consideration. except in those with very large nodules (> 4–5 cm), or those with acute respiratory compromise.
  - Thus, testing of most thyroid nodules detected (either by palpation or incidentally during other radiology studies) in hospitalized patients can be postponed until after the patient has recovered from any acute illness that resulted in the current hospitalization.
  - This recommendation excludes scenarios in which the thyroid nodule is likely contributing to ongoing symptoms, or preventing recovery.
- The initial evaluation of a thyroid nodule is an assessment of thyroid function.
  - This is most accurately measured by obtaining a serum TSH measurement. Patients with suppressed TSH levels (~ 5% to 10%) may have an autonomously

functioning nodule. This is important because such nodules pose virtually no risk of being cancerous.
  - Patients with TSH values normal or elevated should be considered for fine needle aspiration for full diagnostic evaluation.
- Prior to patient discharge, a follow-up appointment with an endocrinologist should be arranged for further evaluation.

BIBLIOGRAPHY

Alexander EK, Marqusee E, Lawrence J, et al. Timing and magnitude of increases in levothyroxine requirements during pregnancy in women with hypothyroidism. *N Engl J Med.* 2004; 351:241–249.

American Association of Clinical Endocrinologists medical guidelines for clinical practice for the evaluation and treatment of hyperthyroidism and hypothyroidism. *Endocr Pract.* 2002;8(6):457–469.

Bartalena L, Bogazzi F, Pecori F, et al. Graves' disease occurring after subacute thyroiditis: report of a case and review of the literature. *Thyroid.* 1996;6:345–348.

Cooper DS. Drug therapy: antithyroid drugs. *N Engl J Med.* 2005; 352:905–917.

Fatourechi V, Aniszewski JP, Fatourechi GZ, et al. Clinical features and outcome of subactue thyroiditis in an incidence cohort: Olmsted County, Minnesota. *J Clin Endocrinol Metab.* 2003;88:2100–2105.

Fish LH, Schwartz HL, Cavanaugh J, et al. Replacement dose, metabolism, and bioavailability of levothyroxine in the treatment of hypothyroidism. Role of triiodothyronine in pituitary feedback in humans. *N Engl J Med.* 1987;316:764–770.

Holm IA, Manson JE, Michels KB, et al. Smoking and other lifestyle factors and the risk of Graves' hyperthyroidism. *Arch Intern Med.* 2005;165:1606–1611.

Ringel MD. Management of hypothyroidism and hyperthyroidism in the intensive care unit. *Crit Care Clin.* 2001; 17:59–74.

Surks MI, Ortiz E, Daniels GH, et al. Subclinical thyroid disease. Scientific review and guidelines for diagnosis and management. *JAMA.* 2004;291:228–238.

Toft AD. Thyroxine therapy. *N Engl J Med.* 1994;331:174.

Wartofsky L. Acute presentation of thyroid disease. In: Wachter RM, Goldman L, Hollander H, eds. *Hospital Medicine.* Baltimore, MD: Williams & Wilkins; 2005.

Woeber K. Update on the management of hyperthyroidism and hypothyroidism. *Arch Fam Med.* 2000;9:743–747.

GASTROINTESTINAL ILLNESS

38 ABDOMINAL PAIN
Norton J. Greenberger

EPIDEMIOLOGY/OVERVIEW

- Abdominal pain is a very frequent complaint in patients of all age groups. Five percent of all patient visits to a PCP are for abdominal pain.
- In the emergency department (ED) or PCP's office, the goal is appropriate triage.
- The vast majority of patients, particularly those with chronic abdominal pain, will have benign reasons for abdominal pain (such as irritable bowel syndrome) and can most often be evaluated in the outpatient setting.
- Hospitalists are often involved in the care of patients presenting with the acute onset of abdominal pain, as such patients typically require observation or admission to a hospital to rule out or differentiate between various etiologies with potentially high morbidity and mortality if not promptly recognized and treated.
- Abdominal pain can also occur in hospitalized patients, often severely ill, admitted originally for a different diagnosis. For example, acalculous cholecystitis frequently occurs in critically ill or postoperative patients.

CLINICAL PRESENTATION, DIFFERENTIAL, MAKING THE DIAGNOSIS

- Dictums in the approach to the patient with acute abdominal pain:
  - An orderly, painstakingly detailed history is vital, especially the chronologic sequence of events.
    - Have the patient accurately describe the nature of the pain. Supply adjectives of the patient's description, whenever vague.
    - Try to determine if pain is colicky.
    - In addition to location, radiation, precipitants, relievants, ask about other symptoms, that is, anorexia, nausea, emesis, diarrhea, previous similar symptoms, weight loss.
    - The onset, frequency, and duration of pain are important features. For example, the pain of pancreatitis is typically gradual and steady while

rupture of a viscus with resultant peritonitis begins suddenly and is maximal from the onset.
    - Ask about factors that can precipitate, aggravate, or relieve the pain. Eating can trigger pain of mesenteric ischemia. Antacids reduce pain of esophageal reflux. Pancreatitis pain is partially relieved by sitting in a knee-chest position.
    - Does the trip to the hospital by car aggravate symptoms? If yes, suspect a disorder causing peritoneal irritation.
    - Ask about medications such as NSAIDs, acetyl-salicyclic acid (ASA), ethanol, family history (FH) of gallbladder disease, inflammatory bowel disease (IBD), recent travel, meals in restaurants and family members with similar symptoms.
    - In women, ask about menstrual cycle, possible pregnancy, sexual activity, oral contraceptive use.
    - Note the areas where visceral pain can be referred (Fig. 38-1).
  - Abdominal examination
    - Personally check all vital signs, temperature, pulse, respirations, blood pressure, oxygen saturation and pain score.
    - Have the patient try and distinguish between *pressure* and *pain* as you examine all quadrants of the abdomen. Standing over the patient, press firmly on the level of the right humerus as the reference point for pressure and ask the patient to distinguish between pressure and pain as all nine areas of the abdomen are gently palpated.

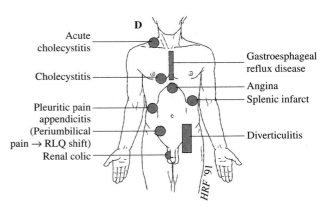

FIG. 38-1 Referred pain.

■ Try to determine if abdominal pain is originating from an intra-abdominal source or the anterior abdominal wall. In Carnett's sign the patient tenses abdominal muscles by flexing the neck and if this maneuver increases pain it is originating from the anterior abdominal wall and vice versa if pain is intra-abdominal. Anterior abdominal wall pain is frequently attributable to a rectus sheath hematoma in patients on anticoagulants.

■ If abnormalities (tenderness, fullness, mass) are found in one area, check the contralateral area of the abdomen to confirm that it is different.

■ Percussion can be used to determine liver size, spleen size, and distended bladder. Solid organs give a dull sound when percussed.

■ Try to determine if palpable bowel is "thickened" in the right upper quadrant (RUQ) and left lower quadrant (LLQ).

■ Listen for bowel sounds, bruits, rubs, and so forth.

■ Listen for a succussion splash; if present suspect gastric outlet obstruction.

○ In addition to a detailed abdominal examination, careful pelvic and rectal examinations are *mandatory* for every patient with acute abdominal pain.

○ The possibility of an intrathoracic lesion must be considered in every patient with abdominal pain, especially if pain is in the upper abdomen.

○ Laboratory and imaging studies may be of considerable value, but they may not establish the diagnosis (eg, WBC count, imaging studies).

○ Sometimes, even under the best of circumstances, a definitive diagnosis cannot be established at the time of the initial examination.

○ Contrary to earlier beliefs, administration of analgesics does not obfuscate the diagnosis and should not be withheld if a patient is experiencing severe pain.

• For the differential diagnosis of abdominal pain and keys to making the diagnosis, please see Tables 38-1 and 38-2.

DISEASE MANAGEMENT STRATEGIES

• Many of the diagnoses causing abdominal pain that are commonly seen by hospitalists are discussed in more detail in other chapters: viral gastroenteritis (Chap. 59; colitis and diarrhea, including *Clostridium difficile* (Chap. 41); Crohn's disease (Chap. 42); ulcerative colitis (Chap. 43); diverticular disease and diverticulitis (Chap. 44); abnormal liver enzymes and acute hepatitis (Chap. 39); pancreatitis (Chap. 45); small bowel obstruction (Chap. 46).

TABLE 38-1 Differential Diagnosis of Acute Abdominal Pain

COMMON CONDITIONS	KEY DIAGNOSTIC TEST(S)
Acute appendicitis*	CT scan (see text)
Acute cholecystitis*	Ultrasound
Acute diverticulitis*	CT scan
Acute pancreatitis*	Serum amylase/lipase CT scan
Perforated peptic ulcer*	CT scan
Ruptured aneurysm*	Imaging procedure
Acute mesenteric ischemia*	CT angiogram
Ischemic colitis	Colonoscopy
Intestinal obstruction*	Flat film, imaging study
Renal colic	CT scan, U/A
IBD	Endoscopy, imaging studies
Anterior abdominal wall pain	Carnett's sign (see text)
Acute infectious enteritis	History; stool studies
Splenic infarct*	Imaging procedure
Nonsurgical disorders simulating an acute abdomen (see text)	See Table 38-2
Acute abdominal pain in women • Pelvic inflammatory disease • Ectopic pregnancy • Adnexal pathology	Pelvic examination, pelvic ultrasound

*Surgical consultation indicated.

• Imaging is used to diagnose the underlying cause of the acute abdomen; however, a targeted history and physical examination is still required to determine the best initial imaging modality.

• In general, plain radiography has limited value. Several studies suggest that plain radiography has contributed to management in only 4% of cases despite important information present in 66% of films.

○ If a patient has diffuse abdominal pain, an erect chest film to diagnosis pneumoperitoneum still appears to have value.

○ *Kidneys, ureter, bladder (KUB) and uprightradiographs (x-rays)*—On supine x-ray intraperitoneal air collects under Morrison's pouch (inferior surface of liver or hepatorenal abscess)

■ Capula sign is air under central tendon of abdomen

■ Rigler's sign is visibility of both sides of the bowel wall

■ *Conditions simulating air under the diaphragm include*—Chilaiditi's syndrome (interposition of colon between liver and diaphragm manifesting as air but bowel markings are present), subphrenic abscess, subdiaphragmatic fat, basal curvilinear atelectasis.

○ Free air is evident in only 70% to 80% of perforated peptic ulcer.

○ A normal KUB does not exclude a small bowel obstruction because it takes up to 24 hours for the changes to develop on KUB.

TABLE 38-2 Nonsurgical Disorders Simulating the Acute Abdomen

NONSURGICAL DISORDERS	KEY DIAGNOSTIC FEATURES
METABOLIC	
• Diabetes mellitus	Elevated blood glucose; ketoacidosis
• Hyperthyroidism	Elevated T4 decreased TSH
• Porphyria	Elevated porphobilinogen, delta amino levulinic acid
• Familial mediterranean fever	Episodes last 1–3 days, may have pleuritis/peritonitis
• Hypercalcemia	Elevated blood calcium
• Hypokalemia	Decreased serum potassium
• Heavy metal poisoning (As, Pb, etc.)	Screen for heavy metals
• Hypophosphatemia	Decreased serum phosphorous
CONNECTIVE TISSUE DISEASES	
• Vasculitis	Systemic multiorgan disease ↑ ESR, (+) ANA, (+) P-ANCA
• SLE	> 4 of 11 criteria for SLE diagnosis are met
• Scleroderma	Skin lesions, Raynaud's phenomenon, visceral involvement
IMMUNOLOGIC	
• Anaphylaxis	Identify insult (drugs, foods, insect sting)
• Hereditary angioneurotic edema	Decrease Cl inhibitor activity
• Hemolytic uremic syndrome	Renal failure, schistocytes on peripheral smear
• Henoch-Schönlein purpura	Skin biopsy → leukocytoclastic vasculitis IgA and C3 deposition
• Systemic mast cell disease	Increased serum tryptase; increased mast cells in biopsies
MISCELLANEOUS	
• Pneumonia	Lower lobes, physical examination, x-ray
• Papillary necrosis	Consider in sickle cell crisis, obstructive uropathy, diabetes with urinary tract infection
• Sickle cell crisis	History, periarticular pain, effusions
• Herpes zoster	Pain and rash in dermatomal distribution
• Pseudo obstruction	Dilated bowel without mechanical process identified
• Lower rib margin syndrome	Reproduction of pain with pressure on rib margin
• Epiploic appendagitis	CT scan

Abbreviations: SLE, systemic lupus erythematosus; ANA, antinuclear antibodies; ANCA, antineutrophil cytoplasmic antibody.

- The amount of gas normally seen on KUB is <2.5 cm in the small bowel and <5.5 cm in the large bowel. The cecum can be somewhat larger, up to 8 cm. If on plain film the diameter of the small bowel is greater than 3 cm, it suggests either an obstruction or an ileus.
- The key to the differentiation of colonic obstruction and paralytic ileus on a plain abdominal film is whether there is dilatation of the cecum. The cecum is the most dilated segment of the colon in obstruction. If the transverse colon is more dilated than the cecum, a diagnosis of ileus is most likely.
- Megacolon refers to a dilatation of the transverse colon greater than 6 cm. When there is acute colonic distention (cecum greater than 9 cm), then there is an imminent risk of perforation. The plain film may be an useful adjunct to serial examinations in patients at risk for megacolon.
- Gas in the inguinal region may suggest a strangulated hernia.
- Omega loop sign suggests sigmoid volvulus (massively dilated loop of colon that looks like an inverted U projecting out of the pelvis toward the RUQ). Sigmoid volvulus is about three times more common than cecal volvulus.
- If dilated small bowel extends to the lower portion of the abdomen, it indicates that the obstruction is at least in the distal small bowel or perhaps in the proximal colon. If air is seen distally in the colon or rectum, either a partial small bowel obstruction or an acute complete small bowel obstruction may be present as some of the air distal to the obstruction site has not been expelled.
- The presence of air-fluid levels are not pathognomic of obstruction. Causes of air-fluid levels include ileus, obstruction, gastroenteritis, ischemia, hypokalemia, uremia, and it is also seen in normal individuals.
  - When kidney stones are suspected, the KUB will only detect 50% of ureteral stones because of low density and small size of many stones.
  - If you are planning to obtain an abdominal CT (CT) anyway in the ED, skip the plain abdominal x-ray.
- Helical CT is very sensitive for identifying the presence and location of a high-grade small bowel obstruction (dilated proximal small bowel >2.5 cm

with normal caliber distal small bowel), the presence of appendicitis as the cause of right lower quadrant (RLQ) pain, when there is a search for metastatic disease or when the differential diagnosis of abdominal pain is broad.

- ○ While ultrasound (US) is a targeted examination looking at the biliary tree or ovarian structures, CT offers a more comprehensive analysis of the liver and extrahepatic abdomen and pelvis.
- ○ CT is better than US for detecting small abscesses as well as for identifying extrahepatic collections. Portal venous air is more readily detected by CT.
- ○ For obstructive jaundice either US or CT can be used to rule out an obstructive lesion of the common bile duct (CBD) and equally reliable in identifying the level of obstruction, but CT is better for evaluation of liver, biliary tree, pancreas, portal and retroperitoneal lymph nodes, and vascular structures.
  - ▪ The upper limit of the CBD is usually <4 mm in diameter.
  - ▪ With age the CBD becomes slightly dilated, up to 7 mm in patients less than 60 years, and up to 10 mm in patients more than 60 years.
  - ▪ The CBD may be up to 6–7 mm if the patient has had a prior cholecystectomy.
- ○ CT is less operator dependent and faster. For nonradiologists, CT is easier to read and understand.
- ○ Contrast-enhanced helical CT is performed with IV, oral, and rectal contrast. Aspiration pneumonitis from vomiting gastrografin is a risk of using oral contrast in high-grade small bowel obstruction and can be severe.
- US is the preferred method for diagnostic imaging of the liver and biliary tree in patients with acute RUQ pain.
  - ○ CT is less reliable for demonstrating gallbladder abnormalities and detecting gallstones, since cholesterol gallstones have the same density as bile.
  - ○ For choledocholithiasis, the sensitivity of US is lower than for gallstones and gas in the duodenum can obscure visualization of the distal CBD. CT has a similar sensitivity.
- Magnetic resonance imaging (MRI) is used to evaluate abdominal pain but not as an initial test.
  - ○ MRI cholangiography is greater than 90% sensitive for detecting choledocholithiasis and is an alternative to endoscopic retrograde cholangiopancreatography (ERCP) in patients unlikely to benefit from a therapeutic intervention such as stone extraction or papillotome. No contrast is administered because of native high signal intensity of fluid on T2-weighted images.

- ○ MRI without contrast enhancement has a 85% sensitivity for detecting liver cancer and about 75% sensitivity for detecting individual lesions. MRI can identify more than 90% of hepatic hemangiomas and the vast majority of cases of focal nodular hyperplasia.

ACUTE APPENDICITIS

- Classical sequence of symptoms (50% to 60% patients)
  - ○ *Abdominal pain*—Almost invariably the initial symptom
    - ▪ Frequently poorly localized to epigastrium and periumbilical area
    - ▪ Reaches peak of intensity 4–6 hours, then may subside
    - ▪ Reappears in RLQ as progressively severe steady pain aggravated by motion or cough
  - ○ *Anorexia, nausea, vomiting (90%)*—Presence of hunger distinctly unusual
  - ○ *Abdominal tenderness*—Found in location corresponding to location of appendix (abdomen, flank, pelvic)
    - ▪ Percussion, rebound tenderness, referred rebound tenderness
  - ○ *Fever*—Typically low grade (99.5°F–100.5°F)
  - ○ Laboratory
    - ▪ WBC of 10,000–16,000
    - ▪ Appendoliths (5%)
- Atypical appendicitis
  - ○ Retrocecal and retroileal appendicitis
    - ▪ Inflamed appendix shielded from anterior abdominal wall; therefore, less pain and less discomfort on walking or coughing.
    - ▪ Classic shift of pain from epigastrium to RLQ may not occur.
    - ▪ Muscular rigidity is absent and abdominal tenderness is minimal.
    - ▪ Pain may remain so poorly localized that diagnosis of appendicitis is overlooked.
  - ○ Pelvic peritonitis
    - ▪ Pain, often severe, is a constant symptom.
    - ▪ Pain begins in epigastrium but quickly settles in lower abdomen.
    - ▪ Pain may localize in LLQ rather than RLQ.
    - ▪ Urge to defecate and urinate are prominent symptoms.
    - ▪ Absence of abdominal tenderness is deceptive.
    - ▪ Tenderness must be sought by rectal and pelvic examinations.

○ *Appendicitis in the elderly*—The diagnosis is often overlooked because symptoms and signs are often mild.
  ▪ Pain is often minimal or even absent.
  ▪ Abdominal tenderness may be deceptively mild.
  ▪ Shift of pain to the RLQ occurs only in 20% of cases.
  ▪ Temperature may be only slightly elevated.
  ▪ Appendicitis can present with a painless mass (appendiceal abscess)
  ▪ *Imaging*—Should diagnostic imaging be performed if the clinical presentation is highly suggestive of the disease?
  ▪ Yes. See Table 38-3. Even in patients with a clinically high probability of acute appendicitis, cross-sectional imaging should be performed because it will accurately detect one-third of patients with another diagnosis or normal findings.

PERFORATED PEPTIC ULCER

• Clinical manifestations of the typical presentation
  ○ In most patients, it is clear that an intra-abdominal catastrophic event has occurred.
  ○ The patient will be tachycardic and hypotensive.
  ○ The pain of perforation begins suddenly and is severe, excruciating, agonizing. Pain initially is epigastric and RUQ, later spreads.
  ○ Abdominal tenderness is marked, abdomen is rigid and board-like, rebound tenderness is usual, and bowel sounds are diminished or absent.
  ○ Classic "lull" may supervene followed by increased signs of peritonitis, bowel and abdominal distention, and hypovolemia.
  ○ *Diagnostic studies*—Elevated WBC and serum amylase (16%), with marked increase in erythrocyte sedimentation rate (ESR) seen with larger perforations; radiographic evidence of pneumoperitoneum (75%).

• Atypical features may be seen when the ulcer seals soon after perforation, resulting in less intense pain and more subtle abdominal findings.
  ○ Pneumoperitoneum must usually be present to establish the diagnosis.
  ○ Spillage from early sealing/slowly leaking perforation may track to the right into the gutter and cecal fossa resulting in RLQ pain simulating acute appendicitis.
  ○ With posterior perforation there is spillage into the lesser sac, resulting in less severe symptoms plus back pain.
  ○ Undiagnosed perforation sometimes occurs in neuropsychiatric patients, especially schizophrenics, and in elderly patients, who may not complain of abdominal pain. Therefore perforated viscus must be included in the differential diagnosis in such patients with unexplained shock.
• Treatment is surgical.

ACUTE CHOLECYSTITIS

• Gallstones, often asymptomatic, are common after the age of 40 (20% of women and 8% of men).
• Typical presentation is acute RUQ pain (pain can also be RLQ, epigastric, or LUQ in 15%), possibly associated with eating, especially fatty foods. Pain may radiate to the back and/or right shoulder.
• Murphy's sign is a diagnostic maneuver on physical examination (while palpating the RUQ in the region of the gallbladder fossa, ask the patient to take a deep breath—increased pain often associated with abrupt cessation of the deep inspiration as the inflamed gallbladder descends to hit the fingertips is a positive Murphy's sign).
  ○ The sensitivity of a positive Murphy's sign is only 27% and imaging is required to diagnose the cause of RUQ pain.

TABLE 38-3   Appendicitis—Should Diagnostic Imaging be Performed if the Clinical Presentation is Highly Suggestive of the Disease?

DEFINITE DX	LOW PROBABILITY N = 109	INTERMEDIATE PROBABILITY N = 97	HIGH PROBABILITY N = 144
Acute appendicitis	11 (10%)	23 (24%)	99 (65%)
Other diagnoses	34 (31%)	37 (38%)	26 (18%)
• IBD	7 (6%)	9 (9%)	6 (4%)
• Enteritis	15 (14%)	8 (8%)	1 (< 1%)
• Acute right-sided diverticulitis	0	1 (1%)	5 (3%)
• Ovarian cyst	3 (3%)	3 (3%)	1 (< 1%)
Normal findings	64 (59%)	37 (38%)	24 (17%)

SOURCE: Data were modified from Rettenbacher T, et al. Appendicitis: should diagnostic imaging be performed if the clinical presentation is highly suggestive of the disease? *Gastroenterology.* 2002;123:992–998.

- Diagnostic testing
  - *Labs*—Serum bilirubin is usually <4 mg/dL unless the patient has choledocholithiasis; liver tests may only be transiently abnormal (aspartate aminotransferase [AST]/alanine aminotransferase [ALT] > 400 U/L in 10% cases, mimicking viral hepatitis).
  - Abnormal RUQ US (95% sensitivity for gallstones).
- Differential diagnosis includes
  - *Mirizzi syndrome*—Distended gallbladder (cystic duct stone) compresses the CBD simulating obstructive jaundice.
  - *Ascending cholangitis*—Jaundice with sepsis picture; urgent need to decompress biliary tree (ERCP, percutaneous cholecystotomy, cholecystectomy).
  - Acalculous cholecystitis (see section Acalculous Cholecystitis).
- Treatment
  - *Rationale for antibiotic use*—In a study of 167 patients, positive bile cultures were found in 22% of patients with symptomatic gallstones and in 46% of patients with acute cholecystitis.
    - The most frequent isolates were *Escherichia coli* (41%), enterococcus (12%), *Klebsiella* (11%), and enterobacter (9%).
    - Appropriate empiric IV antibiotic regimens include piperacillin/tazobactam 3.375–4.5 g q6 hours) or ampicillin/sulbactam (3 g q6 hours); metronidazole (500 mg q8 hours) plus a fluoroquinolone (ciprofloxacin 400 mg q12 hours) particularly in the penicillin-allergic patient. Specific choices are often determined by local formulary availability and should take into account renal dysfunction and relative cost.
    - De-escalate antibiotic therapy after results of blood and/or bile cultures are known.
  - Ketorolac (30–60 mg IM or IV) often provides effective analgesia.
  - The type and timing of definitive management (elimination of gallstones) is determined by surgical risk.
    - In low-risk patients (ASA class I or II), cholecystectomy can be pursued after 24–48 hours of supportive care and antibiotics.
    - In high-risk patients (ASA class III and above), non-surgical options (dissolution therapy, lithotripsy) subsequent to hospitalization may be appropriate. However, if the patient fails to respond to supportive care and antibiotics, or develops complications (gangrenous cholecystitis, perforation), percutaneous cholecystostomy should be considered.
    - Patients with choledocholithiasis (a gallstone in the CBD) may also benefit from endoscopic management.

ACALCULOUS CHOLECYSTITIS

- Risk factors for acalculous cholecystitis include diabetes mellitus, sepsis, cholesterol emboli, immunosuppression, opiates, TPN, infections, major trauma, nonbiliary surgery, burns, mechanical ventilation.
- Clinical presentation
  - In a critically ill patient who may be intubated and sedated, the appearance of unexplained fever and elevated WBC associated with often vague abdominal discomfort may be the only clues.
  - In less critically ill patients the presentation may be similar to that seen in calculous cholecystitis.
  - A RUQ mass and jaundice may provide additional clues to the diagnosis in 20% of patients.
- *Diagnosis is by US*—Findings include an absence of gallstones, thickening of the gallbladder wall (> 5 mm), pericholecystic fluid, positive Murphy's sign with the US probe. Emphysematous cholecystitis is associated with gas bubbles seen in gallbladder fundus ("Champagne sign"). Failure to visualize the gallbladder on hepatobiliary iminodiacetic acid (HIDA) scan is also diagnostic, but this test is not recommended in critically ill patients.
- Treatment
  - Empiric antibiotics (see options under acute cholecystitis) should be initiated as soon as the diagnosis is clinically suspected.
  - Urgent surgical or interventional radiology consultation for more definitive therapy (cholecystectomy, cholecystostomy) should be obtained as soon as the diagnosis is established.

BIBLIOGRAPHY

Greenberger NJ. Sorting through non-surgical causes of acute abdominal pain. *J Crit Illn.* 1992;7:1–6.

Greenberger NJ. Techniques for physician assessment of acute abdominal pain. *J Crit Illn.* 1994;9:397–404.

Greenberger NJ. The abdomen in history taking and physical examination. Essentials and clinical correlates. *Mosby Yearbook.* 1992;199–261.

Rettenbacher T, Hollerweger A, Gritzmann N, et al. Appendicitis: should diagnostic imaging be performed if the clinical presentation is highly suggestive of the disease? *Gastroenterology.* 2002;123:992–998.

Silen W. Abdominal pain. In: *Harrison's Principles of Internal Medicine.* 16th ed. New York, NY: McGraw-Hill: 2005: 82–84.

39 ABNORMAL LIVER ENZYMES AND ACUTE HEPATITIS

Mary Ann H. Sherbondy

EPIDEMIOLOGY/OVERVIEW

- Abnormal liver enzymes encompass the continuum from asymptomatic clinic patient to the patient who presents in fulminant hepatic failure (FHF).
- An estimated 8.1% of population have an abnormal ALT or AST level.
- Acquiring a complete medical history is the most important portion of evaluation.
- Physical examination may help point to a diagnosis.

CLINICAL PRESENTATION, DIFFERENTIAL, MAKING THE DIAGNOSIS

- Patient presentation may range from RUQ pain and jaundice to malaise to no symptoms at all.
- Obtaining a thorough medical history is essential for making a diagnosis, particularly the following:
  ○ Use or exposure to any chemicals or medications, especially over-the-counter and herbal medications
  ○ Duration of abnormalities in liver enzymes
  ○ Associated symptoms, such as jaundice, arthralgias, weight loss, pruritus, fevers
- Obtain a thorough social history, including remote history of illicit drug use and alcohol use.
- Physical examination may narrow the differential diagnosis in a patient.
  ○ Presence of stigmata of chronic liver disease (ie, spider angioma, palmar erythema).
  ○ Tender hepatomegaly, suggesting acute hepatitis secondary to virus or alcohol.
  ○ Other physical findings may help point to a non-hepatic cause of abnormal liver enzymes.
    ▪ Jugular venous distention accompanied by hepatomegaly, pointing toward congestive hepatopathy
    ▪ Lymphadenopathy pointing toward malignancy
- In eliciting the cause of abnormal liver enzymes, a detailed history and physical examination is essential (Fig. 39-1).
  ○ Past medical and surgical history
    ▪ History of diseases associated with liver disease

History and physical examination
Past medical history
Medication history
Social history
FH

Laboratory studies
Viral markers (hepatitis BsAg, hep BcAb, hep C Ab)
Autoimmune markers (ANA, ASMA, ALKM, AMA)
Iron studies (Fe/TIBC, ferritin)
Ceruloplasmin (patients < 40 years of age)
Alpha-1 antitrypsin level

Imaging study
US
Dual phase CT scan
MRI

Liver biopsy

FIG. 39-1 Algorithm for workup of abnormal liver enzymes.

- Ulcerative colitis → Primary sclerosing cholangitis
- Autoimmune disease (ie, rheumatoid arthritis, lupus) → autoimmune hepatitis, primary biliary cirrhosis
- Diabetes and hyperlipidemia → Nonalcoholic fatty liver disease
  ○ Medications, both prescription and over-the-counter medications
    ▪ Imperative to ask about herbal medications as many people do not consider these preparations harmful (Table 39-1)
  ○ Social history
    ▪ History of alcohol use

TABLE 39-1 Herbal Products that may Lead to Acute Liver Failure

Bai-Fang herbs
Chaparral
Comfrey
Germander
Greater celandine
Gum Thistle
Heliotrope
He Shon Wu
Impila
Jin Bu Huan
Kava kava
LipoKinetix
Ma Huang
Pennyroyal
Rattleweed
Senecio
Skullcap
Sunnhemp

TABLE 39-2   Hepatocellular Liver Injury—Elevated Transaminases

Hepatic sources
  Medications
  Alcohol abuse
  Viral hepatitis (hepatitis B and C)
  Hereditary hemochromatosis
  NAFD
  Autoimmune hepatitis
  Wilson's disease
  Alpha-1 antitrypsin deficiency

Nonhepatic causes
  Muscle disorders
  Thyroid disorders
  Celiac disease
  Adrenal insufficiency
  Anorexia nervosa

- History of illicit drug use, including both intravenous drugs and intranasal cocaine
- Sexual history, identifying sexual partners with high-risk behavior (ie, IV drug users) and men having sex with men
- FH
- A history of undefined liver disease could be unrecognized hemochromatosis
- A FH of psychiatric or neurologic disease in younger members could be unrecognized Wilson's disease
- In establishing a differential diagnosis, it is important to establish the pattern of abnormal liver enzymes.
  - Pattern of hepatocellular injury (Table 39-2)
  - Pattern of cholestatic liver disease (Table 39-3)

TRIAGE AND INITIAL MANAGEMENT

ACUTE HEPATITIS

- The patient who presents with acute hepatitis requires the most immediate attention as patients with FHF should be identified early and transferred to a transplant center if necessary.
- Common causes of acute hepatitis
  - Transaminases < 500 U/L
    - Alcoholic hepatitis (AST/ALT ratio often 2:1)
    - Viral hepatitis
    - Transaminases > 500 U/L
    - Viral hepatitis
      - Hepatitis A, B, D, E
      - Herpes hepatitis
      - Cytomegalovirus
      - Epstein-Barr virus

TABLE 39-3   Cholestatic Liver Disease—Elevated Alkaline Phosphatase and Bilirubin

Hyperbilirubinemia
Conjugated
  Extrahepatic cholestasis
    Choledocholithiasis
    Primary sclerosing cholangitis
    AIDS cholangiopathy
    Acute and chronic pancreatitis
    Biliary strictures
    Parasitic infections (i.e., ascaris lumbricoides)
  Intrahepatic cholestasis
    Viral hepatitis
    Alcoholic hepatitis
    Nonalcoholic steatohepatitis
    Primary biliary cirrhosis
    Drugs and toxins
    Sepsis
    Infiltrative diseases
    TPN
    Hepatic crisis in sickle cell disease

Unconjugated
  Increased bilirubin production
    Hemolysis
  Impaired bilirubin uptake
    Congestive heart failure
    Gilbert's syndrome
    Portosystemic shunts
  Medications
  Impaired bilirubin conjugation
    Crigler-Najjar syndrome
    Gilbert's syndrome
    Hyperthyroidism
    Chronic liver disease

Elevated alkaline phosphatase and/or gamma-glutamyl transpeptidase
  Primary biliary cirrhosis
  Primary sclerosing cholangitis
  Bile duct obstruction
  Adult bile ductopenia
  Medications (i.e., steroids, phenytoin)
  Non-hepatic source
    Bone
    Placenta in pregnant women in 3rd trimester

- Autoimmune hepatitis
- Drug-induced liver injury
- Ischemia or hypoperfusion

ACUTE/FULMINANT HEPATIC FAILURE

- Acute liver failure is defined by acute liver injury associated with impaired hepatic synthetic function and encephalopathy developing within 6 weeks in a patient with previous normal liver function.
- An estimated 2000 patients present in FHF in the United States per year.

TABLE 39-4 King's College Criteria for Acute Liver Failure

Acetaminophen toxicity
  Arterial pH < 7.3
    Or
  PT > 6.5
  Serum Cr 3.4 mg/dL
  Grade III/IV encephalopathy

Nonacetaminophen toxicity
  PT > 100 seconds
  Or (any three. of the following)
  Drug toxicity
  Age < 10 years or > 40 years
  Jaundice to coma in 7 days
  PT > 50 seconds
  Serum bilirubin > 17.5 mg/dL

Abbreviation: PT, prothrombin time.

- Most prominent causes of FHF
  - Drug-induced liver injury
  - Viral hepatitis
  - Autoimmune liver disease

Presentation in acute hepatitis
Medical history
Social history
Physical examination

Initial laboratory analysis
Liver enzymes
Chemistry 7
PT/INR
Arterial blood gas
Arterial lactate
CBC
Type and screen
Acetaminophen level
Toxicology screen
Viral serologies
(hepatitis A Ab IgM, hep BsAg, hep BcIgM, hepatitis E Ab, hepatitis C Ab)
Ceruloplasmin
Pregnancy test
Arterial ammonia
Autoimmune markers
HIV status
Amylase and lipase

*Patient monitoring
PT/INR
Mental status

FIG. 39-2 Algorithm for workup of acute liver failure. Abbreviations: PT, prothrombin time; INR, international normalized ratio; CBC, complete blood count.
*If worsening coagulopathy or awareness, transfer patient to a liver transplant center.

TABLE 39-5 Drugs that may Lead to ALF

Isoniazid
Sulfonamides
Phenytoin
Statins
PTU
Halothane
Disulfiram
Valproic acid
Amiodarone
Dapsone
Didanosine
Efavirenz
Metformin
Ofloxacin
PZA
Troglitazone
Diclofenac
Isoflurane
Lisinopril
Nicotinic acid
Imipramine
Gemtuzumab
Amphetamines/ecstasy
Labetalol
Etoposide
Flutamide
Tolcapone
Quetiapine
Nefazodone
Allopurinol
Methyldopa
Ketoconazole
Trimethoprim-sulfamethoxazole
Rifampin-isoniazid
Amoxicillin-clavulanate

- Shock or hypoperfusion
- Unknown (20% of cases)
- King's College Criteria (Table 39-4)
  - Criteria most commonly used and most frequently tested to evaluate poor transplant-free survival
  - Decent specificity but low sensitivity
- Other criteria used include APACHE II (Acute Physiology and Chronic Health Evaluation II) scores and measuring factor V levels (Fig. 39-2 and Table 39-5)

BIBLIOGRAPHY

Ioannou GN, Boyko EJ, Lee SP. The prevalence and predictors of elevated serum aminotransferase activity in the United States in 1999–2002. *Am J Gastroenterol.* 2006;101:76–82.

Polson J, Lee WM. AASLD position paper: the management of acute liver failure. *Hepatology.* 2005;41:1179–1197.

Pratt DS, Kaplan MM. Primary care: evaluation of abnormal liver enzymes results in asymptomatic patients. *N Engl J Med.* 2000;342:1266–1271.

40 CIRRHOSIS

Thomas M. Shehab

EPIDEMIOLOGY/OVERVIEW

- Cirrhosis accounts for approximately 30,000 deaths and 400,000 hospital admissions per year in the United States.
- Cirrhosis is the pathologic term describing advanced hepatic fibrosis that includes the formation of regenerative nodules and distortion of hepatic architecture.
- Patients with cirrhosis present with compensated disease (without obvious symptoms) or decompensated cirrhosis (clinically apparent disease with at least one of the multiple complications of cirrhosis) (Table 40-1).

PATHOPHYSIOLOGY

- Cirrhosis results from the deposition of excess collagen within the liver in response to ongoing liver injury.
- In advanced (histologic) cirrhosis, the level of architectural distortion often precludes diagnosis of the original etiology.
- Decompensation of cirrhosis typically occurs secondary to the physiologic changes resulting from portal hypertension.
- Hepatic scarring leads to increased hepatic stiffness and subsequent portal hypertension. The portal hypertension leads to a number of changes in the mesenteric vasculature and in the renin-angiotensin-aldosterone system (Fig. 40-1).

CLINICAL PRESENTATION, DIFFERENTIAL, MAKING THE DIAGNOSIS

- Cirrhosis can be the consequence of any long-term, persistent injury to the liver. The etiology does not

TABLE 40-1 Decompensated Cirrhosis—Clinical Presentations

1. Portal hypertensive related gastrointestinal bleeding
2. Ascites
3. Hepatic encephalopathy
4. Hepatocellular carcinoma
5. Hepatopulmonary syndrome
6. Spontaneous bacterial peritonitis
7. Hepatorenal syndrome

Portal hypertension ⟶ Splanchnic arterial vasodilation ⟶ Activation of the renin angiotension-aldosterone systems ⟶ Sodium retention ⟶ Pathologic fluid retention and further complications

FIG. 40-1 Physiologic changes in cirrhosis and portal hypertension.

significantly impact the outcome once cirrhosis and portal hypertension have developed (Table 40-2).
- Patients with compensated cirrhosis may come to clinical recognition based on laboratory abnormalities, abnormal imaging, or alternatively cirrhosis can be incidentally noted at the time of surgery.
- Patients with decompensated liver disease come to clinical recognition based on the complications of cirrhosis.
- There are multiple potential benefits of diagnosing the etiology of the cirrhosis including options for therapy, counseling for the family, and prognostic recommendations (Table 40-3). Treatment may decrease the likelihood of the patient developing decompensated liver disease.
- Patients with cirrhosis and portal hypertension may have a number of physical examination, laboratory, and imaging abnormalities suggestive of underlying cirrhosis and portal hypertension (Table 40-4).

DISEASE MANAGEMENT STRATEGIES

MANAGING THE PATIENT WITH COMPENSATED CIRRHOSIS

- Patients with compensated cirrhosis often are eligible for treatments of the underlying disease. Treatment of

TABLE 40-2 Most Common Etiologies Leading to End-Stage Liver Disease and Orthotopic Liver Transplantation in the United States

Hepatitis C	28
Alcohol	16
Other (etiology not classified)	10
Primary biliary cirrhosis/primary sclerosing cholangitis	9
Cryptogenic	8
Hepatitis C and alcohol	6
Miscellaneous	6
Autoimmune hepatitis	4
Hepatitis B	4
NAFD	3
Congenital	2
Metabolic	2
Hepatocellular carcinoma	1
Vascular	1

SOURCE: United Network of Organ Sharing (UNOS). Accessed 2007. www.unos.org.

TABLE 40-3   Common Etiologies of Cirrhosis and Evaluation of these Etiologies

DIAGNOSIS	DIAGNOSTIC EVALUATION
Chronic hepatitis B	Hepatitis B surface antigen positive and positive hepatitis B DNA testing
Hepatitis C	Presence of hepatitis C antibody and hepatitis C RNA
Alcohol-related liver disease	Regular moderate to heavy alcohol use (80 g of alcohol for 10–20 years highly correlated with development of cirrhosis)
Hereditary hemochromatosis	Elevated iron saturations and ferritin. Positive testing for genetic hemochromatosis. Iron overload on liver biopsy
NAFD	History consistent with insulin resistance
Autoimmune hepatitis	Presence of autoantibodies (antinuclear and antismooth muscle antibody), gamma globulin spike on serum protein electrophoresis
Primary sclerosing cholangitis	Biliary tract strictures on ERCP or MRCP
Primary biliary cirrhosis	Positive antimitochondrial antibodies

Abbreviations: ERCP, endoscopic retrograde cholangiopancreatography; MRCP, magnetic resonance cholangiopancreatography.

the underlying disease may decrease their risk of decompensation.
- Patients with compensated cirrhosis should be referred to gastroenterology/hepatology for further evaluation and management.
- Compensated cirrhotics are at increased risk of drug-induced liver injury and dose modification of medications with hepatic clearance should be made.

TABLE 40-4   Physical/Radiologic/Laboratory Findings Suggestive of Cirrhosis and Portal Hypertension

Physical examination findings

1. Spider angiomata: most commonly found on chest and back
2. Terry's nails: changes in nail bed with the proximal one-half of the nail bed appearing white and distal nail bed appearing pink to red
3. Gynecomastia present in up to 70% of cirrhotics
4. Splenomegaly. Patient may have palpable spleen or dullness in Traube's space
5. Dupuytren's contracture: most common in alcohol-related liver disease

Physical examination findings commonly seen in decompensated liver disease

1. Ascites
2. Shifting
3. Dullness
4. Fluid wave on physical examination
5. Jaundice, typically visible in sclera, bilirubin 2.8 or higher
6. Asterixis can also be seen in uremia
7. Proximal muscle wasting

Radiology findings

1. Splenomegaly
2. Nodularity to liver surface. Liver echogenicity may be abnormal in patients with liver disease

Laboratory evaluation

1. Abnormal liver enzymes: Often patients with advanced liver disease will have an AST to ALT ratio of > 1.
2. Thrombocytopenia
3. Elevated bilirubin
4. Low albumin
5. Elevated prothrombin time

Abbreviations: AST, aspartate aminotransferase; ALT, alanine aminotransferase.

- Cirrhotics are at particular risk of therapeutic misadventures with excess doses of acetaminophen. Acetaminophen remains the medication of choice in these patients for short-term treatment of fever or pain (nonsteroidals can increase the risk of gastrointestinal (GI) bleeding and precipitate hepatorenal syndrome). However, acetaminophen doses in these patients should not exceed 2000 mg/day and should not be used on a daily basis.
- Patients with compensated cirrhosis may have decompensation of their liver disease after surgical procedures. The likelihood of decompensation is higher in patients with more advanced liver disease. However, compensated cirrhosis would not be an absolute contraindication for surgery in most settings.
- Patients should be vaccinated for hepatitis A and hepatitis B.

MANAGEMENT OF DECOMPENSATED CIRRHOSIS

- All patients with decompensated liver disease should be managed in collaboration with a gastroenterologist/hepatologist.
- All patients with decompensated cirrhosis should be considered for orthotopic liver transplantation.
- The Childs-Pugh classification is often used to assess the severity of liver disease (Table 40-5).
- Priority for liver transplantation is now based on a Childs-Pugh score of 7 (minimal listing criteria) and severity of liver disease based on the model for end-stage liver disease (MELD) (www.unos.org/ resources/ MeldPeldCalculator.asp?index=98).
- All patients with newly decompensated chronic liver disease should be evaluated for the precipitant of the decompensation (intercurrent infection, development of hepatocellular carcinoma, acute portal vein thrombus).

TABLE 40-5 Childs-Pugh Classification

	POINTS ASSIGNED		
PARAMETER	1	2	3
Ascites	Absent	Slight	Moderate
Bilirubin, mg/dL	< 2	2–3	> 3
Albumin, g/dL	> 3.5	2.8–3.5	< 2.8
Prothrombin Time			
Seconds over control	< 4	4–6	> 6
INR	< 1.7	1.7–2.3	> 2.3
Encephalopathy	None	Grade 1–2	Grade 3–4

Abbreviation: INR, international normalized ratio.

Assessment for new clinical issues should also take place for all cirrhotic patients who have evidence of clinical worsening.

PORTAL HYPERTENSION-RELATED UPPER GASTROINTESTINAL BLEEDING

- Patients with portal hypertension can develop esophageal, gastric, and/or rectal varices. In addition, they can develop bleeding from portal hypertensive gastropathy. Less commonly patients will develop portal enteropathy or portal colopathy.
- Bleeding from esophageal varices accounts for approximately 30% of cirrhosis-related deaths.
- Estimates suggest that only 50% of variceal bleeding will not stop spontaneously. This is in direct contrast to most other sources of upper GI bleeding which stop spontaneously in more than 85% of cases (see Chap. 47).
- Patients with upper GI bleeding and a history of portal hypertension should undergo urgent endoscopy and be started on an intravenous octreotide drip (Table 40-6).

TABLE 40-6 Approach to GI Bleeding in a Patient with Cirrhosis

1. **Hemodynamic resuscitation**
   ○ Two large bore intravenous accesses
   ○ Maintain hemoglobin between 9 and 10 g/dL
2. **Determination of source of bleeding**
   ○ Esophageal varices are not a contraindication to nasogastric lavage.
   ○ Rapid upper GI bleeding can present as bright red blood per rectum.
3. **Management of portal hypertension**
   ○ Octreotide drip
4. **Early endoscopy**
   ○ Given the low rate of spontaneous stopping of bleeding, urgent upper endoscopy with intervention is indicated.
5. **Ongoing bleeding refractory to endoscopic intervention**
   ○ Consider Sengstaken-Blakemore tube placement.
   ○ Consider urgent TIPS placement.

- Twenty-five percent of patients with variceal bleeding will die within 2 weeks of the initial bleeding. There has been only modest improvement in survival rates over the last two decades.

ASCITES

- More than 75% of patients presenting with ascites will have underlying cirrhosis and portal hypertension.
- All patients with new-onset ascites and all patients with ascites who are admitted to the hospital should undergo diagnostic paracentesis the day of admission.
- Serum-ascites albumin gradient (SAAG) should be calculated for all patients with new-onset ascites. In addition, ascites fluid should be evaluated for cell count and differential and culture bottles should be directly inoculated. SAAG > 1.1 g/dL are most often seen in patients with portal hypertension and congestive heart failure. SAAG levels < 1.1 g/dL are seen in association with peritoneal inflammation (malignancy, pancreatitis, peritoneal infection).
- The majority of patients with clinically evident ascites will have resolution of the ascites with strict adherence to a 2-g sodium diet.
- Most patients do not require fluid restriction.
- Patients requiring medication therapy should be started on spironolactone 100 mg and furosemide 40 mg each morning. Doses should be doubled if there is a lack of response after 7 days (Table 40-7).
- Patients with truly refractory ascites should undergo serial paracentesis and/or consideration of a transjugular intrahepatic portosystemic shunt (TIPS) placement.

HEPATIC ENCEPHALOPATHY

- Patients may present with subtle issues related to concentration or day-night reversal (Table 40-8).

TABLE 40-7 Medical Management of Cirrhotic Ascites

1. **Dietary**
   2000-mg sodium restriction
      1. Dietary counseling
      2. Family/caregiver education
2. **Medication therapy**
   Starting doses (both medications used together)
      1. Spironolactone 100 mg orally each day
      2. Furosemide 40 mg orally each day
3. **Recommendations**
   Dose diuretics in the morning
   For insufficient response: double dose of both medications
   Maximal dose: typically 400 mg spironolactone and 80 mg furosemide
   Wait at least 5–7 days before doubling dose

TABLE 40-8 Stages of Encephalopathy

	STAGE			
	1	2	3	4
State of arousal	Day-night reversal	Lethargic	Sleepy	Unarousable
Neurologic	Tremor	Asterixis reflexes	Hyperactive	Unresponsive
examination	Altered handwriting	Ataxia	Rigidity	

- Treatment should include avoidance of sedatives or medications that can cloud the sensorium.
- Standard treatment is with lactulose, with the dose titrated to achieve 2–3 soft bowel movements a day
- For patients who cannot tolerate lactulose, a variety of antibiotics may be helpful. Neomycin is the first antibiotic studied for this purpose, but its long-term use is complicated by ototoxicity and nephrotoxicity. Other oral antibiotics such as metronidazole, vancomycin, and rifaximin are better tolerated than neomycin
- There is no good clinical evidence supporting protein restriction in patients with hepatic encephalopathy. However, oral protein intake should not exceed 70 g/day in a patient with a history of hepatic encephalopathy.
- Patients with acute/semi-acute worsening of must be evaluated for possible precipitants of the worsening encephalopathy, including infection, GI bleeding, or medication effect.

HEPATOCELLULAR CARCINOMA

- Diagnosed typically with classical imaging characteristics on CT or MRI scanning.
- Elevated alpha protein is suggested but not diagnostic.
- Diagnosis is made by liver biopsy.

CARE TRANSITIONS

- Patients with decompensated cirrhosis can be discharged once the factors leading to the episode of acute decompensation have been identified and treated (bleeding, dietary indiscretion, medication effect, etc.).
- The patient should have follow-up with their PPCs within 7–10 days and with gastroenterology/hepatology in 2–4 weeks.

- Ascites patients and their caregivers should be seen by nutrition for counseling on 2-g sodium diet.
- Patients with substance abuse issues should be referred for evaluation and management of substance abuse issues.

BIBLIOGRAPHY

Murphy SL. Deaths: final data for 1998. *Natl Vital Stat Rep.* 2000;48:1.

Runyon BA. Management of adult patients with ascites due to cirrhosis. *Hepatology.* 1998;27:264.

WEB RESOURCE

United Network of Organ Sharing (UNOS). www.unos.org

41 COLITIS AND DIARRHEA, INCLUDING *Clostridium difficile*

Marvin Ryou

EPIDEMIOLOGY/OVERVIEW

- This chapter reviews major causes of colitis and diarrhea, aside from Crohn's disease, covered in Chap. 42, and ulcerative colitis (UC), covered in Chap. 43.
- Common diagnostic entities causing colitis in hospitalized patients are listed in Table 41-1.
  ○ From a global perspective, infectious colitis (Table 41-2) accounts for most diarrheal disease, particularly in developing countries.
    ▪ About 165 million cases of shigellosis are reported annually worldwide, but only 15,000 in the United States.
    ▪ *Campylobacter* species are the most common bacterial enteropathogens in the developed world. The Centers for Disease Control and Prevention (CDC) estimated that *Campylobacter* caused nearly 2 million diarrheal illnesses in the United States in 1999.

TABLE 41-1   Differential Diagnosis of Colitis

DISEASE	CLUES TO DIAGNOSIS/ PRESENTATION	DIAGNOSTIC STUDIES	TREATMENT
Appendicitis See Chap. 38 for details	Most commonly occurs in the second/third decades of life. Signs and symptoms are often nonspecific: indigestion, flatulence, bowel irregularity. Pain in the periumbilical area can subsequently localize to the RLQ. Nausea/vomiting usually follows onset of pain. Fever and leukocytosis follow thereafter.	CT scan may show wall thickening, an appendicolith, phlegmon, abscess, free fluid, and/or fat stranding.	Antibiotics and surgical resection.
Diverticulitis/ diverticular colitis See Chap. 44 for details	Classic presentation for diverticulitis is LLQ abdominal pain, fever, nausea, vomiting, and constipation. Complications include peritonitis and septic shock. A disease of middle-aged and older patients. Diverticular colitis is rarer. Patients with diverticulosis occasionally develop a segmental colitis, usually involving the sigmoid, thought to be secondary to mucosal prolapse, fecal stasis, or local ischemia.	Diverticulitis is diagnosed by abdominal CT showing bowel wall thickening. Diverticular colitis is diagnosed endoscopically and histologically.	Bowel rest, IVF, IV antibiotics. For abscesses, percutaneous drainage vs. surgery.
IBD See Chaps. 42 and 43 for details	Crohn's classically presents with mucus-containing nongrossly bloody diarrhea, abdominal cramping, fevers, malaise, weight loss. Bimodal incidence. Complications include strictures, fistulas, abscesses, and colon cancer. Any segment of GI tract can be affected. UC classically presents in young adults with grossly bloody diarrhea, lower abdominal cramps, and urgency. Complications include fulminant colitis, toxic megacolon, perforation, and colon cancer. Both entities have numerous extracolonic manifestations.	On biopsy, Crohn's has transmural inflammation with noncaseating granuloma. Skip lesions, fissures, ulcerations and cobblestoning seen on endoscopy and barium enema. On endoscopy, UC manifests with rectal involvement and extends proximally and contiguously. The mucosa is grossly granular, friable mucosa with diffuse ulceration and pseudopolyps. On microscopy, there are superficial microulcerations and crypt abscesses.	For mild disease, 5-ASA compounds are used. Metronidazole and ciprofloxacin have also been used. For moderate disease, oral steroids are usually added. For severe disease, AZA, cyclosporine, 6-MP, methotrexate, infliximab, and surgery are all considered.
Pseudomembranous colitis	The prototypic entity associated with *C. difficile* infection. Usually antecedent antibiotic use. Fever, chills, nausea, vomiting, dehydration, tenesmus, diarrhea, and lower abdominal cramping. Peripheral leukocytosis common.	Although usually not necessary, can be confirmed rapidly using sigmoidoscopy revealing characteristic yellow-white raised mucosal plaques or pseudomembranes, confirmed on biopsy. *C. difficile* toxin positive.	Metronidazole and enteral vancomycin. Colectomy for severe cases. See Table 41-4
Infectious colitis See Table 41-3 for more details	Usually presents with acute diarrhea (bloody or watery depending on causative organism) ± abdominal cramping, nausea/vomiting, and fevers.	Stool cultures, stool O&P, *C. difficile* toxin assay.	Antimicrobials
Ischemic colitis	Risk factors: increased age, systemic atherosclerotic disease, hypercoagulability, hypotension, atrial fibrillation. Classic presentation is crampy LLQ pain associated with guaiac positive or frankly bloody stool.	Flexible sigmoidoscopy or colonoscopy.	Bowel rest; IV fluids; consider antibiotics; surgery for infarction, fulminant colitis, or obstruction.
NSAID-induced colitis	Up to 10% of newly diagnosed cases of colitis may be because of NSAID use. Typically patients are older (average age 63) with no gender predilection and present with diarrhea and either occult of gross lower GIB.	Endoscopy (although findings range from mild proctitis to ulcerative pan-colitis); trial of NSAID discontinuation.	Discontinuation of NSAID. Steroids and sulfasalazine have been used.

(Continued)

TABLE 41-1 Differential Diagnosis of Colitis (*Continued*)

DISEASE	CLUES TO DIAGNOSIS/ PRESENTATION	DIAGNOSTIC STUDIES	TREATMENT
Antibiotic-associated noninfectious diarrhea	Quite common. Antibiotic eliminates colonic bacteria that metabolize carbohydrates, causing osmotic diarrhea.	Diagnosis of exclusion. Endoscopy appears generally normal and *C. difficile* test is negative.	Discontinuation of antibiotic; use of probiotics (*Lactobacillus* species) to reestablish normal flora has not been established by large, randomized trials
Miscellaneous drug-induced colitis	1. Colitis associated with enema use (soap, gastrografin, hydrogen peroxide). 2. "Cathartic colon" from laxative abuse. 3. Drugs causing ischemic colonic injury include OCPs (via mesenteric thrombosis), vasopressin, cocaine, ergotamine, alosetron, dextroamphetamine, and neuroleptics. 4. Postcolonoscopy colitis, from inadequate rinsing of glutaraldehyde disinfectant from scope prior to use. 5. Other toxins include gold, isotretinoin, ampicillin, amoxicillin, and erythromycin (antibiotics associated with hemorrhagic colitis), various chemotherapeutic agents such as MTX, 5-FU, and cytosine.	History of medication exposure and clinical suspicion.	Discontinuation of medication and supportive care.
Typhlitis	Acute necrotizing colitis (usually the cecum) seen in severe immunosuppression. Fever, abdominal pain (40%–60% localize to RLQ) and diarrhea (20%–45% bloody) in a neutropenic patient should suggest this diagnosis.	Difficult to diagnose given nonspecific symptoms, signs, and radiographic findings. CT abd classically shows cecal wall thickening with pericecal fluid.	Bowel rest, IVF, and IV antibiotics. Surgery may be required in cases of perforation or persistent GI bleeding.
Diversion colitis	Following fecal diversion, 1/3 of patients develop mucoid discharges that may progress to rectal bleeding and pain in the bypassed segment. The putative cause is luminal nutrient deficiency.	Flexible sigmoidoscopy with biopsies and luminal aspirates for O&P, culture, and *C. difficile* toxin assay.	Usually none required. Reports of 5-ASA compounds used with good effect. Reanastomosis presumably definitive therapy.
Microscopic colitis	Otherwise known as collagenous and lymphocytic colitis. Symptoms include chronic watery (sometimes profuse) diarrhea. Tends to affect females > males. Mean age of onset 50–65. Autoimmune etiology suggested by frequent association of arthritis, thyroid abnormalities, asthma, and diabetes.	Endoscopic biopsy. Histology reveals chronic mucosal inflammation. (Note that endoscopic visualization is normal.) Colonic involvement is usually diffuse.	Bismuth; antidiarrheal agents; 5-ASA compounds; antibiotics (60% of patient respond); steroids and immunosuppresives for more severe disease
Radiation colitis	To be suspected in patients with antecedent abdomino-pelvic radiation, especially >3000 cGy. 1/3 to 1/2 of patients suffer acute injury with diarrhea and tenesmus (the rectum is more susceptible) during the first month of therapy. 15% have chronic symptoms manifested by rectal pain, diarrhea, and bleeding.	Ulcers and friable tissue seen on endoscopy.	No good medical approach. Some efficacy demonstrated with prednisone + oral 5-ASA agents; sucralfate enemas; short-chain fatty acid enemas.

Abbreviations: IBD, inflammatory bowel disease; NSAID, nonsteroidal anti-inflammatory drug; RLQ, right lower quadrant; LLQ, left lower quadrant; GI, gastrointestinal; UC, ulcerative colitis; GIB, gastrointestinal bleeding; CT, computed tomography; IVF, in vitro fertilization; IV, intravenous; 5-ASA, 5-aminosalicylic acid; 6-MP, 6-mercaptopurine; OCPs, oral contraceptive pills; MTX, methotrexate; 5-FU, 5-fluorouracil; O&P, ova and parasites.

TABLE 41-2   Bacterial, Viral, and Parasitic Infections of the Colon

ORGANISM	CLUES TO THE DIAGNOSIS	TESTING	ANTIMICROBIAL THERAPY
C. difficile	The #1 cause of healthcare-associated diarrhea. Feared complications include pseudomembranous colitis and fulminant colitis.	Testing for toxins A and B	Flagyl, oral vancomycin See Table 41-1
Shigella species	Predilection for lower GI tract. Infection can result from inoculation of just 10 organisms. Intestinal complications include toxic megacolon, obstruction, perforation. Non-GI manifestations include neurologic disease, reactive arthritis, and HUS.	Stool culture	Bactrim, fluoroquinolone; avoid antimotility agents
Escherichia coli	Colitis associated with EHEC (bloody) and EIEC (dysentery) strains.	Stool culture	Fluoroquinolone; avoid antimotility agents
Campylobacter jejuni	Most frequently identified cause of acute infectious diarrhea in many industrialized countries. Usually affects jejunum and ileum before progressing to colon, but can occasionally manifest with colitis alone.	Stool culture	Macrolides
Yersinia enterocolitica	Associated with pseudo-appendicitis and mesenteric adenitis. In addition to colitis, GI complications include: suppurative appendicitis, toxic megacolon, perforation, intussusception.	Stool culture	Fluoroquinolones. Doxycycline or bactrim are alternatives. Usually resistant to penicillin, ampicillin, and 1st-generation cephalosporins
Salmonella species	Usually manifests as gastroenteritis. Rare invasive disease can lead to aneurysms, mycotic aneurysm, and osteomyelitis.	Stool culture	Quinolones. Bactrim, amoxicillin, and 3rd-generation cephalosporins are also options
Mycobacterium tuberculosis	Classically involves the terminal ileum and cecum and can mimic Crohn's.	Caseating granulomas, positive culture, or acid-fast bacilli on colonoscopic biopsy	Antituberculous medications
Entamoeba histolytica	Suspect in travelers to Latin America, Southern and Western Africa, India, Far East. Most patients are asymptomatic, and only 10% develop acute invasive disease, usually enterocolitis.	Trophozoites in stool or serologic testing (indirect heme-agglutination vs. ELISA)	Metronidazole + luminal agent for cysts (iodoquinol, diloxanide furoate, or paromomycin)
CMV	May present with a diffuse proctocolitis. Commonly but not always associated with underlying HIV. Sigmoidoscopy will show friable, inflamed rectal mucosa with contact bleeding and superficial mucosal ulcerations. Stool microscopy will show an exudate of mixed inflammatory cells.	CMV inclusion bodies within endothelial and smooth muscle cells on biopsy; viral culture is unreliable; serology, viremia PCRs, and early antigen detection assays are less specific	Ganciclovir induction followed by valganciclovir oral therapy; foscarnet and cidofovir are also options
Giardia lamblia	Most common waterborne illness in the United States Often seen via ingestion of contaminated water after hiking or swimming in the wilderness; also common after travel abroad. Causes flatulence, bloating, mild diarrhea, malaise, and anorexia.	Stool antigen testing, much more sensitive than stool ova and parasites	Metronidazole in adults, albendazole in children

Abbreviations: CMV, cytomegalovirus; GI, gastrointestinal; HUS, hemolytic uremic syndrome; enterohaemorrhagic E. coli (EHEC); enteroinvasive E. coli (EIEC); HIV, human immunodeficiency virus; ELISA, enzyme-linked immunosorbent assays.
Immunosuppressed: *Cryptosporidium, Cyclospora, Isospora belli, Microsporidia, Mycobacterium avium* complex.

○ Intestinal ischemia, especially ischemic colitis, accounts for about 1 in 1000 hospital admissions in the United States. The increasing incidence in recent years is likely because of the aging of the population and the growing number of critically ill patients.

○ Medication-induced colitis is increasingly recognized. Nonsteroidal anti-inflammatory drug (NSAID)-induced colitis may represent almost 10% of all colitis.
○ Of particular concern to hospitalists is antibiotic-induced colitis, primarily *Clostridium difficile*

infection, which is the number one cause of health-care-associated diarrhea (20–60 cases per 100,000 patient days).

CLINICAL PRESENTATION, DIFFERENTIAL DIAGNOSIS

- Elements of the history providing clues to specific diagnoses are summarized in Table 41-3.
- Important physical examination findings include
  - Vital signs (particularly temperature, heart rate, and blood pressure).
  - Abdominal examination findings, including tenderness, distension, altered bowel sounds, guarding, and rebound.
  - In addition, the examiner should look for signs of vascular disease, vasculitis, and immunosuppression, and assess volume status.
- Profound abdominal distention, rebound tenderness, and rigidity suggest severe complications, such as ischemic colitis, fulminant colitis, perforation, or sepsis (see Chap. 80). Surgical consultation should be obtained immediately and transfer to the intensive care unit (ICU) considered.
- Differential diagnosis (Table 41-1) includes appendicitis, diverticular colitis, inflammatory bowel disease (IBD), NSAID-induced colitis, infectious colitis (including *C. difficile* colitis), ischemic colitis, radiation

colitis, and microscopic colitis. Certain diagnoses should be suspected in specific patient populations:
- Colonic involvement by cytomegalovirus (CMV), *Mycobacterium avium*, and non-Hodgkin's lymphoma is common in acquired immunodeficiency syndrome (AIDS) patients.
- Typhlitis should be suspected in neutropenic patients with fever, right lower quadrant (RLQ) pain, and diarrhea.
- Older patients with known or suspected atherosclerotic disease presenting with crampy abdominal pain and bloody diarrhea should be evaluated for ischemic colitis.

TRIAGE AND INITIAL MANAGEMENT/MAKING THE DIAGNOSIS

- If infectious colitis is suspected, patients should be placed on contact precautions pending results of stool cultures and *C. difficile* toxin.
- The following laboratory and radiographic studies should be obtained or considered:
  - Complete blood cell count and differential, liver function tests (LFTs) including albumin, and serum chemistries to assess for electrolyte abnormalities, especially potassium and magnesium.

TABLE 41-3 Clues in the History

CHARACTERISTIC	SUGGESTIVE OF
Type, severity, and location of abdominal discomfort	Pain out of proportion to examination or diffuse, poorly localized pain is suggestive of ischemic colitis. Sometimes, location of discomfort can suggest anatomic location of involvement but is considered nonspecific overall.
Watery vs. bloody diarrhea	Watery suggests osmotic or secretory. Bloody suggests inflammatory or cytotoxic/invasive.
Frequency and volume of diarrhea	High volume suggests small bowel involvement.
Nausea and vomiting	Nausea and vomiting can be nonspecific, but immediately after ingestion suggest preformed toxins (*Staphylococcus aureus* or *Bacillus cereus*).
Tenesmus	Suggests rectal involvement.
Fevers or chills	Can be nonspecific, but can also suggest infectious etiology
Immunosuppression	Expands differential of potential infectious etiologies (see also Table 41-3).
Travel history	Suggests infectious etiology (see Table 41-3).
Recent dietary record	For example, dairy products in lactose-intolerant patients or sorbitol in gum can cause diarrhea.
History of atherosclerosis	Raises the possibility of ischemic colitis.
Medication use	Recent antibiotic use is a risk factor for *C. difficile* infection, and NSAID-induced colitis is common.
Sick contacts	Suggestive of infectious etiology (see Table 41-3).
Recent hospitalization	A risk factor for *C. difficile* infection.
Recent hypotension	Suggestive of ischemic colitis (see Table 41-1).
Prior diverting ostomy	Suggests diversion colitis (see Table 41-1).
Previous abdominal radiation	Suggests radiation colitis (see Table 41-1).

Abbreviation: NSAID, nonsteroidal anti-inflammatory drug.

- Routine stool cultures should be sent in patients with acute diarrheal illnesses, especially if fever or bloody stools are present.
- Stool should be sent for *C. difficile* toxin assay in patients recently hospitalized, treated with antibiotics, or receiving cancer chemotherapy.
- Stool ova and parasites should be checked in travelers, immigrants, the immunocompromised, and those with more than a week of diarrheal symptoms. In these populations, acid-fast staining of stool should also be obtained to exclude *Cyclospora*, *Isospora*, *Cryptosporidium*, and *Mycobacterium*.
- Testing for fecal occult blood should be performed if stools not grossly bloody.
  - In patients who develop diarrhea after more than 3 days of hospitalization, the yield of stool culture and stool ova and parasites is very low. Many authorities advocate obtaining only a stool *C. difficile* toxin in this setting.
  - The utility of fecal leukocytes is debatable and therefore not recommended.
  - Additional stool studies may be helpful in selected patients based on the history of present illness.
  - Blood cultures (two sets from different venous puncture sites) should be obtained prior to the administration of any antibiotics.
- Radiologic studies may help assess the severity of colitis. Plain abdominal films (KUB [kidney, ureter, and bladder] and upright) are notoriously nonspecific, but may help rapidly exclude toxic megacolon or perforation.
  - Occasionally, thumbprinting may be seen, indicating submucosal edema.
  - Distension and pneumatosis are encountered in advanced inflammation or ischemia.
  - Free air under the diaphragm indicates frank perforation.
- Computed tomography (CT) is often obtained in patients with unrevealing plain abdominal x-ray films. Typical findings include wall thickening, either in segmental or continuous. CT is particularly helpful when suspecting fistula or abscess. Similar to plain films, CT can also be unrevealing, especially early in the disease course (or in such disease entities as microscopic colitis, which appears normal even endoscopically).
- Initial patient management focuses on:
  - Rehydration, typically with normal saline or lactated Ringer's.
  - Correction of electrolyte abnormalities, particularly potassium and magnesium. The frequency of repeat blood tests depends on the severity of the electrolyte derangement, and may need to be more than once daily in the initial treatment phase.
  - Bowel rest by making the patient NPO.

- Relief of significant emesis by placement of a NG tube.
- Avoidance of antimotility agents or at least minimized, as they may precipitate ileus or toxic megacolon.
- There are no guidelines for the empiric administration of antibiotics for colitis.
  - Traveler's diarrhea and shigellosis can be treated with 3 days of trimethoprim-sulfamethoxazole or a fluoroquinolone.
  - Routine antibiotic treatment of salmonellosis should be avoided in otherwise healthy people, as it may lead to prolonged stool carriage with *Salmonella*.
  - In patients over the age of 50, with orthopedic or valvular prostheses, or other significant medical comorbidities, *Salmonella* can be treated with 5–7 days of trimethoprim-sulfamethoxazole or a fluoroquinolone.
  - Five days of erythromycin is recommended for *Campylobacter* colitis.
  - Antibiotic treatment of *Escherichia coli* O157:H7 should generally be avoided, as it may lead to release of Shiga toxin and precipitate hemolytic uremic syndrome (HUS).
- If a perforation or abscess collection is suspected, assume that most intra-abdominal infections are polymicrobial and require treatment with empiric broad spectrum antibiotics to cover bowel flora.
  - Beta-lactam/beta-lactamase inhibitor combinations, such as ampicillin-sulbactam or piperacillin-tazobactam, may be useful in this setting.
  - Cephalosporins lack anaerobic coverage, except for cefoxitin. Most cephalosporins should be combined with metronidazole in the treatment of intra-abdominal sepsis.
  - For patients allergic to penicillins, consider fluoroquinolones in combination with metronidazole for anaerobic coverage.
  - Neither fluoroquinolones nor cephalosporins have significant activity against enterococci.
- Gastroenterology consultation should be obtained for
  - Assistance with the decision to start empiric steroids if IBD is strongly suspected, and infectious etiologies are unlikely or have been ruled out.
  - Sigmoidoscopy or colonoscopy, if the diagnosis is unclear and there is no concern for perforation or peritonitis. Endoscopy is superior to contrast enemas, permitting direct mucosal visualization, sampling for cultures, and biopsy if indicated.
- Surgical consultation should be obtained for
  - Abdominal perforation
  - Toxic megacolon (which may require early surgical intervention to avoid perforation)
  - Intra-abdominal abscess that is not responding to appropriate interventional radiology drainage

DISEASE MANAGEMENT STRATEGIES

- *C. difficile* is the most common cause of nosocomial diarrhea. *C. difficile* infections in North America are rising in prevalence and virulence. Risk factors include
  - Exposure to antimicrobials
  - Duration of hospitalization
  - Malnutrition and chronic illness
  - Proton pump inhibitors and H2 blockers may facilitate colonization and infection with *C. difficile* by eliminating the gastric acid barrier. Over-prescribing these drugs in the general medical inpatient setting should therefore be avoided.
- *C. difficile* produces two potent cytotoxins, A and B, which cause a profound inflammatory response. A new fluoroquinolone-resistant strain with toxin hyper-production causes especially severe disease.
- Symptoms typically start 4–9 days after initiation of antibiotic therapy, but can arise after completion of antibiotics in up to 30% of patients. (Many patients develop diarrhea during antibiotics without having *C. difficile* infection.)
- Pseudomembranous colitis because of *C. difficile* infection presents with diarrhea (hematochezia is rare), lower abdominal cramping, fever, nausea, and vomiting. Physical findings are nonspecific, and include diffuse abdominal pain and distention. Leukocytosis is usually present, and may be impressive. Although not necessary, the diagnosis can be confirmed rapidly by sigmoidoscopy, which reveals characteristic yellow-white, raised plaques that can coalesce and cover the entire mucosa.
- *Diagnosis* is usually made by detecting *C. difficile* toxin in stool samples. The gold standard is a tissue culture assay for the cytopathic effects of toxins A and B; this assay is highly sensitive (94% to 100%) and specific (99%), but expensive, and the incubation period is prolonged (24–48 hours). Most hospital labs now use enzyme-linked immunosorbent assays (ELISA) that are less sensitive, but quicker and cheaper.
  - Five to ten percent of cases of *C. difficile* will be missed by ELISA testing.
  - Many of the commonly available ELISA tests only detect toxin A, and some strains of *C. difficile* only produce toxin B.
  - Enterotoxin-producing methicillin-resistant *Staphylococcus aureus* (MRSA) may cause nosocomial antibiotic-associated diarrhea that resembles *C. difficile* infection, and should be considered in the differential if *C. difficile* toxin assays are negative and stool cultures show heavy MRSA.
- Treatment is metronidazole or vancomycin, depending on the severity of illness (Table 41-4).
  - Relapses are common (10% to 25% of cases), and generally respond to retreatment with initial therapy.
  - Adjunctive therapies may include the use of cholestyramine, a resin that theoretically binds up *C. difficile* toxin, and probiotics, which promote reestablishment of normal flora. However, evidence for their efficacy is rather limited.
  - Intravenous (IV) immunoglobulin containing *C. difficile* antitoxin has been used successfully in case reports of severe, persistent colitis. A vaccine is also in development.
- Acute infectious colitis, non-*C. difficile* (Table 41-3)
  - Antimicrobial therapy usually plays little role in treatment, regardless of whether infection is mediated by toxins (*S. aureus*, *Bacillus cereus*, or *E. coli* O157:H7) or tissue invasion (*Campylobacter*).
  - Fluid and electrolyte replacement is of highest priority.
- NSAID-induced colitis (Table 41-1)
  - An under-recognized cause of colitis, particularly prominent in the elderly population.
  - Diagnosed when the patient improves following discontinuation of NSAIDs, and other etiologies have been excluded.
  - Steroids and sulfasalazine have been used in treatment.
- Antibiotic-associated, noninfectious diarrhea (Table 41-1)
  - Caused by elimination of colonic anaerobes that metabolize carbohydrates, Resulting in osmotic diarrhea.
  - Treatment is supportive. The offending antibiotic should be discontinued, if possible.
- Ischemic colitis
  - Predisposing factors include increased age, systemic atherosclerotic disease, hypercoagulability, hypotension, and atrial fibrillation, but often no specific cause is found. Even severe constipation can cause ischemic colitis. Each form of colitis requires an individualized diagnostic and treatment plan. See American Gastroenterological Association (AGA) 2000 guidelines.
  - Classic presentation is crampy left lower quadrant (LLQ) pain associated with guaiac positive or frankly bloody stool. Fever and peritoneal signs raise the specter of infarction.
  - The spectrum of ischemic colitis ranges from reversible colopathy (35%), transient colitis (15%), chronic ulcerating colitis (20%), stricture (10%), and gangrene (15%) to fulminant colitis (< 5%).
  - Diagnosis is confirmed by sigmoidoscopy or colonoscopy.
    - Continuous mucosal friability typically seen in left colon, in the "watershed" area from splenic flexure to sigmoid, usually with rectal sparing (given vascular redundancy).

TABLE 41-4   *C. difficile* Treatment

Treatment

1. For mild-moderate, initial infection
- Metronidazole 500 mg tid or 250 mg qid × 10–14 days
- Cessation of inciting antimicrobial
- Avoidance of antiperistaltic agents (e.g. loperamide)

2. For severe infection (leukocytosis, high fevers, toxic megacolon), the recommendations are not as clear; some suggest
- Initial therapy with vancomycin 125 mg po qid quickly followed by metronidazole 500 mg IV q 8 hours if clinical status fails to improve
- Concomitant vancomycin 125 mg po qid and metronidazole 500 mg IV q 8 hours (metronidazole IV may achieve therapeutic concentrations in the gut because of enterohepatic circulation; this is *not* true of vancomycin IV, which has little efficacy for *C. difficile*)
- Vancomycin enemas as adjunctive therapy
- Decompression colonoscopy
- Colectomy required in some patients
- IV immunoglobulin

3. First relapse (within 1 month)
- Relapses do not generally seem to be related to antibiotic resistance
- Therefore, retreatment with 10- to 14-day course of metronidazole indicated

4. Second relapse (oral vancomycin taper)
- 125 mg/6 h × 7 days
- 125 mg/12 h × 7 days
- 125 mg/d × 7 days
- 125 mg every other day × 6 days (i.e. 3 doses)
- 125 mg every 3 days for 9 days (i.e. 3 doses)

Adjunctive or novel treatments (limited evidence for efficacy)

1. Cholestyramine
- Anion-binding resin which theoretically binds the toxin of *C. difficile*
- 4 g given three–four times daily in combination with vancomycin taper as described above
- Separate doses of vancomycin by 3 hours to avoid neutralization of antibiotic

2. Probiotics
- *Saccharomyces boulardii*, a nonpathogenic yeast, has been used to prevent relapses, when used in combination with metronidazole or vancomycin
- *Lactobacillus* species have been used to re-establish normal flora

3. Vaccine
- Currently being tested in clinical trials

Prevention and control guidelines (from the American College of Gastroenterology)
1. Limit the use of antimicrobial drugs.
2. Wash hands with soap and water between contact with all patients suspected of *C. difficile*—alcohol-based hand rubs are ineffective at killing or eliminating *C. difficile* spores.
3. Use enteric (stool) isolation precautions with *C. difficile* diarrhea.
4. Wear gloves when in contact with patients who have *C. difficile* diarrhea/colitis or with their environment.
5. Disinfect objects contaminated with *C. difficile* with sodium hypochlorite, alkaline glutaraldehyde, or ethylene oxide.
6. Educate the medical, nursing, and other appropriate staff members about the disease and its epidemiology.

TABLE 41-5   *C. difficile*—Clinical Features and Diagnosis

Epidemiology: The most common cause of nosocomial diarrhea, with an incidence ranging from 20 to 60 cases per 100,000 patient days. Rare in outpatients.

Risk factors:
1. Exposure to antimicrobials (disruption of normal colonic flora)
2. Hospitalization (direct correlation between LOS and percentage of patients infected)
3. Host immunity vs. strain virulence (not as well-defined as RFs #1 and #2)

Pathogenesis: Largely the result of the elaboration of 2 potent toxins, A and B, which are cytotoxic and can cause a profound inflammatory response.

Clinical features: Broad, ranging from asymptomatic carriage to fulminant colitis. Symptoms typically start 4–9 days after initiation of antibiotic therapy but can develop even after antibiotic therapy has been halted in up to 30% of patients. Diarrhea is a hallmark of infection but can be seen with antibiotic use anyway, independent of *C. difficile* infection.

Pseudomembranous Colitis: The prototypic entity associated with *C. difficile* infection. Symptoms include diarrhea (hematochezia is rare), lower abdominal cramping, fever, nausea, and vomiting. Physical findings are nonspecific and include diffuse abdominal pain and distension. Leukocytosis is usually present. Although not necessary, the diagnosis can be confirmed rapidly by sigmoidoscopy which reveals characteristic yellow-white, raised plaques that can coalesce and cover the entire mucosa.

Diagnosis: By determining the presence of toxin in stool samples. The gold standard is a tissue culture assay which tests for the cytopathic effects of toxins A and B in the stool; this assay is highly sensitive (94%–100%) and specific (99%) but is expensive and the incubation period is prolonged (24–48 hours). Most hospital labs now use ELISA that are less sensitive but offer same-day results.

Abbreviations: LOS, length of stay.

○ Consider a hypercoagulable workup in younger patients with ischemic colitis and no other risk factors, and in those with recurrent episodes.

○ Treatment consists of supportive care, including bowel rest and IV fluids.

▪ Consider an NG tube if ileus is present.

▪ Consider empiric broad spectrum antibiotics in moderate-to-severe cases.

▪ Follow serial abdominal examinations. Persistent fever, leukocytosis, bleeding, or evidence of perforation/peritonitis should prompt surgical consultation.

▪ Avoid vasodepressors.

▪ Obtain surgical consultation for clinical deterioration, suspected infarction, fulminant colitis or obstruction caused by ischemic stricture.

CARE TRANSITIONS

When discharging patients from the hospital, keep in mind the following points regarding patient education and public health considerations:

• Emphasize proper hydration at home, particularly with fluids containing electrolytes (e.g. Gatorade, broth)

• Educate regarding proper hand-washing as well as safe food-handling practices.

• Many causes of infectious colitis (e.g. *E. coli* O157:H7 or *Shigella*) must be reported to public health officials. Requirements for the reporting of disease can be obtained from the web site of the Council of State and Territorial Epidemiologists: www.cste.org.

BIBLIOGRAPHY

Brandt LT, Boley SJ. The American Gastroenterological Association. Ischemic colitis. *Gastroenterology.* 2000;118: 951.

Guerrant RL, Van Gilder T, Steiner TS, et al. Practice guidelines for the management of infectious diarrhea. *Clin Infect Dis.* 2001;32:331–351.

Hecht G. Bacterial infections of the colon. In: Yamada T, Alpers DH, Laine L, et al., eds. *Textbook of Gastroenterology.* Vol. 2. Philadelphia, PA: Lippincott Williams and Wilkins; 2003: 1864–1882.

Hurley BW, Nguyen CC. The spectrum of pseudomembranous enterocolitis and antibiotic-associated diarrhea. *Arch Intern Med.* 2002;162:2177–2184.

McDonald LC, Killgore GE, Thompson A, et al. An epidemic, toxin gene-variant strain of *Clostridium difficile. N Engl J Med.* 2005;353:2433–2441.

Sreenarasimhaiah J. Diagnosis and management of ischemic colitis. *Curr Gastroenterol Rep.* 2005:7:421–426.

Warny M, Pepin J, Fang A, et al. Toxin production by an emerging strain of *Clostridium difficile* associated with outbreaks of severe disease in North America and Europe. *Lancet.* 2005;366(9491):1079–1084.

42 CROHN'S DISEASE

Jonathan Levine and Robert Burakoff

EPIDEMIOLOGY/OVERVIEW

• Crohn's disease is a disorder of uncertain etiology involving an exaggerated mucosal immune response in the intestinal tract.

• The incidence of Crohn's disease is relatively rare. It affects about 6–7.1 people in 100,000. There has been a steady rise in incidence in the United States between 1950 and 1985 while the incidence of UC has remained steady.

• IBD can present at any age although there is a bimodal age distribution with the peak age for diagnosis between ages 15 and 30 with a second, but smaller, peak between the ages of 50 and 80. The risk for Crohn's disease is equal for both sexes.

• Both Crohn's disease and UC are relapsing and remitting disorders.

• There is an increased incidence of Crohn's disease in first-degree relatives of patients.

• Evaluation of ethnic patterns reveals a higher incidence of Crohn's disease amongst jews of northern European descent and a lower incidence amongst black and Hispanic populations compared to Caucasians.

PATHOPHYSIOLOGY

• Crohn's disease is characterized by transmural mucosal inflammation. The inflammation often leads to fibrosis and microperforations with fistulae.

• In genetically predisposed individuals, an inflammatory response is initiated by putative environmental triggers that are not controlled by normal homeostatic mechanisms.

• Environmental factors, which have been implicated in Crohn's disease in genetically susceptible individuals, include smoking, oral contraceptives, nutritional deficiencies, and certain infectious agents.

- The first major Crohn's disease susceptibility gene, *NOD2/CARD 15* was recently identified.
- Inflammation is characterized by an imbalance in activity between proinflammatory mediators (eg, interleukin [IL]-1, alpha tumour necrosis factor [TNF], IL-6, IL-12/23, gamma interferon) and anti-inflammatory mediators (IL-10, prostaglandin E2).
- Crohn's disease, unlike UC, may involve the entire gastrointestinal (GI) tract. Eighty percent of patients have small bowel involvement, usually in the distal ileum, with one-third of patients having exclusively ileitis.
  - Fifty percent of patients have ileocolitis, which refers to involvement of both the ileum and colon.
  - Twenty percent of patients have disease limited to the colon. Unlike UC, one-half of such patients have sparing of the rectum.
  - A small percentage of patients have predominant involvement of the mouth or gastroduodenal area.
  - One-third of patients have perianal disease.

CLINICAL PRESENTATION

- Clinical manifestations of Crohn's disease are much more variable than those of UC because of the transmural inflammation and extent of disease. Fatigue, prolonged diarrhea with abdominal pain, weight loss, and fever are common features.
  - However, as many as 10% of patients will not have diarrhea.
  - Poor growth is common in children and may be present before other features of the disease become obvious.

- It may be difficult to distinguish ileitis from colitis unless the Crohn's colitis is limited to the left colon. Such patients may present with gross bleeding which mimics UC. Other features suggesting ileitis are small bowel obstruction (SBO) and an inflammatory mass in the RLQ. Appendicitis is sometimes suspected.
- Crampy abdominal pain is common regardless of the location in the GI tract.
- Because of the transmural inflammation, patients often develop fibrotic strictures leading to repeated small bowel and occasionally colonic obstructions.
- Hemoccult positive stools are common in Crohn's disease but gross bleeding is less frequent than in UC. A history of prolonged diarrhea without bleeding but with other features suggestive of IBD such as skin, eye, or joint problems (see extraintestinal manifestations below) or a family history of IBD should suggest the diagnosis of Crohn's disease.
- Transmural inflammation is associated with the development of sinus tracts, which can lead to serosal penetration and bowel wall perforation. This can present acutely as localized peritonitis with fever, abdominal pain, and tenderness with a palpable mass. Diffuse peritonitis is rare but occasionally occurs. Penetration of the bowel wall can also present as an indolent process related to fistulization such as recurrent urinary tract infections (enterovesical fistula), psoas abscesses and/or ureteral obstruction with hydronephrosis (retroperitoneal fistulae), passage of gas/feces through the vagina (enterovaginal fistulae) and cosmetic problems from bowel contents draining to the skin surface (enterocutaneous fistulae).
- Extraintestinal manifestations (Table 42-1) can be varied and include

TABLE 42-1   Extraintestinal Manifestations of IBD

LOCATIONS	MANIFESTATIONS
Musculoskeletal	Arthritis-colitic type, ankylosing spondylitis, isolated joint involvement Hypertrophic osteoarthropathy-clubbing, periostitis Miscellaneous-osteoporosis, aseptic necrosis, polymyositis
Skin and mouth	Reactive lesions: erythema nodosum, pyoderma gangrenosum, apthous ulcers, necrotizing vasculitis Specific lesions: fissures and fistulas, oral Crohn's disease, drug rashes Nutritional deficiency: acrodermatitis enteropathica, purpura, glossitis, hair loss and brittle nails Associated diseases: vitiligo, psoriasis, amyloidosis
Hepatobiliary	Primary sclerosing cholangitis and bile duct carcinoma Associated inflammation: autoimmune chronic active hepatitis, pericholangitis, portal fibrosis and cirrhosis, granulomatous disease Metabolic: fatty liver, gallstones associated with ileal Crohn's disease
Ocular	Uveitis/iritis, episcleritis, scleromalacia, corneal ulcers, retinal vascular disease
Metabolic	Growth retardation in children and adolescents, delayed sexual maturation
Renal	Calcium oxalate stones

- ◦ Oral involvement-apthous ulcers with pain in the mouth and gums.
- ◦ Skin manifestations including erythema nodosum, pyoderma gangrenosum, and psoriasis.
- ◦ Eye involvement including episclerits and uveitis.
- ◦ Musculoskeletal including arthritis and hypertrophic osteoarthropathy including clubbing and periostitis.
- ◦ Peripheral arthritis, primarily involving large joints and ankylosing spondylitis. An undifferentiated spondyloarthropathy or anklyosing spondylitis may be the presenting manifestation in some cases of Crohn's disease.
- ◦ Sclerosing cholangitis.
- ◦ Venous and arterial thromboembolic disease.

MAKING THE DIAGNOSIS

- Crohn's disease and UC can usually be differentiated endoscopically, pathologically, and serologically in most patients.
- Typical endoscopic findings include focal ulcerations adjacent to areas of normal-appearing mucosa along with polypoid mucosal changes that give a typical "cobblestone" appearance. "Skip lesions" are characteristic with normal segments of bowel interrupted by large areas of obvious disease.
- Biopsy is usually confirmatory rather than diagnostic. Major findings include focal ulcerations, and acute and chronic inflammation. Noncaseating granulomas are found in 30% of patients.
- An upper gastrointestinal (UGI) series or barium enema may be useful in documenting the length and location of strictures and be useful in reaching areas of the GI tract, otherwise inaccessible by endoscopy.
- More than 60% of patients have anti-*Saccharomyces cerevisiae* antibodies (ASCA). Less than 10% of patients have perinuclear antineutrophil cytoplasmic antibodies (p-ANCA) as compared to nearly 75% of UC patients. The combination of these two tests has been proposed as a means for diagnosing IBD and for distinguishing Crohn's disease from UC. For example, studies have demonstrated that a combination of a positive ASCA with a negative p-ANCA is more likely to identify a Crohn's patient. Conversely, patients with a negative ASCA and a positive p-ANCA are more likely to have UC.

DIFFERENTIAL DIAGNOSIS

- The differential is extensive and varies with the site of involvement and the chronicity of the patient's presentation.

- In milder cases, symptoms are often vague and nonspecific. Lactose intolerance, irritable bowel syndrome or other malabsorption syndromes must be considered. Usually, radiologic and endoscopic studies help to clarify this.
- Crohn's with colonic involvement must be distinguished from UC as both medical and surgical treatments differ. Distinguishing factors include small bowel involvement, sparing of the rectum, absence of gross bleeding, focality of gross and microscopic lesions with the presence of granulomas and fistulae.
- Appendicitis, diverticulitis, diverticular colitis, ischemic colitis, and a perforating or obstructing carcinoma can all mimic the clinical presentation of Crohn's disease.
- Infectious etiologies must be considered in patients with voluminous and persistent diarrhea. *Shigella, Salmonella, Campylobacter, E.coli* O157:H7, and amebiasis must be considered and testing is readily available by stool cultures.
- *C. difficile* should always be considered in patients in the setting of recent antibiotic use. Three negative *C. difficile* toxin tests are required to exclude infection and are 90% sensitive for the absence of disease.
- In patients with mainly small bowel involvement, *Yersinia* infection can mimic an acute Crohn's ileitis.

TRIAGE AND INITIAL MANAGEMENT

- In the setting of hospital medicine, two varieties of patients with IBD may present. The first includes patients without an established diagnosis who often present with abdominal cramping, diarrhea, and anorexia with or without malnutrition. A complete history and physical are vital and should be directed toward chronicity of symptoms, past medical history, family history of IBD, NSAID use, tobacco use, and an appropriate review of systems including questions addressing stool frequency and appearance and extraintestinal manifestations.
- A second group includes patients with established Crohn's disease who are now having breakthrough symptoms. Presentation between the two groups can obviously be similar. After stabilizing the patient, the patient's gastroenterologist or primary care physician (PCP) should be contacted to discuss the circumstances of this admission and to compare the patient's past responses to therapies.
- Patients are often both volume depleted and with electrolyte and acid-base abnormalities. Initial triage should be directed at volume and electrolyte repletion. Initial imaging should include an abdominal CT to

TABLE 42-2   Treatment Options for Crohn's Disease

DISEASE BEHAVIOR	PRINCIPAL THERAPIES
Fibrostenotic disease	Surgery
Inflammatory disease	5-ASA, IV or oral corticosteroids, 6-MP/ AZA, methotrexate, infliximab, surgery
Fistulizing disease	6-MP/AZA, metronidazole, infliximab, surgery

Abbreviations: 5-ASA, 5-aminosalicylic acid; 6-MP, 6-mercaptopurine; AZA, azathioprine.

rule out abscess formation and to help localize the colitis anatomically.
- Sigmoidoscopy or colonoscopy may be required to evaluate the colonic mucosa to evaluate extent of disease and to take biopsies ruling out infectious etiologies (see Differential Diagnosis for full list).
- Surgical consultation may be indicated depending on the severity of the presentation.

DISEASE MANAGEMENT STRATEGIES

- Drugs used to treat Crohn's disease include aminosalicylates, corticosteroids, immunomodulating agents, antibiotics, and new biologic agents such as infliximab (Tables 42-2 and 43-3).
- Sulfasalazine is effective only for treating Crohn's colitis, not for small bowel disease. Most adverse effects are because of the sulfapyridine component. As a result sulfa-free 5-ASA agents have been

developed to enable delivery to specific parts of the GI tract.
  ◦ 5-ASA enemas and suppositories are effective for treatment of the rectosigmoid colon. Oral 5-ASA in a pH sensitive release reaches the colon and oral 5-ASA is available in a time-release preparation for release in the colon and small intestine.
  ◦ Both mesalamine and sulfasalazine can induce and may maintain remission in patients with Crohn's disease, especially patients with colitis.
- Corticosteroids quickly reduce inflammation and induce remission. They have no proven role in maintaining remission and long-term treatment is not advised because of serious adverse effects.
- Azathioprine (AZA) and its metabolite 6-mercaptopurine (6-MP) inhibit the synthesis of rapidly dividing cells. Both are steroid sparing and effective in inducing and maintaining remission in Crohn's disease. Important side effects include pancreatitis, allergic reactions, and dose-dependent leukopenia.
- Methotrexate, an antimetabolite, is effective for treating patients with active disease and for maintaining remission. Significant side effects include interstitial pneumonitis and hepatic fibrosis.
- Antibiotics can be effective in subgroups of patients with Crohn's disease, particularly those with fistula formation. They are often used in patients not responding to 5-ASA drugs. For Crohn's ileitis, ciprofloxacin can be started for 6 weeks and then tapered over 6 weeks. Ciprofloxacin and metronidazole have been used successfully in treating ileocolonic Crohn's or Crohn's colitis.

TABLE 42-3   Initial Medication Dosages

DISEASE	MEDICATION AND DOSAGE
Crohn's ileitis	Asacol 2.4 g/d with an increase to a maximum of 4.8 g/d for initial therapy as needed, maintenance dosing is considered the dose which maintains clinical improvement; or pentasa started at 2 g/d increasing to 4 g/d as needed, maintenance considered the dose which produces clinical improvement Ciprofloxacin 500 mg po bid for 6 weeks tapered to 500 mg po qd for 6 weeks; or levaquin 500 mg po qd in combination with metronidazole 1–1.5 g/d Steroids: Prednisone 40–60 mg/d until response (usually 10–14 days), then taper 5–10 mg/week; or budesonide 9 mg/d for 8–16 weeks, then taper 3 mg increments over 2–4 weeks
Ileocolitis and colitis	Sulfasalazine 2 g/d with increase to 4 g/d or asacol 2.4 g/d with an increase to a maximum of 4.8 g/d for initial therapy as needed, maintenance dosing is considered the dose which maintains clinical improvement; or pentasa started at 2 g/d increasing to 4 g/d as needed, maintenance considered the dose which produces clinical improvement Ciprofloxacin 500 mg po bid for 6 weeks tapered to 500 mg po qd for 6 weeks; or levaquin 500 mg po qd in combination with metronidazole 1–1.5 g/d Steroids: Prednisone 40–60 mg/d with tapering as described above
Refractory disease	AZA or 6-MP 50 mg/d: genetic testing is now available to assess an individual's metabolism and doses can be adjusted accordingly with a usual therapeutic dose of 1-1.5 mg/kg for 6-MP and 2–2.5 mg/d for AZA Methotrexate 25 mg weekly IM (always with simultaneous oral folic acid), then 15 mg IM weekly for maintenance Infliximab 5 mg/kg at 0, 2, and 6 weeks, then q8 weeks thereafter

- Probiotics are currently being evaluated for treatment.
- Infliximab, a mouse-human monoclonal chimeric antibody to tumor necrosis factor-alpha, has recently been approved for treatment of patients with fistulous Crohn's disease. In addition to maintaining improvement in patients with fistulous disease, infliximab acts as a steroid sparing agent and results in rapid improvement in severe inflammatory Crohn's and its extraintestinal manifestations. Its long-term use has proven to be efficacious in combination with 6-MP or AZA.
- Patients with IBD have an increased risk of developing colorectal cancer (CRC). This is especially true for Crohn's patients with colitis and requires periodic surveillance by colonoscopy after 8 years of known disease. Findings of dysplasia or cancer warrant proctocolectomy.
- Other indications for surgery include severe disease refractory to medical therapy, toxic megacolon, steroid dependence, abscesses, fibrotic strictures, perforations, and fistula formation.

TRANSITIONS OF CARE

- Patients admitted with a new diagnosis of Crohn's disease should have a gastroenterology consult obtained during the initial admission. This is important in assisting with initial management and in facilitating the transition of care to a gastroenterologist who will manage the patient's long-term care.
- The Crohn's and Colitis Foundation of America are extensively involved in patient education, providing emotional support through support groups and physician referrals. Further information is available at their Web site, http://www.ccfa.org/.

BIBLIOGRAPHY

Boon N, Hanauer SB, Kiseil J. The clinical significance of p-ANCA and ASCA in indeterminate colitis (abstract). *Gastroenterology.* 1999;116:A671.

Burgmann T, Clara I, Graff L, et al. The Manitoba inflammatory bowel disease cohort study: prolonged symptoms before diagnosis—how much is irritable bowel syndrome? *Clin Gastroenterol Hepatol.* 2006;4:614.

Choi PM, Zeliz MP. Similarity of colorectal cancer in Crohn's disease and ulcerative colitis: implications for carcinogenesis and prevention. *Gut.* 1994;35:950.

Farmer RG, Hawk WA, Turnbull RB Jr. Clinical patterns in Crohn's disease: a statistical study of 615 cases. *Gastroenterology.* 1975;68:627.

Hanauer SB, Meyers S. Management of Crohn's disease in adults. *Am J Gastroenterol.* 1997;92:559.

Joossens S, Reinisch W, Vermeire S, et al. The value of serologic markers in indeterminate colitis: a prospective follow-up study. *Gastroenterology.* 2002;122:1242.

Schwartz DA, Loftus EV Jr, Tremaine WJ, et al. The natural history of fistulizing Crohn's disease in Olmsted County, Minnesota. *Gastroenterology.* 2002;122:875.

43 ULCERATIVE COLITIS
Scott Hande and Robert Burakoff

EPIDEMIOLOGY/OVERVIEW

- UC is an idiopathic chronic inflammatory disorder of the gut. Several clinical features distinguish it from the other major IBD, Crohn's disease (see Clinical Presentation below and Chap. 42).
- UC is a relatively uncommon new diagnosis, with a roughly estimated incidence of 10 cases per 100,000 person-years in European and North American studies. Because it is a chronic disorder frequently diagnosed in young patients, the prevalence of UC is significantly larger—approximately 100 patients per 100,000 persons.
- UC is typically diagnosed in the second, third, or fourth decade of life. A second, smaller "peak" in the distribution of incidence occurs around the seventh decade.
- The risk for UC is comparable between men and women.
- The risk appears to be similar between whites and blacks, but lower among Hispanic, Asian, and Native American populations. Jews have a higher rate of UC than other Caucasian ethnicities.
- The incidence and prevalence of UC appears to vary geographically, with higher rates in northern regions, such as Scandinavia. Within the United States, hospitalizations for UC are more common in northern states.
- The rate of UC is higher among people living in an urban environment compared with those who live in a rural setting, and higher among people of higher socioeconomic status.
- Studies on mortality in UC are conflicting, some showing a slightly increased risk of death and others showing no increase in mortality risk.
- The morbidity and healthcare costs of UC, though poorly quantified, are considerable.
  - Patients with UC often require evaluation and therapy for flares of colitis. Less common (but more worrisome) causes for morbidity and admission

include toxic megacolon, colonic adenocarcinoma, or complications related to therapy.
○ UC has a negative impact, albeit difficult to quantify, on subjective measures of morbidity, such as self-reported quality of life (QOL).

PATHOPHYSIOLOGY

• The pathophysiology of UC remains imperfectly understood. Current understanding of the disease process suggests that colonic inflammation results from a dysregulated immune response to gut flora or other antigens in genetically predisposed patients.
• Genetic factors
○ Monozygotic twins have a concordance rate of 10% to 15% for UC, suggestive of a relatively small genetic influence in its pathophysiology.
○ First-degree relatives of a patient with UC have 10-fold relative risk of developing UC.
• Microbial and environmental factors
○ Colitis fails to develop in animal models raised in germ-free environment, indicating that UC pathogenesis requires microbial flora.
○ Antigens from commensal or pathogenic microbial species may trigger an immune response within the colonic mucosa.
○ However, no specific infective agent has been found, and trials of antibiotics have failed to demonstrate a consistent therapeutic benefit in UC. These findings suggest that bacterial infection alone does not explain the etiology of UC.
○ No dietary trigger for UC has been found.
○ Smoking and nicotine appear protective in UC, in contrast with Crohn's disease.
• Immune factors
○ Microbial antigens activate the innate immune system within the colonic mucosa, either by crossing a defective epithelial barrier or by binding specific receptors on the epithelial surface.
○ The adaptive immune system (T cells, macrophages) in the colonic mucosa is activated but fails to downregulate, leading to chronic cytokine production (IL-1, IL-6, TNF) and inflammation. Subsequent tissue damage perpetuates the inflammatory response.

CLINICAL PRESENTATION, DIFFERENTIAL, MAKING THE DIAGNOSIS

• Unlike Crohn's disease, the inflammation in UC is limited to the colon (with the exception of "backwash ileitis" in some patients with colitis extending to the cecum and into the distal ileum).

○ Inflammation is limited to the mucosal layer (except in cases of toxic megacolon).
○ Inflammation typically begins in the rectum and extends proximally in a confluent fashion.
  ▪ Nearly half of patients have UC limited to the rectum or rectosigmoid colon.
  ▪ Twenty to thirty percent of patients have extensive colitis, defined as extending proximal to the splenic flexure.
• The presentation of UC typically depends on the extent of colon involved and the severity of the inflammation. Initial symptoms are often insidious in their onset, and the disease is typically localized in the distal colon and rectum only. A subset of patients develop progressive colonic involvement and thus progressive symptomatology.
• Typical symptoms include
○ *Hematochezia*—This may be the only symptom in patients with disease limited to the rectum. Rectal bleeding is so common in UC that its absence should cause one to challenge the diagnosis.
○ *Diarrhea*—Increased stool frequency and/or decreased stool consistency indicates more extensive colonic involvement with impaired water resorption and rapid transit.
○ *Tenesmus/urgency*—The symptoms signal severe rectal inflammation with impaired compliance.
○ *Abdominal pain*—Pain associated with UC is usually a vague, crampy, hypogastric discomfort. Severe pain suggests transmural inflammation and impending perforation.
○ *Others*—Fever, nausea, weight loss may be present.
• Clinical signs in patients with active flares of UC include weight loss, pallor, abdominal tenderness, and heme-positive (or frankly bloody) digital rectal examination. Worrisome features include fever, tachycardia, abdominal distention, or severe tenderness/guarding.
• Typically, laboratory findings include anemia and iron deficiency. Electrolyte derangements and hypoalbuminemia portend more severe illness.
○ ANCA are frequently present, but have limited value in confirming the diagnosis. They may be useful in distinguishing UC from Crohn's disease.
• The symptoms and signs of relapses are the same as those of the initial presentation.
• Complications of UC flares include hemorrhage, dehydration and electrolytes depletion, and perforation (with or without megacolon).
○ Extraintestinal manifestations of UC include erythema nodosum, pyoderma gangrenosum, arthropathy, sacroiliitis, oral aphthae, episcleritis, uveitis, primary sclerosing cholangitis, osteopenia, and venous thromboembolism (VTE).

○ The feared complication of chronic UC is CRC, principally in patients with extensive colitis. This increased risk becomes apparent ~ 10 years after the onset of disease. Patients with > 15 years of disease have an annual risk of ~ 1% for developing CRC.
• The diagnosis is made on the basis of supportive clinical, colonoscopic, radiographic, and pathologic findings. Other causes of colitis or rectal bleeding must be excluded (Table 43-1). Among those that should be routinely considered are infectious colitis, ischemic colitis, neoplastic disease, diverticular disease, Crohn's disease, and irritable bowel syndrome.
○ Stool collection is helpful to exclude infectious colitides, including *C. difficile* (Table 43-2). The presence of leukocytes in the feces supports the presence of an inflammatory diarrhea, but is nonspecific and adds little information if a colitis is already apparent by clinical or radiographic measures.
○ A plain film or CT of the abdomen may confirm the presence of a colitis, but are not specific for UC.

They are most useful for evaluating for megacolon or perforation, and should be performed in patients presenting with significant pain or fever.
○ Colonoscopy or sigmoidoscopy is required to confirm the diagnosis. Colonoscopy is preferable in most new presentations of UC because it also allows the physician to evaluate the extent of disease. Biopsies should be taken to help exclude alternative diagnoses. Histology demonstrating chronic active colitis in the absence of an alternative etiology supports the diagnosis of UC.

TRIAGE AND INITIAL MANAGEMENT

• A careful history is critical to identifying any precipitating factors for the patient suspected of having active UC. Key questions include prior history of UC, family history of IBD, travel history, recent antibiotic

TABLE 43-1 Conditions that may Mimic UC

CONDITION	DISTINGUISHING FEATURES
Crohn's disease	Skip lesions
	Small bowel or perianal involvement
	Strictures, abscesses, fistulae, or perforations
	Granulomas on histology
Infectious colitis (see Table 43-2)	Typically acute onset
	May involve small bowel
	May spare rectum (exceptions include gonococcus, lymphogranuloma venereum)
	Pain is frequently prominent
	With *C. difficile*, characteristic pseuomembranes may be seen on colonoscopy
	Crypt architecture preserved on histology
Ischemic colitis	Older patients
	"Watershed" region of colon involved with rectal sparing
	Acute onset
	Necrosis without chronic inflammation by histology
Microscopic colitis	Nonbloody diarrhea
	Colon grossly normal by colonoscopy
Diverticular disease	Diverticular bleeding is acute, painless, and usually self-limited
	Diverticulitis is segmental, rarely associated with diarrhea or hematochezia, and responds to antibiotics
Radiation proctitis/colitis	History of radiation
	Telangiectasias by colonoscopy in region of radiation field
Malignancy	Examples: adenocarcinoma of the colon, lymphoma, and metastatic disease
	Typically readily distinguished by endoscopy and biopsy
GI vasculitis	Examples: polyarteritis nodosa, Behçet's syndrome, Henoch-Schönlein purpura—systemic features of these vasculitides are typically present (and absent in UC)
	Vasculitis or ischemic injury seen on histology
Irritable bowel syndrome	Nonbloody diarrhea
	No nocturnal symptoms, weight loss, or fever
	Normal laboratory parameters
	Absence of colitis by imaging or endoscopy
Diversion colitis	History of colonic diversion
Solitary rectal ulcer	Bleeding (not diarrhea)
	Discrete ulcer by colonoscopy
Medication-induced colitis	Examples: NSAIDs, oral contraceptives, chemotherapeutic agents
	History of above medication use
	Typically readily distinguished by endoscopy and biopsy

TABLE 43-2 Infectious Agents Causing Colitis and/or Proctitis

PATHOGEN	RISK FACTORS
Bacterial	
E. coli	
EIEC	Food-borne
EHEC, including serotype O147:H7	Food-borne (meat, lettuce, unpasteurized milk)
Salmonella species (nontyphoid)	Food-borne (poultry, eggs, meat)
Shigella species	Food-borne (dairy)
	Fecal-oral
Camplyobacter species	Food-borne (poultry, other animals, water)
Y. enterocolitica	Food-borne (dairy, meat)
Aeromonas species	Water-borne
Plesiomonas shigelloides	Raw shellfish
C. difficile	Antibiotic exposure
	Hospitalization or institutional care
M. tuberculosis	Immunosuppression
	Travel to (or from) endemic regions
	Need not have pulmonary involvement
Nontuberculous *Mycobacteria*	Immunosuppression
Chlamydia trachomatis	Anal intercourse
Neisseria gonorrhoeae	Anal intercourse
Treponema pallidum	Anal intercourse
Viral	
CMV	Immunosuppression
Herpes simplex	Immunosuppression
Protozoan	
E. histolytica	Water-borne, endemic areas

exposure, other medications (including NSAIDs), and smoking history.

- A history and physical examinations are also essential for evaluating disease severity. Patients should be questioned about stool frequency and appearance, abdominal pain, constitutional symptoms (fever, sweats, weight loss), and extraintestinal manifestations (see above).
- Patients with active colitis are frequently volume depleted because of diarrheal losses. Initial management should be directed toward volume and electrolyte repletion.
- Patients with severe anemia should be transfused packed red blood cells (pRBCs) to avoid undue cardiopulmonary stress. Any patient admitted with a UC flare should have an active type and screen, in anticipation of progressive bleeding or urgent surgery.
- Bowel rest does not reduce inflammation in UC and is not necessary for mild-moderate disease (although patients often have a diminished appetite and avoid food because of the resulting increase in stool frequency). Enteral nutrition should be withheld from patients with severe or fulminant disease who may require urgent surgery.
- As per above, infectious colitis is one of the most common mimics of UC (Table 43-2). An infectious colitis must be excluded by a careful history, examination of the stool, and in some cases by endoscopy and

biopsy. This is particularly critical if steroids or other immunosuppressive therapy is contemplated.
  - Common pathogens which should be routinely tested by stool studies include *Salmonella, Shigella, E. coli, Campylobacter, Yersinia*, and *C. difficile*.
  - Other pathogens should be tested on the basis of clinical suspicion (Table 43-2).
- Surgical consult is appropriate for patients with severe colitis. Signs of systemic toxicity, including toxic megacolon, mandate emergent surgical evaluation. Broad spectrum antibiotics are also appropriate in such patients.
- Gastroenterology consult is also appropriate to help assist with the evaluation, perform a colonoscopic examination, and help guide medical therapy.

DISEASE MANAGEMENT STRATEGIES

- 5-Aminosalicylic acid (5-ASA) is effective for both inducing (~ 70%) and maintaining remission in patients with mild-to-moderate disease through topical anti-inflammatory effects on the colonic mucosa.
  - Sulfasalazine (5-ASA linked sulfapyridine) was the first drug in this class. Side effects from the sulfa moiety limit its clinical use.
  - Numerous preparations of free 5-ASA (mesalamine) or other 5-ASA prodrugs have since been developed

TABLE 43-3   Common 5-ASA Medications

GENERIC NAME	TRADE NAME	FORMULATION	DOSE
Sulfasalazine	Azulfidine	5-ASA linked to sulfapyridine	1000–2000 mg po bid
Mesalamine	Asacol	Coated 5-ASA with release at pH > 7 (distal ileum)	800–1600 mg po tid
Mesalamine	Pentasa	Coated 5-ASA with time-release (small bowel and colon)	500–1000 mg po qid
Mesalamine	Rowasa	5-ASA enema	4000 mg prn qhs
Mesalamine	Canasa	5-ASA suppository	1000 mg prn dhs
Olsalazine	Dipentum	Two linked 5-ASA molecules	1000 mg po bid
Balsalazide	Colazal	5-ASA linked to inert carrier	2250 mg po tid

(Table 43-3). For patients with distal disease, enema or suppository formulations are also an option.

◦ 5-ASA medications are generally well tolerated. Among the uncommon side effects are fever, rash, pneumonitis, interstitial nephritis, pericarditis, and paradoxical worsening of colitis.

- Corticosteroids are effective in inducing remission in patients with moderate-to-severe disease, but their adverse side effects make them unsuitable long-term agents.

◦ Prednisone 40–60 mg daily is a typical starting dose for patients with moderate symptoms. A slow taper ensues.

◦ Most hospitalized patients have severe disease and warrant IV steroids: hydrocortisone 100 mg IV tid or methylprednisolone 25mg IV bid. Oral steroids may be started once fever and tachycardia have resolved and stools are < 4/d.

◦ The use of corticosteroids at doses higher than those described above is discouraged, as it offers only increased risks of steroid-related complications without additional efficacy. Providers should be aware of equivalent dosages of the various corticosteroid agents.

- 6-MP and AZA are useful for maintaining remission in moderate-to-severe disease. Their slow onset of action limits their utility in achieving remission. Patients on these medications are at risk for life-threatening leucopenia, even after years of use. Patients should have a white blood cell (WBC) countchecked within 2 weeks of starting or increasing the dosage of these drugs.

- Cyclosporine (2–4 mg/kg/d IV) can be used as a bridge to 6-MP/AZA in patients with severe disease who have failed steroid therapy. Levels must be carefully monitored to reduce the risk of nephrotoxicity. Patients with low serum cholesterol may be at risk for seizures, and all patients are at increased risk for infections.

- Infliximab (5–10 mg/kg) has recently emerged as an alternative option in patients refractory to steroids. Patients should be screened for latent tuberculosis (prior to receiving infliximab, a recombinant antibody against TNF.

- Unlike Crohn's disease, UC is curable by total proctocolectomy. Therefore, one should avoid prolonged use of potentially toxic medical therapy once remission seems clinically unlikely.

◦ The current preferred surgical option is proctocolectomy with ileal pouch-anal anastomosis (IPAA), which allows a high rate of fecal continence.

◦ Patients with fulminant colitis, megacolon, or perforation require emergent surgery, typically a subtotal colectomy with ileostomy and Hartmann's pouch.

- Conversely, colectomy is not a panacea. In addition to acute surgical complications, chronic pouchitis, pouch failure, and incontinence do occur. Even with optimal results, patients typically will have multiple loose stools daily. Therefore, surgery for refractory UC should be pursued only after a limited trial of all reasonable medical options.

CARE TRANSITIONS

- Patients with UC are typically stable for discharge if they are afebrile, pain-free, have controlled diarrhea (< 4 bowel movements/d) with no or minimal blood, are tolerating adequate enteral nutrition/hydration, and are on oral medications.

- UC is a chronic condition characterized frequently by recurring flares of disease as well as serious long-term sequelae, including colon cancer. As such, all patients with UC should have a gastroenterologist for ongoing outpatient care.

◦ Patients discharged following treatment of a flare should be given an appointment for a follow-up visit with a gastroenterologist, preferably within 2 weeks of discharge.

◦ The primary gastroenterologist should be informed of pertinent inpatient events, including procedures and medication changes.

- The medication plan should be reviewed carefully with patients prior to discharge.

- Providers should educate patients, particularly those with new diagnoses, about the long-term nature of UC. Patients should be counseled about the importance of maintenance therapy—even if feeling well—to prevent future relapses. Patients with extensive colitis should be advised of the increased risk for CRC and the need for a screening regimen within 8 years of their diagnosis.
- Finally, patients with UC should be made aware of the outstanding education and support they can receive by seeking information from the Crohn's and Colitis Foundation of America at their Web site, www.ccfa.org.

BIBLIOGRAPHY

Carter MJ, Lobo AJ, Travis SPL. Guidelines for the management of inflammatory bowel disease in adults. *Gut.* 2004;53:V1.

Forcione DG, Sands BE. Differential diagnosis of inflammatory bowel disease. In: Sartor RB, Sandbown WJ, eds. *Inflammatory Bowel Disease.* 6th ed. London: Saunders; 2004:357.

Jewell DP. Ulcerative colitis. In: Feldman M, Friedman LS, Sleisenger MH, eds. *Gastrointestinal and Liver Disease.* 7th ed. Philadelphia, PA: Saunders; 2002:2039.

Kornbluth A, Sachar DB. Ulcerative colitis practice guidelines in adults (update): American College of Gastroenterology, Practice Parameters Committee. *Am J Gastroenterol.* 2004;99:1371.

Podolsky DK. Inflammatory bowel disease. *N Engl J Med.* 2002;347:417.

Sandler RS, Loftus EV. Epidemiology of inflammatory bowel diseases. In: Sartor RB, Sandbown WJ, eds. *Inflammatory Bowel Disease.* 6th ed. London: Saunders: 2004;245.

Sands BE. Therapy of inflammatory bowel disease. *Gastroenterology* 2000;118:S68.

44 DIVERTICULAR DISEASE AND DIVERTICULITIS

Norton J. Greenberger

EPIDEMIOLOGY/OVERVIEW

- Diverticular disease has increased in prevalence from 5% to 10% in the 1920s to 35% to 50% by 1990.
- Less than 5% of individuals aged less than 40 have diverticular disease, but this increases to 30% at age 60 and 65% at age 85.

- Gender
  - Males less than 50 years predominate.
  - Common for females between the ages of 50 and 70 years, and markedly more common in females more than 70 years of age.
- Diverticular disease is less common in vegetarians.
- Fifteen to twenty-five percent of patients with diverticulosis will develop infection (diverticulitis).

PATHOPHYSIOLOGY

- In diverticulosis, areas of weakness where the vasa recta penetrate the colonic wall are sites for diverticular development.
  - Myochosis, or thickening of the circular and longitudinal muscles, occurs owing in part to elastin deposition.
  - With time, luminal diameter decreases as fibrosis sets in.
  - Alterations in collagen structure, and decreased tensile wall strength are contributing factors that progress with age, leading to the development of diverticular sacs.
- In diverticulitis, increased intraluminal pressure and/or inspissated particulate material within a diverticular sac leads to microperforation, with resulting local inflammation and necrosis.
  - Fecoliths, with obstruction of a diverticular opening, are now thought to be an unusual cause of diverticulitis.
  - Microperforations may be walled off by mesentery and pericolic fat, resulting in a localized abscess.
    - Poor containment of the perforation or free macroperforation can lead to peritoneal soiling and peritonitis.
  - If adjacent organs are involved, fistulae, that is, sigmoidal vesical, can develop.
- The microbiology of diverticulitis reflects normal colonic flora: gram-negative rods and anaerobes (usually *E. coli* and *Bacteroids fragilis*).
- Diverticular bleeding occurs when the vasa recta at the site of a diverticulum become damaged, predisposing to rupture (see also Chap. 48).

CLINICAL PRESENTATION, DIFFERENTIAL, MAKING THE DIAGNOSIS

- Patients often have asymptomatic and incidental findings on imaging tests or endoscopic examinations.
- Symptomatic diverticulosis may be characterized by LLQ pain which is often exacerbated by eating, increased pain before defecation, relief of pain after

defecation (often incomplete), passage of pencil-thin stools, constipation, loose stools, and passage of mucus. These symptoms may be alleviated with bulking agents and/or a high fiber diet.

- *Acute diverticulitis* is a disease of variable severity characterized by lower abdominal pain and tenderness.
  - Diverticulitis is three to four times more frequent in the left vs. the right side of the colon. Right-sided diverticulitis presenting with RLQ pain may lead to diagnostic confusion with other entities such as appendicitis.
    - Right-sided diverticulitis is rare in patients from western countries (1.5% of cases), but is common in Asians (up to 75% of cases).
  - About 50% of patients will report experiencing a similar previous episode of pain, and prior attacks of diverticulitis are helpful in making a diagnosis.
  - Other symptoms include nausea and vomiting (up to 60% of cases), constipation (50%) or diarrhea (30%).
  - Only 20% of patients present with pain that is of less than 24 hours duration.
  - Hematochezia is rare.
- There is usually focal tenderness, and ~ 20% will have a palpable tender mass. Signs of peritoneal irritation and a possibly complicated diverticulitis include fever, abdominal muscle spasm, guarding, and rebound tenderness.
- The WBC count is typically elevated, while other laboratory studies are usually normal, although amylase may be elevated with perforation or peritonitis.
- CT scan is the usual method of confirming the presence of acute diverticulitis and its possible complications (sensitivity and specificity > 95%). CT scan may also help exclude other causes of abdominal pain in the differential diagnosis (Crohn's disease, ischemic colitis, splenic hematoma, carcinoma, renal calculus, appendicitis, ovarian cysts, ectopic pregnancy).
  - Typical CT findings include bowel wall thickening (> 4 mm), increased soft tissue density, masses (phlegmon or abscesses), pericolic fluid collections, fat stranding, and extraluminal air.
  - Gastrografin barium enema may demonstrate whether a contained perforation (abscess) is communicating with the bowel lumen.
- *Diverticular bleeding* presents as painless hematochezia or maroon stools, and is covered in Chap. 48.

TRIAGE AND INITIAL MANAGEMENT

- Uncomplicated acute diverticulitis may be treated in the outpatient setting, but complicated diverticulitis or mild cases with associated comorbidities should be hospitalized for treatment (see Table 44-1).

TABLE 44-1   Decision-Making Regarding the Site of Care for the Patient with Acute Diverticulitis

Consider *outpatient* treatment if	*Inpatient* treatment appropriate for
Mild presentation	Elderly
Tolerating fluids	Immunosuppressed
Compliant	High fever, markedly elevated WBC
Stable home situation	Complications
Stable vital signs	• Perforation
	• Peritonitis
	• Abscess
	• Fistula
	• Obstruction

- Outpatient management consists of
  - *Bowel rest*: A clear liquid diet, advancing slowly after clinical improvement (typically 2–3 days)
  - Oral antibiotics for 7–10 days
    - Ciprofloxacin (500 mg bid) plus metronidazole (500 mg tid)
    - *Or* amoxicillin/clavulanate (875/125 mg bid)
    - *Or* trimethoprim/sulfamethoxazole (160/800 mg bid) plus metronidazole (500 mg tid)
  - Close outpatient follow-up (see Care Transitions below)
- Inpatient treatment consists of
  - *Bowel rest*: Either NPO with IV hydration, or clear liquids
    - Advance the diet slowly after several days once there is clear evidence of clinical improvement to a low residue diet.
  - *IV antibiotics*: Appropriate regimens include
    - Metronidazole (500 mg q 8 hours) plus ciprofloxacin (400 mg q 12 hours) or other fluoroquinolone
    - *Or* metronidazole (500 mg q 8 hours) plus cefotaxime (1–2 g q 6 hours) or other third-generation cephalosporin
    - *Or* ampicillin-sulbactam (3 g q 6 hours) or other beta-lactamase inhibitor combination
    - *Or* imipenem (500 mg q 6 hours) or other carbapenem
  - Monitoring for clinical improvement or the development of complications

DISEASE MANAGEMENT STRATEGIES

- Twenty-five percent of patients diagnosed with a first attack of acute diverticulitis and 60% of recurrences develop complications.
- Complications that require broad-spectrum antibiotics and urgent surgical consultation include
  - Clinical deterioration or failure to improve with medical treatment

∘ Free intraperitoneal macroperforation with diffuse peritonitis—a rare complication with a very high mortality rate (~ 25%), particularly in the setting of fecal soilage—that requires emergent surgery
∘ Abscess that may be drained by percutaneous catheter prior to definitive surgical treatment or as an alternative in patients at high surgical risk
∘ Fistula which typically occurs between adjacent loops of bowel, but may also involve the bladder
  ▪ Enterovesical fistulae suspected clinically when the patient has concomitant urinary tract infection and/or pneumaturia
∘ Complete obstruction—a rare complication of diverticulitis—in the setting of strictures or lesions suspicious for malignancy requiring resection.

CARE TRANSITIONS

• Patients managed medically for uncomplicated diverticulitis may transition to outpatient care once there is clear clinical improvement and they tolerate oral intake.
  ∘ IV antibiotics can be switched to one of the oral outpatient treatment regimens given above to complete a total 7- to 14-day course.
  ∘ Patients should be educated regarding a high-fiber diet once their symptoms have resolved.
    ▪ There is no evidence that avoiding seeds and nuts influences the risk of diverticulitis.
  ∘ Fiber supplements may also be recommended.
• Outpatient follow-up should include
  ∘ Colonoscopy within 4–6 weeks, to exclude malignancy, if not performed within the past 5 years.
  ∘ Patients who have experienced two or more episodes of acute diverticulitis should be considered for elective surgical resection of the involved bowel to reduce the risk of future episodes.

BIBLIOGRAPHY

Biondo S, et al. Acute colonic diverticulitis in patients under 50 years of age. *Br Surg*. 2002;89:1137.
Brook I, Frazier EH. Aerobic and anaerobic microbiology in intraabdominal infections associated with diverticulitis. *J Med Microbiol*. 2000;49:827.
Tursi A. Acute diverticulitis of the colon: current medical therapeutic management. *Expert Opin Pharmacother*. 2004;5:55.

45 PANCREATITIS

Eric R. Schumacher

EPIDEMIOLOGY/OVERVIEW

• Acute pancreatitis (AP) is diagnosed in approximately 185,000 patients in the United States annually, and the incidence has increased during the last decade.
  ∘ The mean age at the time of diagnosis of AP is 52.
  ∘ AP is more common in males, in particular white males.
• AP results in approximately 245,000 hospital admissions annually.
  ∘ Average length of stay (LOS) for patients with AP is approximately 5.9 days.
  ∘ The most recent government statistics report mean charges of ~ $24,000 per case with a countrywide total cost of ~ $5.7 billion.
• In 2002, the CDC reported 3532 deaths because of AP.
  ∘ The majority of these were seen in patients 70 or older.
• Mortality ranges from < 1% in those with mild disease to > 25% in those with severe disease.

PATHOPHYSIOLOGY

• AP is an acute inflammatory process involving the pancreas.
  ∘ Pancreatic enzymes from acinar cells and other toxic materials are released into the surrounding tissue causing chemical irritation and initiation of the inflammatory response.
  ∘ Eighty percent of cases are interstitial pancreatitis with the remaining 20% necrotizing pancreatitis.
• The majority of cases (80%) are related to gallstone (biliary) disease or heavy alcohol consumption.
• Other causes of pancreatitis include
  ∘ Drugs (furosemide, thiazides, valproic acid, pentamidine, AZA, sulfonamides, tamoxifen, tetracyclines, estrogen, didanosine, corticosteroids, NSAIDs, and angiotensin-converting enzyme [ACE] inhibitors)
  ∘ Hyperlipidemia (hypertriglyceridemia or chylomicronemia)
  ∘ Abdominal trauma/surgery
  ∘ Hypercalcemia
  ∘ Vasculitis

◦ Infection (coxsackievirus, CMV, mumps, *Mycoplasma pneumoniae, Campylobacter,* and some parasites)
◦ Endoscopic retrograde cholangiopancreatography (ERCP)
◦ Cystic fibrosis
◦ Peritoneal dialysis
◦ Cardiopulmonary bypass
• "Idiopathic" AP is most commonly related to microlithiasis or sphincter of Oddi dysfunction.

CLINICAL PRESENTATION, DIFFERENTIAL, MAKING THE DIAGNOSIS

• The diagnosis of AP is based on a suggestive history and physical examination and elevation of the amylase and lipase levels.
• The differential diagnosis of pancreatitis most commonly includes peptic ulcer disease, abdominal aortic aneurysm, intestinal obstruction, cholecystitis, cholangitis, mesenteric ischemia, or perforated viscus.
• The history should include
  ◦ Known gallstones, alcoholism, hypercalcemia, previous trauma, autoimmune disease
  ◦ Risk factors for pancreatic disease (elevated triglycerides, positive family history for pancreatic disease)
  ◦ Drug history (thiazide use, human immunodeficiency virus [HIV] drugs, over-the-counter drugs)
  ◦ The classic presentation of AP is upper abdominal pain that may radiate to the back (seen in ~ 50% of cases), usually acute in onset and severe in intensity, commonly associated with nausea and vomiting
• The physical examination is not specific
  ◦ Tachycardia is commonly seen and in some cases hypotension.
  ◦ Fever should precipitate a search for an infectious etiology, although it may also be a sign of the underlying inflammatory process.
  ◦ There may be concomitant multiorgan failure (MOF) or the systemic inflammatory response syndrome.
  ◦ Classic signs, including Cullen's (periumbilical bruising) and Grey Turner's (flank bruising), are uncommon and represent fat necrosis and subcutaneous bleeding. Initial signs of peritonitis are not commonly seen.
• Laboratory studies are required to confirm the diagnosis of AP.
  ◦ Elevated levels of pancreatic enzymes (amylase/lipase) greater than three times the upper limit of normal, in the absence of renal failure, support a diagnosis of pancreatitis. Smaller elevations in the

serum amylase or lipase have a low specificity for AP and may be seen in other causes of abdominal pain.
  ▪ Amylase levels are elevated within 12 hour of onset, peak within 24 hours and remain elevated for 3–5 days. A sensitivity of 80% to 90% and a specificity of 70% have been reported for this test. False elevation may be seen in conjunction with salivary gland abnormalities, renal failure (with normal urine levels), ascites, mesenteric ischemia obstruction, or perforation.
• Lipase is the preferred test as it has fewer false positives (+) than serum amylase. The lipase level tends to remain elevated for a longer duration than amylase. Sensitivity of lipase is 80% to 90% with a specificity of 90% have been reported.
• Other laboratory studies are obtained for multiple severity scoring systems and to assist in triage and management.
  ◦ Liver function panel (including aspartate aminotransferase [AST]/alanine aminotransferase [ALT]) is helpful in screening for biliary involvement.
    ▪ An ALT >150 has a good specificity (96%) for biliary pancreatitis. Alkaline phosphatase levels > 300 and total bilirubin > 2.9 also show specificity of > 90% for biliary pancreatitis. Sensitivities of these studies are < 50%.
    ▪ Overall, elevated levels of liver profile tests are helpful while normal levels do not rule out biliary involvement.
  ◦ A complete blood count (CBC) is routinely obtained.
    ▪ A high or rising hematocrit (Hct) suggests hemoconcentration that carries a poor prognosis if not rapidly reversed with aggressive fluid administration.
    ▪ Leukocytosis is commonly seen and is nonspecific but may aid to diagnosis cholangitis in association with an elevated liver profile and fever.
  ◦ Chemistry profile is also routinely obtained to assess prognosis.
    ▪ Elevated glucose levels may relate to degree of pancreatic dysfunction in those with previous euglycemic values.
• Serum calcium levels may be decreased secondary to saponification, precipitation, and decreased parathyroid hormone (PTH) response.
  ◦ Fever should guide decision-making relating to obtaining blood cultures.
  ◦ Lactate dehydrogenase (LDH) levels may be elevated in the setting of pancreatic necrosis.
  ◦ Triglyceride levels may be helpful in those patients in whom an etiology is not apparently clear; values > 1000 are usually clinically significant.

◦ A C-reactive protein (CRP) level >150 mg/L is an indicator of inflammatory response and is associated with a worse prognosis at 48 hours.
- CT imaging of the abdomen using IV contrast enhancement confirms the diagnosis of pancreatitis and provides information relating to severity.
  ◦ When imaging is required because of diagnostic uncertainty, do not perform plain films of the abdomen. "Sentinel loop" (air-filled small intestine overlying the inflamed pancreas) or "colon cutoff sign" (air-filled transverse colon ending at the area of the pancreas) are suggestive but nonspecific for diagnosis of AP.
  ◦ CT scan is reserved for those patients suspected of having severe pancreatitis (APACHE II [Acute Physiology and Chronic Health Evaluation II] score > 8), those with multisystem failure, those in whom the diagnosis is uncertain, or those who fail to show improvement despite appropriate treatment.
    ▪ There are no data supporting its use in the first 24 hours, except to rule out other causes of abdominal pain if the diagnosis is unclear.
    ▪ CT performed within 72 hours of onset of symptoms of AP may, in fact, underestimate the degree of pancreatic necrosis.
    ▪ After this time frame CT scanning is the imaging modality of choice for grading the severity of pancreatic necrosis. When more than 50% of the pancreas becomes necrotic, the positive predictive value of CT scanning approaches 100%.
    ▪ In patients who have pancreatic necrosis, infection remains a serious complication. These patients may benefit from interventional radiologic aspiration of the area, especially in those who fail to improve with current treatment.
    ▪ The Balthazar-Ranson grading system and CT severity index (Table 45-1) score > 6 correlates with an increased morbidity and mortality. Some studies have shown CT scoring to be superior to Ranson criteria and APACHE II in predicting complications and death in patients with pancreatitis.
  ◦ Ultrasound (US) of the abdomen should be obtained within the first 24–48 hours especially in those who present for the first time with pancreatitis or when the etiology is unclear.
    ▪ US assists with diagnosing cholelithiasis, cholecystitis, or common bile duct disease leading to gallstone pancreatitis.
    ▪ Unfortunately, the sensitivity for detecting common bile duct stones is < 50% (especially stones < 3 mm) and determining pancreatic anatomy is often hindered by overlying bowel loops.
  ◦ Magnetic resonance imaging (MRI) is reserved for those patients who are unable to undergo a

TABLE 45-1   The Balthazar-Ranson Grading System and CT Severity Index

BALTHAZAR-RANSON GRADING SYSTEM	
CT GRADE	DEFINITION
A	Normal appearing pancreas
B	Focal or diffuse enlargement of the pancreas
C	Pancreatic gland abnormalities associated with mild peripancreatic inflammatory changes ("stranding")
D	Fluid collection in a single location, usually within the anterior pararenal space
E	One or more fluid collections near the pancreas (such as within the anterior pararenal space and within the lesser sac) and/or the presence of gas in or adjacent to the pancreas

CT SEVERITY INDEX (0–10)			
CT GRADE	SCORE	NECROSIS	SCORE
A	0	None	0
B	1	< 33%	2
C	2	33%–50%	4
D	3	> 50%	6
E	4		

CT Grade (0–4) + Necrosis (0–6) = Total score

contrast-enhanced CT scan. MRI is less accurate in those patients who are unable to tolerate holding their breath or remaining still for longer periods of time.
  ▪ MRI is superior to CT in detecting cholelithiasis, choledocholithiasis, and anomalies of the pancreatic duct.
  ▪ Magnetic resonance cholangiopancreatography (MRCP) is useful as a noninvasive modality for detecting common bile duct stones.

TRIAGE AND INITIAL MANAGEMENT

RISK ASSESSMENT

- Once the diagnosis is made, several risk factor scoring systems are available to assist in identifying those patients at risk for developing severe pancreatitis. These include Ranson criteria, Glasgow criteria, APACHE II, and the CT severity index.
- Ranson criteria (Table 45-2) comprise 11 clinical signs, 5 of which are measured on admission and the remaining 6 at the end of the first 48 hours.
  ◦ The presence of three or more Ranson criteria on admission has a sensitivity of > 60% in predicting a severe clinical course.
  ◦ Reevaluation at 48 hours looks at systemic effects of the underlying pancreatic process.
    ▪ One to three Ranson criteria represent mild pancreatitis.

TABLE 45-2   Ranson Criteria

On admission
- Age > 55 year
- WBC > 16,000 µL
- Serum glucose > 200 mg/dL
- LDH > 350 IU/L
- AST > 250 IU/L

During first 48 hours
- Drop in Hct of > 10 points
- Serum calcium < 8 mg/dL
- Base deficit > 4 mEq/L
- Increase in BUN > 5 mg/dL
- Fluid sequestration > 6 L
- Arterial PO_2 < 60 mm Hg

Abbreviation: BUN, blood urea nitrogen.

- Morbidity and mortality increase with scores above four. Mortality rates of > 50% have been seen when > 5 criteria are present.
- Glasgow criteria and APACHE II scores are particularly useful in patients with gallstone pancreatitis.
  - The presence of three or more Glasgow criteria predicts a complicated course in the majority of cases (Table 45-3).
- APACHE II scoring uses 12 physiologic variables to predict disease severity. It also takes into account the patient's age and health status in its scoring. Both morbidity and mortality increase with increasing APACHE II scores.
  - APACHE II scores of > 8 indicate a severe case of AP and in most cases a need for ICU care.
  - One advantage of APACHE II scores is the ability to calculate on a daily basis allowing an objective measure of response to treatment course.
  - An easy to use APACHE II calculator can be found at www.globalrph.com/apacheii.htm.
- CT severity index compliments the prognostic information from scoring criteria that may help guide triage for critically ill patients.

INITIAL MANAGEMENT

- Initial management of AP involves supportive care, aggressive fluid resuscitation, pain control, treatment

TABLE 45-3   Glasgow Criteria

- Serum albumin < 3.2 g/dL
- Arterial PO_2 on room air < 60 mm Hg
- Serum calcium < 8 mg/dL
- WBC > 15,000/µL
- AST or ALT > 200 IU/L
- LDH > 600 U/L
- Serum glucose > 180 mg/dL
- BUN > 45 mg/dL

of reversible causes, prevention of organ failure, and minimization of peripancreatic complications.
- Maintaining adequate IV volume is crucial and use of vigorous IV hydration is indicated. IV rates of > 150 cc/h for the first 24–48 hours are not uncommon (5–10 L total) in preventing hypovolemia from third space losses and/or emesis. Scoring systems utilize markers of intravascular depletion in determining severity of the disease process. Serial measurements of the Hct are used to assess adequacy of hydration.
- NG suction is of benefit in those with ileus or severe pancreatitis but is not helpful in mild cases.
- Pain control is commonly achieved with narcotic analgesics.
  - In the past, meperidine was the preferred pain reliever as it was thought that morphine derivatives had a negative effect on Oddi's sphincter. This negative effect has not been substantiated.
  - Thoracic epidural analgesia has also been used successfully to treat pancreatic pain.
- Bowel rest is often used for the first 24–48 hours. In milder cases, oral nutrition can begin once abdominal pain has improved, nausea/vomiting has resolved, vital signs are stable, and bowel function has returned. Clear liquids are used first, then advanced as tolerated to a regular diet. Special pancreatic diets have not been found to be beneficial.

NUTRITION

- In patients with severe pancreatitis who will be without adequate oral nutrition for >7 days, enteral nutrition or total parenteral nutrition (TPN) should be initiated as soon as possible.
  - Enteral nutrition maintains the integrity of the intestinal mucosa that will atrophy if bowel rest is prolonged, increasing morbidity in these patients. Enteral feedings have proven to cost less, have fewer complications, and essentially no difference in mortality rates compared to patients receiving TPN. Jejunal feeding using an elemental or semi-elemental formula eliminates the concern of stimulating the exocrine pancreas.

PANCREATIC NECROSIS

- Antibiotic use is generally reserved for those with severe pancreatitis, sepsis, or in patients with known pancreatic necrosis or abscess.

○ Antibiotic prophylaxis to avoid conversion of sterile necrosis to infected necrosis is controversial.
○ The AGA guideline recommends that patients should have extensive necrosis (> 30% of the gland by CT criteria) to qualify for antibiotic prophylaxis for no more than 14 days.
○ Prior to initiating antibiotics, fine-needle aspiration guided by CT imaging for culture and gram stain is recommended, usually for patients with worsening symptoms, fever, and typically after 7–10 days of being ill.
  ▪ The most common bacterial pathogens isolated are *E. coli, Klebsiella, Enterococcus, Staphylococcus,* and *Pseudomonas.*
  ▪ Antibiotics with good pancreatic tissue penetrance include imipenem, meropenem, clindamycin, fluoroquinolones, cephalosporins, and metronidazole.
  ▪ Utilization of fluoroquinolones with clindamycin is less effective than imipenem or meropenem.
  ▪ There does not appear to be an increased incidence of fungal superinfection associated with prior antibiotic prophylaxis.
• More than 50% of patients will develop fluid collections and usually these resolve over time.
• Symptomatic pseudocysts usually require drainage.
• Drainage of intra-abdominal abscesses via surgical, endoscopic, or percutaneous methods is indicated.
• Patients with infected necrosis will typically require surgical debridement in addition to parenteral antibiotics.

GALLSTONE PANCREATITIS

• Urgent ERCP within 24 hours of initial presentation should be performed in those patients with gallstone pancreatitis complicated by cholangitis or sepsis to alleviate obstruction.
• Although ERCP has *no* role in the initial diagnosis of AP, ERCP should be performed within 72 hours in patients with biliary pancreatitis, that is, a persistent dilated common bile duct or visible common bile duct stone or jaundice.
• The use of ERCP, endoscopic sphincterotomy (ES), and laparoscopic surgical techniques have changed the options for patients with gallstone pancreatitis. For patients at high risk for surgery such as advanced age, ERCP, and sphincterotomy are reasonable alternatives.
○ Patients with mild biliary pancreatitis who undergo laparoscopic cholecystectomy and cholangiogram have improved outcomes.
○ In individuals who have had ERCP with ES, AGA institute recommends cholecystectomy ideally within the same hospitalization or within 2–4 weeks post discharge.

DISEASE MANAGEMENT STRATEGIES

• Hospitalists should lead or participate in initiatives that assure adherence to evidence-based practices that assure the highest standard of care for the patient with pancreatitis.
• There may be opportunities for hospitalists to develop order sets and guidelines for managing AP in collaboration with gastroenterologists, surgeons, and interventional radiologists.
• Patient and family education about the course of pancreatitis should begin at the time of admission.
○ Pain management, nutrition, and the role of antibiotics should be reviewed with the patient.
○ Advance directives should be noted at the time of admission.
○ A free and useful patient information sheet is available at www.patient.co.uk/showdoc/479/.
• See Chap. 70 for more information on alcohol withdrawal prophylaxis.
• VTE prophylaxis is recommended in all hospitalized patients.

CARE TRANSITIONS

• Patients may be discharged when they are tolerating an oral diet and their pain is controlled on oral analgesics. Patients with a more severe course may need to be discharged on enteral feeds or even TPN.
• If the underlying cause of the pancreatitis is determined, care plans can be made to help prevent recurrence.
○ Eliminate medications that may cause pancreatitis.
○ Alcohol cessation and referral to alcoholics anonymous or other support groups.
○ Prompt outpatient cholecystectomy in those patients with biliary disease who did not undergo the procedure while hospitalized.
○ Dietary and lifestyle modification should be encouraged in those patients with hypertriglyceridemia and drug therapy may be necessary as well.
○ Additional workup of hypercalemia may be indicated and need not require continued hospitalization.
• Timely and accurate communication with the patient's PCP is essential for a successful transition to outpatient management.

BIBLIOGRAPHY

American Gastroenterological Association (AGA) institute medical position statement on acute pancreatitis. *Gastroenterology.* 2007;132:2019–2021.

Balthazar EJ, Robinson DL, Megibow AJ, et al. Acute pancreatitis: value of CT in establishing prognosis. *Radiology.* 1990; 174:331–336.

Banks PA. Practice guidelines in acute pancreatitis. *Am J Gastroenterol.* 1997;92:377–386.

Bolek T, Baker M, Walsh RM. Imaging in practice: L imaging's role in acute pancreatitis. *Cleve Clin J Med.* 2006;73:857–862.

Corfield AP, Cooper MJ, Williamson RC, et al. Prediction of severity in acute pancreatitis: prospective comparison of three prognostic indices. *Lancet.* 1985;2:403–407.

Deaths from 358 Selected Causes, by 5-Year Age Groups, Race, and Sex: United States 2002. 18 Nov. 2004. 01 Mar. 2006. http://www.cdc.gov/nchs.

HCUPnet: a Tool for Identifying, Tracking, and Analyzing National Hospital Statistics. HCUPnet. 2003. 01 Mar. 2006. http://hcup.ahrq.gov.

Heinrich S, Schafer M, Rousson V, et al. Evidenced-based treatment of acute pancreatitis: a look at established paradigms. *Ann Surg.* 2006;243:154–168.

Larvin M, McMahon MJ. APACHE-II score for assessment and monitoring of acute pancreatitis. *Lancet.* 1989;2:201–205.

Nathens AB, Curtis JR, Beale RJ, et al. Management of the critically ill patient with severe acute pancreatitis. *Crit Care Med.* 2004;32:2524–2536.

Ranson JH. Etiological and prognostic factors in human acute pancreatitis. *Am J Gastroenterol.* 1982;77:633–638.

Tenner S. Initial management of acute pancreatitis: critical issues during the first 72 hours. *Am J Gastroenterol.* 2004;99: 2489–2494.

Whitcomb DC. Acute pancreatitis. *N Engl J Med.* 2006;354: 2142–2150.

Yadav D, Agarwal N, Pitchumoni CS. A critical evaluation of laboratory tests in acute pancreatitis. *Am J Gastroenterol.* 2002;97:1309–1318.

46 SMALL BOWEL OBSTRUCTION

Lynn Wilkinson

EPIDEMIOLOGY/OVERVIEW

- SBO is the most common surgical disorder of the small intestine accounting for as many as 12% to 16% of surgical admissions annually.

Expert reviewer: David C Brooks, MD, Director of Minimally Invasive Surgery, Brigham and Women's Hospital.

- According to most surgical series, SBO is managed surgically in 50% to 75% of patients admitted.
- The overall mortality rate for SBO is approximately 5%. Rapid and accurate diagnosis and appropriate management that include prompt surgical consultation are essential and can be lifesaving.
  - Mortality for adhesive SBO is currently 1% to 2%.
  - The presence of strangulation increases the mortality rate to about 20%.
- The most common cause of SBO in the United States is adhesions from prior laparotomy, which accounts for about 60% of cases.
  - SBO as a result of adhesions may occur after any type of laparotomy, though is most common following surgery of the lower abdomen and pelvic cavity.
  - Overall, adhesions have been shown to develop in 6% to 11% of all patients who undergo laparotomy.
  - In 1994, all abdominal adhesion procedures were identified in a study of hospital discharges using a national hospital discharge database. The study showed that there were more than 300,000 hospitalizations for adhesiolysis (most relating to SBO), resulting in over 800,000 days of inpatient care and $1.3 billion in expenditures.
- Malignant tumors account for about 20% of cases of SBO. Metastatic disease is more common than primary small bowel malignancies as a primary cause for SBO.
- Hernias account for approximately 10% of cases of SBO in the United States and are more often associated with strangulation than are adhesions.
- Crohn's disease causes 5% of all cases of SBO in the United States. SBO may be the first manifestation of Crohn's disease.
- Miscellaneous causes (Table 46-1) for SBO account for only 2% to 3% of cases in the United States.

PATHOPHYSIOLOGY

- It is important to differentiate complete SBO from partial SBO, pseudo-obstruction, and adynamic ileus.
  - Complete SBO is commonly managed operatively.
  - Partial SBO is most often managed nonoperatively.
- Complete SBO occurs when normal intestinal flow is interrupted.
  - Ingested fluid, food, gas, and digestive secretions accumulate above the site of obstruction leading to distention of the bowel proximal to the obstruction.
  - Distention stimulates peristalsis above and below the level of obstruction often leading to several

TABLE 46-1   Causes of SBO

Extrinsic
Adhesions
Masses
Hernia
Carcoinomatosis
Volvulus
Diverticular disease
Superior mesenteric artery syndrome
Intestinal malrotation
Familial mediterranean fever

Intramural
Tumors
Strictures (such as those caused by IBD and radiation injury)
Intussusception such as those caused by neoplasm or Meckel's
    diverticulum
Traumatic hematoma

Intraluminal
Gallstones (gallstone ileus)
GI bezoars
Neoplasms

loose bowel movements in the initial hours after onset of obstruction.
  ○ As the bowel distends, intramural and intraluminal pressure rise leading to bowel wall edema and congestion that ultimately compromise blood flow to the intestine resulting in intestinal ischemia.
    ▪ If the process continues to progress with luminal pressure exceeding venous hydrostatic pressure bowel infarction, or strangulation, ensues.
    ▪ Strangulation is reported to occur in between 20% and 40% of patients with complete obstruction.
• Closed loop obstructions occur when both entrance and exit to a segment of small bowel becomes occluded.
  ▪ For example, it happens typically in torsion around an adhesion.
  ▪ When this is suspected or proven, immediate operation should be undertaken to prevent an ischemic segment.
• If the SBO is partial, only a portion of the bowel lumen becomes occluded and there is continued passage of intestinal contents distally.
  ▪ This process occurs more slowly and there is minimal risk of strangulation.
  ▪ Partial SBO may be managed nonoperatively.
• Intestinal pseudo-obstruction is a chronic condition where the normal peristaltic mechanism is impaired. These patients can have massive abdominal distention but no obstruction. It affects the colon more often than the small intestine.
• Adynamic ileus can be distinguished clinically from mechanical SBO by the presence of large amounts of gas in the colon. The peristaltic activity of the small

bowel is lost and leads to progressive dilatation and stasis of intestinal contents.
  ○ Adynamic ileus can occur as a result of intra-abdominal infection, postoperative ileus, electrolyte abnormalities, and pancreatitis.

CLINICAL PRESENTATION, DIFFERENTIAL, MAKING THE DIAGNOSIS

• There are four key considerations in the evaluation of patients with SBO.
  ○ Recognize mechanical obstruction.
  ○ Distinguish partial from complete obstruction.
  ○ Distinguish simple (nonstrangulating) from strangulating obstruction.
  ○ Identify the underlying cause for obstruction.
• It is important to keep in mind when evaluating the patient with suspected SBO that early, reversible ischemia is not clinically discernible.
• In addition, clinical indicators of strangulation such as fever, tachycardia, peritoneal signs, leukocytosis, acidosis, and/or continuous abdominal pain are not sensitive, specific, or accurate when it comes to diagnosing strangulating obstruction. This is especially true in elderly patients with SBO.
• History should note the hallmark presenting complaints of SBO.
  ○ Nausea and vomiting
  ○ Paroxysmal crampy or colicky abdominal pain
    ▪ Abdominal pain may be constant and severe, particularly in more advanced cases where there is a strangulating obstruction.
  ○ Inability to pass flatus
    ▪ Passage of loose stool and flatus can occur for 12 hours or longer after complete SBO whereas continued passage beyond this time increases suspicion for partial rather than complete SBO.
  ○ Obtaining the past history of prior abdominal surgeries, GI disease, and other medical illnesses is imperative in evaluating a patient with suspected SBO.
    ▪ Prior surgery is the most significant risk factor for the development of SBO because of adhesion formation.
• Physical examination
  ○ Physical examination may reveal fever and signs of volume depletion, especially with strangulation.
  ○ Abdominal examination should note whether the following signs are present:
    ▪ Scars from prior abdominal surgeries
    ▪ Bowel sounds which may be hyperactive, hypoactive, or high-pitched

○ Bowel sounds that may be hyperactive, hypoactive, or high-pitched are generally not helpful in making the diagnosis of SBO but provide important baseline information.
  ▪ Abdominal distention
○ Especially if the blockage causing abdominal symptoms is more proximal, abdominal distention may not be present.
○ Distal SBO such as one that involves the ileum almost always causes significant distention.
  ▪ Hernias at incision, inguinal, and femoral sites
  ▪ Masses as this may sometimes help to reveal the cause of SBO
  ▪ The location of abdominal tenderness, both focal and diffuse
  ▪ Peritoneal signs indicating strangulation
○ Peritoneal signs should prompt immediate surgical consultation and treatment.
  ▪ Abnormal rectal examination
○ Gross or occult blood should raise suspicion for strangulation.
○ A mass may be consistent with malignancy or acute infection.
• Laboratory evaluation is generally not helpful in making the specific diagnosis of SBO but is helpful in determining the severity of illness.
○ A CBC with differential and complete metabolic panel should be performed.
  ▪ Mild leukocytosis is common in simple obstruction but can be marked and/or with bandemia in strangulating obstruction.
  ▪ Hemoconcentration may be present with increased Hct.
○ Electrolyte abnormalities are often seen such as hypokalemia and abnormal levels of magnesium, calcium, and phosphate.
○ There is often elevated blood urea nitrogen (BUN) and possibly creatinine reflecting volume depletion.
○ Metabolic alkalosis is often seen in patients with frequent emesis.
○ Mild elevations in serum amylase are a common though nonspecific finding.
○ Elevated lactate levels should raise concern for strangulation.
  ▪ There are no laboratory studies that accurately predict simple vs. strangulated obstruction prior to the onset of irreversible intestinal ischemia.
• Radiographic evaluation includes plain films and abdominal CT.
○ Plain films of the abdomen, including an upright chest film and a flat and upright plain abdominal radiograph (KUB), are often performed initially, and used to be a routine test for all patients with abdominal pain.

▪ Plain abdominal radiography is diagnostic for SBO in about 50% to 60% of cases.
▪ The flat and upright KUB identifies air-fluid levels, dilatation of bowel proximal to the site of obstruction, bowel wall thickening, and lack of gas distal to the site of obstruction.
▪ Plain films may also be normal in appearance in patients with SBO.
▪ Plain radiography of limited value, as several studies suggest,that obtaining these studies contributed to management in only 4% of cases, despite important information was present in 66% of films.
▪ The place of the erect chest film for the diagnosis of pneumoperitoneum, however, still appears to be of value.
▪ For bowel obstruction, plain abdominal radiology has a positive likelihood ratio of 10 and a negative likelihood ratio of 0.
○ The most significant advances in the evaluation of abdominal pain for the possibility of SBO have involved contrast-enhanced CT imaging in making the diagnosis, determining the cause and location and also identifying signs of strangulation.
  ▪ CT imaging has mostly supplanted UGI studies with small bowel follow through in diagnosing SBO. It is the most sensitive and specific radiographic study for identifying SBO.
  ▪ If you are planning to obtain an abdominal CT in the emergency department (ED) anyway, skip the plain abdominal x-ray.

TRIAGE AND INITIAL MANAGEMENT

• Most patients with partial SBO and no signs of strangulation should initially be managed conservatively.
• Studies show that 20% to 73% of cases of SBO can be successfully managed with a conservative, nonoperative approach.
• The patient is given nothing by mouth and is treated aggressively with IV fluids to correct volume depletion. A Foley catheter is placed in order to monitor the urine output. The minimum urine output desired is 0.5 mL/kg/h.
• A NG tube is placed in the stomach to suction the fluid from the stomach.
○ In uncomplicated cases with enteric fluid baking up behind an obstruction, considerable amounts of fluid can be decompressed from the stomach and small bowel.
○ This decompression may be the process that allows a loop of bowel to untwist or move and thus release the obstruction.

○ In addition, NG tubes are placed to help prevent aspiration from recurrent emesis and for patient comfort by preventing further abdominal distention. Serial abdominal examination is performed to monitor for significant changes in abdominal examination or peritoneal signs.

• Electrolyte replacement is an important part of nonoperative management of these patients. Hypokalemia can slow down bowel motility. Adequate correction of any electrolyte abnormalities is important in managing these patients appropriately.

• It remains unproven whether antibiotics have a definitive role in the preoperative management of simple (nonstrangulating) SBO.

• Resolution of obstruction is identified when the patient's symptoms are improving including decreasing abdominal distension, passing of flatus or bowel contents, decreasing NG outputs and ability to tolerate oral intake. If further difficulty ensues then further evaluation and imaging such as CT scan should be undertaken.

• A surgical consultation is warranted on any patient suspected of having a SBO and should never be delayed.

○ Several retrospective studies report that a 12–24 hours delay of surgery in patients with complete SBO is safe, however the incidence of strangulation and other complications such as need for bowel resection significantly increases after longer periods of nonoperative management.

■ There has long been debate in the literature about how long a patient with SBO can safely be treated conservatively and there are differing schools of thought among surgeons about how long to wait before surgical treatment is undertaken.

■ There are no clear sensitive markers that indicate how long it is safe to wait to surgically treat patients with simple (nonstrangulating) SBO since early reversible strangulation is not clinically apparent.

■ In a recent study by Williams et al. (2005), surgically treated patients had fewer recurrences and longer time to recurrence than those patient treated conservatively. Surgically treated patients also had a longer hospital stay.

■ The use of supplementary diagnostic tools such as CT scanning can be useful to pinpoint patients needing early operative management.

• The prompt surgical treatment of patients with strangulating obstruction is not debatable. Patients with clear evidence of bowel compromise, hernia incarceration, peritonitis, or sepsis should be operated on without delay.

○ One or more of the following variables should suggest the need for operative intervention; tachycardia, fever, significant abdominal pain, leukocytosis, metabolic acidosis, and peritoneal signs.

○ Also, any patient with SBO with no prior history of abdominal surgery and no history of malignancy should also be considered for surgical management.

DISEASE MANAGEMENT STRATEGIES

• Diagnostic and therapeutic laparoscopic techniques including laparoscopic adhesiolysis are becoming more common in the treatment of SBO. Studies are demonstrating that intestinal obstruction can be approached safely and effectively by laparoscopy, and this approach can be used to provide diagnosis as well as treatment. Laparoscopy may lead to

○ Decreased hospital stay for the patient

○ Reduced complications including decreased formation of postoperative intra-abdominal adhesions

○ Earlier resumption of bowel function

• Bioresorbable membranes such as Seprafilm adhesion barrier hold promise for prevention but have yet to become established as standard treatment.

○ This product has been tested by randomized, controlled clinical trials and has been shown to safely and significantly reduce the extent, severity, and frequency of the incidence of early adhesion formation after abdominal surgery.

○ A more recent randomized, single blind, controlled trial in patients undergoing intestinal resection demonstrated that although the overall bowel obstruction rate was unchanged, there was a reduction in adhesive-related SBOs requiring reoperation.

BIBLIOGRAPHY

Bickell NA, Federman AD, Aufses AH Jr, et al. Influence of time on risk of bowel resection in complete small-bowel obstruction. *J Am Coll Surg.* 2005;201(6):847–854.

Fazio VW, Cohen Z, Fleshman JW, et al. Reduction in adhesive small-bowel obstruction by Seprafilm adhesion barrier after intestinal resection. *Dis Colon Rectum.* 2005;49:1–11.

Fevang BT, Jensen D, Svanes K, et al. Early operation or conservative management of patients with small bowel obstruction? *Eur J Surg.* 2002;168:475–481.

Franklin ME, Gonzalez JJ, Miter DB, et al. Laparoscopic diagnosis and treatment of intestinal obstruction. *Surg Endosc.* 2004;18:26–30.

Hayanga AJ, Bass-Wilkins K, Bulkley GB. Current management of small-bowel obstruction. *Adv Surg.* 2005;39:1–33.

Maglinte DDT, Kelvin FM, Sandrasegaran K, et al. Radiology of small bowel obstruction: contemporary approach and controversies. *Abdom Imaging.* 2005;30(2):160–178.

Paterson-Brown S, et al. Review: modern aids to clinical decision-making in the acute abdomen. *Br J Surg.* 1990;70:3–18.

Ray NF, Denton WG, Thamer M, et al. Abdominal adhesiolysis: inpatient care and expenditures in the US in 1994. *J Am Coll Surg.* 1998;186(1):1–9.

Williams SB, Greenspon J, Young HA, et al. Small bowel obstruction: conservative vs. surgical management. *Dis Colon Rectum.* 2005;48(6):1140–1146.

47 UPPER GASTROINTESTINAL BLEEDING

Naresh T. Gunaratnam

EPIDEMIOLOGY/OVERVIEW

- UGI bleeding is a common GI emergency and results in 300,000–350,000 hospital admissions annually in the United States.
- Bleeding from the UGI tract is approximately five times more common than lower GI bleeding and men are affected twice as commonly as women.
- The mortality rate associated with UGI bleeding is approximately 7% to 10%. However, patients developing GI hemorrhage while hospitalized for other reasons carry a much higher mortality rate of about 33%.
- Endoscopic assessment and treatment of UGI bleeding has evolved over the past three decades from a purely diagnostic role to one where it is the standard for definitive therapy.

CLINICAL PRESENTATION

- *Hematemesis* is vomiting of blood and is the most common presentation of an UGI bleed and the source is almost always proximal to the ligament of Treitz.
- This may be bright red indicating a recent or active bleed or "coffee ground" representing older blood reduced by acid in the stomach.
- *Melena* is black, tarry, and sticky stool with a specific foul odor by degradation of blood in the intestines and colon. This mostly represents an UGI source, however blood from the right colon may also present as melena.

- A massive UGI bleed can present as hematochezia (bright red blood per rectum) in 15% of the cases and carries a worse prognosis.

INITIAL EVALUATION

- A focused history assessing NSAID use, risk factors or history of liver disease, and dyspeptic symptoms can help in patient management. Those with known liver disease or risk factors for liver disease (eg, alcohol abuse or IV drug use) should be presumed to have and treated for a variceal bleed till proven otherwise.
- Initial evaluation should focus on vital signs and orthostatic changes as postural hypotension > 10 mm Hg represents a significant volume loss (> 15%) and is a predictor of poor outcomes (Table 47-1).
- A peripheral IV access with two large bore (at least18 gauge) catheters or a central venous access must be achieved in patients with an acute bleed especially if hemodynamically unstable.
- Colloids (normal saline or lactate Ringer's) are the initial fluids of choice and administered rapidly to restore intravascular volume. Continuous monitoring is required, especially for fragile patients with comorbid cardiopulmonary disease.
- Supplemental oxygen should be administered routinely.
- NG tubes can be very helpful in the localization of bleeding, as a bloody NG aspirate confirms the source to be from the upper tract.
  - Bright red blood from the NG tube that does not clear with lavage is an indication for emergent endoscopy, while coffee ground material which clears with lavage in a patient who is hemodynamically stable allows for a more elective endoscopy.
  - A negative NG aspirate, however, does not rule out an UGI bleed as brisk duodenal bleeding or an incorrectly placed tube (e.g, coiled in the esophagus) may result in false negative aspirates.

TABLE 47-1 Hemodynamics, Vital Signs, and Blood Loss

HEMODYNAMICS VITAL SIGNS	BLOOD LOSS (%) FRACTION OF INTRAVASCULAR VOLUME LOSS	SEVERITY OF BLEED
Shock (hypotension)	20–25	Massive
Postural hypotension	10–20	Moderate
Normal	< 10	Minor

SOURCE: From Feldman M, Friedman LS, Sleisenger MH. *Sleisenger and Fordtran's Gastrointestinal and Liver Disease.* Philadelphia, PA: WB Saunders; 2003:212.

- The color of aspirate has been correlated with mortality, clear aspirate 6%, red blood 18%, and red blood with hematochezia had 30% mortality in a national survey.
  - A CBC, prothrombin time (PT) and partial thromboplastin time (PTT), and BUN/creatinine are all helpful in evaluating and treating an acute UGI bleed.
  - The initial hemoglobin (Hgb) may be falsely elevated as it may take up to 72 hours for hemodilution to take place.
  - BUN level is elevated in GI bleed as blood proteins are degraded by the bacteria and released urea is reabsorbed.
  - A raised BUN/creatinine ratio (> 36) may an UGI source of bleeding with a sensitivity of 90% and specificity of 27%.
- An increased PT and low platelets are common in patients with advanced liver disease and may need to be corrected in order to control bleeding.
- Cardiac enzyme analysis and a baseline electrocardiogram (ECG) are recommended in those at risk for coronary disease, as acute blood loss can precipitate myocardial ischemia.

RISK STRATIFICATION

- The majority of GI bleeds stop spontaneously without any recurrence. Approximately 20% of bleeds can continue or recur leading to patient morbidity and mortality.
- Old age (> 65 years), shock, comorbid illnesses, low Hgb on evaluation, melena, multiple transfusions (> 4 U), hematochezia, fresh blood emesis or NG aspirate, and need for emergency surgery are clinical predictors resulting in increased risk of rebleeding (see Table 47-2).
- Severity of bleeding may be based on clinical criteria (see Table 47-3).

TABLE 47-2 Statistically Significant Predictors of Persistent or Recurrent Bleeding

RISK FACTOR	ODDS RATIO FOR INCREASED RISK
Age	
> 65 yr	1.3
> 70 yr	2.30
Shock (systolic BP < 100 mm Hg)	1.2–3.65
Comorbid illness	1.6–7.63
Initial Hgb < 10 g/dL	0.8–2.99
Coagulopathy (prolonged INR)	1.96 (1.46–2.64)
Melena	1.6
Blood in NG or stomach	1.1–11.5
Hematemesis	1.2–5.7
Continued bleeding	3.14 (2.4–4.12)

TABLE 47-3 Severity of Bleeding Based on Clinical Criteria

Bleeding criteria	
Mild	≤ 1 g/dL drop in Hgb
	Minimal or no anemia
	Stable hemodynamics
	Infrequent melena
	Coffee ground hematemesis
Moderate	1–2 g/dL drop in Hgb
	Anemia ≥ 10 g/dL
	Stable hemodynamics or tachycardia only
	Melena
	Hematemesis
Severe	≥ 2 g/dL drop in Hgb
	Profound anemia (< 10 g/dL)
	Hemodynamic instability (orthostatism, shock)
	Hematochezia or large volume (> 350 cc)
	Frequent melena
	Repeated hematemesis
Rebleeding criteria	≥ 1.5 g/dL drop in Hgb
	Recurrent hematemesis
	Recurrent or increased frequency melena/hematochezia

CLINICAL AND ENDOSCOPIC CRITERIA TO PREDICT BLEEDING SEVERITY

- Rockall et al. (1996) have developed a scoring system involving both clinical and endoscopic criteria to predict risk of both rebleeding and mortality. A total score of < 3 was associated with excellent prognosis while a score > 8 carried a high mortality. For cases with a score < 3, rebleeding occurred in < 5% and mortality was 0% (see Table 47-4).

PROGNOSTIC VALUE AND TIMING OF ENDOSCOPIC FINDINGS

- Previous endoscopic guidelines and studies have demonstrated endoscopic findings referred to as stigmata of recent hemorrhage.
- Active bleeding and a visible vessel in an ulcer base carry the highest risk of rebleeding, while a clean base ulcer or flat spot have minimal risk (see Table 47-5). In a prospective study over 6 years, Laine and Peterson (1994) have demonstrated that peptic ulcer with a clean base or a Mallory-Weiss tear has a < 2% risk of rebleeding. These patients could therefore be safely fed and discharged early from the hospital.

ROLE OF ENDOSCOPY

- About 80% of patients with ulcers stop bleeding spontaneously, and it can be debated if endoscopy in these

TABLE 47-4   Rockall Scoring System for Risk of Rebleeding and Death after Admission to Hospital for Acute GI Bleeding

VARIABLE	SCORE			
	0	1	2	3
Age (year)	< 60	60–79	> 80	
Shock	No shock (systolic BP > 100, pulse < 100)	Tachycardia (pulse > 100, BP > 100)	Hypotension (systolic < 100, pulse > 100)	
Comorbidity	None		Cardiac failure, ischemic heart disease, any major comorbidity	Renal failure, liver failure, disseminated malignancy
Diagnosis	Mallory-Weiss, no lesion or no stigmata of hemorrhage	All other diagnoses	Malignancy of UGI tract	
Major SRH	None or dark spot		Blood in UGI tract, adherent clot, visible or spurting vessel	

patients will alter patient outcome. However, endoscopy findings provide vital additional information to effectively triage both high- and low-risk patients.

- Approximately 21% of the patients with bleeding peptic ulcers had a clean base ulcer with a 3% risk of recurrent bleeding. They concluded that these patients can be discharged safely after endoscopy for outpatient management.
- Early endoscopy decreased the costs of care of patients with acute GI bleeding.
  - Patients were prospectively randomized to receive endoscopy in the emergency room while the control group underwent endoscopy in 1–2 days.
  - Patients with low-risk findings were discharged from the emergency room. "Endoscopy triage" lead to early discharge of patients with low risk of rebleeding, without increasing morbidity and mortality.
  - Median cost saving were $2068.
- Based on multiple studies confirming the beneficial effects of endoscopic therapy, urgent endoscopy has been recommended by National Institute of Health (NIH) and American Society of Gastrointestinal

TABLE 47-5   Risk of Recurrent Bleeding by Endoscopic Criteria

ENDOSCOPIC FINDING	RISK OF RECURRENT BLEEDING	MORTALITY
Active bleeding	55%	11%
Visible vessel	43%	11%
Adherent clot	22%	7%
Flat spot	10%	3%
Clean base	5%	2%

SOURCE: Laine L, Peterson W. Bleeding peptic ulcer. *N Engl J Med.* 1994;331:717–727.

Endoscopy for patients who have active bleeding or who have clinical findings categorizing them at high risk for rebleeding.
- The definition of urgent endoscopy varies widely in various studies, from 2 to 24 hours after presentation to the hospital.
- It has been determined that 76% to 78% of the patients with acute GI bleeding undergo endoscopy within the first 24 hours.

CAUSES OF UGI BLEEDING

GASTRIC AND DUODENAL ULCERS

- Gastroduodenal ulcer disease is the most common cause of acute GI bleeding. Ulcer disease is responsible for up to 50% of patients presenting with UGI bleeding. Hospitalization rate for ulcer-related GI bleeding has remained the same (40–60 cases per 100,000 patients) over the last two decades (see Table 47-6).

TABLE 47-6   American Society of Gastrointestinal Endoscopy Bleeding Survey—Endoscopic Diagnosis for UGI Bleeding in 2225 Patients

DIAGNOSIS	FREQUENCY (%)
Duodenal ulcer	24.3
Gastric erosions	23.4
Gastric ulcer	21.3
Varices	10.3
Mallory-Weiss tear	7.2
Esophagitis	6.3
Erosive duodenitis	5.8
Neoplasm	2.9
Stomal ulcer	1.8
Esophageal ulcer	1.7
Miscellaneous	6.8

- Most ulcer disease is attributed to *Helicobacter pylori* infection (*H. pylori*) or NSAIDs.
  - With awareness and aggressive therapy there has been a decline in the prevalence of *H. pylori* in the western world.
  - The epidemiology of peptic ulcer has changed with a much higher percentage of *H. pylori* negative ulcer disease now being reported.
- Endoscopic therapy has been associated with reduction in the rates of rebleeding, blood transfusion, length of hospital stay, need for other therapeutic interventions, costs, and mortality; therefore the need for surgical intervention to treat UGI bleeding is now rare.

STRESS ULCER PROPHYLAXIS

- Not all hospitalized patients benefit from stress ulcer prophylaxis simply because they are acutely ill. Risk factors for stress ulcers in critically ill patients include
  - Mechanical ventilation > 48 hours
  - Coagulopathy
  - Shock, severe sepsis, MOF
  - Head trauma, neurosurgery
  - > 30% burns
  - Quadriplegia
- There is no evidence that anticoagulated patients or patients receiving glucocorticoids benefit from stress ulcer prophylaxis unless they have other risk factors. Steroids do increase the risk of stress ulceration in patients receiving nonsteroidal anti-inflammatory therapy.
- Hospitalists can play a role ensuring that patients appropriately received H2 blockers and proton pump inhibitors.

TREATMENT

- Along with resuscitation, endoscopy is part of the initial care to triage patients in low- and high-risk categories.
- Endoscopic hemostasis is indicated to treat ulcers with major stigmata of recent hemorrhage.
  - Patients who have active bleeding, spurting or oozing from the ulcer, a nonbleeding visible vessel in the ulcer base, and a densely adherent clot should receive endoscopic therapy.
  - In a recent meta-analysis by Bardou et al., endoscopic treatment was associated with statistically significant absolute decreases in rates of rebleeding, surgery, and mortality.
- Acid suppression therapy has been shown to be of benefit to patients with bleeding peptic ulcers.

- The role of gastric acid inhibition to stop bleeding or to prevent recurrent bleeding is related to stability of blood clot, which is favored by a higher gastric pH.
  - A pH of > 6 is required for platelet aggregation while clot lysis occurs at pH < 6.
- Proton pump inhibitors appear to be more effective than H2-receptor antagonists in preventing persistent or recurrent bleeding (Lau et al). Their data suggested that beneficial effect of proton pump inhibitors were mainly observed in those patients not having adjunct endoscopic therapy.
- Although no head-to-head studies are available at present, data are suggestive that proton pump inhibition is a class effect and that the improvement in rebleeding can be achieved by using omeprazole or pantoprazole, 80 mg bolus followed by 8 mg/h for 72 hours after endoscopic therapy.
- Those patients with suspected or established esophageal or gastric varices should be treated with IV octreotide initially with a 50 μg bolus followed by 50 μg/h for up to 48 hours.
  - Definitive endoscopic treatment with ligation or sclerosis of the bleeding varix should be performed emergently.
  - Failure of endoscopic treatment associated with continued bleeding is an indication for a transjugular intrahepatic portosystemic shunt (TIPS). This procedure is performed by interventional radiologists where an expandable metal stent is placed between the hepatic and portal veins to reduce portal pressure.

DEALING WITH RECURRENT BLEEDING

- Primary endoscopic hemostasis can be achieved in > 95% of patients with bleeding peptic ulcers and ulcers with non-bleeding visible vessel. Rebleeding can occur in up to 10% to 20% of these patients and a mortality in 4% to 10%. If rebleeding occurs, it typically occurs within 48–72 hours.
- A repeat endoscopy with repeated therapy in the absence of massive rebleeding has become accepted practice. Recurrent bleeding after a second endoscopic intervention should initiate plans for alternative interventions including angiographic embolization of the bleeding vessel and surgery.
- In a prospective randomized trial, Lau et al. (2000). randomized 92 patients with recurrent bleeding after endoscopic hemostasis, 48 patients were assigned to repeat endoscopic therapy and 44 patients were assigned to emergency ulcer surgery.

- Seventy-three percent (35 of 48) of patients had long-term control of bleeding by repeat endoscopic therapy.
- Twenty-seven percent required surgery, and there were 11 endoscopic failures with two perforations secondary to thermocoagulation.
- Overall fewer complications (14.6% vs. 36.4%) were noted in the repeat endoscopy group. This study suggests that a repeat endoscopy is effective in controlling rebleeding and in reducing the need for surgical intervention and its associated complications.

FAILURE OF ENDOSCOPIC THERAPY

- Active nonvariceal GI hemorrhage that overwhelms endoscopic intervention requires an urgent surgical operation. It is therefore imperative to obtain surgical consultation in all patients presenting with a major GI hemorrhage.
- Hypotension, Hgb < 10 g/dL, fresh blood in the stomach, ulcer with active bleeding, and large ulcers > 2 cm were independent risk factors predicting poor control of bleeding with endoscopy alone. In a prospective study by Chung et al., the presence of blood spurting and ulcers > 2 cm were significantly related to failure of endoscopic therapy.
- Therapeutic angiography is an alternative option for patients who have failed endoscopic therapy and are not candidates for surgery. Therapeutic options include selective intra-arterial vasopressin infusion or embolotherapy with microcoils, and gelatin or polyvinyl alcohol particles.
  - Embolization has been shown to stop bleeding in massive gastroduodenal ulcers. Detection of bleeding site at the time of endoscopy provides vital information to the interventional radiologist to select the target area for catheterization. Technical success rates have been reported to be from 50% to 90%.
  - Known complications of embolization are bowel ischemia, necrosis with perforation, abscess formation, and hepatic infarction, especially in patients with poor hepatic reserve.

PREVENTION OF RECURRENT BLEED

- There are convincing data that treatment with proton pump inhibitors prevents ulcer rebleeding. Follow-up endoscopy is warranted to exclude malignancy in patients with large gastric ulcers.

- The data linking persistent *H. pylori* with recurrent ulcer hemorrhage are compelling, making eradication of infection the best approach for these patients.
  - Most tests of active infection may exhibit increased false-negative rates in the setting of acute bleeding.
  - The optimal diagnostic approach may include testing for *H. pylori* by serology or antral biopsy at the time of endoscopy, with reconfirmation of negative results by repeat testing when the bleeding resolves.
  - Oral therapy can be started immediately or during follow-up in patients found to have *H. pylori* infection.
- Patients with peptic ulcer bleeding should be encouraged to discontinue NSAIDs usage. If this is not possible, therapy with misoprostol (200 µg four times daily) or omeprazole both appear to be effective in prevention of gastroduodenal ulcers and erosions.

BIBLIOGRAPHY

Adang RP, Vismans JF, Talmon JL, et al. Appropriateness of indications for diagnostic upper gastrointestinal endoscopy: association with relevant endoscopic disease. *Gastrointest Endosc.* 1995;42:390.

Baradarian R, Ramdhaney S, Chapalamadugu R, et al. Early intensive resuscitation of patients with upper gastrointestinal bleeding decreases mortality. *Am J Gastroenterol.* 2004; 99:619.

Consensus development panel. Therapeutic endoscopy and bleeding ulcers. *JAMA.* 1989;262:1369–1372.

Corley DA, Stefan AM, Wolf M, et al. Early indicators of prognosis in upper gastrointestinal hemorrhage. *Am J Gastroenterol.* 1998;93:336.

Das A, Wong RC. Prediction of outcome of acute GI hemorrhage: a review of risk scores and predictive models. *Gastrointest Endosc.* 2004;60:85.

Feldman M, Friedman LS, Sleisenger MH. *Sleisenger and Fordtran's Gastrointestinal and Liver Disease.* Philadelphia, PA: WB Saunders; 2003:212.

Gralnek IM, Dulai GS. Incremental value of upper endoscopy for triage of patients with acute non-variceal upper GI hemorrhage. *Gastrointest Endosc.* 2004;60:9.

Laine L, Peterson W. Bleeding peptic ulcer. *N Engl J Med.* 1994;331:717–727.

Lau JY, Sung JJ, Lee KK, et al. Effect of intravenous omeprazole on recurrent bleeding after endoscopic treatment of bleeding peptic ulcers. *N Engl J Med.* 2000;343:310.

Rockall TA, Logan RF, Devlin HB, et al. Selection of patients for early discharge or outpatient care after acute upper gastrointestinal haemorrhage. National audit of acute upper gastrointestinal haemorrhage. *Lancet.* 1996;347:1138.

48 LOWER GASTROINTESTINAL TRACT BLEEDING

Naresh T. Gunaratnam

EPIDEMIOLOGY/OVERVIEW

- Lower gastrointestinal (LGI) bleeding refers to blood loss through the rectum originating distal to the ligament of Treitz.
- Approximately 95% originates in the colon; remainder originates distal to the ligament of Treitz and the ileocecal valve.
- Typically, patients experience hematochezia, but may also have melena or test positive for occult blood loss when there is slow bleeding from the right colon.
  - UGI bleeding presenting with hematochezia is nearly always associated with hemodynamic compromise.
  - Hematochezia confined to the surface of the stool or toilet tissue suggests a perianal source like hemorrhoids or fissures.

CLINICAL PRESENTATION

DIVERTICULOSIS

- The prevalence of diverticula, sac-like protrusions in the bowel wall, increase with age (65% at age 85; most common presentation during sixth and seventh decades).
  - Arterial vessels lining diverticula are progressively traumatized, leading to weakness and bleeding.
  - Three to five percent of patients with diverticulosis are at risk for bleeding.
  - Fifty percent of patients will have a history of previous diverticular bleeding.
  - Diverticular bleeding and acute diverticulitis are not typically concurrent.
- Bleeding related to diverticulosis accounts for 30% to 50% of acute rectal bleeding. The symptoms include
  - *Acute blood loss, bright red or maroon stools*— occult or minor bleeding not characteristic
  - Typically painless
  - Abdominal pain and bloating as a result of increased colonic motility related to cathartic effect of blood
  - Spontaneous resolution (75% of cases)
  - Rebleeding after the first episode (25% of cases)

ANGIODYSPLASIAS

- Dilated, tortuous, endothelium-lined submucosal vessels predisposed to bleeding, given the absence of smooth muscle in the vessel.
  - Bleeding is from a venous source; less brisk than diverticuli.
  - Typically, angiodysplasias are < 5 mm and are usually found in the right colon (cecum and ascending colon) in up to 3% to 6% of those undergoing colonoscopy.
  - Incidence increases with age; bleeding most common in those > 65 years.
  - Common cause of GI bleeding in elderly patients with renal failure.
- Bleeding related to angiodysplasias accounts for 20% to 30% of acute lower GI bleeds. The symptoms include
  - Typically occult blood loss; often patients have a history of previous bleeding from angiodysplasia.
  - Brisk bleeding presenting as hematochezia possible, especially if on platelet inhibitors or blood thinners.
- Lesions can be effectively treated using endoscopic techniques, including argon plasma coagulation (APC), thermal probes, and injection sclerotherapy.

ISCHEMIC COLITIS

- Left colon is most often involved and there are multiple identified risk factors.
  - Patients at higher risk if history of abdominal vascular surgery, vasculitis, clotting disorders or estrogen use; in most cases no clear etiologic factor.
  - Arrhythmia or heart failure-associated hypotension is often a trigger event.
  - Even severe constipation has been associated with ischemic colitis.
  - In cases without identifiable cause, recovery usually complete in a few days.
- Symptoms typically include abdominal pain and low-volume hematochezia.
- Workup for large vessel disease with angiography is not indicated.
- Therapy is directed at addressing the underlying cause if one is identified.

INFECTIOUS COLITIS

- Acute infections with *Salmonella*, *Shigella*, and *Campylobacter* are most common cause of infectious diarrhea in the United States, and all can present with bloody diarrhea.
  - History of travel and evidence of systemic signs such as fevers, rashes, arthralgias, or eosinophilia may suggest infectious colitis.

○ *Patients with HIV*—Increased risk for CMV colitis and lymphoma.
• Stool testing to isolate pathogen is valuable in early diagnosis and treatment.

INFLAMMATORY BOWEL DISEASE

• UC and Crohn's disease can both present with acute bloody diarrhea as their initial presentation; UC more likely to present with hematochezia.
  ○ History of chronic diarrhea may be helpful, but there is great overlap between infectious colitis and ischemic colitis in presentation.
• Workup including stool cultures and sigmoidoscopy with biopsies is very helpful in differentiating between IBD, ischemia, and infectious colitis.

NEOPLASMS

• Neoplasms account for 10% of rectal bleeding in those > 50 years.
• Bleeding occurs from erosion or ulceration of tumor.
• Cancers of rectum and sigmoid are more likely to present with hematochezia; right-sided neoplasms more commonly associated with maroon stools.
• Treatment aimed at surgical resection; endoscopic treatment has a limited role.

HEMORRHOIDS

• Dilated submucosal veins in the anus; associated bleeding is nearly always painless.
  ○ Blood may coat the stool or toilet paper or drip into the toilet bowl.
  ○ Serious bleeding is rare; patients on blood thinners, platelet inhibitors, and advanced liver disease at greatest risk for severe bleeding.
• Therapy directed at increasing dietary fiber to decrease trauma to the hemorrhoids during defecation; surgical ligation reserved for those who fail conservative management.

SOLITARY RECTAL ULCERS

• Rectal ulcers can develop in chronically constipated individuals as consequence of pressure necrosis on the rectal mucosa by impacted stool.
• Hematochezia with brisk arterial bleeding is common.

• Endoscopy reveals an ulcer in the rectal vault; if bleeding vessel is identified, endoscopic therapies are effective.
• Treatment of constipation vital to promote healing and decrease risk of recurrence.

RADIATION PROCTITIS

• Patients with a history of radiation therapy for treatment of prostate or pelvic malignancies are at increased risk for bleeding from rectum.
• *Most common presentations*—Early bleeding within 6 weeks of treatment or late bleeding after approximately 1 year after treatment.
• Effective therapies include endoscopic treatment with APC, thermal probes, and surgical or endoscopic application of formaldehyde.

POSTENDOSCOPIC INTERVENTION

• Patients presenting up to 2 weeks after an endoscopic polypectomy or biopsy are at risk of bleeding from the site of polypectomy or biopsy.
• Episodes are usually self-limiting; persistent bleeding associated with a falling Hgb is indication for repeat endoscopy with a therapeutic intervention.

MECKEL'S DIVERTICULUM

• Meckel's diverticulum is remnant of the vitelline duct, usually located 100 cm proximal to the ileocecal valve. Autopsy series suggest prevalence of 0.3% to 3%.
• Approximately 50% contain gastric mucosa; may present with bleeding, typically in a child or young adult.

EMERGENCY DEPARTMENT TRIAGE

• It is important to rule out an UGI bleed which could be life-threatening and influence immediate treatment and triage to an ICU.
  ○ Melena and hematochezia can be seen with both UGI and LGI bleeding.
  ○ NG lavage where bile is aspirated in the setting of a normal BUN: creatinine ratio (in patient with normal renal function, typically 20:1) very helpful in excluding an UGI bleed.

○ A BUN to creatinine ratio > 36 (in a patient with normal renal function) raises concern for an UGI bleed even if NG lavage is reportedly negative.
  - A malpositioned NG tube or lavage that fails to obtain bile may yield a false-negative NG lavage.
  - Bleeding distal to a closed pylorus may not reveal blood in the stomach.
- Young patients with self-limited bleeding without hemodynamic compromise can be evaluated as outpatients.
- Patients with hemodynamic instability, transfusion requirements, persistent bleeding, and multiple comorbid medical problems should be admitted with consultations to a gastroenterologist and general surgeon. Patients with hemodynamic compromise should be admitted to an ICU or monitored floor.
- See Fig. 48-1 for diagnostic algorithm.

INITIAL MANAGEMENT

- Place two large bore IV catheters or a central venous catheter to enable rapid infusion of volume expanders or blood, used immediately to correct hemodynamic instability.
- Correct coagulopathy and thrombocytopenia with fresh frozen plasma (FFP) and platelets with aim of correcting the international normalized ratio (INR) < 1.5 and platelets > 50,000.
- Hgb should be corrected to at least 10 g in patients with coronary disease, compromised respiration, or multiple comorbidities. Lower levels acceptable in asymptomatic, healthy individuals.
- Suspect active, ongoing bleeding if the Hgb does not rise with transfusion as predicted.

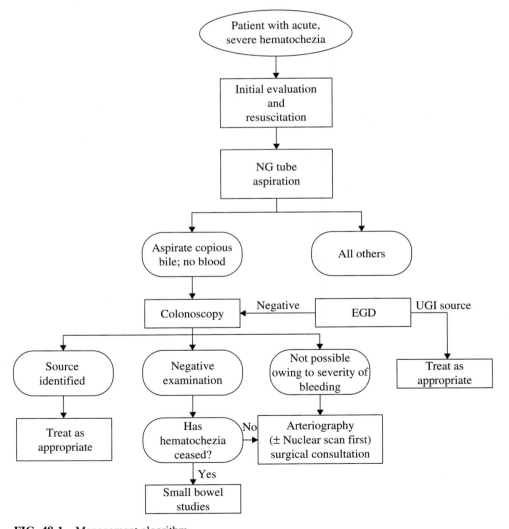

FIG. 48-1 Management algorithm.
SOURCE: Adapted from Zuccaro G. Management of the adult patient with acute lower gastrointestinal bleeding. *Am J Gastroenterol.* 1998;93:1202.

DIAGNOSTIC EVALUATION

COLONOSCOPY

- Once UGI bleed has been ruled out, colonoscopy is initial test for further evaluation. Patients who are hemodynamically stable should be prepped with at least 4–6 L of oral polyethylene glycol (PEG) lavage (orally or via NG tube over 2 hours) to optimize yield of the examination.
- Metoclopramide 10 mg can be given before lavage to reduce nausea and vomiting and improve bowel motility.
- Colonoscopy can help localize site of bleeding, obtain tissue, and treat bleeding lesion if identified. Bleeding from diverticuli, angiodysplasia, post polypectomy sites, radiation proctitis, and stercoral ulcers can all be effectively treated endoscopically. Actively bleeding diverticuli are hard to identify, are rarely treated endoscopically.

RADIONUCLIDE IMAGING AND ANGIOGRAPHY

- Radionuclide imaging to localize lower active GI bleeding if not well localized by endoscopy. Bleeding must occur at rate of 0.1–0.5 mL/min to be localized; scans are best done when the patient is actively bleeding to improve the yield. Endoscopy should be performed prior to radionuclide imaging if the patient is hemodynamically stable.
- The test can be repeated in 12–24 hours if negative, but is not reliable to identify the site of bleeding.
- If the radionuclide scan is positive, then angiogram is performed to localize the bleeding site and possibly provide treatment (requires a bleeding rate of 1–1.5 mL/min to be positive). Fifty to eighty percent of lower GI bleeds occur in the distribution of the superior mesenteric artery (diverticular and angiodysplasia), therefore this artery is evaluated first.
- Patients with a positive angiography can be treated surgically, with vasopressin infusion or with selective embolization of the bleeding vessel.

UPPER GASTROINTESTINAL EVALUATION FOR LOWER GASTROINTESTINAL BLEEDING

- If the bleeding site is not localized with colonoscopy, and radionuclide imaging and angiography, then assessment of potential UGI and small bowel bleeding sources should commence.
- An esophagogastroduodenoscopy (EGD) with push enteroscopy should be performed to rule out UGI bleeding lesions to the level of the proximal jejunum. If negative, capsule endoscopy should be performed to assess for small bowel lesions.
- If capsule endoscopy is negative, dedicated CT enterography should be performed to rule assess for small bowel lesions. Standard enteroclysis (a small bowel tube is passed and a double contrast study is performed) is superior to a small bowel follow through to detect small bowel lesions associated with bleeding.
- Meckel's scan should be performed in a young person with unlocalized, recurrent UGI or LGI bleeding to rule out Meckel's diverticulum.

CARE TRANSITIONS

- Stable patients whose bleeding site has been isolated and controlled should follow up with a specialist who can oversee future evaluation or treatment for that condition.
- In a patient with significant diverticular bleeding, referral to surgeon is appropriate to discuss the role of surgery in the management of their diverticulosis.
- Patients with significant bleeding from colonic angiodysplasia should be considered for elective endoscopic treatment with thermal ablative therapies.
- Patients with obscure GI bleeding can be worked up electively as an outpatient.

BIBLIOGRAPHY

Davies NM. Toxicity of nonsteroidal anti-inflammatory drugs in the large intestine. *Dis Colon Rectum.* 1995;38:1311–1321.

Gostout CJ. The role of endoscopy in managing acute lower gastrointestinal bleeding. *N Engl J Med.* 2000;342:125–127.

Gostout CJ, Wang KK, Ahlquist DA, et al. Acute gastrointestinal bleeding. Experience of a specialized management team. *J Clin Gastroenterol.* 1992;14:260.

Lewis BS. Small intestinal bleeding. *Gastroenterol Clin North Am.* 2000;29:67–95.

Van Cutsem E, Piessevaux H. Pharmacologic therapy of arteriovenous malformations. *Gastrointest Endosc Clin N Am.* 1996;6:819–32.

Zuccaro G. Management of the adult patient with acute lower gastrointestinal bleeding. *Am J Gastroenterol.* 1998;93:1202.

Zuckerman GR, Prakash C. Acute lower intestinal bleeding. Part II. Etiology, therapy, and outcomes. *Gastrointest Endosc.* 1999;49:228–238.

HEMATOLOGICAL DERANGEMENTS

49 ANEMIA IN THE HOSPITALIZED PATIENT

Eric Kupersmith, Susan Coutinho McAllister, and Alpesh Amin

EPIDEMIOLOGY/OVERVIEW

- Anemia is defined as reduced RBC mass.
- The World Health Organization (WHO) has specified criteria for anemia in men and women as follows:
  ◦ *Adult men*—Hgb < 13 g/dL, Hct < 39%
  ◦ *Adult women*—Hgb < 12 g/dL, Hct < 36%
- Hgb concentration, Hct, and RBC count are calculated by using the RBC mass and blood volume.
  ◦ Hct % = mean corpuscular volume (MCV) (femtoliter) × RBC count (× 10^6 μL) × 10
  ◦ RBC count = # of RBC in millions/μg/L of whole blood
- Red cell distribution (RDW) is a measure of the variation in RBC size (%).
  ◦ Patients with both a microcytic and macrocytic anemia may have a normal MCV but increased RDW because of variation in RBC size.
- Reticulocytes are precursors of mature RBCs. They are
  ◦ Larger than mature RBC
  ◦ Usually 3 days in bone marrow, 1 day in peripheral blood
  ◦ Usually 1% of total circulating RBC
  ◦ Reticulocytes move from the bone marrow to the periphery in response to anemia, upward of 2 days
- The reticulocyte production index (RPI) corrects the reticulocyte count for the degree of anemia.
  ◦ Hct 45%, maturation factor 1.0
  ◦ Hct 35%, maturation factor 1.5
  ◦ Hct 25%, maturation factor 2.0
- A low RPI < 2 suggests a hypoproliferative anemia (impaired production in response to anemia)
  ◦ Iron, folate, B_{12} deficiency
  ◦ Decreased erythropoietin secondary to renal failure
  ◦ Endocrine disorders (thyroid, pituitary)
  ◦ Chemotherapy, bone marrow failure, infiltration of bone marrow
- A high RPI > 3 suggests a hyperproliferative anemia

  ◦ Hemolysis
  ◦ Bone marrow response to acute blood loss
  ◦ Bone marrow recovery from acute injury, infection
- In the steady state, RBC production equals RBC loss.
  ◦ Mature RBCs circulate for 110–120 days before removal by macrophages.
  ◦ The life span of transfused RBC is shorter.
- The prevalence of anemia in hospitalized patients ranges from 30% to 90% depending on the patient population and may be exacerbated by frequent blood draws.
- Many factors are associated with anemia in the hospitalized patient. The average RBC—the MCV classifies the type of anemia as follows:
  ◦ Microcytic (< 80 fL)
  ◦ Normocytic (80–100 fL, the size of the nucleus of a lymphocyte on peripheral smear)
  ◦ Macrocytic (> 100 fL)
- Since the MCV is an average measure of RBC, the MCV may be normal with combined processes, but the RDW will be increased.
- Microcytic anemia results from impaired Hgb synthesis in the RBC.
  ◦ Iron deficiency
  ◦ Lead poisoning
  ◦ Sideroblastic anemia
  ◦ Thalassemia
- Normocytic anemia has many causes including
  ◦ Chronic renal failure
  ◦ Myelodysplasia
  ◦ Bone marrow infiltration
  ◦ Anemia of chronic disease
- Macrocytic anemia also has many causes including
  ◦ Defects in DNA synthesis (folate, B_{12}, myelodysplasia)
  ◦ Hypothyroidism
  ◦ Liver disease and alcoholism
  ◦ Drugs such as zidovudine, hydroxyurea
- Anemia is a sign of another underlying disease process and should prompt an evaluation to uncover and treat the primary cause.

PATHOPHYSIOLOGY

- Anemia causes decreased oxygen-carrying capacity.
- Anemia may result from decreased RBC production, increased RBC destruction, and blood loss.

○ Decreased RBC production (iron deficiency, endocrine disorders, heavy metal or chemical toxicity, infection or renal disease, B_{12} and folic acid deficiencies, thalassemia, sideroblastosis, myelodysplasia)

○ Increased RBC destruction or hemolysis (immuno-hemolytic disease states, trauma, spherocytosis, RBC enzyme deficiencies, hemoglobinopathies, destruction of RBC in the reticuloendothelial system and spleen associated with transfusion reactions, infections with malaria or *Clostridium perfringens,* burns, or fresh-water drowning)

○ Acute and chronic blood loss, most commonly, menstrual or from the GI tract.

• Anemia of chronic disease, notably chronic infection, malignancy, inflammation and systemic disorders, has the following features:

○ Decreased RBC life span

○ Abnormal response to erythropoietin

○ Increased uptake and retention of iron by the reticuloendothelial cells

○ Microcytic or normocytic morphology of RBCs

CLINICAL PRESENTATION, DIFFERENTIAL, MAKING THE DIAGNOSIS

• Initial workup begins with the history.

○ Symptoms and signs are nonspecific and less likely with anemia that is chronic and mild.

○ Exercise and illness may precipitate symptoms, especially if there is preexisting coronary artery disease.

• Physical examination should look for signs indicating the severity of anemia.

○ Evidence of acute blood loss and hypovolemia

• Other clues to the specific etiology of the anemia may include

○ Icterus (hemolysis, liver disease)

○ Cyanosis of the ears, nose, and digits (cold antibody usually IgM or C3 autoimmune hemolytic anemia)

○ Koilonychia or spoon nail or Plummer-Vinson syndrome, namely, glossitis, dysphagia, esophageal webs (severe iron deficiency)

○ Smooth beefy red tongue (B_{12} deficiency)

○ Petecchiae, conjunctival hemorrhage (thrombocytopenia)

○ Splenomegaly (portal hypertension from cirrhosis, idiopathic thrombocytopenia purpura [ITP], warm antibodies usually IgG autoimmune hemolytic anemia, extravascular hemolysis)

○ Positive stool guaiac (blood loss)

○ Neurologic symptoms and signs (B_{12} deficiency)

• Initial laboratory evaluation should always include CBC, RBC count, RBC indices, and examination of peripheral smear for abnormal cells along with reticulocyte count. In addition, routine chemistries, checking renal and liver function should be obtained.

○ See Fig. 49-1 and Table 49-1 for RBC morphology in the diagnosis of anemia.

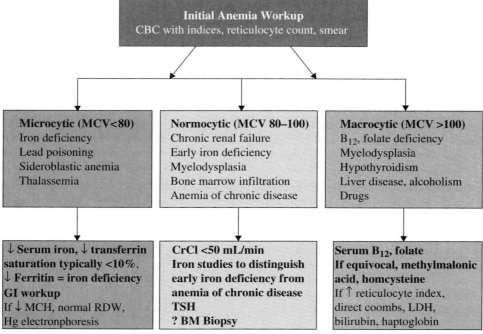

FIG. 49-1 Anemia workup.

TABLE 49-1 RBC Morphology in the Diagnosis of Anemia

MORPHOLOGY	CAUSE	SYNDROMES
Spherocytes	Loss of membrane	Hereditary spherocytosis, immunohemolytic anemia
Target cells	Increased ratio of RBC surface area to volume	Hgb disorders: thalassemias, Hgb S; liver disease
Schistocytes	Traumatic disruption of membrane	Microangiopathy, intravascular prostheses
Sickled cells	Polymerization of Hgb S	Sickle cell syndromes
Acanthocytes	Abnormal membrane lipids	Severe liver disease (spur cell anemia)
Agglutinated cells	Presence of IgM antibody	Cold agglutinin disease
Heinz bodies	Precipitated Hgb	Unstable Hgb, oxidant stress
Howell-Jolly bodies	Nuclear fragments	Hemolytic and megaloblastic anemias, splenectomy
Basophilic stippling	Aggregated ribosomes	Lead poisoning, thalassemia, hemolytic states
Heinz bodies	Denature Hgb	Unstable hemoglobinopathies, some hemolytic anemias
Cabot ring	Nuclear remnants	Megaloblastic anemia
Pappenheimer bodies	Degenerating cellular remnants containing iron	Post-splenectomy, hemolytic, sideroblastic, and megaloblastic anemias
Rouleaux formation	Artificial (because of preparation), or increased cathodal proteins	Multiple myeloma, Waldenstrom's macroglobulinemia
Presence of parasites	Parasitic infection	*Plasmodium* (malaria), *Babesia* (babesiosis)
Nucleated RBC	Regenerative/pathologic response of bone marrow	Extramedullary hematopoiesis, hypoxia, hemolysis

SOURCE: Adapted from *Harrison's Principles of Internal Medicine*. 16th ed. McGraw-Hill; 2005.

○ The presence of a microangiopathic smear in the setting of acute renal insufficiency would alert the clinician to the possibility of thrombotic thrombocytopenia purpura (TTP) or HUS.
  ▪ RBC fragments, helmet cells, microspherocytes, decreased platelets, large platelets consistent with destruction.
  ▪ These patients may suffer irreversible renal failure and death without emergency plasmapheresis.
○ The presence of reticulocytosis, helmet cells, schistocytes, spherocytes, Howell-Jolly bodies, and basophilic stippling would prompt the clinician to check hemolysis laboratory tests.
  ▪ Serum haptoglobin (which binds free Hgb) ≤ 25 mg/dL and ↑ LDH (from hemolyzed RBC) has a specificity of 90% for hemolysis.
  ▪ ↑ Unconjugated bilirubin also supports the diagnosis of hemolysis which should prompt hematology consultation.
• Further diagnostic testing is determined by initial test results.

TRIAGE AND INITIAL MANAGEMENT

• The focus of initial management is based on the severity of the anemia, and whether urgent hematologic consultation or transfusion is required. See Chap. 52.

• If the anemia is stable and chronic, incidental to the hospitalization, then appropriate evaluation without transfusion should proceed based on whether the anemia is microcytic, normocytic, or macrocytic.
• Identification of the underlying condition causing anemia is required for appropriate treatment.
• Iron treatment is indicated for iron deficiency anemia and anemia of chronic disease with coexistent iron deficiency.
  ○ Parenteral iron can enhance the response to erythropoietic agents in patients with cancer and in patients on chronic hemodialysis.
  ○ Although iron dextran is associated with anaphylaxis, the newer agents (iron sucrose or sodium ferric gluconate, Venofer and Ferrlecit) are extremely safe and do not require a test dose.
  ○ Iron should not be prescribed for patients with anemia of chronic disease who have a high or normal ferritin (above 100 ng/mL).
• Erythropoietic agents are indicated in anemic patients with chronic kidney disease, zidovudine-treated HIV, selected cancer patients on chemotherapy, and for surgical patients to reduce the risk of allogeneic blood transfusions.
  ○ Erythropoietic stimulating proteins stimulate iron uptake and heme biosynthesis in erythroid progenitor cells.
  ○ Poor results are associated with high levels of proinflammatory cytokines and poor iron availability.

- Target Hgb is about 11 g/dL for maximum incremental gain in QOL markers and avoidance of adverse outcomes.
- Overcorrection to normal levels and insufficient treatment are associated with unfavorable outcomes.
- In the preoperative period for patients undergoing orthopedic surgery with moderate anemia (Hgb 10–13 g/dL), erythropoietic-stimulating proteins have been shown to be safe and as effective as preoperative autologous blood donation.
- Before starting therapy, iron deficiency must be ruled out.
- If minimal response (Hgb improved by < 1 g/dL) after 1 month, then iron status should be re-evaluated and iron supplementation considered.
- If no response in a replete patient after 8 more weeks, the patient is nonresponsive.
- Blood transfusion is indicated in bone marrow failure syndromes and in acute hemorrhage and may be required for patients with thalassemia and other forms of chronic hemolysis.
  - Transfusions are a rapid and possibly effective intervention, but have been associated with increased LOS, increased cost, and increased morbidity and mortality in critically ill and surgical patients.
  - At this time, there is no one Hgb value that should trigger transfusion. Ongoing studies continue to evaluate the risk-benefit ratio of transfusion based solely upon Hgb value. See Chap. 52.
- Splenectomy is an option in select circumstances.
  - Thalassemia major
  - Hereditary spherocytosis
  - TTP purpura or immune thrombocytopenia purpura (ITP) with autoimmune anemia (Evans syndrome) treatment failures

DISEASE MANAGEMENT STRATEGIES/ CARE TRANSITIONS

- Hospitalists need to ensure that the receiving physician is aware of the presence of anemia, pending tests at the time of discharge, and recommendations of consultants.
- Iron deficiency in particular requires a complete GI workup unless other causes of acute blood loss have been identified.
- The presence of anemia may be associated with worse long-term outcomes in patients with cancer, chronic kidney disease, HIV, and congestive heart failure (CHF).
- A management plan that incorporates dietary changes, repletion, and/or erythropoietic stimulating proteins needs to be communicated to patients, families, and PCPs.

BIBLIOGRAPHY

Cella D. Factors influencing quality of life in cancer patients: anemia and fatigue. *Semin Oncol.* 1998;25(3 suppl 7):43–46.

Goodnough LT, Shander A, Spivak JL, et al. Detection, evaluation, and management of anemia in the elective surgical patient. *Anesth Analg.* 2005;101:1858–1861.

Greenburg AG. Pathophysiology of anemia. *Am J Med.* 1996;101(suppl 2A):7S–11S.

Ludwig H, Fritz E. Anemia in cancer patients. *Semin Oncol.* 1998;25(3 suppl 7):2–6.

Mercadante S, Gebbia V, Marrazzo A, et al. Anaemia in cancer: pathophysiology and treatment. *Cancer Treat Rev.* 2000;26:303–311.

Strauss DJ, Riggs SA. Quality of life and health benefits of early treatment of mild anemia. *Cancer.* 2006;107(8):1909–1917.

Weiss G, Goodnough LT. Anemia of chronic disease. *N Engl J Med.* 2005;352:1011–1023.

50 SICKLE CELL DISEASE
Andrew D. Campbell

EPIDEMIOLOGY

- Sickle cell trait—one hemoglobin S gene (Hbg S) with normal Hgb (Hbg A)—is generally asymptomatic, affecting approximately 8% of the African American population in the United States.
- Sickle cell disease (SCD)—homozygous for Hbg S (SS) or Hbg S and Hbg C or beta thalassemia with Hbg S > 50% of total Hgb—has a prevalence of 1 in 500 African American newborns in the United States.
  - There are 90,000 sickle cell patients in the United States (17,000 pediatric patients).
  - The median age of survival (national sickle cooperative study 1995):
    - *For Hbg SS SCD*—42 years (males), 48 years (females)
    - *For Hbg SC SCD*—60 years (males), 68 years (females)

CLINICAL FEATURES

- Hematologic abnormalities include
  - Moderate (Hgb 8–10) to severe (Hgb 5–7) anemia, which is usually normocytic and normochromic.

The presence of microcytosis should prompt a search for concomitant beta or alpha thalassemia or iron deficiency.

- Often prominent (> 5%) reticulocytosis.
- Neutrophilia, resulting from activated marrow and from functional hyposplenism. The presence of neutrophilia can make it difficult to identify coexisting infection.
- Thrombocytosis.
- Hyperbilirubinemia, resulting from premature sickle cell destruction.

- Aplastic crisis is defined as an acute drop in baseline Hgb with a substantially reduced reticulocyte count (usually < 1%) without involvement of the WBC or platelet count. Complete cessation of RBC production can last up to 10–14 days. Aplastic crisis is commonly associated with
  - Parvovirus B19 ("fifth's disease")
  - Symptoms of upper respiratory infection (40% of patients).
- Vaso-occlusive conditions are painful episodes resulting in the following:
  - Bone pain from acute vaso-occlusion of vessels resulting in local hypoxia and pain. Common target pain sites include arms, legs, chest, and lower back.
  - *Hand-foot syndrome (dactylitis)*—Painful swelling of hands and feet, occurring most often in children < 2 years old.
  - *Splenic sequestration crisis*—Defined by acute drop in Hgb > 2 g/dL from baseline with an acute enlarging spleen and a retic count ≥ baseline. This condition is most common in children < 5 years old.
  - Acute chest syndrome (ACS) that is defined as the presence of a new pulmonary infiltrate in combination with fever or respiratory symptoms (cough, tachypnea) in a patient with SCD. Keep in mind the following:
    - Patients present with pleuritic chest pain, dyspnea, shortness of breath (SOB), fever, and hypoxia.
    - Chest pain is not necessary for diagnosis of ACS.
    - It can be impossible to distinguish from pneumonia, so should always treat presumptively with antibiotics covering gram positives and mycoplasma for patients over the age of 4 years old.
    - Chest x-ray (CXR) may initially be negative, although crackles may be appreciated on examination.
    - If no infiltrate initially on CXR, repeat 6–12 hours later after hydration.
  - Abdominal pain caused by vaso-occlusion of mesenteric blood supply, sometimes associated with microinfarction of liver, spleen, or lymph nodes. There are usually no signs of peritoneal inflammation.

Do not overlook other common causes—right upper quadrant (RUQ) pain—gallbladder pain, increased jaundice, cholelithiasis/cholecystitis, or liver intrahepatic crisis.

- Up to 40% SCD patients will develop gallstones by 18 years of age because of chronic hyperbilinemia which causes scleral icterus.
- The features of *intrahepatic crisis* include sudden, painful liver enlargement (intrahepatic sickling) with elevated direct bilirubin and LFTs, commonly including coagulopathy.
- *Liver sequestration* is characterized by engorgement of liver sinusoids by sickled cells, generally chronic with mild ALT/AST elevations (2–3 × upper limit of normal).
- Painful erection is caused by the inability of sickled cells to traverse the tortuous vessels of the penis.
  - Stuttering is a partial erection.
  - Priapism, a complete erection, requires inpatient admission, if prolonged > 4–6 hours, because of the risk of impotence.
- Renal dysfunction affects up to 30% of sickle cell patients by age 30 and 5% of adults develop chronic renal insufficiency.
  - Painless and usually mild, hematuria indicative of papillary necrosis.
  - Microalbuminia, usually preceding proteinuria, an early marker of glomerular injury.
- Acute, clinically apparent neurologic events (stroke) occurs in 8% to 11% of children suffering from SCD; mean age of incidence of 7.7 years old.
  - Common presenting symptoms and signs include: hemiparesis, monoparesis, aphasia or dysphasia, seizures, severe headache, cranial nerve palsy, stupor, and coma.
  - Stroke may occur without warning as an isolated event or may complicate other complications of SCD such as ACS or aplastic crisis.
- In the setting of high WBC (> 15,000/mm^3), tenderness, local swelling, and fever, osteomyelitis can mimic bone infarct as a complication of SCD.
  - CRP may be more useful than erythrocyte sedimentation rate (ESR) which can be normal in the presence of osteomyelitis.
  - Obtain blood cultures, MRI as the preferred imaging modality.

TRIAGE

- Aplastic crisis, vaso-occlusive complications mentioned above, and severe pain all are indications for inpatient admission. The PCP or hematologist who knows the patient and family best should assist with triage decision-making and treatment plans. All patients < 5 years old with fever > 101.5°F will be admitted.

- Additional criteria for sickle cell patients requiring inpatient hospitalization with fever > 101.5°F include
  - History of sepsis or bacteremia (including strep pneumonia)
  - Any patient with a history of splenectomy
  - Any toxic appearing patient
  - Temp > 39°C, WBC > 30K or WBC < 5000
  - Evidence of acute complications including
    - Acute drop in Hgb, enlarging spleen
    - ACS/pneumonia
    - Concerns about follow-up/compliance

TREATMENT

APLASTIC CRISIS

- Check CBC daily with reticulocyte count at least every other day.
  - Order blood transfusion for any hemodynamic unstable patient or Hgb < 4–5 g/dL. Give 5 cc/kg initially and no more than 5 cc/kg/h to raise Hbg 1–2 g.
- Spontaneously remits after about 10 days, with massive reticulocytosis (20%).

SPLENIC SEQUESTRATION

- Serial abdominal examinations every 4 hours initially, then q shift.
- Transfuse for any hemodynamically unstable patient or if Hgb < 4–5 g/dL. Exchange transfusion may be needed.
- Splenectomy usually reserved for recurrent cases or severe cases that do not respond to chronic blood transfusions.

ACUTE CHEST SYNDROME

- This is an emergency in patients who are hypoxic, or have > 1 lobar involvement, and should be treated as soon as possible with RBC transfusions in an effort to reduce percentage of sickle Hgb.
- Very sick patients may require intensive care with exchange transfusion ± intubation.
- Obtain CBC/diff, retic count, and type and screen. Blood culture if febrile.

- Prescribe antibiotics
  - Cefuroxime, cefotaxime (150 mg/kg/d) or ceftriaxone (50–100 mg/kg/d) + macrolide (azithromycin, biaxin, or erythromycin) in all patients 5 years or older because mycoplasma and chlamydia are common organisms in ACS.
  - Add vancomycin if clinical deterioration since resistant *Streptococcus pneumoniae* is very possible.
  - Consider additional gram-negative coverage if severely ill.
- Administer IV fluids 1–1.25 times maintenance, no more than 1.5 times maintenance (risk of pulmonary edema). If history of cardiac dysfunction (current digoxin or Lasix), or if S_3 gallop, development of new rales or peripheral edema on examination, decrease IV fluids and consider furosemide (Lasix).
- Prescribe a trial of bronchodilators for all patients with history of asthma; continue all other asthma medications. Consider short course of steroids if significant asthma.
- Cardiopulmonary monitoring, including heart rate, respiratory rate, and O_2 saturation with a low threshold for obtaining arterial blood gases (ABG)—is required for all patients.
  - Administer O_2 by cannula or mask to maintain O_2 saturation > 95%.
- Blood transfusions can prevent clinical deterioration.
  - Indications for blood transfusion in ACS include
    - Hypoxia, O_2 saturation < 92% to 93%
    - More than one lung lobe involved
    - History of recurrent of ACS or ACS in the past requiring ICU stay or exchange transfusion
    - Worsening symptoms (acute SOB, more hypoxia, dropping Hgb)
  - Transfuse to achieve Hgb ≈ 10 g/dL; if Hgb > 10–11 g/dL, do not transfuse (prevent hyperviscosity). Consider leukopoor, sickle-negative packed RBCs (C, E, Kell-matched if available) which raises Hgb 2–3 g/dL.
  - Laboratory monitoring includes daily CBC and Hgb electrophoresis before and after blood transfusions.
  - If evidence or history of CHF or pulmonary edema, consider furosemide during or after blood transfusion.
  - Transfer to ICU for exchange transfusion (single volume) if
    - PaO_2 < 70 mm Hg
    - Rapidly progressive pneumonia
    - Marked dyspnea, acute CHF develops
  - Monitor these patients closely, because they can get sick very, very quickly!
- Adequate pain control is essential. PCA (principal component analysis) commonly required for

associated chest, rib, or abdominal pain that can be severe.

○ *Do not undertreat pain*—Further hypoventilation can worsen ACS.

PAINFUL EPISODE MANAGEMENT

- Moderate/severe painful crises requiring hospitalization should be treated with hydration (1–1.5 times maintenance IV fluids), analgesics, and close monitoring.
- Morphine sulfate 0.05–0.15 mg/kg per dose IV q2 hours or 0.05–0.1 mg/kg/h continuous infusion or via PCA.
  ○ For PCA give 1/3–1/2 of total maximum dose by continuous infusion, with 1/2–2/3 via PCA boluses.
  ○ Total morphine dose > 0.1 mg/kg/h may occasionally be required but should be used with caution.
  ○ Alternative analgesics including hydromorphone (dilaudid) 0.015–0.02 mg/kg IV q 3–4 hours may be appropriate in selected cases.
  ○ In most cases, prn analgesic orders are not appropriate. Strongly consider consultation with Pain Service if available.
  ○ Analgesics may be weaned as tolerated by decreasing dose, not by prolonging interval between doses. Discuss analgesic changes with patient, designated family member, and the patient's primary physician in the outpatient setting.
  ○ Prescribe a bowel regimen to avoid narcotic-induced constipation.
- Consider ketorolac (Toradol) 0.5 mg/kg (30 mg maximum dose) IV q 6–8 hours in addition to opioid analgesia if no contraindication present (ie, gastritis, ulcer, coagulopathy, dehydration, or renal impairment).
  ○ Do not use ibuprofen with ketorolac.
  ○ Ibuprofen 10 mg/kg po q 6–8 hours or other anti-inflammatory agent if no contraindication present (ie, ketoroalac, gastritis, ulcer, coagulopathy, or renal impairment). Limit more frequent dosing to 72 hours maximum duration.
- The etiology of a new or increasing O_2 requirement should be investigated.
  ○ Provide O_2 by nasal cannula or face mask as needed to keep pulse oximetry > 92% or > patient's baseline value, if > 92%. Avoid excessive or unnecessary O_2, which may suppress the reticulocyte count and exacerbate anemia.
  ○ Offer heating pads or other comfort measures. Avoid ice or cold packs.
- Reassess pain control on a regular basis (at least twice daily) by discussing efficacy and side effects with patient/family.

INTRAHEPATIC CRISIS

- Monitor LFT and coagulation studies.
- Order abdominal US.
- Simple blood or exchange transfusion may be critical since these patients can decompensate quickly.

GALLBLADDER DISEASE (ACUTE CHOLECYSTITIS)

- Obtain gallbladder US. Start antibiotics to cover *Salmonella*.
- Consider transfusion to lower Hbg S percentage.
- Cholecystectomy needed in most patients in future.
- Bentyl, actigall, and low-fat diet are options other than cholecystectomy.

PRIAPISM

- Unlike stuttering, priapism requires inpatient monitoring when prolonged > 4–6 hours. Priapism is more severe and more painful.
- Hydration with 1.5 × normal and pain control. PCA is sometimes needed.
- Pseudoephedrine may be used acutely.
- *Strongly consider blood transfusion*—With goal of reducing Hgb S percentage < 30%.
- Consult urology for possible irrigation/aspiration (corpus cavernosum) to achieve detumescence if priapism continues > 6 hours.

PAPILLARY NECROSIS

- *Treatment*—Bed rest and high urinary flow with fluids ± diuretics.

PROTEINURIA

- ACE inhibitors have been shown to decrease renal protein loss in a randomized controlled trial in adults.
- Obtain urine protein/creatinine studies.

STROKE

- For diagnosis obtain head CT without contrast immediately if MRI cannot be obtained quickly. Then get an MRI of brain as soon as possible later.
- Initiation of transfusion therapy should not be delayed by arrangements for imaging.

- Treatment of choice is *exchange transfusion* to decrease Hgb S percentage < 30.
- Since exchange transfusion can take a few hours (3–6 hours) to start, a simple blood transfusion if Hgb < 9–10 is a temporizing measure to increase Hgb to 10–11 g/dL to suppress the endogenous Hbg S reticulocytosis and decrease the anemia.
- Do not administer simple blood transfusion if Hgb is > 10 g/dL or do not transfuse to a target > 11 g/dL, because hyperviscosity can worsen stroke.
- Rapid ICU triage, neurology consultation, and neurosurgery consult, especially if large intracranial shift or hemorrhagic stroke on imaging.
- If the Hgb drops < 8 g/dL after the exchange blood transfusion, another simple blood transfusion is probably required to initiate discharge planning.
- Begin a chronic blood transfusion protocol (approximately every 3–4 weeks) to keep Hgb S < 30% to 40% for stroke prophylaxis.

EMPIRIC ANTIBIOTIC COVERAGE FOR INPATIENTS WITH SICKLE CELL DISEASE

- Prescribe cefuroxime or cefotaxime or ceftriaxone until cultures are negative for 48 hours.
- Highly consider mycoplasma coverage (erythromycin, azithromycin, or clarithromycin) if pneumonia/ACS is present.
- If patient is very ill appearing or not responding to the cephalosporins, would strongly consider adding vancomycin for resistant *S. pneumoniae*.
- If central line present, consider adding vancomycin for gram-positive *Staphylococcus*.

GENERAL TRANSFUSION GUIDELINES FOR SICKLE CELL DISEASE

- Acute indications
  - Stroke, MOF, hepatic crisis, ACS, aplastic crisis, splenic sequestration crisis, symptomatic anemia
- Simple transfusion (< 10 g/dL)
  - *Goal*—Reduce Hgb S percentage < 30%.
  - Give 10 cc/kg of antigen matched blood (C, E, Kell) leukopoor, packed RBCs over 2–3 hours. If Hbg > 10, perform exchange transfusion if clinically needed.
  - *Erythrocytapheresis (exchange transfusion)*—Recommended for acute stroke, worsening ACS, or splenic sequestration, MOF. Need double lumen central line.

SPECIAL CONSIDERATIONS RELATING TO SURGERY

PREOPERATIVE/ANESTHESIA MANAGEMENT

- Recommend simple transfusion to achieve a Hgb of 10–11 g/dL.
  - If Hgb > 10 (which is rare in these patients), exchange transfusion may be advised to decrease Hbg S < 40%.
  - Transfusion or exchange should occur within 5 days of procedure.
  - If surgery is high risk, it may be necessary to perform exchange transfusion to avoid complications associated with hyperviscosity.
  - Alloimmunization should be minimized by giving antigen-matched blood (matched at least for Kell, C, E antigens).
- Recommend 2–4 hours of presurgical hydration.
- Patients with asthma should adhere to maintenance medications prior to surgery.

POSTOPERATIVE/ANESTHESIA MANAGEMENT IN SCD

- Check postoperative CBC and reticulocyte count. Type and screen are performed in case of postoperative anesthesia complications.
  - If ACS develops postoperative/anesthesia and Hgb < 10, simple transfusion.
  - If Hgb > 10, consider exchange transfusion.
- Cardiopulmonary/O_2 monitoring on all patients. Administer O_2 for saturation < 95%.
- IV fluid hydration—1–1.5 × maintenance.
- Provide incentive spirometry.
- Adequate pain control, workup fevers, empiric antibiotic coverage if needed postoperatively.

DISCHARGE PLANNING

- The following criteria should be met:
  - Adequate pain relief on oral analgesics
  - Adequate oral fluids intake and ability to take other oral medications
  - Afebrile for 24 hours, with negative cultures
  - Resolution of any pulmonary symptoms and adequate oxygenation on room air
  - Stable Hgb
  - Appropriate follow-up arranged (primary care, SCD clinic) within 1–2 weeks

BIBLIOGRAPHY

Adams R, McKie V, Nichols F, et al. The use of transcranial ultrasonography to predict stroke in sickle cell disease. *N Engl J Med.* 1992;326:605–610.

Charache S, Terrin M, Moore R, et al. Effect of hydroxyurea on the frequency of painful crises in sickle cell anemia. Investigators of the multicenter study of hydroxyurea in sickle cell anemia. *N Engl J Med.* 1995;332:1317–1322.

Gaston MH, Verter JI, Woods G, et al. Prophylaxis with oral penicillin in children with sickle cell anemia: a randomized trial. *N Engl J Med.* 1986;314:1593–1599.

Lane P, Buchanan G, Hutter J, et al. Sickle cell disease in children and adolescents: diagnosis, guidelines for comprehensive care, and care paths and protocols for the management of acute and chronic complications. Sickle Cell Disease Care Consortium Publication, September 2002, pp. 1–37.

National Heart, Lung and Blood Institute; National Institutes of Health. *Management and Therapy of Sickle Cell Disease.* 4th ed. NIH Publication No 02-2117, June 2002.

Miller ST, Sleeper LA, Pegelow CH, et al. Prediction of adverse outcomes in children with sickle cell disease. *N Engl J Med.* 2000;342:83–89.

Platt O, Brambilla D, Rosse W, et al. Mortality in sickle cell disease—life expectancy and risk factors for early death. *N Engl J Med.* 1994;330:1639–1644.

Powars D, Chan L, Hiti A, et al. Outcome of sickle cell anemia. *Medicine.* 84(6):363–376.

Steinberg M. Management of sickle cell disease. *N Engl J Med.* 1999;340(13):1021–1029.

The role of hydroxyurea in sickle cell disease. *Br J Haematol.* 2003;120:177–186.

Vichinsky EP, Haberkern CM, Neumayr L, et al. A comparison of conservative and aggressive transfusion regimens in the preoperative management of sickle cell disease. *N Engl J Med.* 1995;333:206–213.

Vichinsky EP, Styles LA, Colangelo LH, et al. Acute chest syndrome in sickle cell disease: clinical presentation and course. *Blood.* 1997;89:1787–1792.

51 THROMBOCYTOPENIA

Rovie Mesola

EPIDEMIOLOGY/OVERVIEW

- The normal adult platelet count is 150,000–400,000/mm^3.
- A platelet count below 150,000/mm^3 is defined as thrombocytopenia, however clinical signs and symptoms of thrombocytopenia may not be evident until the platelet count falls well below 100,000/mm^3.

- Bleeding risks occur with following platelet count ranges:
  - *Surgical bleeding:* < 50,000/mm^3
  - *Self-limited bleeding:* < 40,000/mm^3
  - *Clinical spontaneous bleeding requiring attention:* < 12,000/mm^3
  - *Spontaneous severe life-threatening bleeding:* < 6000/mm^3; the most common cause of death associated with severe thrombocytopenia is intracerebral hemorrhage.
- Isolated, mild asymptomatic thrombocytopenia (counts above 75,000/mm^3), often uncovered incidentally on a CBC, can be worked up in the outpatient setting with a repeat platelet count in 1–2 weeks.
- When encountered in the hospital setting, thrombocytopenia is usually part of a systemic dysfunction or treatment complication. In the ICU, thrombocytopenia may be multifactorial, and is a poor prognostic sign as it is usually secondary to severe infection. Causes of thrombocytopenia of particular concern to the hospitalist include
  - Drug-induced, often because of antibiotics or heparin-induced thrombocytopenia (HIT) (see the section on HIT in Chap. 90)
  - Disseminated intravascular coagulation (DIC)
  - Thrombotic thrombocytopenic purpura-hemolytic uremic syndrome (TTP-HUS)
  - Pregnancy-related syndromes, including preeclampsia and HELLP (Hemolytic anemia Elevated Liver enzymes and Low Platelet count) syndrome (hemolysis, elevated liver enzymes, and low platelets).

PATHOPHYSIOLOGY

- True thrombocytopenia may be because of one of three possible mechanisms.
  - Decreased platelet production (Table 51-1)
  - Increased peripheral destruction or consumption (Table 51-2)

TABLE 51-1 Causes of Decreased Platelet Production

- Postviral syndrome (eg, rubella, mumps, varicella, parvovirus, hepatitis C, EBV)
- HIV (via direct destruction of megakaryocytes)
- Postchemotherapy and postradiation therapy
- Congenital or acquired bone marrow aplasia or hypoplasia
- Alcohol and other drugs
- Vitamin B$_{12}$ and folic acid deficiency

Abbreviation: EBV, Epstein-Barr virus.

TABLE 51-2   Causes of Increased Peripheral Platelet Destruction

- ITP
- DIC
- SLE
- Post-transfusion, post-transplantation (alloimmune destruction)
- TTP-HUS
- Antiphospholipid syndrome
- HELLP syndrome
- Drug-induced (eg, quinine, heparin, quinidine, valproic acid)
- Postinfectious (eg, IM, CMV)
- HIV (similar mechanism to ITP)
- Physical destruction (eg, cardiopulmonary bypass)

Abbreviation: SLE, systemic lupus erythematosus; IM, intramuscular.

- ○ Splenic sequestration (the overall platelet mass remains normal, and patients rarely present with bleeding)
  - Seen in patients with chronic liver disease, portal hypertension, and splenomegaly
- Pseudothrombocytopenia is encountered in two settings.
  - ○ Blood obtained with inadequate anticoagulant leading to clumping.
  - ○ EDTA (ethylene diamine tetraacetic acid)-dependent agglutinin mediated clumping in patients where the blood sample was collected with EDTA-coated tubes leading to falsely decreased platelet count and elevated WBC count (clumped platelets are read as leukocytes by the machine).
  - ○ Always examine the peripheral smear if pseudothrombocytopenia is a concern. A platelet count can be repeated using collection tubes with citrate or heparin as anticoagulant.

CLINICAL PRESENTATION, DIFFERENTIAL, MAKING THE DIAGONSIS

- Bleeding is the most common presentation of thrombocytopenia. It is usually superficial (eg, gingival bleeding, epistaxis, petechiae, purpura), occurring after minor cuts, and rarely delayed. Patients may also present with menorrhagia and metrorrhagia. Petechiae are usually seen on the dependent areas of the body (feet and ankles or sacral area in bed-bound patients).
- History (including a medication review) and physical examination are key points in evaluating thrombocytopenia.
- Approach to the thrombocytopenic patient (Fig. 51-1)
  - ○ History (including a review of both prescribed medications, and herbal supplements) and physical examination to determine if the thrombocytopenia is an isolated finding or related to a systemic process.

- ○ Peripheral smear and CBC to examine all cell lines.
- ○ Bone marrow aspirate and biopsy, indicated in all patients with significant thrombocytopenia of unclear etiology. An exception may be the patient < 60 years old with isolated thrombocytopenia. Bone marrow aspiration/biopsies can be safely performed with platelet counts below 10,000/mm^3.
- Heparin-induced thrombocytopenia (HIT) can be a life-threatening thrombotic disorder that follows exposure to either unfractionated or low molecular weight heparin.
  - ○ HIT is defined as a decrease in the platelet count by ≥ 50% compared to baseline or the new onset of otherwise unexplained thrombocytopenia within 2 weeks of starting heparin therapy.
  - ○ Onset of HIT typically occurs between 5 and 14 days but may occur earlier in patients previously exposed to heparins.
  - ○ See Chap. 90 for more information on making this diagnosis and therapeutic options.
- The list of drugs other than heparin that are commonly associated with drug-induced thrombocytopenia is extensive. Common culprits include
  - ○ Quinidine
  - ○ Quinine
  - ○ Rifampin
  - ○ Trimethoprim-sulfamethoxazole
  - ○ Acetaminophen
  - ○ Digoxin
  - ○ Vancomycin

TRIAGE AND INITIAL MANAGEMENT

- The principal goal of treatment is prevention of bleeding by maintaining a safe platelet count; the underlying disease process and the need to perform procedures determines the actual number that is considered "safe."
- When faced with a patient presenting with thrombocytopenia, the first consideration is to determine whether the thrombocytopenia is isolated thrombocytopenia or part of a multisystem disorder. Most cases of thrombocytopenia seen in the hospital setting are usually associated with underlying systemic illness.
- Low platelet counts secondary to an underlying multisystem disorder will require treatment of the primary disease entity (eg, DIC, sepsis, HIV/AIDS, HELLP) as the main consideration.
- Patients with life-threatening bleeding, significant thrombocytopenia and impending septic shock (patients with DIC) will require urgent therapeutic intervention, transfer to a critical care setting, and comanagement with an intensivist.

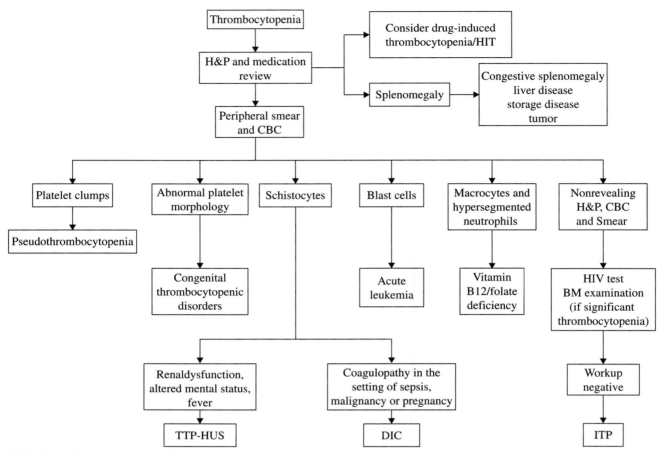

FIG. 51-1 Clinical evaluation of patients with thrombocytopenia.

- The presence of thrombocytopenia and microangiopathic hemolytic anemia (schistocytes in the peripheral smear) should lead the hospitalist to strongly consider TTP-HUS and a hematology consult.
- Indications for platelet transfusion in thrombocytopenia
  - Critical bleeding regardless of cause
  - Prior to surgical or invasive procedures to maintain the platelet count at $\geq 50,000/mm^3$
  - Asymptomatic patients with platelet counts $< 10,000/mm^3$
- Anticoagulants, aspirin, and NSAIDs are relatively contraindicated in thrombocytopenic patients.

DISEASE MANAGEMENT STRATEGIES

- Definitive treatment of the thrombocytopenia is dependent upon the underlying etiology.

THROMBOTIC THROMBOCYTOPENIC PURPURA-HEMOLYTIC UREMIC SYNDROME

- Request a hematology consult to arrange for plasma exchange (1.0–1.5 plasma volumes per day).
- If plasma exchange is not readily available, FFPs should be given immediately.
- Treat idiopathic TTP-HUS with prednisone 1 mg/kg/d or methylprednisolone 125 mg IV q 12 hours.
- Avoid platelet transfusion if there is no significant bleeding.
- Monitor hemolysis (LDH, haptoglobin), platelet count, BUN/creatinine.

DISSEMINATED INTRAVASCULAR COAGULOPATHY

- Treat the underlying disease.
- Provide hemodynamic support.

- Transfuse platelets as warranted.
- Transfuse FFP and/or cryoprecipitate (if fibrinogen < 50 mg/dL) for active bleeding with coagulopathy.
- Monitor PT/PTT, fibrinogen levels, platelet count, other signs of MOF.

HEPARIN-INDUCED THROMBOCYTOPENIA

- Stop all heparin exposure (including heparin flushes).
- Hematology consult may be warranted to diagnosis this condition and to advise management.
- See Chap. 90.

IMMUNE THROMBOCYTOPENIA PURPURA

- The specific treatment of ITP depends on the platelet count and whether hemorrhage is present. Consider hematology consultation to advise treatment and follow the patient post discharge:
  - ◦ The presence of hemorrhage requires the administration of
    - Platelet transfusion
    - IV immune globulin (1 g/kg/d for 2–3 days)
    - Methylprednisolone (1 g/d for 3 days)
  - ◦ Decline in platelet count without bleeding
    - *Less than 30,000/mm³*—Consider hematology consultation to advise optimal treatment, usually prednisone (1–1.5 mg/kg/d) and anti-D immune globulin (75 µg/kg).
    - *30,000–50,000/mm³*—Prednisone may be prescribed or close monitoring of platelet count.
    - *Less than 50,000/mm³*—No treatment required other than avoidance of antiplatelet agents and NSAIDs.

PRIMARY HIV-ASSOCIATED THROMBOCYTOPENIA

- Infectious disease consultation is advised to optimize care, including diagnosis because many of these patients may have multiple reasons for thrombocytopenia.
  - ◦ Patients who are currently not on antiretroviral medications should be started on a multidrug regimen of antiretroviral drugs that includes zidovudine (AZT) at a minimum dose of 600 mg/d.
  - ◦ Patients already on highly active antiretroviral therapy (HAART) should have AZT added to the regimen.

- ◦ Additional therapy will be dependent on the severity of the thrombocytopenia and is similar to that of ITP (ie, IVIg, steroids).

CARE TRANSITIONS

- In general, it is advisable to discharge patients only after the platelet count has stabilized or is rising. Spontaneous bleeding rarely occurs with counts above 12,000/mm³. The patient's home situation, comorbidities, and occupation should also be considered in discharge planning.
- TTP-HUS
  - ◦ Parameters
    - Hgb/Hct, platelet count, LDH/indirect bilirubin, BUN/creatinine, neurologic status
- HIT
  - ◦ Parameters
    - Platelet count, INR (for patients on coumadin)
    - Inform all future healthcare providers against subsequent heparin exposure
- ITP
  - ◦ Parameters
    - Platelet count
    - Patients on steroids should be monitored for osteopenia and cataracts

BIBLIOGRAPHY

Ballem PJ, Segal GM, Stratton JR, et al. Mechanisms of thrombocytopenia in chronic autoimmune thrombocytopenic purpura. Evidence of both impaired platelet production and increased platelet clearance. *J Clin Invest.* 1987;80:33.

Cines D, Blanchette V. Immune thrombocytopenic purpura. *N Engl J Med.* 2002;346:1003.

George JN, Raskob GE, Rizvi Shah S, et al. Drug-induced thrombocytopenia: a systematic review of published case reports. *Ann Intern Med.* 1998;129:886–890.

Schiffer CA, Anderson KC, Bennett CL, et al. Platelet transfusion for patients with cancer: clinical practice guidelines of the American Society of Clinical Oncology. *J Clin Oncol.* 2001;19:1519.

Strauss R, Wehler M, Mehler K, et al. Thrombocytopenia in patients in the medical intensive care unit: bleeding prevalence, transfusion requirements, and outcome. *Crit Care Med.* 2002;30:1765.

Vanderschueren S, De Weerdt A, Malbrain M, et al. Thrombocytopenia and prognosis in intensive care. *Crit Care Med.* 2000;28:1871.

Warkentin TE. Heparin-induced thrombocytopenia: recognition, treatment and prevention. The seventh ACCP conference on anti-thrombolytic therapy. *Chest.* 2004;126(3 suppl): 311s–337s.

52   TRANSFUSION MEDICINE

Susan Coutinho McAllister, Eric Kupersmith, and Alpesh Amin

EPIDEMIOLOGY/OVERVIEW

- The most common cause of anemia requiring transfusion in the hospital is blood loss.
  - Bleeding may be intraluminal (ie, GI), postsurgical, retroperitoneal, spontaneous thoracic/abdominal/pelvic cavity, trauma-related, and/or because of an underlying bleeding diathesis (congenital or acquired).
  - Many hospitalized patients acquire anemia from frequent blood draws.
  - 1–2 L of acute blood loss can result in iron deficiency.
- Inpatient transfusion practice should be based upon the acuity, volume, and duration of blood loss, each patient's underlying condition and ability to compensate for the loss, as well as the inherent risks associated with blood transfusion and availability of this scare resource.
- The clinician has available
  - *RBCs*—Packed, autologous, washed, leukopoor
  - *Platelets*—Irradiated, leukoreduced, pheresed (single donor)
  - Cryoglobulin
  - FFP
  - Immunoglobulin IgG
  - Donor lymphocytes
  - Granulocytes
  - CD34+ (stem cells)
- Risks of transfusion include
  - Transfusion reactions
  - Blood-borne infections
- Hospitalists should minimize the iatrogenic blood loss that occurs from excessive blood testing, lead initiatives that promote the appropriate use of RBCs, FFP, and platelet concentrates, and identify and report transfusion reactions in a timely manner.

PATHOPHYSIOLOGY

- Massive blood loss may cause anemia because of limited bone marrow reserve. Consequences depend upon volume and duration of bleeding.
- Individual tolerance to anemia varies based upon oxygen delivery to the tissues and the compensatory mechanisms for maintaining delivery (Table 52-1).
- Acute blood loss causes physiologic changes owing to hypovolemia as well as anemia. Volume lost is generally replaced with crystalloid or colloid resulting in acute normovolemic anemia.
- The physiologic response to acute normovolemic anemia is regulated by the autonomic nervous system at the levels of the central, regional, and microcirculatory distribution of blood flow. Additionally, Hgb affinity for oxygen is lessened because of a shift to the right on the Hgb oxygen dissociation curve. This shift is because of an increase in RBC 2, 3-DPG (3-diphosphoglycerate) in response to anemia.
- Central blood flow changes are associated with an increase in cardiac output (CO). CO increases because of both an increase in stroke volume (SV) and heart rate. SV is increased because of an increased preload and decreased afterload which results from the decrease in blood viscosity, as well as increased inotropy from sympathetic stimulation.
- Regional blood flow is shunted from nonvital organs to vital organs, such as the heart and brain. This increased flow to the heart aids in meeting cardiac oxygen demand since myocardial oxygen extraction cannot fully compensate for the decrease in oxygen delivery resulting from anemia.

TABLE 52-1   Physiologic Response to Acute Anemia

BLOOD FLOW	MECHANISMS OF COMPENSATION
Central	Increased CO
	Oxygen dissociation curve shifted to the right (facilitates delivery)*
Regional	Nonvital to vital organ redistribution of blood flow
	Brain oxygen extraction increases in acute anemia
Microcirculatory	Oxygen extraction is increased via capillary recruitment and homogeneous blood flow

*Hgb delivery of oxygen remains the same until Hgb level is < 7g/dL. *The prior belief that delivery of oxygen was maximal at Hgb of 10 g/dL is not valid.*
Source: Adapted from Madjdpour C, Spahn DR, Weiskopf RB. Anemia and perioperative red blood cell transfusion: a matter of tolerance. *Crit Care Med.* 2006;34S:S102; Hebert PC, Wells G, Blajchman MA, et al. A multicenter, randomized, controlled clinical trial of transfusion requirements in critical care. Transfusion requirements in critical care investigators, Canadian critical care trials group. *N Engl J Med.* 1999;340:409; Morisaki H, Sibbald WJ. Tissue oxygen delivery and the microcirculation. *Crit Care Clin.* 2004;20:213.

• Microcirculatory blood flow becomes homogeneous through the capillary bed facilitation increased oxygen extraction (Table 52-1).

RISKS OF TRANSFUSION

• The frequency of transfusion reactions (see Table 52-2).
  ◦ *Mild reactions (febrile, nonhemolytic, or allergic reactions)*—1/100 per units transfused
  ◦ *Transfusion-related acute lung injury or TRALI*—1/2000–5000 per units transfused
  ◦ *Anaphylaxis*—Approximately 1/20,000-50,000 per units transfused
  ◦ *Acute hemolytic transfusion reactions*—Approximately 1/60,000–250,000 per units transfused
  ◦ *Delayed hemolytic transfusion reactions*—1/1000 per units transfused
• In patients with compensated heart failure, excessive use of pRBCs can trigger CHF.

• The frequency of blood-borne infections has declined owing to advances in testing and technology. Nevertheless, the risks must be taken into account when prescribing blood products.
  ◦ Risk of HIV or hepatitis C virus (HCV) is 1/2,000,000 per unit transfused.
  ◦ Risk of hepatitis B virus (HBV) is 1/60,000–200,000 per unit transfused.
  ◦ Risk of bacterial contamination of platelets resulting in sepsis is 1/10,000 platelet transfusions.
  ◦ The risks of other transfusion-transmitted infections such as Chagas' disease or babesiosis are unknown.
• The risk of anaphylaxis is 1/20,000 per unit transfused. The risk of urticarial transfusion reactions is 1/100 per unit transfused.
• Other disadvantages to frequent transfusions are iron overload, alloantibody production, posttransfusion purpura, and transfusion-related graft vs. host disease. Nonimmune mediated hemolysis, hyperkalemia, metabolic alkalosis and hypokalemia, hypothermia.

TABLE 52-2 Acute Adverse Effects of Transfusion

Transfusion risks vary among various blood components. Acute reactions occur within 24 hours of blood product transfusion. The components with the highest risk and the associated signs and symptoms are listed. When an adverse effect of transfusion occurs, the first step is to *stop* the transfusion. Urticaria is the only circumstance when a patient may be treated symptomatically and transfusion continued.

Hemolysis (immune, intravascular): RBC, WBC (including granulocytes and platelets) may cause hemolysis. Patients may develop fever, chills, dyspnea, and hypotension, as well as pain in the chest and back, and along the IV infusion line. Bleeding, oozing, and oliguria occur. Urinalysis will reveal hemoglobinuria. After stopping transfusion, IV fluids must continue infusing and the blood product should be returned to the blood bank for investigation. Supportive care with aggressive treatment of hypotension is the key. When severe, DIC may occur and must be treated as such.

Hemolysis (immune, extravascular): RBC, WBC (including granulocytes and platelets) may cause this type of reaction. Patients are often asymptomatic and diagnosis is from a positive direct antiglobulin test, crossmatch incompatibility, hyperbilirubinemia, or no change in the posttransfusion Hgb concentration. Incompatible components should be avoided.

Hemolysis (nonimmune): RBC may cause this reaction. Urinalysis will reveal hemoglobinuria, but patients are otherwise without symptoms. After stopping transfusion, the unit of blood must be returned to the blood bank for investigation to exclude immune hemolysis.

Simple allergic: All blood components may cause simple allergic reactions. Patients may develop urticaria or hives. Transfusion should be stopped temporarily to provide symptomatic relief with antihistamine therapy before resuming transfusion.

Anaphylaxis: All blood components may cause anaphylaxis. Patients develop hypotension, shock, respiratory stridor, wheezing, abdominal pain, diarrhea, nausea, and cardiovascular collapse. After stopping transfusion, airway management and supportive care, which may indicate epinephrine, should be instituted.

Sepsis: Platelets and RBC may cause sepsis. Patients develop high fever or hypothermia, rigors, hypotension, tachycardia, bleeding, oozing, as well as nausea and diarrhea. After stopping transfusion, the unit of blood must be returned to the blood bank for investigation and Gram stain. Blood cultures should be obtained before starting antimicrobial therapy. Supportive care for sepsis should be provided.

Febrile, nonhemolytic: RBC, WBC, and platelets may cause these reactions. Patients develop fever and/or chills. This is a diagnosis of exclusion; hemolytic reaction and sepsis must be excluded. After stopping transfusion and returning blood product to blood bank for investigation, symptomatic relief may be provided with antipyretics, as well as parenteral meperidine for rigors. Transfusion should not be restarted given the possibility of hemolysis or sepsis.

TRALI: All blood components except cryoprecipitate may cause TRALI. Patients develop acute respiratory distress, chest radiographs show pulmonary interstitial infiltrates when there is not another cardiogenic or pulmonary cause. Supportive care with oxygen and/or mechanical ventilation should be provided. The prognosis of TRALI is better than acute respiratory distress syndrome if treated appropriately in the first 24–48 hours.

Hypervolemia: All blood components except cryoprecipitate may cause hypervolemia; WBC rarely cause. Patients develop increased central venous pressure, dyspnea, and pulmonary edema. After stopping the transfusion, patients should be positioned upright and treated with oxygen and diuretics, like furosemide, as needed.

SOURCE: Sazama K, DeChristopher PJ, Dodd R, et al. Practice parameter for the recognition, management, and prevention of adverse consequences of blood transfusion: *Arch Pathol Lab Med.* 2000;124:61.

INDICATIONS FOR TRANSFUSION

PACKED RED BLOOD CELLS

- The indications for transfusion depend on whether the patient is actively bleeding and whether the patient being cared for is in the operating room or postanesthesia care unit.
- The "transfusion trigger" has been under increasing scrutiny over the last decade and the verdict is still not known.
- In the surgical literature there has been a rough guideline of the "10/30 rule" (ie, pRBC transfusion indicated for Hgb less than 10 g/dL or Hct less than 30%); this has fallen out of favor as a growing body of literature has strongly suggested worse outcomes in patients with transfusions than without.
- Recent data demonstrate that there may be no mortality benefit in critically ill patients receiving prophylactic transfusions to maintain their Hgb above 10 g/dL.
- The patient should be considered for a transfusion based on current guidelines (Table 52-3).
- The clinician needs to assess for signs and symptoms relating to the presence of anemia and the acuity of the process:
  - Hypotension, postural hypotension, tachycardia, exertional dyspnea, lightheadedness, confusion, lethargy.

TABLE 52-3 Guidelines for Red Cell Transfusions and Volume Replacement in Adults

Need based on estimation of lost blood volume
> 40% loss (> 2000 mL): rapid volume replacement, including RBC transfusion, is required.
30%–40% loss (1500–2000 mL): rapid volume replacement with crystalloids or synthetic colloids is required; RBC transfusion will probably be required.
15%–30% loss (800–1500 mL): transfuse with crystalloids or synthetic colloids; RBC transfusion is unlikely, unless underlying anemia, continued blood loss, or reduced cardiovascular reserve.
≤ 15% loss (≤ 750 mL): no RBC transfusion need unless preexisting anemia, or inability to compensate because of severe cardiac or respiratory disease.

Need based on Hgb concentration
Hb < 7 g/dL: RBC transfusion indicated. If the patient is otherwise stable, 2 units of packed RBC should be transfused and clinical status and Hb should be reassessed.
Hb 7–10 g/dL: correct strategy is unclear.
Hb > 10 g/dL: RBC transfusion not indicated.
High-risk patients: those > age 65 years, and/or with cardiovascular or respiratory disease may tolerate anemia poorly. Such patients may be transfused when Hb < 8 g/dL.

SOURCE: Adapted from Guidelines for the clinical use of red cell transfusions. *Br J Haematol.* 2001;113:24.

- Initially if a patient is actively bleeding and hemodynamically unstable, volume resuscitation and transfusion are clearly warranted.
- Comorbidity also determines the target transfusion Hct.
  - Patient with coronary artery disease, systolic heart failure, cerebrovascular disease, chronic lung disease, acute respiratory failure, or impaired oxygen transport may not tolerate a significant anemia.
  - Some evidence has demonstrated a higher mortality and morbidity with lower Hgb in cardiac disease states.
- In women of childbearing age, the presence of pregnancy should be determined.
- The target Hct should then be determined as follows:
  - No signs or symptoms of anemia and no comorbidity— 21%
  - Either a sign or symptom or a comorbidity risk— 26%
  - Ongoing chemotherapy, acute myelogenous leukemia (AML) treatment, bone marrow transplant service— 26%
  - Both a sign or symptom and a comorbidity risk— 29%
  - Acute coronary syndrome—30% to 33%
- Current transfusion guidelines suggest indications based upon clinical evidence to support the use of pRBC transfusions (Table 52-3).
- While these include Hgb-based transfusion guidelines, individual transfusion decisions should be based upon each unique situation and the clinical gestalt (Table 52-3).
- Factors to consider are the likelihood of continued bleeding, multiple comorbidities (specifically coronary artery disease and CHF), and clinical evaluation.
- Each unit of pRBC should raise the Hct by 3% to 4% and the Hgb by 1 g/dL in the absence of active bleeding or hemolysis.

PLATELET TRANSFUSIONS

- The indications for transfusion depend on the clinical situation, whether the patient is actively bleeding or about to undergo a surgical procedure (Table 52-4).
- Special circumstances include patients who are actively bleeding 24 hours after cardiopulmonary bypass.
- Patients with HIT have a low incidence of bleeding and platelet transfusion is a relative contraindication.
- Multiple platelet transfusion reactions merit a washed platelet restriction.

TABLE 52-4   Platelet Transfusion Triggers

CLINICAL SETTING	ACCEPTABLE PLATELET COUNT
1. Thrombocytopenia without bleeding, anticipated surgery, risk factors, or platelet defects	5000
2. Thrombocytopenia because of chemotherapy or other acute leukemic treatment but otherwise as 1	10,000
3. Microvascular bleeding, minor procedure, risk factors	30,000
4. Platelet dysfunction or drug-induced platelet defect but otherwise as 3	50,000 or clinical response
5. Active bleeding or major surgical procedure	50,000
6. Active bleeding or major surgical procedure and platelet dysfunction or a drug-induced platelet defect	100,000 or clinical response
7. Major neurosurgical procedure	100,000

SOURCE: Sazama K, DeChristopher PJ, Dodd R, et al. Practice parameter for the recognition, management, and prevention of adverse consequences of blood transfusion. *Arch Pathol Lab Med.* 2000;124:61.

- Alloimmunization should be suspected when patient appears refractory to transfusion (ie, failure of platelet count to rise adequately following two or more independent platelet transfusions).
  - The clinician should check the percent reactive AB (PRA)—If > 80% react, then the patient is alloimmunizing and will need HLA-matched platelets.

FRESH FROZEN PLASMA

- FFP is often indicated to urgently reverse warfarin when a patient is either actively bleeding or about to undergo emergency surgery.
- Appropriate specialty consultation (stroke specialists, hematologists, or neurosurgeons) should be performed when a patient has a life-threatening hemorrhage, intracranial hemorrhage, or extremely high INR with active bleeding.
- Other special circumstances include
  - Massive bleeding (> 1 blood volume or 10 RBC units)
  - TTP
  - Plasmapheresis
- Reversal of warfarin (coumadin) target INR < 1.5
  - Vitamin K to supplement FFP unless the goal of INR is temporary with a plan to resume warfarin within a couple of days postoperatively.
  - Weight-based FFP dosing should be used to provide optimal reversal.

CLINICAL PRESENTATION, DIFFERENTIAL, MAKING THE DIAGNOSIS

This section will focus on the workup for specific transfusion reactions.

- Shock, hypotension, angioedema, or respiratory distress occurring within seconds to minutes of a transfusion with plasma, pRBC, platelets, granulocytes, cryoglobulin, or IgG suggests anaphylactic transfusion reaction.
  - The transfusion must be stopped, and the patient treated with epinephrine.
  - See Chap. 24.
- Fever, chills, and dyspnea within 1–6 hours of a transfusion of pRBC or platelets also occur within seconds to minutes of the start of a transfusion with any blood product.
  - Atopic patients at increased risk.
  - The patient requires monitoring for the possibility of anaphylaxis.
  - Administer diphenhydramine.
  - Discontinue transfusion. If urticaria dissipates and there is no associated dyspnea, hypotension, or anaphylaxis, then the transfusion may be resumed after maximal premedication with H1 blocking antihistamine.
  - If urticaria recurs, reduce plasma content of transfused blood product through cell washing, centrifuging.
- The symptoms of TRALI typically occur within 2–4 hours and range from cough, dyspnea, acute respiratory distress syndrome (ARDS) with hypoxemia, hypotension, fever, and pulmonary edema secondary to any blood product.
  - Treatment is supportive.
- Fever, chills, dyspnea within 1–6 hours following a transfusion of pRBC or platelets suggests a febrile, nonhemolytic immune transfusion reaction related to recipient antibodies to donor WBC, and donor cytokines.
  - Stop transfusion and assess to see if hemolytic reaction is occurring.
  - Administer acetaminophen. Avoid aspirin in patients with thrombocytopenia.

○ Although benign, infection and hemolysis should be ruled out. Bacteria or endotoxin is more common with platelet transfusions because platelets are stored at room temperature. If suspect, culture donor unit and blood.

○ Leukocyte poor pRBC and platelets in the future to avoid or minimize reaction.

• Acute hemolytic transfusion reactions from pRBC related to ABO incompatability, anti-Rh, or anti-Jk occur within 24 hours of transfusion and may present with fever alone or DIC.

○ Maintain vital signs.

○ If the patient is receiving the transfusion, stop the transfusion and alert the blood bank immediately. Every hospital has a protocol for evaluating transfusion reactions which must be followed meticulously.

○ Administer normal saline to maintain urinary output. Avoid Ringer's lactate solution because Ca^{2+} may initiate clotting of any blood in line. Avoid dextrose-containing solutions which may hemolyze any of the remaining red cells in the line.

○ Laboratory tests include direct antiglobulin test, plasma free Hgb, type and crossmatch, hemolysis workup, serum K^+, and urine sample for Hgb testing.

• Delayed hemolytic transfusion reactions to pRBC from antibody to the Kidd or Rh system occur 2–10 days following transfusion and require a high index of suspicion because many of these patients have other reasons for being anemic.

○ If no brisk hemolysis, no treatment is required.

○ Avoid transfusions containing the RBC antigen.

• Posttransfusion purpura in women (95%) related to anti-HPA1a presents with severe thrombocytopenia 5–10 days posttransfusion of pRBC, platelets, and granulocytes. The incidence is unknown.

○ Treatment is supportive.

• Transfusion associated with graft vs. host disease, because of donor lymphocyte immune-mediated reaction, causes dysfunction of the skin, liver, GI, and bone marrow, occurring 4–30 days posttransfusion.

○ The only way to prevent this usually fatal complication is to gamma irradiate all lymphocyte-containing components.

TRIAGE AND INITIAL MANAGEMENT

ACUTELY BLEEDING PATIENT

• Concomitantly, supplemental oxygen should be provided, IV access should be obtained, lab studies drawn, and crystalloid or colloid prepared and infused.

• Pertinent standard labs should be obtained: CBC, PT/INR, PTT, and type and cross.

• Place two large bore peripheral IV catheters for volume resuscitation or in combination with a large bore central catheter.

○ A common misconception is that a standard triple lumen catheter can be used in isolation. The standard triple lumen is 18 gauge and has a long tip slowing the flow into the vein. Also, the three ports, while useful for hanging varied medications, do not allow for swifter volume administration.

PATIENT WITH SUBACUTE OR CHRONIC BLOOD LOSS ANEMIA

• If the patient is not severely symptomatic, consider alternatives to transfusion, such as iron therapy for iron deficiency (consider IV iron for profound deficiency and/or intolerance to oral iron) or erythropoietin for patients with chronic renal disease. These may also be used as adjuvant therapies even if transfusion is necessary.

• Appropriate specialists should be consulted to assist with the evaluation and definitive treatment of the underlying cause of blood loss.

DISEASE MANAGEMENT STRATEGIES

• If a patient is clinically stable, despite a "drop" in the blood count, and the patient is not still actively bleeding and the underlying cause is understood, the patient's clinical picture should influence the decision to transfuse more than an absolute number.

• The clinician should review trends in heart rate, ECGs, oxygen saturation, functional status changes and reported symptoms of chest discomfort, dyspnea on exertion, dizziness, weakness, and fatigue. If these signs and/or symptoms are new or worsening and are attributable to the anemia, it may be reasonable to ordertransfusion.

• Other key factors to consider include the likelihood of recurrent bleeding and self-containment.

○ The majority of retroperitoneal bleeding will self-tamponade and only require supportive care. These patients will reabsorb the lost iron through the reticuloendothelial system.

○ Other sources of intercavitary bleeding often require surgery as well as transfusion because of hemodynamic instability.

○ Patients with subacute blood loss often will not require blood products after triage and initial management is complete (with or without transfusion).

○ Transfusion guidelines should assist clinical decision-making to identify which patients will benefit more from transfusion vs. iron supplementation along with other specific intervention(s) for their underlying process(es).

○ Potential nontransfusion therapies for blood loss anemia, depending on underlying causes, include iron supplementation (oral or IV) and erythropoietic stimulating protein injection(s). Iron repletion is required prior erythropoietic stimulating protein therapy.

• Another important aspect of treatment of anemia with transfusions is patient preference. Patients may decline transfusion for a variety of reasons, including religious belief (Jehovah's Witnesses), or fear of blood-borne infections such as HIV (Table 52-5).

○ If the reason is fear, an explanation of the relative safety of donated blood may allay fears. If the fear is based on a prior transfusion reaction, discussion of preventative measures that can be taken may be beneficial in achieving patient agreement to a life-saving transfusion.

• In patients for whom refusal is absolute (typically based on cultural or religious beliefs), a "bloodless medicine" approach becomes the only treatment option. The complexities of the medical, legal, and ethical ramifications of refusal of transfusion are beyond the scope of this chapter, but are based on shared decision-making and fully informed consent. Strategies for bloodless medicine include

○ Steps to reduce blood loss, including early definitive intervention in actively bleeding patients, the use of blood salvaging systems during surgery and limiting blood loss from phlebotomy.

○ Autologous blood donation may be an option for patients other than Jehovah's Witnesses.

TABLE 52-5 Patients Refusing Transfusion

Jehovah's Witness patients do not accept most blood products. Treatment of individuals refusing transfusion may be difficult. Management strategies include reducing patient's oxygen requirement and determining acceptable options to increase oxygen-carrying capacity.

Sedation, mechanical ventilation, and induction of mild hypothermia are interventions which may be used to decrease oxygen requirements in these patients.

Alternative oxygen carriers, erythropoietin, and IV iron are acceptable to some patients and may be used to increase oxygen-carrying capacity. Providing 100% oxygen, hyperbaric oxygen therapy, and an autologous transfusion may also be utilized to increase oxygen-carrying capacity.

Blood loss should be minimized. Careful attention by providers to limit phlebotomy and decreasing ongoing loss are the key.

○ Many patients refusing blood products, including Jehovah's Witnesses, will accept iron infusion, albumin, or coagulation factor concentrates or recombinant coagulation products and erythropoietin.

○ Blood substitutes, currently in clinical trials, may be available on a compassionate use basis.

○ Reduction of oxygen demand, through hypothermia and/or sedation (up to therapeutic paralysis and mechanical ventilation).

○ Improvement of oxygen carrying capacity by use of a hyperbaric chamber.

○ For web-based resources and more information, see www.bloodlessmed.com.

CARE TRANSITIONS

• Access to healthcare and/or medication side effects may impact on a patient's ability to comply with treatment plans.

○ Lack of insurance may preclude a surgical option.

○ Intolerance to medication may lead to noncompliance and hospitalization.

○ For example, a young woman with menorrhagia may develop a severely symptomatic/profoundly iron deficiency anemia despite treatment with oral iron because of GI side effects precluding compliance with oral therapy. Definitive care (hysterectomy) may not be an option if she does not have health insurance. IV iron prior to discharge may be one important aspect of an appropriate care strategy.

• Sometimes the hospitalist, PCP, and/or specialist consultant do not agree regarding the need for transfusion therapy. At this juncture, the hospitalist should discuss the risks vs. benefits with the patient, the healthcare team, and with the physician who will be responsible for outpatient follow-up and come to an agreement based on the patient's best interests and preferences.

• Many patients are at continued risk for recurrence of bleeding and therefore need to be alerted to signs and symptoms of bleeding, and a plan needs to be discussed and put in place with the patient and PCP or subspecialist.

○ The plan may include follow-up Hgb counts for comparison to the inpatient laboratory data at specified intervals, depending on the source of bleeding and likelihood of occult rebleeding.

• It is essential that the primary care doctor is aware of the hospital course and rationale for changes in previous therapies or for new therapies.

BIBLIOGRAPHY

Corwin HL, Gettinger A, Pearl RG, et al. The CRIT study: anemia and blood transfusion in the critically ill—the current clinical practice in the United States. *Crit Care Med.* 2004;32:39.

Guidelines for the clinical use of red cell transfusions. *Br J Haematol.* 2001;113:24.

Hebert PC, Van der Linden P, Biro G, et al. Physiologic aspects of anemia. *Crit Care Med.* 2004;20:187.

Hebert PC, Wells G, Blajchman MA, et al. A multicenter, randomized, controlled clinical trial of transfusion requirements in critical care. Transfusion requirements in critical care investigators, Canadian critical care trials group. *N Engl J Med.* 1999;340:409.

Madjdpour C, Spahn DR, Weiskopf RB. Anemia and perioperative red blood cell transfusion: a matter of tolerance. *Crit Care Med.* 2006;34S:S102.

Marcucci C, Madjdpour C, Spahn DR. Allogeneic blood transfusions: benefits, risks and clinical indications in countries with a low or high human development index. *Br Med Bull.* 2004;70:15.

Morisaki H, Sibbald WJ. Tissue oxygen delivery and the microcirculation. *Crit Care Clin.* 2004;20:213.

Sazama K, DeChristopher PJ, Dodd R, et al. Practice parameter for the recognition, management, and prevention of adverse consequences of blood transfusion. *Arch Pathol Lab Med.* 2000;124:61.

Spahn DR, Dettori N, Kocian R, et al. Tranfusion in the cardiac patient. *Crit Care Clin.* 2004;20:269.

Spahn DR. Strategies for transfusion therapy. *Best Pract Res Clin Anaesthesiol.* 2004;18:661.

Vincent JL, Baron JF, Reinhart K, et al. The ABC (anemia and blood transfusion in critical care) investigators. Anemia and blood transfusion in critically ill patients. *JAMA.* 2002;288:1499.

INFECTIOUS DISEASES

53 FEVER OF UNKNOWN ORIGIN

David Oxman and Harry Schrager

EPIDEMIOLOGY/OVERVIEW

- *Definition*—The original criteria for fever of unknown origin (FUO) by Petersdorf and Beeson in 1961 was fever greater than 38.3°C (101°F) on several occasions, persisting without diagnosis for at least 3 weeks, in spite of 1 week of investigations in the hospital. This classic definition of FUO has been revised to a febrile illness of 3 weeks, duration that has not been diagnosed after at least three outpatient visits or 3 days of hospitalization.
- *Etiology*—Over 200 different causes of FUO have been reported, but all fall into four broad categories. The relative importance of each category varies with different patient populations and geographic locales. Up to 30% of FUO remain undiagnosed after intensive workup.
- *Infectious*—Although the proportion of FUO associated with infection has fallen in recent decades, many case series still report undiagnosed infections as the commonest cause of FUO.
  - ○ The most common bacterial causes of FUO are
    - ▪ TB, most often from reactivation of latent disease.
      - • Purified protein derivative (PPD) testing and chest radiography are helpful but may miss cases in the immunosuppressed or those with extrapulmonary infection.
    - ▪ Occult intra-abdominal abscesses.
      - • Includes diverticular, hepatic, biliary, splenic, and subphrenic abscesses.
      - • More common with history of prior abdominal surgery or predisposing conditions such as Crohn's disease.
      - • Splenic abscess may occur with intravenous (IV) drug users with preceding bacteremia.
    - ▪ Subacute bacterial endocarditis, which may present with negative blood cultures if prior antibiotics have been given (see Chap. 54).
      - • True culture-negative endocarditis is rare, less than 5% of cases.
      - • HACEK group (*Haemophilus aphrophilus, Actinobacillus actinomycetemcomitans, Cardiobacterium hominis, Eikenella corrodens,* and *Kingella kingae*)

- *Bartonella* sp. require prolonged incubation; if suspected, the microbiology laboratory should be notified.
  - Vertebral osteomyelitis is common in the elderly and should be considered in the patient with fever and back pain.
  - Common viral causes include
    - Cytomegalovirus (CMV) and Epstein-Barr virus (EBV). Diagnosed by serum IgM antibodies and/or PCR.
    - In returning travelers from endemic areas infections such as dengue or chikungunya fever should be considered.
- *Neoplastic*—With the advent of better diagnostic imaging and earlier detection, the percentage of malignancies presenting as FUO has declined.
  - Fever in malignancy results from either tissue necrosis or the release of pyrogenic cytokines.
  - Hematologic malignancies, such as lymphoma, leukemia, and myeloma, are much more likely to cause FUO than solid organ malignancies.
  - Among solid organ tumors, renal cell carcinoma is most often associated with FUO. Hematuria is absent in many patients. Other solid tumors occasionally presenting with FUO are hepatocellular, breast, and colon cancer.
- *Inflammatory, rheumatologic, and autoimmune*—The percentage of FUO attributable to rheumatologic disease has risen over time, probably because of greater awareness of these entities.
  - Local or systemic vasculitides, such as temporal arteritis or polyarteritis nodosa, may present as FUO. Temporal arteritis is an especially common cause of FUO in the elderly, and in 10% of elderly patients with temporal arteritis present with fever alone.
  - Other inflammatory conditions such as polymyalgia rheumatica or inflammatory bowel diseases may also present initially with fever.
  - Still's disease (transient rash, arthritis, fever, leukocytosis, and extremely high ferritin levels), rheumatic fever, sarcoidosis, and systemic lupus erythhematosus are also in the differential diagnosis.
- *Miscellaneous*
  - *Drug fever* (Table 53-1)—Many drugs can cause fever, by a variety of mechanisms.
    - Beta-lactam antibiotics, cardiac medications (including amiodarone, procainamide, quinidine, nifedipine, captopril, and hydralazine), antitubercular drugs (isoniazid and rifampin), and anticonvulsants are common culprits.
    - Rash and eosinophilia may be present, but often are not.
    - Drug fever may develop in a patient who has been taking the offending agent chronically over a long period of time.
  - Drug fever is a diagnosis of exclusion and is only confirmed when the fever resolves with stopping the suspected agent.
  - *Factitious fever*—One review put the incidence of factitious fever causing FUO as high as 10%. Fever may be simulated by manipulation of thermometers, or self-induced by the injection of pyrogenic materials. Typically, the patient is a young adult female with experience working in healthcare.
  - *Thromboembolic disease*—In the right clinical setting, for example, hypercoagulable state, evaluation for deep venous thrombosis or subacute pulmonary embolism should be considered.
  - *Other considerations*—Other considerations include hyperthyroidism, familial Mediterranean fever (a genetic disease in persons predominantly of Mediterranean descent, presenting with short-lived, recurrent attacks of sterile peritonitis, pleurisy, or arthritis), and Kikuchi's disease (FUO with necrotizing cervical lymphadenitis, especially in young Asian women).

CLINICAL PRESENTATION, DIFFERENTIAL, MAKING THE DIAGNOSIS

- Many FUO patients can be evaluated as outpatients. Select patients may be admitted for evaluation, most often because of the severity of clinical illness. The hospitalist may admit outpatients with FUO, or treat patients developing FUO in the hospital. The latter patients are considered to have nosocomial FUO.
- FUO is not merely any febrile illness without an immediately apparent cause. Before making the diagnosis of FUO, the following initial evaluation must fail to find a source for the fever:
  - A careful medical history and physical examination are the most important parts of any FUO evaluation.
    - Prior illnesses, past surgical procedures, medication lists, and vaccination histories should be thoroughly reviewed.
    - Particular attention should be paid to travel and sexual history, recreational activities, occupational exposures as well as exposure to pets and other animals and culinary habits (eg, handling and consuming raw and unpasteurized foods).
    - The timing and pattern of fever is generally nonspecific and unhelpful, perhaps with the exception of the characteristic tertian or quartan fevers of malaria (fever periodicity is usually absent in falciparum malaria, which is the most lethal form of malaria).
    - Ophthalmologic examination should be performed if the initial general examination is unrevealing.
    - Repeated evaluations over time may be necessary.

TABLE 53-1   Mechanisms of Drugs Frequently Causing Fever

MECHANISM OF DRUG FEVER	COMMON DRUGS CAUSING FEVER
Hypersensitivity • Most common cause. • Offending drug or metabolite elicits the formation of antibody-antigen complexes or a T-cell-mediated immune response. • Most commonly occurs within the first 3 weeks of starting a medication, but may occur after years of use. • Fever may or may not be accompanied by rash/hives, liver, kidney, or hematologic abnormalities, or mucosal or respiratory involvement. • Fever resolves within 3–7 days of stopping the offending drug.	**Anticonvulsants,** especially • Carbamazepine • Phenytoin **Antimicrobials,** including • Beta-lactams • Sulfonamides • Nitrofurantoin • Minocycline **Miscellaneous** • Allopurinol • Heparin
Altered thermoregulation • Drugs that increase metabolic rate and heat production • Drugs that alter hypothalamic thermoregulatory centers via production of cytokines/endogenous pyrogens	**Exogenous thyroid hormone** (increases metabolism) **Anticholinergics** (alter hypothalamic thermoregulation) • Phenothiazines • Tricyclic antidepressants • Atropine • Antihistamines **Sympathomimetics** (alter hypothalamic thermoregulation and cause peripheral vasoconstriction) • Amphetamines, cocaine, MDMA (ecstasy)
Drug administration • Drugs may be contaminated with exogenous pyrogens • Drugs may have intrinsic pyrogenic properties **Secondary to the pharmacologic effect of the drug** • Cell lysis/tumor necrosis following chemotherapy • Jarisch-Herxheimer reaction caused by release of pathogen endotoxins following use of cidal antimicrobials **Idiosyncratic** • May be associated with genetic factors	**Intrinsic pyrogens** • Amphotericin • Bleomycin Associated with multiple drugs, tumors, and pathogens **Malignant hyperthermia** associated with anesthetics • Succinylcholine • Halothane **Neuroleptic malignant syndrome** • Major tranquilizers such as haloperidol **Serotonin syndrome** • Serotonin reuptake inhibitors • Monoamine oxidase inhibitors • L-tryptophan • Lithium **Glucose-6-phosphate dehydrogenase deficiency** • Primaquine • Quinine sulfate • Sulfonamides

○ Several routine diagnostic tests are helpful and should be ordered as part of an initial evaluation.
  ▪ Complete blood count (CBC) with differential
  ▪ Blood chemistries, liver function tests, and lactate dehydrogenase (LDH)
  ▪ Urinalysis and urine culture
  ▪ Blood cultures (ideally three sets drawn from different sites over a period of at least several hours, in a patient who is not on antibiotics)
  ▪ Erythrocyte sedimentation rate (ESR) and C-reactive protein (CRP) (which may be elevated in a wide variety of conditions and is not specific)
  ▪ Human immunodeficiency virus (HIV) testing
  ▪ PPD
  ▪ Chest x-ray

○ Serologic tests for infectious causes may be helpful but should not be ordered routinely. Rather, they should be ordered only if the patient has a suggestive epidemiologic background. Lyme disease, babesiosis, and ehrlichiosis are tick-borne diseases common in some parts of the United States for which serologic testing should be considered with the right exposure history.
○ Similarly, routine rheumatologic tests, such as antinuclear antibody (ANA) titers and rheumatoid factor, should also only be ordered in a suggestive clinical setting.
○ Additional testing, including imaging studies or biopsies, should only be undertaken as part of the initial evaluation of a possible FUO based on

clinical suspicion because of signs and symptoms uncovered by the history and physical examination.
- Special situations
  - *Immunosuppressed*—The percentage of FUO caused by infections is even higher in this group.
    - Impaired immune responses may lead to absence of typical signs on physical examination or radiography.
    - Decreased cell-mediated immunity may lead to disseminated viral or fungal disease.
    - Febrile neutropenic patients are at high risk of sepsis, and should receive empiric broad-spectrum antibiotics after appropriate cultures have been obtained.
  - *HIV*—The vast majority of FUO in patients with advanced HIV are caused by infections, with mycobacterial infection—TB and *Mycobacterium avium*—and *Pneumocystis carinii* pneumonia being the most common.
    - Disseminated viral infections, such as CMV, should also be considered. A common noninfectious cause of FUO in these patients is lymphoma.
    - Primary HIV infection often leads to a self-limited mononucleosis-like febrile illness, and should be considered as a cause of FUO in the patient with appropriate risk factors.
    - AIDS (acquired immunodeficiency syndrome) patients with FUO should, in addition to standard evaluations, have isolator blood cultures sent for fungal and mycobacteria. Serum cryptococcal antigen should be checked. The threshold for bronchoscopy in a patient with AIDS and pulmonary symptoms is lower.
  - *Nosocomial FUO*—A hospital-associated fever for at least 3 days with no identifiable cause.
    - These fevers often result from iatrogenic causes, such as intravascular or urinary catheter-related infections, blood transfusions, thromboembolic disease from immobilization, or drug therapy.
    - Postoperative fevers are particularly common, and may be a normal physiologic response not related to underlying infection.
  - *Returning travelers or immigrants* (Table 53-1)—Careful consideration should be given to diseases present in the area visited, as well as specific exposures that may predict the cause of fever.
    - The fever may be because of common illnesses like urinary tract or respiratory infections, but infections less commonly seen in the United States, such as malaria, typhoid fever, dengue fever, amebic liver abscess, and rickettsial infections are seen in travelers to developing countries.
    - Acute HIV infection and other sexually transmitted diseases (STDs) should be considered. Up to 20% of returning travelers reported a new sexual

contact during their trip, and for some travelers the purpose of their trip was sexual tourism.
- Certain infections rarely seen in the United States are common causes of FUO in other countries, and should be considered in immigrants from endemic areas. Brucellosis is very common in the Middle East, Spain, and parts of South America. Q fever (*Coxiella brunetti*) is a common cause of FUO and culture-negative endocarditis in Australia and New Zealand. Melioidosis commonly causes FUO in Southeast Asia.

TRIAGE AND INITIAL MANAGEMENT

- Empiric treatment for FUO is not recommended. Undirected treatment may not only delay the diagnosis, but also cause considerable harm.
  - Empiric antibiotics can obscure laboratory testing such as blood cultures.
  - Routine administration of corticosteroids can worsen such conditions as TB or parasitic disease.
- Major exceptions to this rule include
  - FUO in an immunocompromised patient or a potentially septic immunocompetent patient. In these cases, empiric therapy with an antimicrobial must be initiated, typically in the hospital setting.
  - Patients strongly suspected to have temporal arteritis, where starting corticosteroids may prevent blindness and other vascular complications.

DISEASE MANAGEMENT STRATEGIES

- If the diagnosis of FUO has not been established based on the initial evaluation above, additional testing may be warranted.
- In the absence of a specific diagnosis to explain FUO, CT (computed tomography) scans of chest, abdomen, and pelvis should be performed to assess for adenopathy, lymphoma, and other malignancies, TB, and occult intra-abdominal or hepatic abscess.
- Some authorities have advocated the use of nuclear medicine testing, such as white blood cell (WBC) scanning or gallium scanning when initial tests and CT imaging are negative, but their role is poorly defined. Some of the literature supporting the use of nuclear medicine tests in the diagnosis of FUO is from an era in which CT scanning was of poorer quality than today. Positron emission tomography (PET) has been shown to be helpful in some studies, but its limited availability makes routine use impractical.

- Magnetic resonance imaging (MRI) can be helpful for the diagnosis of systemic vasculitis. One study showed a significant increase in the diagnosis of systemic vasculitis when MRI of the aortic arch and cervical arteries were performed.
- *Biopsies*—Examination of tissue is often required to diagnose an FUO. Localized abnormalities on physical examination or diagnostic imaging (eg, enlarged lymph nodes or pulmonary nodules) may be targeted for biopsy. In general, biopsies should be directed toward abnormal findings, and not be done routinely and blindly.
  - The exception is in elderly patients with suspected temporal arteritis, where temporal artery biopsy should be done despite the absence of physical findings.
  - The role of bone marrow aspiration and liver biopsy in the diagnosis of FUO is debatable. Some studies suggest a diagnostic yield of about 15% for each. We recommend pursuing bone marrow and liver biopsies only if there are suggestive abnormalities (cytopenias or abnormal peripheral smears, abnormal liver function tests), and a thorough diagnostic evaluation has been otherwise unrevealing.
- As diagnostic imaging and CT-guided biopsy have become more sophisticated and accessible, the need for invasive procedures such as laparotomy to diagnose the cause of FUO has become rare.

CARE TRANSITIONS

- Discharge planning for the patient with FUO will vary with the underlying etiology.
- Older patients and those with malignancies have the worst prognosis.
- For the 10% to 30% of patients with FUO who will not receive a more specific diagnosis and for whom no underlying etiology will be found, the prognosis is still quite good.
  - More than 80% will have their fevers resolve spontaneously.
  - The mortality rate is quite low (~ 3% at 5 years).
  - Careful ambulatory follow-up is warranted.

BIBLIOGRAPHY

Blair J. Evaluation of fever in the international traveler. *Postgrad Med.* 2004;116:13–20.

Blockmans D, Knockaert D, et. al. Clinical values of [18F] fluoro-deoxyglucose positron emission tomography for patients with fever of unknown origin. *Clin Infect Dis.* 2001;32:191–196.

Castillo JR, Armstrong WS. Fever of unknown origin in adults. *Infect Med.* 2006;23:6–15.

Durack DT, Street AC. Fever of unknown origin—reexamined and redefined. *Curr Clin Top Infect Dis.* 1991;11:35–51.

Knockaert DC, Vanderschuerne S, Blockmans D. Fever of unknown origin in adults. *J Intern Med.* 2003;253:263–275.

Knockaert DC, Dujardin KS, Bobbaers HJ. Long-term follow-up of patients with undiagnosed fever of unknown origin. *Arch Intern Med.* 1996;156:618–620.

Mackowiak PA, Durack DT. Fever of unknown origin. In: Mandell GL, Bennett JE, Dolin R, eds. *Principles and Practices of Infectious Diseases.* 2005.

Ryan ET, Wilson ME, Kain KC. Illness after international travel. *N Engl J Med.* 2002;347(7):505–516.

Wagner AD, Andersen J, Raum E, et al. Standardized work-up programmed for fever of unknown origin and contribution of magnetic resonance imaging for diagnosis of hidden systemic vasculitis. *Ann Rheum Dis.* 2005;64:105–110.

54 BACTERIAL ENDOCARDITIS

John J. Ross

EPIDEMIOLOGY/OVERVIEW

- Approximately 15,000 new cases of endocarditis occur in the United States annually.
- Endocarditis is a serious and not uncommon condition on inpatient general medicine wards.
  - In-hospital mortality is 22% for *Staphylococcal aureus* endocarditis, compared to 15% for non-*S. aureus* cases.
  - Many patients require valve surgery, despite optimal medical management.
- Over the last several decades, the average patient with endocarditis has become sicker and older, with a greater burden of comorbid medical conditions such as diabetes mellitus and chronic renal failure.
  - In developed countries, 24% of endocarditis overall and 39% of *S. aureus* endocarditis arise as a complication of hospitalization, hemodialysis, central venous catheterization, and other healthcare interventions.
- As a result of these developments, *S. aureus* is now the most common cause of endocarditis, at least in academic medical centers, with viridans streptococci playing a secondary but still important role.

PATHOPHYSIOLOGY AND MICROBIOLOGY

- Risk factors for endocarditis include
  - Structural heart disease
  - Prosthetic heart values (with 100,000 new heart valves implanted annually in the United States)
  - IV drug use, both hospital-acquired and substance abuse
  - Prior endocarditis
- Two events are required for the development of infective endocarditis (IE):
  - The formation of sterile platelet-fibrin thrombi on the heart valves, or nonbacterial thrombotic endocarditis. These may arise either after valvular endothelial damage from turbulent blood flow around regurgitant or stenotic valves, or less often from the hypercoagulability of malignancy or inflammatory states.
  - Transient bacteremia that seeds the thrombus. Bacterial colonization stimulates further platelet-fibrin deposition, eventually resulting in vegetation formation.
- Potential sources of transient bacteremia include the oropharynx, the respiratory , gastrointestinal (GI) and genitourinary (GU) tracts, skin wounds, ulcers, vascular catheters, and intravenous drug use (IVDU).
- The causative role of dental work in endocarditis is grossly exaggerated.
  - Many more cases of endocarditis from viridans streptococci probably arise from the low-grade bacteremias associated with daily activities such as brushing teeth or chewing food, rather than from dental manipulations and extractions.
  - According to the American Heart Association (AHA), "only an extremely small number of cases of IE might be prevented by antibiotic prophylaxis even if it were 100% effective." (Wilson et al., 2007)
- A wide variety of cardiac lesions increase the risk for endocarditis. Degenerative valvular and congenital heart abnormalities include
  - Any acquired valvular stenosis and insufficiency
  - Prosthetic heart valves with an incidence of 1% to 4% of valve recipients during the first year after initial replacement and approximately 1% per year subsequently
  - Rheumatic heart disease (now uncommon in developed countries)
  - Bicuspid aortic valves
  - Mitral valve prolapse, especially when mitral regurgitation is present, estimated as five times the risk of the general population

- Prior endocarditis with a recurrence rate of 4.5% in survivors of the first episode who are not substance abusers
- Congenital cyanotic heart disease such as ventricular septal defect, ostium primum atrial septal defects, patent ductus arteriosus, coarctation of the aorta, and tetralogy of Fallot.
- However, up to 47% of patients with endocarditis have no previously known heart disease.
  - Unusual organisms such as *Listeria* or *Salmonella* can cause endocarditis in HIV patients.
  - Liver, heart, and heart lung transplant patients also have a higher risk of endocarditis as a complication of immunosuppression than the general population.
  - Patients with arteriovenous fistulae for hemodialysis, central venous pressure or pulmonary arterial catheters, peritoneovenous shunts for ascites, or ventriculoarterial shunts for hydrocephalous have an increased risk of endocarditis.
- In most patients, endocarditis involves the atrial surface of the mitral valve and the ventricular surface of the aortic valve, presumably because these surfaces are downstream from regurgitant jets that damage the endothelium.
  - One prominent exception is the IV drug user, in whom tricuspid valve involvement typically predominates.
  - Although IVDU is the most serious risk factor for right-sided endocarditis, left-sided valvular endocarditis is also common in drug users, notably because of *S. aureus*.
- Only 5% to 7% of patients diagnosed by strict criteria as having bacterial endocarditis (without prior antibiotic treatment) have sterile blood cultures.
- Blood culture results are more specific if separate cultures are all positive for the same organism.
- Gram-positive bacteria are far more likely to cause endocarditis than gram-negative bacteria and fungi (Table 54-1). This probably relates to the "stickiness" of gram-positive bacteria, or their superior ability to bind to connective tissue.
- In academic medical centers, *S. aureus* is now the most common cause of endocarditis. In community-based series of endocarditis, and in rural areas, viridans streptococci still predominate.
- Coagulase-negative staphylococcal endocarditis is rare on native valves, but is the second most common cause of prosthetic valve endocarditis (PVE), after *S. aureus*.
- Approximately 10% of patients with endocarditis have negative blood cultures. This is usually because of administration of antibiotics prior to performing blood cultures.

TABLE 54-1   Microbiology of Endocarditis

Staphylococcus	
S. aureus	23%–45%
Coagulase-negative staphylococci	6%–14%
Streptococcus	
Viridans group streptococci	9%–18%
Streptococcus bovis	2%–25%
Other streptococci	5%–7%
Enterococci	8%–11%
HACEK	0%–2%
Non-HACEK gram-negative bacteria	0%–2%
Fungi	0%–2%
Polymicrobial	1%–3%
Miscellaneous	2%–5%
Culture-negative	5%–14%

Source: Fowler VG Jr, Miro JM, Hoen B, et al. Staphylococcus aureus endocarditis: a consequence of medical progress. *JAMA.* 2005;293:3012–3021; Hoen B, Alla F, Selton-Suty C, et al. Changing profile of infective endocarditis: results of a 1-year survey in France. *JAMA.* 2002;288:75–81; Bouza E, Menasalvas A, Munoz P, et al. Infective endocarditis: a prospective study at the end of the twentieth century. *Medicine (Baltimore).* 2001:80:298–307.

○ Historically, culture-negative endocarditis was sometimes caused by nutrient-variant streptococci (now known as *Granulicatella adiacens* and *Abiotrophia defectiva*). Current blood cultures techniques are usually successful at isolating these bacteria, as well as the HACEK group of fastidious gram-negative periodontal bacteria, which are
  ▪ *Haemophilus aphrophilus*
  ▪ *Actinobacillus actinomycetemcomitans*
  ▪ *Cardiobacterium hominis*
  ▪ *Eikenella corrodens*
  ▪ *Kingella kingii*
○ In culture-negative endocarditis, clinicians should speak to the technicians in the microbiology laboratory to ensure that blood culture bottles are incubated for at least 2 weeks to optimize the yield for fastidious pathogens.
○ Serology, valve culture, and valve polymerase chain reaction (PCR) may help diagnose additional cases of culture-negative endocarditis, especially in patients with specific risk factors, such as
  ▪ Kitten and cat exposure (*Bartonella henselae*)
  ▪ Homelessness, alcoholism, body lice (*Bartonella quintana*)
  ▪ Exposure to livestock and other animals (*Coxiella burnetii* or Q fever)
  ▪ Consumption of unpasteurized goat milk (brucellosis)
  ▪ Bird exposure (psittacosis)
  ▪ Prosthetic valve (legionellosis)
• Cases of endocarditis caused by methicillin-resistant *S. aureus* (MRSA) have increased in recent years, especially among chronically ill and frequently hospitalized patients. Endocarditis caused by community-acquired methicillin-resistant S. aureus (CA-MRSA) is rare at present, but may be more frequent in the future.
• Rates of mortality and valve replacement are similar with methicillin-sensitive *S. aureus* (MSSA) and MRSA endocarditis, although patients with MRSA endocarditis are more likely to have persistent bacteremia (43% for MRSA vs. 9% for MSSA). This most likely reflects the slow bactericidal action of vancomycin.

CLINICAL PRESENTATION, DIFFERENTIAL, MAKING THE DIAGNOSIS

• The history should identify risk factors for and clinical features suggestive of bacterial endocarditis.
  ○ Unfortunately, patients with endocarditis are notorious for presenting with nonspecific complaints and false localizing signs, and are often misdiagnosed with viral syndromes and the like prior to arrival at the hospital.
  ○ Patients ultimately diagnosed with endocarditis may complain of fever, malaise, weakness, dyspnea, sweats, weight loss, cough, nausea, headache, myalgias, arthralgias, chest pain, abdominal pain, and back pain.
  ○ Patients with fever and varied complaints should be questioned carefully about shaking chills. *Clinicians must strongly suspect bacteremia and endocarditis in patients with fever and true rigors.* Blood cultures are mandated in all such patients.
  ○ IV drug users with tricuspid valve endocarditis often have septic pulmonary emboli, with cough, dyspnea, and chest pain, and radiographic findings of infiltrates and effusions.
• The physical examination may be unremarkable in patients with endocarditis. Cardiac murmurs are often present, although these are often because of underlying valvular pathology.
  ○ New regurgitant and changing murmurs are fairly specific but not sensitive for the diagnosis of endocarditis.
  ○ The peripheral stigmata of left-sided endocarditis described in the preantibiotic era—Osler's nodes; Janeway lesions; nonblanching, linear reddish brown splinter hemorrhages; exudative, edematous, retinal Roth's spots; and petechiae on the conjunctivae, palate, and extremities—are absent in most contemporary patients with endocarditis, presumably because of the relatively prompt institution of antibiotic therapy. Immunologic vascular phenomena are more characteristic of subacute bacterial endocarditis.

○ According to conventional wisdom, Janeway lesions are painless, macular, blanching, violaceous hemorrhagic emboli in the palms and soles, while Osler's nodes are painful, violaceous nodules in the finger and toe pads, caused by immune complexes. However, no basis exists for this clinical distinction in the original accounts of Osler and Janeway, and pathologic descriptions of these lesions overlap substantially. One expert on physical diagnosis has flatly stated "I cannot tell the difference between the two." (Sapira, 1990)

• The complications of endocarditis in descending order of frequency include
  ○ *Cardiac*—Congestive heart failure (CHF) secondary to valvular regurgitation, and perivalvular abscess.
  ○ *Neurologic*—Encephalitis, meningitis, stroke, brain abscess, cerebral hemorrhage, and seizures.
  ○ *Renal*—Infarct secondary to embolism, interstitial nephritis from antibiotics, glomerulonephritis secondary to immunoglobulin and complement deposition, and renal abscess.
  ○ *Vertebral*—Osteomyelitis, epidural abscess
  ○ *Joint*—Acute septic arthritis.
  ○ Metastatic abscess formation in the kidney, brain, and spleen.
  ○ Occasional patients with endocarditis present with embolic manifestations, including stroke, splenic infarction with left upper quadrant (LUQ) and left shoulder pain, hematuria from renal infarction, visual loss from retinal artery embolism or endophthalmitis, and mycotic aneurysm.

• The modified Duke criteria are used to classify cases of suspected endocarditis as definite, possible, or rejected (Tables 54-2 and 54-3).

TABLE 54-2 Modified Duke Criteria for the Diagnosis of IE

Definite IE (must meet either pathologic or clinical criteria)

Pathologic criteria

• Microorganisms demonstrated by culture or histological examination of a vegetation, a vegetation that has embolized, or an intracardiac abscess specimen; *or*
• Pathologic lesions; vegetation or intracardiac abscess confirmed by histologic examination showing active endocarditis

Clinical criteria

• 2 major criteria; *or*
• 1 major criterion and 3 minor criteria; *or*
• 5 minor criteria

Possible IE

• 1 major criterion and 1 minor criterion; *or*
• 3 minor criteria

Diagnosis of endocarditis rejected

• Firm alternative diagnosis explaining evidence of IE; *or*
• Resolution of IE syndrome with antibiotic therapy for < 4 days; *or*
• No pathologic evidence of IE at surgery or autopsy, with antibiotic therapy for < 4 days; *or*
• Does not meet criteria for possible IE as above

TABLE 54-3 Definition of Terms Used in the Modified Duke Criteria for the Diagnosis of IE

Major criteria

Blood culture positive for IE

• Typical microorganisms consistent with IE from 2 separate blood cultures: viridans streptococci, S. bovis, HACEK group, S. aureus; or community-acquired enterococci in the absence of a primary focus; *or*
• Microorganisms consistent with IE from persistently positive blood cultures defined as follows: at least 2 positive cultures of blood samples drawn > 12 h apart; or all of 3 or a majority of ≥ 4 separate cultures of blood (with first and last sample drawn at least 1 h apart); *or*
• Single positive blood culture for *C. burnetii* or anti–phase 1 IgG antibody titer > 1:800

Evidence of endocardial involvement

• Echocardiogram positive for IE: oscillating intracardiac mass on valve or supporting structures, in the path of regurgitant jets, or on implanted material in the absence of an alternative anatomic explanation; or abscess; or new partial dehiscence of prosthetic valve; new valvular regurgitation (worsening or changing or preexisting murmur not sufficient)

Minor criteria

• Predisposition, predisposing heart condition, or IDU
• Fever, temperature > 38°C
• Vascular phenomena, major arterial emboli, septic pulmonary infarcts, mycotic aneurysm, intracranial hemorrhage, conjunctival hemorrhages, and Janeway's lesions
• Immunologic phenomena: glomerulonephritis, Osler's nodes, Roth's spots, and rheumatoid factor
• Microbiologic evidence: positive blood culture, but does not meet a major criterion as noted above, or serologic evidence of active infection with organism consistent with IE

Abbreviation: IDU, injection drug use.

• The blood culture is the single most important diagnostic test in IE.
  ○ When endocarditis is suspected, three sets of aerobic and anaerobic blood cultures should be drawn from separate sites prior to starting antibiotics.
  ○ Ideally, each set should be obtained at least 1 hour apart, if the patient is stable enough to delay antibiotics for that long.
  ○ More than 3–5 blood cultures will not increase the diagnostic yield.
• The AHA now recommends transesophageal echocardiography (TEE) as a first-line screening test, when the suspicion for endocarditis is at least moderate. TEE has a greater degree of spatial resolution than transthoracic echocardiogram (TTE) and is more sensitive for detecting small vegetations and valvular abscesses.
  ○ This would include all bacteremic patients with cardiac risk factors for endocarditis, as well as patients with any bacteremia caused by S. aureus, viridans streptococci, and the HACEK group, community-acquired enterococcal bacteremia, and any patient with high-grade bacteremia of uncertain source.

○ Transthoracic echocardiography is still an acceptable screening test in low-risk patients with a low clinical suspicion for endocarditis but the diagnostic yield is low as it is for TEE for these patients.

○ If the initial TEE is negative and the clinical suspicion for endocarditis remains high, TEE may be repeated after 7–10 days. False-negative results may occur with TEE if vegetations are small or have embolized; false-positive TEE may be produced by myxomatous deterioration, valvular scarring, and other degenerative changes.

• Laboratory findings in endocarditis are nonspecific. WBC counts tend to be elevated with left shift, but may be normal, especially in subacute bacterial endocarditis caused by viridans streptococci and HACEK bacteria. Anemia of chronic disease is often present. The ESR is usually at least moderately elevated and is often greater than 100 mm/h. Mild hematuria, thrombocytopenia, and hepatic transaminitis are also common.

• Contact with the microbiology laboratory in cases of suspected endocarditis is crucial, as supplemental testing of isolates is often necessary.

○ For endocarditis with viridans streptococci, the minimum inhibitory concentration (MIC) should be determined by E-test or other method, as the duration and intensity of therapy is dependent on the MIC (see Table 54-4).

○ In enterococcal endocarditis, synergy testing should be performed for aminoglycosides (see Table 54-4).

TRIAGE AND INITIAL MANGEMENT

• If the suspicion for endocarditis is high, it is reasonable to start antibiotics empirically while awaiting results of blood cultures. For native valve endocarditis, an appropriate initial regimen is nafcillin or oxacillin plus gentamicin (see Table 54-4 for dosing). Vancomycin can also be added if the patient has risks for MRSA, such as extensive healthcare exposure or IVDU. For PVE, an

TABLE 54-4 Antibiotic Therapy for Native Valve IE

Highly penicillin-susceptible viridans streptococci and *S. bovis* (MIC ≤ 0.12 μg/mL)	Penicillin G 12–18 million U/24 h IV continuously, or divided q4–6 h × 4 weeks; *or* Ceftriaxone 2 g IV once daily × 4 weeks; *or* Penicillin or ceftriaxone as above, combined with gentamicin 3 mg/kg IV once daily, each for 2 weeks (not recommended for patients with > 65 years, renal dysfunction, 8th nerve dysfunction, or infection with *Abiotrophia*, *Granulicatella*, and *Gemella*); *or* Vancomycin 15 mg/kg IV q12 h × 4 weeks, not to exceed 2 g daily unless serum levels are low; recommended only for patients allergic or intolerant to penicillin and ceftriaxone
Relatively penicillin-resistant viridans streptococci and *S. bovis* (MIC > 0.12 to ≤ 0.5 μg/mL)	*Either* penicillin G 24 million U/24 h IV continuously or divided q4–6 h × 4 weeks; *or* Ceftriaxone 2 g IV once daily × 4 weeks, *plus* Gentamicin 3 mg/kg IV once daily for 2 weeks Alternatively, can give vancomycin monotherapy × 4 weeks as above, but recommended only for patients allergic or intolerant to penicillin and ceftriaxone
Penicillin-sensitive *Streptococcus pneumoniae* and group A streptococci	Penicillin or ceftriaxone in above doses for 4 weeks
Group B, C, and G streptococci, or pneumococci and group A streptococci with higher penicillin MICs	Relatively uncommon, and definitive data on management lacking; group B, C, and G streptococci often display moderate penicillin resistance; infectious diseases consultation recommended
MSSA	Nafcillin or oxacillin 2 g IV q4 h × 6 weeks Some clinicians add gentamicin 1 mg/kg IV q8 h for the first 3–5 days to hasten resolution of bacteremia; evidence of improved outcomes not established, risk of nephrotoxicity higher Cefazolin 2 g IV q8 h × 6 weeks can be substituted for nafcillin or oxacillin in patients with mild penicillin allergy; for penicillin anaphylaxis, use vancomycin × 6 weeks as above
MRSA	Vancomycin 15 mg/kg IV q12 h × 6 weeks; adjust dose to achieve peak serum concentration of 30–45 μg/mL 1 hour after dose, and trough concentration of 10–15 μg/mL
Tricuspid valve endocarditis caused by MSSA	Nafcillin or oxacillin 2 g IV q4 h × 4–6 weeks In IVDU with MSSA tricuspid valve endocarditis, rapid clinical response to antibiotics, no evidence for left-sided involvement, normal renal function, and low suspicion for metastatic complications such as vertebral osteomyelitis, can use short-course combination therapy with nafcillin or oxacillin dosed as above, plus gentamicin 1 mg/kg IV q8 h, both for 2 weeks
HACEK bacteria	Ceftriaxone 2 g IV once daily × 4 weeks
Other gram-negative bacteria	Therapy individualized according to sensitivity data, and with infectious diseases consultation; beta-lactam and aminoglycoside combination therapy typically administered for a minimum of 6 weeks; cardiac surgery usually required
Fungal endocarditis	Traditional treatment is valve replacement surgery with amphotericin B-based antifungal regimen, followed by prolonged, perhaps lifelong, oral azole therapy; infectious diseases consult mandated

TABLE 54-5 Antibiotic Therapy for PVE

Penicillin-susceptible viridans streptococci and *S. bovis* (MIC ≤ 0.12 μg/mL)	Penicillin G 24 million U/24 h IV continuously or divided q4–6 h × 6 weeks, *or* ceftriaxone 2 g IV once daily × 6 weeks *plus* Gentamicin 3 mg/kg IV once daily for 2 weeks
Relatively or fully penicillin-resistant viridans streptococci and *S. bovis* (MIC > 0.12)	Penicillin G 24 million U/24 h IV continuously or divided q4–6 h × 6 weeks, *or* ceftriaxone 2 g IV once daily × 6 weeks *plus* Gentamicin 3 mg/kg IV once daily for 6 weeks
Methicillin-sensitive coagulase-negative staphylococci and *S. aureus*	Nafcillin or oxacillin 2 g IV q4 h × for a minimum of 6 weeks, *plus* Rifampin 300 mg IV/po q8 h, for a minimum of 6 weeks, *plus* Gentamicin 1 mg/kg IV q8 h for 2 weeks
Methicillin-resistant coagulase-negative staphylococci and *S. aureus*	Vancomycin 15 mg/kg IV q12 h for at least 6 weeks; adjust dose to achieve peak serum concentration of 30–45 μg/mL 1 hour after dose, and trough concentration of 10–15 μg/mL, *plus* Rifampin 300 mg IV/po q8 h, for a minimum of 6 weeks, *plus* Gentamicin 1 mg/kg IV q8 h for 2 weeks

appropriate initial regimen is vancomycin, gentamicin, and rifampin (see Table 54-5 for dosing).

- All patients diagnosed with bacterial endocarditis should have infectious disease consultation to help optimize the antibiotic regimen, anticipate and identify complications of therapy, advise the duration of treatment, and to assist in outpatient follow-up.
- Cardiology and possibly cardiac surgery consultation should be obtained in all patients with proven endocarditis to help identify the need for surgery and to facilitate operation if needed. The need for surgery is unpredictable in these patients, and may be sudden; even if patients respond to medical therapy, valve replacement is often necessary down the road, especially in aortic or mitral valve endocarditis.

DISEASE MANAGEMENT STRATEGIES

- Successful treatment of endocarditis hinges upon prolonged high-dose IV antibiotics. Why should this be necessary?
  - The numerical burden of bacteria in endocarditis is relatively small, compared to infections such as pneumonia and pyelonephritis that respond to shorter courses of therapy.
  - Bacteria in vegetation are densely packed and in low metabolic state, and hence less sensitive to the bactericidal activity of antibiotics.
  - While endocarditis is an intravascular infection, the host response is ineffective, and cure in endocarditis is far more reliant on antibiotics than most other infections.
  - As well, the vegetation itself acts as a physical barrier to antibiotic penetration.
- Recommended regimens for IE are listed in Tables 54-4, 54-5, and 54-6, respectively. These are more fully discussed in AHA 2005 guidelines by Baddour et al. (2005).

- Great confusion arises about the role of aminoglycosides in gram-positive endocarditis. Aminoglycosides alone are not active against gram-positive bacteria. However, they augment the killing of cell-wall active antibiotics, such as beta-lactams and glycopeptides.
- This synergistic killing is of highest value in enterococcal endocarditis. Enterococci are inherently resistant to most antibiotics, and may display tolerance to ampicillin and vancomycin, especially in the setting of endocarditis. Cure rates in enterococcal endocarditis with ampicillin or vancomycin alone are unacceptably low, but are markedly increased when combined with gentamicin. Enterococcal isolates from patients with endocarditis should be tested for synergy to gentamicin and streptomycin (it may be necessary to call the microbiology laboratory to ensure that this is done). If synergy is absent, infectious consultation should be obtained. Cure rates are much lower in this setting, and therapy is empiric. Courses of ampicillin or vancomycin monotherapy of long duration (eg, 8–12 weeks) are sometimes used.
- In endocarditis associated with viridans streptococci, combining a beta-lactam with an aminoglycoside

TABLE 54-6 Antibiotic Therapy for Native Valve and PVE with Enterococci

Penicillin- and gentamicin-susceptible strains	Ampicillin 2 g IV q4 h × 6 weeks, *plus* Gentamicin 1 mg/kg IV q8 h × 6 weeks If major penicillin allergy: vancomycin 15 mg/kg IV q12 h for at least 6 weeks; adjust dose to achieve peak serum concentration of 30–45 μg/mL 1 hour after dose, and trough concentration of 10–15 μg/mL, *plus* gentamicin 1 mg/kg IV q8 h × 6 weeks
Resistance to penicillin, aminoglycoside, or vancomycin	Infectious diseases consultation

allows for shorter total antibiotic courses, although cure rates are similar.

○ The value of aminoglycosides in staphylococcal endocarditis is much less certain. In native valve *S. aureus* endocarditis, the addition of gentamicin for the first 3–5 days of therapy reduces the duration of bacteremia by 24 hours, but does not affect overall cure rates, and increases the risk of nephrotoxicity. Gentamicin is often used for synergy in staphylococcal and streptococcal PVE, primarily based on retrospective data.

• Vancomycin is a slowly bactericidal antibiotic, and is not a first-line choice for endocarditis, except in cases of serious beta-lactam allergy or resistance to methicillin, as in MRSA. One exception is PVE caused by coagulase-negative staphylococci, where isolates may appear more sensitive to oxacillin or nafcillin than they really are; vancomycin is the preferred backbone of therapy for coagulase-negative staphylococcal PVE, unless there is conclusive evidence of methicillin sensitivity.

• Rifampin seems to have a particular value when used for synergy in the treatment of staphylococcal PVE.

• If there is any question about the interpretation of sensitivity testing and the appropriate choice of antibiotic regimen, infectious diseases consultation is appropriate. This also facilitates outpatient follow-up.

• Persistent fever in endocarditis should initiate a search for complications, including perivalvular abscess, mycotic aneurysm, splenic abscess, and vertebral osteomyelitis, and septic pulmonary emboli (in tricuspid endocarditis).

• Clinical and echocardiographic features suggesting potential need for surgery are listed in Table 54-7.

○ An increasing body of data suggest that early surgery reduces mortality, especially in patients with moderate-to-severe CHF or perivalvular complications.

TABLE 54-7   Clinical and Echocardiographic Features Suggesting Potential Need for Surgical Intervention

Vegetation factors conferring higher embolic risk
• Persistent vegetation after systemic embolization
• Anterior mitral valve leaflet vegetation, especially > 10 mm
• ≥ 1 embolic events during first 2 weeks of antibiotic therapy
• Increase in vegetation size on therapy

Valvular dysfunction
• Acute aortic or mitral insufficiency with signs of CHF
• CHF unresponsive to medical therapy
• Valve perforation or rupture

Perivalvular extension
• Valvular dehiscence, rupture, or fistula
• New heart block
• Large abscess or extension of abscess despite appropriate antibiotic therapy

○ Periannular abscess is most common as a complication of aortic valve endocarditis, where it may be heralded by new atrioventricular (AV) node block.

○ Myocardial and perivalvular abscesses are rarely cured without surgery, and these patients often do poorly if surgery is delayed.

○ Fungal and gram-negative endocarditis (except for HACEK bacteria) generally require surgery for cure.

• No data exist to show that anticoagulation in native valve endocarditis decreases the risk of embolic complications. The management of anticoagulation in PVE is controversial.

○ If complications are not present, many physicians recommend to continue it cautiously, avoiding supratherapeutic coagulation.

○ If patients with PVE develop stroke, it is generally recommended to stop anticoagulation for 2 weeks, to reduce the risk of hemorrhagic transformation.

• Duration of antibiotic therapy is calculated from *the first day on which blood cultures were negative*, when blood cultures are initially positive. Two sets of blood cultures should be obtained every 24–48 hours, until resolution of bacteremia is documented.

• When patients with native valve endocarditis undergo prosthetic valve replacement, the postoperative regimen should be changed to one appropriate for PVE. If valve cultures from the operating room are positive, the patient should receive a full course of postoperative antibiotics.

• Presumed *culture-negative endocarditis* is treated empirically with prolonged broad-spectrum antibiotics, in conjunction with infectious diseases consultation.

CARE TRANSITIONS

• Medically stable patients with endocarditis can often complete IV antibiotic therapy on an outpatient basis. This should not be attempted in patients with unstable CHF, perivalvular complications, neurologic complications, persistent fever and bacteremia, AV block, or active IVDU.

• Patients should be instructed to seek medical care promptly if they develop fever, rigors, or dyspnea.

• Patients with IVDU should be referred for drug rehabilitation.

• After discharge, patients should be closely monitored for relapse of infection, decompensated CHF, and antibiotic toxicity, including *Clostridium difficile* colitis. Patients on aminoglycosides and glycopeptides should be monitored for nephrotoxicity and hearing loss. While antibiotics continue, it is reasonable to check weekly CBC, creatinine, and liver transaminases to assess for the possibility of drug-related cytopenias, interstitial nephritis, and hepatitis. Some clinicians also follow the ESR occasionally over the course of treatment.

PREVENTION

- In 2007, AHA revised its guidelines for antibiotic prophylaxis for endocarditis, taking into account the rarity of endocarditis after dental and other procedures and the lack of proof of benefit.
- Antibiotic prophylaxis is now recommended only for patients with these cardiac conditions:
  - Prosthetic heart valve
  - Previous endocarditis
  - Unrepaired cyanotic congenital heart disease
  - Completely repaired congenital heart defect with prosthetic material (for the first 6 months after the procedure)
  - Repaired congenital heart disease, with residual defects at the site, or adjacent to the site, of a prosthetic patch or device
  - Cardiac transplantation recipients with cardiac valvulopathy
- Patients with these conditions should be given antibiotic prophylaxis before gingival or periapical manipulation or perforation of oral mucosa, or incision and biopsy of the respiratory tract mucosa. Acceptable regimens include amoxicillin 2 g or clindamycin 600 mg, taken orally 30–60 minutes before the procedure.
- Patients with these conditions undergoing surgery involving infected skin, soft tissue, or musculoskeletal tissue should receive an antistaphylococcal penicillin or cephalosporin prior to the procedure. Vancomycin may be substituted if the patient is penicillin allergic, or if MRSA is known or suspected.
- In the absence of evidence either for or against its use, antibiotic prophylaxis is no longer recommended solely to prevent endocarditis in patients undergoing GU or GI tract procedures.

BIBLIOGRAPHY

Baddour LM, Wilson WR, Bayer AS, et al. AHA scientific statement. Infective endocarditis: diagnosis, antimicrobial therapy, and management of complications. *Circulation.* 2005;111:e394–e434.

Bouza E, Menasalvas A, Munoz P, et al. Infective endocarditis: a prospective study at the end of the twentieth century. *Medicine (Baltimore).* 2001:80:298–307.

Farrior JB, Silverman ME. A consideration of the differences between a Janeway lesion and an Osler's node in infectious endocarditis. *Chest.* 1976;70:239–243.

Fowler VG Jr, Miro JM, Hoen B, et al. Staphylococcus aureus endocarditis: a consequence of medical progress. *JAMA.* 2005;293:3012–3021.

Hoen B, Alla F, Selton-Suty C, et al. Changing profile of infective endocarditis: results of a 1-year survey in France. *JAMA.* 2002;288:75–81.

Sapira JD. *The Art and Science of Bedside Diagnosis.* Baltimore, MD: Williams & Wilkins; 1990:440.

Wilson W, Taubert KA, Gewitz M, et al. Prevention of infective endocarditis: a guideline from the American Heart Association. *Circulation.* 2007 April 19; [epub ahead of print].

55 COMMUNITY- AND HOSPITAL-ACQUIRED URINARY TRACT INFECTION

John J. Ross

EPIDEMIOLOGY/OVERVIEW

- Urinary tract infections (UTIs) are very common, both in the community and the hospital setting.
- Over half of all women will develop at least one UTI during their lifetime.
- Nosocomial catheter-associated UTI is the most frequent type of nosocomial infection, comprising about 35% to 40% of all hospital-acquired infections.

PATHOPHYSIOLOGY

- The vast majority of UTIs arise by the ascending route.
- A minority of UTIs arise from bacteremia. This is most common with *S. aureus.* Although *S. aureus* can infect the urine of patients with Foley catheters by the ascending route, in patients with staphylococcal pyelonephritis from the community, the possibility of underlying bacteremia and endocarditis should be strongly considered.
- Most UTIs are caused by uropathogenic strains of *Escherichia coli.* These strains possess surface filaments, known as pili or fimbriae, which permit binding to urinary epithelium.
  - Type 1 fimbriae on *E. coli* are associated with cystitis.

○ *E. coli* strains with P fimbriae are associated with pyelonephritis and bacteremia.
• The normal human urinary tract has robust anatomic and physiologic protections against infection. These include
  ○ The normal flushing mechanism of the bladder
  ○ Urinary Tamm-Horsfall protein, which binds uropathogenic strains of *E. coli*
  ○ Chemical properties of urine, such as low pH, high osmolality, and high urea concentration, which inhibit bacteria
  ○ Bladder epithelial mucopolysaccharide, which prevents bacterial binding
  ○ IgA secretion
  ○ Neutrophil surveillance of the bladder mucosa
• In the community, cystitis and pyelonephritis are much more common in women, because of the shorter female urethra.
  ○ In women under the age of 50 years, the predominant risk factor for UTI is frequency of sexual intercourse, which facilitates movement of bacteria into the bladder.
  ○ Other significant risks include
    ▪ History of recent UTI
    ▪ Diabetes mellitus
    ▪ The use of spermicide, which increases periurethral *E. coli* colonization
    ▪ New sexual partners, which may reflect sexual acquisition of uropathogenic strains of *E. coli*.
  ○ Genetic factors likely also play a role: women with frequent cystitis are more likely to have a history of maternal UTIs.
• Several host abnormalities increase vulnerability to UTI. These include
  ○ Urinary stasis from obstruction or neurologic disease
  ○ Vesicoureteral reflux
  ○ Urinary calculi, which may cause local irritation, obstruction, and serve as a nidus for persistent infection
  ○ Diabetes mellitus, caused by glucosuria which makes the urine more hospitable for bacteria, and impaired host inflammatory response
• For the purposes of the hospitalist, there is one overwhelmingly important cause of UTI: placement of an indwelling urinary catheter.
  ○ The rate of acquisition of bacteriuria after placement of a urinary catheter is 5% per day. Essentially, 100% of patients have bacteriuria 1 month after placement of an indwelling urinary catheter.

CLINICAL PRESENTATION, DIAGNOSIS, AND MANAGEMENT

ASYMPTOMATIC BACTERIURIA

• Asymptomatic bacteriuria is very common. It is found in up to 50% of elderly patients in long-term care facilities, and in most patients with spinal cord injury. Rates approach 100% in patients with chronic indwelling Foley catheters and permanent ureteric stents.
• Asymptomatic bacteriuria is grossly overdiagnosed and overtreated. Even the presence of pyuria or cloudy urine by itself does not warrant antibiotic treatment. In most groups studied, treatment of asymptomatic bacteriuria is associated with increased antibiotic side effects, increased acquisition of antibiotic-resistant organisms, and no long-term benefits.
• Similarly, treatment of asymptomatic candiduria has not been associated with clinical benefit, and long-term eradication rates are disappointing.
• Therefore, patients with asymptomatic bacteriuria need not be treated, with three notable exceptions
  ○ *Pregnancy*—Pregnant women with asymptomatic bacteriuria should receive 3–7 days of antibiotic therapy, and should have urine cultures repeated later in pregnancy
  ○ Prior to transurethral resection of the prostate, or other urologic procedures involving mucosal bleeding
  ○ Preschool children with vesicoureteral reflux
• Screening and treatment of asymptomatic bacteriuria has been studied, and *not* found to be helpful in the following groups:
  ○ Premenopausal, nonpregnant women
  ○ Diabetic women
  ○ Older persons living in the community
  ○ Elderly, institutionalized subjects
  ○ Persons with spinal cord injury
  ○ Catheterized patients while the catheter remains in situ

CYSTITIS

• The diagnosis of cystitis is straightforward in otherwise well women presenting with dysuria and urinary frequency, and with pyuria on urinalysis, or positive leukocyte esterase or nitrites on dipstick testing.
• Women with vaginal irritation or discharge should be assessed for genital herpes and vaginitis.
• If urine cultures demonstrate less than 10^5 organisms/mL patients may have bacterial urethritis (without cystitis).
• Gonorrhea or chlamydia should also be considered in this setting.
• Three days of antibiotic therapy with trimethoprim-sulfamethoxazole or fluoroquinolones is standard for uncomplicated cystitis.
  ○ Studies have shown that relapse rates are lower with trimethoprim-sulfamethoxazole or fluoroquinolones, compared to beta-lactam antibiotics.
  ○ Because of increasing resistance of community isolates of *E. coli* to trimethoprim-sulfamethoxazole,

some clinicians advocate using fluoroquinolones as empiric first-line therapy for cystitis.

○ Trimethoprim-sulfamethoxazole is still preferred if local resistance rates in *E. coli* are low (ie, less than 20%), because of its lower cost and the desire to forestall the emergence of resistance to fluoroquinolones from overuse.

• *Nitrofurantoin* is a time-honored urinary anti-infective, whose active metabolites damage bacterial ribosomes and DNA. As resistance in the community to both trimethoprim-sulfamethoxazole and fluoroquinolones increases, nitrofurantoin may be increasingly important for first-line therapy for cystitis.

○ Courses of 7 days are recommended for cystitis; in one trial, a 3-day course of nitrofurantoin for cystitis was less effective than 3 days of trimethoprim-sulfamethoxazole.

○ Nitrofurantoin is generally active against *E. coli* and *Citrobacter*, as well as many strains of vancomycin-resistant enterococci. However, it is less useful against many gram-negative rods (GNR), causing urinary catheter-associated UTI, including *Pseudomonas*, *Providencia*, *Serratia*, *Proteus*, *Enterobacter*, and *Klebsiella*.

○ Nitrofurantoin is not effective in the treatment of pyelonephritis, and it should be avoided in patients with creatinine clearances of less than 40 mL/min.

• *Fosfomycin* is an older urinary anti-infective, given as a single 3-g dose. It is a structural analog of phosphoenolpyruvate that inhibits the initial step in bacterial cell wall synthesis. It is generally less effective than trimethoprim-sulfamethoxazole and fluoroquinolones, but may still be useful as another relatively inexpensive treatment for cystitis because of vancomycin-resistant enterococci (VRE).

• Despite popular wisdom, there is no evidence that hydration is beneficial in treating or preventing UTIs. Hydration has been recommended as a means of rapidly reducing bacterial counts by dilution. However, dilutional effects on antibiotics and urinary antibacterial factors, such as Tamm-Horsfall protein, probably negate this. Hydration may be useful in minimizing the potential nephrotoxicity of aminoglycosides.

• Urinary analgesics, such as phenazopyridine (Pyridium) are generally unnecessary, and may cause GI upset, headache, and rarely methemoglobinemia.

PYELONEPHRITIS

• Upper UTI in healthy adults presents with fever, flank pain, malaise, and anorexia, usually, but not invariably, combined with lower tract symptoms of urinary frequency and dysuria. Pyuria and serum leukocytosis are almost always present.

○ In healthy young women with appropriately treated pyelonephritis, fever may be impressive and sustained, taking up to 4 days to resolve. Resolution of fever is more rapid in older adults with pyelonephritis.

○ Older adults with pyelonephritis often have atypical symptoms, such as malaise, mental status change, and vague abdominal pain. Fever is usually lower grade, and flank pain often absent.

• Pyelonephritis is the most common cause of gram-negative bacteremia. Up to 61% of older adults with pyelonephritis are bacteremic.

• *Imaging studies* are unnecessary in acute pyelonephritis when the diagnosis is straightforward, and the patient is not critically ill. Ultrasound (US) or CT is appropriate in pyelonephritis when

○ Patients are not responding appropriately after 72 hours of antibiotics.

○ Patients are severely ill or immunocompromised.

○ The presentation is atypical and the diagnosis is unclear.

○ Structural abnormalities or obstruction of the urinary tract are suspected.

• Patients with pyelonephritis should receive 14 days of antibiotic therapy. Most, if not all, antibiotic therapy can be delivered orally. For patients from the community, preferred regimens include ampicillin plus an aminoglycoside, or a fluoroquinolone. Most antibiotics are excreted in the urinary tract, and achieve high concentrations in urine. As aminoglycosides and fluoroquinolones display concentration-dependent killing, compared to the time-dependent killing of beta-lactam antibiotics, they may be theoretically superior to beta-lactams in the treatment of pyelonephritis.

• When patients with prior UTI are admitted to hospital with pyelonephritis, antibiotic therapy should take into account prior culture and sensitivity data, and broader empiric therapy prescribed if the patient has a previous history of antibiotic-resistant organisms.

• Patients who develop pyelonephritis in the hospital or chronic care setting may also require broader empiric therapy, possibly with an antipseudomonal beta-lactam in combination with an aminoglycoside or fluoroquinolone.

NOSOCOMIAL CATHETER-ASSOCIATED URINARY TRACT INFECTION

• The presence of a Foley catheter increases the risk of UTI in several ways.

○ Bacteria are able to migrate outside the catheter and the urethral mucosa to gain entry to the bladder; less often, they ascend through the lumen of the catheter.

○ Bacteria produce biofilm (glycocalyx) on the catheter, protecting them from antibiotics and host defenses. In time, they may also deposit biofilm directly on the bladder uroepithelium.
○ Urinary catheters may damage the protective glycosaminoglycan layer of the bladder mucosa
○ Foreign bodies such as urinary catheters depress neutrophil function.

• Errors in catheter care contribute to infection risk. These include elevating the tubing above the bladder, or allowing the tubing to droop below the collecting bag.

• While *E. coli* is still the most common microbe in catheter-associated UTI, it is less predominant than it is in the bacteriology of community-acquired cystitis and pyelonephritis. *Enterococcus*, *Pseudomonas*, *Enterobacter*, *Providencia*, *Citrobacter*, and *Candida* each cause significant proportions of catheter-associated UTI.

• Bacteremia from catheter-associated UTI is uncommon, occurring in less than 1% of cases, but because of the large number of hospitalized patients with Foley catheters, up to 15% of nosocomial bacteremias may be urinary in origin.

• *Removal of the urinary catheter and bag* is an essential component of treatment for these infections. Ideally, the urinary catheter should be removed permanently, or if this is not possible, it should be left out for as long as possible.

• Data are lacking to make definitive recommendations regarding duration of therapy. However, 7 days of treatment is customary, based on culture and sensitivity data. If bacteremia is documented, or flank pain is present to suggest pyelonephritis, 14 days of total therapy is indicated.

PROSTATITIS

• *Acute bacterial prostatitis* presents with fever, rigors, perineal discomfort, dysuria, and urinary urgency and frequency. The prostate is swollen and often exquisitely tender on examination. Acute prostatitis is generally seen in older men, with *E. coli* as the usual culprit. In the younger and/or sexually venturesome, the possibility of *Neisseria gonorrhoeae* should be entertained. Pelvic CT or transrectal US sometimes demonstrates a prostatic abscess.

• *Chronic bacterial prostatitis* presents with relapsing dysuria and other urinary symptoms. If perineal discomfort and prostatic tenderness are present, they are usually much milder than in acute prostatitis. *E. coli* and other gram-negatives are usually responsible; rarely, *Cryptococcus neoformans* or other fungi are involved.

• Treatment of acute bacterial prostatitis is 4 weeks of oral antibiotics, based on culture results, with needle drainage of abscesses if present. Chronic prostatitis may require 6–12 weeks of oral therapy; cure rates are often low because of microabscesses or small calculi, which enable infection to persist. Trimethoprim-sulfamethoxazole or fluoroquinolones are preferred for their superior penetration into the prostate.

UNUSUAL URINARY TRACT INFECTION SYNDROMES

EMPHYSEMATOUS PYELONEPHRITIS

• Emphysematous pyelonephritis is a life-threatening form of upper UTI in diabetics. It is associated with gas and tissue necrosis in the renal parenchyma and perinephric soft tissues, and is usually caused by *E. coli*.

• Emergent nephrectomy is the traditional treatment of choice in septic patients. However, percutaneous catheter drainage with medical therapy has been successful in less severely ill patients in case reports, and in the author's experience. Kidney function is often significantly reduced on the affected side.

XANTHOGRANULOMATOUS PYELONEPHRITIS

• Xanthogranulomatous pyelonephritis (XGP) is a chronic variant of pyelonephritis in middle-aged women, associated with nephrolithiasis, obstruction, and prior symptomatic UTIs. Patients present with fever, malaise, and abdominal pain. The renal calyces are dilated, and the parenchyma replaced by necrotic inflammatory tissue, especially lipid-laden macrophages. Kidney stones are usually found within the inflammatory process. Involvement is usually unilateral.

• *E. coli* and *Proteus* are most frequently responsible.

• As the kidney is usually totally destroyed at the time of diagnosis, nephrectomy is customary. Localized disease can be treated with partial nephrectomy and antibiotics.

RENAL TUBERCULOSIS

• Genitourinary tuberculosis is rare in the United States. However, it is a valid diagnostic consideration in patients with urinary symptoms, sterile pyuria, calcification of the renal parenchyma, and risk factors for TB exposure.

• Most patients do not have fever, night sweats, or active pulmonary TB.

• Diagnosis is made on the basis of three early morning urine cultures for acid-fast bacilli.

"Purple Urine Bag Syndrome"

- Occasionally, elderly patients with chronic Foley catheters and drainage bags develop purple urine in the collecting system, provoking consternation on the part of patients and caregivers. The proposed mechanism is bacterial breakdown of tryptophan to indirubin and indigo.
- Urine cultures are usually polymicrobial; multiple gram-negative bacteria are implicated.
- The condition is benign, and responds to antibiotics and removal of the urinary catheter and bag.

Bladder Stones And *Corynebacterium urealyticum*

- Another complication of chronic Foley catheterization is infection with the diphtheroid bacterium *Corynebacterium urealyticum*. This urea-splitting bacterium is associated with struvite stone formation in the bladder and encrusted cystitis. The complication is more common in elderly men with a history of urinary tract manipulation.
- Clinical clues are the presence of alkaline urine, and repeated urine cultures reported as gram-positive rods, or normal flora. Because microbiology laboratories usually assume that urinary diphtheroids are contaminants, the condition may not be diagnosed unless the clinician requests speciation of the isolate.
- Treatment involves bladder stone removal and IV vancomycin (*C. urealyticum* is often resistant to other agents).

COMPLICATIONS

- *Perinephric abscess* occasionally complicates pyelonephritis when urinary tract obstruction is present. The abscess is usually restricted to the perinephric space by Gerota's fascia. Percutaneous catheter drainage is now standard, and avoids the need for surgery in most cases.
- *Intrarenal abscess* is most often seen as a consequence of bacteremia, sometimes in the setting of staphylococcal endocarditis. Patients present with flank pain and fever, with a slow clinical response to antibiotics. Early in the course, contrast-enhanced CT scans may show either intense focal inflammation in a lobe of the kidney (somewhat facetiously termed *lobar nephronia*, by analogy with lobar pneumonia). These patients may respond to antibiotics alone, but if frank suppuration is evident on CT scans, percutaneous catheter drainage is appropriate.

INFECTION CONTROL

- Patients with resistant uropathogens, such as vancomycin-resistant enterococci and extended-spectrum beta-lactamase (ESBL)-producing *Klebsiella*, should be placed on contact precautions. Further details are given in Chap. 60.

PREVENTION

- *Postcoital voiding* may help prevent UTIs in susceptible, sexually active women.
- *Postcoital antibiotics* (single-strength trimethoprim-sulfamethoxazole or ciprofloxacin 100 mg) may also be helpful, and are as effective as daily prophylaxis in premenopausal women.
- *Continuous low-dose antibiotics* are also used as prophylaxis in women with frequent UTIs, particularly when infection is not related to coitus. Trimethoprim-sulfamethoxazole, fluoroquinolones, and nitrofurantoin have all been used in this setting. Clinicians should be aware that both short- and long-term use of nitrofurantoin are associated with uncommon but potentially severe reactions, including pulmonary hypersensitivity, hepatitis, hemolytic anemia, and peripheral neuropathy.
- *Methenamine mandelate* and *methenamine hippurate* are broken down in acidic urine to ammonia and formaldehyde, which denatures proteins and acts as a broad-spectrum antibiotic active against gram-positive bacteria, gram-negative bacteria, and fungi. They are ineffective against urea-splitting bacteria, such as *Proteus*, that produce high urinary pH and prevent formaldehyde formation. Methenamine compounds may be useful in preventing recurrences of UTI, and they are generally well tolerated, aside from occasional GI upset. Urinary acidification with ascorbic acid (vitamin C) may be necessary to ensure acidic urine. They should be avoided in patients with chronic renal insufficiency. They are also not effective in patients with chronic indwelling urinary catheters, because of the lack of buildup of formaldehyde to therapeutic concentrations in the bladder.
- *Cranberry juice* or tablets seem to be at least modestly effective in prophylaxis of UTI in ambulatory women. Polyphenol antioxidant compounds present in cranberry juice prevent the fimbrial adhesion of uropathogenic strains of *E. coli*. Cranberry juice may potentiate the therapeutic effect of warfarin.
- *Vaginal estrogens* in postmenopausal women reduce vaginal overgrowth with gram-negative bacteria, promote protective colonization by lactobacilli, and were

associated with a reduction in UTIs in small clinical trials.

- *Impregnated urinary catheters*, using either silver alloy or the combination of minocycline and rifampin, reduce the short-term risk of UTI in hospitalized patients, but the cost-benefit implications are unclear.

- *Not inserting a urinary catheter*, and prompt removal of the urinary catheter once placed, are the most effective means of preventing UTIs in the hospital. Foley catheters are widely overused in the inpatient setting; up to 50% of urinary catheter insertions are inappropriate. The accepted indications for urinary catheters are as follows:
  ○ Bladder outlet obstruction
  ○ Urinary incontinence in patients with open sacral or perineal wounds
  ○ As a comfort measure in the terminally ill, at the patient's request
  ○ Monitoring of urine output in the critically ill
  ○ During prolonged surgical procedures with general or spinal anesthesia

BIBLIOGRAPHY

Behr MA, Drummond R, Libman MD, et al. Fever duration in hospitalized acute pyelonephritis patients. *Am J Med.* 1996;101:277–280.

Brosnahan J, Jull A, Tracy C. Types of urethral catheters for management of short-term voiding problems in hospitalised adults. *Cochrane Database Sys Rev.* 2004;(1): CD004013.

Jepson RG, Mihaljevic L, Craig J. Cranberries for preventing urinary tract infections. *Cochrane Database Sys Rev.* 2004;(2):CD001321.

Nicolle LE, Bradley S, Colgan R, et al. Infectious Diseases Society of America guidelines for the diagnosis and treatment of asymptomatic bacteriuria in adults. *Clin Infect Dis.* 2005; 40:643–654.

Saint S, Lipsky BA. Preventing catheter-related bacteriuria: should we? Can we? How? *Arch Intern Med.* 1999;159: 800–808.

Scholes D, Hooton TM, Roberts PL, et al. Risk factors associated with acute pyelonephritis in healthy women. *Ann Intern Med.* 2005;142:20–27.

Sobel JD, Kauffman CA, McKinsey D, et al. Candiduria: a randomized, double-blind study of treatment with fluconazole and placebo. *Clin Infect Dis.* 2000;30:19–24.

Warren JW, Abrutyn E, Hebel JR, et al. Guidelines for antimicrobial treatment of uncomplicated acute bacterial cystitis and acute pyelonephritis in women. Infectious Diseases Society of America (IDSA). *Clin Infect Dis.* 1999;29:745–758.

56 HOSPITAL-ACQUIRED BACTEREMIA

Danielle Scheurer

EPIDEMIOLOGY/OVERVIEW

- Nosocomial bloodstream infections are classified as primary (64%) or secondary (36%) if arising from infections at other sites.
- Intravascular catheters usually cause primary bloodstream infections.
  ○ Central venous lines cause 90% of catheter-related bacteremias.
  ○ Catheter-related bloodstream infections arise at a rate of 5 per 1000 catheter days, with 50,000–120,000 cases occurring annually in the United States.
  ○ Crude in-hospital mortality is 35%, and age-adjusted death rates have risen 78% in the last two decades.
  ○ Most cases are monomicrobial (87%), as in Table 56-1.
- Certain patient characteristics predispose to nosocomial bacteremia (Table 56-2).
- Some catheter factors also increase the risk for bloodstream infections (Table 56-3).

TABLE 56-1 Microbiology of Bloodstream Infections

CATEGORY	ORGANISM
Gram-positive 65%	CoNS 31%
	S. aureus 20%
	(> 50% MRSA)
	Enterococci 9%
Gram-negative 25%	*E. coli* 6%
	Klebsiella sp. 5%
	Pseudomonas sp. 4%
	Enterobacter sp. 4%
	Serratia sp. 2%
	Acinetobacter baumannii 1%
Fungi 9.5%	*Candida* sp. 9%

Subpopulations: most common organisms (Wisplinghoff et al., 2004)
Burn patients, *Pseudomonas aeruginosa*
HIV patients, *S. aureus*
Hemodialysis patients, gram-positive organisms
Patients with cancer, gram-negatives
Patients with needleless devices, hydrophilic gram-negative pathogens
(*P. aeruginosa*, *Stenotrophomonas maltophilia*, *A. baumannii*, and *Serratia marcescens*)

TABLE 56-2 Patients at High Risk for Nosocomial Bloodstream Infections

Extremes of age
Number and severity of comorbid conditions
Immunosuppression (especially neutropenia)
Malnutrition
Loss of skin integrity (such as burns)

CLINICAL PRESENTATION, DIFFERENTIAL, MAKING THE DIAGNOSIS

- Bloodstream infection should be suspected in any hospitalized patient with an intravascular catheter and signs or symptoms of infection (fever, leukocytosis, or hemodynamic instability).
- In many patients with infected vascular catheters, infection is only present within the lumen of the catheter, and the external catheter site appears normal.
- The clinical definition of the National Nosocomial Infections Surveillance System (NNIS) is helpful for research purposes, but is rarely used in clinical practice (Table 56-4).
- In a patient with a suspected bloodstream infection, blood cultures must be obtained prior to instituting empiric antibiotic therapy.
  ○ Two sets of blood cultures must be obtained from two different peripheral veins.
  ○ The yield of positive cultures increases with the amount of blood inoculated (should be at least 10 cc/bottle).
  ○ Blood cultures should also be drawn from the central venous catheter, if present.
  ○ Place the catheter tip in a sterile container and send for culture at the time of central venous catheter removal if infection is suspected.

TRIAGE AND INITIAL MANAGEMENT

- All initial antimicrobial therapy should be given IV as soon as possible after blood cultures are drawn.

TABLE 56-3 Catheter Factors that Increase the Risk of Bloodstream Infection

Duration of placement
Lower extremity placement > upper extremity placement
Repeated access
Internal jugular placement > subclavian placement
Nontunneled catheters > tunneled catheters > totally implantable catheters
Polyvinyl chloride and polyethylene > Teflon
For arterial catheters, cut down at insertion and presence of local inflammation

TABLE 56-4 NNIS Definition of Bloodstream Infection

Criterion 1	Recognized pathogen from blood culture not related to an infection at another site
Criterion 2	Fever
At least one of the following:	Chills
	Hypotension
And at least one of the following:	Common skin contaminant from 2 or more cultures from different occasions*
	Skin contaminant from at least one culture in a patient with an intravascular line
	Positive antigen test on blood, not related to infection at another site

*Diphtheroids, *Bacillus sp.*; coagulase-negative staphylococcus, *Propionibacterium sp.*; or micrococci.

  ○ First-line treatment is with vancomycin. Linezolid or daptomycin should be considered in vancomycin-allergic patients.
  ○ Gram-negative coverage with a third- or fourth-generation cephalosporin should be added for severely ill or immunocompromised patients.
  ○ Amphotericin B, fluconazole, or caspofungin should be added for suspected fungemia.
- The duration of treatment should be as follows:
  ○ Ten to fourteen days for immunocompetent patients without valvular heart disease, and without an intravascular prosthetic device, as long as they promptly respond to therapy
  ○ Four to six weeks if the patient has persistent bacteremia after catheter removal, endocarditis, septic thrombophlebitis, or other metastatic seeding
  ○ Six to eight weeks with osteomyelitis
- Higher risk of death from bloodstream infections is associated with older age, longer hospital stay before bloodstream infection, cancer or digestive system diseases, pneumonia as the source of bacteremia, polymicrobial infection, and candidemia.

DISEASE MANAGEMENT STRATEGIES

- *Catheter removal*—Although there are no published randomized, double-blind, clinical trials to dictate the management for removal of devices in catheter-related infections, the following guidelines are endorsed by the IDSA (Infectious Diseases Society of America) and SHEA (The Society for Healthcare Epidemiology of America):
  ○ Infected short-term peripheral catheters should be removed.
  ○ In nontunneled catheter-related bacteremia or fungemia, the catheter should be removed.
  ○ For tunneled catheters, such as the Hickman, Groshong, and Broviac catheters, the decision to

remove is based on the severity of illness, presence of complications (endocarditis, septic thrombosis, tunnel infection, or metastatic seeding), and documentation that the catheter is infected.

- If the infection is associated with severe systemic disease, erythema/purulence over the exit site, or clinical signs of unexplained sepsis, it should be removed.
- If the infection is associated only with fever or mild-to-moderate systemic disease in the absence of complications, it need not always be removed.
- Tunneled catheters infected with coagulase-negative staphylococci can usually be salvaged with a combination of parenteral and indwelling antibiotics ("antibiotic lock" technique).
- In patients with mild-to-moderate bloodstream infections of tunneled catheters with *S. aureus*, GNR, and *Candida* sp., and limited options for catheter replacement, an attempt may be made to salvage the catheter with combined systemic and antibiotic lock therapy, with guidance from infectious diseases consultation.
- Hospital-associated bloodstream infections with *S. aureus* are associated with rates of endocarditis as high as 25%. Transesophageal echocardiogram (TEE) should be strongly considered in all patients with nosocomial *S. aureus* bacteremia.

- Prevention strategies should lower the incidence of central venous catheter infection.
  ○ Standardized procedures for insertion and maintenance of the line by a skilled team using maximal barrier precautions.
  ○ *Preferential site insertion*—Upper extremity > lower extremity and subclavian > internal jugular.
  ○ Preferential selection of totally implantable catheters or tunneled catheters for long-term use (avoiding nontunneled catheters).
  ○ Identify factors that are clearly associated with increased risk of infectious complications and develop procedure-specific protocols.
    - Use antiseptics at the site for insertion and maintenance. Chlorhexidine is better than alcohol or povidone-iodine.
    - Use antimicrobial or antiseptic-impregnated catheters in patients at high risk for acquiring nosocomial bloodstream infections.
    - Use prophylactic antibiotic-lock solutions in immunocompromised patients.
    - Avoid cut down method for arterial catheters.
    - Avoid unnecessary repeated access of catheters.
    - Do not routinely replace central venous catheters over guidewires.
    - Discontinue catheters as soon as possible.

BIBLIOGRAPHY

Carratala J, Niubo J, Fernadez-Sevilla A, et al. Randomized, double-blind trial of an antibiotic-lock technique for prevention of Gram-positive central venous catheter-related infection in neutropenic patients with cancer. *Antimicrob Agents Chemother.* 1999;43(9):2200–2204.

Henrickson KJ, Axtell RA, Hoover SM, et al. Prevention of central venous catheter-related infections and thrombotic events in immunocompromised children by the use of vancomycin/ciprofloxacin/heparin flush solution: a randomized, multicenter, double-blind trial. *J Clin Oncol.* 2000;18(6): 1269–1278.

Mermel LA. Prevention of intravascular catheter-related infections. *Ann Intern Med.* 2000;132(5):391–402.

Mermel LA, Farr BM, Sherertz RJ, et al. Guidelines for the management of intravascular catheter-related infections. *Clin Infect Dis.* 2001;32:1249–1272.

Pittet D, Li N, Woolson RF, et al. Microbiological factors influencing the outcome of nosocomial bloodstream infections: a 6-year validated, population-based model. *Clin Infect Dis.* 1997;24(6):1068–1078.

Pittet D, Wenzel RP. Nosocomial bloodstream infections. Secular trends in rates, mortality, and contribution to total hospital deaths. *Arch Intern Med.* 1995;155(11):1177–1184.

Schwartz C, Henrickson KJ, Roghmann K, et al. Prevention of bacteremia attributed to luminal colonization of tunneled central venous catheters with vancomycin-susceptible organisms. *J Clin Oncol.* 1990;8(9):1591–1597.

Wisplinghoff H, Bischoff T, Tallent SM, et al. Nosocomial bloodstream infections in US hospitals: analysis of 24,179 cases from a prospective nationwide surveillance study. *Clin Infect Dis.* 2004;39(3):309–317.

WEB RESOURCES

Centers for Disease Control and Prevention. http://www.cdc.gov/ncidod/dhqp/pdf/nnis/2004NNISreport.pdf
Centers for Disease Control and Prevention. http://www.cdc.gov/ncidod/dhqp/pdf/nnis/NosInfDefinitions.pdf

57 INFLUENZA

John J. Ross

EPIDEMIOLOGY/OVERVIEW

- Annual influenza epidemics contribute to as many as 50,000 excess deaths each winter in the United States. About 85% of fatal influenza occurs in those > 65 years of age. Most deaths actually result from superimposed bacterial pneumonia, decompensated CHF, and/or chronic obstructive lung disease.

- From year to year, influenza strains usually differ only slightly in their major antigenic determinants, a process known as *antigenic drift*. Individuals exposed to influenza strains circulating in recent years are often somewhat immune to new strains arising from antigenic drift.
- Novel strains arise at unpredictable intervals, perhaps from genetic recombination events involving mammalian and avian influenza viruses. Such antigenic shift creates radically different strains to which there is little or no population immunity. If the resultant virus is highly pathogenic for humans, the dreaded scenario of a worldwide influenza pandemic could ensue.
- Avian influenza A (H5N1) might trigger such a pandemic, if it better adapts to human-to-human transmission.

PATHOPHYSIOLOGY

- Influenza in humans generally spreads person to person by aerosols.
- Influenza virus replicates in both the upper and lower respiratory epithelium. Influenza has a limited ability to replicate outside the respiratory tract, suggesting that the systemic symptoms of influenza are usually caused by cytokines and other components of the host immune response.
- The major surface proteins and antigenic determinants of influenza virus are hemagglutinin (H) and neuraminidase (N).
- Hemagglutinin binds to sialic acid residues on the surface of respiratory ciliated columnar cells, allowing virus entry by receptor-mediated endocytosis.
- Neuraminidase cleaves sialic acid, facilitating release of new virions from infected cells.
- Neuraminidase also severs sialic acid from the mucin barrier of the respiratory epithelium. This may facilitate viral invasion, as well as bacterial superinfection.

CLINICAL PRESENTATION, DIFFERENTIAL, MAKING THE DIAGNOSIS

- Influenza infection is associated with a broad variety of clinical presentations, from minimally symptomatic upper respiratory tract infection to life-threatening viral pneumonia and adult respiratory distress syndrome (ARDS).

- Influenza outbreaks typically occur in the winter months in the northern and southern hemispheres.
  - There is no seasonality to the prevalence of flu in the tropics, and there have been outbreaks of flu on cruise ships during summer months. This should be kept in mind in travelers who present with flu-like illness.
- Classic influenza often begins abruptly within 1 or 2 days of exposure to a sick contact, with fever, chills, malaise, headache, arthralgias, and anorexia. Myalgias are particularly bothersome, and typically involve leg and back muscles.
- Respiratory symptoms, with dry cough, sore throat, and nasal congestion and drainage, are usually present at the onset of illness, but may be overshadowed by systemic complaints.
- This presentation is so characteristic of influenza that any sickness with prominent systemic symptoms is often referred to as a "flu-like illness."
- High-grade fever, from 100°F to 104°F, is present at the onset of illness, usually abating in 3–5 days.
- The throat and nasal passages are hyperemic, but exudates are absent, and nasal discharge is clear and runny. Minor cervical lymphadenopathy may be present.
- Less than 20% of patients have scattered crackles or wheezes on lung auscultation. The frequency of pulmonary involvement increases with age.
- After fever subsides, patients often have fatigue and malaise for 1 or 2 weeks before returning to their usual state of well-being.
- Because many respiratory pathogens cause "flu-like syndromes," suspected influenza cases should be confirmed by laboratory testing.
  - Viral cultures are highly sensitive and specific for the diagnosis of influenza, and are important for epidemiologic and surveillance purposes. However, they are of little clinical utility, as results require 5–10 days.
  - Serology and PCR are also of limited use in suspected influenza, because of the relatively long turn around time.
  - A variety of tests are available for the rapid diagnosis of influenza. These can detect influenza A and B antigens within 30 minutes from throat swabs, nasopharyngeal swabs, or nasal washings and aspirates. Many of these are approved for use outside the laboratory setting.
  - Rapid tests are > 90% specific, but only about 70% sensitive.

TRIAGE AND INITIAL MANAGEMENT

- *Infection control*—Recommendations for hospitalized patients with known or suspected influenza are summarized in Table 57-1.

TABLE 57-1   Infection Control Measures for Influenza

Type of isolation

Seasonal influenza

- Droplet precautions: standard surgical mask and gloves; door can be kept open; negative pressure room not required

Pandemic/avian influenza

- Air-borne isolation precautions with negative-pressure room, if available
- If not available: single room with door closed, or designated multibed room or ward
- Healthcare workers should wear high-efficiency masks (NIOSH-certified N-95 or equivalent), long-sleeved cuffed gowns, face shields, or gloves

Duration of isolation

Seasonal influenza

- In adults, virus shedding falls rapidly 48 h into the course of illness, and ends completely when clinical illness is resolved, typically after 5–10 days total
- Virus may be shed for longer in children

Pandemic/avian influenza

- Maintain precautions for 7 days after resolution of fever, or possibly up to 21 days

Healthcare worker exposures

Seasonal and pandemic/avian influenza

- Persons caring for infected patients should monitor their temperature
- If they develop fever and flu-like symptoms, oseltamivir treatment should be initiated, if no other explanation of symptoms is found
- Postexposure chemoprophylaxis with oseltamivir 75 mg once daily for 7–10 days should be considered after inadvertent exposure to aerosols or body fluids

Abbreviation: NIOSH, National Institute for Occupational Safety and Health.

- Only four drugs are currently available for the treatment and prophylaxis of influenza (Table 57-2). All are pregnancy category C (risk cannot be ruled out—human studies are lacking and animal studies are either positive for fetal risk or lacking as well; however, potential benefits may justify the potential risks).
- Older influenza drugs, the adamantanes, prevent viral replication of influenza A only, by blocking the viral M2 ion channel and inhibiting fusion of the viral and host cell membranes. These drugs have a high incidence of central nervous system (CNS) side effects,

including insomnia, dizziness, and confusion, and require dosage adjustment in renal or hepatic failure.

- ○ Resistance to amantidine and rimantidine has risen steeply worldwide in recent years, perhaps in part owing to their availability over the counter in many countries.
- ○ The Centers for Disease Control and Prevention (CDC) announced in January 2006 that 90% of influenza isolates in the United States were resistant to amantidine and rimantidine.
- ○ *Amantidine and rimantidine are therefore no longer recommended for the treatment or prophylaxis of influenza.*
- Neuraminidase inhibitors are active against both influenza A and B, and inhibit the release of new virions from infected cells.
- ○ Neuraminidase inhibitors shorten the duration of influenza symptoms by 1–2 days in healthy persons, if treatment is begun within 36–48 hours after onset of symptoms.
- ○ The treatment effect is less pronounced in elderly and high-risk patients.
- ○ No effect of therapy is observed if therapy is initiated > 48 hours after symptoms onset.
- As treatment effect of neuraminidase inhibitors in uncomplicated influenza is modest, and the therapeutic window is brief, the mainstay of therapy is supportive care—fluids, acetaminophen cough suppressants, and rest. Avoid salicylates, especially in patients under the age of 18, due to the risk of Reye's syndrome.
- Updated treatment recommendations from the CDC can be found at http://www.cdc.gov/flu/professionals/treatment/.

DISEASE MANAGEMENT STRATEGIES

- Complications of influenza
- ○ Viral pneumonia from influenza is presently rare, but is more common in the setting of pandemic influenza.

TABLE 57-2   Antiviral Agents for Influenza

DRUG	DOSAGE	DOSE ADJUST FOR RENAL INSUFFICIENCY	SIDE EFFECTS AND CONTRAINDICATIONS
Oseltamivir	75 mg po twice daily for 5 days	75 mg po once daily	Nausea, vomiting, hepatitis
Zanamivir	10 mg (2 inhalations) twice daily for 5 days	No	Cough, allergy, sinusitis, bronchitis, bronchospasm; contraindicated in underlying airways disease. Not FDA-approved for influenza prophylaxis

Abbreviation: FDA, Food and Drug Administration.

- Neuraminidase inhibitors are widely recommended for the treatment of influenza pneumonia. However, there are no published studies to support their efficacy.
- Treatment of influenza pneumonia should focus on meticulous respiratory and other supportive care, aggressive treatment of complications such as bacterial pneumonia, and stringent infection control practices to limit spread of influenza within the hospital.
  ○ Hospital admissions for bacterial pneumonia typically double during influenza season. Common causes of secondary bacterial pneumonia after influenza are *Streptococcus pneumoniae*, *Haemophilus influenzae*, and *S. aureus*.
- Several cases of severe necrotizing pneumonia associated with CA-MRSA after influenza A have recently been reported in the United States.
  ○ Exacerbations of cardiac disease and chronic bronchitis are common with influenza.
  ○ Toxic shock syndrome (TSS) occasionally occurs in children and adults after influenza, presumably because damage to the respiratory epithelium allows overgrowth of toxin-producing staphylococci.

○ Reye's syndrome, with hepatic steatosis and encephalopathy, may occur in children and teens with influenza who receive aspirin or other salicylates.
○ Other rare complications of influenza include myositis, pericarditis, myocarditis, encephalitis, transverse myelitis, and Guillain-Barré syndrome.
- Prevention of influenza
  ○ The goal of influenza vaccination is to induce virus-neutralizing antibodies to prevent infection and/or lessen the severity of clinical illness (Table 57-3).
    - Vaccination should occur throughout the fall and winter months (September–March in the northern hemisphere).
    - Travellers should receive influenza vaccine once annually based on where they live.
    - Patients diagnosed with influenza A or B should still be vaccinated, as this will protect them from infection with the other influenza type.
  ○ Types of vaccine
    - Inactivated intramuscular vaccines may be used in healthy persons and also in immunocompromised patients.
    - Low-dose intradermal immunization with inactivated vaccines has been shown to offer seroprotection, but has not yet been demonstrated to prevent influenza. In times of short vaccine

TABLE 57-3 Target Groups for Vaccination

Annual influenza vaccination is recommended for the following groups, consult the CDC Web site for updated prioritization recommendations should vaccine shortfalls occur: http://www.cdc.gov/flu/professionals/vaccination/recommendations.htm

Vaccination with inactivated influenza vaccine is recommended for the following persons who are at increased risk for severe complications from influenza:

- Children aged 6–23 months
- Children and adolescents (aged 6 months–18 years) who are receiving long-term aspirin therapy, and, therefore, might be at risk for experiencing Reye's syndrome after influenza virus infection
- Women who will be pregnant during the influenza season
- Adults and children who have chronic disorders of the pulmonary or cardiovascular systems, including asthma (hypertension is not considered a high-risk condition)
- Adults and children who have required regular medical follow-up or hospitalization during the preceding year because of chronic metabolic diseases (including diabetes mellitus), renal dysfunction, hemoglobinopathies, or immunodeficiency (including immunodeficiency caused by medications or by HIV)
- Adults and children who have any condition (eg, cognitive dysfunction, spinal cord injuries, seizure disorders, or other neuromuscular disorders) that can compromise respiratory function or the handling of respiratory secretions or that can increase the risk for aspiration
- Residents of nursing homes and other chronic care facilities that house persons of any age who have chronic medical conditions
- Persons aged ≥ 65 years.

Vaccination with inactivated influenza vaccine is also recommended for the following persons because of an increased risk for influenza-associated clinic, emergency department, or hospital visits, particularly if they have a high-risk medical condition:

- Children aged 24–59 months
- Persons aged 50–64 years

In addition, to prevent transmission to persons identified above, vaccination with TIV or LAIV is recommended for persons who live with or care for persons at high risk for influenza-related complications, unless contraindicated.

- Healthy household contacts and caregivers of children aged 0–59 months and persons at high risk for severe complications from influenza
- Healthcare workers

Abbreviation: TIV, trivalent influenza vaccine; LAIV, live attenuated influenza vaccine.

supply, low-dose intradermal vaccination offers a promising strategy to increase immunization rates.
- There is also an intranasal live attenuated influenza vaccine (LAIV), licensed for use in healthy persons aged 5–49 years.
- LAIV is contraindicated in those < 5 years and ≥ 50 years old; patients with chronic medical conditions; patients who are immunocompromised, including those because of HIV; those under the age of 18 on chronic salicylate therapy; and pregnant women.
- Expedited efforts are underway to develop a vaccine for avian influenza.
  - Contraindications to vaccination include allergy to eggs, or previous Guillain-Barré syndrome within 6 weeks of influenza vaccination.
  - Influenza chemoprophylaxis should not be used as a substitute for influenza vaccination in the prevention of flu.
    - Influenza prophylaxis with oseltamivir (75 mg daily starting within 2 days of exposure and continuing for 7–10 days) should be considered for unvaccinated persons in certain high-risk settings, such as flu outbreaks in hospitals and long-term care facilities.

BIBLIOGRAPHY

Centers for Disease Control and Prevention. High levels of adamantane resistance among influenza A—H3N2) viruses and interim guidelines for use of antiviral agents(United States, 2005–2006 influenza season. *MMWR Morb Mortal Wkly Rep.* 2006;55(2):44.

de Jong MD, Thanh TT, Khanh TH, et al. Oseltamivir resistance during treatment of influenza A (H5N1) infection. *N Engl J Med.* 2005;353:2667.

Falsey AR, Walsh EE. Viral pneumonia in older adults. *Clin Infect Dis.* 2006;42:518.

Jefferson T, Demicheli V, Rivetti D, et al. Antivirals for influenza in healthy adults: systematic review. *Lancet.* 2006;367:303.

Moscona A. Neuraminidase inhibitors for influenza. *N Engl J Med.* 2005;353:1363.

Writing Committee of the World Health Organization (WHO) Consultation on Human Influenza A/H5. Avian influenza A (H5N1) infection in humans. *N Engl J Med.* 2005;353:1374.

WEB RESOURCE

Centers for Disease Control and Prevention. http://www.cdc.gov/flu/

58 SKIN AND SOFT TISSUE INFECTIONS

Ranjan Chowdhry and Harry M. Schrager

EPIDEMIOLOGY/OVERVIEW

- Skin infections run the spectrum (Fig. 58-1) from infections involving
  - Superficial layers (impetigo)
  - Deep dermal and subcutaneous tissue (cellulitis)
  - Deeper skin structures with abscess (furunculosis) formation
  - Fascia (necrotizing fasciitis [NF]) and muscle (myonecrosis)
- Cellulitis is the most common skin infection requiring hospitalization and is defined as "an acute suppurative infection of the epidermis, dermis, and subcutaneous tissue."
  - The incidence of cellulitis is 24.6/1000 person-years.
  - The incidence of cellulitis is higher in males of all ages and in the elderly.
- Although the majority of patients with cellulitis (78%) receive treatment in the outpatient setting, moderate-to-severe skin and soft tissue infections often require hospitalization for parenteral therapy.
  - Diabetic foot infections account for the largest number of diabetes-related hospital bed-days.
- For more severe cases, hospitalists play a critical role in triage. Outpatient parenteral antimicrobial therapy for some of these patients may be a cost-effective alternative to an inpatient admission and provide superior outcomes and enhanced patient satisfaction. Appropriate triage to intensive care unit (ICU) or to the surgical service may be life saving.

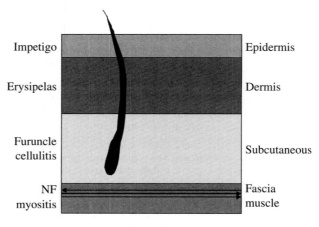

FIG. 58-1 Anatomic correlations of skin and soft tissue infections.

- This chapter will focus on the most common and serious skin and soft tissue infections seen on inpatient wards and ICUs.

PATHOPHYSIOLOGY AND MICROBIOLOGY

- Bacteria enter the skin through cracks, fissures, or punctures (eg, bites) of the epidermis and dermis. They attach, multiply, and cause localized infection or invade and produce deeper infection and bacteremia (Fig. 58-1).
- *S. aureus* and groups A, B, C, and G, beta—hemolytic streptococci are the most common causes of skin and soft tissue infections and should generally be covered in most empiric regimens of all types of skin infection.
  - Most uncomplicated cellulitis is a monomicrobial beta-hemolytic streptococcal or staphylococcal infection.
  - The latter arise most often from overt trauma or superficial abscess or ulcers but occasionally mimic typical streptococcal cellulitis.
  - MRSA is a common colonizer in patients recently admitted to the hospital, persons residing in long-term care facilities, dialysis patients, and IV drug abusers.
  - CA-MRSA is rising in incidence. In one recent report, MRSA was isolated from 59% of patients presenting to the emergency room with skin and soft tissue infections. The large majority of these strains were CA-MRSA strains.
  - Although these infections are more common in certain populations—IV drug abusers, correctional facility inmates, competitive sports participants (especially contact sports), military personnel, children in day care and homeless persons—many cases have no known contact with these groups or with prior healthcare.
  - CA-MRSA is more virulent than hospital-acquired MRSA and has now become endemic in the general population.
- Infections with GNR tend to occur in patients with chronic decubitus ulcers, chronic foot ulcers associated diabetes, and ischemic ulcers related to peripheral vascular disease. Exposure to antibiotics targeting *S. aureus* and streptococci selects these organisms unless the underlying condition is corrected.

CLINICAL PRESENTATION, DIFFERENTIAL, MAKING THE DIAGNOSIS

- The differential diagnosis of cellulitis includes drug reactions, insect bites (hypersensitivity reactions), gout, thrombophlebitis, contact dermatitis, Sweet's syndrome, stasis dermatitis, viral exanthems, vasculitic lesions, herpes zoster, anthrax, tularemia, and plague.
- The purpose of the history and physical examination is to make the correct diagnosis and to assess the severity of the infection. The history should inquire about
  - The characteristic symptoms of cellulitis (tenderness, fever, chills, erythema, warmth, swelling or induration, abscess formation)
  - The possibility of other conditions that might mimic cellulitis
  - Abruptness or rapidity of progression, inability to bear weight, severe pain (as an indication of severity)
  - Chronicity (for complications such as osteomyelitis)
  - Antecedent injury (to guide antibiotic therapy or surgical intervention)
  - Any comorbidities that would affect management and prognosis (presence of immunosuppression, peripheral vascular disease, alcohol and substance abuse) (see Table 58-1)
  - Recent hospitalization and recent antibiotic use (suggesting treatment failures or other diagnoses)
  - Obtaining a history of MRSA colonization is important because these patients may require empiric treatment for MRSA initially
- The clinician should perform a skin examination specifically noting the presence of
  - A raised or indurated border or lymphangitis (as an indication of a superficial group A *Streptococcus* (GAS) infection often treated in the outpatient setting)
  - Fluctuance, gas gangrene (clostridial myonecrosis), and crepitus (NF, pyomyositis) requiring additional imaging and/or surgical consultation

TABLE 58-1 Predisposing Factors

Obesity
Edema in extremities caused by CHF, venous insufficiency
  (e.g., after saphenous venectomy), lymphatic insufficiency (e.g., after lymph node dissection), or radiation therapy
Acute and chronic skin ulcers (portal of entry and generally colonized with bacteria)
Fissured toe web space from maceration or fungal infections
Inflammatory dermatoses, e.g., atopic eczema
Diabetes and its complications, e.g., peripheral neuropathy

○ Pain out of proportion to skin findings or skin anesthesia around the wound (NF, myonecrosis)

○ Violaceous bullae, cutaneous hemorrhage, "hardwood" induration, sloughing of skin (as an indication of deeper infection)

○ Location of infection (digits, genitals, thigh, and head likely require hospitalization)

○ Size of infection (extensive skin involvement is an indicator of severity especially in immunocompromised or diabetic patients)

• In addition, in an infection involving an extremity, the clinician should perform a targeted physical examination specifically noting:

○ Unstable vital signs (evidence of systemic toxicity)

○ Presence of severe peripheral vascular disease (which may alter presentation of cellulitis and preclude eradication of infection without appropriate intervention)

○ Presence of ulceration (for possible surgical debridement or underlying osteomyelitis)

TRIAGE AND INITIAL MANAGEMENT

• The first step is determination of the need for hospitalization after the diagnosis of cellulitis has been made. The need to admit patients would depend on the underlying comorbid and predisposing conditions and the severity of the infection. The Eron classification system for patient with skin and soft tissue infections defines the following four levels of severity:

○ *I*—Absence of fever, comorbidities (outpatient, oral antibiotics)

○ *II*—More severely ill, febrile (outpatient parenteral or inpatient parenteral antibiotics)

○ *III*—Septic physiology, limb-threatening infection, unstable comorbid illness (inpatient)

○ *IV*—Sepsis syndrome, deep-tissue infection, or NF (inpatient ICU)

• For consideration of possible outpatient treatment, inquire about compliance and ability to follow up, the possibility of substance abuse, and current insurance (to cover parenteral or oral therapy).

• Evidence of toxicity, immunosuppression, spreading lymphangitis, suspicion for deep infection, failure of outpatient antibiotic therapy, and extensive area of involvement should prompt admission.

• Location of the infection, the possibility of a foreign object in the wound, or human or animal bite also helps guide triage admission decision.

LABORATORY TESTING

• The following laboratory tests should be performed initially:

○ A CBC (marked leukocytosis, leucopenia, abnormalities in the differential, thrombocytopenia for severity, immunosuppression)

○ Chemistry profile (metabolic disturbances suggesting sepsis syndrome, hypoperfusion, more severe infection)

○ Creatine kinase (myonecrosis)

• Cultures to guide antimicrobial therapy should be performed for all hospitalized patients.

○ In moderate-to-severe disease and in the immunocompromised host the clinician should attempt to obtain the infecting organism by culture and sensitivity testing (blood cultures or wound or ulcer material or swab).

○ For patients undergoing wound debridement, request that the surgeon culture from nonsurface tissue to avoid finding the myriad superficial colonizing organisms that frequently are unrelated to invasive infection.

○ Aspirate skin and soft tissues, or biopsy of skin lesions for culturing (typically in immunocompromised hosts).

○ Consider swabbing the nares for culture to screen for MRSA as an adjunctive method that may help infer whether the infecting organism is MRSA.

• The clinical manifestations of deep infection may not be present initially and require repeated detailed examinations.

○ Imaging in the form of x-rays, CT scans with IV contrast, and MRI with gadolinium may aid in diagnosis.

INDICATIONS FOR PROMPT SURGICAL CONSULTATION

• Once the diagnosis of deep infection is suspected or made, a surgical consultation is essential for exploration and drainage.

SELECTION OF EMPIRIC ANTIBIOTICS

• For deep infections, empiric antibiotic regimens need to be broad with coverage for *S. aureus* including MRSA, Streptococci, gram-negative

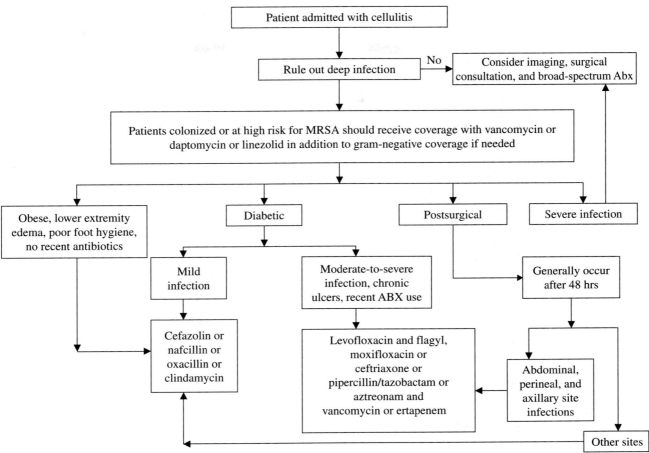

FIG. 58-2 Empiric antibiotic selection.

bacilli (rods), clostridia and other anaerobes such as *Bacteroides fragilis*. Refer to Fig. 58-2 and Table 58-2.
- Once the patient has been stabilized and operative culture results are available, in consultation with the infectious disease service, the antibiotic regimen should be narrowed down appropriately.

ADJUNCTIVE THERAPIES

- In addition to surgical consultation and empiric antibiotics, adjunctive therapy should be implemented promptly.
- The affected limb must be kept elevated at least above the waist.

TABLE 58-2 Guide to Empiric Antibiotic Selection for Skin and Soft Tissue Infection

S. aureus (MSSA)	Oral agents: cephalexin, dicloxacillin, doxycycline, minocycline, amoxicillin/clavulanic acid, clindamycin, linezolid trimethoprim/sulfamethoxazole
	IV: cefazolin, nafcillin/oxacillin, ampicillin/sulbactam, vancomycin, daptomycin, linezolid (last two agents are uncommonly indicated)
S. aureus (MRSA)	Oral agents: doxycycline, minocycline, clindamycin, linezolid, trimethoprim/sulfamethoxazole
	IV: vancomycin, daptomycin, linezolid
GAS	100% susceptible to penicillin and cephalosporins
	Other agents: clindamycin, vancomycin, daptomycin, linezolid
Gram negatives	Predicated on susceptibility pattern in the region.
	Fluoroquinolones, 3rd-generation cephalosporins, carbapenems, piperacillin/tazobactam, aztreonam (for severely penicillin allergic)

Antibiotic change may be required once susceptibility pattern is available.
Empiric therapy should always cover *S. aureus* and GAS.

- Diuretic therapy may be considered in select patients who have substantial lymphedema.
- Venous thromboembolism (VTE) prophylaxis.

DISEASE MANAGEMENT STRATEGIES

COMMUNITY-ACQUIRED METHICILLIN-RESISTANT *S. aureus*

- Skin and soft tissue infections are common with CA-MRSA, but NF and osteomyelitis, as well as other clinical entities (necrotizing pneumonia, septicemia, and endocarditis) have been associated with these staphylococci.
- CA-MRSA can be distinguished from the traditional healthcare associated MRSA on the basis of
  - Sensitivities to clindamycin, macrolides, and fluoroquinolones
  - The Panton-Valentine leukocidin (PVL) genes These genes produce toxins that can cause tissue necrosis and leukocyte destruction and are associated with CA-MRSA skin infections and necrotizing pneumonia.
- Treatment options include vancomycin, linezolid, moxifloxacin, levofloxacin (high dose, 750 mg), clindamycin, trimethoprim-sulfamethoxazole, doxycycline, and combinations with rifampin.
  - An emerging CA-MRSA clone known as USA300 typically carries PVL, and is resistant to beta-lactams and erythromycin, but it is sensitive to clindamycin, trimethoprim-sulfamethoxazole, and fluoroquinolones.
  - An important feature to note about using clindamycin to treat CA-MRSA is that approximately one in five strains that appear susceptible will fail treatment owing to inducible resistance.
    - The marker for this inducible phenotype (clindamycin resistance) is an antibiotic resistance profile reporting resistance to erythromycin and susceptibility to clindamycin. Before discharging a patient home on clindamycin it is important to request that the microbiology laboratory perform the "D" test to exclude inducible clindamycin resistance.

DIABETIC FOOT INFECTIONS

- Optimal management of diabetic foot infections can reduce the associated morbidity and need for hospital admission and related expenses.
- The care of these patients requires a multidisciplinary approach involving surgery (vascular, podiatric,

orthopedic), infectious diseases, wound care nursing staff, and endocrinologists or internists. Antibiotics alone will not heal diabetic neuropathic ulcers.
- Therapy aimed solely at aerobic gram-positive cocci usually will be sufficient for mild to moderate infections in patients who have not recently received antibiotics (see Fig. 58-3 for antibiotic choices). In all other patients, a broad-spectrum regimen covering gram negatives and anaerobes should be included pending culture results.
- Duration of treatment has to be individualized, but in the absence of abscess collections or deep infection a 1- to 2-week course should suffice.
- Neuropathy is usually the underlying cause for these ulcers.
  - Disturbances in sensory and autonomic function leads to unrecognized ulceration from trauma or excessive pressure on a deformed foot.
  - The ulcer becomes colonized by microflora and then eventually infection begins.
  - Many infections could be prevented with good local wound care of noninfected ulcers.
- Arterial perfusion of the affected limb should be carefully evaluated and vascular surgery consultation obtained if insufficient.
  - In the presence of moderate-to-severe peripheral vascular disease, the following may occur:
    - Less erythema on physical examination despite extensive infection
    - Slower cure time
    - Incomplete ulcer healing even in the absence of infection
  - In patients with severe vascular disease who are not surgical candidates, amputation often is required for infected nonhealing ulcers and osteomyelitis.
- Nonhealing, chronic ulcers are a common problem in diabetics.
  - Among other interventions, it is essential to off-load local foot pressure to promote healing.
  - X-ray films should be obtained to rule out osteomyelitis. Plain films are inexpensive, and, if abnormal, they are diagnostic in the absence of previous surgery, trauma, or osteomyelitis.
  - If the suspicion for osteomyelitis is high and x-rays are not diagnostic, an MRI with gadolinium can be useful.
  - Avoid MRI if there is a relatively low pretest probability as the MRI can be misleading because of ultra-high sensitivity for signal abnormalities that may mimic osteomyelitis.
- If osteomyelitis is diagnosed, débridement is important for microbiologic diagnosis and cure; bone should be sent for pathology and microbiology.
- Chronic osteomyelitis related to nonhealing ulcers does not generally cause high fevers and/or significant leukocytosis (systemic inflammatory response

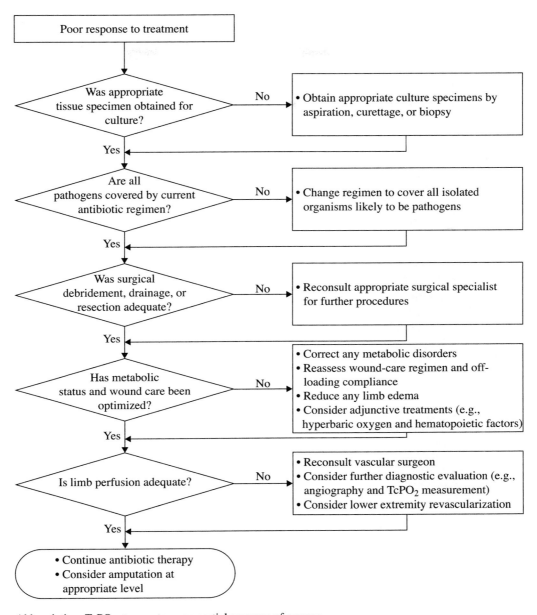

Abbreviation: TcPO₂, transcutaneous partial pressure of oxygen.

FIG. 58-3 Approach to assessing a diabetic patient with a foot infection who is not responding well to treatment. SOURCE: Copied with permission from Lipsky BA, et al. Diagnosis and treatment of diabetic foot infections. *Clin Infect Dis.* 2004.39(7):885–910.

syndrome [SIRS]); other causes of sepsis should be investigated in such patients with chronic ulcers without marked cellulitis. Occasionally, acute cellulitis overlying chronic osteomyelitis could present with sepsis.
• Generally, antibiotic therapy should be continued only until the infection has resolved but not necessarily until the wound or ulcer has completely healed.

• Glycemic control plays a key role in the resolution of infection. Hyperglycemia is a major predisposition for infection, not diabetes mellitus itself. See Chap. 36 for more on management of hyperglycemia in hospitalized patients.
• Inadequate response to therapy—Refer to Fig. 58-3 for management strategies in such cases.

GAS GANGRENE

- Consider this diagnosis with infections associated with severe penetrating trauma or crush injuries associated with interruption of blood supply. It is primarily caused by *Clostridium perfringens* and a few other *Clostridium* species.

NECROTIZING FASCIITIS

- NF may be monomicrobial (GAS also called *Streptococcus pyogenes*, *Vibrio vulnificus*, *Aeromonas hydrophila*) developing with no clear source or portal.
- In 2005, a report from UCLA was published describing a newly recognized entity of monomicrobial NF caused by CA-MRSA (see above).
- NF may be polymicrobial, which tends to occur in patients with diabetes mellitus, peripheral vascular disease, decubitus ulcers, perianal abscesses, status post abdominal surgeries, and intravenous drug abuse (IVDA).

SURGICAL SITE INFECTIONS

- Fevers less than 48 hours after surgery are generally not because of infection.
  - Exceptions to this rule are mainly hyperacute clostridial and group A streptococcal infection.
- Surgical site infections (SSI) typically develop on postoperative day 5 and most are caused by *S. aureus*.
- The surgical site should be carefully examined and if signs of infection are identified, the wound should be opened to drain the infection and most often antibiotics should be administered.
- For more on SSI, see Chap. 104.

HUMAN BITES

- The microorganisms involved include aerobes—viridans group streptococci, *S. aureus*, *Eiknella*—and anaerobes—*Peptostreptococcus*, *Fusobacterium* sp. and *Prevotella* sp.
- Wounds may be occlusive (in which teeth actually bite the body part) or clenched fist injuries (occur when the fist of one person strikes the teeth of another).
- An expert in hand surgery should evaluate clenched fist injuries for penetration into tendon, joint, or bone. These patients generally need to be admitted for IV antibiotics and close monitoring. The duration of therapy would depend on the depth of infection.

Ampicillin/sulbactam, ertapenem, or clindamycin plus a fluoroquinolone are appropriate choices.

CAT AND DOG BITES

- Cat bites become infected in the majority of cases. These also tend to be deeper than dog bites because of the sharp nature of their teeth, and tend to cause osteomyelitis and septic arthritis more often than dog bites.
- The bacteria involved are *Pasteurella*, *Fusobacterium*, *S. aureus*, and *Capnocytophaga*.
- In the acutely hospitalized patient, IV ampicillin/sulbactam or ertapenem are the drugs of choice. In the penicillin-allergic patient, a fluoroquinolone (or trimethoprim-sulfamethoxazole in children) plus clindamycin is the preferred regimen.

WATER-RELATED INFECTIONS

- In patients with fresh water injury or exposure one needs to consider covering the aggressive GNR *A. hydrophila*.
- Salt water exposure, particularly warm waters of the Gulf of Mexico, is a risk for *Vibrio* (GNRs) infection that may produce violatious bullous cellulitis (necrotizing infection). There have been recent reports of *Vibrio* infections in the North-East part of the United States as well.
- Meat packers and butchers and shellfish handlers may develop *Erysipelothrix rhusiopathiae* (gram-positive rod) infection.
- Hot tub folliculitis is caused by *Pseudomonas aeruginosa* contamination of inadequately chlorinated hot tubs/whirlpool baths.

TOXIC SHOCK SYNDROME

- Divided into staphylococcal TSS and streptococcal TSS.
- The triad of fever, hypotension, and flat macular diffuse erythroderma characterizes staphylococcal TSS and occurs typically without invasive infection but rather with absorption of exotoxin from a mucocutaneous site including colonized clean wounds.
  - Although initially recognized in females using tampons, now nonmenstrual cases comprise at least 50% of cases. Nonmenstrual cases occur in patients with postsurgical and postpartum wounds, sinusitis, and subcutaneous lesions of the perianal and axillary region.

- Streptococcal TSS occurs in the setting of invasive, typically necrotizing soft tissue infection or pneumonia. The diagnosis of this entity is mostly clinical and the patients are frequently not bacteremic.
  - Staphylococci and streptococci may be seen in the Gram stain and cultures of the involved site, but the signs of inflammation may be unimpressive.
  - Patients may present with a macular rash and diarrhea and then rapidly go into shock.
- Antibiotic regimens should include clindamycin, which primarily inhibits toxin production (inhibiting protein synthesis) as well as a beta-lactam or vancomycin although MRSA is uncommonly a producer of TSS.

FACIAL CELLULITIS

- Erysipelas and impetigo tend to occur on the face.
- In both cases *S. aureus* and streptococci should be covered.
- Herpes zoster can initially appear as facial cellulitis especially in patients who are immunocompromised. A dermatomal lesion that does not cross the midline is a clue to zoster.

ORBITAL CELLULITIS

- Preseptal (periorbital) and orbital (postseptal) cellulitis are often difficult to distinguish clinically. An orbital CT is frequently required to distinguish these two entities.
  - Orbital cellulitis is localized posterior to the orbital septum, and involves infection of the fat and muscle contained within the bony orbit.
  - In contrast, preseptal cellulitis is a soft tissue infection, localized anterior to the orbital septum.
  - Orbital cellulitis commonly produces proptosis, painful and restricted eye movements, double vision or vision loss whereas preseptal cellulitis does not.
- Sinusitis is the most common risk factor for orbital cellulitis.
- Management should be in consultation with otolaryngologists and ophthalmologists.
- Broad-spectrum IV antibiotics (nafcillin/cefazolin/vancomycin, and ampicillin-sulbactam, ertapenem, piperacillin-tazobactam, ceftriaxone) should be administered.

IMMUNOCOMPROMISED HOSTS

- Skin infections are common in this population of patients.
- Identifying a microbiologic etiology is important. Infection in patients with cell-mediated immune deficiency (HIV) can be caused by bacteria, fungi, helminths, protozoa, and viruses.
- Skin lesions may be a manifestation of a systemic infection, such fungemia with embolic lesions.
- Prompt biopsy should be considered in cases with atypical findings.
- In patients appearing systemically ill, broad-spectrum antibiotics including MRSA and gram-negative coverage should be administered.

CARE TRANSITIONS

- Timing of discharge has to be individualized for each patient. In general, once systemic signs of infection have resolved and the local signs and symptoms of inflammation have begun to subside, discharge should be considered if the patient can continue to keep the limb elevated and can be relied upon to take medications as prescribed.
  - When the above criteria are met, most patients can be switched to an oral regimen based on the clinical and microbiologic data available.
  - In certain special circumstances (eg, slow response to treatment or difficult to treat organisms), one may consider continuing IV antibiotics as an outpatient in consultation with an infectious diseases consultant.
- Close outpatient follow-up is the key to ensure eradication of infection in patients with any type of skin infection.
  - Although not validated in controlled studies, eradication of MRSA colonization can be attempted. Commonly used strategies include
    - Mupirocin ointment applied to the nares three times per day for a week, and
    - Bathing with chlorhexidine soap for 1 week
    - Followed by screening cultures to document eradication (screening cultures of the nares plus one other site such as wound site, perineum, axilla, or catheter exit sites; done on three different days).
  - Ideally, diabetics and patients with complicated infections should be seen in clinic within 2–5 days of discharge.
  - Subsequent care should be carefully coordinated between the surgeon, infectious disease service, and primary care physician in patients with complicated deep infections.
- Foot hygiene, daily foot examinations, and institution of protective measures in patients with neuropathy are extremely important for prevention of new infections. Patients with foot deformities and nonhealing ulcers may benefit from custom-made orthopedic shoes.

BIBLIOGRAPHY

Ellis Simonsen SM, et al. Cellulitis incidence in a defined population. *Epidemiol Infect.* 2006;134(2):293–299.

Erin LJ. Key decision points in evaluating and treating cellulites. Expert Panel Recommendations on Managing Cellulitis from Hospital to Home.

Eron EJ. Infections of skin and soft tissue: outcomes of a classification scheme. *Clin Infect Dis.* 2000;31:287.

Eron LJ, Passos S. Early discharge of infected patients through appropriate antibiotic use. *Arch Intern Med.* 2001;161:61–65.

Home Health Care Consultant, Annals of Long-Term Care, and Clinical Geriatrics, Supplement. December 2002.

Lipsky BA, et al. Diagnosis and treatment of diabetic foot infections. *Clin Infect Dis.* 2004;39(7):885–910.

Moran GJ, et al. Methicillin-resistant *S. aureus* infections among patients in the emergency department. *N Engl J Med.* 2006;355(7):666–674.

Reiber GE. The epidemiology of diabetic foot problems. *Diabet Med.* 1996;13(suppl 1):S6–S11.

Stevens DL, Bisno AL, Chambers HF, et al. Practice guidelines for the diagnosis and management of skin and soft-tissue infections. *Clin Infect Dis.* 2005;41(10):1373–1406.

Tice A. Outpatient parenteral antimicrobial therapy as an alaternative to hospitalization. *Int J Clin Pract.* 1998;95(suppl):4–8.

59 VIRAL GASTROENTERITIS
Harry Schrager

EPIDEMIOLOGY/OVERVIEW

- Viral gastroenteritis is extremely common, causing significant morbidity in developed countries and significant mortality in the developing world.
- Most cases of acute gastroenteritis are viral. While the mortality rate is low, morbidity is significant, and results in ~ 700,000 hospital admissions yearly in the United States.
- *Norovirus* (previously known as Norwalk-like viruses) causes the majority (~ 90%) of epidemic gastroenteritis, with 23 million cases, 612,000 hospitalizations, and 3000 adult deaths annually in the United States.
- At least half of all food-borne illness is caused by noroviruses.
  - In addition to restaurants (39%) and catered events, the most common settings for outbreaks of noroviruses are hospitals and long-term care facilities (29%). Outbreaks on cruise ships are also common.

- *Rotavirus* is the most common diarrheal illness in children under the age of 2. It occurs both as an endemic and epidemic disease, and results in 400,000 physician visits, 200,000 emergency department (ED) visits, and 55,000–70,000 hospitalizations annually in the United States, at a cost of $300,000,000.
- Viruses primarily associated with sporadic gastroenteritis include
  - Enteric adenovirus, predominantly seen in children under the age of 2
  - Astrovirus, largely a pediatric illness, but also seen in the elderly and immunocompromised

NOROVIRUS

- Norovirus infects the jejunum (sparing stomach and colon), resulting in an intact mucosa with blunting of the microvilli, widening of the intercellular spaces, and leukocytic infiltration of the lamina propria. These histologic changes underlie the clinical features of
  - Malabsorption
  - Increased intestinal fluid secretion
  - Gastroparesis and delayed gastric emptying, promoting nausea and vomiting
- Noroviruses survive temperatures ranging from freezing temperatures to 60°C, and tolerate levels of chlorine in excess of that typical of public water supplies.
- Norovirus is shed in the stool for 1–2 weeks following the onset of clinical symptoms. Norovirus is spread is by fecal-oral contamination, contaminated water (including swimming pools), food (steamed oysters have caused several outbreaks), and fomites.
- Norovirus is highly infectious. Up to 80% of those exposed acquire the disease, although one-third of infections may be asymptomatic. As few as 10 virus particles can be infectious.

CLINICAL PRESENTATION, DIFFERENTIAL, MAKING THE DIAGNOSIS

- Norovirus infection presents after an incubation period of 1–2 days. Symptom onset is abrupt, with abdominal cramps, nausea, and vomiting. Although norovirus was once known as "winter vomiting disease," there is no confirmed seasonality to outbreaks of norovirus.
- Diarrhea, more common in adults than children with norovirus, is loose and watery, without blood or mucus.

Malaise, myalgia, headache, and low-grade fever are common. The illness is self-limited, lasting 1–3 days.

- There are no commercially available tests for norovirus, although sensitive and specific assays are available through the CDC for outbreak investigations (contact your local public health authorities). Diagnosis is typically based on clinical and epidemiologic features:
  - Stool cultures negative for bacterial pathogens or parasites
  - More than 50% of cases associated with vomiting
  - Mean duration of illness 12–60 hours
  - Mean incubation period 24–48 hours
- *Treatment*—The mainstay of treatment is supportive care with hydration and replacement of electrolyte losses. Bismuth and other antidiarrheals (eg, loperamide) may provide relief from abdominal cramping and frequency of stools, but do not significantly impact fluid and electrolyte losses.
  - Antidiarrheals are not recommended for children under the age of 5.
  - No vaccine is currently available for norovirus. Infection confers only temporary strain-specific immunity.
  - Prevention consists of infection control measures.
    - Food-borne and water-borne disease may be prevented by correct handling of foods, strict handwashing by food-handlers after using the bathroom and before handling food items, and paid sick leave for food-handlers who are ill.
    - In healthcare facilities, in addition to strict adherence to standard precautions including hand hygiene and environmental decontamination, strategies should include the use of private rooms or cohorting of sick patients. Contact precautions to prevent staff contamination while caring for and/or cleaning up after patients with vomiting or diarrhea should be implemented.

ROTAVIRUS

- Histologically, the jejunum and duodenum in rotavirus infection show patchy blunting of the microvilli and monocytic infiltration of the lamina propria, and rotavirus can be detected by electron microscopy in the epithelium.
- Enterotoxins in acute rotavirus infection damages the mucosa and the brush-border enzymes involved in sugar metabolism, resulting in malabsorption and increased intestinal fluid secretion.
- Rotavirus is shed in the stool for 1–4 weeks following the onset of clinical symptoms, as well as in asymptomatic patients.

CLINICAL PRESENTATION, DIFFERENTIAL, MAKING THE DIAGNOSIS

- Patients with rotavirus present after an incubation period of 2 days with vomiting and watery diarrhea, without mucus or blood, lasting 3–8 days. Fever and abdominal pain are frequent features.
- Diagnosis can be confirmed by enzyme-linked immunosorbent assays (ELISAs) or latex agglutination tests of stool specimens. PCR assays and cultures are other options, but they may be less widely available.
- *Treatment*—The mainstay of treatment is supportive care with hydration and replacement of electrolyte losses.
  - Once rehydration is complete, refeeding may commence. Contrary to past popular belief, clear liquids or other limited diets (such as bananas, rice, applesauce, toast [BRAT]) are not necessary and are inadequate nutritionally. The avoidance of high-fat foods and lactose is prudent.
  - Antidiarrheal agents and most antiemetics should not be used, especially in young children, because of lack of proven efficacy and/or potential for significant adverse side effects. Ondansetron may be a reasonable option for protracted emesis.
  - Prevention of rotavirus consists of infection control measures analogous to those for norovirus.
  - *Vaccine development*—Universal immunization with pentavalent human-bovine rotavirus reassortant vaccine (approved by the Food and Drug Administration [FDA] in 2006) is recommended by the CDC and the American Academy of Pediatrics (AAP), and is effective in preventing ~ three-fourths of cases and significantly reduces ED visits and hospitalizations. It is administered as a series of three oral doses at ages 2, 4, and 6 months. Unlike a previous tetravalent human-rhesus rotavirus reassortant vaccine withdrawn from the US market in 1999, the newer vaccine has not been associated with an increased risk of intussusception.

BIBLIOGRAPHY

Centers for Disease Control and Prevention. Norwalk-like viruses: public health consequences and outbreak management. *MMWR Morb Mortal Wkly Rep.* 2001;50(No. RR-9): 1–17. Available at: www.cdc.gov/ncidod/dvrd/revb/gastro/norovirus.htm

Guerrant RL, Van Gilder T, Steiner TS, et.al. Infectious Diseases Society of America guidelines: practice guidelines for the management of infectious diarrhea clinical infectious diseases. *Clin Infect Dis.* 2001;32:331–351. Available at: www.idsociety.org.

Kapikian AZ, Estes MK, Chanock RM. Norwalk group of viruses. In: Fields BN, Knipe DM, Howley PM, eds. *Fields Virology.* 3rd ed. Vol. 1. Philadelphia, PA: Lippincott-Raven; 1996: 783–810.

King CK, Glass R, Bresee JS, et al. Managing acute gastroenteritis among children: oral rehydration, maintenance, and nutritional therapy. *MMWR Recomm Rep.* 2003;52(RR16):1–16. Available at: www.cdc.gov/mmwr/preview/mmwrhtml/ rr5216a1.htm.

Koo D, Maloney K, Tauxe R. Epidemiology of diarrheal disease outbreaks on cruise ships, 1986 through 1993. *JAMA.* 1996;275:545–547.

Mounts AW, Holman RC, Clarke MJ, et al. Trends in hospitalizations associated with gastroenteritis among adults in the United States, 1979–1995. *Epidemiol Infect.* 1999;123:1–8.

Musher DM, Musher BL. Contagious acute gastrointestinal infections. *N Engl J Med.* 2004;351:2417–2427.

Richardson S, Grimwood K, Gorrell R, et al. Extended excretion of rotavirus after severe diarrhoea in young children. *Lancet.* 1998;351:1844.

Rockx B, de Wit M, Vennema H, et al. Natural history of human calicivirus infection: a prospective cohort study. *Clin Infect Dis.* 2002;35:246–253.

White KE, Osterholm MT, Mariotti JA, et al. Foodborne outbreak of Norwalk virus gastroenteritis: evidence for post-recovery transmission. *Am J Epidemiol.* 1986;124:120–126.

Widdowson M-A, Sulka A, Bulens SN, et al. Norovirus and foodborne disease, United States, 1991–2000. *Emerg Infect Dis.* [serial on the Internet]. January 2005 [date cited]. Available at: http://www.cdc.gov/ncidod/EID/vol11no01/04-0426.htm.

WEB RESOURCE

Centers for Disease Control and Prevention. www.cdc.gov/rotavirus/

60 ANTIBIOTIC RESISTANCE

John J. Ross

EPIDEMIOLOGY/OVERVIEW

- The prevalence of antibiotic-resistant organisms in both hospital and community has mushroomed in the last 20 years.
- This crisis of resistance has been compounded by a dearth of new antibiotics.

- As antibiotic resistance mounts, many pharmaceutical companies have actually shrunk their anti-infective drug discovery programs, in favor of developing more profitable agents for chronic conditions, such as cardiovascular disease and erectile dysfunction.

PATHOPHYSIOLOGY

- Much antibiotic resistance is an inevitable consequence of widespread antibiotic use, particularly as many bacterial mechanisms of resistance antedate the antibiotic era.
- However, potentially preventable causes of antibiotic resistance include antibiotic overprescription by physicians and misuse, as well as the massive usage of antibiotics in agriculture, which is 10–30 times greater than human consumption in the United States.
- There are several clinically relevant mechanisms of antibiotic resistance (Table 60-1).
  - *Beta-lactamases* are the major source of resistance to beta-lactam antibiotics, such as penicillins, cephalosporins, and carbapenems.
    - Some beta-lactamases are evolutionarily ancient, having perhaps evolved from penicillin-binding proteins (PBPs) as long as two billion years ago, but beta-lactamases have markedly increased in diversity, distribution, and prevalence in the decades since the clinical introduction of antibiotics.
    - Minor mutations may significantly widen the spectrum of activity of beta-lactamases, accounting for the rapid expansion in resistance owing to this mechanism in recent years. Over hundreds of beta-lactamases have been characterized, grouped into four major classes.
    - In the healthcare setting, genes for beta-lactamases and other resistance mechanisms may be widely disseminated among bacteria via plasmids, transposons, and integrons.
    - The presence of chromosomal beta-lactamases may only become apparent after exposure to a broad-spectrum beta-lactam drug. This type of inducible gram-negative beta-lactamase production is especially common in *Pseudomonas* and *Enterobacter*, in which the initial clinical isolates may be deceptively sensitive, with resistance emerging only during treatment.
  - *Altered target site*—Modifications in several antibiotic targets have become common as a result of antibiotic use. These include:
    - Altered PBPs in pneumococci
    - Ribosomal methylation, conferring resistance to macrolides and clindamycin

TABLE 60-1 Mechanisms of Antibiotic Resistance

RESISTANCE MECHANISM	IMPORTANCE	EXAMPLES
Enzymatic inactivation of antibiotic	High	Beta-lactamases, aminoglycoside-modifying enzymes
Altered target site	High	Ribosomal methylation (macrolides, clindamycin); alterations in PBPs (beta-lactams); mutations in DNA gyrase (quinolones)
Protection of target site	Moderate	*tetM* ribosomal protection protein (tetracyclines)
Diminished permeability	Moderate	Loss of porin proteins (beta-lactams, aminoglycosides, quinolones)
Efflux pumps	Moderate	Pseudomonal resistance to beta-lactams, streptococcal and staphylococcal resistance to macrolides
Overproduction of target site	Low	Hyperproduction of dihydropteroate synthase (sulfas)
Bypass of metabolic pathway	Low	Dependence on external thymine source (sulfas, trimethoprim)

- Mutations in DNA gyrase of gram-negative bacteria and topoisomerase IV in gram-positive bacteria, resulting in high-level fluoroquinolone resistance
  ○ *Efflux pumps*—They are energy-dependent membrane proteins that prevent intracellular accumulation of antibiotics. They are important in resistance to macrolides, beta-lactams, fluoroquinolones, and especially tetracyclines.
  ○ *Decreased permeability*—Penetration of beta-lactam antibiotics into gram-negative bacteria is partly dependent upon the presence of outer membrane channels known as porins. Mutations leading to loss of function or repression of production are major causes of gram-negative resistance to cephalosporins and carbapenems.
  ○ Pathogenic bacteria may combine multiple resistance mechanisms to evade the action of antibiotics. For example, it is not unusual for resistant strains of *Pseudomonas* in the healthcare setting to possess inducible beta-lactamases, efflux pumps, and diminished membrane permeability.

RISK FACTORS FOR ANTIBIOTIC-RESISTANT INFECTION

- Exposure to the healthcare system is the major risk factor for acquisition of most antibiotic-resistant bacteria. This risk increases with
  ○ Duration of hospitalization
  ○ Intensity of antibiotic exposure
  ○ Severity of illness
  ○ Malnutrition
  ○ Immunosuppression
  ○ Degree of instrumentation, such as placement of urinary catheters and central venous catheters
- Poor caregiver adherence to handwashing and other infection control practices is also a major risk factor.

- Chronically ill patients in long-term care facilities repeatedly treated with antibiotics and frequently readmitted to acute care hospitals are an important reservoir for antibiotic-resistant organisms.
- Strains of some resistant organisms, including *P. aeruginosa*, *Acinetobacter baumannii*, and VRE, are remarkably hardy, persisting in the hospital environment for weeks despite desiccation. This underscores the role of disinfection of patient rooms after discharge.

CLINICAL MANIFESTATIONS OF MAJOR ANTIBIOTIC-RESISTANT PATHOGENS

METHICILLIN-RESISTANT *Staphylococcal aureus*

- *S. aureus* is unique among virulent bacteria, being common in both community and hospital settings.
- Most hospital isolates of *S. aureus* in the United States are methicillin resistant.
- MRSA is an important cause of wound infection, cellulitis, bacteremia, and central-line sepsis in the hospital.
- MRSA is an increasingly important pathogen in diabetic foot infections and in other patients with osteomyelitis.
- MRSA causes about 25% of hospital-acquired pneumonia.
- MRSA is also an occasional cause of UTI in patients with Foley catheters.
- MRSA is, by definition, not susceptible to any beta-lactam antibiotics. Vancomycin is the most widely used antibiotic to treat serious MRSA infections in the hospital, and it is a bactericidal antibiotic with the best

track record in the treatment of MRSA bacteremia. It should be noted that although vancomycin is bactericidal, it is relatively slow-acting in this respect, and is clearly inferior to beta-lactams in the treatment of MSSA bacteremia.

- Vancomycin should be administered with caution to patients with unstable renal function, and elderly patients on long-term vancomycin should be monitored for ototoxicity.
- Oral bactrim is acceptable step-down therapy in many situations, excepting bacteremia.
- Linezolid is a useful alternative to bactrim in the oral therapy of MRSA. Limitations of linezolid include its expense and GI intolerance in up to 10% of patients. Like bactrim, it is bacteriostatic and should not be used to treat MRSA bacteremia. Linezolid also has a propensity to cause serotonin syndrome in patients taking selective serotonin reuptake inhibitors (SSRI), such as fluoxetine. Thrombocytopenia does not seem to be as common with linezolid therapy as initial reports suggested, but patients on linezolid should still be monitored for hematologic toxicity.
- Daptomycin is a relatively new, once-daily IV antibiotic approved for the treatment of skin and soft tissue infections caused by MRSA. Although daptomycin is bactericidal, there are at present limited data on its efficacy in the treatment of MRSA bacteremia.

COMMUNITY-ACQUIRED METHICILLIN-RESISTANT Staphylococcus aureus

- It has long been anticipated that MRSA would eventually become prevalent in the community, as well as the hospital setting. Although this proved to be correct, the exact manner in which this transpired was unforeseen.
  ○ It was erroneously predicted that MRSA would leach out of the healthcare system to cause community-acquired infections. However, a novel, virulent strain of MRSA, the USA300 strain, recently evolved in the community, quite distinct from nosocomial strains of MRSA.
- CA-MRSA has a smaller and more easily transferable version of the genetic element for methicillin resistance. CA-MRSA strains are also notable in usually having genes for PVL, a toxin producing neutrophil death and tissue necrosis. Strains of CA-MRSA positive for PVL are capable of causing serious infections in healthy individuals, including extensive boils and furunculosis, cellulitis, NF, and necrotizing pneumonia.
- CA-MRSA infections have been associated with athletes, soldiers, prisoners, men who have sex with men, HIV-positive persons, and IV drug users. However, they are on the rise among children and adults without traditional risk factors, and CA-MRSA has become a common pediatric pathogen in many regions of the United States.
- At least for the present, CA-MRSA in the United States is usually susceptible to clindamycin (most nosocomial strains of MRSA are resistant to clindamycin). CA-MRSA strains are also generally sensitive to bactrim, vancomycin, and linezolid.
- It has been suggested that clindamycin or linezolid might be particularly beneficial in the treatment of necrotizing infection because of PVL-positive strains of CA-MRSA, as these drugs inhibit protein synthesis and toxin production. However, there is little clinical evidence at present to back this assertion.

METHICILLIN-RESISTANT S. AUREUS CARRIER STATE

- About 31% of Americans are carriers for MSSA, and 1% are carriers for MRSA. Persons 65 years of age or older, women, persons with diabetes, and those who were in long-term care in the past year are more likely to have MRSA colonization. The major reservoir for human colonization is the anterior nares. S. aureus is not "normal skin flora," although it is able to colonize regions of skin breakdown in persons with surgical wounds, venous stasis ulcers, IVDU, psoriasis, eczema, and other skin conditions. There is no protective benefit of staphylococcal colonization. Persons colonized with MSSA or MRSA not only spread the bacteria to others, but they are also more likely to acquire active infection.
- Attempts may be made to eradicate the MRSA carrier state. The most popular and probably most effective strategy is intranasal mupirocin ointment twice daily for 5–7 days. The use of chlorhexidine liquid soaps in the shower or bath daily for 1 week may also be helpful in those with recurrent staphylococcal skin abscesses, or with axillary and perineal colonization.
- Elimination of MRSA carriage is less likely when MRSA reexposure is frequent or in the patient with a heavy burden of organisms, such as seen in decubitus ulcers or severe skin disease.

VANCOMYCIN-RESISTANT ENTEROCOCCI

- The rise in the prevalence of VRE over the past two decades has paralleled the increase in C. difficile infections.
  ○ The use of oral vancomycin to treat C. difficile is associated with VRE colonization.

○ VRE and *C. difficile* have several risk factors in common, including duration and intensity of antimicrobial exposure, exposure to specific agents (including third-generation cephalosporins, clindamycin, fluoroquinolones, and imipenem), patient age, length of hospitalization, and severity of underlying illness.

• Enterococci have relatively low virulence for healthy people. However, they are important nosocomial pathogens for several reasons.

○ Resistance to most commonly used antibiotics, including all cephalosporins, conferring a large selection advantage in the hospital setting. Even "sensitive" enterococci are only highly sensitive to penicillin, ampicillin, and vancomycin among older antibiotics.

○ The massive enterococcal cell wall helps it to survive dehydration and persists in the hospital environment on bedrails, fabrics, call buttons, and other fomites.

○ Biofilm production allows enterococci to adhere to and infect central venous catheters, Foley catheters, and other devices.

• VRE are important for two reasons.

○ VRE bacteremia is associated with increased mortality, especially in patients with neutropenia.

○ There are also grave concerns that the high prevalence of both VRE and MRSA in the hospital setting will facilitate the transfer of the enterococcal *VAN-A* genes for vancomycin resistance to staphylococci, resulting in vancomycin-resistant *S. aureus* (VRSA). Although strains of VRSA have been reported in the United States, they are presently rare.

• VRE in the healthcare setting most commonly causes UTI and vascular catheter-associated bacteremias. Prior to the availability of newer antibiotics with specific activity against VRE (Table 60-2), it was noted that some patients with VRE infections improved without antibiotics with the removal of a nidus of infection, such as a Foley catheter or central venous catheter. Therefore, removal of such foci is an essential component of the treatment of VRE infection.

• In asymptomatic patients with Foley catheters and positive urine cultures for VRE, it is acceptable to remove the urinary catheter, and await the results of repeat urine cultures before treating.

• Clinical isolates of VRE from some sites are of doubtful significance, especially when recovered as one of many bacterial species. Examples include decubitus ulcers, sputum, and intra-abdominal drainage. VRE isolates are more likely to require treatment if isolated in high quantity, and if the patient has a higher burden of acute and chronic illness.

• Specific management of VRE infection depends on the results of susceptibility testing. Ampicillin has useful activity against many strains of VRE. Tetracyclines and fluoroquinolones have marginal activity for some strains of VRE. Nitrofurantoin may be successful in patients with cystitis caused by VRE and normal renal function. The older, underused oral antibiotic fosfomycin, given as a single 3-g dose, may also be useful for VRE cystitis.

• The newer antibiotics, linezolid, tigecycline, and daptomycin, may be useful in the treatment of serious VRE infection. Of these three, only daptomycin is bactericidal.

• Quinupristin-dalfopristin is generally active against *Enterococcus faecium*, but not *E. faecalis*.

• The management of endocarditis caused by VRE is poorly defined, and should only be undertaken in conjunction with infectious diseases consultation.

EXTENDED SPECTRUM BETA-LACTAMASE-PRODUCING GRAM-NEGATIVE RODS

• *Klebsiella pneumoniae* is an encapsulated gram-negative pathogen associated with pyelonephritis, cholangitis, and less often pneumonia in the community. *Klebsiella* infections are more common in diabetics, probably

TABLE 60-2   Some Newer Antibiotics Potentially Useful in the Treatment of Drug-Resistant Bacteria

ANTIBIOTIC	ADVANTAGES	DISADVANTAGES
Linezolid	Active against MRSA and VRE	Bacteriostatic, hence limited utility in bacteremias and endocarditis; may cause serotonin syndrome if used with SSRIs; GI upset; cost
Tigecycline	Active against MRSA, VRE, some strains of ESBL-producing bacteria	Bacteriostatic; GI upset common; *Pseudomonas* and *Proteus* are resistant; cost
Colistin	Active against many highly resistant gram-negative pathogens	Not a new antibiotic; its use was abandoned in the 1970s because of nephrotoxicity and neurotoxicity
Daptomycin	Bactericidal antibiotic against MRSA and VRE	Pathogens may become less sensitive during treatment; cost
Telithromycin	Active against many strains of macrolide-resistant pneumococcus	May cause blurred vision, exacerbations of myasthenia gravis, and hepatotoxicity

reflecting impaired neutrophil phagocytosis of the luxuriant *Klebsiella* capsular polysaccharide.

- Recent years have seen a dramatic increase in strains of *Klebsiella pneumoniae* resistant to all beta-lactam antibiotics except for carbapenems, such as imipenem and meropenem. They are usually sensitive to amikacin, but often resistant to other aminoglycosides, such as gentamicin and tobramycin. Resistance to fluoroquinolones is also common in these isolates.

- These strains are sometimes colloquially known as "killer *Klebsiella*," in reference to the higher associated-mortality in many series.

- The hydrolytic enzyme responsible for this high-grade resistance is known as an extended-spectrum beta-lactamase (ESBL).

- ESBL genes are carried on plasmids, integrons, and transposons, and are typically accompanied by other antibiotic resistance genes, explaining the resistance to multiple drug classes commonly encountered in these isolates.

- The presence of an ESBL may be missed by an unwary technician in the microbiology laboratory, underscoring the importance of a careful review of antibiotic sensitivity data by clinicians.

- An important clue to the presence of an ESBL is sensitivity to a second-generation cephamycin, such as cefoxitin, and simultaneous resistance to a third-generation cephalosporin, such as ceftriaxone or ceftazidime. This laboratory artifact should prompt confirmatory testing to detect the presence of an ESBL.

- Healthcare-associated strains of *Proteus mirabilis* and *E. coli* may also possess ESBLs.

- ESBL-positive *Klebsiella* is presently a nosocomial pathogen, associated with pneumonia, UTI, intra-abdominal infection, bacteremias, and wound infection. Risk factors are similar to those for acquisition of other resistant nosocomial pathogens, including severity of illness, length of stay (LOS), ICU admission, hemodialysis, central venous catheter, urinary catheter, and intensity and duration of antibiotic exposure.

- When the microbiology laboratory confirms the presence of an ESBL, these strains should be considered functionally resistant to all beta-lactams, aside from carbapenems. Although they sometimes appear sensitive to cefepime and piperacillin-tazobactam in vitro, treatment failures have been reported with these agents.

PANDRUG-RESISTANT
Acinetobacter baumannii

- Another disturbing trend in recent years has been the emergence of *A. baumannii* strains resistant to

carbapenems and indeed all conventional antibiotics. Several outbreaks of pandrug-resistant *Acinetobacter* have occurred in US hospitals.

- *Acinetobacter* is ubiquitous in the environment. It has low virulence for healthy persons, and requires a breakdown in host defenses for pathogenicity, such as a tracheostomy site, IV catheter, or devitalized wound.

- *Acinetobacter* was a common cause of gram-negative wound infection in the Vietnam War, and has recently caused serious infections in wounded soldiers returned from the Middle East.

- Other gram-negative bacteria with resistance to all conventional antibiotics are becoming more prevalent as well, especially *P. aeruginosa*.

- Optimal management in unclear. Favorable results have been reported in some cases with the use of colistin (polymyxin E). Colistin is a cyclic, cationic polypeptide detergent with moderate specificity for bacterial cell membranes. Systemic IV use is associated with substantial nephrotoxicity and neurotoxicity, usually reversible after drug discontinuation. The safety profile of colistin is much more favorable when administered as an aerosol to patients with respiratory infection with pandrug-resistant GNR.

- Such cases are best managed in conjunction with infectious diseases consultation.

INFECTION CONTROL ISSUES

- Depending on resources, screening of high-risk patients for MRSA (nasal swabs) and VRE (rectal swabs) should be considered.

- Patients known to have infection or colonization with MRSA, VRE, or highly resistant GNR should be placed on contact precautions, including
  - A private room. If a private room is not available, the patient can be cohorted with another patient known to be colonized or infected with the same organism.
  - Gloves for all persons entering the room, regardless of whether they intend to have direct contact with the patient, followed by immediate removal of gloves and handwashing on leaving the room.
  - Gowns should be worn by all persons entering the room who anticipate substantial contact with the patient or the room environment, or if the patient is incontinent or has an open, undressed wound.
  - Patients on contact precautions should have dedicated items for personal care, such as stethoscopes, thermometers, and sphygmomanometers. When this is not possible, items should be thoroughly disinfected between patients.

THE ROLE OF HOSPITALISTS IN ANTIBIOTIC RESISTANCE PREVENTION

- Unfortunately, there is little cost to bacteria of acquiring and maintaining antibiotic resistance genes and potentially great survival benefit.
- Although some antibiotic resistance may be inevitable, its spread can be curtailed by concerted efforts to curb antibiotic overuse in agriculture, pediatrics, and hospital medicine.
- Multidisciplinary antibiotic stewardship programs seek to limit antibiotic resistance in hospitals by rationalizing and restricting antibiotic use. Ideally, hospitalists and infectious diseases physicians should collaborate in developing local guidelines for antibiotic use and restriction.
  ○ Diminishing the intensity and duration of antibiotic use reduces spread of resistance within the hospital.
  ○ Hospital antibiograms help to determine appropriate empiric therapy based on local patterns of antibiotic resistance.
- Narrow antibiotic coverage as soon as culture and sensitivity data are available.
- Observe meticulous contact precautions for patients with resistant organisms, especially the use of gloves.
- *Patient-to-patient transmission of resistant organisms within the hospital most commonly occurs via the hands of healthcare workers.* Handwashing is a simple and effective means to limit the spread of resistant bacteria by caregivers, but compliance rates are typically low. Handwashing compliance is typically worse among physicians than nurses, and lower in the hectic ICU setting than on general medical wards. Periodic surveillance of handwashing compliance by infection control practitioners is a useful means of education and reinforcement.
  ○ Alcohol-based handwashing is at least as effective as soap and water in clearing bacteria from hands, with much higher rates of compliance.
  ○ Hospitalists should wear gloves whenever exposure to *C. difficile* is likely, and hands should be washed afterward with antimicrobial soap and water, given the limited effect of alcohol-based handwashing on *C. difficile* spores.
- Invasive devices such as urinary catheters and central venous lines provide a foothold for the entry of resistant pathogens and should be removed whenever feasible.
- Some specialists treat *Pseudomonas* and similarly resistant GNR with two active antibiotics, such as a beta-lactam and an aminoglycoside, in the hope of forestalling the development of antibiotic resistance. A recent meta-analysis of clinical trials found no evidence to support this practice. However, treating serious *Pseudomonas* infections with two antibiotics prior to the availability of sensitivity data may improve outcomes, by making it more likely that the patient is receiving at least one effective antibiotic.
- Some hospitals have used "crop rotation" strategies of antibiotic use, periodically changing the workhorse antibiotics within an institution to limit selection pressures for resistance among hospital flora. Evidence supporting this approach is not robust, and one mathematical model predicts it may actually produce more antibiotic resistance.

CARE TRANSITIONS

- There is no uniform standard for removing patients with resistant organisms from contact precautions.
- In general, repeatedly negative cultures are required to assure resolution of active colonization. Most hospitals and long-term care facilities require two or three consecutive negative cultures of nares (for MRSA) or perineum (for VRE) and at least two consecutive negative cultures of previously positive sites, obtained after completion of antibiotic therapy and collected 5–7 days apart.
- When patients colonized or infected with resistant organisms are discharged to rehabilitation or long-term care facilities, it is reasonable and beneficial psychologically to allow them to participate in group meals and activities if wounds are covered, bodily fluids are contained, and they observe good hygienic practices.
- Healthy family members should be reassured that their risk from resistant nosocomial organisms is low. When patients are discharged to home, family members should wash hands after contact and when leaving the house. Gloves should be worn for contact with body fluids, and the patient's linen and environment cleaned on a regular basis.

BIBLIOGRAPHY

Bliziotis IA, Samonis G, Vardakas KZ, et al. Effect of aminoglycoside and beta-lactam combination therapy versus beta-lactam monotherapy on the emergence of antimicrobial resistance: a meta-analysis of randomized, controlled trials. *Clin Infect Dis.* 2005;41:149–158.

Centers for Disease Control and Prevention. *Acinetobacter baumannii* infections among patients at military medical facilities treating injured US service members, 2002–2004. *MMWR Morb Mortal Wkly Rep.* 2004;53:1063–1066.

Falagas ME, Kasiakou SK. Colistin: the revival of polymyxins for the management of multidrug-resistant gram-negative bacterial infections. *Clin Infect Dis.* 2005;40:1333–1341.

Jacoby GA, Munoz-Price LS. The new beta-lactamases. *New Engl J Med.* 2005;352:380–391.

Macdougall C, Polk RE. Antimicrobial stewardship programs in healthcare systems. *Clin Microbiol Rev.* 2005;18:638–656.

Magee JT. The resistance ratchet: theoretical implications of cyclic selection pressure. *J Antimicrob Chemother.* 2005;56:427–430.

Moellering RC Jr, Fishman, NO eds. Antimicrobial resistance prevention initiative: proceedings of an expert panel on resistance. *Am J Med.* 2006;119(6A):S1–S70.

Spellberg B, Powers JH, Brass EP, et al. Trends in antimicrobial drug development: implications for the future. *Clin Infect Dis.* 2004;38:1279–1286.

Zirakzadeh A, Patel R. Vancomycin-resistant enterococci: colonization, infection, detection, and treatment. *Mayo Clin Proc.* 2006;81:529–536.

WEB RESOURCE

http://www.hospitalmedicine.org/AM/Template.cfm?Section=Home&Template=/CM/HTMLDisplay.cfm&ContentID=7542

NEUROLOGIC ILLNESS

61 CONFUSION: EXAMINATION AND DIFFERENTIAL DIAGNOSIS

Zeina Chemali

EPIDEMIOLOGY/OVERVIEW

- Confusion is a mental state characterized by the lack of a clear and orderly thought process. The patient is not able to maintain a stream of coherent thoughts.
- Confusion is a common symptom and is frequently seen in multiple medical, neurologic, and psychiatric disorders including delirium, neurodegenerative diseases, schizophrenia (or dementia precox), and depression. Confusion can be acute or chronic.
  - Delirium affects 10% to 30% patients hospitalized with medical illness and can reach up to 50% in the elderly population.
  - Depression affects ~ 25% of the population at a given time.
  - Neurodegenerative diseases, most commonly Alzheimer's disease (AD), affect up to 25% of the aging population > 85 years of age.
- Confusion is one of the diagnoses for which processes of care are measured and reported, more so in hospital and residential settings. This is done to improve clinical outcomes and restrict patient harm and organizational liability.
- For the sake of clarification, the main categories of confusion will be discussed separately. Delirium is discussed at length in Chap. 62.

PATHOPHYSIOLOGY

- Confusion has a large number of underlying causes. With an acute change of mental status, life-threatening conditions need to be ruled out. However, chronic causes leading to confusional states are also common. Causes of confusion may be because of
  - The underlying medical condition and its treatment
  - Drug use or withdrawal
  - Drug side effects
  - Underlying neurologic conditions such as cerebrovascular accidents, seizure, migraine, neurodegenerative disorders, tumors, CNS infections, head trauma
  - Underlying psychiatric conditions, including schizophrenia, depression, panic attacks, and anxiety disorders
- The first step in dealing with confusion is to recognize it and look for its causative agent. Once the cause is known, treatment and management can be instituted.

CLINICAL PRESENTATION, DIFFERENTIAL, MAKING THE DIAGNOSIS

- An alteration in cognition and behavior should be recognizable right away at least to those who know the patient best. Inpatient physicians who have no baseline when they see a confused patient for the first time might overlook mild confusion. Because early changes in cognition may be subtle, hospitalists should consult with family members and caregivers to obtain an accurate picture of the patient's baseline mental status and any current change in mental status or behavior.
  - Behavior is the expression of the underlying mood and emotions coupled to cognitive processes leading to the understanding of a certain situation and providing accuracy in judgment and insight.
  - Thought processes and perception can be disrupted by confusion, and psychiatric and other disorders. Delusions are not only because of psychiatric diseases. Neurologic conditions can present with psychosis and delusions as seen in multiple sclerosis, AD, and seizures with postictal psychosis.
- Questions should address functional dependence, level of activity, history of falls, pain, and terminal illness.
- Moreover, individual factors should be taken into consideration, namely, the developmental history, any previous history of mental retardation or learning disability, the level of education, and relevant past psychiatric or neurologic history.
- The onset of the change should be noted.
  - Acute pathologies include trauma, infections, drug toxicity, or withdrawal.
  - Slowly progressive pathologies include dementia, slowly growing tumors, and psychiatric disorders.
  - If the illness has a fluctuating course (a hallmark of delirium), it should be noted as well.
- Symptoms of lethargy, fatigue, and weakness should be noted.
- Taking a detailed history and performing a thorough examination will help differentiate between an altered cognition caused by a chronic disease or aging and one resulting from serious metabolic or neuropsychiatric problem.
- The bedside examination should include a general and neurologic examination, as well as a detailed mental status examination assessing the higher mental functions (Table 61-1).

- Be sure to test for the level of alertness, attention, memory, language, and praxis.
- Other executive functions such as planning, initiation, motivation, insight, and judgment are assessed as part of the higher mental status functions. The frontal lobes are the primary sites for these functions. Any alteration or disease affecting the frontal lobes will be manifested by symptoms in the domains cited above.
- When a patient presents with a change in cognition, establish a baseline cognitive examination and monitor for changes. In the older hospitalized patient, the differential is often between delirium, dementia, and depression (Table 61-2) but may include structural disease that requires neuroimaging.
  - If acute changes are noted, perform a delirium assessment (see Chap. 62 for more details on delirium assessment and management).
  - If chronic changes are noted without the coexistence of delirium, perform a neurocognitive evaluation as stated above (see also Chap. 98 for more details on, section on dementia and Table 98-2).
- Major categories of neurologic and psychiatric disorders that may feature confusion in the clinical presentation are found in Table 61-3.

INITIAL EVALUATION

- The American Academy of Neurology's 2001 practice parameter for the evaluation of confusion and specifically dementia entails a CBC and complete metabolic profile (including magnesium and calcium), fasting blood sugar, cholesterol, triglycerides, thyroid-function tests, toxin screen, B_{12}, rapid plasma reagin (RPR), folate, cortisol level, urinalysis, electrocardiogram (ECG), and arterial blood gas to assess for conditions such as infections and metabolic disorders that can cause or contribute to cognitive dysfunction.
- Neuroimaging can be performed to rule out acute events such as stroke or subdural hematoma leading to confusion.
  - Performing an anatomic imaging study of the brain (CT with contrast or MRI) is highly recommended as part of the diagnostic workup of patients with cognitive impairment, particularly of recent/acute onset.
  - *Nuclear imaging*—Fluorine-18-labeled fluorodeoxyglucose (FDG) PET can document the

TABLE 61-1   Neurologic Examination of Confused Patients

Step 1: Attention

Establish the diagnosis of confusion (ie, abnormal attention). The inability to sustain attention is an indicator of delirium and needs to be assessed promptly. It is absolutely necessary to test attention before moving on to testing language and memory.
- Consciousness
  - Assess the level of arousal (awake, drowsy, lethargic, comatose)
  - Assess the level of awareness: The degree of orientation to person, space, and time is noted.
    - *Note: Orientation is not sensitive enough to pick up confusion and disorientation is nonspecific (as patient could also be psychotic, amnestic, aphasic).*
- Days of the week or months of the year forwards and backwards
  - *Note: Serial sevens and spelling words backwards are not good tests, particularly for patients who are illiterate/uneducated.*
- Have the patient play a game that requires attention. Examples include
  - Examiner taps once, patient taps twice on the table; examiner taps twice, patient does not tap on the table.
  - Patient taps the examiner's palm every time a certain letter of the alphabet is mentioned.

Step 2: Language

If attention is normal, proceed with testing language. When assessing the patient's language ability, he/she is asked to name, repeat, read, and write (if literate). The patient's comprehension is tested by his/her ability to follow commands.
- Start with speech. Engage the patient in a conversation, listen for output (assesses for aphasia and fluency).
- Test comprehension with following of simple commands (such as nodding yes or no answers), progressing to more complex commands involving multiple steps.
- Test repetition ("no ifs and/or buts"; "if I were to come, she would go").
- Test naming of objects.
- Ask the patient to read a sentence ("raise your right hand") out loud and perform the task in the sentence: tests reading and comprehension together.
- Have the patient write his name, address, and a sentence about the weather.

Step 3: Memory

If language is normal, test for amnesia. Memory is the ability to collect information, store, and retrieve it as needed.
- Immediate memory: digital span (also tests attention), repeat three words/objects (and ask the patient to remember them).
- Short-term memory: Ask them to recall the three words/objects given to them earlier.
- Long-term memory
  - Test recent memory by asking the name of the president. Ask the patient to remember what he/she had for breakfast (as long as this can be independently verified).
  - Have a conversation with the patient about something the patient is interested in, for example, if the patient is interested in football, ask about the local football team.
  - Assess remote memory: List presidents in reverse order, ask about other significant historic events and/or personal (verifiable) history such as names and ages of grandchildren.

Step 4: Calculation

- Ask the patient to perform simple computations ($2 + 5 = 7$)
- Ask the patient to solve word problems ("how many nickels are there in $1.65?")

Step 5: Construction

- Have the patient draw a clock with all the numbers and placing the hands at a particular time of day.

Step 6: Abstraction

- Ask the patient to explain similarities and differences.
  - What distinguishes a giraffe from other animals? A long neck.
  - What is similar about apples and oranges?

Step 7: Look for focal neurologic deficits by screening cranial nerve, reflex, motor, and sensory examinations.

- Note visuospatial neglect and anosognosia (lack of awareness of the deficit).
- Note any apraxias: the inability to carry out learned movements/tasks because of an acquired brain disease. Apraxias are common in neurodegenerative diseases.

Note: Do not use the Mini-Mental State Examination (MMSE)—the numbers do not mean anything without a baseline.

TABLE 61-2   Differentiating Between Depression, Delirium, and Dementia at the Bedside

PARAMETER	DEPRESSION	DELIRIUM	DEMENTIA
Onset	Weeks	Abrupt, hours/days	Months to years
Duration	3–6 months, may be chronic	Days to 3 weeks	Years
Orientation	Intact	Disorientation, but usually not to person	Disoriented
Level of consciousness	Intact	Disturbed	Intact
Symptoms	Apathy, hopelessness, sadness, little effort to perform task	Impaired attention, inconsistent performance, difficulty to understand task	Impaired cognition in multiple domains, intact effort at performing task
Judgment	Poor judgment, fear of making a decision	Impaired	Impaired, may lack insight
Diurnal pattern	Worse in morning	Day drowsiness	"Sundowning"
	Sleep impaired	Frequent hallucinations, nightmares	Impaired sleep
Psychosis	Delusions	Delusions	Late delusion

TABLE 61-3   Major Categories of Neurologic and Psychiatric Disorders That May Feature Confusion in the Clinical Presentation

Inherited disorders and developmental disorders	• Mental retardation caused by static encephalopathy from congenital or inherited disorders • Fragile X • Huntington's disease • Wilson's disease • Leukodystrophies • Porphyrias

Neurodegenerative disorders	• AD is the most prevalent dementia.
	  ○ It affects 6% of people at 65 years, and its prevalence doubles every 5 years.
	  ○ It presents with memory complaints affecting short-term memory, semantic memory, and later on procedural memory. Visuospatial deficits are noted. Personality changes occur later in the disease.
	  ○ AD is caused by an abnormal degeneration of neurons with the presence of neuritic plaques with beta-amyloid cores and neurofibrillary tangles of phosphorylated tau proteins. Beta-amyloid deposition causes cell damage and cell death giving rise to the symptoms of AD (Nussbaum and Ellis, 2003).
	  ○ Cholinergic neuronal transmission is the earliest neurotransmitter casualty in AD. By the first year of diagnosis, 40%–90% of choline acetyltransferase is decreased in the cortex and the hippocampus with the nucleus basalis of Meynert showing a slow and progressive neuronal loss throughout the disease state.
	• Vascular dementia, affecting men more than women over the age of 50, is the second most common dementia and classically presents with a stepwise deterioration.
	  ○ Confusion may develop because of an acute intercurrent illness or acute strokes or intracerebral hemorrhages (associated with focal neurologic findings), or as a dementia-like syndrome characterized by white matter changes and chronic cerebral ischemia.
	  ○ Risk factors include hypertension and rhythm abnormalities (Knopman, 2006).
	• Frontotemporal dementia presents at a younger age with personality changes.
	  ○ Depression and psychosis could be prominent.
	  ○ The patient shows deficits in executive function early on.
	  ○ Memory and visuospatial disturbances occur late in the disease (Sjogren and Andersen, 2006).
	• LBD is a neurodegenerative disorder that is characterized by cognitive impairment, fluctuating mental status, Parkinsonian features and visual hallucinations.
	  ○ The behavioral aspects of the disorder are common and poorly responsive to antipsychotic medication.
	• Corticobasal ganglionic degeneration
	• Parkinson's disease and dementia
	• Prion diseases
	• Progressive supranuclear palsy

CNS infections	• Although less common than structural lesions, CNS infections, including brain abscesses, are equally dangerous. Patients present with acute or subacute confusion. • CNS infections causing acute or chronic mental status changes should be considered as a neuropsychiatric emergency and treatment instituted as soon as possible. • Common infectious agents causing confusion include HIV, HSV, VZV, West Nile Virus, Lyme disease, syphilis, Listeria *S. pneumoniae* and *Neisseria meningitidis*. See Chap. 65.
Inflammatory and autoimmune disorders	• Systemic lupus erythematous with CNS involvement • Whipple's disease • Multiple sclerosis. Being among the most devastating neurologic disorders affecting young patients and causing cognitive and emotional problems. Confusion can be the only presentation of the demyelinating illness.
Neoplastic lesions and paraneoplastic syndromes	• All types of primary cancers and metastasis to the brain and the meninges can present with confusion (Washburn, 2005). • In addition, the paraneoplastic limbic encephalitis presents with a profound memory deficit where the information is lost as soon as it is encoded.

Trauma	• Head injury is the most common cause of neuropsychiatric syndromes causing confusion and alteration in higher mental functions.
	  ○ Especially in the elderly population, one should elicit the history to rule in or rule out chronic subdural collections.
	  ○ For any acute change in mental status, subarachnoid hemorrhage and epidural collection should be ruled out by performing a head CT and if clinically indicated a spinal tap, by checking for xanthochromia.

(Continued)

TABLE 61-3   Major Categories of Neurologic and Psychiatric Disorders That May Feature Confusion in the Clinical Presentation (*Continued*)

Endocrine and metabolic disorders	Patients can present with symptoms of confusion, agitation, mood and behavioral changes, memory problems, and so on with the following diagnoses: • Diabetes • Thyroid disorders • Pheochromocytoma • Any electrolyte imbalance (Bazakis and Kunzler, 2005), particularly hypo- and hypernatremia • Illicit drug use and alcohol intake • Wernicke's encephalopathy is a neuropsychiatric emergency requiring IV thiamine. • B_{12} deficiency may present with cognitive abnormalities even before significant macrocytosis and anemia are present.
Seizures	• These attacks are generally brief, stereotyped, and recurrent. They can occur in relation to the sleep cycle, the menstrual cycle or because of a structural or developmental lesion. • Although often in adults, seizures may be the first manifestation of CNS primary structural lesions, be it a tumor, a vascular malformation, or a cerebrovascular accident, idiopathic seizures are common. • A transient disturbance in memory or behavior may be the only sign for temporal lobe epilepsy. Patients sometimes complain of accelerated forgetting. Symptoms should not be attributed to a de novo psychiatric disorder unless seizures have been entertained and ruled out. • The EEG is often normal. • A 24-hour recording or long-term monitoring may be needed to rule out this diagnosis.
Migraine	• A common neurologic disorder, with a female predominance. The disability ranges from moderate to severe and the frequency of attacks depends on gender and socioeconomic context with women from low-income households between the ages 30 and 49 years being especially high risk. • Migraine is experienced as a paroxysmal headache, often unilateral, associated at times with nausea and visual distortions. Migraine is classified according to the Headache Classification Committee into many subgroups. • Confusion is often seen as a prodrome or part of the migraine with aura. • A good history, in a young patient, is generally sufficient to rule in or rule out this disorder.
Sleep disorders	Patients with chronic sleep disorders may present with confusion, and they are more prone to psychiatric disorders (Lieberman et al. 2005). The most common sleep disorders are • OSA is suggested by a history of snoring in an obese patient. • RLS is suggested by a history of an urge to move the legs in the evening and at rest. • Narcolepsy is suggested by a history of a sudden attack of sleepiness triggered by an emotional stimulus. These disorders may present with symptoms of excessive daytime sleepiness, tiredness, and confusion. Patients may present with complaints of executive dysfunction with deficits in organizational skills, attention, and planning.
Psychiatric diseases	Depression, psychosis, anxiety, and panic disorders. A small but significant percentage of patients presenting with confusion have a primary psychiatric disorder. • A prior history of psychiatric disease is important in making this diagnosis. • It is uncommon to have a de novo psychiatric illness, presenting as confusion, especially if the patient is past the critical time for illness declaration, ie, early twenties for schizophrenia, 20–30 years old in affective disorders. • In a young population, drug withdrawal or intoxication is a prime factor presenting as an acute change of mental status. • In the elderly population, drug-drug interactions are common causes of confusion. The examiner should assess for a thought disorder, inquire about reality distortions as in delusions and perceptual abnormalities as in hallucinations. Keep in mind that comorbid psychiatric disorders are more frequent in a medically sick population and in neurologic patients (Butler et al., 2005). Examples: • The high incidence of affective disorders, panic attacks, and hallucinations in epilepsy • The high incidence of depression in multiple sclerosis and Parkinson's disease • Apathy in neurodegenerative disorders

Abbreviations: LBD, Lewy body dementia; HSV, herpes simplex virus; VZV, varicella zoster virus; EEG, electroencephalography; OSA, obstructive sleep apnea; RLS, restless legs syndrome.

presence of an anatomic deficit in the evaluation of patients with cognitive impairment. Single-photon emission computed tomography (SPECT) assesses brain metabolism indirectly by imaging the regional distribution of blood flow. The presence of the characteristic biparietal-temporal flow defects in a subject with no vascular disease would be highly suggestive of AD.

- *Electroencephalography (EEG)*—EEG is used to rule out seizures and to check on background brain activity. If positive, it is helpful. The physician should always base the diagnosis of seizure and seizure-related disorders on history and push for long-term monitoring if needed.
- Lumbar puncture may be indicated for some patients to rule out a reversible cause of dementia or chronic confusional state. Otherwise cerebrospinal fluid biomarkers have no diagnostic advantage over a competent clinical diagnosis in patients with cognitive dysfunction.
- Neuropsychological testing, performed in the outpatient setting, is likely to provide more complete information regarding the nature of the cognitive impairments in addition to providing a quantitative and qualitative baseline useful in evaluating future change.

DISEASE MANAGEMENT STRATEGIES

- The treatment of confusion and altered mental status, whether it is acute or chronic, starts by treating the underlying cause leading to the perturbation of cognition, behavior, and affect. For chronic changes in mental status, a dementia evaluation is performed usually in the outpatient setting after reversible causes of chronic confusion are ruled out.
- When a dementing disorder or a confusional state is accompanied by severe symptoms such as psychosis, agitation, and violent or disinhibited behavior putting the patient and his environment at risk, other treatment modalities are used, such as medications.

Medications used to manage confusional states.

- Neuroleptics
  - Caution is given to the development of a metabolic syndrome, hypertension, diabetes, obesity, prolactin elevation, and QTc prolongation.
  - The medications include aripiprazole, olanzapine, quetiapine, risperidone, and ziprasidone.

  - They can increase the risk of cerebrovascular adverse events including strokes and transient ischemic attacks as evidenced in studies comparing these agents to placebo.
  - Typical antipsychotics like haloperidol have a high incidence of extra pyramidal syndrome (EPS) and can cause confusion owing to their anticholinergic properties.
- Benzodiazepines are less effective than antipsychotics in the treatment of agitation in the elderly. They can cause paradoxical agitation, confusion, memory problems, and excessive sedation. When used with other CNS agents, they may precipitate respiratory depression. They also increase the risk of falls in the elderly. Their use is recommended on a short-term basis only.
- *Anticonvulsants*—When used to treat agitation, the patients should be monitored for drug-drug interactions. Titration should be slow. Most commonly used agent in emergency settings is valproic acid with easy IV access.
- Caregivers are assisted and supported.

CARE TRANSITIONS

- Patients are prescribed medications targeting symptoms (see above) in addition to addressing their needs for assistance in their activities of daily living (ADL).
- Patients may require at least temporary placement in a secure and supervised environment such as a transitional care unit or skilled nursing facility, depending on their other medical needs.
- Family, particularly those in caregiver roles, need assistance and support, especially if the patient comes home while still confused, such as with patients suffering from dementia.
- Dementia cannot be diagnosed in the inpatient setting, although a new diagnosis of dementia may be suspected. Such patients need referral for outpatient evaluation once the acute medical issues that brought them to the hospital have resolved.
  - So far, curative treatment for AD is not available. The most successful approach to treat AD is to boost acetylcholine available to the cells by inhibiting its destruction by acetyl cholinesterase, hence the development of acetyl cholinesterase inhibitors (Table 61-4).

TABLE 61-4 Medications for Slowing the Progression of Dementia

DRUG	ACTION	DOSE	SIDE EFFECTS
Donepezil	An acetyl cholinesterase inhibitor	The dose range is 5–10 mg daily	To prevent GI side effects, nausea and diarrhea, titration should be slow, often starting with the lowest dose every other day. GI effects decrease when the drug is taken with food. It may also cause insomnia, fatigue, muscle cramps, fatigue, tremor, and anorexia.
Galantamine	An acetyl cholinesterase inhibitor with dual action matching cholinesterase inhibition with direct nicotinic agonist actions causing acetylcholine release	Usual dose range is 8–32 mg daily	GI side effects necessitate slow titration of the. dose It should be used with caution in patients with moderate hepatic impairment and the dose should be decreased.
Rivastigmine	Long-acting agent with selectivity for acetylcholinesterase and butyrylcholinesterase inhibition Studies have shown its efficacy in LBD	Initiate at 1.5 mg bid and then increase by 1.5 mg every month	Because of severe GI side effects, a long titration phase is necessary.
Memantine	Memantine is an NMDA antagonist. Recent studies show that memantine has small beneficial effects at 6 months in moderate-to-severe AD (Areosa et al. 2006)	Maximum dose of 20 mg/d	Physicians should monitor for side effects, agitation, and visual hallucinations.

Abbreviation: NMDA, N-methyl-D-aspartate.

BIBLIOGRAPHY

Areosa SA, Sherriff F, McShane R, et al. Memantine for dementia. *Cochrane Database Syst Rev.* 2006;(2):CD003154.

Bazakis A, Kunzler C. Altered mental status due to metabolic or endocrine disorders. *Emerg Med Clin North Am.* 2005;23:901–908.

Budson A, Price B. Memory dysfunction. *N Engl J Med.* 2005;352:692–699.

Butler C, Zeman A. Neurological syndromes which can be mistaken for psychiatric conditions. *J Neurol Neurosurg Psychiatry.* 2005;76 (suppl 1):i31–i38.

Cockrell JR, Folstein MF. Mini-mental state examination (MMSE). Psychopharmacol Bull. 1988;24(4):689–692.

Cummings JL, Frank JC, Cherry D, et al. Guidelines for managing Alzheimer's disease: Part II. Treatment. *Am Fam Physician.* 2002;65:2525–2534.

Daffner KR, Mesulam MM, Scinto LFM, et al. The central role of the prefrontal cortex in directing attention to novel events. *Brain.* 2000;123:927–939.

Gleason O. Delirium. *Am Fam Physician.* 2003;76(5):1027–1032.

Inouye S. Delirium in older persons. *N Engl J Med.* 2006;354:1157–1165.

Knopman DS. An overview of common non-Alzheimer dementias. *Clin Geriatr Med.* 2001;17(2):281–301.

Knopman DS. Dementia and cerebrovascular disease. *Mayo Clin Proc.* 2006;81(2):223–230.

Lieberman et al. Severe decrements in cognition function and mood induced by sleep loss, heat, combat, dehydration and undernutrition during simulated combat. *Biol Psychiatry.* 2005;57(4):422–429.

Milisen K, Braes T, Fick DM, et al. Cognitive assessment and differentiating the 3Ds (dementia, depression, delirium). *Nurs Clin North Am.* 2006;41(1):v1–v22.

Nussbaum RL, Ellis CE. Alzheimer's disease and Parkinson's disease. *N Engl J Med.* 2003;348(14):1356–1364.

Sjogren M, Andersen C. Frontotemporal dementia—a brief review. *Mech Ageing Dev.* 2006;127(2):180–187.

Washburn L. Altered mental status: cause determines treatment. *JAAPA.* 2005;18(2):16–22.

62 DELIRIUM

Jatin K. Dave, Colleen M. Crumlish,
and James Rudolph

EPIDEMIOLOGY/OVERVIEW

- Delirium is a syndrome characterized by the acute onset of impaired attention that fluctuates, together with altered consciousness and impaired cognition.
- Delirium can be the sole indicator of serious illness and should be treated as a medical urgency.
- In hospitalized older adults, the prevalence of delirium is 10% to 31% upon hospital admission and the incidence is 3% to 29% after admission.
- Delirium is associated with as high as a 10-fold increase in in-hospital mortality.
- Patients are at increased risk for falls, infections, and pressure ulcers. Additionally, patients with delirium have increased LOS, staff time requirements, and rates of nursing home placement and loss of independence, all of which represent significant costs to the healthcare system.
- Despite the incidence of delirium and its associated morbidity, mortality, and costs, more than 50% of cases go unrecognized by physicians.
- There is evidence to suggest that delirium can be prevented with cost-effective intervention protocols that address delirium risk factors.
- Delirium can be classified by the affected population: *postoperative delirium, ICU delirium, and terminal delirium,* or by the subtype: hypoactive (50%), hyperactive (25%), or mixed (25%) delirium. Delirium can last for days to months.

PATHOPHYSIOLOGY

- The pathophysiology of delirium is poorly understood. A widespread cerebral metabolic dysfunction as a result of systemic processes such as electrolyte/ acid-base disturbances, hypoxia, or hypotension is a commonly proposed mechanism for the development of delirium.
- The exact nature of such metabolic disturbance needs further investigation. Three proposed mechanisms for metabolic failure include cholinergic failure, serotonin deficiency, and inflammatory pathways.
- Drugs with anticholinergic activities are common precipitants of delirium. Several small studies have demonstrated a strong association between serum anticholinergic activity levels and delirium in medical

and surgical patients. Recent research focuses on designing biomarkers for delirium.

CLINICAL PRESENTATION, DIFFERENTIAL, MAKING THE DIAGNOSIS

- Initial assessment in all patients (Fig. 62-1).
  1. Symptoms of delirium
     - Common symptoms of delirium include confusion/agitation, inability to focus/concentrate, disorientation, hallucinations, sleep disturbances, and decreased appetite. Other symptoms

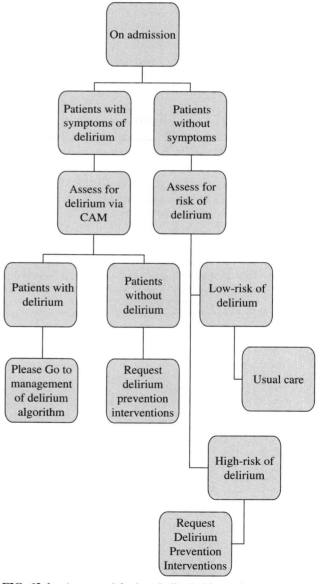

FIG. 62-1 A protocol for hospitalized older patients.

include functional decline, unsteady gait, recurrent falls, and tremor.
- Hypoactive delirium is more common than hyperactive delirium. The lack of behavioral disturbances in these patients is one explanation for high nondetection rates.
2. Risk assessment
   - The development of delirium involves the complex interrelationship between a vulnerable patient with predisposing risk factors and exposure to precipitating events (see Table 62-1).
   - Patients with many predisposing factors are at high risk for delirium with mild stress. The presence of more than one risk factor has a multiplicative rather than additive effect on delirium risk (Inouye 1998). For example, an older male patient with advanced dementia and visual impairment may develop delirium with a single administration of a medication with high anticholinergic activity (such as diphenhydramine) or even with a simple change in environment such as hospitalization. Conversely, a patient with few predisposing risk factors will develop delirium only when exposed to multiple or severe precipitating factors (eg, major surgery, severe illness, ICU admission, multiple psychoactive medications).
3. Diagnosing delirium via a Confusion Assessment Method (CAM)/Diagnostic and Statistical Manual of Mental Disorders, Fourth Edition (DSM-IV) criteria and differentiating delirium from depression
   - Delirium is a clinical diagnosis often based on observed changes in mental status. Acute onset, fluctuating levels of consciousness, and impaired attention are the hallmarks of delirium (see Table 62-2).

TABLE 62-1 Risk Assessment

PREDISPOSING FACTORS	PRECIPITATING FACTORS
Cognitive impairment	> 6 total medications
Increased comorbidity	> 3 new inpatient medications
Sensory impairment	Psychotropic medication
Age	Infection
Male gender	ICU admission
Depression	Dehydration (BUN-creatine ratio > 18)
Alcohol abuse	Environmental change
	Restraint use
	Malnutrition
	Use of bladder catheter
	Iatrogenic event (falls, hospital-acquired infections, complications of diagnostic procedures, or medication toxicity)

Abbreviation: BUN, blood urea nitrogen.

- Two commonly used validated instruments include the DSM-IV and the CAM. In combination with mental status testing, the CAM has become the preferred tool for diagnosis of delirium.
- Differentiating delirium from dementia and depression is highlighted in Table 62-3. This is especially challenging for hospitalists because of
  - A lack of baseline cognitive assessment
  - The higher prevalence of undiagnosed dementia and depression
  - A possible coexistence of two disorders (delirium and dementia)
- In patients with an acute change in mental status, the diagnosis of delirium should be presumed until proven otherwise.

TABLE 62-2 CAM versus DSM-IV

DSM-IV	CAM (the diagnosis of delirium requires the presence of 1 and 2 and either 3 or 4)
Disturbance of consciousness with reduced ability to focus, sustain, or shift attention.	1. Acute change in mental status and fluctuating course
A change in cognition or the development of a perceptual disturbances that is not better accounted for by a preexisting, established, or evolving dementia.	2. Inattention
The disturbance develops over a short period of time (usually hours to days) and tend to fluctuate during the course of the day	3. Disorganized thinking
There is evidence from the history, physical examination, or laboratory findings that the disturbance is caused by direct physiologic consequences of a general medical condition.	4. Altered level of consciousness

TABLE 62-3   Differentiating Dementia from Delirium and Depression

	DEMENTIA	DEPRESSION	DELIRIUM
Onset	Insidious (years)	Subacute (weeks to months)	Abrupt (days)
Consciousness	Clear	Clear	Altered
Primary defect	Memory	Mood	Attention
Hallmark	Progression	Response to Rx	Fluctuation
Patient may report	"I do not have memory problems" (reflecting lack of insight)	"I have very serious memory problems" (reflecting hopelessness)	Why do we care about memory? (reflecting disorganized thinking)

4. Assessment of delirious patients (Fig. 62-2)
   • Common causes of delirium are listed in Table 62-4.
   • Delirium is typically multifactorial in the elderly and requires a comprehensive approach to management.
   • Common causes of delirium include medications (both reaction and withdrawal), pain, electrolyte disturbances, urinary retention/stool impaction, and infections.
   • History focusing on the onset of symptoms, baseline cognition and function, symptoms of sensory impairment, malnutrition, new medications, falls, environmental change, bowel/bladder habits is helpful in patients with/at risk for delirium.
   • The physical examination should focus on vital signs, volume status, cardiopulmonary, skin, abdomen, and neurologic assessment.
   • Laboratory testing should include a CBC with differential, urinalysis, electrolyte testing, and ECG on all patients. Additional laboratory and radiology studies should be directed by the history and physical examination.
   • A CT scan of the the brain should be performed if there is a focal neurologic deficit, a history of trauma, or if the delirium etiology is unclear after the primary evaluation.

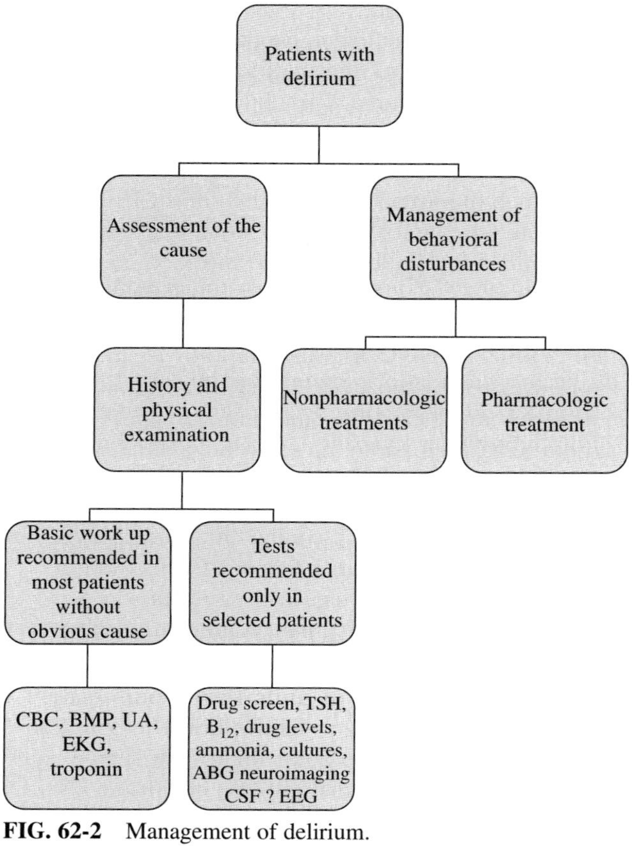

FIG. 62-2 Management of delirium.

TRIAGE AND INITIAL MANAGEMENT

• Delirium is a medical urgency and should be promptly assessed and treated.
• Initial assessment involves the determination of the patient's risk to harm oneself and the search for occult critical illnesses (eg, hypoglycemia, myocardial infarction [MI], sepsis).
• The treatment of behavioral disturbances using the lowest possible dose of medications and avoiding restraints are important strategies in providing quality care in hospitalized patients with delirium.
• Supportive care (eg, nutrition, skin care) and the prevention of complications (eg, falls, deep venous thromboses) are necessary while searching for the underlying causes.

DISEASE MANAGEMENT STRATEGIES

• Hospitalists are often involved in or lead initiatives to develop and/or implement clinical guidelines or care pathways for prevention, early detection, and management of delirium.

TABLE 62-4   Common Causes of Delirium

D	Drugs	Opioids, benzodiazepines
E	Electrolytes	Hyper-/hyponatremia, hyper-/hypoglycemia, and so forth.
L	Lack of drugs, water, or food	Pain, withdrawal, dehydration, and so forth.
I	Infection	Sepsis, UTI, aspiration pneumonia
R	Reduced sensory input	Impaired vision, impaired hearing, neuropathy
I	Intracranial causes	Subdural hematoma, meningitis, seizure
U	Urinary retention/fecal impaction	Drugs, constipation
M	Myocardial	MI, CHF, arrhythmia

- Delirium is considered a poor marker of overall quality of care in hospitalized older adults. Optimal inpatient care involves assessing delirium risk on every elderly patient, instituting prevention and early detection strategies, reducing hospital complications, and implementing evidence-based treatment guidelines.
- Protocols for risk assessment, risk factor modification, and nonpharmacologic and pharmacologic management of delirium may improve the care provided to hospitalized older adults.

TREATMENT

- Effective treatment of delirium requires
  - Prompt identification and management of the underlying causes focusing on predisposing and precipitating factors (as described above)
  - Nonpharmacologic measures, and
  - Timely pharmacologic measures to manage agitation
- One of the key steps in treating delirium is a careful review of the medication list and elimination of unnecessary medications.
- Removing unnecessary medical devices is another important step in treatment of delirium. Both formal restraints and informal restraints (such as IV catheters, oxygen tubing, urinary catheters, and ECG leads) are associated with delirium. Limiting the use of restraints to selected patients at risk of compromising their safety is essential.
- Nonpharmacologic strategies include
  - *Reorientation*—Using clocks, calendars, message boards, and when possible, family members
  - *Improving sensory input*—Restoring eyeglasses, hearing aids, and/or amplifiers
  - *Maintenance of sleep-wake cycle*—Increasing daytime activities and avoiding unnecessary night time interruptions (signs with "no vitals between 11 PM and 6 AM" in stable patients)
  - *Maintenance of nutrition*—Monitoring and providing assistance with meals if needed
  - *Maintenance of function*—Out of bed/ambulation schedule

- History, physical, laboratory, and diagnostic studies should guide other simultaneous treatments such as an appropriate bowel regimen to avoid constipation.

MANAGEMENT OF AGITATION

- Treatment of symptoms should coincide with identifying risk factors and searching for a precipitating cause of delirium.
- Pharmacologic therapy should be considered when nonpharmacologic management strategies have failed and agitated symptoms present a risk to the patient or others.
- While antipsychotic medications are the agents of choice, there is no drug with FDA approval for the treatment of delirium.
- The best existing evidence for the initial treatment of psychosis symptoms associated with delirium is for haloperidol.
- When feasible, a baseline ECG should be obtained before therapy to assess the QT interval. If the corrected QT interval is greater than 500 msec, an alternative agent is necessary. The QT interval should be monitored daily if therapy is continued.
- In addition to QTc prolongation, other contraindications to haloperidol include Parkinson's disease and dementia with Lewy bodies.
  - The lowest possible dose should be used and for the shortest duration. The recommended initial dosing in the elderly is 0.25–0.50 mg every 4 hours as needed intravenously or orally and 1–2 mg every 2–4 hours as needed in the general population (American Psychiatric Association).
    - The peak oral effect is 4–6 hours.
    - The peak IV effect is 20–40 minutes.
  - Dosing can be titrated for continued agitation. A single dose for the older, frail patient should not exceed 2 mg.
  - Older patients should be monitored for extra pyramidal, anticholinergic, and parkinsonian side effects.
  - Once symptoms are controlled, the drug should be tapered as soon as possible.

- Newer atypical antipsychotic medications (eg, olanzapine, quetiapine, risperidone, ziprasidone) have been tested only in small uncontrolled studies, are expensive, and are associated with increased mortality in patients with dementia.
- Benzodiazepines can cause/worsen delirium, but may be necessary for refractory agitation.
  ○ Lorazepam, starting at doses of 0.5–1.0 mg intravenously or orally, is recommended.
  ○ Benzodiazepines are also recommended in patients with Parkinson's disease and Lewy body dementia (LBD) who cannot tolerate neuroleptics and in alcohol/ sedative withdrawal.

PREVENTION

- Since over half the cases of delirium occur after hospital admission, it is important to consider iatrogenic and preventable causes of delirium.
- There is compelling evidence to support the efficacy of multicomponent strategies to prevent delirium. These strategies require risk assessment and modification, minimizing precipitating factors, appropriate medication prescribing, and surveillance methods.
- In a nonrandomized, controlled trial of 852 general medical patients greater than 70 years of age, a multi component strategy reduced the incidence of delirium (9.9% vs. 15% in usual care group) (Marcantonio et al. 2006).
  ○ Intervention protocols addressed cognitive impairment, sleep deprivation, immobility, visual and hearing impairment, and dehydration.
  ○ The nonpharmacologic sleep-enhancement protocol involved a warm drink at bedtime, relaxation music, and a back massage.
  ○ Fluorescent lights were turned off and unit-wide noise-reduction strategies were implemented.
  ○ With this intervention, many patients fell asleep spontaneously and the use of medication for sleep declined significantly.
- In a randomized controlled trial of proactive geriatric consultation in 126 hip fracture patients, the intervention group had reduced incidence (32% vs. 50% in usual care group) and severity (12% severe delirium vs. 29% in usual group) of delirium (McCusker et al. 2002). Recommendations focused on
  ○ Adequate oxygen delivery
  ○ Fluid/electrolyte balance
  ○ Pain management
  ○ Elimination of unnecessary medications
  ○ Regulation of bowel/bladder function
  ○ Nutrition

  ○ Early mobilization and rehabilitation
  ○ Prevention, early detection, and treatment of postoperative complications
  ○ Environmental stimuli
- Recent smaller studies evaluating haloperidol or donepezil preoperatively did not reduce the incidence of delirium (Sampson, 2006 #408; Kalisvaart, 2005 #159).

CARE TRANSITIONS

- Patients are often discharged to another level of care before their delirium is completely resolved. The hospitalist plays a critical role in this transition of care.
- Careful communication with the primary care provider and subacute care facility should focus on medications, patients' cognitive status on discharge, and hospital lab and study results. Attention should be given to continued supportive care and complication prevention.
- Patients with delirium are at higher risk of medication errors because of not being able to participate in medication reconciliation and the higher number of comorbidities/medications in frail older patients.
- Familiy and care taker education about delirium is also a key part of the care transition.

CONCLUSION

- Delirium is a common syndrome in hospitalized older adults that is under-recognized and often inappropriately managed.
- A systematic approach to all hospitalized patients focusing on delirium risk assessment and delirium diagnosis via CAM or *DSM-IV* criteria may allow early detection and proper management of delirium.
- Because of the morbidity and mortality associated with delirium, it should be considered a medical urgency.
- Hospitalists should identify delirium early and treat the underlying causes.
- The history, physical examination, and targeted ancillary testing can help identify the potential precipitating stressors.
- Appropriate nonpharmacologic measures and supportive care should be instituted. Pharmacologic treatment may be necessary to treat agitation.
- Strategies to prevent delirium are effective and should be implemented.

BIBLIOGRAPHY

American Psychiatric Association (APA): Practice guidelines for the treamtment of patients with delirium. *Am J Psychiatry.* 156;5 May 1999 Supplement.

Arfken C, Lichtenberg P, Tancer M. Cognitive impairment and depression predict mortality in medically ill older adults. *J Gerontol A Biol Sci Med Sci.* 1999;54:M152–M156.

Australian Society for Geriatric Medicine Position Statement No. 5 Orthogeriatric Care—Revised 2005doi:10.1111/j.1741-6612. 2005.00103.x. *Australas J Ageing.* 2005;24: 178–183.

Casarett DJ, Inouye SK. Diagnosis and management of delirium near the end of life. *Ann Intern Med.* 2001;135: 32–40.

Elie M, Rousseau F, Cole M, et al. Prevalence and detection of delirium in elderly emergency department patients. *CMAJ.* 2000;163:977–981.

Fields SD, MacKenzie CR, Charlson ME, S, et al. Cognitive impairment. Can it predict the course of hospitalized patients? *J Am Geriatr Soc.* 1986;34:579–585.

Hustey FM, Meldon SW. The prevalence and documentation of impaired mental status in elderly emergency department patients. *Ann Emerg Med.* 2002;39:248–253.

Inouye SK, Bogardus ST Jr, Charpentier PA, et al. A multicomponent intervention to prevent delirium in hospitalized older patients. *N Engl J Med.* 1999;340:669–676.

Inouye SK, Charpentier PA. Precipitating factors for delirium in hospitalized elderly persons. Predictive model and interrelationship with baseline vulnerability. *JAMA.* 1996;275: 852–857.

Inouye SK. Delirium after hip fracture: to be or not to be? *J Am Geriatr Soc.* 2001;49:678–679.

Inouye SK. Delirium in hospitalized elderly patients: recognition, evaluation, and management. *Conn Med.* 1993;57: 309–315.

Inouye SK. Delirium in hospitalized older patients: recognition and risk factors. *J Geriatr Psychiatry Neurol.* 1998;11: 118–125.

Inouye SK. Delirium: a barometer for quality of hospital care. *Hosp Pract (Minneap).* 2001;36:15–16, 18.

Inouye SK. Delirium in older persons. *N Engl J Med.* 2006;354:1157–1165.

Inouye SK. Prevention of delirium in hospitalized older patients: risk factors and targeted intervention strategies. *Ann Med.* 2000;32:257–263.

Kalisvaart KJ, de Jonghe JFM, Bogaards MJ, et al. Haloperidol prophylaxis for elderly hip-surgery patients at risk for delirium: a randomized placebo-controlled study. *J Am Geriatr Soc.* 2005;53:1658–1666.

Levkoff SE, Evans DA, Liptzin B, et al. Delirium. The occurrence and persistence of symptoms among elderly hospitalized patients. *Arch Intern Med.* 1992;152: 334–340.

Marcantonio ER, Flacker JM, Wright JR, et al. Reducing delirium after hip fracture: a randomized trial. *J Am Geriatr Soc.* 2001;49:516–522.

Marcantonio ER, Rudolph JL, Culley D, et al. Serum biomarkers for delirium. *J Gerontol A Biol Sci Med Sci* 2006;61: 1281–1286.

McCusker J, Cole M, Abrahamowicz M, et al. Delirium predicts 12-month mortality. *Arch Intern Med.* 2002; 162:457–463.

Sampson EL, Raven PR, Ndhlovu PN, et al. A randomized, double-blind, placebo-controlled trial of donepezil hydrochloride (Aricept) for reducing the incidence of postoperative delirium after elective total hip replacement. *Int J Geriatr Psychiatry.* 2007;22:343–9

Siddiqi N, House AO, Holmes JD. Occurrence and outcome of delirium in medical in-patients: a systematic literature review. (10.1093/ageing/afl005.) *Age Ageing.* 2006;35: 350–364.

63 ISCHEMIC STROKE/ TRANSIENT ISCHEMIC ATTACKS

Susan L. Hickenbottom

EPIDEMIOLOGY/OVERVIEW

- *Stroke* is a clinical syndrome characterized by rapidly developing symptoms or signs of focal neurologic dysfunction due to a vascular cause. Therefore, stroke includes both ischemic and hemorrhagic cerebrovascular events.

- *Cerebral infarction* or *ischemic stroke* is used when radiological or pathological confirmation of the suspected stroke is obtained.

- *Transient ischemic attack (TIA)* is an abrupt, focal loss of neurologic function caused by temporary ischemia. Although in the past it was thought that TIAs could persist up to 24 hours, modern imaging techniques have shown that deficits lasting > 1 hour usually represent irreversible cerebral infarcts and that most true TIAs typically last < 15 minutes.

- Approximately 70 to 75% of strokes are ischemic in nature; the remainder result from intracranial and subarachnoid hemorrhage.

- Over 700,000 strokes and over 165,000 deaths from stroke occur each year in the United states. Stroke is the number three killer of Americans and is the number one cause of long-term disability and nursing home placement among adults. There are over 4.5 million stroke survivors in the United states.

- In 2006, the estimated annual cost of stroke in the United States was > $51,000,000,000.
- African Americans and Hispanic Americans carry a disproportionate share of the burden of stroke at all ages, with more than double the incidence and mortality of non-Hispanic whites.

PATHOPHYSIOLOGY

- Ischemia is caused by transient or permanent occlusion of a cerebral blood vessel. The possible causes of cerebrovascular occlusion are myriad and will be described below.
- After occlusion, there is impaired cerebral blood flow (CBF) resulting in a central area (core) of severely reduced perfusion and a peripheral area of less reduction (ischemic penumbra). In the core, CBF is so low that it will invariably succumb to infarction. The cells in the penumbra lose electrical function but retain structural integrity. The penumbra thus represents a potentially salvageable area, but the time window for intervention appears to be brief. Thus, it is imperative to rapidly reestablish blood flow in acute stroke in order to minimize the cerebral injury.
- Impaired cerebral perfusion sets into motion a series of events called the ischemic cascade. Neurons become unable to maintain aerobic respiration, and with resulting anaerobic respiration, neurons are no longer able to maintain ionic balance.
- Excitotoxicity occurs, in which glutamate and other excitatory neurotransmitters worsen the neuronal injury via excessive stimulation of neurons during their energy-depleted state. These neurotransmitters depolarize the neuronal cell membrane, which is followed by an influx of sodium, chloride, and water, resulting in cytotoxic edema.
- Influx of calcium follows and may lead to neuronal death. Increased intracellular calcium activates several enzymatic pathways that cause proteolysis, destruction of cell wall lipids, free radical formation, further release of intracellular calcium, and increased production of nitric oxide.
- The enzymatic disturbances and free radical production lead to widespread disruption of neuronal and endothelial integrity. In addition, in the ischemic zone a series of cytokines are released, some of which may promote an inflammatory response and disrupt the microcirculation, thereby worsening the ischemic injury.
- Lastly, cell death may occur in a delayed fashion by apoptosis, a genetically programmed form of cell death that may be induced by neuronal ischemia.
- Potential etiologies for ischemic stroke or TIA include

  - *Large artery disease (15%–25%):* The most common cause is atherosclerosis, but other causes include arterial dissection, vasculitis, fibromuscular dysplasia, and moyamoya disease. Vessels involved may include the extra- and intracranial carotid and vertebral arteries, the basilar artery and the middle, anterior, and posterior cerebral arteries.
  - *Small vessel disease (15%–30%):* These infarcts are < 1 cm in size and are caused by the occlusion of a single small penetrating artery supplying the deep areas of the brain such as the internal capsule, thalamus, basal ganglia, and brainstem. Small vessel disease is most often associated with long-standing hypertension or diabetes.
  - *Cardioembolism (20%–25%):* Emboli may arise from the heart or proximal aorta. Common sources of emboli include mural thrombi from atrial fibrillation, dilated cardiomyopathy, and wall motion abnormalities after myocardial infarction (MI), and valvular heart disease.
  - *Other less common causes (5%):* Hypercoaguable states and other hematologic abnormalities, drug-related, infections, migraine.
  - *Cryptogenic stroke (20%–30%):* In most series, approximately 25% of strokes do not have an identifiable cause, with a higher percentage of cryptogenic stroke in patients < 45 years old.

CLINICAL PRESENTATION, DIFFERENTIAL, MAKING THE DIAGNOSIS

- The presenting signs and symptoms of stroke are entirely dependent upon the location of brain tissue involved in the vascular process. Figures 63-1 and 63-2 provide a review of the intracranial vascular anatomy and the main arterial territories supplied by the cerebrovascular circulation.
- The major arterial syndromes and their typical signs and symptoms are outlined in Table 63-1.
- While stroke signs and symptoms are helpful in localizing the stroke to a specific region of the brain or arterial territory, it is important to remember that the clinical presentation typically does not provide any information about stroke etiology.
- While headache, vomiting, and decreased level of consciousness are somewhat more common with hemorrhagic stroke, ischemic stroke can present with similar symptoms, especially if the vertebrobasilar arterial system is involved, or if a hemispheric stroke is large enough to cause mass effect and increased intracranial pressure. Likewise, thrombotic and embolic strokes cannot be distinguished from each

Circle of Willis

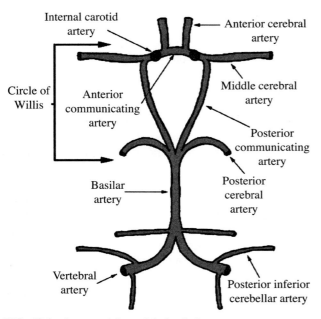

FIG. 63-1 Intracranial arterial circulation.

TABLE 63-1 Presenting Signs and Symptoms of Stroke by Vascular Distribution

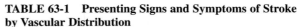

ARTERY	CLINICAL FEATURES
Anterior circulation	
ICA	Ipsilateral monocular vision loss (*amaurosis fugax*)
	± Contralateral weakness or sensory changes
MCA	Contralateral weakness, sensory changes (face/arm > leg)
	± Contralateral visual field deficit
	Aphasia (dominant hemisphere)
	Neglect and other visuospatial difficulties (nondominant hemisphere)
ACA	Contralateral weakness, sensory changes (leg > face/arm)
	Personality changes (disinhibition, lack of motivation, disinterest)
Posterior circulation	
PCA	Contralateral visual field deficit ± other visual phenomena
VB	Ipsilateral cranial nerve deficits ± ataxia
	Contralateral or bilateral weakness or sensory changes
	Contralateral or bilateral sensory changes
	Diplopia
	Dysarthria
	Dysequilibrium or vertigo (not in isolation)
	Altered level of consciousness

Abbreviations: ACA, anterior cerebral artery; ICA, internal carotid artery; MCA, middle cerebral artery; PCA, posterior cerebral artery; VB, vertebrobasilar system.

other based merely on presenting signs and symptoms alone.

• The differential diagnosis of stroke includes various other neurologic and medical entities. Keys to distinguishing stroke from other diagnoses include its acute onset (as opposed to subacute onset or chronic progression) and the focality of the presenting neurological signs and symptoms. In most cases, careful history taking, physical examination, and diagnostic testing can establish the correct diagnosis. Table 63-2

lists the differential diagnoses for acute ischemic stroke and diagnostic tests that can be used to help confirm this diagnosis.

• Many acute stroke patients are initially evaluated in the emergency department (ED). After attention to the issues of oxygenation and hemodynamic stability, a medical history and physical examination should focus on specific stroke risk factors and etiologies, followed by clinical localization of the ischemic territory (Table 63-1).

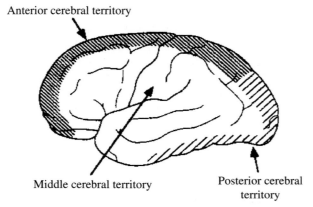

FIG. 63-2 Major arterial territories of the brain.

TABLE 63-2 Differential Diagnoses of Acute Ischemic Stroke

DISORDERS THAT MIMIC AIS	DIAGNOSTIC TOOLS
Intracerebral hemorrhage	CT/MRI
Subarachnoid hemorrhage	CT, lumbar puncture, cerebral angiography
Subdural/epidural hematoma	History of trauma, CT/MRI
Structural lesion (neoplasm, etc.)	CT/MRI
Hypo- or hyperglycemia	Fingerstick glucose
Other metabolic derangements	Routine chemistry studies
Seizure	Clinical history, EEG
Complicated migraine	Clinical history
Conversion disorder	Clinical history, psychiatric evaluation

Abbreviations: AIS, acute ischemic stroke; CT, computed tomography; MRI, magnetic resonance imaging; EEG, electroencephalogram.

- Other disorders that may resemble ischemic stroke must be considered and excluded if possible given the available information (Table 63-2).
- Laboratory studies, including a complete blood count (CBC), electrolytes, glucose, and coagulation parameters, should be obtained.
- Electrocardiography (ECG) is needed to assess for evidence of arrhythmia or cardiac ischemia.
- Emergent computed tomography (CT) is required to identify intracerebral hemorrhage (ICH) and early signs of cerebral ischemia.

TRIAGE AND INITIAL MANAGEMENT

- Some ischemic stroke patients may be candidates for thrombolytic therapy with tissue-type plasminogen activator (tPA). To be eligible for tPA, patients must have a clinical syndrome consistent with acute stroke, a noncontrast head CT scan (HCT) that reveals no hemorrhage or alternate explanation for the symptoms, and the drug must be given *within 3 hours of stroke symptom onset.*
- Numerous exclusion criteria for treatment exist and adherence to protocol is necessary to avoid complications. Thorough discussion of use of tPA for acute ischemic stroke is outside the scope of this text, but interested readers are referred to the references Adams et al (2007) and Albers et al (2004).
- Initial ED and hospital management should include efforts to avoid fever (goal body temperature < 99.5°F), maintain normoglycemia (glucose < 140 mg/dL), and maintain adequate oxygenation (oxygen saturation > 92%).
- The initial management of blood pressure (BP) in the acute stroke patient has been controversial; however, consensus guidelines have now emerged.
  - Elevated BP in acute stroke tends to be a transient phenomenon, as the brain demands higher arterial pressures to ensure adequate cerebral perfusion pressure to maintain blood flow to the ischemic penumbra.
  - Precipitous lowering of BP using sublingual calcium channel blockers or other similar agents should be avoided. In general, patients with ischemic stroke (who have *not* been treated with thrombolytic therapies) can be allowed BP readings up to 220/115 for the first 48 hours after stroke, as long as no other end-organ damage is present (eg, MI, hypertensive encephalopathy). For patients with TIA, BP control can be initiated immediately, as long as symptoms do not recur.
- Heparin is no longer routinely used in patients with acute ischemic stroke (except subcutaneous heparin for venous thromboembolism [VTE] prophylaxis), as there is no evidence that it reduces morbidity, mortality, or stroke recurrence. This includes all heparin types and applies to all stroke subtypes.
- Diagnostic studies are needed to determine the risk factors and cause of the stroke, since specific treatments are available for specific stroke etiologies (Fig. 63-3).
- There is no true "standard" approach to the evaluation of all stroke patients, and consideration must be given to each patient's medical and neurological condition, prognosis, and the possible risks and benefits of the interventions that are being considered.
- For example, some patients are very poor candidates for carotid revascularization procedures (ie, carotid endarterectomy [CEA] or angioplasty/stenting [CAS]) because of their other medical problems, and therefore they have no need of carotid diagnostic studies.
- Patients with severe (70%–99%) carotid stenosis ipsilateral to the side of an anterior circulation stroke gain excellent risk reduction for secondary stroke from CEA, as long as they are good surgical candidates. Selected patients may also benefit from CAS, especially if they are considered high risk for CEA. Specialists from neurology, neurosurgery, vascular surgery, and/or interventional radiology should be consulted to assist in decisions regarding carotid revascularization.
- Prevention of in-hospital complications of stroke should be emphasized, including
  - *VTE prophylaxis:* For any patient not ambulatory within 48 hours, prescribe low-molecular-weight heparin or unfractionated heparin in prophylaxis doses, and/or sequential compression devices. Sequential compression devices alone are recommended only for patients at high risk of bleeding. See Chap. 88.
  - *Aspiration pneumonia:* All patients should receive a bedside swallowing screen prior to taking anything by mouth, including medications. If necessary, a formal swallowing evaluation can be performed.
  - *Urinary tract infection:* Indwelling urinary catheters should be avoided if possible.
  - *Decubitus ulcers:* Immobile patients should be turned at frequent intervals.
  - *Falls:* Fall precautions should be taken in any stroke patient with altered mental status, weakness, numbness, and balance or visual disturbances.
  - *Malnutrition:* Efforts should be made to initiate early nutrition. If a patient is unable to swallow safely, a nasogastric or Dobhoff tube should be inserted and enteral nutrition begun.

DISEASE MANAGEMENT STRATEGIES

- After the hyperacute period of the first few hours after stroke onset, secondary prevention therapy should be

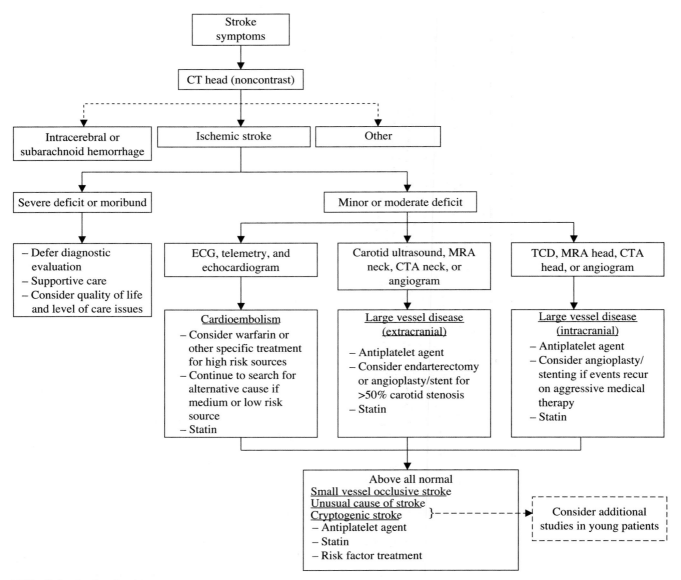

FIG. 63-3 Stroke algorithm.

initiated for all ischemic stroke patients. Stroke risk factors are listed in Table 63-3.

• *Hypertension is the most important modifiable stroke risk factor, and it is estimated that over half of all strokes (both ischemic and hemorrhagic) can be attributed to uncontrolled hypertension.* Goal blood pressure should be < 140/85 in patients with uncomplicated hypertension and < 130/80 in patients with diabetes or chronic kidney disease.

• Oral antihypertensive agents can be initiated 24–48 hours into the acute stroke hospitalization, as long as the patient is neurologically stable. Choice of initial

TABLE 63-3   Risk Factors for Stroke

NONMODIFIABLE	MODIFIABLE
Age	Hypertension
Sex	Diabetes
Race/Ethnicity	Hyperlipidemia
Family history	Cardiac disease (atrial fibrillation and others)
	Smoking
	Excessive alcohol use
	Physical inactivity

antihypertensive agent is flexible, and should be made based on patient comorbidities and degree to which BP needs to be lowered. Reaching target BP goal as an outpatient is likely more important than the agent selected; many patients will require multiple agents for successful control. In general, avoid agents that can unpredictably, suddenly drop blood pressure such as sublingual nifedipine or hydralazine, agents that can cause excessive sedation such as clonidine, or agents that can interfere with cerebral autoregulation such as hydralazine.

- All diabetic patients with stroke or TIA should have a glycohemoglobin checked to assess glycemic control. Patients without a known history of diabetes should have fasting blood glucose checked; hyperglycemia should be aggressively controlled during the hospitalization.

- All patients with stroke or TIA should have a fasting lipid profile checked within 48 hours of stroke onset. Outpatient goal low-density lipoprotein (LDL) cholesterol should be < 100 mg/dL, and < 70 mg/dL for patients with ongoing or multiple vascular risk factors. Statin agents should be first-line therapy, as they have been demonstrated to effectively lower cholesterol and yield non–cholesterol-lowering effects in patients with stroke and other vascular disease. The recent SPARCL trial (stroke prevention by aggressive reduction of cholesterol levels) demonstrated significant secondary stroke prevention for stroke/TIA patients, even in those with normal or borderline normal cholesterol levels. This trial used 80 mg of atorvastatin, but it is unknown whether other doses or statins would work equally well.

- Atrial fibrillation (AF) creates high risk for primary or secondary stroke, with stroke recurrence rates as high as 10% annually if untreated. Rate/rhythm control does not reduce risk of stroke. Oral anticoagulation with warfarin (international normalized ratio [INR] 2.0–3.0) is the preferred treatment, as it is greatly superior to antiplatelet therapy for reducing stroke risk. Several clinical stroke risk stratification schemes have been developed to help determine which patients with AF could be treated with aspirin alone and which would require full anticoagulation.

- Most patients with AF-associated stroke do not need to be treated with intravenous unfractionated heparin in the acute phase, as the risk for recurrent cardioembolic stroke is estimated to be only about 1% per week. Initiation of systemic oral anticoagulation may need to be delayed for days to weeks if a patient has a large stroke, as the risk for hemorrhagic transformation can be high.

- All current smokers, defined as anyone who has smoked in the past 12 months, should be counseled on quitting and given appropriate educational and support materials. Pharmacologic intervention to treat nicotine withdrawal can be given during the acute stroke hospitalization.

- Information regarding other lifestyle changes, such as reducing heavy alcohol intake, or increasing physical activity should also be provided.

- In addition to risk factor modification, antithrombotic therapy is the mainstay of secondary stroke prevention. Five antithrombotic agents are Food and Drug Administration (FDA)-approved for secondary stroke prevention: aspirin (ASA), ticlopidine, clopidogrel, extended-release dipyridamole/aspirin (ER-DP/ASA) combination, and warfarin (Table 63-4).

- Warfarin should be reserved for patients with AF or other specific cardiac abnormalities that yield a high risk for stroke (atrial myxoma, severe cardiomyopathy, etc.)

- Most stroke/TIA patients can be managed with antiplatelet therapy. Ticlopidine is not used frequently secondary to potential for severe hematologic side effects. According to the most recent guidelines, ASA (50–325 mg daily), clopidogrel (75 mg daily), or ER-DP/ASA (200/25 mg twice daily) are all acceptable as first-line therapy. The combination of ASA and clopidogrel is not recommended in stroke/TIA patients, as it appears to increase the risk for serious hemorrhagic complications without lowering stroke risk more than either single agent alone. A head-to-head trial of clopidogrel and ER-DP/ASA is currently ongoing.

CARE TRANSITIONS

- Selected patients with TIA may be admitted to an observation unit for expedited workup and treatment. These patients are usually discharged home within 24–48 hours, and should have timely follow-up with their primary care provider (PCP), ideally within a few days.

- Many patients with stroke will require some type of rehabilitation, which may take place in an inpatient setting ("acute rehab"), an extended care facility ("subacute rehab"), or in the outpatient setting. A plan for rehabilitation should be initiated early during the hospital stay, ideally within the first 48 hours. Consulting a physiatrist, along with physical, occupational, and speech therapists, will be useful in determining the proper disposition for the stroke patient.

- Education about stroke diagnosis, warning signs, risk factor modification and secondary stroke prevention, and rehabilitation should be provided to all stroke or TIA patients and their families during the acute hospitalization or at discharge.

TABLE 63-4 Medications Commonly Used in Stroke

MEDICATION	STANDARD DOSE	DRUG INTERACTIONS	ADVERSE EFFECTS
tPA	0.9 mg/kg (maximum 90 mg); 10% as IV bolus over 1 minute, then remainder as IV infusion over 1 hour	Anticoagulants, including heparin and warfarin	Systemic and intracranial hemorrhage
Aspirin	50–325 mg qd	Other antiplatelet agents, NSAIDs, heparin, warfarin	Dyspepsia, tinnitus, gastrointestinal bleeding
Ticlopidine	250 mg bid	Aspirin and other antiplatelet agents, NSAIDs, heparin, warfarin, cimetidine, theophylline	Diarrhea, nausea, vomiting rash, gastrointestinal bleeding, neutropenia, thrombotic thrombocytopenic purpura, aplastic anemia
Clopidogrel	75 mg qd	Aspirin and other antiplatelet agents, NSAIDs, heparin, warfarin At high concentrations, may inhibit certain hepatic enzymes and decrease metabolism of various medications	Rash, diarrhea, dyspepsia, gastrointestinal bleeding
Dipyridamole	Extended-release formulation (200 mg) given in combination with 25 mg aspirin bid	None	Headache, dizziness, flushing, abdominal distress, diarrhea, vomiting
Warfarin	Individualized according to patient response as measured by international normalized ratio (INR). Usual dosages vary from 1–10 mg qd and titrated to keep INR between 2.0 and 3.0	Aspirin and other antiplatelet agents, NSAIDs, ticlopidine, clopidogrel, heparin. Interacts with multiple other medications through pharmacokinetic mechanisms. Consult literature before initiating therapy	Gastrointestinal and other systemic bleeding, warfarin necrosis syndrome, systemic atheromatous embolization ("purple toe" syndrome)

NSAIDs, nonsteroidal anti-inflammatory drugs.

Bibliography

Adams HP, del Zoppo G, Alberts MJ, et al. Guidelines for the early management of adults with ischemic stroke. *Stroke.* 2007;38:1655.

Albers GW, Amarenco P, Easton JD, et al. Antithrombotic and thrombolytic therapy for ischemic stroke: the seventh ACCP conference on antithrombotic and thrombolytic therapy. *Chest.* 2004;126(suppl 3):483S.

Alberts MJ, Hademenos G, Latchaw RE, et al. Recommendations for the establishment of primary stroke centers. Brain attack coalition. *JAMA.* 2000;283:3102.

Amarenco P, Bogousslavsky J, Callahan A 3rd et al. High-dose atorvastatin after stroke or transient ischemic attack. *N Engl J Med.* 2006;355:549.

American Heart Association (AHA). 2006 *Heart and Stroke Statistical Update.* Dallas, TX: AHA; 2006.

Rothwell PM, Buchan A, Johnston SC. Recent advances in management of transient ischaemic attacks and minor ischaemic strokes. *Lancet Neurol.* 2006;5:323.

Sacco RL, Adams R, Albers G, et al. Guidelines for prevention of stroke in patients with ischemic stroke or transient ischemic attack: a statement for healthcare professionals from the American Heart Association/American Stroke Association Council on Stroke. *Stroke.* 2006;37:577.

The National Institute of Neurological Disorders and Stroke rt-PA Stroke Study Group. Tissue plasminogen activator for acute ischemic stroke. *N Engl J Med.* 1995; 333:1581.

Web Resources

Society of Hospital Medicine Quality Improvement Resource Room
http://www.hospitalmedicine.org/AM/Template.cfm? Section=Quality_Improvement_Resource_Rooms&Template=/ CM/HTMLDisplay.cfm&ContentID=6566

64 CEREBRAL HEMORRHAGE

Galen V. Henderson

EPIDEMIOLOGY/OVERVIEW

- Currently 88% of all strokes are ischemic, 9% cerebral hemorrhage, and 3% subarachnoid hemorrhage (SAH).
- The worldwide incidence of intracerebral hemorrhage ranges from 10 to 20 cases per 100,000 population and increases with age.
- Annually 37,000–52,400 people in the United States have an *intracerebral hemorrhage.*
- Thirty eight percent of affected patients survive the first year.
- Types of cerebral hemorrhage are as follows:
  ○ Primary intracerebral hemorrhage, accounting for 78% to 88% of cases, originates from the spontaneous rupture of small vessels damaged by chronic hypertension or amyloid angiopathy.
  ○ Secondary intracerebral hemorrhage occurs in a minority of patients in association with vascular abnormalities (such as arteriovenous malformations and aneurysms), tumors, or impaired coagulation.

PATHOPHYSIOLOGY

- Intraparenchymal bleeding results from the rupture of the small penetrating arteries that originate from basilar arteries or the anterior, middle, or posterior cerebral arteries.
- Chronic hypertension induces degenerative changes in the vessel wall, thereby reducing vessel compliance and increasing the likelihood of spontaneous rupture near the bifurcations, where the most prominent degeneration of the media and smooth muscles is seen.

CLINICAL PRESENTATION, DIFFERENTIAL, MAKING THE DIAGNOSIS

- Risk factors
  ○ Hypertension is the most important risk factor for spontaneous intracerebral hemorrhage.
  ○ Intracerebral hemorrhage is more common in men than women, those older than 55 years of age, and more in certain populations, such as blacks and Japanese.
  ○ Improved control of hypertension appears to reduce the incidence of intracerebral hemorrhage.
  ○ Excessive use of alcohol by impairing coagulation and directly affecting the integrity of cerebral vessels increases the risk of cerebral hemorrhage.
  ○ Cerebral amyloid angiopathy, which is characterized by the deposition of beta-amyloid protein in the blood vessels of the cerebral cortex and leptomeninges, is associated with cerebral hemorrhage.
- Clinical presentation
  ○ Patients with a large hematoma usually have a decreased level of consciousness as a result of cerebral tissue shifts (cerebral herniation) as a result of compartmentalized intracranial pressure (ICP) gradients.
  ○ These cerebral shifts cause distortion of the thalamic and brain stem reticular activating system. Patients with a supratentorial intracerebral hemorrhage involving the putamen, caudate, and thalamus have contralateral sensory motor deficits.
    ■ Signs such as aphasia, neglect, gaze deviation, and hemianopia may occur as a result of the disruption of connecting fibers in the subcortical white matter and functional suppression of overlying cortex.
  ○ In patients with an infratentorial intracerebral hemorrhage, signs of brain stem dysfunction include disconjugate gaze, cranial nerve abnormalities, and contralateral motor deficits.
  ○ Ataxia, nystagmus, and dysmetria are prominent when the intracerebral hemorrhage involves the cerebellum or its connections.
  ○ Common nonspecific symptoms seen in supratentorial and infratentorial hematomas include headache and vomiting as a result of increased ICP and meningismus resulting from blood in the ventricles.
  ○ Suspect SAH if the patient complains of sudden, severe headache (the worst headache in the patient's life).
    ■ Nausea and vomiting, loss of consciousness, obtundation, stiff neck, ocular hemorrhage, and cranial nerve deficits, especially involving the third nerve, are characteristics of spontaneous SAH.
    ■ Risk factors include trauma (majority); spontaneous secondary to aneurysms, arteriovenous malformations (AVMs), vasculitis, and carotid or vertebral dissection; or idiopathic associated with cigarette smoking, birth control pills, hypertension, and alcoholism.
- Diagnosis
  ○ With the rapid onset of neurological symptoms, an initial cranial computed tomography (CT) scan is necessary to distinguish between a cerebral infarction and intracerebral hemorrhage (ICH).

- Vomiting, early change in level of consciousness, and high elevation of blood pressure in a patient with acute stroke suggest ICH.
  - On the initial CT scan, the location and size of the hematoma, the presence of ventricular blood or herniation, and the occurrence of hydrocephalus should be noted.
  ○ Lumbar puncture should be performed if the initial CT scan is negative and the history and physical examination suggest spontaneous SAH.
  - High opening pressure, blood that persists in subsequent tubes, xanthochromia if more than 6 hours since the onset of symptoms, and white blood cell (WBC) count may be elevated.
  - The presence of blood in the spinal fluid may last 2 weeks and that of xanthochromia longer.
  ○ Emergent angiography should be considered for all patients without a clear cause of hemorrhage who are surgical candidates, particularly young, normotensive, and clinically stable patients.
  ○ Angiography is not required for older hypertensive patients who have a hemorrhage in the basal ganglia, thalamus, cerebellum, or brain stem and in whom CT findings do not suggest a structural lesion.
  ○ Magnetic resonance imaging (MRI) and magnetic resonance angiography (MRA) are helpful and may obviate the need for contrast cerebral angiography in selected patients. They should also be considered to look for cavernous malformations in normotensive patients with lobar hemorrhages and normal angiographic results who are surgical candidates.

TRIAGE AND INITIAL MANAGEMENT

- All patients with a new diagnosis of cerebral hemorrhage should be monitored in a dedicated intensive care unit (ICU) for at least 24 hours after the clinical event because the risk of neurologic deterioration and cardiovascular instability is highest during the first 24 hours after the onset.
- The patient's neurologic status should be assessed hourly with the use of a standard evaluation such as the Glasgow Coma Scale or National Institute of Health Stroke Scale (NIHSS).
  http://rnbob.tripod.com/glascow.htm
  http://www.ninds.nih.gov/doctors/NIH_Stroke_Scale.pdf
- Consider intubation if the patient cannot protect their airway or the Glasgow Coma Scale is < 9. (Remember, this is an arbitrary number and the patient may still be able to protect their airway below this value.)
  ○ A delay in protecting the airway can lead to secondary injury from aspiration, hypoxemia, and hypercapnia.

- Fluid management
  ○ The goal of fluid management is euvolemia to prevent and manage cerebral edema.
  - Use only isotonic solutions and avoid hypotonic medications.
  - If signs of brainstem herniation or mass effect (dilated pupil, decreased consciousness, or worsening examination), then the patient should be transferred to ICU for aggressive management of increased ICP.
  ○ For critically ill patients invasive monitoring is performed in the ICU.
  - Optimal central venous pressure (CVP) should be maintained between 5 mm Hg and 12 mm Hg or pulmonary wedge pressure at ≈ 10–14 mm Hg.
- Management of blood pressure
  ○ Continuous blood pressure monitoring of systemic arterial pressure should be considered in patients who require intravenous administration of antihypertensive medications and/or hyperosmolar agents.
  ○ Cardiovascular instability is associated with increased ICP and needs immediate attention.
  ○ Elevated blood pressure is common after intracerebral hemorrhage and is associated with expansion of the hematoma and a poor outcome. It remains unclear whether elevated blood pressure predisposes patients to expansion of the hematoma or is a consequence of this event.
  ○ Elevated blood pressure can also be a protective response (referred to as the Cushing-Kocher response) whose aim is to preserve cerebral perfusion.
  ○ There is considerable controversy regarding the initial treatment of blood pressure after an intracerebral hemorrhage. Recommendations for hypertensive management in this setting are given in Table 64-1.
- Rapid deterioration or clinical and/or CT evidence of transtentorial herniation or hydrocephalus should mandate an urgent neurosurgical consultation.
  ○ The presence of blood in the ventricles is associated with a higher mortality rate.
  - Ventricular blood interferes with the normal egress of cerebral spinal fluid via the ventricular foramen and/or arachnoid granulations; therefore, external drainage of cerebrospinal fluid through ventricular catheters reduces ICP and ventricular blood.
  ○ For supratentorial hemorrhages, craniotomy does not alter the outcomes compared to medical management.
  ○ Cerebellar hematomas have high morbidity and mortality that are related to compression of the brain stem and surgical decompression may be required.
  ○ A mass effect resulting from the volume of the hematoma, the edematous tissue surrounding the

TABLE 64-1 Hypertension Management in ICH

Medication choices for elevated blood pressure control

Nicardipine*	5 mg/h increased by 2.5 mg/h to a max amount of 15 mg/h
Labetalol*	5–100 mg/h by intermittent bolus doses of 10–40 mg or continuous drip (2–8 mg/min)
Esmolol	500 µg/kg as a load; maintenance use, 50–200 µg/kg/min
Nitroprusside	0.5–10 µg/kg/min
Hydralazine	10–20 mg q4–6 h
Enalapril	0.625–1.2 mg q6 h as needed

1. If *systolic* BP is 180–230 mm Hg, *diastolic* BP 105–140 mm Hg, or mean arterial BP ≥130 mm Hg on two readings 20 minutes apart, treat the patient to a MAP goal < 130 mm Hg.
2. If *systolic* BP is < 180 mm Hg and *diastolic* BP < 105 mm Hg, defer antihypertensive therapy.
3. If ICP monitoring is available, cerebral perfusion pressure should be kept at > 70 mm Hg.

Medication choices for low blood pressure control

Volume replenishment is the first line of approach. Isotonic saline or colloids can be used and monitored with central venous pressure or pulmonary artery wedge pressure. If hypotension persists after correction of volume deficit, continuous infusions of pressors should be considered, particularly for low systolic blood pressure such as < 90 mm Hg.

Phenylephrine†	2–10 µg/kg/min
Dopamine	2–20 µg/kg/min
Norepinephrine	Titrate from 0.05 to 0.2 µg/kg/min

Abbreviation: ICH, intracerebral hemorrhage; MAP, mean arterial pressure; ICP, intracranial pressure.
*Most commonly used in neurointensive care units to obtain blood pressure control in the acute phase.
†Most commonly used in neurointensive are units to maximize cerebral perfusion pressure without inducing cerebral vasoconstriction or tachycardia.
SOURCE: Adapted from *Stroke*. 1999;30:905–915 and Brigham and Women's Blood Pressure control policy in the NeuroICU.

hematoma, and obstructive hydrocephalus with subsequent herniation remains the chief secondary cause of death in the first few days after intracerebral hemorrhage. Strategies for management in consultation with neurosurgery and neurology include

- Transient hyperventilation.
- Use of hyperosmolar agents such as mannitol or hypertonic saline.
- Placement of an intraventricular catheter for the drainage of cerebrospinal fluid to lower ICP may be undertaken by the neurosurgical consultant.
- Corticosteroids should be avoided, because randomized trials have failed to demonstrate their efficacy in patients with an intracerebral hemorrhage.

- Seizures
  - Most seizures occur at the onset of intracerebral hemorrhage or within the first 24 hours.
    - All patients with spontaneous SAH should receive seizure prophylaxis.
    - Subdural and parenchymal bleeding probably do not require prophylaxis.
  - Anticonvulsants can usually be discontinued after the first month in patients who have had no further seizures.
  - Patients who have a seizure more than 2 weeks after the onset of an intracerebral hemorrhage are at higher risk for further seizures and may require long-term prophylactic treatment with anticonvulsants.

- Management of body temperature
  - Body temperature should be maintained at normal levels.
  - Acetaminophen 650 mg and/or cooling blankets should be used to treat hyperthermia > 38.5°C. Fevers in the patient population, regardless of the etiology, has been associated with higher morbidity.
  - A diligent search for underlying infectious causes of fever, particularly for possible nosocomial infections such as aspiration and/or ventilator-associated pneumonia (see Chap. 78) and urinary catheter-related UTI (see Chap. 55), should be undertaken.
- Management of warfarin-related cerebral hemorrhages
  - The frequent use of long-term anticoagulation in patients to prevent stroke in individuals with atrial fibrillation (AF) has resulted in an increase in warfarin-associated hemorrhage.
  - Half of patients die within 30 days with warfarin-associated hemorrhage. Despite treatment options, outcomes have not been improved.
  - No consensus exists about the optimal short-term treatment of this lethal, iatrogenic form of stroke. A recommended algorithm is given in Fig. 64-1.
  - See Table 64-2 for a review of medications that can be used to reverse an elevated international normalized ratio (INR).

See Chap. 63 for secondary prevention and care transitions.

TABLE 64-2   Review of Medications that can be Used to Reverse an Elevated INR

ADVANTAGES	DISADVANTAGES/LIMITATIONS
Fresh frozen plasma (FFP): FFP alone is insufficient and not fast enough for adequate warfarin reversal (Goldstein, 2006)	
• Readily available in most emergency departments and hospitals	• Requirement of testing for ABO Compatibility and thawing before administration • Variable content of vitamin K-dependant factors • Effect of dilution that may delay immediate reversal • Reports that 800 mL (4 U) of FFP did not reverse warfarin-induced coagulopathy (Makris, 1996) • Prohibitive volume load (up to 3500 mL needed) that takes time to finish infusion and increases the risk of congestive heart failure
Vitamin K (intravenous)	
• Ready availability • Ease of administration • Predictable effect • Longer duration of action than FFP	• Delayed effect (ie, 4–6 hours) • Small risk of anaphylactic reaction (3/10,000: Riegert-Johnson, 2002) • Reduced effect in patients with hepatic insufficiency.
Prothrombin complex concentrate (PCC)	
• Reliable content of factors II, VII, IX, X, proteins C, S • Faster administration of small volume without waiting for compatibility testing and thawing with less risk of CHF • Complete reversal of INR more rapidly (within 10–15 min) compared with FFP (Fredriksson, 1992; Makris, 1997; Boulis, 1999; Cartmill, 2000; Preston, 2002; Lubetsky, 2004; Yasaka, 2005) • Optimal dose for administration: 500 IU for INR < 5 (Yasaka, 2005), 50 IU/kg (UK guideline, 1998), 30 IU/kg regardless of INR (Hanley, 2004), 25–50 IU/kg (Australasian guideline, 2004)	• Potential thrombogenicity, exacerbation of DIC, especially with high dose (Fredriksson, 1992; Kohler, 1990, 1998, 1999; McNeill, 1998; Roddie, 1999; Hellstern, 1999; Leissinger, 1999; Cartmill, 2000; Preston, 2002) • No adverse events with doses of 25 IU/kg • Expensive

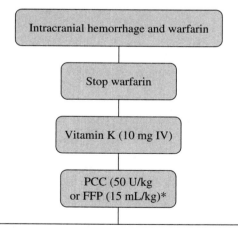

Abbreviations: PCC, prothrombin complex concentrate; FFP, fresh frozen plasma.

FIG. 64-1   Algorithm for emergency treatment of cerebral hemorrhage and warfarin.
*Caution: FFP may not fully reverse the effects of warfarin. For example, Factor IX does not rise 20% post FFP and is not reflected in the INR.

BIBLIOGRAPHY

Ansel et al. Managing oral anticoagulation therapy. Sixth ACCP consensus conference on antithrombotic therapy. *Chest.* 2001;119:22a–S38.

Broderick JP, Adams HP Jr, Barsan W, et al. Guidelines for the management of spontaneous intracerebral hemorrhage: a statement for healthcare professionals from a special writing group of the stroke council, American Heart Association. *Stroke.* 1999;30(4):905–915.

Brott T, Broderick JP, Kothari R, et al. Early hemorrhage growth in patients with intracerebral hemorrhage. *Stroke.* 1997;28(1): 1–5.

Hanley JP. Warfarin reversal. *J Clin Patho.* 2004;57:1132–1139.

Huttner HB, Schellinger PD, Hartmann M, et al. Hematoma growth and outcome in treated neurocritical care patients with intracerebral hemorrhage related to oral anticoagulant therapy: comparison of acute treatment strategies using vitamin K, fresh frozen plasma, and prothrombin complex concentrates. *Stroke.* 2006;37(6):1465–1470.

Juvela S, Kase CS. Advances in intracerebral hemorrhage management. *Stroke.* 2006;37(2):301–304.

Mayer SA, Brun NC, Begtrup K, et al. Recombinant activated factor VII for acute intracerebral hemorrhage. *N Engl J Med.* 2005;352(8):777–785.

Mendelow AD, et al. Early surgery versus initial conservative treatment in patients with spontaneous supratentorial intracerebral haematomas in the international surgical trial in intracerebral haemorrhage (STICH): a randomised trial. *Lancet.* 2005;365(9457):387–397.

Qureshi AI, Tuhrim S, Broderick JP, et al. Spontaneous intracerebral hemorrhage. *N Engl J Med.* 2001;344(19):1450–1460.

65 MENINGITIS/ENCEPHALITIS

Susan L. Hickenbottom

EPIDEMIOLOGY/OVERVIEW

- The presence or absence of normal brain function is the important distinguishing feature between meningitis and encephalitis. Patients with meningitis may be lethargic, uncomfortable, or complain of headache, but cerebral function remains normal. On the other hand, in encephalitis, patients will also usually have focal neurologic deficits.
- However, the clinical distinction between the two entities is sometimes blurred, and the patient is usually diagnosed as having meningitis or encephalitis based upon which features predominate, although the term "meningoencephalitis" is also a common term used when clinical features overlap.
- Bacterial meningitis has an annual incidence of 4–6 cases per 100,000 adults. Cases are usually sporadic, though close contact may play a role in some, especially in *Neisseria meningitidis* meningitis.
- The term "aseptic" meningitis is used to describe patients who have clinical and laboratory evidence of meningeal inflammation with negative routine bacterial cultures. There are about 15,000 cases of aseptic meningitis each year in the United States. The summertime predominance of aseptic meningitis is largely due to the seasonal transmission of enteroviruses.
- There are about 30,000 cases of encephalitis each year in the United States.

PATHOPHYSIOLOGY

- Bacterial meningitis: *Streptococcus pneumoniae* and *N. meningitides* are responsible for 80% of all cases. Less common causes of bacterial meningitis include parameningeal sources, such as epidural or subdural abscesses, and sinus or ear infections. Bacterial meningitis can also result from bacterial endocarditis with hematogenous seeding of the cerebrospinal fluid (CSF) and meninges.
- *Aseptic meningitis:* Numerous infectious agents and other conditions can cause aseptic meningitis; these are summarized in Table 65-1.
- *Encephalitis:* In recent exhaustive attempts to determine the cause of encephalitis, in 63% of cases no etiology was determined. Viruses cause the largest proportion of encephalitis cases in which a cause is found. Neurotropic viruses include herpes simplex virus (HSV) (types 1 and 2), eastern and western equine encephalitis viruses, St. Louis encephalitis virus, Japanese B encephalitis virus, and West Nile virus.

CLINICAL PRESENTATION, DIFFERENTIAL, MAKING THE DIAGNOSIS

- Bacterial and aseptic meningitis often have a similar initial presentation with fever, headache, stiff neck, photophobia, altered mental status, nausea/vomiting, and, less commonly, seizures. Less than 50% of patients present with the classic triad of fever, neck stiffness, and altered mental status, but almost all patients have at least two of the symptoms listed above. Physical examination will often reveal nuchal rigidity in both conditions.
- Patients with encephalitis often will present with the same symptoms as meningitis, but brain function abnormalities are also common and may include language dysfunction (difficulty speaking, reading, or comprehending language); altered behavior or personality change; focal motor, sensory, or visual deficits; or movement disorders. Differential diagnosis for these patients will include brain abscess, brain neoplasm, stroke, and subdural or epidural hematoma. Of these only brain abscess would routinely present with fever.
- The most important focus of differential diagnosis should be distinguishing between bacterial and aseptic meningitis/viral encephalitis. Bacterial meningitis should be considered a life-threatening but treatable medical emergency, whereas aseptic meningitis has a self-limited course that resolves without specific medical therapy. While encephalitis can also be life threatening, limited interventions are available and most patients can be treated only with supportive measures.
- Lumbar puncture (LP) is mandatory in any patient in whom meningitis or encephalitis is suspected, as the CSF profile is the key in distinguishing between bacterial meningitis and other conditions (Table 65-2).
- Brain herniation is a rare, but much feared, complication of LP and may occur in patients with increased intracranial pressure from diffuse cerebral edema or

TABLE 65-1 Pathogens Causing Aseptic Meningitis

PATHOGEN	COMMON	UNCOMMON
Viral	Enteroviruses (echo, coxsackie) Herpes simplex virus Arboviruses	Epstein-Barr virus Cytomegalovirus Varicella zoster virus Adenovirus Measles Mumps Rubella HIV Poliovirus Mollaret's (recurrent) meningitis (most cases probably due to reactivation of HSV-2 in sacral nerve roots)
Other bacterial	Mycobacterium tuberculosis Borrelia burgdorferi (Lyme disease)	*Treponema pallidum (syphilis)* *Leptospira* sp. *Mycoplasma pneumoniae* *Rickettsia* sp. *Ehrlichia* sp. *Brucella* sp.
Fungal		*Cryptococcus neoformans* *Histoplasma capsulatum* *Coccidioides immitis* *Candida* sp. *Aspergillus* sp.
Parasitic		*Toxoplasma gondii* *Taenia solium* (cysticercosis)
Malignancy	Lymphoma Leukemia Metastatic carcinomas (breast, lung)	Melanoma
Drugs	Nonsteroidal anti-inflammatory drugs	Intravenous immunoglobulins Trimethoprim-sulfa Azathioprine
Autoimmune		Sarcoid Behcet disease Systemic lupus erythematosus

from rapidly expanding masses (brain abscess, subdural empyema, or cerebral necrosis in aggressive encephalitides). Thus, brain imaging with computed tomography (CT) or magnetic resonance imaging (MRI) is almost always undertaken prior to LP to detect brain shift or severe diffuse cerebral edema. One study, however, reported that 41% of head CTs for suspected meningitis are not necessary. Head CT is required when patients are > 60 years of age, immunocompromised, have coexisting central nervous system (CNS) disease, a recent seizure history, or have focal neurologic findings on examination. The cause and effect relationship of LP and herniation has also been questioned. Many patients who herniated

TABLE 65-2 CSF Profiles and Differential Diagnosis of Meningitis

	OPENING PRESSURE (cm of H_2O)	PROTEIN (mg/dL)	GLUCOSE (mg/dL)	WBC COUNT AND differential (cells/μL)
Normal	6–18	14–45	45–80	< 5, with no more than 1 neutrophil
Bacterial meningitis	↑ to ↑↑↑ (40% > 40 cm of H_2O)	↑ to ↑↑ (usually > 50; often > 100)	↓ to ↓↓ (< 40)	↑↑ to ↑↑↑ 100–50,000 WBC; > 85% neutrophils
Viral meningitis	Normal to ↑	↑	Normal	↑ to ↑↑ 6–500 WBC; > 85% lymphocytes, monocytes, or histiocytes

Symbols:
↑ = mildly elevated   ↓ = mildly decreased
↑↑ = moderately elevated   ↓↓ = moderately decreased
↑↑↑ = severely elevated

after LP have no characteristics that would have helped predict this prior to the procedure.

- Historical or physical examination clues can sometimes aid in determining the etiology of meningoencephalitis. Hospitalists should be sure to
  - Obtain a comprehensive travel and exposure history (insect/tick bites, rodents, birds, contact with individuals with similar symptoms, medications known to cause aseptic meningitis)
  - Swimming in fresh water is a risk factor for primary amebic meningitis (PAM) due to *Naegleria* and *Acanthamoeba*. Early diagnosis and treatment are essential for the patient to have any chance of survival.
  - Review sexual history (human immunodeficiency virus [HIV], HSV-2, syphilis)
  - Examine patients for any skin rashes, which may be suggestive for a potential etiology (Lyme disease, Rocky Mountain spotted fever, meningococcal infection)
  - Examine the patient for any genital rashes or ulcers (HSV-2, syphilis, Behcet disease)
  - Be aware that asymmetric flaccid paralysis strongly suggests the possibility of West Nile virus meningoencephalitis (or polio, which is now exceedingly rare in developed countries)
- Brain biopsy is an infrequently used diagnostic option for patient with encephalitis in whom less invasive testing has not revealed the pathogen and who have a worsening clinical course.

TRIAGE AND INITIAL MANAGEMENT

BACTERIAL MENINGITIS

- Bacterial meningitis is a *medical emergency*. If neuroimaging or LP will be delayed, empiric antibiotic therapy should be initiated immediately, prior to performing these diagnostic tests. Table 65-3 summarizes empiric antibiotic selection for suspected pathogens based on patient age and other characteristics, and also recommended duration of therapy.
- After LP has been performed (including recording opening pressure), CSF should be sent for the following diagnostic studies: protein and glucose levels, cell counts and differential, Gram stain, and culture. Gram staining of fluid allows for rapid identification of the causative organism (sensitivity 60%–90%; specificity > 97%). Bacterial antigen tests are of limited utility, but they can be used in patients with a CSF profile suggestive of bacterial meningitis, but negative Gram stain and culture. Polymerase chain reaction (PCR) for bacterial strains is an emerging technology for these patients as well.
- On selected patients, CSF analysis may also include cytology, fungal or acid-fast bacilli smear and culture, and bacterial or viral PCR, especially for herpes simplex virus.
- Adjunctive dexamethasone therapy is now also recommended for most adult patients with suspected or confirmed *S. pneumoniae* meningitis, with randomized trials demonstrating reduced morbidity and mortality in the subset of adults with pneumococcal meningitis. Patients should receive dexamethasone 10 mg with or before the first dose of antibiotics and continue for 4 days at a dose of 10 mg every 6 hours. Therapy should be discontinued if the patient is found not to have bacterial meningitis, and some experts recommend discontinuing dexamethasone if the meningitis is found to be caused by any organism other than *S. pneumoniae*.

TABLE 65-3   Empiric Antibiotic Choices by Patient Age or Other Characteristics in Adults with Bacterial Meningitis

	COMMON PATHOGENS	EMPIRIC ANTIBIOTIC
Age 16–50 yrs	*Neisseria meningitidis* *Streptococcus pneumoniae*	Ceftriaxone or cefotaxime, and vancomycin
Age > 50 yrs	*S. pneumoniae, N. meningitidis, Listeria monocytogenes*, aerobic gram-negative bacteria	Ceftriaxone or cefotaxime, and vancomycin, plus ampicillin
Relative immunocompromised state (alcoholism, pregnancy)	*S. pneumoniae, Haemophilus influenza, L. monocytogenes,*	Ceftriaxone or cefotaxime, and vancomycin plus ampicillin
Cranial trauma, CSF shunt, recent neurosurgery	*Staphylococcus aureus*, coagulase-negative staphylococci, *Pseudomonas aeruginosa* and other gram-negative bacilli	Vancomycin and cefepime, ceftazidime or meropenem

Common adult doses: ampicillin 2 g q4 h; cefepime 2 g q8 h; ceftriaxone 2 g q12 h; cefotaxime 2 g q4–6 h; meropenem 2 g q8 h; vancomycin 15 mg/kg q8–12 h adjusted to maintain trough concentrations of 15–20 μg/mL.

- The safety of adjunctive dexamethasone therapy has not been adequately studied in patients with meningitis and septic shock, or in those with septic shock and adrenal insufficiency.
- Monitoring in an intensive care unit (ICU) setting is often recommended for patients with bacterial meningitis, in order to recognize changes in the patient's level of consciousness and the development of new neurological signs, monitor for subtle seizures, and treat severe agitation effectively. Practical recommendations and admission criteria are outlined in Table 65-4.
- Bacterial meningitis is often associated with septic shock, adrenal insufficiency, seizures, and hyponatremia. Bacterial meningitis patients need to be closely monitored for these conditions and treated aggressively if they develop these conditions.
- Decline in level of consciousness may arise for several reasons including development of meningoencephalitis with brain edema, acute hydrocephalus, seizures, or cerebral infarcts arising from vasculitis. Evaluation for these conditions should include CT or MRI of the brain and electroencephalogram (EEG).
- Once hemodynamically and neurologically stable, close monitoring is not indicated. Follow-up or neuroimaging may be useful in patients with uncommon pathogens or whose clinical course does not improve as expected. These tests may aid in evaluation of a possible parameningeal focus of infection and complications such as subdural empyema or cortical vein thrombosis.

TABLE 65-4 Management of Bacterial Meningitis in Adults in the Intensive Care Unit

Neurocritical care

For patients increased intracranial pressure and risk of brain herniation:
Consider intracranial pressure monitoring and intermittent administration of osmotic diuretics (mannitol or hypertonic saline) to maintain intracranial pressure < 15 mm Hg and a cerebral perfusion pressure > 60 mm Hg
Initiate repeated lumbar puncture, lumbar drain, or ventriculostomy in patients with acute hydrocephalus
EEG monitoring in patients with clinical seizures or fluctuating neurologic exam

Airway and respiratory care

Intubate patients with worsening level of consciousness or inability to protect airway
Maintain ventilatory support

Circulatory care

In patients with septic shock, administer low doses of corticosteroids; continue if adrenal insufficiency is diagnosed
Initiate inotropic agents to maintain blood pressure (mean arterial pressure 70–100 mm Hg)
Initiate crystalloids or albumin to maintain adequate fluid balance
Consider use of Swan-Ganz catheter to monitor hemodynamic status

Gastrointestinal care

Initiate tube feeding of a standard nutritional formula
Initiate prophylaxis with proton pump inhibitor

Other supportive care

Administer subcutaneous heparin or other agent as DVT prophylaxis
Maintain normoglycemic state with use of sliding scale insulin or continuous IV insulin administration
In patients with hyperthermia (> 39°C), use antipyretic agents or cooling by conduction

SOURCE: Adapted from Van de Beek D, de Gans J, Tunkel AR, et al. Community-acquired bacterial meningitis in adults. *N Engl J Med.* 2006;354:44.

ASEPTIC MENINGITIS

- Treatment for most cases of aseptic meningitis is supportive and should address pain control, relief of fever, and gentle hydration. Many patients can be treated symptomatically at home, but others require admission. Criteria for admission may include severe headache or neck pain, nausea/vomiting, or CSF pleiocytosis with some neutrophilic presence that may require empiric treatment for bacterial meningitis.
- Patients with suspected viral meningitis (CSF cell count < 500/µL, > 75% CSF lymphocytes/monocytes, protein concentration < 80–100 mg/dL, normal CSF glucose concentration, and negative Gram stain) can be observed without antibiotic therapy.
- When it is not clear whether the patient has a viral or bacterial process, the treating physician should choose appropriate empiric antibiotics after obtaining blood and CSF cultures, making the decision to continue after culture results are available in 24–48 hours. Repeat LP may be needed in patients with persistent symptoms who do not have a clear diagnosis.
- Treatment of fungal, tuberculous, and other rarer meningitides is outside the scope of this review, but should focus on identifying the pathogen and initiating appropriate antifungal therapy. Patients with fungal and/or tuberculous meningitis may require up to 12 months of therapy or more, and relapses are common.

ENCEPHALITIS

- Treatment for encephalitis is also supportive in most cases, as no specific therapy is available except for a few pathogens. In milder cases, care focuses on control of headache/neck pain, fever and gentle hydration.
- Seizures are not uncommon in encephalitis and should be managed with standard anticonvulsant therapy.
- Comatose patients require ICU care with ventilation, aggressive pulmonary toilet, hydration, nutrition, and deep venous thrombosis (DVT) prophylaxis. Patients with suspected increased intracranial pressure should be managed with hyperventilation, hyperosmolar agents, and dexamethasone.
- The following antiviral or antibacterial agents can be used for these infectious entities:
  - *Herpes simplex virus 1 or 2:* Acyclovir 10 mg/kg IV q8 h or foscarnet 60 mg/kg IV q8 h for 10–14 days
  - *Varicella zoster virus:* Acyclovir 10 mg/kg IV q8 h for 10–14 days
  - *Cytomegalovirus:* Ganciclovir 5 mg/kg IV q12 h for 14 days
  - *Rocky Mountain spotted fever, ehrlichiosis, Lyme disease:* Doxycycline 100 mg IV q12 h for 7–10 days
  - *Leptospirosis:* Penicillin G 4 million units IV q4 h for 7–10 days

DISEASE MANAGEMENT STRATEGIES

- Patient and family expectations regarding the expected outcome, especially with regard to neurological outcomes, should begin early in the hospital course.
  - Overall mortality rates in adults with bacterial meningitis range from 3% to 10% in meningococcal meningitis and up to 20% to 35% in patients with streptococcal meningitis. Major morbidity occurs in approximately 20% to 30% of adults with streptococcal meningitis.
  - In patients with aseptic meningitis prognosis is dependent on underlying etiology: viral and chemical meningitis have excellent prognosis with no neurological sequelae, while fungal, tuberculous, and carcinomatous meningitis all have worse prognosis.
  - The course and prognosis for encephalitis is highly variable, depending upon the pathogen. The clinical course may range from mild with no sequelae to rapidly deteriorating with death or severe neurologic disability. Fatality rate is highest for eastern equine encephalitis, with reported rates as high as 50% to 75%.
- Patients treated with antibiotic or antiviral therapy must understand that they will be required to complete a prolonged course of intravenous (IV) therapy (7–21 days).
- Patient and family information is available from the Meningitis Foundation of America, Inc. Phone 800-668-1129; Web site www.musa.org

CARE TRANSITIONS

- Duration of IV antibiotic therapy for bacterial meningitis is typically 7–10 days for *N. meningitidis* and *H. influenza*; 10–14 days for *S. pneumoniae*; and at least 21 days for gram-negative bacilli and *Listeria*. Patients cannot be transitioned to oral antibiotics and so may require IV antibiotics outside the inpatient setting to complete their full course.
- Patients left with neurological sequelae from meningitis or encephalitis often will require physical, speech, and/or occupational therapy after illness, and a few will have massive neurologic deficits, which may require transition to an extended care facility.
- Patients should follow up with their primary care provider (PCP) in 1–2 weeks after discharge.

BIBLIOGRAPHY

De Gans J, van de Beek D. Dexamethasone in adults with bacterial meningitis. *N Engl J Med.* 2002;347:1549.

Kupila L, Vuorinen T, Vainionpaa R, et al. Etiology of aseptic meningitis and encephalitis in adult population. *Neurology.* 2006;66:75.

Redington JJ, Tyler KL. Viral infections of the nervous system, 2002: update on diagnosis and management. *Arch Neurology.* 2002;59:712.

Roos KL. Mycobacterium tuberculosis meningitis and other etiologies of aseptic meningitis syndrome. *Semin Neurol.* 2000;20:329.

Rothbart HA. Viral meningitis. *Semin Neurol.* 2000;20:277.

Straus SE, Thorpe KE, Holroyd-Ledue J. How do I perform a lumbar puncture and analyze the results to diagnose bacterial meningitis? *JAMA.* 2006;296:2012.

Tunkel AR, Hartman BJ, Kaplan SL, et al. Practice guidelines for the management of bacterial meningitis. *Clin Infect Dis.* 2004;39:1267.

Van de Beek D, de Gans J, Tunkel AR, et al. Community-acquired bacterial meningitis in adults. *N Engl J Med.* 2006;354:44.

66 SEIZURE

Susan L. Hickenbottom

EPIDEMIOLOGY/OVERVIEW

- Seizures are episodes of temporary brain dysfunction secondary to abnormal electrical activity.
- Approximately 10% of the population will suffer a seizure at some point in their life.
- Around 25% of seizures will have a clearly identified, temporally linked cause. These seizures are referred to as "provoked" or "acute symptomatic" seizures, and do not have a tendency to recur, unless the provoking condition recurs.
- In contrast, epilepsy is defined as two or more *unprovoked* seizures. Individuals with epilepsy have a high rate of seizure recurrence if not treated with anticonvulsant medications.
- *Status epilepticus* is defined as the occurrence of a single unremitting seizure of longer than 10–20 minutes, or frequent recurrent seizures without interictal return to baseline clinical state.
- Over 2.5 million people in the United States have been diagnosed with epilepsy, and an estimated 185,000 people are diagnosed with the disorder each year.
- Epilepsy has an age-specific distribution, with higher rates in the very young and the very old: >140/100,000 at the two extremes of age, compared to approximately 60/100,000 for those aged 10–65 years. Disorders seen in the extremes of age, including cerebral palsy/mental retardation, stroke, and Alzheimer disease, raise the risk of seizures ten fold. As the population ages, the prevalence of epilepsy is expected to rise.
- To date, clinicians have no way to prevent the development of epilepsy in high-risk patients, and in two-thirds of persons with epilepsy no identifiable cause is found.

PATHOPHYSIOLOGY

- Epileptic seizures result from hypersynchronization of neuronal networks in the cerebral cortex. *Epileptogenesis* is defined as the process by which, over time, focal regions of the brain become hyperexcitable and develop the ability to spontaneously generate seizures.
- Some regions of the brain appear to be more vulnerable to the epileptogenic process—including the hippocampus, entorhinal cortex, and amygdala, which together make up the mesial temporal lobe.
- While the pathophysiology of epileptogenesis is not well understood, current research has focused on the molecular level, with studies examining voltage-gated ion channels, neurotransmitters, neuronal proteins, and alteration of gene expression within neurons.

CLINICAL PRESENTATION, DIFFERENTIAL, MAKING THE DIAGNOSIS

- Seizure classification is made through the clinical phenomenology of the seizure episode (seizure *semiology*). The main seizure types are *partial* (arising from one area of the brain, with or without spread to other areas) and *generalized* (involving both hemispheres of the brain simultaneously). Table 66-1 outlines a simplified version of seizure classification.

PARTIAL SEIZURES

- Partial seizures are further divided into simple partial seizures (with no alteration in level of awareness) and complex partial seizures (with impairment of level of awareness). With complex partial seizures, patients typically report amnesia for all or part of the episode.
- Partial seizures typically last only for a few minutes, but can be sustained ("partial status epilepticus").
- If the abnormal focal electrical discharge associated with partial seizures spreads to involve both hemispheres,

TABLE 66-1 Simplified Version of International League Against Epilepsy (ILAE) Classification of Seizures

Localization-related seizures (partial onset)

Simple partial seizures (no impairment of awareness)
- With motor symptoms
- With sensory symptoms
- With autonomic symptoms
- With psychic symptoms

Complex partial seizures (with impaired awareness)
- Beginning as simple partial onset
- With impaired awareness from onset

Primary generalized seizures

Absence
- Typical absence
- Atypical absence

Myoclonic
Clonic
Tonic
Tonic-clonic (primary)
Atonic ("drop attacks")

Unclassifiable

the event is then described as a *secondary generalized* seizure (usually tonic-clonic). If the preceding partial seizure is brief, or the patient is amnestic for the episode, it may be difficult to distinguish between secondarily generalized seizure and primary generalized seizures (discussed below) without the use of electroencephalogram (EEG).

• An *aura* is the patient's subjective experience of the onset of a seizure, and is in fact, a simple part seizure itself.

• The clinical presentation of a partial seizure (or aura) depends on the area of the cortex that is involved, which may include the temporal, frontal, occipital, or parietal lobe.

○ *Temporal lobe* seizures are the most common type of partial seizure, and were previously referred to as "psychomotor seizures." Common auras associated with these seizures are listed in Table 66-2.

■ Individuals who witness a patient having a temporal lobe partial seizure will often describe oral or manual *automatisms* (lip smacking or chewing, picking at clothes, patting); subtle dystonic posturing of a hand or limb; or, most often, staring or unresponsiveness for a period of time.

■ *Frontal lobe* partial seizures generally have prominent motor manifestations. The patient will often describe involuntary rhythmic jerking of the fingers, followed by the hand and arm, and then the face, all on the same side of the body (*jacksonian march*). Because preplanned motor programs are located in the prefrontal, or supplementary, motor cortex, patients may have complex and bilateral motor manifestations, such as bicycling movements, while still maintaining awareness and consciousness throughout the seizure.

■ *Occipital lobe* partial seizures manifest with sudden onset of positive visual phenomena rather than visual loss. These visual changes may include poorly formed colored lights, complex figures or scenes, or other visual hallucinations, which are usually stereotyped.

■ *Parietal lobe* partial seizures are associated with subjective numbness, tingling, or rarely pain, on the contralateral side of the body. These sensory symptoms may also follow a jacksonian march pattern.

GENERALIZED SEIZURES

• The most common type of generalized seizure is the *generalized tonic-clonic* (GTC), previously referred to as a "grand mal" seizure.

• GTC seizures can occur as primary (generalized from the onset) or as a secondarily generalized seizure after a partial onset seizure.

○ Primary GTC seizures do not begin with any aura or warning.

○ They begin with an abrupt loss of consciousness, which may be accompanied by a shriek or yelp.

○ The *tonic* phase of the seizure typically lasts 10–30 seconds and extension of the back and limbs with upward deviation of the eyes; the patient may appear cyanotic during this phase.

○ The *clonic* phase follows with rhythmic, often violent, jerking of the extremities with possible tongue or cheek biting, with frothy or bloody sputum coming from the mouth, possible loss of bladder, or bowel control. This phase typically lasts from 30 to 90 seconds.

• Patients may also have elevated heart rate or blood pressure, dilated pupil(s), and respiratory or metabolic acidosis with GTC seizures.

• Both GTC and complex partial seizures are typically followed by a postictal period, which typically lasts for 5–30 minutes, but can be more prolonged, especially if the ictal event itself is of longer than usual duration. Table 66-3 outlines typical postictal symptoms.

• *Absence seizures* usually occur during childhood, and were previously referred to as "petit mal" seizures. They manifest with sudden behavioral arrest, staring, and unresponsiveness, lasting between 5 and 10 seconds. There is usually no postictal confusion.

TABLE 66-2 Classic Presentation of Temporal Lobe Simple Partial Seizures (Auras)

SYMPTOM	ANATOMIC LOCALIZATION
Sense of epigastric rising areas	Cortex with projection to autonomic
Stereotyped sense of fear/panic	Amygdala/limbic cortex
Déjà vu/Jamais vu	Hippocampus
Odors (usually foul)	Olfactory cortex
Depersonalization/derealization	Unknown/limbic cortex

TABLE 66-3 Common Postictal Symptoms

Confusion
Headache
Exhaustion/sleep
Nausea
Memory loss
Generalized weakness
Thirst
Fear
Embarrassment
Loneliness
Depression
Perceptual alterations
Psychosis

DIFFERENTIAL DIAGNOSIS

- Because seizures are paroxysmal, often lead to loss of consciousness and are usually not witnessed by the examining physician; the diagnosis often relies on third-party witnesses and their ability to describe the event. Thus, other paroxysmal neurologic disorders may be confused with seizures. These include
  - ◦ *Syncope:* Associated with transient decrease of global cerebral blood flow, resulting in loss of consciousness.
    - Syncope can often be differentiated from seizures by identifying typical provoking factors, such as position change, exertion, dehydration, micturition/defecation, or environmental factors (hot room, pain, sight of blood).
    - Patients with syncope may report a prodrome of light-headedness, diaphoresis, and/or palpitations; whereas patients with seizures would report one of the typical auras described above, or may be amnestic for the spell.
    - Witnesses will often describe syncopal patients as being pale and sweaty, while those with seizures have staring, shaking of the limbs, or oral or manual automatisms.
    - Occasionally, patients with syncope may have a few brief, generalized convulsive movements (especially if they are prevented from assuming a flat position)—this is referred to as "convulsive syncope."
    - Finally, syncopal episodes tend to be briefer than seizures, lasting only 10–30 seconds with rapid return to normal mental status as compared to 1–3 minutes for seizures, which are often followed by a longer postictal period.
  - ◦ *Transient ischemic attack (TIA):* TIAs are brief episodes of focal neurologic dysfunction secondary to decreased perfusion of a particular region of the brain.
    - Most TIAs last 10–20 minutes, but their duration may be briefer. TIAs are usually not associated with confusion or loss of consciousness.
    - As a general rule, TIAs present with "negative" phenomena such as weakness, numbness, or loss of vision; seizures tend to have "positive" phenomena such as limb shaking, paresthesias, or visual hallucinations.
    - However, if patients have prolonged partial seizures, they may develop a "Todd phenomenon," in which the cortical neurons involved in the seizures remain depolarized and nonfunctional for minutes to hours. If the seizure is unwitnessed in a patient with Todd phenomenon, it could be mistaken for a TIA or stroke.
    - Finally, multiple, recurrent, stereotyped episodes are more suggestive of seizures, as one would expect that multiple TIAs would eventually result in permanent neurologic deficits.
  - ◦ *Migraine:* Some patients suffer from "complicated migraines," with which they may develop focal neurologic symptoms, and many patients have an aura preceding their typical headaches.
    - Although migraine auras may be similar to seizure auras in quality, auras associated with migraines tend to develop over minutes rather than seconds.
    - Of course, most migraine aura are accompanied or followed by a typical migraine headache.
  - ◦ *Psychogenic nonepileptic spells ("pseudoseizures"):* These spells can be easily mistaken for epileptic seizures, but they are not associated with any change on electroencephalogram (EEG).
    - Pseudoseizures are often difficult to distinguish from epileptic seizures, but may have some suggestive characteristics, including maintaining consciousness despite generalized shaking, nonrhythmic/alternating shaking of limbs, pelvic thrusting, or prolonged duration (hours).
    - Pseudoseizures are thought to represent a conversion disorder and are more common in patients with a history of other psychiatric disorders or a history of physical or sexual abuse. However, in some series, up to 50% of patients with pseudoseizures also have epileptic seizures. These patients often eventually require referral to a tertiary epilepsy center where they can undergo continuous EEG/video monitoring to determine the nature of their spells.

MAKING THE DIAGNOSIS

- EEG can be used to diagnose seizures, but often is unrevealing unless one of the patient's typical spells occurs during the recording. Nevertheless, EEG should be ordered for most hospitalized patients with seizures, if for no other reason than to establish a baseline study.
- If an episode is not captured on EEG, the diagnosis must be made based on clinical history and by ruling out potential mimickers of seizure.

TRIAGE AND INITIAL MANAGEMENT

- Initial workup should include a detailed history, including family history of "seizures, fits, or convulsions," and a physical and neurological examination, which should focus on identifying any lateralizing signs (weakness, hyperreflexia, or positive Babinski sign) that could suggest a contralateral brain lesion.

- A neuroimaging study should be done in all patients following a first seizure, in order to rule out an underlying brain lesion. In the emergency setting, a noncontrast head CT (HCT) will likely be done to evaluate for large mass lesion, hemorrhage, or large stroke. However, MRI scanning with contrast is much more sensitive than HCT in identifying a subtle lesion that could serve as a focus for seizure. MRI could be deferred until after discharge, depending on clinical characteristics. In up to 70% of patients with seizure, neuroimaging is normal.
- All patients with any type of seizure should undergo evaluation for provoking conditions, including:
  ○ Hypo- or hyperglycemia
  ○ Hypo- or hypernatremia
  ○ Hypocalcemia
  ○ Hypomagnesemia
  ○ Hyperthyroidism
  ○ Renal failure/uremia
  ○ Acute drug/alcohol intoxication or withdrawal
  ○ Noncompliance with antiepileptic regimen in patients with epilepsy
  ○ Environmental factors such as sleep deprivation and menstrual cycle
  ○ Systemic infection
- Any underlying metabolic abnormalities should be corrected as rapidly as is safe for the patient. Care must be taken to avoid too-rapid correction of hyponatremia, as this may lead to central pontine myelinolysis.
- Lumbar puncture (LP) is an essential step in the evaluation of seizure if the clinical presentation is suggestive of an acute infectious process that involves the central nervous system (CNS) or in any immunosuppressed patient, and it may also be needed in patients with a history of cancer known to metastasize to the CNS. In other settings, LP is unlikely to be helpful, and may even cloud the diagnostic picture, as prolonged seizure may lead to elevated protein and pleiocytosis in the cerebrospinal fluid (CSF). LP should only be performed after ruling out a space-occupying brain lesion with neuroimaging.
- EEG should be performed in all patients with a first seizure; it may be performed during the acute hospitalization or can be deferred until after discharge. The diagnostic limitations of EEG are noted above; a normal EEG does not rule out a seizure, and a "positive" EEG may show only nonspecific abnormalities.
- The decision to initiate antiepileptic drugs (AEDs) is often difficult. These medications are not required in patients with provoked seizures, as long as the provoking condition is brought under control. Adult patients with an unprovoked first seizure and a normal workup may or may not require AEDs; most prospective studies demonstrate a 33% to 50% chance of seizure recurrence after a first unprovoked seizure. However, seizure recurrence increases dramatically after a second or third unprovoked seizure, so these patients will need to be started on AEDs. Seizure recurrence is also higher in patients with a structural brain abnormality, a history of serious brain injury, partial seizure as first seizure, focal abnormalities found on neurologic examination, mental retardation, and/or interictal epileptiform abnormalities on EEG; patients with these characteristics may need to be started on AEDs after a first seizure.

- Patients with a single, brief seizure do *not* require administration of benzodiazepines; this treatment is reserved for patients with status epilepticus (see below). Administration of benzodiazepines or other sedatives may cloud consciousness, prolong the postictal phase, or depress respiratory status to the point of requiring intubation, all of which make the diagnostic evaluation of the seizure more difficult.
- Patients with a first seizure may or may not require hospitalization. Many of these patients can be discharged from the emergency setting if laboratory workup and neuroimaging is normal, and the postictal state has cleared. They should have follow-up with their primary care provider (PCP) or a neurologist within a few days of discharge. Patients should be hospitalized if they have a prolonged postictal phase, incomplete recovery, systemic illness that requires other treatment, a history of head trauma, or other significant medical conditions.

MANAGEMENT OF GENERALIZED CONVULSIVE STATUS EPILEPTICUS IN ADULTS

- Status epilepticus is defined in the overview section above; while it may occur with any seizure type, only generalized convulsive status epilepticus (GCSE) is considered a medical emergency. It carries a 20% mortality rate for a first episode, and may cause neuronal cell death, rhabdomyolysis/ renal failure, lactic acidosis, aspiration pneumonitis, neurogenic pulmonary edema, respiratory failure, and myocardial injury from massive release of catecholamines.
- Diagnosis of GCSE is usually made on clinical grounds, although EEG will reveal continuous seizure activity. EEG is required to diagnose GCSE in patients who have been pharmacologically paralyzed, and is also of use in patients with nonconvulsive status epilepticus.

TIME	ACTION
0–5 min	Diagnose Maintain airway, breathing, and circulation Give supplemental oxygen Obtain IV access ECG continuous monitoring Draw blood for complete blood count, electrolytes and glucose, calcium, magnesium, phosphorus, liver function tests, antiepileptic drug levels (if appropriate), arterial blood gas, toxicology screen Give thiamine 100 mg IV, followed by 50 mL of 50% dextrose IV
6–10 min	Give lorazepam 2–4 mg or diazepam 5 mg IV over 1–2 minutes If seizures persist, repeat in 5–10 minutes. If patient is not already intubated, consider rapid sequence intubation
10–20 min	Give phenytoin 20 mg/kg IV at no more than 50 mg/min *or* fosphenytoin 20 PE/kg IV at 150 PE/min (monitor for hypotension, arrhythmias)
20–60 min	Draw phenytoin level (total and/or free) 20 min after infusion done If seizures persist, intubate patient and give one of the following: • *Continuous IV midazolam*: Load 0.2 mg/kg; repeat 0.2–0.4 mg boluses every 5 min until seizures stop, up to a maximum of 2 mg/kg. Initial continuous infusion rate 0.1 mg/kg/h; range 0.05–0.2 mg/kg/h • *IV phenobarbital*: 20 mg/kg IV at 50–100 mg/min. Draw phenobarbital level about 20 min after loading infusion done • *Continuous IV propofol*: Load 1 mg/kg; repeat 1–2 mg/kg boluses every 3–5 min until seizures stop, up to a maximum of 10 mg/kg. Initial continuous IV rate 2 mg/kg/h; range 1–15 mg/kg/h • *IV valproate*: 40 mg/kg over 10 min. If seizures persist, additional 20 mg/kg over 5 min. Draw valproate level (total or free) 20 min after infusion is complete • If seizures persist with any of the above, proceed to pentobarbital
> 60 min	Give continuous IV *pentobarbital*: load 5–10 mg/kg up to 50 mg/min Repeat 5 mg/kg boluses until seizure stops. Initial continuous IV rate 1 mg/kg/h; range 0.5–1.0 mg/kg/h. Titrate to burst-suppression on EEG. Begin EEG monitoring asap

FIG. 66-1   Treatment protocol for management of GCSE.

• Treatment of GCSE is outlined in Fig. 66-1. The goals of treatment are to stabilize the patient, to break the status seizure activity, and to prevent its recurrence.
• Benzodiazepines remain the first-line treatment of GCSE because they can rapidly control seizures. Diazepam quickly crosses the blood-brain barrier, but its acute anticonvulsant effect is only about 20–30 minutes. Lorazepam may take up to 2 minutes to reach clinical effectiveness, but its duration is 4–6 hours.
• Phenytoin is one of the most commonly used agents for GCSE, and its main efficacy is in preventing recurrence of GCSE for an extended period of time. Fosphenytoin is a prodrug of phenytoin; it is highly water soluble and will not precipitate during intravenous (IV) administration. There is also a much lower rate of local irritation than with phenytoin, and because it does not use propylene glycol as a diluent, cardiovascular side effects may be less frequent as well.
• Refractory GCSE occurs when seizure does not stop after administration of benzodiazepines and phenytoin/fosphenytoin. In general continuous IV infusions are required to manage refractory GCSE, and consultation to neurology or critical care medicine may be needed to assist in managing these patients.

DISEASE MANAGEMENT STRATEGIES

• For patients with epilepsy (two or more unprovoked seizures), management with AEDs will be needed. For nonemergency treatment, AED therapy should be started with a single agent (monotherapy) with a gradual increase in dosage as needed to produce optimal seizure control ("start low and go slow"). Treatment should be monitored regularly, either by AED levels or by clinical parameter, or both.
• Combination therapy (polytherapy) should only be attempted if at least two additional adequate sequential trials of monotherapy have failed.
• In general, AEDs are divided into older drugs (phenobarbital, phenytoin, carbamazepine, and valproate) and newer drugs (gabapentin, lamotrigine, topiramate, levetiracetam, oxcarbazepine, and zonisamide). Newer AEDs have several potential advantages over older ones, including lower side effect rates, little or no need for serum monitoring, once or twice daily dosing, and fewer drug interactions. The older and newer AEDs do not show significant differences in effectiveness and most newer AEDs cost more than the older drugs.

TABLE 66-4   Common Starting AED Regimens for Hospitalized Patients with Seizures

SEIZURE TYPE	INITIAL DOSING REGIMEN
Primary GTC	Phenytoin 300 mg at bedtime Carbamazepine 100 mg twice daily, increase to 200 mg twice daily after 3–4 days* Valproate 250 mg twice daily Topiramate 25 mg at bedtime with moderate titration (3 weeks) to 50 mg twice daily
Partial seizure with or without secondary generalization	Phenytoin, carbamazepine, valproate as above Oxcarbazepine 150 mg twice daily, with rapid titration (1 week) to 300 mg twice daily Lamotrigine 25 mg twice daily with slow (5 week) titration to 100 mg twice daily† Levetiracetam 250 mg twice daily with rapid titration (1 week) to 500 mg twice daily Topiramate 25 mg at bedtime with moderate titration (3 weeks) to 50 mg twice daily

*Carbamazepine autoinduces its own metabolism and must be started at a low dose to avoid toxicity.
†Lamotrigine must be titrated very slowly to avoid development of rash, which can be severe (Stevens-Johnson syndrome).

- For the newer AEDs, lamotrigine and oxcarbazepine have well-documented effectiveness as monotherapy; the other agents have less consistent data.
- While many drug options are available in the outpatient setting, most hospitalists will want to start AED therapy with a medication that will become more rapidly therapeutic. Common treatment options for starting AEDs in the hospitalized patient are outlined in Table 66-4.
- Common side effects of the AEDs are outlined in Table 66-5.

CARE TRANSITIONS

- For female patients of childbearing age, there are additional issues to consider when initiating AED therapy.
  - Folate 0.4–1.0 mg daily should be prescribed to all women of childbearing age who will be started on AEDs. If the patient plans to become pregnant within the next 3 months, folate dose should be increased to 4 mg daily.
  - Women should be counseled on the potential interactions between AEDs and oral contraceptives.
  - Pregnancies should be planned. The risk of major and minor birth defects on AEDs is 6% to 8% (two-three times higher than the risk in mothers without epilepsy).

TABLE 66-5   Common Side Effects of Selected Antiepileptic Drugs

DRUG	SIDE EFFECTS
Carbamazepine	Nausea, vomiting, diarrhea Rash, pruritis Drowsiness, dizziness, lethargy Dysequilibrium Blurred or double vision Hyponatremia Anorexia
Lamotrigine	Nausea Rash (potentially severe) Drowsiness, dizziness
Levetiracetam	Fatigue, drowsiness Anxiety, agitation
Oxcarbazepine	Nausea Rash Drowsiness, dizziness Dysequilibrium Blurred or double vision Hyponatremia
Phenytoin	Drowsiness, dizziness Rash Blurred or double vision Dysequilibrium Gingival hypertrophy Increased body hair growth Neuropathy (long-term use)
Topiramate	Fatigue, drowsiness Difficulty concentrating, word-finding difficulties Paresthesias Taste change Weight loss Renal stones Tremor Mood disruption
Valproate	Nausea, vomiting Fatigue, drowsiness Tremor Weight gain Hair loss Easy bruising (thrombocytopenia)

- Patients with generalized or partial complex seizures will need to be counseled on driving restrictions, which vary widely from state to state. Patients should also be instructed not to swim alone or pursue other activities during which they could suffer serious harm if a seizure were to occur.
- Family members should be educated on what to do if a seizure occurs and when the emergency medical system would need to be activated.
- Patients newly started on AEDs will need timely follow-up with their PCP, within about 1 week. AED serum levels should be drawn at the visit if clinically available (mostly the older AEDs).

BIBLIOGRAPHY

Brodie MJ, Dichter MA. Antiepileptic drugs. *N Engl J Med.* 1996;334:168.

Chang B, Lowenstein DH. Epilepsy. *N Engl J Med.* 2003;349:1257.

Marson A, Jacoby A, Johnson A, et al, for the Medical Research Council MESS Study Group. Immediate vs. deferred antiepileptic drug treatment for early epilepsy and single seizures: a randomized controlled trial. *Lancet.* 2005;365:2007.

Vazquez B. Monotherapy in epilepsy: role of the newer antiepileptic drugs. *Arch Neurol.* 2004;61:1361.

Walker M. Status epilepticus: an evidence-based guide. *BMJ.* 2005;331:673.

PSYCHIATRIC ILLNESS

67 ASSESSING CAPACITY FOR MEDICAL DECISION MAKING

David F. Gitlin and Ajita Mathur

BACKGROUND/OVERVIEW

- In caring for medically ill patients, the hospitalist must endeavor to develop a working therapeutic relationship with the hospitalized individual, so that effective decision making may occur.
- The hospitalist should attempt to provide the patient with adequate information regarding their condition and potential etiologies so that the patient may understand the physician's recommendations regarding tests, procedures, and treatment.
- Generally, this alliance between patient and hospitalist is a successful partnership despite the reality that, typically, no previous treatment relationship existed.
- However, there are some situations in which the patient appears unable to make decisions in concert with the medical team, despite the best efforts of the hospitalist.
- In such cases, concern may be raised that the patient lacks the decision-making ability necessary to decide about the medical treatment, that is, whether the patient is *competent* or not.
- The hospitalist must be prepared to assess the patient's capacity for decision making independent from optimal efforts to provide care for the individual.

- Frequently, the hospitalist will employ the expertise of other consultants for this assessment, including psychiatrists, social workers, and ethicists.
- This chapter will look at the various situations in which questions may arise regarding patient decision making, how to adequately assess whether patients have the ability to make medical decisions, and how the hospitalist should proceed once decision making has been assessed (Fig. 67-1). Lastly, we will consider alternative approaches to resolving medical decision-making concerns that may arise.

HISTORY OF THE COMPETENCY CONSTRUCT

- Physicians have not always struggled with the idea of competent patient decision making.
- Prior to the latter half of the twentieth century, patients were often only passively included in the process of their own medical care.
  - Physicians often did not explain to patients the details of their illness or treatment.
  - The patient was expected to comply with the doctor's interventions, and only when the patient actively disagreed did the physician engage him/her in the process of decision-making.
  - The patient's lack of questioning was taken as agreement, a process known as *simple consent*.
- More recently, advocates argued that individuals should have the right to participate in their own medical treatment.

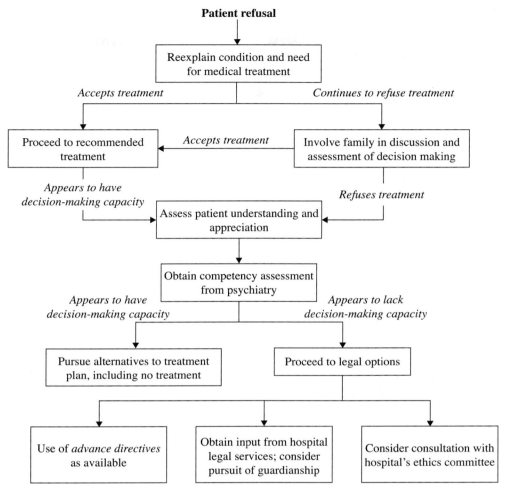

FIG. 67-1   Algorithm for treatment refusal.

○ Several important legal cases most notably Natanson vs Klein (Kansas 1960) supported this position, providing that patients should be involved in the decisions regarding their own medical care.

• Gradually, the doctrine of *informed consent* has become the standard of care in medicine. This doctrine implies that individuals have certain rights and expectations when it comes to making decisions regarding their own medical care.

  ○ First, patients have the right to be informed.

    ▪ This information includes an understanding of their medical condition.

    ▪ In addition, the information should describe the nature of the proposed tests, procedures, and treatments, and the risks and benefits of those interventions.

    ▪ This should include any alternatives to treatment, including no treatment.

  ○ Second, patient decision making should be voluntary.

    ▪ This implies that the physician should not coerce the patient to make specific decisions that might be preferable to the physician.

    ▪ While the physician may be under no obligation to engage in treatment he/she does not agree with, the clinician must allow the patient to reach a decision without undue influence.

  ○ Lastly, the doctrine of informed consent suggests the patient must be *competent* to make adequate medical decisions.

ASSESSMENT OF COMPETENCY

• Competency is primarily a legal term rather than a medical one. Over the past quarter century, both legal and medical scholars have written extensively about what makes a patient competent to engage in medical decision making. This has been supported by a variety of legal verdicts.

- Most scholars now agree that competent decision making is founded on four basic capacities.
  1. Capacity to consistently voice a decision
  2. Capacity to understand relevant information
  3. Capacity to appreciate the relevant information and its potential consequences
  4. Capacity to make rational decisions
- These capacities are somewhat hierarchical. Generally, the clinician begins with the first capacity evaluation, and only progresses with furthor capacity evaluation if the patient appears capable of understanding relevant information.

CAPACITY TO CONSISTENTLY VOICE A DECISION

- This is the simplest of the individual capacities. It basically implies that a person is able to state what they want done in any given situation. This may be as basic as "yes/no" decision making when a specific treatment is recommended. Most patients have this ability.
- It is typically lost when cognitive ability is so impaired as to prevent even the ability to respond. This includes cognitive states such as stupor and coma, expressive aphasias, and severe mental retardation and developmental disorders.
- Occasionally, a cognitively intact individual is so paralyzed with indecision that they are unable to even state a decision consistently, and in the most disabling of these situations may be incapable of decision making.

CAPACITY TO UNDERSTAND RELEVANT INFORMATION

- In general, this is the capacity that most physicians think about when they are considering whether a patient is competent. It is the fundamental task for any individual who is faced with making an informed decision.
- The physician should provide *the amount of information that a reasonable person would want to know.*
  ○ This gives the hospitalist some room depending on the patient's education and cognitive levels as well as his or her emotional ability to handle difficult information.
  ○ The physician should be expected to explain the medical condition, describe the recommended tests or treatments, identify the potential risks and benefits of each of these, and to compare this to other options, including no treatment.
  ○ The physician should allow the patient to demonstrate understanding by repeating what he or she has heard. This will permit the physician to then clarify misunderstandings and provide time for questions.

  ○ Patients with mental retardation, dementia, or other cognitive disorders may have impairments in this capacity.
- Patients with the capacity to understand may appear not to understand information for a variety of reasons.
  ○ English may not be the primary language of the patient, and this language barrier may be the source of miscommunication. The physician should attempt to use an interpreter whenever this concern arises.
  ○ Patient may have a very limited understanding of medical jargon.
    ▪ The hospitalist should always endeavor to use words that the patient knows rather than medical terminology.
    ▪ While all physicians understand "a 90% occlusion of the left anterior descending coronary artery (LAD) and other major coronaries necessitating a four-vessel cabbage," most patients will understand this better if told that they have "a serious blockage of some of the arteries that supply blood to the heart, and that we need to bypass those blocked vessels with four new arteries to fix this problem."
  ○ Simple misunderstandings can occur, leading to patient refusal of care.
    ▪ When the physician allows the patient to describe what he/she understands, this provides the opportunity to recognize misunderstandings and clarify them, often resulting in patient agreement.

CAPACITY TO APPRECIATE RELEVANT INFORMATION AND ITS POTENTIAL CONSEQUENCES

- There is a wide gulf between factual knowledge and the ability to apply it to one's own life circumstances.
- While many patients may understand the basic information regarding their illness and the recommended interventions, they may have very poor appreciation of how this information applies to their personal situation. They may know the facts about the risks of a heart attack but not believe that the chest pain they are having means they are now at risk.
- A lack of appreciation may be due to one of several causes, including
  ○ *Denial:* Denial is a very common human behavior. The ability to deny the existence of some common dangers is part of what allows most people to get through the day.
    ▪ For example, contemplation about the thousands of traffic fatalities that occur each year with each car trip might lead being unable to drive due to fear of the consequences. Denial allows us to make this awareness unconscious.

- Denial of risk contributes to many destructive health behaviors, such as smoking, overeating, and alcoholism.
- When the risks are not immediate, this may be understandable. However, when the risk is more imminent, such as a potentially new diagnosis of cancer or an acute myocardial infarction (MI), denial can become dangerous and interfere with treatment.
- For example, the patient may refuse to stay in the hospital or to have critical tests or treatments. When this occurs, the hospitalist should attempt to assess whether the patient appreciates the risks associated with refusal of care.
- If a patient's appreciation of the risks is in question, then he or she might be considered to lack the capacity for decision making.
  - ○ *Cognitive impairment:* Similar to the ability to understand, patients with cognitive impairments may not appreciate the risks associated with treatment refusal. Conditions such as delirium, dementia, traumatic brain injury, and mental retardation may sufficiently impair appreciation to affect decision-making ability.
  - ○ *Psychiatric illness:* When psychiatric illnesses impair the ability to make medical decisions, it is usually due to the impact on appreciation.
    - Patients with psychotic disorders such as schizophrenia generally understand the information presented to them, but their psychosis may interfere with appreciating that the information relates to them. For example, the psychotic patient will understand all the information about pneumonia, but he/she may believe that the x-rays have been fabricated as part of a governmental plot.
    - Depression may also affect a patient's ability to appreciate the importance of the information available. The depressed patient has complete understanding but may reject treatment as "too much trouble" or feel that he/she "does not deserve help."
  - ○ *Personality issues:* For some individuals, their typical approach to difficult situations may not be entirely functional. Certain personality styles may result in poor appreciation of acute medical illness, which can complicate the ability of the hospitalist to care for these patients.
    - *Narcissistic* persons may experience the development of illness as a personal failure or weakness, or may find the need to comply with the rules of medical environments intolerable. In both cases, their reaction to this loss of control of their lives may lead to anger and conflict with the medical providers, including refusal of care.

- Patients with excessive *dependent* styles may feel quite inadequate when faced with medical illness. Often they will struggle with fearfulness and indecision, deferring excessively to the providers for direction. Hospitalists need to exercise caution and make sure that these patients understand what they are agreeing to.
- *Obsessional and paranoid* individuals will struggle with care providers around issues of trust, fearing that tests and treatment may not be the correct approach. These patients may question everything that the hospitalist attempts to explain to them, and ultimately may be unable to agree to any care.
- Finally, the patient with *borderline* personality traits can be extremely difficult to care for. These patients may have an inability to develop adequate trusting relationships with the care providers, have tendencies to see medical staff as harmful, can be impulsive and irrational, and even exhibit a propensity for self-injurious thinking and behavior.
  - ○ Decision making is often complicated by these features, leading the hospitalist to question the patient's capacity to make medical choices.

CAPACITY TO MAKE RATIONAL DECISIONS

- Even when patients appear to understand information and appreciate its relevance to their personal situation, they may not make decisions in a rational manner. A variety of emotional or cognitive derangements may interfere with their processing of the information.
  - ○ Fear, anxiety, and hopelessness may also obscure the patient's otherwise rational considerations.
  - ○ Conversely, some people have a history of risk-taking behavior or impulsive decision making. For these individuals, "irrationality" may be their standard approach to difficult decision-making situations.
  - ○ When these people become patients, they are likely to continue in this manner. If the pattern of behavior is an enduring one rather than a sudden deviation from previous patterns, then this should be considered their normal processing, and thus *rational* for them.
- The concept of rational decision making is complicated, and as such many courts do not use it for the assessment of legal competence.

DECISION MAKING FOR INCOMPETENT PATIENTS

- Once it has been clinically determined that the patient lacks decision-making ability, an alternate decision-maker must be identified.

- In emergent medical situations, the physician must decide on behalf of the patient. In all other situations, a substitute must be identified.
  - Typically, this will be the closest family member, often referred to as the "next of kin."
  - Most often this is the spouse but may also include parents, siblings, and children.
  - If unclear, the family will often designate an identified member to act on the patient's behalf.
  - Where no family exists, a friend may also be considered.
- The identified decision maker should be instructed to consider *what the patient would have decided if the patient was competent,* rather than what he or she believes is best for the patient or what the decision-maker might choose for him or herself. This is known as "substituted judgment." Unfortunately, too often the family member or friend has never had a conversation with the patient about wishes during lack of capacity.
- The hospitalist should always attempt to discuss future decision making with patients during the course of the hospitalization. Unfortunately, several factors may interfere with this.
  - First, the hospitalist typically does not have an established relationship with the patient on admission.
  - It is often difficult to discuss potential negative outcomes when this prior relationship is limited, especially if a poor outcome is likely.
- Where patients do make their advanced wishes known, the hospitalist should document this information in the medical record.

ADVANCE DIRECTIVES

- Most states now offer the patient and family the ability to document how decisions will be made if the person becomes incapacitated. These documents are known as "advance directives," although terms such as "living will" and "durable power of attorney" may also be used.
- While the specific laws vary from state to state, most allow the patient to designate a specific individual to make decisions on behalf of the patient in the event of loss of capacity to make informed decisions. These are called "proxy" directives, and the designated person the "proxy agent." In addition, many states also permit the individual to document specific directions regarding future care, such as *do-not-resuscitate (DNR)* directives. This may aid the proxy agent as the substitute decision maker.
- Whenever possible, the hospitalist should attempt to identify the existence of an advanced directive, or to have the patient complete one upon admission.

IMPAIRED DECISION MAKING AS A MEASURE OF CONFLICT

- Medical decision making should be seen as a process resulting from positive relationships with family and caregivers, which allows for effective communication and consideration.
- When conflicts exist between any of these spheres of influence (Fig. 67-2), the patient may be unable to make adequate choices.
- Many patients may have problems with decision making due to personality factors as described above that may predispose them to conflict.
- Others will struggle with decision making when no deficit can be identified for a variety of reasons. In some of these cases, the trouble may be the result of conflicts the patient is having with one or more individuals. Conflicts that may exist between the patient and family can also affect medical decision making.
  - Parents, spouses, and children may try to influence the decision based upon their own needs and emotions rather than the patient's.
  - Family members may feel conflicted toward the providers. This may result from their anger or fear about the illness and its potential effect upon their loved one.
  - Family members may undermine the relationship between the hospitalist and patient, further impairing the patient's ability to make decisions. The hospitalist must recognize these conflicts and attempt to help the family members consistently support the patient in their choices.
- Although conflicts between patients and the medical team may occur due to personality issues that interfere with trust and promote conflicts among family members, sometimes, it is the medical team who is conflicted with the patient.
  - Some physicians are less receptive to alternative approaches beyond their recommended treatment,

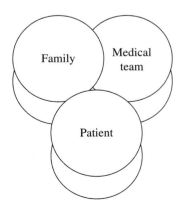

FIG. 67-2 Spheres of influence.

and may not tolerate when patients ask for more information about alternatives.

- ◦ Religious and ethical conflicts between the provider and patient may also be sources of conflict.
- Conflicts may also exist within these spheres. Family members may be at odds with one another, struggling for the affection of the patient, or have ulterior motives regarding the patient's outcome.
  - ◦ At times, well-meaning family members may simply disagree about the approach to care. These conflicts may result in the patient getting caught between competing factions, unable to decide what to do.
  - ◦ Similarly, different members of the medical team may be in conflict regarding the appropriate medical course of action.
    - ▪ Consultants may cause conflict if they communicate recommendations that differ from the primary medical team, sometimes without prior discussion with the attending of record.
    - ▪ While the hospitalist may provide the patient with information and encourage treatment, nurses, social workers, and/or trainees or consultants may communicate different opinions.
- Any of these conflicts—whether among family members or the medical team—can confuse the patient and may diminish the patient's ability to come to an ultimate decision regarding care and treatment.
- In all of these situations, the patient's diminished ability to come to a decision regarding medical care may lead the hospitalist to question the patient's decision-making capacity.
  - ◦ However, if the hospitalist can recognize that the particular conflict exists, he/she may be able to obviate the question of capacity.
  - ◦ Meeting with the involved parties may help to develop alliances around patient care, providing the patient with cohesive rather than adversarial input. This may, in turn, allow the patient to effectively make decisions.
  - ◦ Involving psychiatry or social work, where appropriate, may also help in addressing the conflicts at hand, ultimately helping the patient to successfully consider the choices at hand.

USE OF AN ETHICS COMMITTEE

- Sometimes, the patient's decision-making efforts are complicated because of the difficult nature of the decision. Many medical decisions are affected by personal issues, religious and spiritual issues, or social pressures.
- The patient may come to a decision that appears irrational, or at least in conflict with usual patterns of decision making. Particularly when life or death decisions are involved, patients may either make choices that leave the medical providers uncomfortable, or be unable to make any decision at all.

- Such decisions include DNR/DNI (do not resuscitate/do not intubate) choices, fetus continuation or termination, dialysis or chemotherapy discontinuation, or refusal of life-saving surgery.
- Consultation to psychiatry may help elucidate the specifics of the patient's cognitive and emotional ability to make decisions, but this may not help resolve the situation. In these cases, the primary issue affecting the patient may be more moral than clinical.
- Consultation to the hospital's ethics committee may help both the patient and medical team sort out the relevant issues so that reasonable decisions can be reached.

BIBLIOGRAPHY

Berg JW, Appelbaum PS, Lidz CW, et al. *Informed Consent: Legal Theory and Clinical Practice.* New York: Oxford University Press; 2001.

Dunn AB, Nowrangi MA, Palmer BW, et al. Assessing decisional capacity for clinical research or treatment: a review of instruments. *Am J Psychiatry.* August 2006;163(8):1323–1334.

Grisso T, Appelbaum PS. *Assessing Competence to Consent to Treatment.* New York: Oxford University Press; 1998.

Gutheil TG, Appelbaum PS. *Clinical Handbook of Psychiatry and the Law.* 3rd ed. Philadelphia, PA: Lippincott, Williams, and Williams; 2000.

President's Commission for the Study of Ethical Problems in Medicine and Biomedical/Behavioral Research. Washington, DC: US Government Printing Office; 1982.

Quill TE, Brody H. Physician recommendations and patient autonomy: finding a balance between physician power and patient choice. *Ann Intern Med.* 1996;125(9):763–769.

68 BEHAVIORAL DISTURBANCES THAT INTERFERE WITH MEDICAL CARE

Michelle Nichols and Bernard Vaccaro

OVERVIEW

- Behavioral disturbances are a common problem in the inpatient medical setting, but the true frequency of such disturbances is not recorded.

- Multiple causes of behavioral disturbances exist, and can roughly be divided into behavioral disturbances due to medical conditions, those due to major psychiatric disorders, and those due to difficult interpersonal styles.
- Evaluating the patient and clinical situation is essential in generating a differential diagnosis and subsequent treatment plan.

MEDICAL CAUSES OF BEHAVIORAL DISTURBANCES

- Common medical causes of behavioral disturbances include: delirium, dementia, substance intoxication and withdrawal syndromes, and side effects of medical treatments.
- Delirium is a common cause of behavioral dysregulation and can present in several ways. Its hallmark features include: onset of symptoms over hours to days, waxing and waning course throughout the day, impairments of cognition (i.e., memory, attention, executive function) and emotion (i.e., mood lability, sadness, anxiety), and impairments of consciousness (i.e., paranoia, hallucinations).
- See *Delirium* chapter for further discussion.
- With an aging population, dementia is another common cause of behavioral disturbances. Dementia is defined as the development of cognitive deficits with both memory impairment and one or more of the following: aphasia, apraxia, agnosia, or disturbance of executive functioning.
- Individuals with dementia can have agitation as part of their dementia, be easily confused by changes in environment, exhibit paranoia or delusions as a part of their agitation, and are predisposed to developing delirium as a consequence of their medical conditions.
- Treatment of agitation in delirium and dementia should include management of the patient's environment. Encourage frequent visits by friends and family, place calendars and clocks in prominent locations, encourage interactions with others, provide frequent reassurance, and reinforce diurnal rhythms with bright lights during the day and minimization of external stimuli at night.
- Medication treatment for dementia includes continuation of anticholinesterase treatments and judicious use of psychotropics. In the acute setting, preference is generally given to low-dose high-potency typical neuroleptics;[1] however, when long-term management is required, atypical antipsychotics (i.e., risperidone, olanzapine, quetiapine, ziprasidone) are favored for their reduced rates of parkinsonism and tardive dyskinesia compared with typical neuroleptics.[2,3]

- Of notable exception are patients with Parkinson's and parkinson-like dementias. Antipsychotics should be *avoided* in patients with Lewy body type dementia, as this subgroup displays particular neuroleptic sensitivity with not only adverse motoric side effects but increased mortality.[4,5] In Parkinson's disease, where much of observed psychosis and behavioral abnormalities are deemed iatrogenically precipitated or exacerbated, adjustments of patients' anticholinergic agents and dopamimetic doses are favored prior to neuroleptic trial.[6,7,8]
- Use of other psychotropic agents for the treatment of agitation in dementia is largely empiric. Randomized controlled trials of anticonvulsant medications in this population have yielded largely unimpressive results with regard to behavior control, and antidepressants have shown little behavioral benefit apart from treatment of underlying depression.[9]
- With few exceptions, benzodiazepines and sedative-hypnotics should be avoided with dementia.[2]
- Whenever possible, avoid restraints, indwelling catheters, and iatrogenic sleep deprivation.
- For complicated cases of behavioral disturbances of dementia and delirium, consider psychiatric consultation.
- Substance abuse is a commonly encountered problem in the medical setting. Studies suggest that over $1/2$ to $2/3$ of emergency room visits involve the use or abuse of alcohol or illicit drugs or misuse of prescription drugs; this figure can be even higher in select patient populations.[10,11]
- Substances may be both illegal (e.g., heroin, cocaine, hallucinogens or legal (e.g., alcohol, benzodiazepines, narcotics), including chronic use of sedative-hypnotics as sleep agents or anxiolytics.
- Careful screening on admission for alcohol/sedative-hypnotic use including amount, frequency, and use duration can begin to identify patients at risk for withdrawal syndromes.
- When patients may be confused or unreliable historians, obtain collateral history from family and friends. In some circumstances, calling the pharmacy may be warranted to obtain accurate medication doses.
- Treat alcohol/sedative-hypnotic withdrawal with cross-reactive agents (i.e., lorazepam, oxazepam) in medically compromised individuals or with longer-acting agents (i.e., diazepam, chlordiazepoxide) in non-medically compromised individuals.
- Treat patient's signs and symptoms and do not necessarily give prophylaxis to every individual; this can avoid iatrogenically-induced substance toxicity states.
- In patients with suspected heavy alcohol use, always remember to give multivitamins, and *parenteral* thiamine and folate to prevent Wernicke-Korsakoff syndrome.[12]

- See *Substance Abuse* and *Drug Toxicity* chapters for further discussion.

PATIENTS WITH PRIMARY PSYCHIATRIC DISORDERS

- When patients with major psychiatric disorders such as schizophrenia, bipolar disorder, major depression and substance use disorders get medically ill, they are at risk for receiving less than optimal care because of their mental illness.
- The first step in treating the medical problems of psychiatric patients is close and careful collaboration with the patient's psychiatrist or hospital psychiatric consultant.
- Patients with co-morbid psychiatric illness and major medical illness need ongoing treatment for their mental illness and, if at all possible, their psychotropic medication must be continued.
- Psychiatric patients with psychotic disorders such as schizophrenia, who may present actively paranoid, may respond to the same interventions listed below for the paranoid personality. They should be approached in a straightforward, direct manner. As they may be hesitant about receiving particular procedures or interventions, it is useful to advocate for the treatment in a matter-of-fact manner. [Example: "Getting this procedure is the standard of care for evaluating/treating this illness."]
- Depression is another common problem in the general hospital that can interfere with medical care. It is often difficult in the acute care setting to determine if the depression is due primarily to other medical problems (i.e., delirium, substance abuse) or is an endogenous mood disorder.
- See *Depression* chapter for further discussion.
- Sometime neurological injuries such as stroke, traumatic brain injury, and Parkinson's disease can present with apathy syndromes distinct from depression. These apathy syndromes are more diseases of motivation and initiation of behavior, not primary mood disorders, and are treated differently. A psychiatric consultation can be helpful in these circumstances.

DIFFICULT INTERPERSONAL STYLES

- Perhaps most frustrating to the internist is not the presence of florid primary psychiatric illness, but the encounter of difficult interpersonal styles in patients that can threaten compliance with treatment and undermine medical management of illness.

- While the *Diagnostic and Statistical Manual of Mental Disorders* (DSM) has attempted to operationalize personality dysfunction, these classifications are neither static nor equivalently validated. In addition, the use of terms such as "borderline" or "histrionic" are frequently pejorative, eliciting countertransference reactions among providers to the moniker alone, and potentially negatively impacting health care delivery and disease management.
- Personality is dynamic. In addition to changing with age, illness, interpersonal resources, historical context, and psychosocial stressors can all impact a patient's observed personality.
- Patients who pre-morbid to their medical illness may not have been diagnosed with a personality disorder per se, may regress to more primitive levels of coping as disease may precipitate feelings of helplessness, lost autonomy, shame, and guilt.[13]
- More useful to the internist in managing the patient with "difficult" personality is to refrain from diagnostic labels and to describe a patient's coping mechanisms as he/she attempts to achieve a psychological homeostasis.[14]
- Interventions can be tailored to the patient's style of coping without supposing a more encompassing characterlogic disturbance whose treatment is both outside the internist's capacity of time and scope of expertise.
- While no discussion of coping is atheoretical, the hierarchical classification of coping mechanisms described by Vaillant as more or less mature may be the most pithy and conceptually intuitive to the medical clinician.[14]
- Helpful in identification of the patient's utilized coping mechanisms is the physician's negative reaction toward the patient (i.e., the countertransference); the clinician's awareness of his own emotional barometer can facilitate understanding as well as intervention.[15,16]
- However, before embarking on strategies to manage patient's reactions, it is important that other causes for disruptive behavior be ruled out. The prudent clinician should first assess:[17]
  ○ Is the problem secondary to miscommunication or misunderstanding between the patient and medical staff which could be resolved through clarification?
  ○ Are practical, negotiable issues perturbed by emotional conflict? Can these issues be disassociated and addressed separately?
  ○ Is there an intercurrent medical etiology (i.e., delirium, dementia, CNS inflammatory disease, seizure, etc.), substance use/withdrawal (i.e., alcohol, illicit drugs), primary Axis I psychiatric disorder (i.e., major mood disorder, chronic psychotic disorder), or iatrogenic source (i.e., influence of prescribed

medications, esp. analgesics, steroids, neuroleptics) which could account for, in whole or part, observed behavior? If so, this should be evaluated and addressed appropriately.
  ○ How is the physician-patient relationship regarded in the patient's sociocultural context?
  ○ Is problem behavior being misattributed to the patient? Is the "difficult" personality a member of the medical or nursing team?
- Subsequent approach to the patient should focus on brief psychotherapeutic maneuvers which aim to bolster the patient's adaptive defenses and strengthen the therapeutic alliance. Use of psychotropic medications (esp. low-dose typical neuroleptics) and/or physical restraints should be reserved *only* for those patients most acutely disruptive or dangerous.
- More primitive ways of coping (i.e., "psychotic" and "immature" levels) should be acknowledged but not condoned or overtly challenged. [Example (of a patient s/p orthopedic procedure reticent to engage in physical therapy): "Illness often makes people feel anxious and not want to try things. It is important to know that despite physical therapy sometimes being difficult, it is precisely this treatment which will allow you to regain the strength you need to be able to return home."]
- For paranoid individuals and those personalities who use the least mature, "psychotic" means of coping, clinicians should approach the patient with consistency, humility, and in a manner that maximizes the patient's autonomy. Consistency involves a minimization of change in treatment plan and personnel as well as scrupulous communication among caregivers; change, when necessary, should be disclosed to the patient in a timely fashion. An attitude of courteousness that respects interpersonal boundaries and emotional distances can mitigate much of the querulousness that these patients initiate.[17,18,19]
- The patient utilizing "immature" defenses and who appears detached or aloof should be approached considerately with minimal demands for interpersonal engagement and without requirement for social reciprocity.[18] [Example: "It can be upsetting when there are delays in the surgery schedule, especially for an individual of your sensitivity going through such a trying illness. It is important, though, that you continue to refrain from eating for the next few hours so that we can keep your breathing safe during the procedure."] As with patients who exhibit a more "hysterical" personality, straightforward, regular interactions with schizoid or avoidant patients facilitate normalization of their interpersonal dynamic.[17]

- As regressive behavior escalates, especially in those patients exhibiting Cluster B personality traits, limit-setting and staff "anti-splitting" measures should be applied.
- If there is knowledge of prior attempts by the patient to sabotage treatment, manipulate, or engage in anti-social behavior, formulation of an *a priori* treatment contract with the patient that sets realistic goals of treatment, offers protection of the treatment effort from threats, and outlines contingencies can obviate the need for what can be deemed as more punitive setting of limits following behavioral escalations.[20,21]
- Implementation of administrative policies (i.e., detox protocols, urine screens) and contracting (outlining expected behaviors and graduated consequences for infractions) have been a mainstay of treatments for chemical dependency. While the general hospital setting poses some unique difficulties for implementation, institutional standards in combination with patient negotiation, can ameliorate much of the treatment non-compliance and dangerous/disruptive behavior that may ensue in the drug-dependent population.[22]
- The same principles can be utilized for containment of behavioral problems in the general medical patient. Behavioral contracts which seek to educate, co-opt the participation of all involved parties, and provide supportive buttresses for patients and staff have the greatest chance of being effective.[23]
- Central to the development of any contract with the patient (or family) is the preservation of a working therapeutic relationship. [Example: "When your spouse and five children call throughout the day to check on your status, hours of my day are diverted from direct care of yourself and other patients to answer the phone. By designating one family member as spokesman, all updates can be relayed to and all concerns notified through a single individual. This will permit us to give you and others the greatest opportunity to obtain the best medical care that we can give you."]
- Often times the hospital's patient relations or hospital administrative office can be useful in terms of contract design and execution.
- When limit-setting is employed following a destructive act or threat, a sympathetic approach to the patient that ideally allows him/her to "save face" has the greatest likelihood of being effective.[17,24] [Of note, in the patient who displays avoidant or Cluster A personality traits, a matter-of-fact approach is more effective as it doesn't imply closeness.][17]
- Splitting of staff may occur via deliberate manipulation of select staff, actual differences in affect and

TABLE 68-1   Matching of Defense Level to *DSM-IV*[25] Personality Disorders and Interventions

LEVEL OF DEFENSE	PSYCHOTIC	IMMATURE	NEUROTIC
Diagnostic correlates	Paranoid	Schizoid Avoidant Schizotypal	Obsessive-compulsive
		Borderline Antisocial	
		Narcissistic Histrionic Dependent	
Intervention Strategies	Maximize autonomy Consistency Assume humility Limit-set Employ "anti-splitting" maneuvers Negotiate contracts	Straightforwardness Matter-of-fact relationship	Strategic reframing Personal leverage

SOURCE: Adapted from Fogel BS, Stoudemire A. Personality disorders in the medical setting. In: Stoudemire A, Fogel BS, Greenberg D, eds. *Psychiatric Care of the Medical Patient.* 2nd ed. Oxford: Oxford University Press; 2000:443–458.

behavior secondary to variable patient transference, or different countertransference to the patient among staff. If staff splitting has not been prevented by aforementioned efforts at consistency and uniform communication, "anti-splitting" efforts in the form of multidisciplinary team meetings involving consultants and nursing (with or without family) are imperative for arriving at a consensus on the patient's treatment.[17]

- For those patients with less primitive "neurotic" defenses, interventions utilizing strategic reframing and/or personal leverage are most likely to promote treatment compliance.[17]

- When paired with appeals to the patient's discernment or reasoning, the intellectualizing compulsive personality is more likely to be actively participant in his medical decision-making [Example: "Following this treatment can save you money in the long-run."] Similarly beneficial is the clinician who genuinely acknowledges the narcissistic patient's achievements while encouraging collaboration in the execution of his treatment plan. [Example: "Illness can sometimes cause people to want to give up, but you've been a fighter. Sometimes though, that fighting spirit comes out negatively in your interactions with your doctors. You're right; you're entitled to the best medical care we can give you, but to give you the good treatment that you deserve, we need your cooperation with these tests so we know how best to proceed."][15,17,18]

- Personal leverage is an especially useful intervention in persons with poor self-image or a damaged sense of self-efficacy. By placing treatment recommendations in the context of a revered or valued relationship (i.e., with a particular physician, a family member, a community), treatment compliance and patient's health can be positively impacted. [Example: "Doing this would mean a lot to your children."][17]

- Table 68-1 provides a quick reference to interventional strategy based on identification of the patient's level of coping. [As DSM-IV personality disorder categories may be more familiar to the internist, these are also included for assistance in identification of patients' prominent modalities of defense.]

REFERENCES

1. Howell T, Watts DT. Behavioral complications of dementia: a clinical approach for the general internist. *J Gen Int Med.* 1990;5:431–437.
2. McKeith I, Cummings J. Behavioural changes and psychological symptoms in dementia disorders. *Lancet Neurol.* 2005;4:735–742.
3. Katz IR. Optimizing atypical antipsychotic treatment strategies in the elderly. *J Am Geriatrics Soc.* 2004;52:S272–S277.
4. McKeith I, Fairbairn A, Perry R, Thompson P, Perry E. Neuroleptic sensitivity in patients with senile dementia of Lewy body type. 1992;305:673–678.
5. McKeith I, Ballard CG, Harrison RW. Neuroleptic sensitivity to risperidone in Lewy body dementia. 1995;346:699.
6. Hui JS, Murdock GA, Chung JS, Lew MF. Behavioral changes as side effects of medication treatment for

Parkinson's disease. In Anderson KE, Weiner WJ, Lang AE eds. *Behavioral neurology of movement disorders,* 2nd ed. Philadelphia, PA: Lippincott Williams & Wilkins; 2005:114–129.

7. Fernandez HH, Trieschmann ME, Friedman JH. Treatment of psychosis in Parkinson's disease. *Drug Safety.* 2003;26: 643–659.

8. Kuzuhara S. Drug-induced psychotic symptoms in Parkinson's disease: problems, management and dilemma. *J Neurol.* 2001;248(suppl 3):III/28–III/31.

9. Sink KM, Holden KF, Yaffe K. Pharmacological treatment of neuropsychiatric symptoms of dementia: a review of the evidence. *JAMA.* 2005;293:596–608.

10. Rockett IRH, Putnam SL, Jia H, Smith GS. Declared and undeclared substance use among emergency department patients: a population-based study. *Addiction.* 2006;101: 706–712.

11. Perrone J, de Roos F, Jayaraman S, Hollander JE. Drug screening versus history in detection of substance use in ED psychiatric patients. *Am J Em Med.* 2001;19:49–51.

12. Cook CC. Prevention and treatment of Wernicke-Korsakoff syndrome. *Alcohol Suppl.* 2000;35:19–20.

13. Ursano RJ, Epstein RS, Lazar SG. Behavioral responses to illness. In JL Levenson ed. *Textbook of psychosomatic medicine.* Washington, DC: American Psychiatric Press, 2004:107–125.

14. Vaillant GE. Ego mechanisms of defense: a guide for clinicians and researchers. Washington, DC: American Psychiatric Press, 1992.

15. Groves JE. Taking care of the hateful patient. *New Engl J Med.* 1978;298:883–887.

16. Strain JJ. Psychological Interventions in Medical Practice. New York: Appleton-Century-Crofts, 1978.

17. Fogel BS, Stoudemire A. Personality disorders in the medical setting. In A Stoudemire, BS Fogel, D Greenberg eds. *Psychiatric care of the medical patient,* 2nd ed. Oxford: Oxford University Press, 2000; 443–458.

18. Kahana RJ, Bibring GL. Personality types in medical management. In NE Zinberg ed. *Psychiatry and medical practice in a general hospital.* New York: International Universities Press; 108–123.

19. David DS. Humility and the physician. *J Chronic Dis.* 1979;32:541–542.

20. Selzer MA, Koenigsberg HW, Kernberg OF. The initial contract in the treatment of borderline patients. *Am J Psychiatry.* 1987;144(7):927–930.

21. Sansone RA, Sansone LA. Borderline personality disorder: Interpersonal and behavioral problems that sabotage treatment success. *Postgrad Med.* 1995;97(6):169–179.

22. Peteet JR, Evans KR. Problematic behavior of drug-dependent patients in the general hospital: a clinical and administrative approach to management. *Gen Hosp Psych.* 1991;13:150–155.

23. Liberman A, Rotarius T. Behavioral contract management: a prescription for employee and patient compliance. *Health Care Manager.* 1999;18:1–10.

24. Groves JE. Management of the borderline patient on a medical or surgical ward: The psychiatric consultant's role. *Int J Psychiatry Med.* 1975;6:337–348.

25. American Psychiatric Association: *Diagnostic and Statistical Manual of Mental Disorders,* 4th edition. Washington DC: American Psychiatric Association, 1994.

69 DRUG OVERDOSE

A. Rebecca Daniel

EPIDEMIOLOGY/OVERVIEW

- Approximately 2–5 million overdoses (intentional and accidental) occur annually.
- 2004 emergency department data (Drug Abuse Warning Network, 2004): 1.3 million drug-related visits due to abuse or misuse
  - 30% illicit drugs only
  - 25% pharmaceuticals only
  - 15% illicit drugs + alcohol
  - 8% pharmaceuticals + alcohol
  - 14% alcohol + illicit drugs + pharmaceuticals
- Overall mortality for overdoses is 0.05%; 1% to 2% if hospitalization needed.
- Highest drug-related mortality reported from Poison Control include analgesics, antidepressants, stimulants, sedatives, cardiovascular drugs, and alcohol.

TRIAGE AND INITIAL MANAGEMENT

- See Fig. 69–1.
- A detailed history should be obtained from the patient (if stable and alert) or anyone accompanying the patient, regarding
  - Approximate time of ingestion.
  - All medications and illicit drugs ingested and a review of medicine bottles if available.
  - Any interventions prior to presentation at emergency room or arrival of ambulance

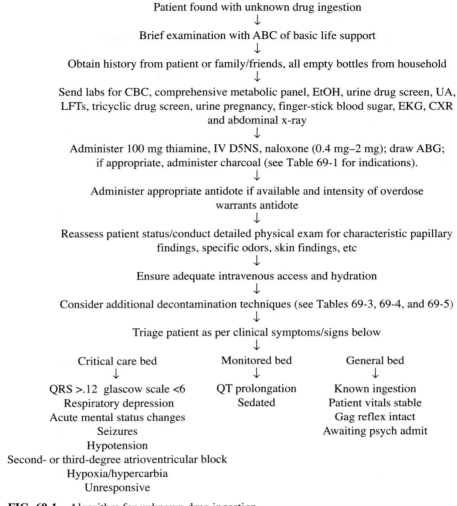

FIG. 69-1 Algorithm for unknown drug ingestion.

○ Previous history of similar occurrence or substance abuse

○ Comorbidity that would affect drug clearance (eg, renal or liver dysfunction)

• Perform a focused physical examination followed by a comprehensive examination when patient is stabilized. (Refer to substances below for key distinguishing symptoms/ signs.)

• Initial management may involve acute resuscitation; remember the basics of ABCs (airway, breathing, circulation). Only after this has been evaluated should you move on to further management.

• Patients with a Glasgow Coma Scale score < 6, or unable to protect their airway due to sedation, should be intubated and admitted to a critical care unit.

• Most steps in the management occur concurrently and consist of decontamination of the patient via cathartics, dilution, adsorbents, bowel irrigation, and/or endoscopic/ surgical removal. Most patients should be given activated charcoal, unless contraindicated (Table 69-1 for specific decontamination strategies).

• If there is an antidote available for the particular drug ingestion then it should be administered emergently; efforts to decontaminate should not interfere.

• Subspecialty consultation is critical for patients with organ failure for possible transplant evaluation.

TABLE 69-1 Modes of Decontamination in Overdose

TECHNIQUE	INDICATION	CONTRAINDICATION	COMMENTS/SIDE EFFECTS/ COMPLICATIONS
Forced acid diuresis Dilution	Increases amphetamine elimination Acidic or alkaline corrosives, must be done within minutes of ingestion	Not routine	No benefits of this modality 250 mL of water or milk
Urine alkalization	Controversial, but used in the past for salicylate, barbiturate, and phenoxyacetate herbicide poisoning	Relative contraindication: severe electrolyte imbalances, fluid overload, renal failure	Pulmonary edema
Charcoal therapy	Most effective if given within 1 hour of drug ingestion; give in all drug ingestions unless it is nontoxic or will not bind to charcoal. Anticholinergic drugs delay gastric emptying and charcoal may be beneficial even > 1 hour after ingestion in these cases	Bowel obstruction or perforation, obtunded patients until intubated, acidic or alkaline corrosives, low viscosity hydrocarbons	1 g/kg (adult 25–100 g mixed with water or sorbitol, PO or NG), do not dilute or multiple small doses. Side effects/complications: Aspiration pneumonia, diarrhea. Cramps, nausea and vomiting common when used with sorbitol. Bowel obstruction can occur when mixed with water and given repeatedly. Aspiration pneumonia.
Gastric lavage	No longer recommended by American Academy of Clinical Toxicology or the European Association of Poisons Centers and Clinical Toxicologists; use *only* if toxic amount of ingestion and < 1 hour of ingestion.	Corrosive agent, noncooperative patient, low-viscosity carbons, obtunded patients, risk for hemorrhage, perforation, esophageal or recent gastric surgery	May be more effective followed by charcoal in preventing absorption of drug. Side effects/complications: Aspiration, laryngospasm, arrhythmias, GI bleed, pneumothorax, accidental pulmonary lavage, hypothermia, electrolyte imbalances
Syrup of ipecac	Use < 30 minutes of ingestion, use in home, prehospital, pediatric patients	Controversial, emesis can delay charcoal administration, mental status changes, seizures, obtunded patients, corrosive agents, low-viscosity hydrocarbons, intractable vomiting, recent GI surgery, elderly, third trimester of pregnancy, severe HTN	Not as efficacious as charcoal Dose: 30 cc by mouth with 8 oz glass of water. Side effects/complications: Vomiting which occurs 20–30 minutes after, can persist, CNS depression, seizures
Cathartics	*Only* as adjunct to activated charcoal to enhance passage of charcoal-poison complex Types: saline cathartics and magnesium citrate cathartics No more than one dose	Magnesium citrate should not be used in renal failure, ileus, obstruction, electrolyte imbalances	Dose: 1 g/kg (1 to 2 mL/kg) of 70% sorbitol or 250 mL of magnesium citrate or 15 to 20 g of magnesium citrate Side effects/complications: Hypernatremia, hypermagnesemia, diarrhea, hypotension
Endoscopic or surgical removal	Endoscopy for pharmaco-bezoars, lethal heavy metals seen on x-ray; surgery for cocaine packets.	Illicit drug packets not recommended for endoscopy	If emergent endoscopy anticipated, avoid administration of charcoal.
Bowel irrigation	Toxic foreign bodies (disc batteries), substance not bound by charcoal, sustained-release drugs, illicit drug packets, pharmaco-bezoars.	Bowel obstruction, ileus, GI bleeding, obtundation	Dose: PO or NG 2 L until clear can range from 5 to 50 L. Quick clean of GI tract with polyethylene glycol (golytely), more effective than gastric lavage and ipecac. If substance can be bound by charcoal, then it is less effective than charcoal therapy Side effects/complications: not well documented

Abbreviations: GI, gastrointestinal; HTN, hypertension.

LABORATORY TESTING

- Not all patients require comprehensive (quantitative) laboratory testing prior to initiation of management.
- Consider when quantitative testing vs. qualitative (screening) is appropriate.
  - Will lab test change management?
  - Is the lab test more reliable than clinical presentation?
  - Is the ingestion unknown/toxicity unidentifiable on examination?
- Toxicology tests are available for the following: acetaminophen, salicylates, theophylline, lithium, digoxin, ethanol, carboxyhemoglobin, methhemoglobin, iron, methanol, ethylene glycol, lead, mercury, arsenic, organophosphates, tricyclics, anticonvulsants, and some "designer" drugs.
  - False negatives 10% to 30% of all drug screens
  - False positives 0% to 10% of all drug screens
- Physicians are more accurate in the clinical diagnosis of ethanol and gamma-hydroxybutyrate (GHB) overdose than when correlating the clinical judgment to laboratory testing in overdoses of ecstasy, amphetamine, cocaine, opiates, benzodiazepines, and cannabis.

GENERAL PATHOPHYSIOLOGY

- Drug toxicity depends on pharmacokinetics and route of ingestion.
- Many drugs are used illicitly in alternative routes (eg, inhalation) to hasten onset of action.
- Emerging trends in drug use include rectal alcohol enemas, intranasal "snorting" of crushed oral meds, subcutaneous injection "skin popping" (eg, heroin), vaginal narcotic troches, and buccal placement of transcutaneous medicines (eg, fentanyl patch).
- Awareness of the route may effect your management of decontamination.
- Ingestion routes include the following:
  - Oral/gastrointestinal (GI) tract
  - Intravenous
  - Intramuscular
  - Sublingual
  - Intranasal
  - Subcutaneous
  - Cutaneous or mucous membrane
  - Rectal
  - Vaginal

DRUG-SPECIFIC PRESENTATIONS AND MANAGEMENT*

ACETAMINOPHEN

- The drug is the leading cause of acute liver failure in the United States (51% of cases in 2003)
- Absorbs rapidly in the gut; half-life is 2–4 hours, longer with extended release formulations.
- The liver metabolizes acetaminophen, but in certain chronic states or with concomitant liver enzyme metabolizing drugs, depletion of glutathione stores results in toxic metabolites of acetaminophen, thereby destroying hepatic cells or in liver failure. This is why chronic alcoholics are more susceptible to hepatoxicity from acetaminophen.
- High mortality is associated with ingestion of 15–25 g; doses > 10 g can cause liver damage.
- Treatment with *N*-acetylcysteine increases glutathione, prevents accumulation of toxic metabolites, and functions as an antioxidant and anti-inflammatory agent.
- Increased risk for toxicity and hepatic injury (depleted glutathione stores) include
  - Children
  - Women
  - Obesity
  - Malnutrition
  - Elderly > 65 years
  - Chronic ingestion of acetaminophen with liver dysfunction
  - Excessive acute ingestion without acute alcohol intoxication (alcohol may be protective in this situation)
  - Alcoholics with acetaminophen use > 4 g daily (controversial)
  - Concomitant use of drugs that cause hepatic enzyme induction
- *Clinical manifestations*
  - *0–24 hours:* Nausea/vomiting, diaphoresis, pallor, lethargy, malaise
  - *24–48 hours:* Resolution of symptoms, patient seems to feel better
  - *48–72 hours:* Right upper quadrant (RUQ) pain, liver function tests (alanine aminotransferase [ALT]) elevated, abnormal coagulation tests (prothrombin time [PT], partial prothrombin time [PTT], international normalized ratio [INR])

---

*For quick comparative summary of common drug and designer drug ingestions, see Tables 69-2 and 69-3.

TABLE 69-2 Common Drug Ingestions and Management

DRUG/POISON	ANTIDOTE	PEARLS OF MANAGEMENT
Acetaminophen (glutathione precursor)	Oral therapy: N-acetylcysteine, 140 mg/kg and then 70 mg/kg q4 hours × 17 doses, discontinue if 4-hour l drug level < 150 mg/dL. Intravenous (IV) therapy: 150 mg/kg in 200 mL 5% dextrose over 15 min IV, then 50 mg/kg in 500 mL over 4 hours then 100 mg/kg in 1000 over 16 hours, discontinue if 4-hour l drug level < 150 mg/dL.	Get LFTs; consider specialist (hepatologist) if patient has increased PT, elevated LFTs, or initial high acetaminophen level. If available, IV N-acetylcysteine therapy can be considered in severe cases. Use acetaminophen nomogram
Ethylene glycol	Ethanol 0.6 g/kg IV then 100 mg/kg/h	HD if ingested more than 30 g or high serum levels; see also Table 69-1
Isopropanol		Check serum isopropyl alcohol level serum acetone; see also Table 69-1
Methanol	Ethanol	HD may be helpful; see also Table 69-1
Digoxin	Digibind 6 mg/kg, use in severe toxicity especially when arrhythmias present	Very expensive drug, look at cost vs. benefit, use in situations where patient profoundly symptomatic Correct electrolytes Check digoxin level Renal function: impaired or prerenal states such as dehydration can precipitate digoxin toxicity
Aspirin	Alkalinization of urine if plasma concentration > 500 mg/L, gastric lavage if < 24 hours from ingestion, activated charcoal	Check serum levels of salicylate HD may be helpful
Tricyclic antidepressants	Supportive care, one dose activated charcoal, correct acidosis	If arrhythmias or prolonged QT, QRS intervals, transfer to ICU (Hall et al, 2004)
Opioid	Naloxone (0.4–2.0 mg IV up to 10 mg total)	
Benzodiazepine	Flumazenil 0.2 mg IV q1 minute to response or 3 mg maximum, supportive care	Risk of seizures, don't use in increased ICP, head trauma
Cyanide	Amyl nitrate, then sodium nitrite	Supportive care with 100% oxygen
Beta-blockers	Glucagon 1mg/mL ampule, 5–10 mg IV	If no improvement consider concomitant poisoning, attempt decontamination if appropriate
Iron	Deferoxamine mesylate	Remember iron overload in patients that receive frequent blood transfusions (eg, sickle cell disease)
Lead	Dimercaprol/sodium calcium edetate	Look at fingernail beds which have characteristic findings
Organophosphates	Atropine/pralidoxime	
Mercury/Arsenic	Dimercaprol 2.5–5 mg/kg IM q4 hour × 2 days, then 2.5 mg/kg IM q12 hours × 2 weeks	
Valproic acid	Supportive care; naloxone (0.8–2 mg) has been shown to reverse CNS depression; carnitine supplementation (50 mg/kg/d)	
Copper	Penicillamine 0.25–2.0 g/d orally	
Warfarin	Vitamin K	Fresh frozen plasma in situations where immediate reversal needed (eg, acute intracranial hemorrhage or urgent procedure or surgery required)
Heparin	Protamine	
Thallium	Prussian blue 10 g q12 hours po	
Phenobarbital		HD may be helpful

Abbreviation: ICP, intracranial pressure; ICU, intensive care unit; LFI, liver function tests.

TABLE 69-3   Designer Drugs Ingestion and Management

DESIGNER DRUG	COMMENTS	CLINICAL EFFECTS	STREET NAMES
Methylenedioxymethamphetamine	Used in obesity, narcolepsy	Hallucinogen, stimulant, serotonin mediated, hepatic failure	Ecstasy, lover's speed, essence, stacy, clarity
Methamphetamine	Used in attention deficit disorder	Lead poisoning	Speed, crank, crystal meth, ice (smoked)
Fentanyl analogs			Persian white, Mexican brown, China white
Arylhexylamine analogs, phencyclidine, ketamine	Supportive care, benzodiazepines	Dose-related effects, euphoria depersonalization, decreased pain perception, severe intoxication rhabdomyolysis, seizures, respiratory depression, hyperacusis	PCP, powder (oral and nasal route), liquid (IV, IM, SQ: popping, smoked)
Methaqualone analogs	Supportive care	Lethargy, obtundation	Quaalude
Methcathinone analogs	Supportive care	Amphetamine-like, euphoria, sexual arousal, hallucinations, hyperreflexia, hypotension	Cat, Jeff
Herbal designer drugs	Supportive care	Has dextromethorphan and diphenhydramine, tachycardia and hypertension, seizures	Green hornet, herbal ecstasy

- ○ *> 72–96 hours:* The rise in abnormal liver function tests peak, nausea, vomiting, diaphoresis, pallor, lethargy, malaise, jaundice, confusion, lactic acidosis, PT/INR elevation, hypoglycemia, hepatic failure, renal failure (acute tubular necrosis), multiorgan failure, and death
- ○ *4 days–2 weeks:* Recovery phase, but can have persistent morbidity associated with renal failure
- • *Management strategies*
  - ○ With drug-induced hepatotoxicity, consult GI/hepatologist emergently.
  - ○ Evidence supports *N*-acetylcysteine as treatment of choice in acetaminophen poisoning; other methods (charcoal, gastric lavage, and ipecac) are not beneficial. Ipecac may be detrimental since it reduces the absorption of *N*-acetylcysteine.
  - ○ There is no benefit from methionine in place of *N*-acetylcysteine.
  - ○ Plasma concentrations of acetaminophen above the normal treatment line are given intravenous *N*-acetylcysteine (Fig. 69-2).

NONSTEROIDAL ANTI-INFLAMMATORY DRUGS

- • Nonsteroidal anti-inflammatory drugs (NSAIDs) are highly protein bound except in renal or liver dysfunction or hypoalbuminemia.
- • Mechanism of action is through inhibition of prostaglandin synthesis.

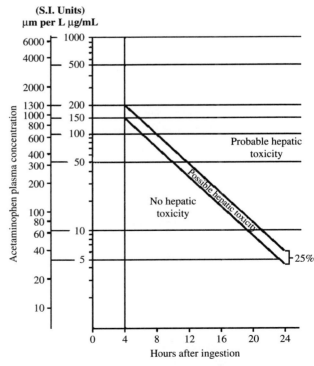

FIG. 69-2 Acetaminophen plasma nomogram utilized in overdose management. Management can be guided by serum levels and time of ingestion. If level is in the "no hepatic toxicity area," do not treat the patient. If the patient has a level beyond that area, treatment is more beneficial.

- NSAIDs interact with anticoagulants and may potentiate GI bleeding.
- Ibuprofen doses < 100 mg/kg are likely benign.
- Usually central nervous system (CNS) is affected at > 3 g ingestion, while renal complications occur at ~ 6 g or more. In the elderly or patients with underlying chronic disease, lower levels of ingestion may still cause significant toxicity.
- Symptoms usually correlate with ibuprofen blood levels.
- *Clinical manifestations*
  - Hypotension, tachycardia
  - Abdominal pain, nausea/vomiting, GI bleeding
  - Confusion, headache, blurred vision, seizures, coma
  - *Laboratory findings:* Metabolic acidosis with increased anion gap, acute interstitial nephritis, nephritic syndrome, renal failure, hepatic injury, thrombocytopenia, pancytopenia, agranulocytosis, hemolytic anemia
- *Management strategies*
  - Charcoal and gastric lavage may be beneficial if ingestion < 4 hours.
  - Adequate hydration to improve renal perfusion and bicarbonate may be administered if there is significant acidosis with pH < 7.1.
  - Check urine for hematuria, proteinuria, cell casts, and eosinophilia.
  - Check complete blood count (CBC), coagulation studies, blood urea nitrogen (BUN), and creatinine as well as liver function tests.
  - If patient develops bleeding, correct coagulopathy with fresh frozen plasma and vitamin K.
  - Hemodialysis is reserved for cases of severe renal failure.
  - Ibuprofen assay may be helpful to correlate likelihood of developing toxicity and help with disposition.

SALICYLATES (ASPIRIN)

- Plasma salicylate level 40–50 mg/dL correlates with clinical findings described below.
- *Clinical manifestations*
  - Tinnitus, agitation, confusion, coma (rare, at levels > 100 mg/dL)
  - Nausea/vomiting, flushing, diaphoresis
  - Tachypnea, hyperventilation, acute pulmonary edema
  - Hyperpyrexia
  - *Laboratory findings:* Initial metabolic alkalosis followed by metabolic acidosis; renal failure, hypokalemia (which must be corrected before alkalinization)
- *Management strategies*
  - Consider gastric lavage if < 12 hours after ingestion.
  - Provide intravenous fluid hydration.

TABLE 69-4 Indications for Hemodialysis in Salicylate Ingestion

- Renal failure
- Congestive heart failure (CHF)
- Acute lung injury
- Persistent CNS disturbances
- Progressive deterioration in vital signs
- Severe acid-base or electrolyte imbalance, despite appropriate treatment
- Hepatic compromise with coagulopathy
- Acute salicylate concentration > 100 mg/dL

Flomenbaum, Goldfran, Hoffman, Howland, Lewin, Nelson *Goldfrank's Toxicologic Emergencies.*

  - Alkalinize with sodium bicarbonate to aim for pH > 7.5.
  - Refer to Table 69-4 for indications for hemodialysis
  - Check acetaminophen level to rule out concomitant overdose.
  - If salicylate level persists or fluctuates with no clinical improvement, consider a pharmacological bezoar.
  - Force diuresis is suspected to increase renal tubular flow and elimination, but it is not sufficient to use this alone.
  - Check electrolytes and arterial blood gas (ABG) to calculate anion gap.
  - Assess acid base status and monitor for an increased anion gap metabolic acidosis and respiratory alkalosis.
  - Check electrocardiogram (ECG) to evaluate for QT prolongation.
  - Examine chest x-ray to assess for pulmonary edema.
  - Use serum levels to help assess prognosis with serum levels < 150 mg/kg more likely is a benign course.

ETHANOL ALCOHOL AND ALCOHOL WITHDRAWAL

- Fifteen to thirty percent of hospitalized and primary care patients have an alcohol problem.
- Alcohol withdrawal can be fatal; intoxicated patients with chronic abuse or dependence histories should be monitored closely for signs and symptoms of withdrawal. Withdrawal can occur within 2–10 days but typically 48–72 hours after last drink. See Chap. 70.
- Clinical presentation is the primary diagnostic tool but blood serum levels and breath analyzers can be helpful in diagnosis of intoxication; false-negative breath analysis can result after use of inhalers, Primatene Mist, mouthwashes, or chewing gum.
- Intoxication in many states is defined as 0.08–0.1 g/dL (serum level), where cerebellar dysfunction becomes apparent.
- Toxic ingestion has been estimated to be 5 g/kg in adult.

- *Clinical manifestations of intoxication*
  - *Extremely intoxicated:* Can be comatose or have respiratory depression
  - Loss of inhibitions, slurred speech, ataxia, confusion
  - Tachycardia, flushing, hypotension
  - Nystagmus, mydriasis
  - Nausea/vomiting
  - *Laboratory findings:* Hypoglycemia, hypokalemia, hypo-phosphatemia, hypomagnesemia, hyperuricemia
- *Management strategies for intoxication*
- Consider intubation and hemodialysis in the comatose, severely intoxicated patient.
- Start IV hydration (D5NS), thiamine 100 mg daily for 3 days, and folic acid 1mg daily.
- Correct electrolytes aggressively.
- Check urine drug screen for concomitant drug ingestion and administer flumazenil and naloxone as appropriate.
- Consider computed tomography (CT) scan of head in patients not improving or those with low ethanol blood levels but persistent neurologic deficits.
- Monitor for alcoholic ketoacidosis.
  - Dehydrated, tachycardia, hypotension
  - Metabolic acidosis with anion gap

ETHYLENE GLYCOL

- Refer to Table 69-5.
- Rapidly absorbed from the GI tract.

- Onset of symptoms is usually 4–12 hours after ingestion.
- Many poison centers do not have specific guidelines for ethylene glycol and the management is variable.
- Hepatic alcohol dehydrogenase metabolizes the ethylene glycol to toxic acid metabolites (glycolic acid, glyoxylic acid, oxalic acid), which results in the anion gap metabolic acidosis.
- Glycolic acid is toxic to the tubular cells in the kidney.
- Oxalate crystals are formed by the combination of oxalic acid and calcium and cause hypocalcemia.
- Treatment relies on administration of fomepizole or ethanol (alcohol dehydrogenase inhibitors).
- *Clinical manifestations*
  - Nausea/vomiting, ataxia, myoclonus, nystagmus, seizures, altered mental status, coma
  - Abdominal pain
  - Tachycardia, dysrhythmias, myocarditis, cardiovascular collapse
  - *Laboratory findings:* Acute renal failure, hypocalcemia, crystalluria (monohydrate—needle-shaped); serum level ≥ 20 mg/dL is considered toxic.
- *Management strategies*
  - Negative urine study for crystals does not exclude ethylene glycol ingestion.
  - If the patient ingested antifreeze, a Wood's lamp will make the urine fluorescent.
  - If history supports ingestion but no metabolic acidosis, patient should still be admitted to a telemetry unit, further confirmatory testing should be obtained.

TABLE 69-5   Summary Comparison of Presentation and Management for Toxic Alcohol Ingestions

TOXIC ALCOHOL	ONSET OF ACTION	METABOLIC DISORDER	ANION GAP	TOXIC LEVEL	DISTINGUISHING CLINICAL MANIFESTATIONS	DIAGNOSIS	ANTIDOTE
Ethylene glycol	> 4–12 hours	Metabolic acidosis	↑	> 20 mg/dL	Crystalluria, nystagmus, acute renal failure, hypocalcemia, and intoxicated	Urinalysis Wood's Lamp fluorescence Gas chromatography for ethylene glycol level	Ethanol/fomepizole Treat with cofactors: thiamine magnesium, pyridoxine
Isopropanol	< 30 minutes serum levels peak, but acetone peaks at > 4 hours and onset can be variable	Ketosis without metabolic acidosis	—	Too variable; fatalities can occur at any level, or can be alert and oriented at > 400 mg/dL	Odor of acetone (fruity), renal tubular acidosis, central nervous system depression	Acetone Isopropanol Level	Supportive care IV fluids with dextrose Thiamine
Methanol	< 30 hours, very variable	Metabolic acidosis	↑	Based on ingestion quantity	Blindness, papilledema, mydriasis, vs. intoxicated	Gas chromatography for methanol level	Ethanol Treat with cofactors: folinic acid

○ If patient was confirmed to have ingested any of the toxic alcohols, they would warrant admission with triaging, if necessary, to a critical care unit because of the variable rapid deterioration involved with this toxic ingestion.

○ Confirmatory lab studies such as gas chromatography should be performed on serum when ethylene or methanol ingestion is suspected, and must be specifically requested. Results are not available immediately.

○ *Start loading dose of ethanol:* 0.8 g/kg (1mL/kg) of 100% diluted 5% to 10% in D5W.

○ Simultaneously administer initial dose 130 mg/kg/h of 100% ethanol dilute to 5% to 10% in D5W

○ Check ethanol level every hour and goal at 100–150 mg/dL with partial loading doses if the level falls below 100 mg/dL.

○ Monitor vitals, blood sugar, and electrolytes (particularly sodium).

○ Administer thiamine 100 mg/day IV, magnesium pyridoxine 100 mg/day IV.

○ *Recommendations for dialysis*
  ▪ Ethylene glycol level > 50 mg/dL
  ▪ End-organ damage
  ▪ Continued metabolic acidosis
  ▪ If amount of intake unknown and could be potentially high

○ Initial symptoms do not always correlate with toxicity and early diagnosis and treatment is crucial in reducing morbidity and mortality.

ISOPROPANOL

• Absorption within < 30 minutes of ingestion.
• Hepatic alcohol dehydrogenase converts isopropanol to acetone, which creates ketosis.
• Ingestion commonly seen in alcoholic patients unable to obtain ethanol, or in patients with suicidal intent.
• Isopropanol levels should be checked but may not be evident until 3–4 hours after ingestion. Serum level does not correlate with level of toxicity.
• 2.7 times more intoxicating than ethanol, but breathalyzer can give false positive for isopropanol as ethanol.
• *Clinical manifestations*
  ○ Tachycardia, hypotension
  ○ *CNS depression:* Areflexia, hypothermia, respiratory depression, muscle weakness, seizures
  ○ Odor of acetone
  ○ Hemorrhagic tracheobronchitis
  ○ *Lab findings:* Renal tubular acidosis, rhabdomyolysis, hemolytic anemia

• *Management strategies*
  ○ Check serum isopropanol level in cases where diagnosis is not absolute. If serum isopropanol not readily available at your institution, check acetone first.
  ○ Check electrolyte abnormalities, hypoglycemia, and creatinine.
  ○ Provide supportive care with intubation if displaying respiratory depression.
  ○ Other supportive measures include intravenous fluids, thiamine administration, and benzodiazepines for seizures.
  ○ Other decontamination methods are not effective unless coingestion is suspected.
  ○ Consider hemodialysis if no improvement with supportive management.
  ○ Sequelae are limited if patient responds to supportive care through the metabolism of isopropanol.
  ○ On discharge the patient should have received education and referral to detoxification center and rehabilitation. Patients with intention of suicide should be assessed by a psychiatric professional.

METHANOL

• See Table 69-6.
• Peak absorption 30–60 minutes; onset < 30 hours, which is variable.
• *Fatal dose:* 15–30 mL of 40% solution.
• Hepatic alcohol dehydrogenase metabolizes methanol to formic acid (formate), which leads to the metabolic acidosis with increased anion gap.

TABLE 69-6   Methanol Toxicity

MAJOR SYMPTOMS/ SIGNS	LABORATORY FEATURES
Early	
Inebriation	May have detectable serum ethanol and methanol levels
Drowsiness	Systemic acidosis with low bicarbonate
Delayed (6–30 hours)	
Vomiting vertigo	Lactic acidemia
Upper abdominal pain ± pancreatitis	↑ Hematocrit
Dyspnea	↑ Anion gap
Acidosis ± Kussmaul respirations	↑ Mean corpuscular volume
Blurred vision	Formic acidemia
Hyperemia of optic disk	↑ Blood glucose
Blindness	↑ Serum amylase
Dilated pupils/absent light reflex	↑ Osmolal gap
Urinary formaldehyde smell	Methanol > 30 mg/dL

Source: Adapted from Haddad S. *Clinical Management of Poisoning and Drug Overdose.* 3rd ed. Winchester: W.B. Saunders Company; 1998.

- Significant neurological sequelae can occur.
- *Clinical manifestations*
  - Tachycardia or bradycardia, hypotension
  - Tachypnea
  - Basal ganglia infarcts or hemorrhages, seizures, initial normal vision followed by blurred vision, blindness and papilledema, cerebral edema, photophobia, mydriasis
  - Abdominal pain, pancreatitis
- *Management strategies*
  - Ethanol is used as in treatment and should be administered as stated in the ethylene overdose section.
  - Check electrolytes, ABG, liver function tests.

BETA-BLOCKER (BB) AND CALCIUM CHANNEL BLOCKER (CCB) OVERDOSE

- Usually overdose is related to unintentional ingestion or medication errors. Toxic exposure surveillance system reported in 2004 that 3% of all exposures are due to cardiovascular drugs.
- Beta-blocker and CCB overdose presentations are similar; often treat for both at same time.
- *Clinical manifestations*
  - Bradycardia refractory to atropine, atrioventricular block, QRS prolongation, hypotension
  - Lethargy; seizures (beta-blockers)
  - Hypothermia
  - Hyperglycemia induced by blocking calcium influx into pancreatic cell and blocking insulin release (calcium channel blockers)
- *Management strategies*
  - *Decontamination:* If ingestion < 1 hour, should give charcoal and consider gastric lavage (although efficacy questionable with extended release formulations).
  - Provide supportive care of hypotension with IV normal saline and atropine 0.5–1 mg IV (efficacy minimal in significant overdose).
  - Glucagon is first-line therapy for beta-blocker overdose (Glucagon stimulate beta-receptor complex, resulting in transient improvement within 5 minutes), but not all beta-blocker preparations respond.
  - Follow the initial dose with glucagon 50–150 μg/kg IV, then 2–5 mg/h to max of 10 mg/h in 5% dextrose, to be tapered as patient improves.
  - In CCB overdose: Initial therapy should be 10–20 mL of 10% calcium gluconate IV with epinephrine 1μg/min IV; if no response, you can attempt high-dose insulin with supplemental dextrose and potassium in refractory cases.

SEDATIVES AND HYPNOTICS

BENZODIAZEPINES
- Amnesic, anxiolytic, anticonvulsant; absorbed quickly through the GI tract. Mechanism of action: enhancing function of gamma-aminobutyric acid (GABA) (inhibitory neurotransmitter in the brain).
- Lipophilic drug accumulates in lipid-rich tissue and can lead to progressive sedation.
- Abrupt discontinuation can cause potentially fatal withdrawal syndrome, with autonomic instability and seizures.
- *Half-life:* 1–200 hours, depending on benzodiazepine. Toxic range 1–9 μg/mL; but most patients are alert within 12–36 hours of ingestion.
- Categorized by duration of action
  - Short-acting (eg, midazolam)
  - Intermediate acting (eg, alprazolam)
  - Long-acting (eg, clonazepam)
  - Very long-acting (eg, chlorazepam)
- *Clinical manifestations*
  - Dysarthria, ataxia, vertigo, CNS depression, sedation
  - Blurred vision
  - Hypothermia
- *Management strategies*
  - Administer gastric lavage and charcoal if ingestion < 1 hour.
  - Avoid forced diuresis/ hemodialysis as not effective.
  - *Flumazenil:* 0.2 mg IV q1 minute to response or 3 mg maximum
    - This is contraindicated in head injury and raised intracranial pressure
    - Watch for seizures, especially in those with co-ingestion
    - It is safe and useful in patients with mixed overdose and in those presenting in coma
    - Most common side effects include facial erythema, headache, and anxiety

BARBITURATES
- Barbiturates replaced by benzodiazepines due to the relative safety.
- *Phenobarbital:* Inducer of hepatic cytochrome system; results in increased metabolism of specific drugs such as corticosteroids, doxycycline, theophylline.
- Categorized by duration of action
  - Ultra-short active (eg, thiopental)
  - Short-acting (eg, pentobarbital)
  - Intermediate acting (eg, allobarbital)
  - Long-acting (eg, phenobarbital)

- *Clinical manifestations*
  - Cardiovascular collapse; vasodilation greater than with benzodiazepines
  - Central nervous depression
  - Hypothermia
  - Bullous cutaneous lesions
- *Management strategies*
  - Administer gastric lavage and charcoal if ingestion < 1–2 hours.
  - Provide supportive care: Intravenous fluids, check electrolytes, liver function tests, and renal function
  - Treat for coingestion

OPIOIDS

- Harrison Narcotic Act of 1914 made the nonmedical use of opioids illegal.
- *Examples of opioids:* Opium, codeine, fentanyl, heroin, hydrocodone, methadone, morphine, oxycodone, paregoric, sufentanil.
- *Clinical manifestations*
  - Vasodilation, orthostatic hypotension, bradycardia
  - Bronchospasm, acute lung injury, antitussive
  - Pruritus (histamine-mediated)
  - Decreased antidiuretic hormone (ADH) secretion
  - Miosis
  - Decreased gastric secretion
  - Coma
- *Management strategies*
  - Administer gastric lavage if ingestion < 1–2 hours.
  - Administer charcoal 1 g/kg po/ng.
  - Hemodynamic/ventilator support.
  - Provide naloxone (0.4–2.0 mg IV up to 10 mg total); may need infusion if large ingestion/synthetic opioids.
  - *Goal of reversal:* Ability to ventilate spontaneously.
  - *Avoid total reversal:* Can lead to acute withdrawal; if this occurs, naloxone infusion should be discontinued.
  - Because of the increased potency opioid in fentanyl patches, it has been a significant drug for diversion and abuse. (Refer to recent Food and Drug Administration [FDA] warnings: http://www.fda.gov/cder/drug/advisory/fentanyl.htm)

COCAINE

- Derived from the leaves of *Erythroxylum coca* (found in Columbia, Peru, Bolivia, West Indies, Indonesia).
- High abuse potential because of quick onset, short duration, and increasing tolerance
- The route of ingestion affects onset; can be self-administered IV, nasal, smoking or GI tract. Fastest onset through IV and smoking.
- Drug "mules" or "body packers/body stuffers" transport drugs (cocaine/opioids, hashish, etc) by ingesting them in small packets.

  - Toxicity occurs when packets rupture and release large amounts of drug into the blood.
- *Lethal dose:* 750–800 mg.
- *Snorting peak effect:* 10 minutes, duration 30 minutes.
- *Intravenous or smoking peak effect*—2 minutes, duration 5–10 minutes.
- *Clinical manifestations*
  - Adrenergic effects, including tachycardia, hyperthermia, hypertension
  - Myocardial infarction (MI), rhabdomyolysis, transient ischemic attack/cerebrovascular accident (TIA/CVA), renal infarction, other tissue ischemia (and related end-organ toxicity)
  - Lactic acidosis
  - Seizures
  - Altered mental status
  - Mydriasis
  - Tachypnea
  - Madarosis (eyelash loss due to smoking cocaine)
  - Hypoglycemia can occur from catecholamine release
  - With adrenergic presentation, consider pheochromocytoma and thyrotoxicosis in the differential diagnosis
  - Psychiatric disturbance due to cocaine toxicity is short lived; schizophrenia and mania should be considered in the differential diagnosis
- *Management strategies*
  - X-ray/CT scan imaging for diagnosis.
    - Charcoal multiple dose, golytely
  - Can test serum, urine, hair saliva for cocaine. Urine test will remain positive for 2–3 days after last use.
  - Admit patients with seizures, intracranial bleed, and strokes for supportive management and monitoring.
  - Admit patients with chest pain to rule out MI.
  - Provide supportive care for hyperthermia as a critical sign of cocaine toxicity. Use rapid-cooling methods.
  - Sedation is required for severe agitation and increased anxiety.

TRICYCLIC ANTIDEPRESSANTS

- Tricyclic antidepressants are absorbed from the GI tract; peak concentrations 2–8 hours after ingestion
- First pass metabolism; thus delayed GI decontamination recommended
- *Clinical manifestations*
  - QRS prolongation, atrioventricular (AV) block (second or third degree), supraventricular tachycardia, torsades de pointes, ventricular fibrillation
  - Hypotension
  - Altered mental status, psychosis, seizures, myoclonus, urinary retention, paralytic ileus
  - Hyperthermia

○ Acute lung injury aspiration

○ Quantitative serum testing is limited and does not correlate with clinical manifestations, except at very high levels *(Flomenbaum et al)*

• *Management strategies*

○ If patient has QRS > 100 millisecond, wide complex tachycardia/ventricular tachycardia, start sodium bicarbonate 1–2 mEq/kg IV boluses every 3–5 minutes

○ Additional agents include magnesium sulfate, lidocaine for ventricular arrhythmias, benzodiazepines or barbiturates for seizures.

○ Recommend patient monitoring and serial ECGs for at least 6 hours; but not all patients with overdose presenting in a delayed fashion need be admitted for monitoring. Most patients have clinical symptoms within several hours of presentation.

○ If cardiac toxicity evident with arrhythmias, then patient will need monitoring for at least 12–24 hours.

HERBAL AND DIETARY SUPPLEMENTS

• The World Health Organization (WHO) estimates that four billion people use herbal therapies.

• Table 69-7 includes some common herbal preparations and their known toxicities

TABLE 69-7   Alternative Medicine and Herbal Supplements: Uses and Toxicity

SOURCE OR ACTIVE INGREDIENT	COMMON OR PURPORTED USE	CLINICAL EFFECTS AND POTENTIAL TOXICITY
Bufotoxin/(toad venom) Love stone	Purported aphrodisiac, hallucinogen	Cardiac glycosides
Chromium picolinate	Body building, athletic enhancement	GI irritation & niacin-like flushing reaction
Comfrey/symphytum officinale	Anti-inflammatory gastritis; diarrhea	Hepatic veno-occlusive disease, possible teratogen/carcinogen
Creatine (monohydrate, creatine monophosphate)	Athletic performance enhancement	GI irritation
DHEA dehydroepiandrosterone	Anticancer, antiaging	Androgenic effects in females; possible stimulation of prostate cancer
Echinacea (angustifolia, Echinacea pallida, Echinacea purpurea)	Immune stimulation	CNS stimulant, allergic dermatitis, anaphylaxis
Garlic/allium sativum	Hyperlipidemia, hypertension	GI irritation, rash, asthma
Ginko, extract of ginko biloba	Alzheimer disease	GI irritation, allergic dermatitis
Ginseng, panax ginseng, panax quinquefolia	Fatigue, immune stimulation, many ailments	Decreases serum glucose, increases cortisol, nervousness, insomnia, GI distress
Glucosamine (glucosamine chondroitin)	Osteoarthritis	Unknown
Goldenseal (hydrastis Canadensis)	Dyspepsia, postpartum bleeding, drug test adulterant	Nausea, vomiting, diarrhea, paresthesia, seizures, hypo- or hypertension
Ji bu huan (tetrahydropalmatine)	Chinese traditional medicine	Acute CNS depression and bradycardia, chronic hepatitis
Ma Huang (ephedrine: various ephedra sp.)	Stimulant athletic performance enhancement, appetite suppressant	Hypertension, tachycardia
Melatonin (source: pineal gland)	Sleep aid	Sedation, headache, loss of libido
Pennyroyal oil (pulegone, menthofuran	Abortifacient	Coma, hepatic necrosis
Rattle snake powder	Hispanic traditional remedy	Salmonella sepsis
Spirulina (blue green algae)	Body building	Niacin-like flushing reaction
Saw palmetto (extract of saw palmetto berry)	Prostatic hypertrophy	Unknown
St. John's wort (hypericum perforatum)	Antidepressant	MAO inhibition, photosensitivity
Tea tree oil (melaleuca alternifolia	Topical antifungal, vaginitis, acne	Sedation, ataxia, contact dermatitis
Valerian root (valeriana officinalis; valeriana edulis)	Sleep aid	Sedation, vomiting
Vanadium (vanadyl sulfate; ammonium vanadyl tartrate)	Body building	Intestinal cramps, diarrhea, black stools
Yohimbine (corynan yohimbe)	Stimulant, purported aphrodisiac	Hallucinations, MAO inhibition, hypertension, irritability, GI irritation
Zinc (zinc gluconate lozenges)	Flu/cold symptoms	Nausea, mouth and throat irritation

SOURCE: Adapted from Olson KR, ed. Clinical management of poisoning and drug overdose. In: *Poisoning and Drug Overdose.* 3rd ed. Stamford, CT: Appleton & Lange; 1999.

- For more information regarding herbal supplements or dietary supplements, refer to the Web site: http://www.ods.od.nih.gov

CARE TRANSITIONS

- Discharge criteria include
  - No ECG abnormalities such as QRS prolongation
  - Electrolyte abnormalities corrected
  - Counsel patient on substance abuse if appropriate
  - Mental status changes resolved
- Provide patient with contacts for rehabilitation, detoxification, and support groups. Alcoholics anonymous/narcotics anonymous are 12-step support groups that enable a patient to address character faults and stressors as well as the acknowledgement of addiction.
- Patients who will be discharged directly to a psychiatric facility should have a detailed discharged summary with any medical complications from the drug overdose described. (eg, renal failure or liver failure as a consequence of the drug overdose → follow-up visit(s) should be scheduled).
- Assess patient financial status (common stressor) and involve social workers/case manager to assist patient.
- Ensure that patients being discharged have follow-up with their primary care physician (PCP) and if necessary a psychiatrist and or addiction specialist. The patient should not be given prescriptions for sedatives, narcotics, or tricyclic medications that the patient could potentially abuse or overdose with.
- Discuss with PCP the management that ensued while hospitalized and the necessity for follow-up in 1–2 weeks.
- Discuss plan of management with family/friends of patients with his/her consent so that patient continues to have support as an outpatient. Suggest support group therapy for the family/friends and an option to help cope with stressors and recent hospitalization of the patient.
- Dual diagnosis groups are available for those patients that have underlying psychiatric diagnosis that may be responsible for the patient "self-treating" with alcohol, illicit, or prescription drugs.
- If you do send a patient home on narcotics for chronic pain control, make sure that the patient is adequately educated.
- Provide patient with the opportunity to self-educate on their disease process. Those with concurrent substance abuse history should be referred to the following websites:
  - National institute on drug abuse, www.nida.nih.gov
  - National council on alcoholism and drug dependence (800 622-2255), www.ncadd.org
  - American Psychiatric Association, www.psych.org
  - Patient education handouts can also be printed from www.jama.com, the patient page link (eg, cocaine addiction, treating drug dependency, etc)
- If you note that a particular drug has side effect that is an atypical presentation, you can also report this to the FDA: www.fda.gov/medwatch
- National poison control center: 1-800-222-1222
- World Health Organization's international poison center Web site: www.who.int/ipcs/poisons/centre/directory/en

BIBLIOGRAPHY

Bailey B. Glucagon in beta-blocker and calcium channel blocker overdoses: a systematic review. *J Toxicol Clin Toxicol.* 2003;41:594–602.

Bjornaas MA, Hovda KE, Mikalsen H, et al. Clinical vs. laboratory identification of drugs of abuse in patients admitted for acute poisoning. *Clin Toxicol.* 2006;44:127–134.

Brok J, Buckley N, Gluud C Interventions for paracetamol (acetaminophen) overdose. *Cochrane Database Syst Rev.*

Caravati EM, Erdman AR, Christian G, et al. Ethylene glycol exposure: an evidence based consensus guideline for out of hospital management. *Clin Toxycol.* 2005;43(5): 327–345.

Center for Medical Consumers. *Healthfacts.* 239 St. New York, NY: Thompson; April 2006:10012.

Chan KM, Wong ET, Matthews WS. Severe isopropanolemia without acetonemia or clinical manifestations of isoprapanol intoxication. *Clin Chem.* 1993, Sept; 39(9):1922–1925.

Drug Abuse Warning Network, 2004 National estimates of drug-related emergency department visits, US department of health and human services, substance abuse and mental health services administration.

Eugene RS, Michael FS, Willis CM. *Diseases of the Liver.* 9th ed. Vol. 2. Lippincott Williams & Wilkins; 2003: 1093–1096.

Fabbri A, Marchesini G, Morselli-Labate AM, et al. Comprehensive drug screening in decision making of patients attending the emergency department for suspected drug overdose. *Emerg Med J.* 2003;20:25–28.

Ford M, Delaney K, Ling L, eds. *Clinical Toxiology.* 1st ed. W.B Saunders; 2001.

Green R, Sitar DS, Tenenbein M. Effect of anticholinergic drugs on the efficacy of activated charcoal. *Clin Toxicol.* 2004;42(3):267–272.

Haddad S. *Clinical Management of Poisoning and Drug Overdose.* 3rd ed. Winchester: W.B. Saunders Company; 1998.

Hall J, Murphy P. *Handbook of Critical Care.* Hoboken, NJ: Science press; 2004.

Kerns W II, Kline J, Ford MD. Beta-blocker and calcium channel blocker toxictity. *Emergency Med Clin North Am.* 1994;12:365–390.

Kline JA, Raymond RM, Schroeder JD, et al. The diabetogenic effects of acute verapamil poisoning. *Toxicol Appl Pharmacol.* 1997;145:357–362.

Lee WM. Acute liver failure in the United States. *Semin Liver Dis.* 2003;23(3):217–226.

Navarro V, Senior J. Drug-related hepatotoxicity. *N Engl J Med.* 2006;354:731–739.

Olson KR, ed. Clinical management of poisoning and drug overdose. In: *Poisoning and Drug Overdose.* 3rd ed. Stamford, CT: Appleton & Lange; 1999.

Shepherd G. Treatment of poisoning caused by B adrenergic and calcium channel blockers. *Am J Health Syst Pharm.* 2006;63(19):1828–35.

Thomas RK, Parick GO. Management of drug and alcohol withdrawal. *N Engl J Med.* 2003;348;18.

Weinbroum A , Rudick V, Sorkine P, et al. Use of flumazenil in the treatment of drug overdose: a double blind and open clinical study in 110 patients. *Crit Care Med.* 1996;24(2):199–206.

Wood DM, Daragan PI, Jones AL. Measuring plasma salicylate concentrations in all patients with drug overdose or altered consciousness: is it necessary? *Emerg Med J.* 2005;22:401–403.

Yeates PJA, Thomas SHL. Effectivess of delayed activated charcoal administration in simulated paracetamol (acetaminophen) overdose. *Br J Clin Pharmacol.* 2000 Jan: 49(1):11–14.

70 MANAGEMENT OF PATIENTS WITH ALCOHOL ABUSE

Sylvia C. McKean

EPIDEMIOLOGY/OVERVIEW

- In the United States, there are an estimated 10–15 million people who heavily use and abuse alcohol.
- Alcohol abuse and dependency cost an estimated 100 billion dollars a year through hospitalization and related medical services.
- Dependent patients who are not treated for withdrawal suffer significant complications in the hospital and 15% will experience seizures and 5% delirium tremens (DTs).
- DTs are associated with a mortality rate of 1% to 5%.

- The hospitalization provides an opportunity to identify alcohol abuse, initiate prophylaxis to prevent withdrawal syndromes, and begin counseling.
- In their role as medical consultants seeing postoperative and trauma patients and as leaders of medical teams, hospitalists may be able to improve patient outcomes by taking an evidence-based approach, including reducing:
  ○ Mortality
  ○ The development of withdrawal syndromes
  ○ Duration of agitation and delirium
  ○ Complications from treatment
- Hospitalists should lead, coordinate, or participate in initiatives to improve the care of this vulnerable population and work with their colleagues specializing in addiction and psychiatry.

PATHOGENESIS

- Alcohol is a general sedative which interacts with many regulatory systems through its action on lipids in cell membranes.
  ○ ↑ release of endogenous opiates
  ○ Activation of gamma-aminobutyric acid A (GABA-A) receptor
    ▪ Binding to this receptor leads to an influx of chloride ions that causes relaxation or relief of anxiety, sedation, and impaired motor skills.
    ▪ During withdrawal of chronic alcohol intake, decreased chloride influx causes tremors, paroxysmal sweating, agitation, and seizures
  ○ Inhibition of *N*-methyl-D-aspartate (NMDA) receptor
    ▪ Binding to this receptor leads to inhibition of the postsynaptic excitatory effects of glutamate.
    ▪ During withdrawal, unopposed excitatory effects of glutamate may lead to seizures and DTs.

TREATMENT OF PATIENTS ACUTELY INTOXICATED WITH ALCOHOL

- Acute toxicity depends on the total dose, pattern of use, concurrent food ingestion, the presence of other drugs, comorbid disease, and tolerance.
  ○ A chronic alcoholic may function normally at a blood alcohol concentration of 500 mg/dL that would cause death in a nonalcoholic, such as a college student on a binge.
  ○ See Table 70-1.
- Alcohol blocks gluconeogenesis, and the combination of alcohol consumption, even at moderate levels, and fasting may result in hypoglycemia and loss of consciousness.

TABLE 70-1   Clinical Signs Correlated with Blood Alcohol Levels

BLOOD ETHANOL CONCENTRATION (mg/dL)	CLINICAL EFFECTS
30–100	Mild euphoria, talkativeness
	Decreased inhibitions
	Impaired attention, judgment
	Mild incoordination, nystagmus
100–200	Emotional instability
	(excitement; withdrawal)
	Impaired memory, reaction time
	Loss of critical judgment
	Conjunctival hyperemia
	Ataxia, nystagmus, dysarthria
	Hypalgesia
200–300	Confusion, disorientation,
	dizziness
	Disturbed perception, sensation
	Diplopia, dilated pupils
	Marked ataxia, dysarthria
300–400	Apathy, stupor
	Decreased response to stimuli
	Vomiting, incontinence
	Inability to stand or walk
> 400	Unconsciousness, coma
	Anesthesia,
	Decreased or absent reflexes
	Hypothermia
	Hypoventilation
	Hypotension
	Death (respiratory arrest)

SOURCE: From Melmon KL, Morrelli HF, Hoffman BB, et al. eds. *Clinical Pharmacology: Basic Principles in Therapeutics.* 3rd ed. New York, NY: McGraw-Hill, Inc; 1992:772.

- Alcohol is rapidly absorbed from the stomach so that lavage and charcoal have no value. Hemodialysis will clear alcohol but is not normally used.
  ○ A 70-kg male will clear approximately one can of beer or 10 g of ethanol per hour.
  ○ An alcoholic can clear alcohol much faster.
- Treatment of acute alcoholic intoxication is primarily supportive, maintaining a patent airway, assisting ventilation if necessary, and treatment of hypoglycemia.
- The hospitalist needs to be vigilant for the development of signs of alcohol withdrawal in the chronic alcoholic as blood alcohol levels fall.

ALCOHOL WITHDRAWAL RISKS

- Validated screening instruments such as the CAGE questionnaire for alcoholism effectively identify patients at risk.[1]
  ○ Can you cut down on your drinking?
  ○ Are you annoyed when asked to stop drinking?
  ○ Do you feel guilty about your drinking?
  ○ Do you need an eye-opener drink when you get up in the morning?
- Physicians should also ask the time of the last drink and specifically inquire about alcohol for all patients, including those who abuse other substances.
  ○ Concurrent use of benzodiazepines may increase tolerance and risk of serious withdrawal, requiring higher benzodiazepine dosages and more prolonged taper.
- Assume patient is at risk of developing withdrawal symptoms if reported alcohol consumption is daily or near-daily drinking of 100 g of ethanol per day (approximately eight standard drinks). See equivalents
  ○ 1 oz 40% (80 proof) spirits
  ○ 4 oz 10% wine
  ○ 8 oz 5% beer
- In addition, suspect dependency if the patient shows evidence of tolerance—few signs of intoxication—when blood alcohol level is high or signs of withdrawal when blood alcohol is still high.
- Inquire about prior history of withdrawal, morning tremor, diaphoresis, anxiety, seizure, and DTs for all patients suspected of dependency.

ALCOHOL WITHDRAWAL SYNDROMES

- Fifty percent of patients in withdrawal will have masked or modified symptoms because of acute illness, comorbidity, trauma, or therapeutic drugs.
- Alcoholics show similar patterns of behavior each time they withdraw from alcohol.

EARLY WITHDRAWAL SYNDROME

- Early withdrawal syndrome is defined within 48 hours of abstinence or reduction in intake.
- Symptoms start approximately 8 hours from abstinence and peak at 24–36 hours.
- Morning hangover is the mildest form and occurs when alcohol consumption is interrupted by 8–12 hours of sleep.
- Eighty-eight percent of chronic alcoholics will experience the following symptoms when they abruptly stop drinking.
  ○ *12 hours*—Jitters/shakes, intense craving, insomnia, vivid dreams, anxiety, nausea/vomiting, paroxysmal sweating, weakness, myalgias.
  ○ Insomnia can last for months after last drink.
  ○ *24 hours*—Agitation, irritability, hypervigilence, tachycardia, hypertension, coarse tremor of hands and tongue. Tremor can last up to 14 days.

- Alcoholic hallucinosis and withdrawal seizures can develop during this time, although some experts consider these manifestations as signs of a separate clinical syndrome.

ALCOHOLIC HALLUCINOSIS

- Alcoholic hallucinosis starts at 24 hours from abstinence and ends by the second or third day.
- Eighteen percent of chronic alcoholics will experience the following symptoms when they abruptly stop drinking:
  - Visual symptoms such as bugs crawling on walls
  - Less commonly auditory symptoms such as buzzing or accusatory voices
- Unlike the DTs, patients are not confused and the electroencephalogram (EEG) is normal.

WITHDRAWAL SEIZURES

- The onset of seizures typically starts 12 hours from abstinence and peak at 24 hours.
- Falling alcohol level may induce the seizure.
- The onset may be delayed by the administration of sedative hypnotic or anesthetic drugs.
- Twenty-three percent of chronic alcoholics will experience withdrawal seizures, typically major motor tonic clonic as a single seizure or rapid burst of several seizures. Three percent develop status epilepticus.
- The probability of seizures is in proportion to the amount of alcohol consumed and whether the patient has had a prior history of withdrawal seizures.
- Alcoholic patients who experience their first seizure or have multiple seizures, or those presenting with focal seizures require a workup for structural central nervous system (CNS) lesions.
- Seizures in alcoholic patients do not usually indicate epilepsy and do not require prolonged anticonvulsant therapy.

LATE WITHDRAWAL SYNDROME

- Late withdrawal syndrome is defined as occurring 48 hours after abstinence.
- This syndrome usually occurs in patients with a long and intense history of alcohol exposure and rarely in patients under 30 years of age.
- This syndrome, notably clouding of consciousness and delirium, can begin after apparent clinical improvement from early withdrawal symptoms and is characterized by

- Confusion, disorientation, hyperactivity
- Profound autonomic hyperactivity (hypertension, tachycardia, fever, diaphoresis, dehydration)
- Increased levels of catecholamines, cardiac output, stroke volume, and oxygen consumption
- Clouding of sensorium can persist 2 weeks or longer after the last drink.

DELIRIUM TREMENS

- DTs is considered to be a late withdrawal syndrome that starts around 48 hours from abstinence up to 14 days later.
- Eighty percent of patients with the DTs have resolution of their symptoms by 72 hours.
- Usually patients have a long and intense history of alcohol abuse and it is uncommon in patients less than 30 years old.
- The risk increases if there is a prior history of DTs.
- Pancreatitis, alcoholic gastritis, trauma, or infections are common precipitants. Other etiologies to consider include sepsis, meningitis, hypoxia, seizure, hypoglycemia, thiamine deficiency, toxic ingestion, and subdural hematoma.
- Symptoms of DTs include
  - Delirium, hallucinations, hyperactivity, agitation
  - Hypertension, tachycardia, fever, tremor, sweats
  - Dilated pupils, disordered sensory perception

WERNICKE'S ENCEPHALOPATHY

- Wernicke's syndrome is characterized by the acute onset of ocular symptoms, confusion, and ataxia.
- Ocular involvement includes (in order of frequency)
  - Horizontal and vertical nystagmus
  - Unilateral or bilateral cranial nerve VI paresis
  - Gaze palsies, less commonly
  - Retinal hemorrhages, occasionally
  - Pupillary changes and complete ophthalmoplegia rarely
- Confusion (disorientation, inattentiveness, disinterest, and sometimes coma) is associated with withdrawal symptoms of alcohol (agitation, delusions, hallucinations).
  - Korsakoff's syndrome (80% of patients who survive Wernicke's syndrome)
- Ataxia is notable for
  - Inability to stand (mild or severe)
  - Lower limb (heel to shin) ataxia with sparing of upper limbs
  - Polyneuropathy (80% of cases)
  - Associated autonomic dysfunction (commonly) and
  - Vestibular derangement (occasionally)

- Overall mortality is 15% caused by complications from coma.
- Laboratory abnormalities may include
  - Hematologic and chemical evidence of alcohol and nutritional deficiency (elevated mean corpuscular volume [MCV], abnormal liver function tests [LFTs], elevated gamma-glutamyltransferase [GGT])
  - Decreased erythrocyte transketolase, indicative of decreased thiamine levels
  - Elevated blood pyruvate
  - Mammillary body atrophy apparent on magnetic resonance imaging (MRI)

KORSAKOFF'S SYNDROME

- Korsakoff's syndrome results from thiamine deficiency which causes a disturbance of memory in which new information cannot be stored.
- Disturbance in the normal temporal sequence of established memories results in confabulation by the patient.
- Testing for this syndrome should not happen until the confusion of Wernicke's syndrome has resolved.

BEDSIDE EVALUATION FOR WITHDRAWAL

- The Clinical Institute Withdrawal Assessment (CIWA) for alcohol is used to determine the severity of withdrawal and assist in treatment. For a free reproducible CIWA tool go to: http://images2.clinicaltools.com/images/pdf/ciwa-ar.pdf
- The CIWA score quantifies symptoms of withdrawal with a range from normal (0) to severe (7) within each category.
  - Agitation
  - Anxiety
  - Auditory disturbances
  - Disorientation
  - Headache
  - Nausea or vomiting
  - Paroxysmal sweats
  - Tactile disturbances
  - Tremor
  - Visual disturbances
- The scoring system is most helpful for clinicians determining inpatient vs. outpatient alcohol detoxification and in facilities for this purpose.
  - This symptom-based approach may require significantly less medication and therefore lead to more rapid detoxification.
  - It may not be useful in the hospital setting for patients with significant comorbid disease, which may impact on symptoms of alcohol withdrawal, and for whom there may be many reasons for altered states. Examples include coronary artery disease (CAD), hypertension, chronic obstructive lung disease, liver disease, human immunodeficiency virus (HIV), general debility, and psychiatric issues.
  - It requires nursing expertise and dedicated time to administer.
- Total CIWA scores of > 15 on admission or a past medical history of withdrawal seizures should trigger prompt prophylactic administration of medication (see Table 70-2).

WITHDRAWAL PROPHYLAXIS

- Treatment should be individualized with frequent monitoring to avoid the emergence of agitation, delirium and complications from oversedation.[2]
- Patients currently drinking and at risk for withdrawal with minimal symptoms (CIWA < 8) should receive withdrawal prophylaxis
  - Orders should be written for no longer than 24 hours at a time with particular attention to whether doses are held or additional "as needed" doses actually administered.
  - Anticipated duration of prophylaxis is 72 hours.
  - Avoid prophylaxis in patients with hepatic insufficiency.
  - Nurses should frequently assess sedation and the presence of withdrawal symptoms (increasing CIWA score > 8).

TABLE 70-2   Drug Equivalency[2]

	HALF-LIFE	INITIAL FREQUENCY OF ADMINISTRATION
Lorazepam (Ativan) 1 mg	10–20 hours	Every 4 hours, then every 6 hours
Chlordiazepoxide (Librium) 25 mg	50–100 hours	Every 6 hours
Diazepam (Valium) 5 mg	30–100 hours	Every 6 hours
Oxazepam (Serax) 30 mg	8–12 hours	Every 3–4 hours, then no less than every 6 hours
Phenobarbital 30 mg		
Ethyl alcohol 25 g (2 drinks)		

- Guiding principles of prophylaxis include
  - ○ Early identification of *all* patients at risk of alcohol withdrawal to prevent progression.
  - ○ The need for more aggressive treatment if factors present that might increase the risk of bad outcomes if withdrawal develops.
  - ○ Use of cross-tolerant medications (preferably benzodiazepines).
  - ○ Frequent bedside assessment and monitoring to assess adequacy of prophylactic dose by best route at appropriate intervals with timely adjustment. Increase dosage if deteriorating vital signs with symptoms of withdrawal.
    - Agitation
    - Tremor
    - Diaphoresis
    - Seizure
  - ○ Administration of thiamine 100 mg, initially IM or IV every day for 1–3 days, and then by mouth with multivitamins, folic acid 1 mg daily orally.

TRIAGE

- Alcohol withdrawal is a dynamic syndrome requiring frequent assessments.
- Patients with severe withdrawal (CIWA score > 25) or requiring high doses of benzodiazepines should have constant observation in an intensive care unit (ICU) or step down with particular attention to pulmonary status.

TREATMENT OF ALCOHOL WITHDRAWAL

- Guiding principles of treatment include
  - ○ Relief of symptoms to achieve the endpoint of "light somnolence"[2] and pharmacotherapy to replace alcohol with a sedative drug that can be tapered in a controlled manner.
  - ○ Clear and reassuring communication that guides the patient and family to participate in care.
  - ○ A quiet environment with lighting consistent with the time of day.
  - ○ Least restrictive intervention to maintain patient safety, including avoiding restraints that can increase patient agitation and immobility.
- Benzodiazepines are the mainstay of treatment[2] (see Table 70-3).
  - ○ Prescribe a single agent and titrate as needed.
  - ○ Lorazepam (Ativan) is preferred (rather than diazepam or chlordiazepoxide) for elderly patients; those with liver disease, and when withdrawal is severe and escalating, requiring frequent IV dosing (see Table 70-4).

TABLE 70-3   Alcoholic Syndromes: Example of Initial Treatment

Prophylaxis

In general, start with lorazepam 1–2 mg q4 hours with prn dosing and titrate according to symptoms of withdrawal, need for supplemental dosing, or evidence of depressed respiration.

Note: Factor in polysubstance abuse, amount of daily consumption, timing of last drink, and comorbid conditions to determine best initial dose. Individualize treatment with frequent bedside monitoring to avoid the emergence of withdrawal symptoms and over sedation.

Acute withdrawal symptoms

Mild	Lorazepam 3 mg q4 hours
Moderate	Lorazepam 4 mg q2 hours
Severe	Lorazepam 4 mg q15 min
	IV to stabilize patient as initial treatment, then individualize with decreased doses.

Note: Regarding efficacy and safety, no one route (IV vs. oral), dosing regimen, or specific benzodiazepine has been determined to be superior. It is important not to mix benzodiazepines because of different half-lives. Lorazepam 0.5 mg IV may be roughly equivalent to lorazepam 1 mg po. Some experts, however, recommend a 1:1 conversion from IV therapy to po in order to avoid over sedation when a patient is able to take oral therapy with additional dosing prescribed on a prn basis to avoid re-emergence of withdrawal. Consider pharmacy and psychiatry or addiction consultation to assist with dosing.

Hold if somnolence or evidence of depressed respiration.

Withdrawal seizures

Benzodiazepines
Dilantin ineffective

Alcoholic hallucinosis

Haloperidol (Haldol) 0.5–2.0 mg every 2 hours with monitoring of QT interval.

Note: Concurrent benzodiazepines provide prophylaxis against seizures and other withdrawal syndromes and neuroleptics should not be prescribed alone.

When vital signs and symptoms are controlled for 24 hours, taper lorazepam slowly (not more than 25% of 24-hour dose per day)

SOURCE: For a free reproducible CIWA tool go to: http://images2.clinicaltools.com/images/pdf/ciwa-ar.pdf

- Advantages of lorazepam (Ativan) include intermediate half-life, relatively straightforward hepatic metabolism, and availability of multiple routes of administration.
- Do not prescribe more than 4 mg of lorazepam in a single bolus.
- Check vital signs before each IV dose and 15 minutes after administration.
  - ○ Diazepam (Valium) or chlordiazepoxide (Librium) may be preferred for prophylaxis, for mild or moderate withdrawal, and for outpatients undergoing detoxification.
    - Advantages of diazepam (Valium) include fast onset of action, relatively long half-life with consequent reduced frequency of administration, self-tapering effect (because of active metabolites and long half-life), and availability of multiple routes of administration.

Table 70-4   Prophylactic Dosing*

	< 1 PINT PER DAY	1 PINT PER DAY	1 QUART PER DAY
Lorazepam	4–6 mg daily	8–12mg daily	16 mg daily
Chlordiazepoxide	100–150 mg daily	200–300 mg daily	400 mg daily
Diazepam	20–30 mg daily	40–60 mg daily	80 mg daily
Oxazepam	120–180 mg daily	240–360 mg daily	480 mg daily

*Clinical judgment is required especially in the elderly, patients with liver disease and other co-morbidities.

- Potential disadvantages of diazepam (Valium) include the risk of a cumulative effect, especially in patients with liver disease because of an active metabolite, desmethyldiazepam with a half-life of several days or longer, and vein irritation.
- When autonomic symptoms are adequately treated with benzodiazepines, haloperidol (Haldol) 1 mg IM, IV, or po q1 hour prn (usually not more than 5 mg per day) may be required to control agitation, disorientation, hallucinations, or delusions resulting from alcohol withdrawal.
  - Check electrocardiogram (ECG) QT intervals and optimize K^+ and Mg^{3+} levels.
- When severe withdrawal cannot be controlled with benzodiazepines and haloperidol, propofol, an intravenous drug used for the induction and maintenance of anesthesia, or phenobarbital is sometimes used in the ICU setting. Both drugs cause respiratory depression, especially when used in combination with other sedating drugs.
  - Benzodiazepines activate the GABA receptors but do not inhibit the NMDA receptors. Perhaps lack of inhibition explains why sometimes severe withdrawal from alcohol cannot be controlled with benzodiazepines.
  - Propofol's mechanism of action on the CNS is similar to that of alcohol. Propofol directly activates the GABA receptors and inhibits the NMDA receptors.
  - Advantage of propofol is less cross-tolerance than benzodiazepines, easy ability to titrate, and rapid clearance so that even when used for days, the patient becomes conscious within 10–15 minutes after discontinuation of the drip. It is, however, expensive.
  - A less expensive alternative than propofol with a different mechanism of action, phenobarbital has been shown to be superior to diazepam for Grade 3 (tremor, hallucinations, disorientation) withdrawal but not for Grade 1 (tremor) or Grade 2 (tremor and hallucinations) withdrawal.
- Intravenous alcohol should be avoided because of the short half-life, toxicity, interactions with other drugs, the need for frequent administration, and the mixed message it sends to the patient about the need to abstain.

- Adjunctive drugs include beta-blockers and alpha-agonists.
  - One study compared atenolol dosed according to heart rate vs. placebo for 120 alcoholics between the ages of 16 and 65. Oxazepam (Serax) was given as needed. This randomized controlled trial excluded combative patients, patients with seizures, polysubstance abuse, diabetes, chronic obstructive pulmonary disease (COPD), asthma, and hypertension.
    - Atenolol was superior to placebo in normalizing vital signs but there was no difference in tremor, seizure, loss of consciousness, anxiety, agitation, or hallucination.
    - The study reported statistically significant reduction in length of stay (LOS, 0.7 days), decreased need for oxazepam, and more rapid normalization of vital signs. Beta-blockers may reduce alcohol cravings.
  - Another study compared clonidine, an alpha-agonist, to librium.
    - Although there were significant limitations to this study, clonidine appeared superior to librium in improving heart rate, systolic blood pressure (BP), and self-rating of alcohol withdrawal scale.
    - Clonidine can mask symptoms of alcohol or sedative withdrawal in polysubstance abusers, and without additional medication for sedative withdrawal these patients can progress to seizures.
- Guidelines for pharmacologic management do not eliminate the need for individualized treatment.[2]
  - Medications and comorbidities may alter symptoms and signs of alcohol withdrawal and need to be factored in the decision-making relating to treatment doses.
  - Clinicians should prescribe lower benzodiazepine dosages for patients who are elderly, frail, or cachectic, or who have renal or hepatic insufficiency, severe pulmonary disease or obstructive sleep apnea, or neurologic disease.
- Benzodiazepines should be tapered to avoid withdrawal seizures and emergence of alcohol withdrawal.
  - Vital signs and symptoms should be stable for at least 24 hours prior to initiating a taper.

○ Tapering benzodiazepines for treatment of acute alcohol withdrawal must be more gradual than when used for prophylaxis.
  ▪ In general, do not taper more than 25% of the prescribed dosage in 24 hours including as needed supplementation.
○ Psychiatric consultation should be considered for treatment of alcohol withdrawal and for taper suggestions.
○ Addiction service consultation, if available, will also assist clinicians in appropriate use of treatment guidelines and provide patients and families with resources for recovery.

CARE TRANSITIONS

• Hospitalists play a crucial role in approaching these patients in a nonjudgmental manner and in insuring optimal care transitions.
• Detoxification from alcohol is only the first step in initiating abstinence.
• Ongoing treatment in the outpatient setting is essential.
• For patients receiving a benzodiazepine taper, consider consultation with an addiction service prior to discharge to explore options.
• For patients who want to remain free of alcohol and can be safely transitioned to home, the taper can be completed in the outpatient setting. Sometimes a family member or significant other administers the taper.
• For patients who do not want to abstain and plan to drink alcohol, discharge can occur without a taper because of assumed ongoing alcohol consumption.

REFERENCES

1. Kitchens JM. Does this patient have an alcohol problem? *JAMA*. 1994;272(2):1782–1787.
2. Mayo-Smith MF. Pharamcological management of alcohol withdrawal: a meta-analysis and evidence-based practice guideline. *JAMA*. 1997;278:144–155.
3. Sullivan JT, Sykora K, Schneiderman J, et al. Assessment of alcohol withdrawal: the revised clinical institute withdrawal assessment for alcohol scale (CIWA-Ar). *Br J Addict*. 1989;84:1353–1357.
4. Kosten TR, O'Connor PG. Management of drug and alcohol withdrawal. *N Engl J Med*. 2003;348(18):1786–1794.
5. Holbrook A, Crowther C, Lotter A, et al. Meta-analysis of benzodiazepine use in the treatment of acute alcohol withdrawal. *CMAJ*. 1999;160:649–655.
6. Baumgartner GR. Randomized control trial comparing clonidine to Librium. *Arch Intern Med*. 1987;147:1223.
7. Kraus ML, Gottlieb LD, Horwitz RI, et al. Randomized clinical trial of atenolol in patients with alcohol withdrawal. *N Engl J Med*. 1985;313(15):905–909.
8. Marik PE. Propofol: therapeutic indications and side effects. *Curr Pharm Des*. 2004;10(29):3639.
9. Melmon KL, Morrelli HF, Hoffman BB, et al. eds. *Clinical Pharmacology: Basic Principles in Therapeutics*. 3rd ed. New York, NY: McGraw-Hill; 1992:772.

71 MANAGEMENT OF PATIENTS WITH DRUG ABUSE

Mohammad Salameh

EPIDEMIOLOGY/OVERVIEW

• Up to 40% of patients presenting to the hospital have drug abuse listed as either a primary or secondary diagnosis.
• Prevalence varies by geographic area (more common in large urban hospitals than in small suburban or rural areas).
• Prevalence is also more common for men than women. Women with partners who abuse drugs are at increased risk of substance abuse.
• There may be a familial or genetic component to the disorder.
• Drug abuse is more common in patients with a history of mental or psychiatric illness. Patients with bipolar disorder and schizophrenia are at particular risk.

CLINICAL PRESENTATION, DIFFERENTIAL, MAKING THE DIAGNOSIS

• There are few specific signs and symptoms; physicians must often sort through a nonspecific presentation to identify the drug abuser.
• Patient denial is often a barrier to effective recognition and treatment.

- Patient history should be obtained in a nonjudgmental manner.
  - The history can be especially helpful if the patient reports or admits to a history of drug abuse and is specific about type of drug used, amount used, method of use, and length of time used.
  - Family and friends can often be helpful in interviewing a patient with a history or suspicion of drug use. However, be mindful of HIPAA (Health Insurance Portability and Accountability Act) compliance issues when speaking to anyone but the patient or DPOA.
  - Patient's history of mental illness, other family members with substance abuse, and erratic employment and problems with interpersonal relationships may suggest drug use and abuse.
  - If the patient does not offer a history of substance abuse, screening questions (eg, CAGE questions—see Chap. 70) can be utilized.
  - Any history regarding substance abuse must include a history of all substances used, the amount used, the mode of use, and a comment on the use of prescription and/or over-the-counter medications.
- Signs and symptoms are often nonspecific and may include chills, anxiety, constipation, confusion, headache, chest pain, lethargy, palpitations, changes in level of consciousness and alertness, sweating, insomnia, erectile dysfunction, hallucinations and delusions, and focal neurologic complaints such as numbness, parasthesias, blurry vision, or ataxia.
- Symptoms of abuse must be balanced with the nonspecific symptoms of withdrawal that may include any of the above plus nausea, vomiting, abdominal pain and cramping, diarrhea, tremor, and severe agitation.
- Signs of drug abuse that are seen on physical examination include several nonspecific findings and others that are dependent on the type of drug used and the mode of delivery of the drug—tachycardia, hypertension, fever, sweating, tremor, papillary changes, ataxia are common.
- Other more specific findings are discussed below with an inventory of the most common types of drugs abused.
- Diagnostic evaluation
  - Urine toxicology screens with confirmatory blood testing may identify the presence of drugs of abuse. Acetaminophen and alcohol levels should always be checked on patients who are suspected of drug abuse.
  - Liver panel may show elevated transaminase levels.
  - Amylase and lipase levels are often elevated, as is the white blood cell (WBC) count and total creatinine kinase levels.
  - Although not necessarily helpful in making a diagnosis, brain imaging with computed tomography (CT) scanning can rule out other causes of agitation and mental status changes in patients with positive drug screens.

TRIAGE AND INITIAL MANAGEMENT

The treatment of drug abuse or withdrawal is mainly supportive in nature. Once a patient is stabilized, strategies for long-term treatment can then be implemented.

- On initial presentation, patients may be agitated, tremulous, and acutely intoxicated.
  - If the drug of abuse is a stimulant, sedation with neuroleptics or benzodiazepines may be indicated.
  - If sedation is the presenting complaint, reversal of the potential agent may be attempted with naloxone or flumezanil.
- Intravenous fluid administration with normal saline to control tachycardia, supplement fluid losses, and treat hypotension or shock may also be indicated.
  - Polysubstance abuse should be assumed and therefore administer thiamine, folate, and multivitamins.
- Induction of vomiting is not helpful, but gastric lavage may decrease absorption of some drugs if the drug is taken orally (check with Poison Control).
- Drug overdoses require frequent checks on neurologic and cardiac status.
  - All patients should be placed on telemetry to monitor cardiac rhythm.
- Patients who are sedated and unable to protect airway require intubation until they are alert and awake.
- Patients who present with alcohol, barbiturate, or benzodiazepine abuse will require barbiturate or benzodiazepine tapers to prevent withdrawal seizures or DTs (see Chap. 70).
- Any patient presenting to the hospital with drug abuse or withdrawal should be seen by a social worker early in hospital stay to help plan and execute long-term therapy. Informing patients of support groups, rehabilitation programs, and education regarding coping is essential to prevent relapse.
- Close communication with primary care physicians is also vital in attempting to prevent relapse. Close follow-up with primary care physicians is especially vital for patients who abuse prescription drugs.

DISEASE MANAGEMENT STRATEGIES

CONSIDERATIONS SPECIFIC TO CERTAIN DRUGS OF ABUSE

COCAINE
- Symptoms of acute intoxication: headache, chest pain, anxiety, palpitations, syncope, sudden cardiac death, seizures, and stroke.

- Physical examination: tachycardia, hypertension, dilated pupils, focal neurologic deficit(s), nasal septum rupture, and abnormal sweating.
- Additional evaluation: thyroid-stimulating hormone (TSH) to rule out hyperthyroidism; ECG to rule out myocardial ischemia; consider CT scan to rule out intracranial hemorrhage; consider EEG to assess seizure activity.
- Treatment: agitation and withdrawal of cocaine can be treated with benzodiazepines, plus longer-acting neuroleptics such as risperidal or olanzapine.
- Hypertensive urgency or emergency from cocaine use should be treated in the ICU; preferred agents for treatment are nitroprusside or phentolamine. Beta-blockers should be avoided since they can potentiate vasospasm and decreased coronary blood flow in patients with cocaine toxicity.
- Lidocaine is the preferred agent in patients who develop arrhythmias.

AMPHETAMINES
- Intoxication is very similar in presentation and sequelae as cocaine use with similar physical examination findings, clinical presentation, and treatment. Chronic use can be associated with violent and aggressive behavior.
- Treatment: high-dose sedatives may be needed to control agitation.
- Induction of vomiting is contraindicated (may precipitate seizures).
- Prescription medications for attention deficit hyperactivity disorder (ADHD) have similar effects and must be considered in this category.

OPIATES
- Symptoms: acute overdose usually presents with severe sedation or obtundation. Respiratory and neurologic depression often requires intubation and aggressive supportive care.
- Physical examination findings: pinpoint pupils; in severe cases, bradycardia and pulmonary edema may be present. If patients inject opiates (eg, heroin), skin markings are often present; if patients with an opiate history present with fever, a detailed skin examination looking for splinter hemorrhages and cardiac examination looking for cardiac murmurs is clearly indicated for suspected endocarditis.
- Additional evaluation: ECG to evaluate for prolonged QT interval; transesophageal echo in patients with fever, blood cultures to evaluate for endocarditis; all patients should have a hepatitis panel and HIV test done.
- If opiate toxicity is in the form of prescription pills, a liver panel and international normalized ratio (INR) are critical, as is an acetaminophen level.

- Treatment: naloxone (0.1–0.4 mg IV, IM, or SC; repeated at 2-minute intervals. Up to 10 mg naloxone maximum; can be administered via endotracheal (ET) tube. If no response with 10 mg, the condition is not likely to be an opiate overdose). Dosing depends on the half-life of the opiate that is used—longer treatment courses need for those drugs with longer half-lives.
- Withdrawal signs and symptoms: agitation, tachycardia, abdominal cramping, diarrhea, nausea, and vomiting.
- Treatment of withdrawal: benzodiazepines to treat agitation; antiemetics; intravenous fluids to prevent dehydration; longer-acting opiates (eg, buprenorphine or methadone) that can be later tapered in the outpatient setting. Buprenorphine is the preferred agent as it has less potential for withdrawal as it is being tapered and overdose with this agent is not as dangerous as it is with methadone.

BARBITURATES AND BENZODIAZEPINES
- Symptoms: similar to that of opiates (obtundation, cardiac depression, and respiratory collapse).
- If toxicology screens are not immediately available, absent deep tendon reflexes, hypotension, and hypothermia are clues to this diagnosis.
- Treatment: supportive care and reversal of the drugs' actions—ventilator support and flumezanil (small doses of 0.2 mg IV or via ET tube; only if the benzodiazepine is high enough to cause respiratory collapse). This drug is not effective for barbiturates.
- For barbiturate overdose, alkaline diuresis is effective in helping drug clearance.
- More commonly, patients abusing these two agents present with withdrawal rather than overdose; treatment similar to alcohol withdrawal including supportive care with benzodiazepine tapers, IV fluids, and beta-blockers or clonidine to control hypertension.

GAMMA-HYDROXYBUTYRATE
- Symptoms of overdose: ataxia, visual changes, vomiting, and somnolence. Drug is undetectable on standard toxicology screen, use should be suspected based on history (recent notoriety as the "date rape" drug, given to unsuspecting individuals).
- Treatment: supportive, including airway support, atropine for bradycardia, and IV fluids.
- Half-life is short; patients generally require only very short hospital stays.

HALLUCINOGENS
- This group includes a wide variety of drugs, namely, lysergic acid diethylamide (LSD), mescaline, psilocybin, mushroom, and ketamine.

- Symptoms of acute intoxication: violent behavior, paranoia, severe hallucinations, ataxia, and anxiety. Patients often have nystagmus on examination and tachycardia.
- Treatment: supportive, including reassurance and placing the patient in a safe environment until the effect of the drug wanes. Benzodiazepines may be helpful to reduce agitation and anxiety; but neuroleptics should be avoided.

PHENCYCLIDINE (PCP)

- Symptoms of intoxication: very aggressive, violent behavior, paranoia, and tachycardia. A very unique and characteristic vertical nystagmus is seen in these patients.
- Treatment: acidify the urine with ammonium chloride or ascorbic acid. Neuroleptics can help control the agitation and hallucinations.

TOXIC INHALANTS

- Recent trend by youth/young adults to use readily available inhalants as a way to obtain a "high" or euphoria.
- Symptoms of intoxication: confusion, ataxia, tachycardia, hypotension, and in severe cases, respiratory and cardiac failure.
- Treatment: supportive; if patients survive the acute episode, long-term sequelae are limited.

METHHYLENEDIOXYMETHAMPHETAMINE (ECSTASY)

- This drug is very popular among American youth, with up to 40% of college students trying it at least once.
- Symptoms: most of its effects are caused by serotonin release; symptoms may include hypertension, tachycardia, dilated pupils, diaphoresis, and trismus (jaw muscle spasm). Severe intoxication may involve ventricular tachycardia, rhabdomyolysis, acute renal failure, seizures, and hyperthermia.
- Laboratory findings include elevated creatine kinase (CK) and hyopnatremia secondary to SIADH (syndrome of inappropriate antidiuretic hormone).
- Standard toxicology screens are not helpful and like GABA, the diagnosis is made based on history and clinical presentation.
- Treatment: supportive, including aggressive IV hydration, beta-blockers to control hypertension and tachycardia, airway support, benzodiazepines for seizures and agitation, and dialysis if acute renal failure is severe and associated with excessively elevated CK levels.

TETRAHYDROCANNABINOL

- Marijuana or Cannabis sativa is a commonly used drug of abuse, but sole use is unlikely to lead to inpatient hospitalization. However, since it is so commonly used, there should be an inquiry about its use.
- It can complicate other medical problems, such as asthma and COPD.
- It can also cause paranoia, tachycardia, hypertension, and dry mouth.
- Therefore, if a toxicology screen shows tetrahydrocannabinol (THC) presence, use and avoidance should be discussed with patients.

ALCOHOL INTOXICATION AND WITHDRAWAL

- See Chap. 70—Management of Patients with Alcohol Abuse

BIBLIOGRAPHY

Beebe DK, Walley E. Substance abuse: the designer drugs. *Am Fam Physician.* 1991;43:1689.

Carroll ME. PCP and other hallucinogens. *Adv Alcohol Sub Abuse.* 1990;9(1–2):167–190.

Comings DE. Genetic factors in drug abuse and dependence. *NIDA Res Monogr.* 1996;159:16–38; discussion 39–48.

Glantz MD, Gordon H. Individual differences in the biobehavioral etiology of drug abuse. *NIDA Res Monogr.* 1996;1–16.

Goldman E, Goldman V, Goldman J, et al. Drug abuse and dependence. *Cecil's Textbook of Medicine.* Philadelphia, PA: W.B. Saunders;2004.

Koesters SC, Rogers PD, Rajasingham CR. MDMA ('Ecstasy') and other 'Club Drugs'. The new epidemic. *Pediatr Clin North Am.* 2002;49:415.

Lange RA, Cigarroa RG, Flores ED, et al. Potentiation of cocaine-induced coronary vasoconstriction by beta-adrenergic blockade. *Ann Intern Med.* 1990;112(12):897–903.

Leri F, Bruneau J, Stewart J. Understanding polydrug use: review of heroin and cocaine co-use. *Addiction.* 2003;98(1):7–22.

Regier DA, Farmer ME, Rae DS, et al. Comorbidity of mental disorders with alcohol and other drug abuse. Results from the Epidemiologic Catchment Area (ECA) Study. *JAMA.* 1990;264:2511.

The Economic Costs of Drug Abuse 1992–2002. Executive Summary. Office of National Drug Control Policy;2002.

The National Institute of Drug Abuse. Research Report Series. Etiology and prevention of drug use: the US National Institute of Drug Abuse Research Monographs: 1991–1994, Updated 2006.

72 MANAGEMENT OF SUICIDAL PATIENTS

Christine K. Kim, Meghan Kolodziej, and David F. Gitlin

EPIDEMIOLOGY/OVERVIEW

- Patients who have attempted suicide may be initially admitted to a general medical service for monitoring and/or treatment following a toxic ingestion.
- In addition, because of reimbursement issues and a shortage of inpatient psychiatry beds, hospitalists may be called upon to manage acutely suicidal patients with psychiatric consultation or comanagement.
- Rarely, patients attempt suicide in the hospital setting.
- Unfortunately, the phenomenon of suicide in a general hospital is not well studied.
- Suicide is a complex phenomena involving voluntary self-destructive acts or thoughts that ranges from passive, fleeting wishes to die to completed suicide.
- Although suicide rarely occurs in a hospital setting, reports of suicidal ideation are much more common. Dealing with suicidal patients often leads to distress among the hospital staff and has complicated medical-legal consequences.
- While suicide is not completely preventable, it is crucial to thoroughly assess patients with suicidal thoughts. Comorbid psychiatric illnesses must be identified and treated.
- About 31,484 people died by suicide in 2003, making it the 11th leading cause of death in the United States, with a rate of approximately 13/100,000. Nearly 53% of these suicides were committed with a firearm.[1]
  - In the general hospital, the rate of suicide ranges from 9.8 to 32 per 100,000.[2]
  - A study at a Veterans Administration (VA) facility showed an even higher rate of suicide at 150 per 100,000 over a 4-year period.[3]
- There are many more suicide attempts than completed suicides. In 2002, 132,353 individuals were hospitalized following suicide attempts and 116,639 individuals were treated in emergency departments and released.[4] The clinical profile of suicide attempters often differs from that of individuals who complete suicide (Table 72-1).
- This chapter reviews the general epidemiology of suicide, clinical presentations of suicidal patients, and management of such patients in a general medical setting.

TABLE 72-1   Typical Characteristics of Suicide Attempters Compared with Suicide Completers

	ATTEMPTERS	COMPLETERS
Gender	Female	Male
Method	Overdose, wrist cutting	Firearms
Age	< 30	> 65
Presence of others at time of attempt	With others	Alone
Intent	Low	High
Likelihood of rescue	High	Low
Presence of stressors	Recent stressors	Recent stressors

CLINICAL PRESENTATION, DIFFERENTIAL, MAKING THE DIAGNOSIS

- Risk factors for suicide (see Table 72-2)
  - Age. The risk of suicide varies over the lifespan.
    - National Vital Statistics Reports: While the mean age range for suicide is 45–54 years old, the rate of suicide increases throughout life with the highest rates seen in individuals over 65 years old.
    - Older victims are more likely to be widowed and suffering from physical illness than their younger counterparts. They are also less likely to have talked about suicide or to have made prior attempts.[5]
    - Adolescence is another period of high risk for suicide and represents the third leading cause of death among young people aged 15–24. Males account for 86% of the suicide victims in this age group.[6]
  - Gender.
    - Women are three times more likely to attempt suicide than men. Women are more likely to use nonviolent means to attempt suicide such as medication overdose and cutting.
    - Men are four times more likely to succeed in suicide. Men are more likely to use violent means such as firearms, hanging, or stabbing.

TABLE 72-2   Risk Factors for Suicide in the General Population

Male gender
Age > 65
Native American highest; Caucasian
Substance abuse
Psychiatric disorders
Prior suicide attempt
Unmarried, separated, divorced, widowed
Social isolation
Loss—relationship, job, or financial

○ Psychiatric illness—general points.
  ▪ It is estimated that 95% of patients who complete suicide have psychiatric diagnoses, with depression and alcoholism the two most common.[7]
  ▪ About 40% of patients who have completed suicide had mood disorders (unipolar or bipolar depression), 20% to 25% chronic alcoholism, 10% to 15% schizophrenia, and 20% to 25% severe personality disorder.[8]
○ Mood disorders.
  ▪ Although suicidality is associated with many psychiatric illnesses, it is most commonly seen in patients with mood disorders. Detecting depressive symptoms is an essential part of evaluation of the suicidal patient (see Table 72-3).
  ▪ In hospitalized patients, many physical symptoms of their medical illness overlap with the symptoms of depression and create a diagnostic challenge. For example, hospitalized patients may experience poor appetite, low energy level, and sleep disturbances related to their illness or the hospital environment.
  ▪ Nonsomatic symptoms such as anhedonia, hopelessness, feelings of guilt, and depressed mood may be more reliable signs of a depressive disorder in hospitalized patients.
○ Substance use disorders.
  ▪ Obtaining a thorough substance use history, particularly that of alcohol use is important. Use of the CAGE questionnaire is sensitive in screening for a diagnosis of alcohol abuse and dependence. At a cutoff point of two positive responses, the sensitivity is 71% and specificity is 90%.[9]
  ▪ Patients in alcohol withdrawal are at higher risk of suicidal behavior as the withdrawal symptoms may be the driving force behind agitation or impulsivity.
  ▪ Suicidal thinking and behavior increases during periods of intoxication with many substances, including alcohol, sedatives, cocaine, and opiates. The underlying mechanism may be disinhibition of otherwise controlled impulses.
  ▪ See Chaps. 70 and 71 for more information.

TABLE 72-3 Diagnosing Depression

Depressed mood
Suicidal ideation
Interest increased or decreased
Guilt or feelings of worthlessness
Energy level decreased
Concentration impaired or indecisiveness
Appetite increased or decreased
Psychomotor agitation or retardation
Sleep increased or decreased

○ Psychotic disorders. Psychosis poses an additional risk factor for suicide.
  ▪ Patients without a primary psychotic illness may become psychotic in a hospital setting. This maybe because of delirium, adverse effects of medication, or secondary to medical problems.
  ▪ Patients with psychosis may become suicidal in response to command hallucinations or persecutory delusions.
○ Personality factors. Personality factors play a role in suicide, and recognizing it in suicidal patients is important.
  ▪ Patients with personality disorders may have interpersonal difficulties with the hospital staff as well as their families. Patients with personality disorder are often viewed as the problematic patients, frequently demanding and difficult. With low frustration tolerance and poor impulse control, these patients may react to a perceived loss of support by the hospital staff by impulsive suicidal gestures.[10]
○ Medical illness. Patients with medical problems that are chronic, terminal, or painful are at a higher risk of developing depression and suicidality.
  ▪ The presence of medical illness is an independent risk factor for suicide. Having more than one medical illness was associated with a 2.4 times increased odds of a suicide attempt.[11]
  ▪ In one study, diagnosis of cancer or asthma increased odds of a suicide attempt by more than fourfold after adjusting for psychiatric covariates.[11]
  ▪ While medical illness increases risk for suicide, it is important to note that increased risk is not necessarily correlated with the severity of illness.
  ▪ It is the presence of comorbid psychiatric illness that appears to be linked to suicidality as the majority of terminally ill individuals do not suffer from depression or become suicidal.[12]
○ Detection of delirium. Reports of suicidal thoughts in a delirious patient are unreliable. However, delirious patients should be assessed completely, as they are often impulsive and may respond to frightening perceptual distortions. Delirious patients have been known to attempt suicide by jumping.[13] If suicidal ideation is present, a delirious patient may be more likely to act upon it.
○ Role of pain. Pain is a significant contributor to suicidality. Many suicidal patients cite pain as a precipitant for the act.
  ▪ Adequate management of pain and eliciting a patient's preference for pain management will not only provide pain relief but also diminish

the fear of losing control over their care. See Chap. 93.

- For patients facing end-of-life care, involvement of palliative care is essential part of the management of their illness. See Chaps. 94, 95, and 96 for more information on palliative care.
  ○ Biologic factors.
    - Research into biologic etiologies for suicide has focused on the serotonergic system. Individuals who commit suicide have been found to have low levels of cerebrospinal fluid serotonin and low levels of serotonin metabolite 5-hydroxyindoleacetic acid (5-HIAA).
    - Although these findings may indicate a biochemical vulnerability to suicide, there is no useful clinical application of these findings.
  ○ Other factors.
    - Other risk factors include ethnicity, with the highest rates in Caucasians and Native Americans.
    - Social factors that put individuals at higher risk for suicide include being unmarried, widowed, or divorced, having poor social supports, and having a family history of suicide.
- Patients who need evaluation for suicidality in the medical hospital setting include survivors of suicide attempts, patients who express thoughts about suicide, patients who express hopelessness, and patients who deny suicidality but whose actions indicate risk for suicide. Unusual behavior or abnormal affect may be an indication of emotional distress. All threats of suicide, suicidal gestures, and suicide attempts should be taken seriously and investigated.
  ○ Suicidal ideation may take a variety of forms, ranging from passive suicidal thoughts—"I wish I weren't here" to active suicidal ideation with a plan and intent. The nature of the patient's suicidal ideation should be elucidated and the patient's access to means determined.
  ○ While suicide attempts are often thought to result from depression, they may actually be impulsive acts rising out of anger, rising tension, or perceived loss of emotional support from either medical personnel or family members.[10]
  ○ However, these impulsive suicide attempts may actually represent a small percentage, as warning signs and indications of potential danger were present in most of patients who attempted suicide in a general hospital.[2]
- Assessment (see Table 72-4)
  ○ Psychiatric consultation should be obtained early. For many patients with concerning presentations who later completed suicide, psychiatric consultations were not obtained.[2]

TABLE 72-4 Suicide Assessment

Ask about suicidal ideation
Assess whether there is a suicide plan and intent to act on the plan
Determine access to lethal means, including whether there are firearms in the house
Are there current precipitants
Determine if the suicidal ideation is acute or chronic
Is there a past history of suicide attempts
Screen for psychopathology
Ask about family history of suicide and psychopathology
Does the patient have risk factors for suicide
What supports does the patient have
Perform a mental status examination
Obtain collateral history from the patient's friends or family

  ○ A number of suicide assessment screens exist but do not have proven validity, and there is no reliable means of recognizing those who are on the brink of suicide.[14] The lack of a valid measure does not, however, relieve the clinician of the obligation to perform a thorough assessment.
    - A history including the patient's risk factors for suicide should be done and any findings should be documented. Not asking certain questions does not relieve the clinician from the need to know.
    - If a patient is being evaluated after a suicide attempt, the risk of the attempt should be assessed from both a medical perspective and from the patient's perspective. A suicide attempt that the patient expected to die from should be more worrisome to the clinician.
    - The probability of rescue from the suicide attempt should be investigated, including whether the patient was alone or with people and if he/she took measures to prevent themselves from being found.
    - If the suicide attempt occurred in response to stressors, it is important to determine whether the stressors are still present.
  ○ It is important for the clinician to directly ask the patient about suicide or intent to self-harm. In one study, asking about "thoughts of death" was 100% sensitive and 81% specific in detecting suicidality. Similarly, asking about "feeling suicidal" was 83% sensitive and 98% specific.[15]
    - It is important to note that probing about suicidality does not contribute to suicidality.
    - Asking about suicidality should be done in a series of mounting questions, including eliciting precipitant factors. For patients with no prior psychiatric history, a premature question about suicidality may be too abrupt and may lead to denial of the symptoms. A series of expanding questions that start with some acknowledgement that the

clinician is aware of the present difficult situation will help to build an alliance.[16]

○ Patients may minimize symptoms of depression or other psychiatric conditions, particularly substance abuse. Thus, collateral information should be gathered from friends and family. Patients may or may not give consent to contact outside sources. However, if the outside information is critical in making the appropriate suicide assessment or if the situation is deemed to be of potential life-threatening nature, patient confidentiality can be overridden. The rationale for this should be carefully documented in the chart. The evaluating clinician should consult the hospital attorney or risk management if serious confidentiality concerns arise.[16]

MANAGEMENT STRATEGIES

• Initial management
  ○ Any patient with active suicidal ideation or any patient who has attempted suicide should be evaluated by a psychiatric consultant.
  ○ While the patient's safety is being assessed, precautions should be taken to keep them safe in the hospital, including a thorough search of the room and the patient's personal belongings to remove potentially harmful materials. This includes medications, sharp objects, and hidden weapons, including firearms.
  ○ Rooms in the general medical hospital generally do not provide an environment that safeguards patients from self-destructive behaviors, and the culture of the medical unit differs significantly from that of a psychiatric unit.
    ▪ The patient may require constant observation to ensure safety. Permitting privacy for the sake of politeness, or inattentiveness by the staff providing constant observation, can result in a potentially lethal outcome, as only a short time is needed to carry out a suicide plan.
    ▪ The majority of suicides that occur in the hospital are by jumping from a height. In one study, of those who completed suicide, the percentage of deaths from jumping was over 75%.[2]
    ▪ If the patient is a potential elopement risk by overpowering a staff, it maybe necessary to utilize a security officer.
    ▪ The decision to discontinue constant observation in a potentially suicidal patient, or in those who are admitted following a suicide attempt, should be carefully documented with the rationale for such a decision.

    ▪ In an overtly suicidal patient, physical restraints and/or chemical restraints may be required to manage the underlying source of agitation or impulsivity.
• Treatment of the suicidal patient is generally focused on contributing factors associated with the suicide attempt. It may include psychotherapy and/or somatic therapies to treat any psychiatric conditions that are found, treatment of substance abuse disorders, and increasing social supports and psychotherapy to improve coping strategies.
  ○ Antidepressants may be effective in decreasing suicidal ideation or behavior associated with a depressive illness. However, an antidepressant's full efficacy may not be evident for 4–6 weeks.
  ○ In addition to managing depressive symptoms, anxiety and insomnia should be addressed as they have been demonstrated to be associated with completed suicide.
  ○ A "suicide contract" is not legally binding and clinicians should not rely on this for patient safety. This type of contract is sometimes used to manage chronic suicidality in the outpatient setting, when a therapeutic alliance exists between a patient and his or her clinician. In the general hospital setting, this does not substitute for a thorough assessment and the use of constant observation when needed.
• Suicide prevention
  ○ The first step in preventing suicide is the early detection and treatment of comorbid psychiatric disorders. Early involvement of the psychiatric consultant is needed to provide an ongoing assessment and to facilitate management.
  ○ There must be a high degree of clinical awareness and staff education to prevent self-destructive behaviors in patients considered to be at high risk. Encourage staff communication and alertness for possible suicidal behavior. Discourage indifference toward the patient by demonstrating concerns for the patient as a person.
  ○ Recognition of delirium, underlying mood or personality disorders, and the presence of substance abuse or withdrawal is essential.
  ○ Treat pain symptoms aggressively and consider comorbid psychiatric issues if the pain appears to be out of proportion with its etiology.
  ○ Maximize social supports by recruiting family, friends, social worker and community resources, and spiritual supports.
• Medicolegal issues
  ○ Hospitals have a legal obligation to provide a safe environment to patients admitted after suicide attempts or those who express suicidality while

hospitalized. Failing to provide reasonable care can have considerable legal liability. While it is not possible to foresee all suicides, the standard of care dictates that clinicians take reasonable steps to assess the risk factors and to provide appropriate treatment to prevent suicide.[17]

○ It is important to document all clinical encounters with suicidal patients including collateral data obtained and the justification for the recommended treatment.

CARE TRANSITIONS

• Involving the suicidal patients in their own management and treatment can be helpful. Patients who demonstrate future orientation by accepting psychotherapy or other types of psychiatric interventions are typically at less risk than those who remain hopeless about the future.

• If the patient has attempted suicide, he or she needs to be medically stabilized and the risk for suicide reassessed throughout the hospital stay.

○ If it has been determined that a patient is not an active suicide risk at the time of discharge, he or she may be sent home with appropriate outpatient follow-up. Outpatient treatment options include psychopharmacology therapy, group therapy, and partial hospital programs.

○ If the patient is actively suicidal with a plan and has access to lethal means, he or she will require inpatient psychiatric admission to a locked facility. While arranging for transfer, the patient should be monitored for safety.

▪ If a patient is refusing psychiatric hospitalization and it has been determined that he or she requires hospitalization for safety, the patient may need to be involuntarily committed to a psychiatric hospital. Each state has different laws and regulations that govern the involuntary commitment of psychiatric patients. The law may require the attestation of a psychiatrist and documentation of the patient's mental illness and risk to themselves.

REFERENCES

1. Hoyert DL, Heron MP, Murphy SL, et al. Deaths: final data for 2003. *Natl Vital Stat Rep.* 2006;54:13.

2. Shapiro S, Waltzer H. Successful suicides and serious attempts in a general hospital over a 15-year period. *Gen Hosp Psychiatry.* 1980;2:118–126.

3. Farberow N. Suicide prevention in the hospital. *Hosp Community Psychiatry.* 1981;32(2):99–104.

4. Centers for Disease Control and Prevention, National Center for Injury Prevention and Control (producer). Web-based Injury Statistics Query and Reporting System (WISQARS) [Online]. (2004). Available online from URL: http://www.cdc.gov/ncipc/wisqars/default.htm.

5. Carney SS, Rich CL, Bruke PA, et al. Suicide over 60: The San Diego study. *J Am Geriatr Soc.* 1994;42:2.

6. Anderson RN, Smith BL. Deaths: leading causes for 2001. *Natl Vital Stat Rep.* 2003;52:9.

7. Dirk D, Asim U, Wajiha S. A retrospective study of general hospital patients who commit suicide shortly after being discharged from the hospital. *Arch Intern Med.* 2001;161: 991–994.

8. Litman RE. Suicides: what do they have in mind? In: Jacobs D, Brown HN, Madison CT, eds. *Suicide: Understanding and Responding.* International Universities Press; 1989: 143–154.

9. Aertgeerts B, Bunntinx F, Kester A. The value of the CAGE in screening for alcohol abuse and alcohol dependence in general clinical populations: a diagnostic meta-analysis. *J Clin Epidemiol.* 2004;57:30–39.

10. Reich P, Kelly M. Suicide attempts by hospitalized medical and surgical patients. *N Engl J Med.* 1976;294: 298–301.

11. Druss B, Pincus H. Suicidal ideation and suicide attempts in general medical illnesses. *Arch Intern Med.* 2000;160: 1522–1526.

12. Brown J, Henteleff P, Barakat S, et al. Is it normal for terminally ill patients to desire death? *Am J Psychiatry.* 1986;143:208–211.

13. White R, Gribble R, Corr M, et al. Jumping from a general hospital. *Gen Hosp Psychiatry.* 1995;17:208–215.

14. Hughes D. Management of suicidal and aggressive patients in the medical setting. In: Stoudemire A, Fogel B, Greenberg D, eds. *Psychiatric Care of the Medical Patient.* New York, NY: Oxford University Press; 2000.

15. Broadhead WE, Leon AC, Weissman MM, et al. Development and validation of the SD DS-PC screen for multiple mental disorders in primary care. *Arch Fam Med.* 1995;4:211–219.

16. Goldberg R. The assessment of suicide risk in the general hospital. *Gen Hosp Psychiatry.* 1987;9:446–452.

17. Berman A, Cohen-Sandler R. Suicide and the standard of care: optimal vs. acceptable. *Suicide Life Threat Behav.* 1982;12(2):114–122.

PULMONARY ILLNESS/CRITICAL CARE MEDICINE

73 SHORTNESS OF BREATH

Andrew S. Karson and
Sylvia C. McKean

EPIDEMIOLOGY/OVERVIEW

• Acute shortness of breath, or dyspnea, is one of the most common complaints that physicians encounter in the ambulatory and inpatient setting.
• Although two-thirds of all cases stem from respiratory and cardiovascular diseases, the differential diagnosis is broad (see Table 73-1).
• Patients report shortness of breath using a variety of descriptors, which can be helpful in identifying potential causes of their symptoms.
• Hospitalists must recognize the importance of assessing the "ABCs" (Airway, Breathing, and Circulation) in a patient with new shortness of breath or a new oxygen requirement.
• Hospitalists should also maintain a clinical suspicion for
  ○ Pulmonary embolism (PE) in acutely ill, hospitalized patients with dyspnea
  ○ Pneumothorax in an acutely dyspneic patient, who has had placement of a central venous catheter

TABLE 73-1   Differential Diagnosis of Acute Dyspnea

Anaphylaxis
Pneumothorax
Pulmonary edema
PE
Cardiac ischemia
Cardiac arrhythmia
Asthma/COPD
Acute mucous plug
Pericardial disease
Pneumonia
Aspiration
Pleural effusion
Primary metabolic acidosis
Withdrawal syndromes/anxiety/pain
Foreign body inhalation
Mechanical chest wall restriction
Deconditioning
Neuromuscular weakness
Anemia
Malignancy

○ Aspiration of oral secretions or food in a patient with dysphagia or recent stroke
○ Cardiogenic pulmonary edema in an acutely dyspneic patient, who has received intravenous hydration
○ Respiratory compensation through hyperventilation for metabolic acidosis, severe anemia, or end-stage liver disease
○ Psychogenic causes from anxiety, pain, and withdrawal syndromes
○ Anaphylaxis from IV contrast or antibiotic therapy
○ Reactive airway diseases in a patient who is scheduled for surgery
• After a targeted history and physical examination, the physician should be able to assign a general pretest probability relating to acute diagnoses under consideration (low, moderate, or high) to direct appropriate diagnostic testing.
• Before obtaining a chest x-ray (CXR), hospitalists should initiate therapy based on clinical suspicion for acutely ill patients with falling oxygen saturation.
• An arterial blood gas (ABG) should be obtained in all patients with acute shortness of breath that have rapidly deteriorating respiratory status or altered mental status.

PATHOPHYSIOLOGY

• Acute respiratory failure (ARF) may occur through failure of the respiratory system because of CNS dysfunction (stroke, sedatives, narcotics), interference with the mechanical function of the chest (flail chest from trauma, pneumothorax), interference of the neuromuscular junction, as well as from airways disease.
• Respiratory depression may develop gradually, and may not be apparent by routine vital signs, and may be present despite normal oxygen saturation.
• Breathing difficulty experienced more often during inspiration rather than expiration suggests the role of respiratory muscles in the experience of dyspnea.
• Patients with neuromuscular disease often report rapid and shallow inhalation as making them feel short of breath.
  ○ Inspiration requires active inspiratory muscle and diaphragmatic contraction.
  ○ Expiration is passive because of elastic recoil.

- Patients with COPD can develop dynamic hyperinflation during exertion that creates a threshold for inspiration and also shortens the vertical muscle fibers.
- "My chest feels tight" may reflect abnormal airway tone (asthma and cystic fibrosis).
- An increased elastic load seen in interstitial lung disease may produce rapid breathing.
- Deconditioning may produce a sensation of "heavy breathing" or of "breathing more," unlike the increased "work of breathing (WOB)" seen in COPD.

CLINICAL PRESENTATION, DIFFERENTIAL, MAKING THE DIAGNOSIS

HISTORICAL FEATURES THAT CAN HELP IN MAKING THE DIAGNOSIS

- Standardized dyspnea questionnaires have demonstrated that the way patients describe their shortness of breath can be helpful in identifying potential causes of their symptoms.
- The history of cigarette exposure and the triad of wheezing, coughing, and sputum production suggest COPD.
- Rapid onset of symptoms may be consistent with potential "flash" pulmonary edema, sudden aspiration pneumonitis, PE, or mucous plug.
  ○ A witnessed aspiration event in patients with altered or depressed mental status may be followed by dyspnea, cough, wheeze, cyanosis, hypoxia, pulmonary edema, and potentially acute respiratory distress syndrome (ARDS).
  ○ Mucus plugging is more likely in neurologically impaired, elderly patients and those with chronic lung disease and thick secretions.
  ○ Interstitial lung disease (connective tissue disorders, drug toxicities, bone marrow transplant patients) produces more chronic symptoms of shortness of breath.
  ○ Acutely expanding pleural effusions (trauma, hemorrhage) can cause dyspnea and hypoxia.
- Shortness of breath that comes at night, with certain exposures, and/or after exercise would be consistent with a diagnosis of asthma.
- Symptoms that appear with exercise, especially if with concomitant chest pain, jaw pain, arm pain, nausea, vomiting, palpitations, and/or light-headedness, should raise the possibility of cardiac ischemia, and/or cardiac arrhythmia.
- Symptoms of withdrawal—opposite of those caused by the offending substance—with pupillary or skin changes increase the likelihood of withdrawal as the cause of acute shortness of breath.

- Neuromuscular weakness, such as in patients with myasthenia gravis or Guillain-Barré syndrome, may produce shortness of breath.
- Patients with kyphoscoliosis may suffer from shortness of breath because of the mechanical restriction of chest wall movement.
- Correlating associated symptoms with risk factors for cardiovascular, pulmonary, and neurologic disorders helps focus the physical examination.

THE PHYSICAL EXAMINATION

- Vital signs are part of the initial critical assessment of acute dyspnea and guide the rapidity of diagnostic testing and treatment.
- Check the respiratory rate yourself, heart rate, BP, oxygen saturation, and temperature and, in selected cases, pulsus paradoxus.
- Pulse oximetry is a single tool in the identification of borderline hypoxemia. The best approach is a high index of suspicion. Know the patient, observe respiratory efforts, the degree of sedation, and airway patency.
- Although oximetry is a simple, reliable, readily available, noninvasive way of measuring oxygenation, sources of error include poor perfusion, motion, excessive light, venous pulsation, dyshemoglobins, pigment, and nail polish.
  ○ Because of the shape of the oxygen dissociation curve, assuming a 95% confidence limit of approximately 4%, an oximeter reading of 95% could represent a partial oxygen pressure (PO_2) between 60 mm Hg (sat PO_2 = 91%) and 160 mm Hg (sat PO_2 = 99%). There is greater variation at lower PO_2 saturations (Fig. 73-1).
- Arterial puncture and blood gas analysis is still required if ventilation (the arterial carbon dioxide tension) or acid-base information is needed.
- The pulsus paradoxus has many definitions in the medical literature, but at the bedside it is most useful to think of the pulsus paradoxus as the fall in systolic arterial pressure during inspiration. To measure this properly, note:
  ○ The systolic and diastolic pressures in inspiration and expiration.
  ○ The ventilatory status (rate, rhythm, depth).
  ○ Although an exaggerated pulsus paradoxus is present in 100% of patients with tamponade after heart surgery, it has also been observed in hypovolemic shock, right ventricular (RV) infarction, severe congestive heart failure (CHF), myocarditis, and other heart diseases. In addition, it has been noted in respiratory illness including asthma, emphysema, and

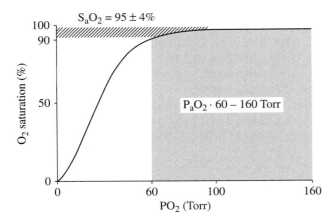

FIG. 73-1   The oxygen dissociation curve.
SOURCE: Adapted from Tobin MJ. Respiratory monitoring in the intensive care unit. *Am Rev Respir Dis.* 1988;138(6):1625–1642.

PE. Extreme obesity and ascites may also be associated with pulsus paradoxus.
  ○ Despite the lack of specificity, checking a pulsus paradoxus in critically ill patients may be a diagnostic clue to the presence of tamponade or other life-threatening causes of acute dyspnea.
• Listen to the patient.
  ○ Assess speech, comprehension, attention (see Chap. 61).
  ○ Clues to possible oropharyngeal swallowing problems include
    ▪ Coughing or choking while drinking, eating, or taking medications
    ▪ Hoarse voice, wet voice quality, or change in voice after swallowing
    ▪ Difficulty managing secretions
    ▪ Facial or tongue weakness, cranial nerve palsies, observed poor motion of the larynx, prolonged time between taking a bite or sip and swallowing
• Be sure to inspect the chest wall and neck veins for an elevated jugular venous pressure (JVP) and the chest wall for abnormalities.
  ○ The presence of a barrel chest (anteroposterior diameter greater than normal) would increase your suspicion of airflow limitation which would be confirmed by auscultation—findings of rhonchi, hyperresonance, forced expiratory time > 9 seconds, and a subxyphoid apical impulse.
  ○ Note use of accessory muscles of respiration and look for paradoxical chest wall motion.
  ○ The presence of a flail chest from multiple rib fractures requires urgent consultation (thoracic surgery).
• Palpate the cardiac region to identify signs of severe CHF (palpable S_3), and/or RV failure (RV heave, tricuspid regurgitation murmur, accentuated P_2, palpable thrill over pulmonic artery).

• Although nonspecific, auscultation for rales, bronchospasm, rhonchi, and absence of breath sounds can confirm your suspected diagnosis.
• A complete cardiac examination requires listening for mitral regurgitant murmurs (louder with acute pulmonary edema, flail mitral leaflet), other valvular heart disease, evidence of RV failure, and pericardial friction rubs.
• A quick neurologic examination begins with simply observing the patient during ordinary conversation since any significant neurologic deficit is likely to affect normal speech, movement, or attention. No other feature of the history or neurologic examination can provide as much information as quickly.

LABORATORY AND RADIOLOGY TESTING

• All patients who complain of shortness of breath or who have an increasing O_2 requirement should have a CXR and ECG.
• Brain natriuretic peptide (BNP) is useful in differentiating heart failure (HF) from other causes of dyspnea, especially in the emergency department setting.
  ○ In the Breathing Not Properly (BNP) Study of patients presenting to the emergency room, BNP levels were found to be more accurate predictors of the presence or absence of HF than any history, physical finding, or other laboratory value.
  ○ Using a BNP cutoff value of 100 pg/mL, investigators observed a sensitivity of 90% and a specificity of 73% for differentiating HF from other causes of dyspnea (see Fig. 73-2).
  ○ In this setting, if BNP is < 100 ng/mL, then HF is highly unlikely with a negative predictive value of 90%. If BNP is > 500 ng/mL, then HF is highly likely with a positive predictive value of 90%.
  ○ For BNP levels between 100 and 500 pg/mL, interpretation should account for the possibility of higher baseline BNP values because of stable underlying cardiac dysfunction, the presence of RV failure from cor pulmonale, the presence of acute PE, and/or renal failure.
  ○ It should also be noted that patients with HF might present with BNP levels that are below what might otherwise be expected, in the setting of flash pulmonary edema, mitral disease, and/or obesity.
  ○ In the inpatient setting, the positive predictive value of BNP is much lower because of comorbid illness. BNP levels rise with age and can be affected by gender and drug therapy as well as cardiovascular, pulmonary, and renal comorbidities.
  ○ In general, as chronic kidney disease worsens, clinicians should use a higher cutoff point of BNP to support the diagnosis of HF.

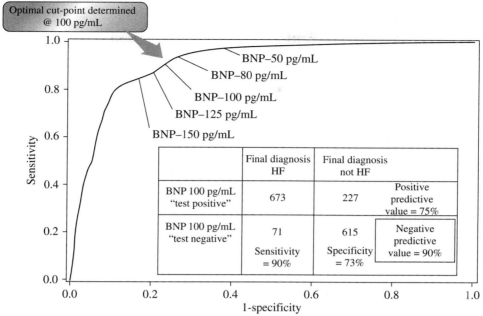

FIG. 73-2 Use of BNP differentiating CHF from other causes of dyspnea.
SOURCE: Used with permission from BNP Consensus Panel 2004.

- D-Dimer has a low positive predictive value and should not be used in the hospital setting to rule out PE. Although the negative predictive value is very high, approaching 96%, hospitalized patients have a high pretest clinical probability of acute PE when they experience new acute shortness of breath with an increasing O_2 requirement.
- Additional directed testing is based on the patient's clinical presentation, your judgment weighing the different diagnostic possibilities, and the urgency of presentation.

TRIAGE AND INITIAL MANAGEMENT: "DO NOT MISS" DIAGNOSTIC CONSIDERATIONS

ACUTE PULMONARY EMBOLISM

- History and physical examination
  - In spite of nonspecific symptoms and signs, clinicians can use this information to assign meaningful probabilities for acute pulmonary emboli.
  - When prospective investigation of pulmonary embolism diagnosis (PIOPED) clinicians assigned a high probability of PE prior to ventilation/perfusion (V/Q) scanning, 67% of patients had emboli. A high clinical probability exists when the clinical symptoms and signs were consistent with pulmonary emboli, an alternative diagnosis was not apparent, such as HF or pneumonia, and the patient had known risk factor(s) for venous thrombosis.
  - The majority of PIOPED patients (64%) had intermediate probabilities for pulmonary emboli for which additional testing is required.
  - When PIOPED clinicians assigned a low probability of pulmonary emboli, only 9% had acute pulmonary emboli. A low clinical probability exists when alternative diagnoses could explain the pulmonary symptoms and signs and the patients had no identifiable risk factors.
- Initial diagnostic studies
  - When PE is considered likely, CT pulmonary angiography (CTA) is usually the first test in the hospital setting unless there is a contraindication or unless the patient has evidence of a DVT. The most common contraindication for CTA is acute or chronic renal insufficiency (not on dialysis). CTA results that are inconsistent with clinical impressions warrant further evaluation.
  - V/Q scanning may also be used to evaluate a patient for a PE if the CXR is essentially normal. The benefit of V/Q scanning is that a normal study excludes the diagnosis of a PE. V/Q scans can be used to evaluate for PE in patients with renal insufficiency.

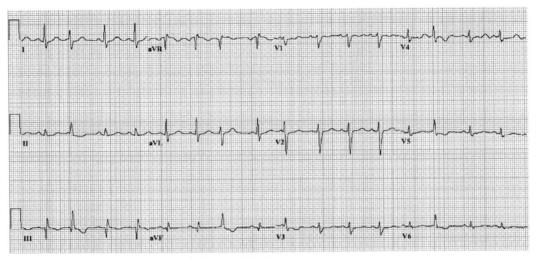

FIG. 73-3 ECG in patient with PE with new S1Q3T3.

○ Because the positive predictive value of a D-dimer assay is so low in the hospital setting, this test should be reserved for healthy patients without comorbid diseases (ie, without cancer, infection, renal failure, CHF, recent surgery).

○ The most common ECG abnormalities seen in patients with PE are nonspecific ST-segment and T-wave changes. ECG findings that have been classically associated with PE, but are infrequently seen clinically, include S1Q3T3 pattern (see Fig. 73-3), evidence of RV strain or dysfunction, and new incomplete right bundle branch block (RBBB).

• Immediate therapeutic maneuvers
  ○ Administer oxygen.
  ○ If there is a high pretest probability of acute PE and there is no contraindication to anticoagulation, start low molecular weight heparin.
  ○ In patients with significant contraindications to anticoagulation (such as active bleeding), expedite the diagnostic workup in anticipation of vena cava filter insertion.

• See Chap. 89.

ACUTE CARDIOGENIC EDEMA

• History and physical examination
  ○ Previous cardiac history, including HF, CAD, cardiac arrhythmia, and certain management features and events experienced to date in the hospital (fluid overload, persistent tachycardia) increase the likelihood of acute cardiogenic edema.
  ○ Physical examination findings the clinician should look for include elevated JVP, bilateral rales, S_3,

which is sometimes easier to palpate than to hear, and peripheral edema.
    ■ The JVP is the most specific physical examination sign for volume overload. The JVP is elevated if seen at the top of the external or internal jugular vein, 3 cm vertical distance above the sternal angle in the 90° upright position.

• Initial diagnostic studies
  ○ CXR typically demonstrates increased interstitial markings with cephalization of pulmonary vessels, Kerley B lines, perihilar infiltrates (classically in a butterfly pattern), and sometimes pleural effusions (see Fig. 73-4 for CXR and CT scan examples of cardiogenic edema). Cardiomegaly may be present in the absence of acute cardiogenic edema.
  ○ ECG should be evaluated and compared to prior ECGs, if possible looking for subtle signs of ischemia. The presence of arrhythmia should guide therapy.
  ○ Laboratory assessment may include cardiac markers and measures of thyroid function. Serum electrolytes including magnesium and liver and renal function should be checked.

• Immediate therapeutic maneuvers
  ○ Administer oxygen.
  ○ Optimize heart rate and BP control.
  ○ Administer IV diuretics for more rapid effect and better absorption because of likely presence of bowel edema. For patients who usually take diuretics, it is important to prescribe a higher dose of a loop diuretic for more immediate effect. The same dose of furosemide in mg IV = 2 times the oral dose of furosemide. IV and po torsemide are equivalent and two times an equivalent dose of furosemide.

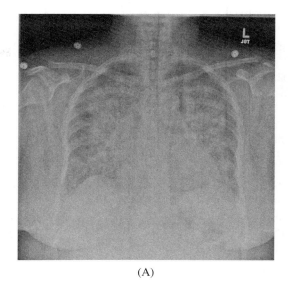

(A)

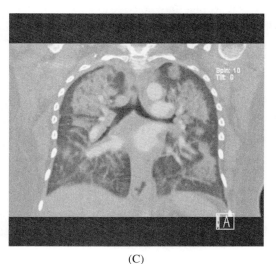

(B)   (C)

FIG. 73-4 (A) CXR of patient with pulmonary edema demonstrating increased interstitial markings, alveolar infiltration, Kerley B lines, and perihilar infiltrates in a classic butterfly pattern. (B) and (C) CT images of same patient.

○ Nitroglycerin and IV morphine also provide symptomatic relief of pulmonary edema.
• See Chaps. 29 and 30.

ASPIRATION PNEUMONIA

• History and physical examination
  ○ Silent aspiration without symptoms can have hypoxia as the only sign.

○ Risk factors for aspiration pneumonia include: advanced age, residence in nursing home, poor dentition, gastroesophageal reflux disease (GERD), and dysphagia secondary to neurologic deficits or anatomic abnormalities or from intubation trauma. Patients with nasogastric tubes, vomiting, or recently begun on oral diets are also at increased risk for aspiration pneumonia.
○ The time course can range from acute presentation to days to weeks with low-grade fevers, cough, malaise, and subsequently purulent sputum.

- Patients may deny any difficulty swallowing because they may not associate a reflex cough after aspiration with difficulty in swallowing.
- Patients who silently aspirate do not have a cough reflex and/or do not show any clinical signs of aspiration at the bedside.
- Initial diagnostic studies
  - Diagnosis is confirmed by characteristic CXR findings along with risk factors
    - Aspiration in supine position: infiltrates in the posterior segments of the upper lobes and/or apical segments of the lower lobes.
    - Aspiration in the semi upright position: infiltrates in the basal segments of the lower lobes.
- Immediate therapeutic maneuvers
  - Administer oxygen and cease po intake. This requires converting oral medications to the IV form.
  - Order aspiration precautions such as elevation of the head of the bed 45 degrees.
  - If the patient has a nasogastric tube, remove whenever possible as this may be contributory.
  - A speech and swallow evaluation may confirm via video swallow that aspiration is occurring and whether food intake is possible. Consultation may be recommended.
    - Mechanical puree diet and thickening of all liquids
    - Chin tuck maneuvers
    - Aspiration precautions (sitting upright during eating with assistance and avoiding lying flat)

PNEUMOTHORAX

- History and physical examination
  - In most cases patients complain of dyspnea and ipsilateral pain.
  - Pneumothorax can be primary, secondary, or iatrogenic.
    - Suspect if history of COPD with bullous disease, tall/thin habitus, chest trauma, infection with pneumocystis, or cystic fibrosis
    - Iatrogenic complications are associated with recent procedures (central lines) with mechanical ventilation treated with positive end-expiratory pressure (PEEP)
  - Patients are typically tachycardic and tachypneic.
  - On affected side listen for decreased chest excursion, decreased breath sounds, and hyperresonance on percussion. A Hammon's crunch might be present. Subcutaneous emphysema may be present. In cases of tension pneumothorax, tracheal deviation toward contralateral side, hypotension, neck vein distention, decreased level of consciousness, and cyanosis may be present.
- Initial diagnostic studies

  - Chest radiograph—a small pneumothorax may be easier to detect on an expiratory film looking at the apices.
- Immediate therapeutic maneuvers
  - Small pneumothroax (≤ 3 cm for primary and ≤ 2 cm for secondary): oxygen therapy and observation may be sufficient
  - Moderate pneumothorax (> 3 cm): tube thoracostomy
  - Tension pneumothorax: needle decompression can be lifesaving and may be required before a CXR can be obtained
    - This should be done in the second rib interspace in the midclavicular line. Place the catheter just above the cephalad edge of the rib because the intercostal vessels are largest on the lower edge.

ANAPHYLAXIS

- History and physical examination
  - Triggers in the hospital are most likely to include drugs, radiocontrast agents, latex, and food.
  - Patients often report pruritis, flushing, urticaria in addition to shortness of breath, and wheezing.
  - Anaphylaxis can rapidly progress to include stridor and severe respiratory distress.
  - Immediately check vital signs as anaphylactic shock occurs in up to 30% of patients.
  - Look for urticaria, angioedema on physical examination.
- Initial diagnostic studies
  - When the diagnosis is unclear, immediately after the reaction, obtain a serum tryptase and 24-hour urinary histamine.
    - Elevations of these markers are seen in anaphylactic or anaphylactoid reactions or very rarely mastocytosis.
    - There may be a role for testing patients with pre-existing reactive airway disease for whom there is a suspicion of possible anaphylaxis. These patients have a significantly higher mortality if they suffer an anaphylactic reaction.
- Immediate therapeutic maneuvers
  - Stop the offending agent.
  - Immediately administer 0.3–0.5 mg of IM epinephrine (1:1000) and fluids.
  - Immediate intubation should be considered if it appears as if angioedema will lead to airway obstruction.
  - Additional therapies include 100% oxygen, albuterol for bronchospasm, IV H1 and H2 antihistamine blockers, and corticosteroids (typically 125 mg of IV methylprednisolone or 20 mg IV of dexamethasone).
- See Chap. 24.

BIBLIOGRAPHY

BNP Consensus Panel 2004. A clinical approach for the diagnostic, prognostic, screening, treatment, monitoring and therapeutic roles of natriuretic peptides in cardiovascular diseases. *Suppl Cong Heart Fail J Clin Hypertens.* 2004;10(5).

Henkind SJ, Benis AM, Teichholz LE. The paradox of pulsus paradoxus. *Am Heart J.* 1987;114(1):198–220.

Hollerman DR, Simel DL. Does the clinical examination predict airflow limitation? *JAMA.* 1995;273(4):313–319.

Mahler DA, Harver A, Lentine T, et al. Descriptors of breathlessness in cardiorespiratory diseases. *Am J Respir Crit Care.* 1996;154:1357–1363.

Maisel AS, Krishnaswamy P, Nowak RM, et al. Rapid measurement of B-type natriuretic peptide in the emergency diagnosis of heart failure. *N Engl J Med.* 2002;347:161–167.

McGee SR. Curriculum in cardiology: physical examination of venous pressure: a critical review. *Am Heart J.* 1998;136:10–18.

Miniati M, Prediletto R, Formichi B, et al. Accuracy of clinical assessment in the diagnosis of pulmonary embolism. *Am J Respir Crit Care.* 1999;159:864.

Scano G, Stendardi L, Grazzini M. Understanding dyspnoea by its language. *Eur Respir J.* 2005;25:380–385.

Schapira RM, Schapira MM, Funahashi A, et al. The value of the forced expiratory time in the physical diagnosis of obstructive airways disease. 1993;270(6):731–736.

The PIOPED Investigators Value of the Ventilation/ Perfusion scan in acute pulmonary embolism. Results of the prospective investigation of pulmonary embolism diagnosis (PIOPED). *JAMA.* 1990;263:2753.

Tobin MJ. Respiratory monitoring in the intensive care unit. *Am Rev Respir Dis.* 1988;138(6):1625–1642.

Turino GM. Approach to the patient with respiratory disease. In: Ausiello D, Goldman L, eds. *Cecil Textbook of Medicine.* 22nd ed. Philadelphia, PA: W.B. Saunders; 2004.

74 ASTHMA
Andrew S. Karson

EPIDEMIOLOGY/OVERVIEW

- Asthma affects more than 17 million adult Americans. Asthma can begin at any age, although most patients develop the condition before age 25.

Expert Reviewer: Rebecca M. Baron, M.D., Pulmonary and Critical Care Division, Brigham and Women's Hospital

- Asthma leads to approximately 500,000 hospitalizations, 15 million office visits, and 2 million emergency room visits annually.
- Disease incidence and prevalence are increasing in industrialized countries for unknown reasons; some postulate that increased prevalence is because of fewer infectious exposures in children.
- The mean hospital LOS for patients with acute asthma exacerbations is 3.7 days with an overall inpatient mortality rate < 0.5%.
- The direct healthcare costs related to asthma are more than 6 billion dollars.

PATHOPHYSIOLOGY

- Asthma is characterized by
  1. Recurrent episodes of airway obstruction that completely resolve spontaneously or as a result of treatment
  2. Bronchial hyperactivity to stimuli that do not typically cause such responses in nonasthmatics
  3. Airway inflammation
- Both genetic and environmental factors influence the development and severity of asthma. See Tables 74-1 and 74-2.
- Asthma represents a disorder of the airways involving inflammatory cell infiltration, smooth muscle cell hypertrophy, and activation of a variety of cell types, including mast cells, T cells, eosinophils, and dendritic cells.
- Various triggers (eg, infections and environmental irritants) cause mast cell degranulation, resulting in activation of the inflammatory cascade and release of preformed mediators (eg, histamine) that promote bronchospasm.
- Airway narrowing that is primarily because of airway smooth muscle contraction, airway edema, and mucus hypersecretion cause symptoms of asthma and physiologic changes.
- Acute exacerbations of asthma are characterized by a progressive increase in shortness of breath, cough,

TABLE 74-1   Risk Factors for Developing Asthma

Genetics (multiple genes felt to be involved in pathogenesis)
Gender (prior to 14 years prevalence higher in boys than girls; after age 40 prevalence higher in females than males)
Chronic rhinitis
Airway hyperresponsiveness
Atopy
Tobacco smoke (both active smoking and second-hand smoke exposure)
Cat, house dust mite, and cockroach allergens
Obesity

TABLE 74-2 Environmental and Irritant Triggers for Asthma Symptoms and Exacerbations

House dust mite feces
Pollen
Fungi (molds and yeasts)
Furred animals
Cockroach allergen
Respiratory infections
Tobacco smoke (both active smoking and second-hand exposure)
Occupational exposures (cleaning solutions, paint, plastics, cooking fumes, among others)
Pollution
Cold air
Exercise
Perfumes

wheezing, and/or chest tightness. There is a measurable decrease in expiratory airflow (peak expiratory flow [PEF] or forced expiratory volume in 1 second [FEV_1]).

• Various environmental triggers, including infections and irritants (Table 74-2), and/or medication noncompliance can trigger exacerbations.

CLINICAL PRESENTATION, DIFFERENTIAL, MAKING THE DIAGNOSIS

• Asthma should be entertained in any patient with episodic cough, wheeze, chest tightness, and/or dyspnea.
  ◦ Asthma should be suspected when symptoms occur in the setting of recent upper respiratory illness, after exercise, or after exposure to various classic environmental and/or irritant triggers (Table 74-2), and/or if the symptoms are typically nocturnal.
  ◦ Not all asthma patients present with wheezing. Up to 15% of patients with new-onset asthma present with chronic cough and no other pulmonary symptoms. Some patients present with "fatigue" related to sleep disturbances that are likely related to nocturnal bronchospasm.
• Physical examination may be relatively normal in the nonacute setting, and evidence of airway obstruction may be subtle.
  ◦ The patient's breathing should be observed at rest, and the clinician should be looking for a prolonged expiratory phase.
  ◦ Patients with acute exacerbations typically demonstrate marked wheezing.
  ◦ Depending on the amount of active airway narrowing, chest auscultation may reveal predominantly expiratory wheezing (high-pitched sounds), and involvement of larger airways may reveal lower frequency rhonchi.

◦ In cases of severe exacerbations, wheezing may be absent because of severely decreased airflow. These patients should have physical findings of tachypnea, tachycardia, cyanosis, hyperinflated chest, use of accessory muscles, and intercostal recession, as well as difficulty speaking in full sentences.
◦ Evidence of focal wheezing, inspiratory stridor, or signs of volume overload should prompt consideration of an illness other than asthma as a cause of the presenting symptoms.
◦ Evidence of atopic dermatitis and/or allergic rhinitis may be present.

• When asthma is suspected, patients should undergo spirometry or PEF assessment to help confirm the diagnosis.
  ◦ Spirometry is the preferred method of measuring airflow limitation and reversibility to help establish a diagnosis of asthma; however spirometry may not be readily available in some settings. An FEV_1 or forced vital capacity (FVC) improvement of ≥ 12% (and ≥ 200 mL) after bronchodilator use supports a diagnosis of asthma.
  ◦ PEF can also be used to help support diagnosis of asthma. While PEF measurements are less sensitive than spirometry, they are more readily obtained and can be used for monitoring purposes.
  ◦ A 60 L/min improvement (or 20% increase in PEF) after bronchodilator use and/or variability in PEF with repeated testing supports a diagnosis of asthma.
• For patients with normal lung function and in whom a diagnostic workup for asthma has been otherwise unrevealing, measurements of airway responsiveness to a provocative challenge (eg, methacholine, exercise, etc.) can help establish or refute a diagnosis of asthma.
• Asthma is strongly associated with allergic diseases and establishing the presence of allergies, typically via history and/or skin testing, can help increase confidence in asthma diagnosis.
• Routine CXRs are usually not helpful in diagnosing asthma, but are often useful in assessing for other diagnoses and in identifying potential causes of asthma exacerbations.
• Acute exacerbations of asthma are characterized by a progressive increase in shortness of breath, cough, wheezing, and/or chest tightness. There is a measurable decrease in expiratory airflow (PEF or FEV_1).
• Attempts should be made to verify potential exposure to environmental and irritant triggers (Table 74-2) and/or medication noncompliance or misuse (eg, poor inhaler technique).
• The differential diagnosis for asthma is listed in Table 74-3.

TABLE 74-3   Differential Diagnosis of Asthma

DIAGNOSIS	SUGGESTIVE FEATURES
Asthma	Onset early in life; symptoms with daily variation, nocturnal symptoms, symptoms after exercise; history of allergy, rhinitis, eczema; family history of asthma; largely reversible airflow limitation
COPD	Onset in midlife; slowly progressive; long history of risk factors for COPD (especially cigarettes); symptoms during exercise; largely irreversible airflow limitation
CHF	Fine basilar crackles; CXR with pulmonary edema and dilated heart; usually without airflow limitation on PFTs; history suggestive of coronary disease and/or previous MI
Gastroesophageal reflux with chronic cough	Chronic cough with little dyspnea; h/o GERD, heartburn, regurgitation, dysphagia, and/or laryngitis
ACE inhibitor–induced cough	Patients on ACE inhibitors
Cystic fibrosis	Young patients; recurrent and persistent pulmonary infections; pancreatic insufficiency
Postnasal drip	
Chronic sinusitis	
Vocal cord dysfunction	
Panic attacks	
Obstructing mass or foreign body	
Hyperventilation syndrome	

Abbreviations: ACE, angiotensin-converting enzyme; MI, myocardial infarction.

TRIAGE AND INTIAL MANAGEMENT OF ACUTE EXACERBATIONS OF ASTHMA

- Assessment of severity of exacerbation and respiratory status includes evaluation of patient's history, symptoms, physical examination, oxygen saturation, CXR, ECG, and potentially ABG measurements (Table 74-4). This evaluation must be made in the context of patient's underlying asthma history and other comorbidities.
- Mild-to-moderate exacerbations (Table 74-4) can often be treated in the community setting.

However, a low threshold should be kept for hospitalization, especially in a patient who has a prior history of requiring intubation for an asthma exacerbation.
- Oxygen therapy should be provided if necessary to achieve goal $SaO_2 \geq 90\%$.
- Often repeated doses of rapid-acting inhaled beta-2-agonist (two to four puffs every 20 minutes for first hour and then decreasing frequency as clinical situation allows) are sufficient to control symptoms. Metered dose inhalers used properly are as effective as nebulized preparations.

TABLE 74-4   Severity of Asthma Exacerbation

SIGN/SYMPTOM	MILD	MODERATE	SEVERE	RESPIRATORY ARREST IMMINENT
Breathlessness	Walking	Talking	At rest	At rest
Position	Can lie down	Prefers sitting	Hunches forward	Hunched forward
Use of accessory muscles/retractions	Not present	Usually	Usually	Paradoxical thoracoabdominal movement
Talks in...	Full sentences	Phrases	Words	Words, or cannot speak
Mental status	Alert, may be agitated	Alert, usually agitated	Alert, usually agitated	Drowsy and/or confused
Respiratory rate	Increased	Increased	Very high > 30	Very high > 30
Pulse	< 100	100–120	> 120	Can be bradycardic or tachycardic
SaO_2% (on air)	> 95%	91%–95%	< 90%	< 90%
PEF after bronchodilator (% predicted or % person best)	> 80%	60%–80%	< 60% and/or < 100 L/min and/or response lasts < 2 hours	Patient unable to perform PEF
Pulsus paradoxus	Absent (< 10 mm Hg)	May be present (10–20 mm Hg)	Often present (> 25 mm Hg)	Often present (> 25 mm Hg); absence suggests respiratory muscle fatigue
Lung auscultation (wheeze)	Moderate, end-expiratory	Loud	Loud	Can have absence of wheeze
PaO_2 (on air)	ABG not necessary	> 60 mm Hg	< 60 mm Hg	< 40 mm Hg
$PaCO_2$	ABG not necessary	< 45 mm Hg	> 45 mm Hg	> 60 mm Hg

SOURCE: Adapted from Global Initiative for Asthma.

TABLE 74-5 Estimated Equipotent Daily Doses of Inhaled Glucocorticosteroids for Adults*

DRUG	LOW DAILY DOSE (mg)	MEDIUM DAILY DOSE (mg)	HIGH DAILY DOSE (mg)†
Beclomethasone dipropionate	200–500	> 500–1000	> 1000–2000
Budesonide‡	200–400	> 400–800	> 800–1600
Ciclesonide‡	80–160	> 160–320	> 320–1280
Flunisolide	500–1000	> 1000–2000	> 2000
Fluticasone	100–250	> 250–500	> 500–1000
Mometasone furoate‡	200–400	> 400–800	> 800–1200
Triamcinolone acetonide	400–1000	> 1000–2000	> 2000

*Comparisons based upon efficacy data.
†Patients considered for high daily doses except for short periods should be referred to a specialist for assessment to consider alternative combinations of controllers. Maximum recommended doses are arbitrary but with prolonged use are associated with increased risk of systemic side effects.
‡Approved for once-daily dosing in mild patients.

- Additional treatment may not be necessary if symptoms improve and patient's PEF returns to > 80% of predicted (or > 80% of personal best).
- If a rapid-acting inhaled beta-2-agonist treatment does not lead to sustained improvement over the first few hours, then initiate a course of oral glucocorticosteroids and consider treatment of potential underlying causes of an exacerbation (eg, infection).
- Triage severe exacerbations, and mild/moderate exacerbations that do not improve rapidly, to acute care facilities (Table 74-4).
- Provide oxygen therapy, if necessary, to achieve goal SaO$_2$ ≥ 90%.
- Treat aggressively with rapid-acting inhaled beta-2-agonists; this is often most easily accomplished with nebulized preparations every 20 minutes for first hour. Some protocols suggest frequent metered dose inhaler with spacer treatment (four puffs every 10 minutes). Critically ill patients may require "continuous" treatment.
- Addition of inhaled or nebulized anticholinergics (such as ipratropium bromide) to inhaled/nebulized beta-2-agonist is more effective than the use of either drug alone.
- Systemic glucocorticosteroids are recommended for patients with severe symptoms and for patients with moderate symptoms who have been slow to respond to augmented beta-2-agonist treatment (especially if patient has recently been treated with steroids and/or if the patient has been intubated or treated in an ICU in the past).
  - Oral glucocorticosteriods are usually as effective as intravenous preparations for patients with a functioning gastrointestinal (GI) tract. Typical starting doses include oral prednisone 60 mg or intravenous methylprednisolone 125 mg.
  - In patients with moderate exacerbations, especially those not receiving systemic glucocorticosteriods, the addition of inhaled glucocorticosteriods might be beneficial. (See Table 74-5.)

- There are little data to support the use of theophylline or oral beta-2-agonists in the setting of acute exacerbations of asthma.
- Epinephrine is not routinely indicated in acute asthma exacerbation, but may be used to treat anaphylaxis and/or angioedema.
- There are no data to support the use of leukotriene modifiers or inhaled helium-oxygen mixtures in the acute setting, and the use of sedatives should be avoided.
- Infectious triggers for asthma exacerbations are typically viral. However, clinicians should consider antibiotic treatment in select patients with signs and/or symptoms of bacterial infection (eg, fever, elevated/ left-shifted white blood count, purulent sputum, infiltrate on imaging).
- Institute mechanical ventilation for patients with ARF (PaO$_2$ < 60 mm Hg, or PaCO$_2$ > 60 mm Hg, or severe acidosis [pH < 7.25]). Patients with signs of hypercapnia or a rising PaCO$_2$, even in the setting of a preserved pH, should be vigilantly monitored for respiratory fatigue. The role of noninvasive mechanical ventilation (NIV) in patients with asthma exacerbations is controversial.
- Triage considerations: general medical unit, see Table 74-6, and ICU, see Table 74-7.

TABLE 74-6 Considerations for Admission to Hospital

Presenting with FEV$_1$ or PEF < 25% of predicted (or personal best)
Posttreatment FEV$_1$ or PEF < 40% of predicted (or personal best)
Posttreatment FEV$_1$ or PEF between 40% and 60% of predicted (or personal best) without good outpatient follow-up
Failure of exacerbation to respond to initial (1–2 hours) management
History of near-fatal asthma requiring incubation
Severe asthma at baseline
Severe comorbidities
Frequent exacerbations, emergency visit, or admission for asthma in past year
Current or recent use of oral glucocorticosteroids
Diagnostic uncertainty
Advanced age
Insufficient home support

TABLE 74-7   Indications for Admission/Transfer to ICU

Changes in mental status
Need for invasive mechanical ventilation
PEF < 30% despite aggressive initial treatment
Persistent or worsening hypoxemia (PaO_2 < 40 mm Hg)
Persistent or worsening hypercapnea ($PaCO_2$ > 60 mm Hg)
Persistent or worsening acidosis pH < 7.25
Hemodynamic instability
Inadequate response to initial emergent management
Inability to provide needed care on general medical floor

DISEASE MANAGEMNT STRATEGIES

ACUTE EXACERBATIONS OF ASTHMA

- As patient respiratory status improves and stabilizes, consideration should be given to decreasing rapid-acting bronchodilators to "as needed" use and to initiating inhaled steroids so that they are "on board" when systemic steroids are completed or tapered.
- Systemic glucocorticosteriods should be continued for 7–10 days (which is as effective as longer courses [and does not typically require a taper]).
- Order venous thromboembolism prophylaxis.
- Symptoms that led up to exacerbation should be reviewed to determine most appropriate outpatient regimen (see disease management strategies for cronic asthma below).
- Disease management strategies listed for chronic asthma should be reviewed and applied as appropriate in the acute exacerbation setting. (For example, smoking cessation counseling and therapy should be recommended for all smokers.)
- Consider specialty consultation for patients with persistent symptoms despite appropriate therapy, for patients who are mechanically ventilated, and for patients in whom there is diagnostic uncertainty.
- There are perioperative considerations for patients with known asthma. (See Chap. 102.)

CHRONIC ASTHMA

- The overall goal of management is to control the airway inflammation and to reverse bronchospasm in order to prevent symptoms.
- Historically, authors classified asthma by severity based on symptoms, airflow limitation, and lung function (as in Table 74-8). Although it is still reasonable

TABLE 74-8   Classification of Asthma Severity by Clinical Features before Treatment

INTERMITTENT

Symptoms less than once a week
Brief exacerbations
Nocturnal symptoms not more than twice a month
- FEV_1 or PEF ≥ 80% predicted
- PEF or FEV_1 variability < 20%

MILD PERSISTENT

Symptoms more than once a week but less than once a day
Exacerbations may affect activity and sleep
Nocturnal symptoms more than twice a month
- FEV_1 or PEF ≥ 80% predicted
- PEF or FEV_1 variability < 20%–30%

MODERATE PERSISTENT

Symptoms daily
Exacerbations may affect activity and sleep
Nocturnal symptoms more than once a week
Daily use of inhaled short-acting beta-2-agonist
- FEV_1 or PEF 60%–80% predicted
- PEF or FEV_1 variability > 30%

SEVERE PERSISTENT

Symptoms daily
Frequent exacerbations
Frequent nocturnal asthma symptoms
Limitation of physical activities
- FEV_1 or PEF ≤ 60% predicted
- PEF or FEV_1 variability > 30%

SOURCE: Global Initiative for Asthma (GINA), National Heart, Lung, and Blood Institute. Pocket guide for asthma management and prevention, revised 2006. Bethesda, MD: Medical Communications Resources, Inc.; 2006.

to base initial treatment decisions on this classification, current recommendations suggest management should be based on a classification system that is based on clinical "level of control" (as in Table 74-9).
- The Global Initiative for Asthma has developed a medication management strategy based on control (Fig. 74-1).
  ○ If patient is "uncontrolled" on his or her current regimen, treatment should be "stepped-up" until controlled; if patient is "partially controlled" then consideration should be given to "step-up."
  ○ If patient maintains control on specific regimen for 3 months then patient should be "stepped-down," with the goal of minimizing side effects of unnecessary medications, using only those needed to maintain control of symptoms.
  ○ In cases where patients are treatment naïve, patients with persistent symptoms should start on step 2 and those with "uncontrolled"-type symptoms should be started on step 3.
- Medications to treat asthma can be classified as "**controllers**" and "**relievers**."

TABLE 74-9 Levels of Control for Asthma

CHARACTERISTIC	CONTROLLED (All of the following)	PARTLY CONTROLLED (Any measure present in any week)	UNCONTROLLED
Daytime symptoms	None (twice or less/week)	More than twice/week	Three or more features of partly controlled asthma present in any week
Limitations of activities	None	Any	
Nocturnal symptoms/awakening	None	Any	
Need for reliever/rescue treatment	None (twice or less/week)	More than twice/week	
Lung function (PEF or FEV$_1$)	Normal	< 80% predicted or personal best (if known)	
Exacerbations	None	One or more/year*	One in any week†

*Any exacerbation should prompt review of maintenance regimen to ensure adequacy.
†By definition, an exacerbation in any week makes that an uncontrolled asthma week.
SOURCE: Adapted From Global Initiative for Asthma.

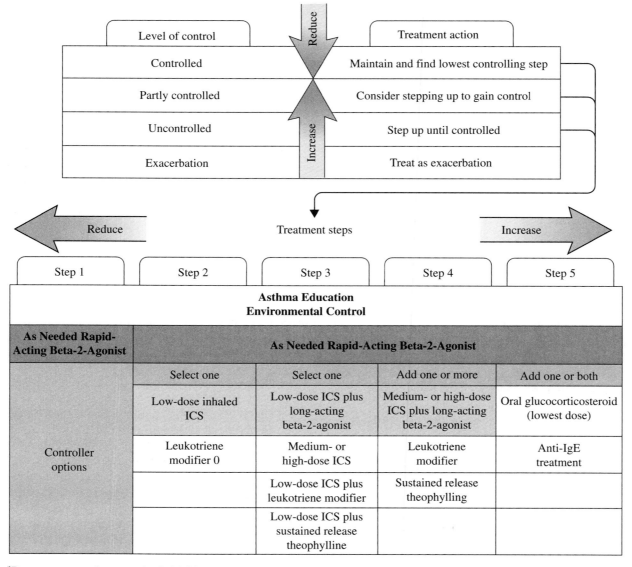

Management Approach Based on Control
For children older than 5 years, adolescents, and adults

Level of control	Treatment action
Controlled	Maintain and find lowest controlling step
Partly controlled	Consider stepping up to gain control
Uncontrolled	Step up until controlled
Exacerbation	Treat as exacerbation

Reduce ← Treatment steps → Increase

	Step 1	Step 2	Step 3	Step 4	Step 5
Asthma Education Environmental Control					
As Needed Rapid-Acting Beta-2-Agonist	As Needed Rapid-Acting Beta-2-Agonist				
Controller options		Select one	Select one	Add one or more	Add one or both
	As Needed Rapid-Acting Beta-2-Agonist	Low-dose inhaled ICS	Low-dose ICS plus long-acting beta-2-agonist	Medium- or high-dose ICS plus long-acting beta-2-agonist	Oral glucocorticosteroid (lowest dose)
		Leukotriene modifier 0	Medium- or high-dose ICS	Leukotriene modifier	Anti-IgE treatment
			Low-dose ICS plus leukotriene modifier	Sustained release theophylling	
			Low-dose ICS plus sustained release theophylline		

*Receptor antagonist or synthesis inhibitor.
Abbreviation: ICS, inhaled corticosteroid.

FIG. 74-1 Management approach based on control.
SOURCE: From Global Initiative for Asthma.

○ *Controllers* are taken on a daily and long-term basis to keep asthma controlled; they act primarily via anti-inflammatory mechanisms.

- Inhaled glucocorticosteroids (ICS) are the most effective and best-studied controller medications available. Most of the benefit of inhaled glucocorticoids occurs at low doses (eg, 400 μg of budesonide daily), but some patients require higher doses for control, especially smokers.
- A leukotriene modifier including cysteinyl-leukotriene 1 receptor antagonists (montelukast, pranlukast, and zafirlukast) or 5-lipozygnase inhibitor (zileuton) can be considered as an alternative monotherapy control agent for patients who have mild persistent asthma and who cannot tolerate ICS.
- Long-acting inhaled beta-2-agonists are the "add-on" drugs of choice if ICS treatment alone does not control symptoms. (Of note, leukotriene modifiers can also be used as add-on therapy to ICS treatment, but are less effective.)
- Long-acting inhaled beta-2-agonists are not known to possess anti-inflammatory properties and therefore should *not* be used as monotherapy in asthma. Of note there is concern for increased mortality in subgroups of asthmatic patients treated with long-acting beta-2-agonists as monotherapy.
- The effective combination of ICS and long-acting inhaled beta-2-agonists (eg, Serevent) has led to the development of combination agents. Combinations including ICS and another long-acting inhaled beta-2-agonist, formoterol, can be used both for control and for relief (given formoterol's relatively rapid onset).
- Theophylline can be added on to ICS treatment if necessary, but has fallen out of favor in preference for long-acting inhaled beta-2-agonists or leukotriene modifiers because of theophylline's toxicity profile and need for monitoring of drug levels.
- The current role of anti-IgE treatment with omalizumab is unclear. It only should be considered in patients with high levels of IgE who have failed standard asthma treatment and after subspecialty referral.
- Long-term use of oral glucocorticoids is discouraged because of side-effect profile, but may be required for severely uncontrolled asthma.
- Cromones do not have an important role in management in adult asthma. However, they could be considered in patients with mild persistent asthma with exercise-induced bronchospasm.

○ *Relievers* are taken as needed to relieve symptoms quickly as they occur; they act primarily via anti bronchospastic mechanisms.

TABLE 74-10 Considerations for Discharge to Home

Condition/regimen stable for at least 12 hours
Patient and/or home care giver able to carry out care plan at home
Inhaled beta-agonist treatment is not more frequent then every 4 hours
Not hypoxic on room air or stable oxygen regimen
Patients who were previously able to ambulate are able to do so

- Rapid-acting inhaled beta-2-agonists are the reliever treatment of choice for patients with acute asthma symptoms (or for the pretreatment of exercise-induced symptoms).
- Inhaled anticholinergics are second-line reliever treatments and are used for the rare patient who cannot tolerate inhaled beta-2-agonists.

- Consultation with an asthma specialist should be considered for all patients with chronic asthma who remain uncontrolled despite step 3 level treatment.
- Many authors stress the importance of the patient-physician partnership in controlling symptoms.
- All patients should have an "asthma action plan" that details how patients and providers should respond to symptoms, including what to do at home, when to call for assistance, and when to seek urgent/emergent medical attention.
- Patients should reduce exposures to known environmental and irritant triggers for their asthma. (See Table 74-2.)
- All smokers should undergo smoking cessation counseling, and pharmacotherapy for smoking cessation should be considered.
- All patients should be trained and evaluated for appropriate medication administration technique.
- Pneumococcal and influenza vaccines should be given.
- Importance of medication compliance should be stressed.

CARE TRANSITIONS

- The optimal duration for patients admitted with asthma exacerbation has not been established. Common discharge criteria are listed in Table 74-10.
- All patients should undergo a follow-up outpatient visit 2–6 weeks after discharge.

BIBLIOGRAPHY

Drazen JM. Asthma. In: Ausiello D, Goldman L, eds. *Cecil Textbook of Medicine*. 22nd ed. Philadelphia, PA: W.B. Saunders; 2004.

GINA Report. Evidence-based guidelines for asthma management and prevention. *Global Strategy for Asthma Management and Prevention.* Global Initiative for Asthma Report. Revised 2006.

Global Initiative for Asthma. www.ginasthma.com

Kallstrom TJ. Evidence-based asthma management. *Respir Care.* Jul 2004;49(7):783–792.

National Asthma Education and Prevention Program. Clinical Practice Guidelines. *Guidelines for the Diagnosis and Management of Asthma.* Expert Panel Report 2. Revised 2002.

75 CHRONIC OBSTRUCTIVE PULMONARY DISEASE

Andrew S. Karson

EPIDEMIOLOGY/OVERVIEW

- COPD affects more than 10 million Americans, is the fourth most common cause of death in the United States (225,000 deaths each year), and mortality from COPD is increasing. The mortality rate for women has doubled in the past 20 years.
- COPD leads to more than 700,000 hospitalizations, 8 million office visits, and 1.5 million emergency room visits annually.
- Disease prevalence correlates with smoking patterns. It is unusual for patients to develop clinically apparent COPD with less than a 20 pack-year smoking history.
- The mean hospital LOS for patients with COPD exacerbations is 4.9 days with an overall inpatient mortality rate of 2% to 4%; mortality is more than 25% in patients requiring mechanical ventilation or ICU admission.
- The direct healthcare costs related to COPD are more than 18 billion dollars.

PATHOPHYSIOLOGY

- COPD is a preventable and treatable disease that is characterized by airflow limitation that is usually progressive and not fully reversible.
- FEV_1 normally declines by about 30 mL/year after age 30 in nonsmokers.

Expert Reviewer: Rebecca M. Baron, M.D., Pulmonary and Critical Care Division, Brigham and Women's Hospital

TABLE 75-1   Risk Factors for Development of COPD

Tobacco smoke
Occupational exposures (dusts, chemicals)
Pollution
Socioeconomic status
Airway hyperresponsiveness
Perinatal and childhood conditions affecting lung growth
Severe childhood respiratory infection
Genetic factors (alpha-1-antitrypsin deficiency)

- Smoking is the most important risk factor for developing COPD (see Table 75-1).
  - In smokers the rate of FEV_1 decline typically is doubled; in approximately 20% of smokers, the decline is even more rapid, approximating 100 mL/year.
  - Smoking cessation reduces rate of FEV_1 loss to that of nonsmokers and lowers mortality rate by 27%. However, loss of FEV_1 is usually not fully reversible.
  - Smoking leads to airway inflammation and neutrophil release of elastase, which contributes to destruction of lung tissue.
- Patients with COPD have varying degrees of three pathologic processes: small airways obstruction, emphysema, and chronic bronchitis.
  - Small airways obstruction refers to an increased resistance to airflow in the distal airways. In smokers, there is typically increased bronchiolar smooth muscle, inflammation, and fibrosis that narrow the airway lumens and thicken their walls. The exact mechanisms involved in these changes are not fully understood.
  - Chronic bronchitis is defined as the presence of chronic cough and sputum production on most days for at least 3 months of the year for at least 2 consecutive years in the absence of any other disease.
    - At least one-third of smokers aged 35–59 have chronic bronchitis, and the prevalence increases with age.
    - Hypertrophy and hyperplasia of the mucus-secreting glands normally found in large airway epithelium lead to narrowing of the smaller airways with accompanying low-grade inflammation. As a result, the airway walls develop squamous metaplasia, ciliary loss and dysfunction, and increased smooth muscle and connective tissue.
    - An increased tendency to develop recurrent episodes of *acute* bronchitis may also contribute to progression of airways obstruction.
  - Emphysema is defined as the enlargement of air spaces distal to the conducting airways. Two important histologic subtypes have been identified

- Centrilobular emphysema is seen almost exclusively in smokers. This form, typically in the upper lobes, primarily involves destruction of respiratory bronchioles, often with normal distal alveoli.
- Panacinar emphysema, occurring anywhere in the lung, but most often in the lower lobes, involves injury and destruction of both respiratory bronchioles and distal alveoli. Some patients develop panacinar emphysema associated with alpha-1-antitrypsin (A1AT) deficiency. Smokers with A1AT deficiency are at high risk of developing panacinar emphysema at a young age.

- In advanced COPD, arterial hypoxemia develops, placing these patients at increased likelihood of developing pulmonary hypertension and cor pulmonale.

CLINICAL PRESENTATION, DIFFERENTIAL, MAKING THE DIAGNOSIS

STABLE CHRONIC OBSTRUCTIVE PULMONARY DISEASE

- COPD should be entertained in any patient with dyspnea, chronic cough, chronic sputum production, and a history of exposure to risk factors (especially cigarette smoke).
- COPD is usually first detected at the time when patients develop dyspnea; this often occurs when the FEV_1 is < 2 L (50% of normal value for most patients). Dyspnea typically becomes severe for most patients at an FEV_1 of about 1 L. See Table 75-2 for disease severity classification.

- Chronic bronchitis and episodes of acute bronchitis often precede the development of dyspnea by years.
- Physical examination abnormalities in the nonacute setting are usually only evident in patients with severe disease. Signs may include
  - An increased respiratory rate and evidence of hyperinflation (including barrel chest appearance)
  - Increased anterior-posterior (AP) diameter
  - Low-lying diaphragms
  - Faint heart sounds
  - Decreased breath sounds often associated with both inspiratory crackles (especially in chronic bronchitis) and expiratory wheezes
  - Secondary pulmonary hypertension and right HF (cor pulmonale) evidenced by an increased second heart sound, jugular venous distention, hepatic congestion, and peripheral edema
- Spirometry confirms the diagnosis of COPD. COPD patients characteristically have FEV_1/FVC < 0.7 and an FEV_1 < "80% predicted." These levels usually are not reversible to normal levels with bronchodilators (in contrast to asthma). It is often not helpful to attempt spirometry studies in the setting of an acute exacerbation of disease.
- Routine x-rays may not be helpful in diagnosing COPD, but are often useful in ruling out other diagnoses and in the evaluation for causes of COPD exacerbations.
  - Hyperinflation, flattened diaphragms, increased AP retrosternal space, and a > 90 degree angle of the sternum and diaphragm are classic COPD CXR findings.

TABLE 75-2 Disease Severity for Stable Disease: Spirometric Classification of COPD Severity*

STAGE	SPIROMETRIC CLASSIFICATION	SIGNS AND SYMPTOMS
Stage I: mild	FEV_1/FVC < 0.70 and $FEV_1 \geq 80\%$ predicted	Possibly chronic cough and chronic sputum production; patient often unaware of pulmonary disease
Stage II: moderate	FEV_1/FVC < 0.70 and $50\% \leq FEV_1 < 80\%$ predicted	Dyspnea on exertion, possibly chronic cough and sputum production
Stage III: severe	FEV_1/FVC < 0.70 and $30\% \leq FEV_1 < 50\%$ predicted	Dyspnea on exertion, reduced exercise capacity, fatigue, and recurrent exacerbations
Stage IV: very severe	FEV_1/FVC < 0.70 and $FEV_1 < 30\%$ predicted or $FEV_1 < 50\%$ predicted plus chronic respiratory failure	Dyspnea impairs quality of life; potentially cor pulmonale

*Respiratory failure: arterial partial pressure of oxygen (PaO_2) < 8.0 kPa (60 mm Hg) with or without arterial partial pressure of CO_2 ($PaCO_2$) > 6.7 kPa (50 mm Hg) while breathing air at sea level.
SOURCE: Adapted from GOLD (Global Initiative for Chronic Obstructive Lung Disease).

SECTION 7 • HOSPITALIST CLINICAL CORE COMPETENCIES

TABLE 75-3   Differential Diagnosis of Stable COPD

DIAGNOSIS	SUGGESTIVE FEATURES
COPD	Onset in mid life; slowly progressive; long history of risk factors for COPD (especially cigarettes); dyspnea during exercise; largely irreversible airflow limitation
Asthma	Onset early in life; symptoms with daily variation, most prominent at night and early morning; history of allergy, rhinitis, eczema; family history of asthma; largely reversible airflow limitation
CHF	Fine basilar crackles; CXR with pulmonary edema and dilated heart; without airflow limitation on PFTs; history suggestive of coronary disease and/or previous MI
Bronchiectasis	Large volumes of purulent sputum; coarse crackles; clubbing; chest imaging shows bronchial dilation and wall thickening
TB	CXR with infiltrate; at risk for previous exposure to TB; microbacterial confirmation
Obliterative bronchiolitis	Onset at younger age; nonsmoker; CT on expiration shows hypodense areas; possible history of rheumatoid arthritis or fume exposure
Diffuse panbronchiolitis	Male; nonsmoker; history of chronic sinusitis; chest imaging with diffuse small centrilobular nodular opacities and hyperinflation

Abbreviation: TB, tuberculosis.
SOURCE: Adapted from GOLD (Global Initiative for Chronic Obstructive Lung Disease).

- CTs are not routinely recommended to make COPD diagnosis. However, they may be indicated for considering advanced treatment options for COPD (eg, lung volume reduction surgery or lung transplantation).
- For the differential diagnosis for stable COPD refer to Table 75-3a.

ACUTE EXACERBATIONS OF CHRONIC OBSTRUCTIVE PULMONARY DISEASE

- COPD exacerbations are characterized by a change in patient's baseline dyspnea, cough, and sputum production, and often include wheezing and change in color of sputum (from white to yellow or green and occasionally with some blood streaking) and volume.
- COPD exacerbations most often occur in the setting of upper respiratory infections or exposure to air pollution, but no clear cause can be found in up to one-third

of cases. Exacerbations are more common in patients who have severe obstruction and/or chronic bronchitis.
- For the differential diagnosis of acute exacerbations of COPD refer to Table 75-4.

TRIAGE AND INITIAL MANAGEMENT OF ACUTE EXACERBATIONS OF CHRONIC OBSTRUCTIVE PULMONARY DISEASE

- Assessment of severity of exacerbation and respiratory status includes evaluation of patient's history, symptoms, physical examination, oxygen saturation, CXR, ECG, and ABG measurements. This evaluation must be made in the context of patient's underlying COPD history and comorbidities.
- See Tables 75-5 and 75-6 for criteria for hospitalization and ICU admission.
- Provide oxygen therapy with goal $SaO_2 \geq 90\%$. Although controversial, some authors warn that CO_2 retention can occur if SaO_2 is raised too high in certain patient populations. Regardless, maintenance of

TABLE 75-4   Differential Diagnosis of Acute Exacerbation of COPD

DIAGNOSIS	SUGGESTIVE FEATURES
COPD exacerbation	Prior history of stable COPD; prior history of COPD exacerbation; smoking history
Asthma exacerbation	Prior history of asthma; prior history of asthma exacerbation; history of allergy, rhinitis, eczema; family history of asthma
CHF exacerbation	Fine basilar crackles; CXR with pulmonary edema and dilated heart; history of HF or suggestive of coronary disease and/or previous MI
Pneumonia	Focal findings on chest auscultation, infiltrate on CXR; high white count with left shift; fever; recent aspiration, history of swallowing disorder
PE	History of thromboembolic disease; tachycardia, hypotension, persistent hypoxia despite high-flow oxygen
Pleural effusion	Focal findings of fluid in pleural space on chest auscultation and imaging
Pneumothorax	Focal findings on chest auscultation; evidence of air in pleural space on CXR; history suggestive of respiratory strain
Cardiac arrhythmia	History of arrhythmia or CAD; palpitations; tachycardia; ECG abnormalities

TABLE 75-5   Indications for Admission to Hospital

Marked increase in severity of symptoms
Failure of exacerbation to respond to initial management
Severe COPD at baseline (or history of previous need for mechanical ventilation)
Severe comorbidities
Frequent exacerbations
Onset of new physical signs (ie, right heat failure)
Diagnostic uncertainty
Advanced age
Insufficient home support

adequate oxygenation is critical, and additional ventilatory support may be necessary for patients with severe hypoxemia or hypercapnea.

- Short-acting inhaled beta-2-agonists are the drugs of choice in acute exacerbations.
- If prompt and robust response does not occur, then add short-acting anticholinergics.
- Nebulized formulations are often preferred in the acute setting.
- Use of methylxanthines is controversial and should be reserved for situations where there has been insufficient response to beta-2-agonists and anticholinergics.
- There are no data to support the use of long-acting beta-2-agonists or long-acting anticholinergics in the acute exacerbation setting.
- Treat with oral or intravenous corticosteriods. Onset of action may be slightly faster for intravenous formulations.
- Antibiotics are generally advised in patients with COPD exacerbations, especially in patients with signs and/or symptoms of infection (eg, fever, elevated/left-shifted white blood count, increased sputum volume, increased sputum purulence, infiltrate on imaging) or in patients requiring mechanical ventilation.
  - Coverage should focus on *Haemophilus influenzae, Streptococcus pneumoniae,* and *Moraxella catarrhalis,* which are the most common bacterial pathogens recovered from the lower airways of COPD patients.
  - Atypical pathogen coverage (*Mycoplasma pneumoniae* and *Chlamydia pneumoniae*) should also be strongly considered.
  - Commonly prescribed antibiotics include doxycycline, levofloxacin, ceftin, and trimethoprim-sulfa

TABLE 75-6   Indications for Admission/Transfer to ICU

Changes in mental status
Need for invasive mechanical ventilation
Persistent or worsening hypoxemia
Persistent or worsening hypercapnea ($PaO_2 > 60$ mm Hg)
Persistent or worsening acidosis pH < 7.25
Hemodynamic instability
Inadequate response to initial emergent management
Inability to provide needed care on general medical floor

with little evidence to support one antibiotic over another.

- Consider NIV for patients who have one or more of the following:
  - Moderate-to-severe dyspnea (with use of accessory muscles and paradoxical abdominal motion)
  - pH ≤ 7.35 and/or $PaCO_2 > 45$ mm Hg
  - Persistently high respiratory rate (> 25 breaths per minute)
  However, avoid using NIPPV in patients with cardiovascular instability, patients at risk for aspiration, and patients with recent facial injury.
- Consider invasive mechanical ventilation for patients who have one or more of the following:
  - NIPPV treatment failure or inability to tolerate NIPPV because of cardiovascular instability, increased risk of aspiration, recent facial injury, or other contraindications to NIPPV
  - Severe dyspnea (with use of accessory muscles and paradoxical abdominal motion)
  - Impending respiratory failure with $PaO_2 < 60$ mm Hg, or $PaCO_2 > 60$, or severe acidosis (pH < 7.25)

DISEASE MANAGEMENT STRATEGIES

ACUTE EXACERBATIONS OF CHRONIC OBSTRUCTIVE PULMONARY DISEASE

- As patient respiratory status improves and stabilizes, consideration should be given to switching from short-acting bronchodilators to longer-acting agents (see disease management strategies for stable COPD below).
- Antibiotic duration should be 7–10 days.
- A 2-week taper of systemic corticosteroid is as effective as an 8-week taper.
- Implement venous thromboembolism prophylaxis. There is an increased incidence of PE in patients presenting with COPD.
- Disease management strategies for patients with stable COPD should be reviewed and applied as appropriate in the acute setting. For example, smoking cessation counseling should be routine and cessation therapy should be offered to all smokers.
- Consider pulmonary consultation for patients with persistent symptoms despite appropriate therapy, for patients who are mechanically ventilated, and for patients in whom there is diagnostic uncertainty.

STABLE CHRONIC OBSTRUCTIVE PULMONARY DISEASE

- Patients should undergo risk factor reduction, and pharmacotherapy aids for smoking cessation should

TABLE 75-7   Pharmacotherapy for Smoking Cessation

Nicotine replacement (nicotine gum, inhaler, nasal spray, transdermal
  patch, sublingual tablet, lozenge)
Bupropion
Nortriptyline
Varenicline

be considered (especially in adults who smoke
heavily) (Table 75-7).
- No medications are known to alter the long-term progression of COPD, but medications can alleviate
symptoms and complications.
- For patients with symptomatic stage 1 (mild) COPD,
bronchodilators can be used singly or in combination.
The choice between beta-2-agonists, anticholinergics,
theophylline, or combination therapy depends on the
individual responses that a patient has in terms of
symptom relief and side affects. In general, beta-2-
agonists and anticholinergics are preferred to methylxanthines based on side-effect profiles. (See Fig. 75-1.)
- Regular treatment with long-acting agents is more
effective than treatment with short-acting agents; for
patients with symptomatic stage 2 (moderate) COPD,
the addition of one or more long-acting bronchodilators should be considered.
- Combination treatments that include bronchodilators
with different mechanisms and durations of action
may increase the amount of bronchodilation with
fewer side effects. The combination of a short-acting
beta-2-agonist and an anticholinergic improves FEV_1
more than either drug alone.
- The addition of ICS to bronchodilator regimen may be
effective for symptomatic COPD patients with FEV_1
< 50% (stage III and IV COPD) and repeated
exacerbations.
- ABGs should be considered in patients with stage III
or IV COPD, and long-term administration of oxygen
is indicated for patients with chronic lung disease and
hypoxemia ($PaO_2 \leq 55$ mm Hg or $SaO_2 \leq 88\%$; *or*
$PaO_2 \leq 59$ mm Hg or $SaO_2 \leq 89\%$ in patients with cor
pulmonale, right HF, or erythrocytosis (haematocrit
[HCT] > 55%).
- All patients using inhaled formulation should be trained
and evaluated for appropriate administration technique.

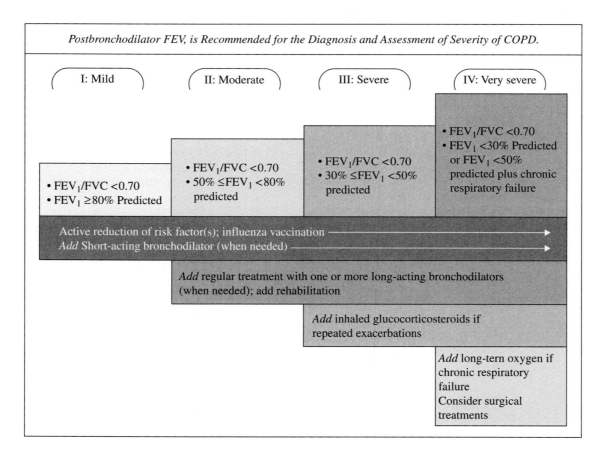

FIG. 75-1   Therapy at each stage of COPD.

TABLE 75-8 Indications for Discharge to Home

Condition/regimen stable for at least 12 hours
Patient and/or home care giver able to carry out care plan at home
Inhaled beta-2-agonist treatment is not more frequent then every 4 hours
Not hypoxic on room air, or on stable oxygen supplementation regimen
Patients who were previously able to ambulate are able to do so

- Influenza vaccines should be offered to all COPD patients and pneumococcal vaccine should be given to all patients more than 65 (and to younger patients with $FEV_1 < 40\%$).
- Exercise training programs (eg, "pulmonary rehabilitation") should be offered to all patients.
- Importance of medication compliance should be stressed.
- Chronic use of systemic glucocorticoids is discouraged.
- End-of-life and advance directive discussions should occur.
- Subspecialty referral for surgical treatments such as bullectomy, lung volume reduction surgery, and lung transplantation can be considered in select patients.
- There are perioperative considerations for patients with known COPD. (See Chap. 102.)

CARE TRANSITIONS

- The optimal duration for patients admitted with COPD exacerbation has not been established. Common discharge criteria are listed in Table 75-8.
- Home visits by a visiting nurse may permit earlier discharge for patients with COPD exacerbations without increasing readmission rates.
- All patients should undergo a follow-up outpatient visit 4–6 weeks after discharge.
- Exercise training programs (eg, "pulmonary rehabilitation") should be recommended to all patients.

BIBLIOGRAPHY

Anthonisen N. Chronic obstructive pulmonary disease. In: Ausiello D, Goldman L, eds. *Cecil Textbook of Medicine.* 22nd ed. Philadelphia, PA: W.B. Saunders; 2004.
Celli BR, MacNee W. Standards for the diagnosis and treatment of patients with COPD. A summary of the ATS/ERS position paper. *Eur Respir J.* 2004:932–946.
Global Initiative for the Diagnosis, Management, and Prevention of Chronic Obstructive Lung Disease. *The Global Initiative for Chronic Obstructive Lung Disease.* National Heart, Lung and Blood Institute; Federal Government Agency (US); 2006.
Global Initiative for Chronic Obstructive Lung Disease. www.goldcopd.com
Pauwels RA, Buist S, Calverly PM, et al. Global strategy for the diagnosis, management and prevention of chronic obstructive pulmonary disease. *Am J Respir Crit Care Med.* 2001;163:1256–1276.

76 ACUTE RESPIRATORY FAILURE
Abigail R. Lara and William J. Janssen

EPIDEMIOLOGY/OVERVIEW

- Respiratory failure is a syndrome of severe impairment in pulmonary gas exchange that results as a final common pathway for a diversity of clinical disorders.
- ARF develops over minutes to hours. In comparison, chronic respiratory failure develops over several days.
- ARF is classified as:
  - Hypoxemic or Type I respiratory failure
    - Characterized by a PaO_2 of < 60 mm Hg with a low or normal $PaCO_2$
    - Most common form of ARF
    - Associated with nearly all types of diseases of the lung
    - Elevated A-a gradient
  - Hypercapnic or Type II respiratory failure
    - Defined by a $PaCO_2$ of > 50 mm Hg
    - pH ≤ 7.30
    - Associated hypoxemia is common
    - Usually a normal A-a gradient (see Table 76-1)
- The incidence of ARF in the United States is 137/100,000 hospitalizations. There is an 88-fold increase between young and older age groups (age 5–17 years vs. age ≥ 80 years).
- Mortality of ARF in all comers is 36%, with increased risk of death found with the following associations:
  - Older age
  - Multiple organ system failure (MOSF)
  - HIV
  - Cancer
  - Chronic liver disease
  - Trauma
  - Drug overdose
- Associated causes of ARF (Table 76-2).

TABLE 76-1   Classification of ARF

HYPOXEMIC RESPIRATORY FAILURE	HYPERCAPNIC RESPIRATORY FAILURE
Other names: • Type I ARF • Respiratory insufficiency	Other names: • Type II ARF • Ventilatory failure • Pump failure
Definition: • The failure of both the heart and lungs to provide adequate O_2 to meet metabolic demands	Definition: • The failure of the lungs to adequately eliminate CO_2
Criteria: • $PaO_2 < 60$ mm Hg on $FiO_2 \geq 50\%$ • $PaO_2 < 40$ mm Hg on any FiO_2 • $SaO_2 < 90$	Criteria: • Acute ↑ in $PaCO_2 > 50$ mm Hg • Acute ↑ above normal baseline in COPD with a ¨ concomitant ↓ in pH < 7.30
Pathophysiologic causes: • R → L shunt • V/Q mismatch • Alveolar hypoventilation • Diffusion defect • Inadequate FiO_2	Pathophysiologic causes: • Pump failure (drive, muscles, WOB) • ↑ CO_2 production • ↑ Dead space • R → L shunt

PATHOPHYSIOLOGY

- Gas exchange occurs primarily across the alveolar capillary units.
- Oxygen diffuses across the alveolar membrane into the capillaries in order to bind to hemoglobin (oxygenation).
- Carbon dioxide diffuses in the opposite direction—traveling from the blood into the alveoli where it is exhaled (ventilation).
- In healthy states, oxygenation, blood flow, and ventilation compliment each other. Thus, there is no alveolar-arterial difference.
- ARF arises when there is a derangement in one or more components of the respiratory system which include:
  ○ CNS
  ○ Chest bellows component
    ▪ Peripheral nervous system
    ▪ Respiratory muscles
    ▪ Chest wall
  ○ Airways
  ○ Alveoli
- There are three major physiologic causes of ARF
  ○ V/Q mismatch: the most common cause of ARF. It occurs when gas exchange becomes ineffective at the alveolar unit because of damage to the alveoli itself, or owing to increased perfusion of blood flow which has occurred because of an obstruction (ie, PE) which diverts blood flow to normally ventilated areas of the lung. V/Q mismatch is characterized by
    ▪ Increased A-a gradient
    ▪ Correction of hypoxemia with administration of 100% FiO_2
  ○ Hypoventilation: implies a decreased drive to breath (often caused by CNS depression) or a decreased inability to breath (caused by diseases affecting the respiratory muscles or chest wall). It is characterized by
    ▪ Hypercapnia
    ▪ Hypoxemia
    ▪ Normal A-a gradient
  ○ Shunt: is defined as the presence of hypoxemia despite administration of 100% FiO_2. It occurs when deoxygenated blood (mixed venous blood) bypasses normally ventilated alveoli and mixed with oxygenated blood, thus leading to a reduction in the arterial blood content of oxygen. Conditions in which shunt should be considered
    ▪ Atrial septal defect
    ▪ Ventricular septal defect
    ▪ Patent ductus arteriosus
    ▪ Arteriovenous malformation in the lung
    ▪ Severe atelectasis, pulmonary edema, pneumonia
    ▪ Hypercapnia occurs only when shunt is $> 60\%$

CLINICAL PRESENTATION, DIFFERENTIAL, MAKING THE DIAGNOSIS

- ARF is a medical emergency, which can pose an immense challenge for healthcare providers. Patients may present with a multitude of signs and symptoms that often do not reflect the severity of the underlying physiologic state.
- Diagnosis of ARF begins with the clinical suspicion of its presence followed by confirmation based on an ABG.
- A careful history can often help lead to the underlying cause of the respiratory failure. (See Table 76-2.)
- Physical examination
  ○ General appearance

TABLE 76-2   Potential Causes of ARF

Pulmonary

Obstructive lung disease
- Aspiration
- Bronchoconstriction (ie, asthma/COPD)
- Edema/inflammation (ie, pneumonia)
- Epiglottis
- Foreign objects
- Secretions

Restrictive lung disease
- Flail chest
- Kyphoscoliosis
- Morbid obesity
- Rib fracture
- Severe burns
- Interstitial lung disease

Disorders of lung parenchyma
- Acute lung injury/ARDS
- Transfusion-related acute lung injury
- Atelectasis
- Pneumonia
- Pulmonary edema
- PE

Intrathoracic abnormalities
- Empyema
- Hemothorax
- Pleural disease/effusion
- Pneumothorax

CNS Depression

Drugs
- Alcohol intoxication
- Anesthetics
- Barbiturates
- Cocaine/heroin
- Methadone
- Narcotics
- Tranquilizers

Primary CNS disorders
- Cerebral ischemia
- Cerebral vascular accidents
- Cerebral tumors/lesions
- CNS infections
- Head trauma
- Central sleep apnea
- Pickwickian syndrome
- Increased intracerebral pressure

Neuromuscular

Drugs
- Antibiotics
- Ca channel blockers
- Anticholinesterases
- Curare/nondepolarizers
- Dexamethonium
- Methyl alcohol
- Paralytics

Primary neuromuscular disorders
- Guillian-Barré syndrome
- High spinal cord injury/disease
- Multiple sclerosis
- Muscular dystrophy
- Myasthenia gravis
- Myotonia
- Phrenic nerve injury
- Polymyositis
- Systemic lupus erythematosus
- Status epilepticus

Poisons/toxins/infections
- Pesticides
- Botulism
- Mushrooms
- Paraquat
- Petroleum distillates
- Rabies
- Tetanus
- Poliomyelitis
- Polymyositis (viral mediated)
- Rabies
- Tetanus

Cardiovascular

- Cardiac arrest
- CHF with pulmonary edema
- Congenital heart disease
- Hypovolemia
- Cardiovascular shock

Other

- Anxiety
- Excess O_2 in chronic CO_2 retainers
- Hypothyroidism
- Malnutrition/fatigue
- Metabolic acidosis
- Metabolic alkalosis
- Postop complications

- Anxiety
- Asterixis
- Tachypnea
- Diaphoresis
- Cyanosis
- Accessory muscle use
  - Intercostal muscle retraction with inspiration
- Head and neck examination
  - Nasal flaring
  - Elevated JVP
- Cardiac examination
  - New heart murmur

- Gallop rhythm
- Pulsus paradoxus
  ○ Pulmonary examination
    - Rales
    - Wheezing
    - Paradoxical respiratory motion
    - Consolidation by percussion
  ○ Neurologic examination
    - Delirium
  ○ Peripheral examination
    - Extremities for perfusion

LABORATORY STUDIES

- ABG measurement is the cornerstone for the initial assessment of ARF. Trends in the values of the ABG are often helpful in determining the pathophysiology. The clinician must know how much oxygen the patient is receiving at the time the ABG is drawn in order to interpret the A-a gradient appropriately. Note that it may take up to 20 minutes before a change in FiO_2 is reflected in the ABG. (See Table 76-3.)
- Initial laboratory studies which should be obtained quickly and help not only in making the diagnosis but also in the triage of the patient include
  ○ Complete blood count which may indicate anemia and/or infection
  ○ Serum chemistry panel, which can be used to define the duration of the event, as well as to provide clues to the etiology of the respiratory failure
  ○ Other: serum creatinine kinase and troponin levels give an indication of cardiac insults. Significant derangements in thyroid function or abnormal urine toxicology screens may explain abnormalities in respiratory drive

IMAGING AND OTHER LABORATORY TESTS

- Chest radiographs (CXR)
  ○ The CXR remains the mainstay for the initial evaluation of ARF. Indicators of disease include
    - Alveolar filling processes: cardiogenic vs. non cardiogenic pulmonary edema
    - Consolidation: pneumonia
    - Loss of costovertebral angles: pleural effusion
    - Tracheal deviation and/or lucency: pneumothorax
  ○ There can be a lag period of 12–24 hours before the disease process becomes evident on the CXR.
  ○ Whenever possible, compare old chest films with current films.
- ECG
  ○ Should be performed in all patients to evaluate the possibility of a cardiovascular etiology or complication from hypoxia (demand ischemia)
- CT scan
  ○ The availability of CT scans, as well as the ease and rapidity of the study, has made it invaluable to helping with the diagnosis. CT scans are most helpful in the acute setting in defining
    - PE
    - Small, but clinically significant pneumothorax
    - Extent of alveolar space disease
    - Interstitial lung disease
- Echocardiogram
  ○ Should be performed in all patients in whom a cardiac source of respiratory failure is suspected.
- Pulmonary function testing (PFTs)
  ○ In the acute setting, PEF may be used to help guide therapy.
  ○ Previous results if available will be helpful in determining the etiology of respiratory failure.

TABLE 76-3   Typical Changes in ABGs in ARF

MECHANISM OF ARF	pH	$PaCO_2$	PaO_2	SERUM HCO_3	$P(A\text{-}a)O_2$
CNS component	↓	↑	↓	WNL	↑*
Chest bellows component	↓	↑	↓	WNL	↑*
Airway Component					
ASTHMA EXACERBATION					
Acute	↑	↓	WNL (or ↓)	WNL	↑
Severe or respiratory muscle fatigue	↓	↑	↓	WNL	↑
COPD EXACERBATION					
No CO_2 retention	↓	↑	↓	WNL	↑
CO_2 retainer	↓	↑↑	↓	↑	↑
Alveolar Component					
Before respiratory muscle fatigue	↑	↓	↓↓	WNL	↑↑
After respiratory muscle fatigue	↓	↑	↓↓	WNL	↑↑

*If atelectasis or an alveolar filling defect is present.
↓, Decreased; ↑, Increased; WNL, within normal limits.

TABLE 76-4 Classification of Pulmonary Abnormalities based on Spirometry

	OBSTRUCTIVE	RESTRICTIVE	MIXED
FEV_1	↓	↓ or normal	↓
FVC	↓ or normal	↓	↓
FEV_1/FVC	↓	Normal or ↑	↓

- Respiratory failure is relatively uncommon in obstructive diseases if the FEV_1 is > 1 L, or in restrictive diseases where the FVC is > 1 L. (See Table 76-4.)
- Pulmonary artery catheterization
  - Utilized in cases where cardiogenic vs. non cardiogenic causes is unclear.
  - Should be performed only in the ICU by personnel who are trained in the insertion and interpretation of the waveforms.
  - Recent data suggest that the use of pulmonary artery catheters in patients with respiratory failure because of acute lung injury did not lead to an improvement in survival and lead to more complications.

TRIAGE AND ADDITIONAL MANAGEMENT

- Once the diagnosis of ARF has been established, the next step is to determine the level of care. In general, most patients with ARF should be admitted to a respiratory care floor or the ICU.
- Triage of the patient to the appropriate level of care is determined by the following:
  - Airway management
  - Delivery of oxygen (nasal canola, high-flow, non invasive positive pressure ventilation (NIPPV), mechanical ventilation)
  - Continuous ECG monitoring
  - Intensity of nursing care
- Initial management should be directed at reversing life-threatening hypoxia and correcting the precipitating clinical condition.
- Supplemental oxygen via nasal cannula or facemask should be administered in attempts to maintain a PaO_2 of ≥ 60 mm Hg; if this cannot be achieved or if hypercapnia develops, then mechanical ventilation should be applied.
  - Types of mechanical ventilation (see Chap. 81)
    - ET intubation
    - Noninvasive position pressure ventilation
      - Bi-level-positive airway pressure (BiPAP)
      - Continuous positive airway pressure (CPAP)
- Drug therapy
  - Bronchodilators

- Are indicated for rapid reversal of airflow limitation from bronchospasm
- Beta-2-agonists are most effective and may be administered by metered-dose inhaler or continuous nebulization
- Albuterol is the inhaled beta-2-agonist of choice Dosing is as follows:
  - Adults: 2.5–5 mg in 4 mL normal saline given via nebulizer every 20 minutes for up to three doses
  - If incomplete response (peak flow 50% to 80% of predicted or personal best), give 2.5–10 mg every 1–4 hours
  - If poor response, then the addition of an anticholinergic or 10–15 mg/h of albuterol by continuous nebulization may be attempted
  - Side effects may be seen at higher doses including, tremor, anxiety, sinus tachycardia, and atrial fibrillation/flutter
    - Inhaled anticholinergics (such as ipratropium) may be used in addition to albuterol to help augment and prolong the bronchodilator effect
  - Corticosteroids
    - Indicated in cases of severe bronchospasm that does not respond to bronchodilators
    - Methylprednisolone and prednisone are the drugs of choice because of their potent glucocorticoid effect
    - Dosing: adults 120–180 mg/d IV in 3–4 divided doses for 48 hours, then 60–80 mg/d until PEF is 70% of predicted/personal best
    - Insufficient data exist for use in causes of ARF other than COPD or asthma
  - Inhaled nitric oxide
    - Used in cases of refractory hypoxemia to help correct the V/Q mismatch
    - Although it is well known to improve oxygenation, no studies demonstrate a benefit in mortality
  - Heliox
    - A low-density gas made of an admixture of nitrogen and oxygen (helium 80% and oxygen 20%), which can improve gas exchange by improving laminar flow through the airways.
    - Most frequently utilized in cases of severe asthmatic bronchoconstriction and may help prevent intubation by buying time for other medications to work.

DISEASE MANAGEMENT STRATEGIES
- Regardless of the causes of ARF, the principles of management should be centered on the following:
  - Treatment of the precipitating cause. For example
    - Antibiotics for pneumonia
    - Bronchodilators and corticosteroids for bronchospasm

- Diuretics for pulmonary edema
- Anticoagulation for PE
  ○ Reduction in WOB
    - Improve airflow by decreasing bronchoconstriction, adding NIPPV, or instituting ET intubation and mechanical ventilation.
    - NIPPV should be considered in all patients with mild-to-moderate respiratory failure. The patient should have an intact airway, intact protective reflexes, and with a clear mental status.
    - NIPPV has been shown to decrease the need for invasive ventilation.
  ○ Maintenance of adequate gas exchange and prevention of further tissue damage by ensuring adequate oxygen delivery to tissues and correction of acidosis
  ○ Relief of suffering (air hunger)
- Evidence-based medicine strategies should be instituted whenever possible. The National Guideline Clearinghouse provides online supplements to a variety of categories at www.guideline.gov.

CARE TRANSITIONS

- All patients with ARF, regardless of underlying etiology, should be admitted to an ICU until they can be stabilized and their clinical course is determined.
- Transfer of patients to the intensive care setting from either the emergency room or the general medicine ward should not occur until the airway has been secured.
- Patients can be considered for transition to lower intensity care using the following guidelines:
  ○ Appropriate treatment of the underlying cause of respiratory failure has been instituted and improvement has occurred
  ○ Return of normal PaO_2 and $PaCO_2$ levels, or to the patient's premorbid baseline
- In those patients who have experienced a prolonged course of respiratory failure, or whose progress is delayed, a long-term care facility with experience in cardiopulmonary rehabilitation should be considered.

BIBLIOGRAPHY

Behrendt CE. Acute respiratory failure in the United States: incidence and 31-day survival. *Chest.* 2000;118:1100–1105.
Holguin F, Folch E, Redd SC, et al. Comorbidity and mortality in COPD-related hospitalizations in the United States, 1979 to 2001. *Chest.* 2005;128:2005–2011.
Honrubia T, Garcia Lopez FJ, Franco N, et al. Noninvasive vs conventional mechanical ventilation in acute respiratory failure:

a multicenter, randomized controlled trial. *Chest.* 2005; 128:3916–3924.
Kramer N, Meyer TJ, Meharg J, et al. Randomized, prospective trial of noninvasive positive pressure ventilation in acute respiratory failure. *Am J Respir Crit Care Med.* 1995;151: 1799–1806.
Nava S, Carlucci A. Non-invasive pressure support ventilation in acute hypoxemic respiratory failure: common strategy for different pathologies? *Intensive Care Med.* 2002;28:1205–1207.
Nicklas RA. National and international guidelines for the diagnosis and treatment of asthma. *Curr Opin Pulm Med.* 1997;3:51–55.
Task Force on Guidelines; Society of Critical Care Medicine. Guidelines for standards of care for patients with acute respiratory failure on mechanical ventilatory support. *Crit Care Med.* 1991;19:275–278.
Wheeler AP, Bernard GR, Thompson BT, et al. Pulmonary-artery versus central venous catheter to guide treatment of acute lung injury. *N Engl J Med.* 2006;354:2213–2224.

77 COMMUNITY-ACQUIRED PNEUMONIA

Adrienne L. Bennett

EPIDEMIOLOGY/OVERVIEW

- Community-acquired pneumonia (CAP) is an acute infection of the lower respiratory tract involving the pulmonary parenchyma in patients who have not been hospitalized during the previous 6 weeks.
- CAP is the leading infectious cause of death and the seventh leading cause of death overall in the United States (National Center for Health Statistics 2003), with a recent increase in mortality rates.
- CAP is diagnosed in ~4 million patients per year, resulting in ~1.4 million hospitalizations annually, and is one of the most common diagnoses cared for by hospitalists.
- The mean hospital LOS for CAP patients is ~5.5 days, with a mean in-hospital mortality of ~5%.
- CAP hospitalizations cost ~$9 billion/year, and the primary determinants of cost are unnecessary admissions and LOS.
- CAP is one of the diagnoses for which processes of care are measured and reported in an effort to improve clinical outcomes.

TABLE 77-1   JCAHO/CMS Pneumonia Core Measures

- All pneumonia patients should have oxygenation assessment (pulse oximetry or ABG) within 24 hours of hospital arrival.
- Blood cultures (two sets from different venous puncture sites) should be collected prior to the first dose of antibiotic.
- The first dose of antibiotic should be given within 8 hours of hospital arrival.
- Initial empiric antibiotic selection should cover prevalent typical and atypical organisms (see Table 77-3).
- Smokers with pneumonia should receive smoking cessation advice/counseling during their hospital stay.
- All pneumonia patients should be assessed for pneumococcal vaccination, which should be administered prior to discharge to patients who meet eligibility criteria.

- ◦ The Joint Commission on Accreditation of Healthcare Organizations (JCAHO) and the Centers for Medicare and Medicaid (CMS) jointly collect and report CAP quality measures.
- ◦ JCAHO/CMS pneumonia core measures are noted in the text in italics (also see Table 77-1).

PATHOPHYSIOLOGY

- CAP most commonly results from microaspiration of pathogens, colonizing or introduced into the nasopharynx. It can also result from hematogenous spread.
- An acute infection of the lower respiratory tract/pulmonary parenchyma, which may cause filling of the alveoli with inflammatory exudate and WBC, is more likely to occur in immunocompromised hosts or with particularly virulent organisms.
- Patient factors influence the risk of CAP and the potential pathogens involved (Table 77-2).
- The causative organism is identified in ≤ 60% of hospitalized cases (Table 77-3), necessitating initial empiric antibiotic treatment that takes into account patient characteristics (risk of aspiration, immunocompromised state) and prevalent pathogens (based on geography, season, known outbreaks, and local antibiotic-resistance patterns).
- Of rising concern are healthcare-associated pneumonia (HCAP) and methicillin-resistant *Staphylococcus aureus* (MRSA) CAP (particularly associated with previous influenza) in patients who may ostensibly present from the community setting with multidrug-resistant (MDR) organisms which are more typical of hospital or ventilator-acquired pneumonia (HAP and VAP). As per the 2005 American Thoracic Society/Infectious Disease Society of America guidelines, patients who have the following risk factors for HCAP should be managed like HAP and VAP patients (see Chap. 78):
  - ◦ Hospitalized for 2 or more days in the past 3 months
  - ◦ Residents of long-term care facilities
  - ◦ Home infusion therapy (including antibiotics) or home wound care
  - ◦ Chronic dialysis within the past month
  - ◦ A family member with a known multidrug-resistant (MDR) pathogen

CLINICAL PRESENTATION, DIFFERENTIAL, MAKING THE DIAGNOSIS

- Signs and symptoms and physical examination findings of CAP are < 50% sensitive for making the diagnosis, but their absence may help exclude the diagnosis.
- Signs and symptoms of CAP may include fever (~ 75% of cases at presentation), fatigue (~ 90%), cough (~ 90%), dyspnea (~ 70%), sputum production (~ 65%), and/or pleurisy (~ 50%).
- In the elderly, CAP may present as mental status changes or generalized malaise without prominent findings of fever or cough.
- Physical examination findings in CAP may include increased tactile fremitus (palpation of chest wall while patient speaking with tactile transmission of speech), dullness to percussion, decreased breath sounds, inspiratory crackles, and whispered pectoriloquy (increased clarity of whispered speech), egophony (when the patient says "e" it is heard as "a" during auscultation).
- The differential diagnosis most commonly includes upper respiratory tract infections such as tracheobronchitis, COPD, or asthma exacerbations. Malignancy, drug-induced pneumonitis (amiodarone and methotrexate are examples), and PE may also present similarly to CAP. Other diagnoses are less frequent, such as pulmonary vasculitides (Wegener's, Goodpasture's), eosinophilic pneumonitis, and bronchiolitis obliterans organizing pneumonia (BOOP).
- An infiltrate on chest radiography (CXR) remains the gold standard for diagnosing CAP, although the pattern of the infiltrate (lobar, interstitial, etc.) is a very nonspecific and insensitive guide to the underlying pathogen.

TRIAGE AND INITIAL MANAGEMENT

- Once the diagnosis of CAP is established, patients should be assessed for evidence of severe (see Table 77-4) or complicated pneumonia (see also Chap. 79), including (but not limited to)
  - ◦ Sepsis, defined as the presence of infection/pneumonia combined with the systemic inflammatory

TABLE 77-2   Sample/Draft Adult CAP Guideline/Order Set

The following assumes the order set includes key elements such as admit to observation or inpatient, principle and secondary diagnoses, patient condition, frequency of vital signs including oxygen saturation and call clinician for orders, allergies and adverse reactions to medications, latex, foods, activity, diet, intravenous fluids if needed, and additional (nonpneumonia-related) medications the patient is on as an outpatient or may need for prophylaxis while inpatient (such as venous thromboembolism prophylaxis—see Chap. 88).

Consider including decision support such as the criteria for severe pneumonia and/or the PORT Calculation Table or a link/easily accessible reference to it (PORT score calculator available free at: www.chestx-ray.com/Practice/PORT/PORT.html).

Give inclusion criteria for using the order set—for this example, principal diagnosis of CAP, admitted inpatient, or observation to the regular medical unit.

List exclusion criteria/when a clinician should not or may not wish to use this order set—such as ICU admission, suspected TB, fungal or nosocomial pneumonia, immunocompromised (HIV/AIDS), etc.

Provide a menu of checkboxes to select from (might include other things, such as CXR or labs, but be sure to include *JCAHO core measures*)

If not already done in the emergency department
    ☐ CXR: ☐ PA and lateral ☐ AP portable ☐ right lateral decubitus   ☐ left lateral decubitus
       reason/diagnosis for CXR: pneumonia
    ☐ *blood cultures times two sets prior to first dose of antibiotic*
    ☐ sputum for Gram stain and culture
    ☐ urine for *Legionella* antigen (consider in patient with severe pneumonia)
    ☐ urine for pneumococcal antigen
    ☐ nasal swab for influenza A&B (September through March)
    ☐ ABG (consider in patient with severe pneumonia or underlying COPD)

    ☐ *Oxygen 2 liters nasal canula, titrate to maintain oxygen saturation ≥ ___%.*

*Many antibiotics require adjustment for creatinine clearance (Clcr) = _____
Clcr = (140 − age in years) × weight in kg ÷ 72 × serum creatinine in mg/dL for women, multiply × 0.85 (creatinine clearance calculator available free at: www.intmed.mcw.edu/clincalc/creatinine.html)

Provide a *menu of checkboxes to guide appropriate antibiotic selection*, based on your hospital formulary and antibiotic resistance patterns, and patient risk factors—for example:

If not already administered in the emergency department, first dose of antibiotic STAT:

Patient at risk for common typical (*S. pneumoniae*, *H. influenzae*) and atypical (*M. pneumoniae*, *Chlamydophila pneumoniae*, *Legionella* species) pathogens:

☐ ceftriaxone 1 g IV every 24 hours *and* azithromycin 500 mg IV or po day 1 followed by 250 mg IV or po every 24 hours

or

☐ for patient with beta-lactam allergy, moxifloxacin 400 mg IV every 24 hours

Patient at increased risk for MRSA (known prior MRSA infection/colonization, resident of an extended care facility):
☐ place on MRSA precautions.
☐ send nasal swab for MRSA screening daily three times.
☐ add to one of the regimens above for usual typical and atypical pathogens above
*vancomycin 1 g IV every _____ hours
*vancomycin dosage adjustment for creatinine clearance:
 Clcr > 60, dose 1 g every 12 hours
 Clcr 40–60, dose 1 g every 24 hours
 Clcr < 40, dose 1 g at longer intervals, based on serum drug levels
☐ check creatinine and trough vancomycin level—draw 30 minutes prior to the fifth dose

Patient at increased risk for Pseudomonas (bronchiectasis, cystic fibrosis, immunocompromised, broad-spectrum antibiotic use for > 7 days in the past month)
☐ *piperacillin-tazobactam _____ g IV every _____ hours
 *piperacillin-tazobactam dosage adjustment for creatinine clearance
 Clcr > 40, dose 3.375 g IV every 6 hours
 Clcr 20–40, dose 2.25 g IV every 6 hours
 Clcr < 20, dose 2.25 g IV every 8 hours
and
*tobramycin 2.5 mg/Kg or ___ mg IV every _____ hours
*tobramycin dosage adjustment for creatinine clearance
 Clcr ≥ 60, dose every 8 hours
 Clcr 40–60, dose every 12 hours
 Clcr 20–40, dose every 24 hours
 Clcr 10–20, dose every 48 hours
 Clcr < 10, dose every 72 hours
and, if patient also at risk for atypical pathogens

(Continued)

TABLE 77-2   Sample/Draft Adult CAP Guideline/Order Set (*Continued*)

☐ azithromycin 500 mg IV or po day 1 followed by 250 mg IV or po every 24 hours

or

☐ for patient at increased risk for Pseudomonas with beta-lactam allergy (regimen also covers atypicals),

    *aztreonam _____ g every 12 hours

    *aztreonam dosage adjustment for creatinine clearance

    Clcr > 30, dose 1 g every 12 hours

    Clcr 10–30, dose 500 mg every 12 hours

    Clcr < 10, dose 250 mg every 12 hours

and

    *tobramycin ___ mg IV every _____ hours (*see dosage adjustment for creatinine clearance above)

and

    moxifloxacin 400 mg IV every 24 hours

☐ check creatinine and trough tobramycin level—draw 30 minutes prior to the fifth dose

☐ notify clinician if patient has a decrease/alteration in hearing while on tobramycin

Patient at increased risk for aspiration (altered levels of consciousness, such as caused by intoxication, stroke, seizure, dementia, often in association with poor dentition, severe debility)

☐ clindamycin 900 mg IV every 8 hours

and, if patient also at risk for atypical pathogens

☐ moxifloxacin 400 mg IV every 24 hours

☐ notify MD (between the hours of ___AM and ___ PM) for oral antibiotics and possible discharge when patient has been afebrile for > 16 hours, mental status is normal or baseline, patient has adequate po intake.

☐ September 1 through March 31, administer influenza vaccine 0.5 mL IM times one dose prior to discharge unless previously received this season or patient allergic (either give inclusion and exclusion criteria for vaccination or an easily accessed reference to help the clinician/RN identify candidates for vaccination)

☐ *Pneumococcal vaccine 0.5 mL IM one dose prior to discharge (either give inclusion and exclusion criteria for vaccination or an easily accessed reference to help the clinician/RN identify candidates for vaccination)*

☐ *Smoking cessation counseling/information packet provided if smoker within past year*

TABLE 77-3   CAP Prevention Strategies

Patients with pneumonia who have smoked within the past year should have smoking cessation advice/counseling during their hospital stay. Smoking cessation advice/counseling includes discussion with the hospitalist, pharmacotherapy, and/or referral to an outpatient smoking cessation program.

Pneumococcal vaccination: *all inpatients with pneumonia 65 years of age or older should be screened for and/or given pneumococcal vaccination when needed.* Pneumococcal vaccination is also appropriate for patients younger than 65 who have functional or anatomic asplenia, other forms of immunocompromise, malignancies, chronic cardiovascular, pulmonary, renal or liver disease, alcoholism, and diabetes mellitus. Revaccination with pneumococcal vaccine is appropriate for patients who were initially vaccinated ≥ 5 years ago and were younger than 65 at the time of the initial vaccination. Asplenic patients should be revaccinated 5 years after the initial dose.

Influenza vaccination: during the months of September to March, inpatients with pneumonia who are age ≥ 50 years and/or who have chronic cardiovascular disease, chronic pulmonary disease, chronic metabolic diseases (including diabetes mellitus), renal dysfunction, hemoglobinopathies, immunosuppression, are residents of long-term care facilities, and women who will be in the second or third trimester of pregnancy during flu season, care for children 6–24 months old, and healthcare providers should also be screened for and/or given influenza vaccination.

Pneumococcal and influenza vaccines may be administered at the same time in different sites without an increase in side effects or a decreased antibody response to either vaccine.

response syndrome (SIRS), which is present if ≥ 2 of the following are present: temperature <96.8°F (36°C) or >100.4°F (38°C); heart rate >90 beats per minute; respiratory rate >20 respirations per minute; $PaCO_2$ < 32; WBC count >12,000 or <4,000 or ≥10% bands.

◦ Septic shock, which is sepsis combined with hemodynamic instability.

◦ Pleural effusions, present in ~ 40% of CAP patients. Any patient with a pleural effusion > 1 cm on a lateral decubitus film, or an effusion which is not free flowing on lateral decubitus film, needs a diagnostic thoracentesis to assess for complicated parapneumonic effusion or empyema and the need for chest tube drainage.

◦ Other sites of infection caused by hematogenous spread, such as meningitis.

• The following laboratory studies should be obtained or considered:

◦ *Blood cultures (two sets from different venous puncture sites) should be collected prior to the administration of the first dose of antibiotic.* Blood cultures are only positive 7% to 16% of the time, and two-thirds of positive blood cultures are *S. pneumoniae.*

TABLE 77-4 Patient Factors Influencing CAP

PATIENT FACTORS/CHARACTERISTICS	ASSOCIATED CAP PATHOGENS
Elderly	More susceptible to CAP, predominantly the common typical (*S. pneumoniae*, *H. influenzae*) and atypical pathogens (especially *C. pneumoniae*, *M. pneumoniae* is increasingly seen in the elderly, also *Legionella* species) and influenza viruses
Extended care facility residents	*S. pneumoniae*, *H. influenzae*, *C. pneumoniae*, *S. aureus*, gram-negative bacteria, anaerobic bacteria, *Mycobacterium tuberculosis*, influenza viruses
Adolescents and young adults	*M. pneumoniae*
Altered levels of consciousness, because of intoxication, stroke, seizure, dementia	Aspiration (chemical) pneumonitis due primarily to lung injury from inhalation of gastric acid. The mainstay of therapy is supportive care, most do not need antibiotics
Altered levels of consciousness, often in association with poor dentition	~ 1/4 of patients who aspirate will develop secondary bacterial pneumonia because of anaerobic bacteria
Alcoholics	Gram-negative bacteria, anaerobic bacteria, *M. tuberculosis*
Diabetes mellitus	Influenza viruses, *Klebsiella pneumoniae*
Smokers, COPD	Influenza viruses, *H. influenzae*, *M. catarrhalis*, *K. pneumoniae*, *Legionella* species
Structural lung diseases (bronchiectasis, cystic fibrosis)	Influenza viruses, *H. influenzae*, *Pseudomonas aeruginosa*
Chronic cardiac disease	Influenza viruses
Chronic renal disease	Influenza viruses
Hemoglobinopathies (sickle cell disease)	Influenza viruses
Foreign-born (11.7% of US residents) and/or of low socioeconomic status	*M. tuberculosis*
Immunosuppressed patients (all causes)	Influenza viruses, *H. influenzae*
Rheumatoid arthritis on etanercept	No increase in the incidence of serious infections compared to placebo, but patients on etanercept who develop sepsis may have a higher mortality rate
Chronic high-dose steroid treatment	*Pneumocystis jiroveci*
HIV	With normal CD4 counts, severe CAP from common typical and atypical organisms, *M. tuberculosis* (incidence increases as CD4 decreases) With CD4 < 200, *P. jiroveci*
Neutropenic	*P. aeruginosa*
Organ transplant recipients	Cytomegalovirus
Acquired/functional asplenia (including sickle cell disease)	Encapsulated organisms: *H. influenzae*, *S. pneumoniae*

Severe pneumonia or ICU patients	• Common typical and atypical pathogens presenting as severe/complicated pneumonia are the most prevalent
	• *Legionella* species (see below) are the second most common pathogens identified (~ 10%)
	• Gram-negative bacteria are the third most common pathogens including
	   ◦ *K. pneumoniae* (most often seen in patients with COPD or diabetes mellitus)
	   ◦ *P. aeruginosa* (most often seen in patients with bronchiectasis, cystic fibrosis, or the immunocompromised)
	   ◦ *P. jiroveci* (in patients with HIV or on chronic high-dose steroid therapy)

Seasonal epidemics	*Influenza* viruses
Epidemic outbreaks (not seasonal)	*Legionella* species
Living in or traveling to certain geographical regions	• Midwestern United States—*Histoplamsma capsulatum* • Desert southwest United States—Coccidiomycosis • Primarily found in the southwest, cases have occurred in 31 states and worldwide—Hantavirus • Southeastern Asian regional epidemics including SARS, avian influenza
Exposure to particular animals/birds	• Bats—*H. capsulatum* • Birds—*Chlamydophila psittaci*, *Cryptococcus neoformans*, *H. capsulatum* • Rabbits—*Francisella tularensis* • Farm animals/parturient cats—*Coxiella burnetii* (Q fever)
Inordinately large number of patients presenting with CAP symptoms	Potential bioterrorism—consider agents such as Influenza, Legionella, Hantavirus, Coccidiomycosis, *Bacillus anthracis*, *Yersinia pestis*, *F. tularensis*, *C. burnetii*, and Ricin.

◦ Complete blood cell count and differential, serum creatinine, blood urea nitrogen, glucose, electrolytes, and LFTs (to aid in risk stratification, see below).
◦ Sputum for Gram stain and culture—a suitable specimen is one that contains fewer than 10 epithelial cells (limited oropharyngeal contamination) and > 25 polymorphonuclear cells (purulent) per low-powered field.
◦ In selected patients (see Table 77-1), appropriate diagnostic studies for legionella, tuberculosis (TB), and HIV should also be undertaken.

- All patients with pneumonia should receive oxygenation assessment by pulse oximetry or ABG (to assess for respiratory failure in patients with severe pneumonia or underlying chronic lung disease).
- Oxygen should be administered as needed to maintain an oxygen saturation > 90% (caution should be exercised in patients with chronic lung disease and the potential for CO_2 retention).
- Patients with severe pneumonia and ARF (refractory hypoxemia and/or acute respiratory acidosis/hypercapnea), particularly those with underlying COPD, should be considered for NIPPV.
- *The first dose of antibiotics should be administered within 8 hours of arrival at the hospital.* In some studies, shortening door-to-antibiotic time to < 4 hours showed increased survival benefits.
- *Initial empiric antibiotic selection that covers prevalent typical (S. pneumoniae and H. influenzae) and atypical (M. pneumoniae, C. pneumoniae, and Legionella) organisms has been demonstrated to reduce mortality rates (Table 77-5). Initial empiric antibiotic selection should also take into account the severity of pneumonia (particularly risk factors for Pseudomonas), other patient characteristics (particularly immunocompromised states, see below), and suspected pathogens, (Tables 77-1 and 77-2) as well as local antibiotic resistance patterns.*
- All patients with evidence of severe or complicated CAP should be admitted to the hospital for treatment, regardless of PORT score (see below).
- The pneumonia patient outcomes research team (PORT) cohort study has provided a useful pneumonia severity index for determining the risk of 30-day mortality to help guide the selection of the appropriate setting for treatment for patients with CAP, especially the elderly who may otherwise look well (see Table 77-6).
- It is estimated that up to one-third to one-half of all patients, who are admitted for treatment of pneumonia, are at low risk for mortality (PORT score ≤ 70) and can potentially be treated safely and effectively as outpatients.
- However, the PORT study excluded patients with HIV/AIDS, and because of a heavy emphasis on patient age in the scoring system, younger patients with severe or complicated pneumonia may have low-risk PORT scores.
- Patients who are not immunocompromised, have no evidence of severe/complicated pneumonia, and have PORT scores ≤ 70 should be considered for outpatient treatment.
- When it occurs, clinical deterioration (worsening hypoxemia/respiratory failure, development of hemodynamic instability) typically happens within the first 24–72 hours after presentation.

- Brief hospitalization/24- to 48-hour observation to initiate antibiotics and assure no clinical deterioration is often the most prudent course for intermediate mortality risk patients (PORT score 71–91).
- Clinical judgment should always inform the application of any prediction rule, such as the PORT score, and psychosocial factors that influence a patient's ability to reliably acquire and take oral antibiotics or the presence of other active comorbid illnesses may necessitate hospitalization.
- Immunocompromised patients are more likely to have severe CAP and should almost always be admitted. Examples include
  ○ Rheumatoid arthritis on immunomodulating therapies
  ○ Conditions requiring chronic high-dose steroids
  ○ HIV/AIDS
  ○ Malignancies, particularly if neutropenic from chemotherapy
  ○ Organ transplants
  ○ Acquired or functional asplenia
- There is a broader range of pathogens and potential empiric treatment options to be considered in immunocompromised patients, based on the type of immunocompromise (examples include *Pneumocystis jiroveci* in patients with HIV/AIDS or chronic high-dose steroid use, Cytomegalovirus in organ transplant recipients, see Tables 77-1 and 77-2).

DISEASE MANAGEMENT STRATEGIES

- Hospitalists are often involved in or lead initiatives to develop and/or implement clinical guidelines or care pathways for diagnoses such as CAP to help assure
  ○ Adherence to evidence-based medicine practices that optimize quality of care and patient outcomes
  ○ Compliance with regulatory agency requirements (such as JCAHO Core Measures)
- One of the most effective and user-friendly ways to present clinical guidelines is in the form of order sets, whether on paper or by computerized physician order entry (CPOE), that help clinicians "do the right thing" (for an example/draft of such a CAP order set, see Table 77-7).
- Patient education and managing patient expectations regarding the expected course of their CAP should begin early in the hospital course
  ○ Patients need to understand that even with appropriate antibiotic therapy, they may remain febrile for several days, and this does not necessarily mean they are not getting better or are on the wrong antibiotic. The fever pattern typically shows a decrease in the maximum temperature of ~ 1°F/d.

TABLE 77-5 CAP Pathogens

PATHOGEN	CLUES TO THE DIAGNOSIS	SPECIAL TREATMENT CONSIDERATIONS
S. pneumoniae	• The most common pathogen, isolated in up to ~ 25% of CAP patients hospitalized on the general medical ward • Sputum Gram stain (purulent with gram-positive diplococci) and culture • Pneumococcal urinary antigen (70%–90% sensitivity/80%–100% specificity in adults) • Two-thirds of positive blood cultures are pneumococcus	• There is an increasing incidence of beta-lactam-resistant pneumococci, particularly in patients age > 65 years, alcoholics, immunocompromised, multiple medical comorbidities, exposure to children who attend daycare centers, use of a beta-lactam antibiotic within the past 3 months • Vancomycin is the rx of choice in areas with a high prevalence of beta-lactam-resistant organisms • With meningeal involvement, a third-generation cephalosporin should be used
H. influenzae	• ~ 5% of hospitalized CAP patients. • Sputum Gram stain (purulent with small, pleomorphic gram-negative rods) and culture	
M. pneumoniae	• ~ 5% of hospitalized CAP patients, increasingly seen in the elderly • ~ 5% have ear pain from hemorrhagic bullous myringitis • Rash, including Stevens-Johnson syndrome • CBC may show hemolysis (confirm with a positive Coomb's test), a normal WBC and thrombocytosis • Complement fixation testing is the most sensitive test • IgM and IgG serologies are available • Cold agglutinins are positive in ~ 50%, but are not sensitive or specific and this test is not cost-effective/recommended	• Azithromycin is the most active treatment against *M. pneumoniae* and there is no reported resistance
C. pneumoniae	• < 5% of hospitalized CAP patients, most commonly elderly • Although not unique, pharyngitis, hoarseness, and sinusitis are common features • Extrapulmonary manifestations may include Guillain-Barré syndrome, reactive arthritis, and myocarditis • Nasopharyngeal swab culture is rarely done as it requires specialized cell culture techniques • IgM and IgG serologies are available but generally do not allow for rapid diagnosis	• Fluoroquinolones are less active against *Chlamydia* than tetracyclines or macrolides • Doxycycline is the treatment of choice in confirmed *Chlamydia* infections
Legionella species	• < 5% of hospitalized CAP patients, but the second most common pathogen in patients in the ICU • Both epidemic and sporadic cases are seen • High mortality rates • Fever, often with minimal respiratory complaints, altered mental status, and GI symptoms are often prominent (nausea, vomiting, diarrhea, abdominal pain) • Laboratory clues to the diagnosis include hyponatremia, abnormal LFTs, and hematuria • The urinary antigen test (only detects serogroup 1, which accounts for ~ 75% of cases) and DFA staining may help make a rapid diagnosis • Sputum or BAL samples should also be obtained for *Legionella* culture on selective media	• Levofloxacin and azithromycin are the drugs of choice in *Legionella,* and should be administered at least initially IV to assure absorption of the drug owing to the prevalence of GI symptoms in these patients
Influenza viruses	• ~ 10% of CAP patients hospitalized on the medical ward • Clinically characterized by the abrupt onset of debilitating fever, headache, myalgia, fatigue, and respiratory tract symptoms • Primary influenza pneumonia is often severe and associated with high fever, dyspnea, and often hypoxemia • Commonly available nasal swab antibody tests allow rapid diagnosis of both influenza A and B • Secondary bacterial pneumonia with typical organisms is the most common complication of influenza infection and is implicated in ~ 25% of influenza mortality	• Neuraminidase inhibitors zanamivir and oseltamivir are active against both influenza A and B • All influenza therapies must be initiated early in the course of illness (24–48 hours) to be of benefit in reducing the duration and severity of symptoms • Amantadine and rimantadine, previously used to treat influenza A, are not recommended because of the very high prevalence (~ 90%) of resistance

(Continued)

TABLE 77-5   CAP Pathogens (*Continued*)

PATHOGEN	CLUES TO THE DIAGNOSIS	SPECIAL TREATMENT CONSIDERATIONS
S. aureus	• Is typically an infrequent cause of CAP, but is the second most frequent pathogen in postinfluenza pneumonia (~ 20% of cases) • Easily recovered from sputum, blood cultures also sometimes helpful	• Many strains, including those acquired in the community, are MRSA, which can be associated with a severe necrotizing pneumonia • Vancomycin is a reasonable choice for initial empiric therapy of postinfluenza pneumonia, given the prevalence of beta-lactam-resistant pneumococcus and MRSA
P. aeruginosa	• Is more common in patients with structural lung diseases (cystic fibrosis and bronchiectasis), immunocompromised or treated with broad-spectrum antibiotics for > 7 days in the past month. Gram-negative bacteria are the third most common pathogens seen in the ICU • Sputum Gram stain (purulent with gram-negative rods) and culture (often initially identified as a nonlactose-fermenting gram-negative rod pending final speciation)	• Classes of antibiotics for the treatment of *Pseudomonas* pneumonia include antipseudomonal penicillins, combination penicillin plus beta-lactamase inhibitor, third- and fourth-generation cephalosporins, monobactam, carbapenems, fluoroquinolones, and aminoglycosides • Although data are somewhat conflicting, most authorities recommend treatment with at least two agents from different classes, because of the prevalence of MDR strains and the potential for emergence of resistance during treatment
M. catarrhalis	• Is more common in smokers and patients with COPD • Sputum culture	
K. pneumoniae	• Is more common in smokers and patients with COPD or diabetes mellitus. Gram-negative bacteria are the third most common pathogens seen in the ICU • Sputum or blood culture	
M. tuberculosis	• Is most commonly seen in foreign-born (immigrants make up ~ 12% of the US population) and/or patients from low socioeconomic backgrounds. It is also seen in patients with HIV whose CD4 count is normal • Fever, typically low-grade, is the usual presenting feature, and respiratory signs/symptoms are only present in ~ 25%–33% of patients with primary TB • Respiratory isolation precautions are mandatory for high-risk patients with CAP until diagnosis ruled out • Hilar adenopathy is the most common chest radiography finding (65%), pleural effusions occur in ~ 33%, and when present, infiltrates (~ 30%) are more common in the right middle lobe, and are only occasionally associated with cavitation • Sputum examination for acid-fast bacilli and culture confirm diagnosis	• MDR TB is prevalent; making directly observed therapy with four-drug regimens more than 26 weeks is the most appropriate treatment
P. jiroveci	• Is seen in immunocompromised patients (HIV and CD4 counts < 200, chronic high-dose steroid treatment) • Indolent onset of fever, nonproductive cough and dyspnea/tachypnea • Hypoxemia, either at rest and/or with exertion, is common • LDH is often elevated, and the level correlates with prognosis/mortality • Immunofluorescent staining of an induced sputum specimen confirms the diagnosis in most patients	• Patients tend to get sicker 2–3 days into therapy because of the inflammatory response to the dying organisms • Steroids reduce respiratory failure and mortality in patients whose PO_2 < 70 or the A-a gradient is > 35 • Trimethoprim-sulfamethoxazole po or IV is the treatment of choice (and is also used for prophylaxis) although other regimens are available for those who experience adverse side effects or are allergic to sulfa
Cytomegalovirus	• Is seen most frequently in organ transplant recipients and patients with HIV and CD4 counts < 50 • Quantitative plasma CMV DNA tests allow the assessment of viral load, which correlates with active disease • Isolation of CMV from blood or BAL cultures is the gold standard for establishing active infection	Gancyclovir IV is the treatment of choice, although resistant strains do exist
Aspiration pneumonia caused by anaerobic bacteria	• Altered levels of consciousness, because of intoxication, stroke, seizure, dementia, often in association with poor dentition. • ~ 1/4 of patients who aspirate will develop secondary bacterial infection necessitating antibiotics, and such patients may account for ~ 25% of all CAP, but anaerobes are not detected in routine sputum cultures	• There is often coinfection with streptococci • Clindamycin is the drug of choice • Metronidazole in combination with a penicillin (to cover streptococci) is an acceptable alternative (single agent metronidazole has a 50% failure rate)

(Continued)

TABLE 77-5 CAP Pathogens (*Continued*)

PATHOGEN	CLUES TO THE DIAGNOSIS	SPECIAL TREATMENT CONSIDERATIONS
	• Indolent symptoms • Pulmonary necrosis or cavitation • Right lower lobe predominance • Putrid sputum	
H. capsulatum	• Is prevalent in the midwestern United States • Findings may include mediastinal or hilar lymphadenopathy or masses, pulmonary nodules, cavitary lesions • The differential diagnosis includes sarcoidosis, TB, and malignancy • Serology is useful in diagnosing acute or active infection • Urinary and blood antigen tests are useful in diagnosing disseminated or diffuse pulmonary disease • Blood, sputum, and BAL cultures are helpful in disseminated or chronic pulmonary histoplasmosis	• Acute pulmonary histoplasmosis in immunocompetent hosts seldom requires antifungal treatment • Chronic pulmonary histoplasmosis should be treated with itraconazole • Fluconazole is less effective in treating histoplasmosis
Coccidiomycosis	• Is found in the desert southwest United States. • Arthralgias and fatigue are common, and skin findings may include erythema nodosum and erythema multiforme • Serologic testing for IgM and IgG antibodies (caveat—detection of antibodies may lag behind illness by weeks, so a negative serology does not exclude the diagnosis)	• Most patients resolve the primary infection without specific treatment • In high-risk patients (immunosuppression, lymphoma, diabetes mellitus, pregnancy) treatment with itraconazole or fluconazole is appropriate • Patients who exhibit severe disease (weight loss > 10%, night sweats persisting > 3 weeks, bilateral infiltrates or involvement of > 1/2 of one lung, symptoms persisting > 2 months) should also be considered for treatment
Hantavirus	• Is primarily found in the southwestern United States, but cases have occurred in 31 states and worldwide • History of exposure to wild rodents • Serologic testing for IgM and IgG antibodies	• The mainstay of therapy is supportive care, no specific antiviral treatment exists
SARS, Avian influenza	• Are examples of regional epidemics with the potential for worldwide spread and high mortality rates	• Neuraminidase inhibitors zanamivir and oseltamivir have activity against avian influenza

Abbreviation: BAL, bronchial alveolar lavage.

○ Patients should be counseled that the signs and symptoms of pneumonia (particularly fatigue and cough) are slow to resolve, particularly in the elderly (typically takes weeks).

○ Patients often ask when they will have a follow-up CXR. In patients who are clinically improving, a follow-up CXR is not necessary. Radiographic changes of pneumonia may persist for many weeks, even in the setting of effective antibiotic therapy, while the lungs heal and the body clears the inflammation from the airways. Radiographic resolution takes even longer in older patients or those with underlying lung disease.

○ Discuss the criteria for discharge home on oral antibiotics (see below) and let the patient and family know that most patients will be ready for discharge in 2–3 days.

○ A free patient information sheet is available at: www.patient.co.uk/showdoc/23069033/.

• If cultures or other diagnostic tests result in a known pathogen and/or antibiotic sensitivities, antibiotic therapy should be narrowed to treat the specific pathogen.

TABLE 77-6 Severe Pneumonia

ATS CRITERIA FOR DIAGNOSING SEVERE PNEUMONIA—PREDICTING THE NEED FOR ICU ADMISSION	

Minor criteria for severe pneumonia
   (at least two present at admission)
Systolic BP ≤ 90 mm Hg
Bilateral or multilobar pneumonia
$PaO_2/FiO_2 < 250$
Respiratory rate ≥ 30 per minute
 	
Diastolic BP 60 mm Hg
	Major criteria for severe pneumonia
	   (any one present anytime from admission through the hospital stay)
	Need for mechanical ventilation
	Septic shock or the need for pressors for > 4 hours
	An increase in the size of infiltrates by > 50% within 48 hours
	Acute renal failure (urine output < 80 mL in 4 hours or serum creatinine > 2 mg/dL in the absence of chronic renal failure)

TABLE 77-7   Initial Empiric Antibiotic Selection: Infectious Disease Society of America and American Thoracic Society Recommendations

PATIENT CHARACTERISTICS	INITIAL EMPIRIC ANTIBIOTIC SELECTION
Immunocompetent, on the general medical wards covers common typical (*S. pneumoniae, H. influenzae*) and atypical pathogens (*C. pneumoniae, M. pneumoniae, Legionella* species)	IV or IM beta-lactam plus IV or po macrolide *or* IV or po fluoroquinolone monotherapy *or* IV or IM beta-lactam plus IV or po doxycycline
Immunocompetent, severe pneumonia, in the ICU	IV beta-lactam plus IV macrolide *or* IV beta-lactam plus IV fluoroquinolone
Patient with beta-lactam allergy	IV quinolone plus IV clindamycin or vancomycin
Patient at risk of *Pseudomonas* (bronchiectasis, cystic fibrosis, immunocompromised state, malnutrition, or broad-spectrum antibiotic use for > 7 days in the past month)	IV antipseudomonal beta-lactam plus IV antipseudomonal fluoroquinolone *or* IV antipseudomonal beta-lactam plus IV aminoglycoside plus either IV antipneumococcal fluoroquinolone or IV macrolide
Patient with beta-lactam allergy and at risk of *Pseudomonas*	IV aztreonam plus IV aminoglycoside plus IV antipseudomonal fluoroquinolone

- Clinical deterioration or failure to show signs of improvement by 72–96 hours should prompt a reassessment for worsening severity or complications of pneumonia, or an alternative diagnosis.
  - Reassess patient factors that might indicate a risk for pathogens not covered by the initial empiric regimen (including risk factors for HIV), and consider the risk of antibiotic-resistant pathogens.
  - Consider a follow-up CXR to rule out new or worsening infiltrates and effusions.
  - Up to 20% of patients initially diagnosed with CAP have other noninfectious causes of their respiratory symptoms and abnormal chest radiographs, such as malignancy, drug-induced changes, or vasculitis. Carefully reviewing the history and clinical course of the illness are key to recognizing these other possible diagnoses.
  - A high-resolution chest CT is also a reasonable diagnostic test in patients thought to have nonresponding CAP. It allows for assessment of infiltrates and effusions, including loculation or abscess formation, and can provide additional information that may point to an alternative diagnosis.

CARE TRANSITIONS

- It is safe to discharge CAP patients home on oral antibiotics once they meet the following clinical stability criteria for 16–24 hours:
  - Afebrile (temperature < 100°F), although discharge can still be considered in a febrile patient if other clinical stability criteria are favorable
  - Improvement in respiratory signs and symptoms

  - Adequate oral intake and able to take oral antibiotics
  - Return to baseline mental status
  - Reasonable resolution of relevant psychosocial barriers to outpatient treatment and follow-up

  For most patients on the general medical ward this will be hospital day 2 or 3.
- Patients who will be transferred to settings with 24-hour skilled nursing care and the option of parenteral therapy if needed (such as skilled nursing facilities and acute rehabilitation hospitals) may be candidates for early discharge if there has been no clinical deterioration in the first 24–48 hours in hospital.
- Prior to discharge, make sure CAP prevention strategies have been implemented (see Table 77-8).
- Duration of antibiotic therapy—evidence-based data to inform this decision are lacking, but many experts recommend
  - In a healthy patient with uncomplicated CAP that responds quickly to therapy, a total of 7–10 days is sufficient.
  - In severe or complicated CAP, a total antibiotic course of 10–14 days, or treatment for at least 5 days after the patient becomes afebrile, is often recommended.
- Have the patient see their primary care physician for outpatient follow-up in 1–2 weeks, or around the time they discontinue antibiotic therapy.
- Be sure to reconcile admission and discharge medications (eg, instruct the patient on when to resume antihypertensive agents that were held for hypotension or acute renal failure).
- Be sure to communicate with the primary care physician in a timely way (ideally within 24 hours of

TABLE 77-8 Assessing the Need for Hospital Admission*

CALCULATING THE PNEUMONIA SEVERITY INDEX (OR PORT SCORE)

PATIENT CHARACTERISTICS	NO. OF POINTS
Demographics	
Male	Age
Female	Age −10
Nursing home resident	+ 10
Comorbid illnesses	
Cancer (active diagnosis within the past year)	+ 30
Liver disease	+ 20
CHF	+ 10
Cerebrovascular disease	+ 10
Renal disease	+ 10
Physical examination findings	
Altered mental status	+ 20
Respiratory rate > 30	+ 20
Systolic BP < 90	+ 20
Temperature < 95°F or > 104°F	+15
Heart rate > 125	+10
Laboratory/CXR findings	
pH < 7.35	+ 30
BUN > 30	+ 20
Na < 130	+ 20
Glucose > 250	+ 10
Hematocrit < 30	+ 10
PO_2 < 60 or pulse oximetry < 90% on room air	+10
Pleural effusion	+10
Total score	

CLASS, RISK, MORTALITY RATES, AND APPROPRIATE SETTING FOR TREATMENT

TOTAL SCORE	CLASS	RISK	% MORTALITY	TREATMENT SETTING
Age < 50 + 0 points	I	Low	0.1%	Outpatient
≤ 70	II	Low	0.6%	Outpatient
71–91	III	Intermediate	2.8%	Outpatient or brief inpatient
91–130	IV	High	8.2%	Inpatient
> 131	V	High	29.2%	Inpatient

*Free PORT calculator available at: http://www.chestx-ray.com/Practice/PORT/PORT.html.

discharge) regarding the patient's hospital course, anticipated antibiotic treatment and other discharge medications, and any special follow-up needs (eg, if the patient is on chronic warfarin therapy and requires more frequent INR checks because of the potential for warfarin-antibiotic interactions).

BIBLIOGRAPHY

Bartlett JG, Dowell SF, Mandell LA, et al. Practice guidelines for the management of community-acquired pneumonia. *Clin Infect Dis.* 2000;31:347–382.

Battleman DS, Callahan M, Thaler HT. Rapid antibiotic delivery and appropriate antibiotic selection reduce length of hospital stay of patients with community-acquired pneumonia. *Arch Intern Med.* 2002;162:682–688.

Fine MJ, Stone RA, Singer DE, et al. Processes and outcomes of care for patients with community-acquired pneumonia. *Arch Intern Med.* 1999;159:970–980.

Fine MJ, Auble TE, Yealy DM, et al. A prediction rule to identify low-risk patients with community-acquired pneumonia. 1997;336:243–250.

Mandell LA, Bartlett JG, Dowell SF, et al. Update of practice guidelines for the management of community-acquired pneumonia in immunocompetent adults. *Clin Infect Dis.* 2003;37:1405–1433.

Marrie TJ, Lau CY, Wheeler SL, et al. A controlled trial of a critical pathway for treatment of community-acquired pneumonia. *JAMA.* 2000;283:749–755.

Niederman MS, Mandell LA, Anzueto A, et al. Guidelines for the management of adults with community-acquired pneumonia. Diagnosis, assessment of severity, antimicrobial therapy, and prevention. *Am J Respir Crit Care Med.* 2001;163:1730–1754.

Rhew DC, Tu GS, Ofman J, et al. Early switch and early discharge strategies in patients with community-acquired pneumonia: a meta-analysis. *Arch Intern Med.* 2001;161:722–727.

78 HOSPITAL-ACQUIRED, VENTILATOR-ASSOCIATED, AND HEALTHCARE-ACQUIRED PNEUMONIA

Nathan J. O'Dorisio

EPIDEMIOLOGY/OVERVIEW

- HAP, VAP, and HCAP are pneumonias in which patients are at risk for infection with multidrug-resistant (MDR) pathogens because of recent direct or indirect exposure to the healthcare system.
- HAP, pneumonia occurring more than 48 hours after hospital admission, is the leading cause of death from nosocomial infection, with mortality rates between 30% and 50%.
- HAP is comprised of two subsets
  - Early onset: within 5 days of admission
  - Late onset: after hospital day 5
- VAP is a subset of HAP developing more than 48–72 hours after ET intubation. VAP occurs in 10% to 25% of patients on mechanical ventilation.
  - VAP increases length of hospital stay by ~ 8 days
  - VAP increases the cost of hospitalization by ~ $40,000

- HCAP is a pneumonia in any patient who
  - Has been hospitalized for 2 or more days within the preceding 90 days (including acute rehabilitation hospitals)
  - Resides in a long-term care facility
  - Has received outpatient intravenous antibiotics, wound care, or chemotherapy within 30 days
  - Attends hemodialysis
  - Lives with someone known to be colonized with MDR pathogens

PATHOPHYSIOLOGY

- The major route of infection is microaspiration. Up to 45% of healthy adults aspirate during sleep. This percentage is increased by severe illness. See Table 78-1.
- HAP, VAP, and HCAP are associated with an increased risk of infection with MDR pathogens. See Tables 78-2 and 78-3.
- In VAP, ET tubes allow some leakage of oral flora and bacteria of gastric origin into the airway. Microorganisms may encase themselves in biofilm on the ET tube; this biofilm may be shed into the distal airways.

CLINICAL PRESENTATION, DIFFERENTIAL, MAKING THE DIAGNOSIS

- Typical diagnostic criteria for pneumonia are often unreliable in HAP, and especially VAP, because of the many causes of dyspnea and pulmonary infiltrates in

TABLE 78-1 Host Risk Factors for Hospital-Acquired Pneumonia

- Age > 70
- Men more likely to get VAP than women, but women are twice as likely to die from HAP
- Chronic lung disease (particularly COPD)
- ARDS
- Decreased mental status, use of intracranial pressure monitors
- Aspiration
- Chest surgery
- Increased gastric pH with H-2 blocker/antacid therapy
- Mechanical ventilation increases risk 6–20-fold
- Prolonged hospitalization prior to intubation, and prolonged intubation
- Reintubation
- Frequent ventilator circuit changes (should be done once weekly, or even less frequently, unless gross soilage occurs)
- PEEP
- Previous antibiotics exposure
- Fall/winter season
- Nasogastric tube
- Transportation to and from the ICU for diagnostic testing/therapeutic interventions

TABLE 78-2 Risk Factors for Infection with MDR Pathogens

Antimicrobial therapy within the past 90 days
Current hospital stay < 5 days
High prevalence of antibiotic resistance in the community/hospital
Immunosuppressive disease
Immunosuppressive therapy
Risk factors for HCAP
- Prior hospital stay > 2 days in preceding 90 days
- Home infusion therapy
- Home wound care
- Chronic dialysis within 30 days
- Nursing home/extended care facility resident
- Household contact with MDR

hospitalized patients, especially mechanically ventilated ones.
  - The presence of a new or worsening infiltrate on CXR, fever, leukocytosis, and purulent airway secretions has a high specificity but low sensitivity (< 50%).
  - The differential diagnosis of respiratory decompensation in critically ill or ventilated patients is broad, and includes HF, pulmonary hemorrhage, ARDS, tracheobronchitis, exacerbation of underlying lung disease, PE, and pulmonary drug reactions.
  - The presence of air bronchograms on x-ray is the most suggestive finding in ventilated patients, but lacks sensitivity.
- The clinical pulmonary infection score (CPIS) may improve the diagnostic accuracy (see Table 78-4).
  - A CPIS score < 6 has good correlation with pneumonia.
- Acquisition of lower respiratory tract samples (via induced sputum, blind bronchial suctioning, or bronchoscopy) for Gram stain and culture is mandatory in the diagnostic workup of suspected HAP, VAP, and HCAP. Such cultures should be obtained in all patients prior to antibiotics, but should not delay the administration of antibiotics.
- Consideration should be given to obtaining these studies in all patients suspected of HAP, HCAP, or VAP: complete blood count, two separate blood cultures, posteroanterior and lateral CXR if possible, and arterial oxygenation status.
- Diagnostic thoracentesis should be performed in all patients suspected of HAP, VAP, and HCAP with pleural effusions in order to rule out complicated parapneumonic effusion or empyema (see Chap. 79).

TRIAGE AND INITIAL MANGEMENT

- Early empiric-appropriate antibiotics in adequate dosages should be initiated promptly in patients

TABLE 78-3 Common Pathogens in HAP, VAP, and HCAP

HAP		VAP	HCAP
EARLY	LATE		
S. pneumoniae	MDR pathogens	MDR pathogens	60% MRSA
H. influenzae	P. aeruginosa	High risk of polymicrobial infection	25% P. aeruginosa
MSSA	K. pneumoniae (extended	9% other staphylococci	
Enterobacter species	spectrum beta-lactamase- producing enterobacteriaceae)	14% P. aeruginosa	
	Acinetobacter species		
	Legionella pneumophilia		
	MRSA		

Abbreviations: MSSA, methicillin-sensitive S. aureus; ESBL, extended spectrum beta-lactamase-producing enterobacteriaceae.

suspected of HAP, VAP, or HCAP (see Table 78-5), taking into account

○ The patient's risk for colonization with MDR pathogens
○ Recent antibiotic treatment
○ Knowledge of local MDR pathogen prevalence and specific patterns of antibiotic resistance

• Supplemental oxygen should be administered to patients with arterial oxygen saturations < 90%.
• Consideration should be given to NIV in patients with respiratory failure.

• Hemodynamic instability, worsening oxygenation status, respiratory failure not responding to noninvasive management, or exacerbation of comorbid conditions may necessitate transfer to an ICU.

DISEASE MANGEMENT STRATEGIES

• All patients being treated for HAP, VAP, and HCAP should be reassessed daily, with special emphasis on

TABLE 78-4 Modified CPIS

BASELINE		NO. OF POINTS
Temperature	> 36.5 and < 38.4	0
	> 38.5 and < 38.9	1
	> 39 and < 36	2
Blood leukocytes (mL)	≤ 4000 and ≤ 11,000	0
	< 4000 and > 11,000	1
	Band forms ≥ 50%	1
Tracheal secretions	Absent	0
	Nonpurulent	1
	Purulent	2
Oxygenation PaO$_2$/FiO$_2$ (mm Hg)	> 240 or ARDS	0
	≤ 240 and no ARDS	2
Pulmonary radiography	No infiltrate	0
	Diffuse or patchy infiltrate	1
	Localized infiltrate	2
DAY 3 SCORE AS ABOVE, AND ALSO		NO. OF POINTS
Pulmonary radiography	No progression	0
	Progression (CHF and ARDS	2
Culture of tracheal aspirate	No or rare growth of pathogenic bacteria	0
	Moderate to heavy growth of pathogenic bacteria	1
	Growth of pathogenic bacteria seen on Gram stain	1
Total score		**Score >6 correlates with pneumonia**

SOURCE: Singh N, Rogers P, Atwood CW, et al. Short-course empiric antibiotic therapy for patients with pulmonary infiltrates in the intensive care unit. A proposed solution for indiscriminate antibiotic prescription. *Am J Respir Crit Care Med.* 2000;162(2 Pt 1):505–511.

TABLE 78-5   Initial Empiric Antibiotics for HAP, VAP, and HCAP

For Patients with no Known Risk Factors for Drug-Resistant Pathogens, Early Onset, and of any Disease Severity

POTENTIAL PATHOGENS	ANTIBIOTIC

S. pneumoniae
H. influenzae
MSSA
Drug-sensitive enteric gram-negative rods (*Escherichia coli*,
   K. pneumoniae, *Enterobacter* species, *Proteus* species,
   Serratia marcescens)
	Ceftriaxone 2 g IV daily
	   or a fluoroquinolone:
	Ciprofloxacin 400 mg IV q 8 hours
	Levofloxacin 750 mg IV daily
	Moxifloxacin 400 mg IV daily
	or
	Ampicillin/sulbactam 3 g IV q 6 hour
	or
	Ertapenem 1 g IV daily

For Patients at High Tisk for Drug-Resistant Organisms and in Late-Onset Disease

POTENTIAL PATHOGENS	COMBINATION ANTIBIOTIC THERAPY

Pathogens listed above, plus MDR pathogens:
P. aeruginosa
K. pneumoniae (ESBL)
Acinetobacter species
L. pneumophilia
MRSA
	An antipseudomonal cephalosporin
	Cefepime 1–2 g IV q 8–12 hour
	Ceftazidime 2 g IV q 8 hour
	   or an antipseudomonal carbapenem
	Imipenem 500 mg q 6 hour or 1 g q 8 hour IV
	Meropenem 1 g IV q 8 hour
	or a beta-lactam/beta-lactamase inhibitor
	Piperacillin-tazobactam 4.5 g IV q 6 hour
	plus
	an antipseudomonal fluoroquinolone
	Ciprofloxacin 400 mg IV q 8 hour
	Levofloxacin 750 mg IV daily
	or
	an aminoglycoside
	Amikacin 20 mg/kg IV daily,
	   target trough level < 4–5 µg/mL
	Gentamicin 7 mg/kg IV daily,
	   target trough level < 1 µg/mL
	Tobramycin 7 mg/kg IV daily,
	   target trough level < 1 µg/mL
	plus
	Vancomycin 15 mg/kg IV q 12 hour,
	   target trough level 15–20 µg/mL, *or*
	Linezolid 600 mg IV q 12 hour

Source: American Thoracic Society, Infectious Diseases Society of America. Guidelines for the management of adults with hospital-acquired, ventilator-associated, and healthcare-associated pneumonia. *Am J Respir Crit Care Med.* 2005;171:388–416.

○ Clinical condition, including oxygenation and ventilation requirements, core temperature, and leukocytosis (repeat the modified CPIS)
○ Lower respiratory tract culture results
• When appropriate and timely initial antibiotics are used, the majority of patients respond within 48–72 hours. Avoid excessive antibiotic utilization that may promote the emergence of MDR pathogens by
○ Discontinuing antibiotics in patients for whom the diagnosis of HAP, VAP, or HCAP is not confirmed within 72 hours
■ Repeat the modified CPIS on day 3, including the two additional criteria (see Table 78-4). A score > 6 on CPIS has high correlation with pneumonia.

○ Narrowing antibiotic therapy based on culture and sensitivity data
○ Limiting the duration of antibiotic treatment—studies indicate that 8 days of therapy is sufficient, and associated with superior outcomes compared to 15 days of antibiotic therapy for VAP (except for culture-proven *Pseudomonas*)
• The failure to respond to appropriate therapy within 72 hours should prompt an investigation for
○ Infectious complications (empyema)
○ Other sources of infection
○ Alternative diagnoses in the differential (CHF, ARDS)
• Follow-up CXRs and respiratory cultures are not routinely indicated in patients with clinically resolving illness.

- Hospitalists can champion initiatives to reduce the incidence of VAP through implementation of patient safety/quality strategies such as ventilator bundles (see www.IHI.org). Care bundles are individual best practices that improve care/outcomes. Ventilated patients should
  - Be in semirecumbent rather than supine position (maintain the head of the bed to between 30 and 45 degrees)
  - Have daily lightening of sedation to assess readiness for removal of the ET tube
  - Receive stress ulcer/GI bleeding prophylaxis
  - Receive deep venous thrombosis prophylaxis (see Chap. 88)
- Although not part of the IHI ventilator bundle, also recommended are
  - Intense blood glucose regulation (80–110 mg/dL)
  - The use of enteral over parenteral feeding, when feasible

CARE TRANSITIONS

- Patients with HAP, VAP, or HCAP often undergo multiple transitions of care during their hospital stay. Accurate and timely communication between the hospitalist and intensivist is essential (see Chap. 13 on hand-offs).
- Discharge readiness for patients with HAP and VAP must include a reassessment of the initial illness that brought the patient to the hospital.
- Timely communication with outpatient providers regarding the hospital course, necessary follow-up, and reconciliation of discharge medications with home medicines (including possible drug–drug interactions, such as between coumadin and many antibiotics) are essential for a smooth transition of care to the outpatient setting.
  - For patients with MRSA, HAP, VAP, or HCAP, follow-up recommendations should include a consideration of colonization eradication strategies and screening cultures to assess clearance of colonization.

Bibliography

American Thoracic Society. Hospital-acquired pneumonia in adults: diagnosis, assessment of severity, initial antimicrobial therapy and preventive strategies. *Am J Respir Crit Care Med.* 1996;153:1711–1725.

American Thoracic Society, Infectious Diseases Society of America. Guidelines for the management of adults with hospital-acquired, ventilator-associated, and healthcare-associated pneumonia. *Am J Respir Crit Care Med.* 2005;171: 388–416.

Fagon JY, Chastre J, Wolff M, et al. Invasive and noninvasive strategies for management of suspected ventilator-associated pneumonia. A randomized trial. *Ann Intern Med.* 2000;132: 621–630.

Fortoukh M, Maitre B, Honore S, et al. Diagnosing pneumonia during mechanical ventilation: the clinical pulmonary infection score revisited. *Am J Respir Crit Care Med.* 2003;168: 173–179.

Mylotte JM. Nursing home-acquired pneumonia. *Clin Infect Dis.* 2002;35:1205–1211.

Singh N, Rogers P, Atwood CW, et al. Short-course empiric antibiotic therapy for patients with pulmonary infiltrates in the intensive care unit. A proposed solution for indiscriminate antibiotic prescription. *Am J Respir Crit Care Med.* 2000;162(2 Pt 1):505–511.

Tablan OC, Anderson LJ, Besser R, et al. Healthcare Infection Control Practices Advisory Committee, Centers for Disease Control and Prevention. Guidelines for preventing healthcare-associated pneumonia, 2003: recommendations of the CDC and the Healthcare Infection Control Practices Advisory Committee. *MMWR Recomm Rep.* 2004;53(RR-3):1–36.

79 COMPLICATIONS OF PNEUMONIA

Karen Catignani

EPIDEMIOLOGY/OVERVIEW

- Delayed or incomplete resolution of pneumonia despite apparently appropriate treatment is common, and may be owing to a noninfectious etiology, unusual pathogens, and/or host factors.
- Noninfectious causes account for up to 20% of the cases of delayed or incomplete resolution of pneumonia. Possibilities include
  - Cancer (bronchogenic carcinoma, bronchoalveolar carcinoma, lymphoma, and bronchial carcinoid tumors)
  - Inflammatory disorders (Wegener's granulomatosis, sarcoidosis, eosinophilic pneumonia, and BOOP)
  - Drug-induced lung injury (amiodarone toxicity, also methotrexate, bleomycin, and nitrofurantoin)
  - Occupational or chemical exposure

- Unusual pathogens should be considered, particularly if the patient has a previously unrecognized risk for multidrug resistance (MDR) pathogens, tuberculosis (TB), or fungi.
- Host factors also directly impact on the time course of resolution such as advanced age, unrecognized immune deficiency, the presence of diabetes, and other comorbidities.
  - The Centers for Disease Control (CDC) recommend routinely testing all patients age 15–54 who are admitted to the hospital for treatment of pneumonia to be tested for HIV status, as 1 in 1000 will be positive for the virus.
  - Primary humoral immune deficiencies, such as X-linked agammaglobulinemia, common variable immune deficiency, and selective IgG subset deficiencies, may require intravenous immune globulin.
  - Diabetic patients with hyperglycemia at the time of admission for community-acquired pneumonia (CAP) have a 5% increase in nosocomial complications as well as increased mortality and hospital length of stay (LOS), even after correcting for other known factors in the Pneumonia Severity Index (see Chap. 77).
- Complications of the pneumonia include parapneumonic effusion, empyema, lung abscess, and trapped lung, respiratory failure, acute respiratory distress syndrome (ARDS), and sepsis.
- Of patients admitted to the hospital with pneumonia, 10% to 15% will have a recurrence within 2 years. The majority of patients have chronic obstructive pulmonary disease (COPD) or aspiration risk factors.

NONRESOLVING PNEUMONIA

- Adequate response to antibiotics in the otherwise healthy adult can be measured by time to defervescence, resolution of symptoms, and normalization of white blood cell count and PO_2 levels, usually seen 3–5 days after initiation of treatment. This time frame is extended in elderly patients with pneumonia.
  - The rate of radiographic resolution is directly related to age and to a lesser degree to the rate of radiographic involvement.
  - About 80% of all patients of 40 years of age have complete radiographic resolution in 6 weeks after the initial diagnosis.
  - About 20% of all patients of 80 years of age have complete radiographic resolution at 6 weeks. (MKSAP *13* Syllabus, Pulmonary and Critical Care, Respiratory Infections).
- Bacteremic pneumonia may take up to 6–7 days to show clinical signs of resolution. See Fig. 79-1 for evaluation of the nonresolving pneumonia.

- Failure to respond to empiric antibiotics 48–72 hours after hospital admission has been associated with current tobacco use, alcohol abuse, or severe pneumonias associated with shock, respiratory failure, multilobar infiltrates, or pleural effusions at presentation. Though infrequent, patients with early failure subsequently have more complicated hospital courses and increased mortality, making it even more important to identify those at risk during initial assessment by history or radiographs (see Chap. 77 for more information on the assessment of pneumonia severity).
- Progression of pneumonia despite empiric broad-spectrum antibiotics has been reported in cases of bacteremic pneumococcal pneumonia, gram-negative pneumonia, and *Legionella* pneumonia.
- Tumor or foreign body causing an obstruction should be considered in patients whose pneumonia reoccurs in the same anatomic location.
- Though it is unreliable to acquire culture data from expectorated sputum once antibiotic treatment has begun, quantitative sputum cultures obtained by bronchoscopy and bronchoalveolar lavage (BAL) have been shown to be helpful up to 41% of the time in evaluation of nonresolving pneumonia.
- Chest x-rays (CXRs) may take several weeks to show radiographic improvement of pneumonia, and should not be done routinely to document resolution, but are often helpful in the diagnosis of parapneumonic effusions and lung abscess in patients who fail to respond to appropriate therapy. There is anecdotal evidence that in patients more than age 40 with a smoking history, a repeat CXR in 7–12 weeks can help rule out an obstructive malignancy.

PLEURAL EFFUSION

- The most common causes of pleural effusion are, in order, congestive heart failure (CHF), pneumonia, cancer, pulmonary embolus, viral disease, postcoronary artery bypass graft surgery (post-CABG), and cirrhosis with ascites. Up to 40% of patients with CAP develop pleural effusions, and roughly 10% will develop complicated parapneumonic effusions (CPE) or empyema.

EVALUATION OF PLEURAL EFFUSIONS

- Clinical judgment does not accurately identify those patients with empyema or significant inflammation that requires pleural drainage to obliterate the pleura

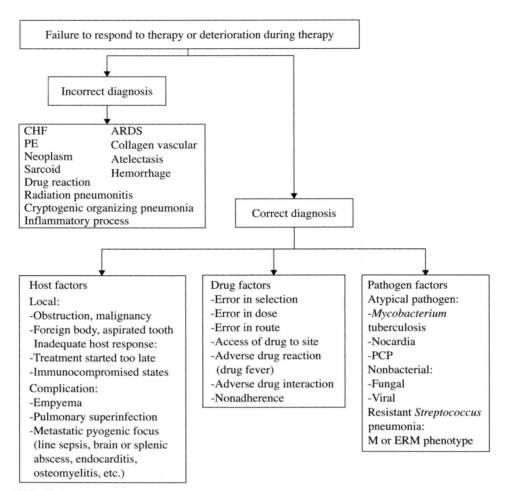

FIG. 79-1 Evaluation of nonresolving pneumonia.
SOURCE: Adapted from Bartlett JG, Dowell SF, Mandell LA, et al. Guidelines from the Infectious Diseases Society of America. Practice guidelines for the management of community-acquired pneumonia in adults. *Clin Infect Dis.* 2000;31:347–382.

space in order to avoid trapped lung. The indications for diagnostic thoracentesis include

○ Effusions that are > 1 cm in depth on a lateral decubitus chest film

○ An increasing pleural effusion or unilateral pleural effusion with persistent fever and tachycardia despite appropriate treatment

○ Radiographic findings that suggest a loculated effusion or an empyema (such as pleural-based opacity with an abnormal contour on CXR or a thickened parietal pleura on contrast chest computed tomography [CT])

• Ultrasonography can distinguish solid from liquid pleural abnormalities with roughly 92% accuracy and can be used to mark the area for the diagnostic tap. Combined with chest radiography, the accuracy increases to 98%.

• Chest CT is useful in identifying parenchymal infiltrates, mediastinal lymphadenopathy, or pleural abnormalities in the persistent undiagnosed pleural

effusion, and can help quantify the extent and loculation of the effusion cavity or the presence of a pleural rind prior to definitive drainage procedures. Spiral CT imaging provides additional information that can help diagnose pulmonary embolus.

• Fluid should be routinely tested for cell counts and differential, bacterial stains and culture, pH, lactate dehydrogenase (LDH), glucose, and protein if an exudative process is suspected (see Fig. 79-2 for the routine evaluation of pleural effusions).

• If pleural fluid (PF) clinically appears to be a transudate, but chemically meets criteria for an exudate, it can be beneficial to compare serum albumin to pleural albumin levels. A serum albumin level at least 1.2 g/dL higher than the albumin of the PF denotes transudative effusion in almost all cases. Otherwise, fluid samples that are "borderline" may prove to be either transudates or exudates.

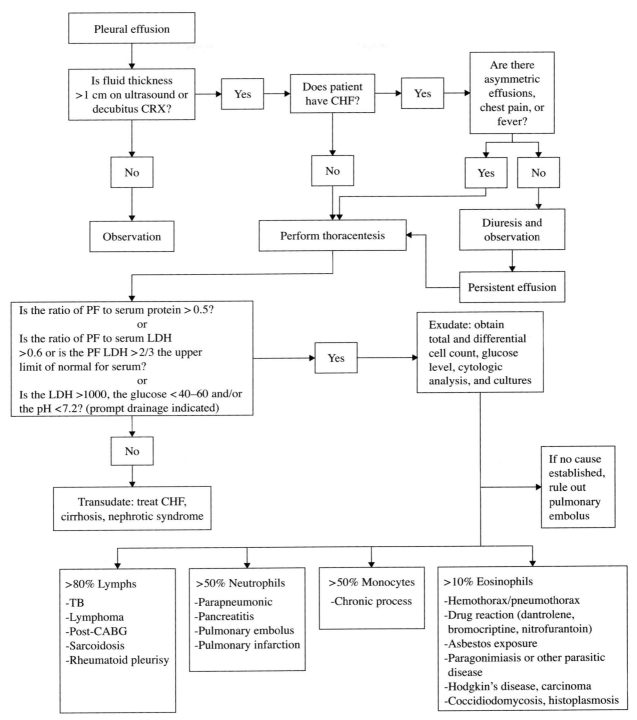

FIG. 79-2 Routine evaluation of pleural effusions.
SOURCE: Adapted from Light RW. Pleural effusion. *N Engl J Med.* 2002;346(25):1971–1977.

- Exudates are most likely the result of an inflammatory, malignant, or infectious condition. PF obtained after diuresis for CHF sometimes meets exudative criteria.

- In the cirrhotic with fever, encephalopathy, ascites, and pleural effusion, aspiration of both peritoneal and PF should be done. Like infected ascetic fluid, PF would have a high leukocyte count but low in protein.

- Bilateral effusions are usually transudates, though bilateral exudative effusions have been reported with malignancy, lupus pleuritis, and yellow nail syndrome.
- *Mycobacterium tuberculosis* (TB) should be suspected in all exudative, lymphocyte predominant pleural effusions. Up to one-third of patients with tuberculous pleuritis will have a false negative purified protein derivative (PPD) skin test. In TB pleural effusion, 50% of cases are reactivation TB with concomitant active TB and appropriate respiratory precautions should be taken in suspected cases. Further testing can be done on PF to establish the diagnosis of tuberculous pleuritis, including levels of adenosine deaminase (> 40 units/L has a high negative predictive value), interferon-γ (>140 pg/mL), acid-fast bacilli (AFB) culture, or performing polymerase chain reaction (PCR) for mycobacterial DNA.
- Low glucose levels in PF (< 60 mg/dL) are found most commonly in malignant or CPE, but can also be consistent with hemothorax, TB, rheumatoid pleuritis, and less commonly with Churg–Strauss syndrome, paragonimiasis, and lupus pleuritis.
- Cytology performed on PF will yield diagnosis up to 70% of the time in cases of metastatic adenocarcinoma. It is much less sensitive in the diagnosis of mesothelioma, lymphoma, squamous cell carcinoma, and sarcoma of the pleura. If malignancy is strongly suspected with negative PF cytology, a diagnostic tissue sample should be obtained by thoracoscopy.
- Generally, routine testing for amylase is not indicated unless there is a high pretest probability of detecting esophageal rupture or pancreatitis-associated effusions. The sensitivity of the test is too low to use as a screen for malignancy.
- Lipid analysis of pleural effusion is not warranted unless there is suspicion for chylothorax or cholesterol effusion by history or clinically by aspiration of milky-white liquid from the pleural space.

PARAPNEUMONIC EFFUSIONS AND EMPYEMA

- Parapneumonic effusions are classically exudative, meeting at least one of the following Light's criteria: PF or serum protein > 0.5, PF LDH or serum LDH > 0.6, or PF LDH > 0.67 of the upper limit of the laboratory's normal serum LDH value. The high sensitivity of these criteria in detecting exudates may classify up to 25% of transudative effusions as exudates. See Table 79-1 for the differential diagnosis of transudates and exudates.
- Uncomplicated parapneumonic effusions typically are minimal to moderate free-flowing effusions < one-third

TABLE 79-1 Differential Diagnosis of Transudative and Exudative Effusions

TRANSUDATE	EXUDATE
CHF	Malignancy
Cirrhosis/hepatic hydrothorax	Parapneumonic, especially anaerobic
Nephrotic syndrome	TB
Pulmonary embolus	Pulmonary embolus
Urinothorax	Viral or fungal disease
Myxedema	Pancreatic pseudocyst
CSF leak to pleura	Intra-abdominal abscess
	Post-CABG or cardiac injury
	Pericardial disease
	Meig's syndrome
	Ovarian hyperstimulation syndrome
	Rheumatoid pleuritis
	Lupus pleuritis
	Drug induced
	Yellow nail syndrome
	Asbestos pleural effusion
	Uremia
	Trapped lung
	Chylothorax/pseudochylothorax

SOURCE: Adapted from Light RW. The undiagnosed pleural effusion. *Clin Chest Med.* 2006;27:309–319.

hemithorax) and resolve with resolution of the pneumonia. Effusions ≥ one-half hemithorax should be drained.
- CPEs result from persistent bacterial invasion of the pleural space with resultant dense fibrin layer on the visceral and parietal fluid. Loculation can result in a condition referred to as trapped lung.
- PF measurements that connote a CPE and therefore warrant prompt drainage include pH < 7.2 (the most discriminative parameter of poor outcome), glucose level < 40–60 mg/dL, LDH > 1000 units, and a positive fluid culture or Gram stain. A white blood cell count > 50,000 per μL is always associated with CPE or empyema.
- Note that pH levels can vary widely between two areas of loculated pleura. It is also important to collect the pH sample directly from the chest cavity into a blood-gas syringe and place it on ice, avoiding using samples collected from other containers used to collect the PF.
- *Streptococcus milleri* is the leading pathogen found in empyema, although PF cultures are positive only 60% of the time. Other pathogens include *Streptococcus pneumoniae*, *Staphylococcus aureus*, gram-negative bacilli, and anaerobes.
- The distinction between CPEs and empyema is difficult, with the latter demonstrating purulence upon drainage as a result of fibroblast activation, scarring, and the accumulation of microorganisms as the infection progresses. Empyema is defined as gross

pus or a positive Gram stain. A positive pleural culture is not necessary to make the diagnosis. Pleural cultures may be negative because of prior antibiotic therapy, difficulty of culturing organisms, and loculation.

- Empyema begins as free-flowing purulent material, becoming more fibrinous and loculated over time, and can eventually form a pleural rind. There is a greater likelihood of treatment success when drainage is accomplished early. Failure to evacuate the fluid generally warrants surgical drainage.
- Empyema is a rare complication of CAP, occurring in 0.7% of cases, with declining mortality owed to improvement in antimicrobials, early detection, and aggressive treatment with chest tubes, image-guided catheters, thoracoscopy or thoracotomy with decortication of the pleural rind.
- For large, loculated, or established empyemas there is evidence that primary treatment with video-assisted thoracoscopic surgery (VATS) is superior to chest tube drainage as far as decreased hospital LOS and duration of chest tube placement.
- Adjunctive intrapleural fibrinolysis to disrupt loculations was thought to decrease the time to defervescence, duration of hospital stay, overall treatment failure, and need for surgical intervention according to several small published trials on CPE. However, in a recent randomized controlled trial (RCT), First Multicenter Intrapleural Sepsis Trial (MIST1) showed neither mortality benefit nor decreased need for surgical drainage in patients treated with intrapleural streptokinase for infected pulmonary fluid collections. There was no improvement on hospital LOS or studies of lung function. This data concurs with the most recent Cochrane Review conducted on the subject.
- After insertion of a chest tube, a chest CT is performed to evaluate chest tube placement. If you suspect malpositioning of the chest tube because of persistent fever, pain, and/or inadequate drainage, the best test remains a chest CT.
- Removal of the chest tube can occur when the pleural effusion has been completely evacuated from the pleural space, the lung is fully expanded, and the daily fluid output < 100–200 mL/d.
- For an excellent and practical guide to chest tube management, please refer to the chapter Chest Tubes in: Elefteriades JA, Cohen LS, Geha AS. House Officer Guide to ICU Care. Second Edition. New York. Raven Press. 1994.
- Therapy should be individualized to the patient, given a lack of definitive evidence-based treatment guidelines for choosing primarily noninvasive vs. surgical drainage.

LUNG ABSCESS

- Patients present with cough productive of foul-smelling sputum, weight loss, night sweats, fever, or digital clubbing. Immunocompromised patients are more likely to have gastrointestinal (GI) complaints, multiple abscesses, or aerobic organisms isolated from the abscess.
- Differential diagnosis includes Wegener's granulomatosis, rheumatoid nodules, pulmonary infarction, cavitation carcinoma, or atypical infections including TB or fungal species.
- Evident by an air-fluid level within a lung cavity, it is formed when a local area of infection and immune response causes damage to the parenchymal structure of the lung.
- Occurs in 4–5 cases per 10,000 hospital admissions.
- Most are multimicrobial and correlate with aspiration risk factors, stroke, alcoholism, epilepsy, dental caries, bronchial carcinoma, bronchiectasis, and post-anesthesia.
- Treatment usually requires 6–8 weeks of antibiotic therapy and should continue until abscess can no longer be seen on radiographic imaging.
- Medical management fails in approximately 10% of cases and should prompt drainage either percutaneously or by lobectomy, depending on practical limitations of size and location.

BIBLIOGRAPHY

Bartlett JG, Dowell SF, Mandell LA, et al. Guidelines from the Infectious Diseases Society of America. Practice guidelines for the management of community-acquired pneumonia in adults. *Clin Infect Dis*. 2000;31:347–382.

Cameron R, Davies HR. Intra-pleural fibrinolytic therapy versus conservative management in the treatment of parapneumonic effusions and empyema. The Cochrane Database of Systematic Reviews. *Cochrane Collab*. 2006;4.

Light RW. Pleural effusion. *N Engl J Med*. 2002;346(25): 1971–1977.

Light RW. The undiagnosed pleural effusion. *Clin Chest Med*. 2006;27:309–319.

Light RW. Parapneumonic effusions and empyema. *Proc Am Thorac Soc*. 2006;3:75–80.

Maskell NA, Davies CWH, Nunn AJ, et al. U.K. controlled trial of intrapleural streptokinase for pleural infection for the first multicenter intrapleural sepsis trial (MIST1) group. *N Engl J Med*. 2005;352:865–874.

Marrie TJ, Campbell GD, Walker DH, et al. Pneumonia. In: Kasper DL, Fauci AS, Longo DL, et al., eds. *Harrison's Priniciples of Internal Medicine*. 16th ed. New York, NY: McGraw-Hill; 2005:1536–1537.

McAlister FA, Majumdar SR, Blitz S, et al. The relation between hyperglycemia and outcomes in 2,471 patients admitted to the hospital with community-acquired pneumonia. *Diabetes Care.* 2005;28:810–815.

Misthos P, Sepsas E, Konstantinou M, et al. Early use of intrapleural fibrinolytics in the management of postpneumonic empyema. A prospective study. *Eur J Cardio-Thorac Surg.* 2005;28:599–603.

Rosón B, Carratalà J, Fernández-Sabé N, et al. Causes and factors associated with early failure in hospitalized patients with community-acquired pneumonia. *Arch Intern Med.* 2004;164:502–508.

80 SEPSIS AND SEPTIC SHOCK

William J. Janssen

EPIDEMIOLOGY/OVERVIEW

- Sepsis is a clinical syndrome that begins with a localized infection followed by systemic inflammation and widespread tissue injury.
  - Sepsis is the leading cause of death in the intensive care unit (ICU). There are more than 750,000 cases of sepsis in the United States each year, resulting in more than 210,000 deaths.
  - More than $16 billion a year are spent on sepsis treatment. The average cost to treat a patient with severe sepsis is $22,000.
  - The incidence of sepsis has doubled in the last two decades. Reasons for this increase include

- Aging of the population
- Development of antibiotic-resistant organisms
- Increased frequency of invasive procedures
- Increased number of immunocompromised patients

- As sepsis progresses, tissue hypoperfusion, hypotension, and organ damage develop. The severity of sepsis is best classified using criteria established by the American College of Chest Physicians and Society of Critical Care Medicine (Table 80-1). Note that mortality correlates with the severity of sepsis.

- It is important to remember that the systemic inflammatory response syndrome (SIRS) is a widespread inflammatory response that results from *any* insult (trauma, pancreatitis, transfusion reaction, etc.). SIRS that results from an infection is known as sepsis.

- The microbiology of sepsis is changing. At one time, gram-negative bacteria were the most common pathogens. Gram-positive bacteria are now more common and cause more than 50% of cases. Gram-negative bacteria comprise 40% of cases while fungi comprise slightly more than 5%. The incidence of fungal sepsis has steadily increased over the last decade.

- The term bacteremia indicates that bacteria have been cultured from the blood. Bacteremia does not have to be present for sepsis to occur.
  - The incidence of positive blood cultures increases with the stage of sepsis.
    - 17% of patients with sepsis have positive blood cultures
    - 69% of patients with septic shock have positive blood cultures
  - Within sepsis categories, the mortality of a patient with severe sepsis is the same, whether blood cultures are positive or negative.

TABLE 80-1 Stages of Sepsis

SEPSIS STAGE	FEATURES	MORTALITY
SIRS	Must have at least two of the following: (1) Temperature > 38°C or < 36°C (2) Heart rate > 90 beats/min (3) Respiratory rate > 20 breaths/min or $PaCO_2$ < 32 mm Hg (4) White blood cell count > 12,000 cells/mm³ or < 4000 cells/mm³, or > 10% immature (band) forms	7%
Sepsis	SIRS plus presumed infection*	16%
Severe sepsis	Sepsis with one of the following: (1) Organ dysfunction (see Table 80-2) (2) Hypoperfusion (3) Hypotension	20%
Septic shock	Sepsis with (1) Hypotension despite adequate fluid resuscitation† (2) Hypoperfusion	46%

*Diagnosis of infection does not require positive cultures. Infection can be presumed from infiltrates on a CXR, white cells in the urine, and so on.
†Patients who require vasopressors or inotropes despite adequate fluid resuscitation are in septic shock.

- Hospitalists may encounter patients with septic physiology at any point during their hospitalization—in the emergency department, on the medical or surgical floors, or through their leadership of rapid response or code teams.
- Hospitalists have an opportunity to improve outcomes by triaging to the best inpatient setting and by developing and expediting initial treatment protocols.

PATHOPHYSIOLOGY

- Sepsis results from complex interactions between the infecting microorganism and the host inflammatory, coagulation, and immune responses.
- Early sepsis is characterized by a proinflammatory state in which neutrophils are activated and high levels of inflammatory cytokines are released.
- Proteases, prostaglandins, and leukotrienes released from inflammatory cells damage the vascular endothelium. This results in leakage of protein-rich fluid from the capillaries and release of nitric oxide, a potent vasodilator.
- Vasodilation of the arterial capillary networks and venous capacitance beds can lead to a drop in the peripheral vascular resistance and relative hypovolemia.
- Patients with sepsis also develop hypovolemia because of
  - Decreased oral fluid intake
  - Insensible losses
    - Increased exhaled moisture from tachypnea and hyperventilation
    - Excess perspiration from fever
  - Urine output (UO) may be increased in early sepsis (even if the kidneys are underperfused) because of high circulating levels diuretic hormones
- In most patients the cardiac output is high (as a result of low peripheral vascular tone). This explains the commonly seen "pink and warm" appearance. As sepsis progresses, myocardial suppression may occur leading to inadequate cardiac output.
- Maldistribution of flow is common in sepsis. Blood flow is preferentially shunted from the myocardium, skeletal muscles, gut, and pancreas to the kidneys and brain. This leads to regional hypoperfusion.
- Perfusion is also impaired on a microscopic level.
  - Injury to the vascular endothelium coupled with a procoagulant state leads to platelet aggregation and microvascular thrombosis. In a severe form this is known as DIC—disseminated intravascular coagulation.

TABLE 80-2 Organ Dysfunction Criteria

Cardiovascular	Systolic BP ≤ 90 mm Hg or MAP ≤ 70 mm Hg for at least 1 hour despite adequate volume resuscitation or vasopressors required to achieve the same goals
Renal	UO < 0.5 mL/kg body weight per hour or acute renal failure
Pulmonary	$PaO_2/FiO_2 ≤ 250$ if other organ dysfunction present
	$PaO_2/FiO_2 ≤ 200$ if no other organ dysfunction present
Hematologic	Platelets < 80,000 per mm^3 or decrease of 50% over 3 days
Metabolic	pH ≤ 7.30 or base deficit > 5.0 mmol/L *and* plasma lactate > 1.5 (upper limit of normal)

Abbreviations: BP, blood pressure; MAP, mean airway pressure.

- Direct blockage of the microvasculature by thrombi impairs downstream flow.
- Erythrocytes become rigid and lose their ability to deform in the microcirculation.
- Cellular metabolism is increased during sepsis. This results in increased oxygen demand. However, the previously described abnormalities result in decreased oxygen delivery (Table 80-2). The end result is cellular hypoxia. Prolonged tissue hypoxia leads to multiorgan failure and death.

CLINICAL PRESENTATION, DIFFERENTIAL, MAKING THE DIAGNOSIS

- A delay in treatment is the biggest factor contributing to poor outcomes. Thus recognizing early sepsis is paramount. One should look for evidence of infection in any patient with SIRS (Table 80-3).
- The history and physical examination should focus on potential sources of infection (Table 80-4).
- Sepsis is a form of distributive shock (Table 80-5).
  - Distributive shock is characterized by vasodilation, low peripheral vascular resistance, and a high cardiac output.
  - Common physical findings include
    - Tachycardia, tachypnea, fever (each are SIRS criteria).
    - Orthostatic hypotension.
    - A hyperdynamic precordium.
    - Extremities that are warm and pink. In severe sepsis and septic shock, the skin can be cool and mottled as a result of hypoperfusion.
    - Encephalopathy/altered mental status.

TABLE 80-3 Factors Contributing to Imbalance between Oxygen Delivery and Demand

DECREASED OXYGEN DELIVERY	INCREASED OXYGEN DEMAND
Hypotension	Increased cellular metabolism
Vasodilation	
Arterial capillary beds	
Venous capacitance beds	
Hypovolemia	
Decreased oral intake	
Insensible fluid losses	
Capillary leak	
Myocardial suppression	
Microvascular thrombosis	
DIC	
Erythrocyte rigidity	
Maldistribution of flow	
Microscopic (capillary level)	
Organ specific	
Anemia	
Bleeding	
Hemodilution following volume	
resuscitation	

TRIAGE AND INITIAL MANAGEMENT

- Resuscitation is the first step in management of a patient with sepsis to assess the airway, respiration, and perfusion.

AIRWAY

- Supplemental oxygen should be supplied to all patients.
- Continuous pulse oximetry should be employed to ensure oxygen saturation > 90%.
- Patients with encephalopathy may require intubation for airway protection.

RESPIRATION

- Mechanical ventilation should be considered in patients with unstable blood pressure (BP), severe sepsis, or septic shock.

TABLE 80-4 Common Sources of Sepsis

Pneumonia
Urinary tract infections
Intra-abdominal infections
Cholecystitis/ascending cholangitis
Diverticulitis
Appendicitis
Peritonitis
GI infections
Clostridium difficile colitis
Catheter-related infections
Septic arthritis
Soft tissue infections
Meningitis
Postsurgical sites

TABLE 80-5 Causes of Distributive Shock

Sepsis
Anaphylaxis and anaphylactoid reactions
Acute adrenal insufficiency (Addisonian crisis)
Thyroid storm
Transfusion reactions
Severe pancreatitis
Toxic shock syndrome
Neurogenic shock after CNS or spinal cord injury
Postcardiopulmonary bypass

Abbreviation: CNS, central nervous system.

- Etomidate is an ultrashort-acting hypnotic agent commonly used as an induction agent for intubation. It should be avoided in sepsis because it can cause adrenal insufficiency and may increase mortality.

PERFUSION

- Restoration of tissue perfusion is paramount. Delays result in tissue ischemia, organ failure, and death.
- Tissue perfusion can be improved by correcting hypovolemia, improving BP, and augmenting oxygen delivery.
- Intravenous fluids should be administered *immediately* after the sepsis syndrome is recognized. Fluid resuscitation can proceed through any available intravenous access; however in patients with severe sepsis or septic shock, a central venous catheter should be placed to facilitate fluid administration and monitoring of venous filling pressures.
- Patients with severe sepsis or septic shock represent a particularly sick group of patients. Early goal-directed therapy has been shown to improve mortality in these individuals. Goals of therapy for the first 6 hours include
  - Central venous pressure (CVP) 8–12 mm Hg
  - Mean arterial pressure > 65 mm Hg
  - UO > 0.5 mL/kg/hr
  - Central venous (S_cvO_2) or mixed venous oxygen saturation ≥ 70%. (A central or mixed venous oxygen saturation < 70% indicates that tissues are starved for oxygen.)
- These goals are best achieved by sequential correction of hypovolemia, hypotension, and oxygen delivery.
- There is no evidence to suggest that colloids are superior to crystalloids.
- The volume of distribution is greater for crystalloids than colloids.
- Larger volumes are therefore required to achieve the same endpoints.
  - Crystalloids (eg, normal saline [NS], Ringer's lactate) should be administered at a rate of 500–1000 mL over 30 minutes.
  - Colloids should be given at a rate of 300–500 mL over 30 minutes.

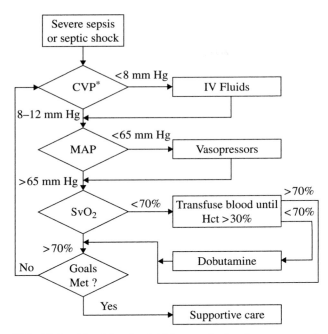

FIG. 80-1 Algorithm for initial resuscitation in severe sepsis and septic shock.
*This algorithm should be instituted immediately after the identification of severe sepsis or septic shock. Goals of care should be met as quickly as possible and in < 6 hours.
*CVP should be measured through a central venous catheter in the internal jugular or subclavian vein.
SOURCE: Adapted from Rivers E, Nguyen B, Havstad S, et al. Early goal-directed therapy in the treatment of severe sepsis and septic shock. *N Engl J Med.* 2001;345(19):1368–1377.

- Resuscitation endpoints (CVP, mean airway pressure [MAP], S_cvO_2, UO) should be assessed immediately after each fluid bolus. Intravenous fluid boluses should be repeated until resuscitation endpoints are met, pulmonary edema develops, or the pulmonary capillary wedge pressure is exceeds 18 mm Hg.
- ○ Most patients require 6–10 L of crystalloid for initial resuscitation.
- ○ Be sure to immediately correct hypovolemia prior to initiating treatment with vasoconstrictors to avoid digital gangrene.

VASOPRESSORS
- ○ Vasopressors are required for patients who remain hypotensive despite adequate fluid resuscitation. Norepinephrine and dopamine should be used as first-line agents.
- ○ *Norepinephrine* is a potent alpha-adrenergic agonist that induces peripheral vasoconstriction with minimal cardiac effects. The starting dose is 0.01 μg/kg/min.

- ○ *Dopamine* is an immediate precursor to norepinephrine and epinephrine. Its effects are dose dependent.
  - At doses < 5 μg/kg/min, the predominant effect is on dopamine receptors in the renal, cardiac, and mesenteric circulation. The result is vasodilation in these organs.
  - Doses between 5 and 10 μg/kg/min cause beta-1-adrenergic receptor stimulation resulting in increased myocardial contractility and heart rate (HR).
  - At doses > 10 μg/kg/min, alpha-adrenergic effects predominate resulting in arterial vasoconstriction and an increase in BP.
- ○ *Vasopressin* is an antidiuretic hormone (ADH) analog with weak vasoconstrictive effects. It is not recommended as a first-line agent for septic shock, but may have a role in refractory cases. Two small studies have suggested that a fixed dose (0.04 U/min) may lower norepinephrine requirements and improve creatinine clearance. More studies are needed to determine if its use is superior to norepinephrine alone. Because of ADH effects, sodium balance must be monitored carefully during drug administration and for several days after cessation.
- ○ *Phenylephrine* is a pure alpha-1-agonist with profound vasoconstricting effects. It has minimal beta-adrenergic activity and is useful in patients with arrhythmias or significant tachycardia. Some concern has been raised about its potential to reduce HR and cardiac output.

INOTROPES
- ○ Myocardial suppression is common in sepsis. In patients who have continued hypoperfusion despite correction of hypovolemia and hypotension, inotropic support may help boost cardiac output and thus improve oxygen delivery.
- ○ *Dobutamine* functions primarily as a beta-1-adrenergic receptor agonist. At doses between 3 and 12 μg/kg/min the cardiac index can be augmented by 20% to 30%. Peripheral vasodilation and tachycardia can result; therefore dobutamine is often used with a vasoconstrictor such as norepinephrine.

DISEASE MANAGEMENT STRATEGIES

CONTROL OF THE SEPTIC FOCUS

- Prompt identification and control of the infection site is essential.
  - ○ A careful history and physical examination often provide clues to the source of infection.

○ Blood cultures, a chest radiograph, and urinalysis with culture are recommended for all patients.

○ Additional diagnostic studies (such as abdominal CT or lumbar puncture) should be driven by clinical clues.

• The time to initiation of antibiotic therapy is the strongest predictor of mortality.

○ Inappropriate initial antibiotic selection is unfortunately common and occurs in up to one-third of cases.

○ When the source of infection is unknown, broad-spectrum antibiotics should be administered. A regimen should be chosen that provides coverage against gram-positive and gram-negative bacteria.

• The rates of methicillin-resistant *Staphylococcus aureus* (MRSA) infections are increasing in both hospitalized patients and in the community. Intravenous vancomycin should be considered in all patients until the possibility of MRSA has been excluded.

• Once a pathogen has been isolated, antibiotic therapy should be tailored to provide more narrow and appropriate coverage.

• Care should be taken with antibiotic dosing. Renal function can deteriorate quickly in septic patients; serum creatinine (SCr) should be measured daily.

STEROIDS AND THE ADRENAL AXIS

• The use of corticosteroids in severe sepsis and septic shock is controversial.

• Evidence suggests that a large proportion of critically ill patients suffer from relative adrenal insufficiency.

○ This defect can result from dysfunction of the hypothalamus, pituitary, or adrenal glands—all of which may be impaired by the high cytokine levels of sepsis.

○ Adrenal impairment can also result from hemorrhage, drug effects (including etomidate), and direct infection (such as HIV).

• Adrenal function is commonly assessed by obtaining serum cortisol levels immediately before administration of adrenocorticotropin-releasing hormone (ACTH) and after 60 minutes.

○ A baseline cortisol level < 15 µg/dL is generally regarded as insufficient in a critically ill patient.

○ The optimum dose of ACTH is unknown. Many experts recommend using 250 µg IV.

○ One multicenter, RCT of patients with septic shock showed a reduction in mortality in patients with relative adrenal insufficiency (defined by a post-ACTH cortisol level increase ≤ 9 µg/dL) who were treated with 200 mg hydrocortisone daily in four divided doses and once daily fludrocortisone (50 µg orally) for 7 days. Treatment with hydrocortisone did not improve outcome in responders to ACTH (ie, change in cortisol > 9 µg/dL).

TABLE 80-6 Guidelines for Determining the Need for Corticosteroids in Septic Shock

Baseline cortisol	< 15 µg/dL	15–34 µg/dL		> 34 µg/dL
Change in cortisol following ACTH		≤ 9 µg/dL	> 9 µg/dL	
Corticosteroids indicated?	Yes	Yes	No	No

○ Two additional small RCTs demonstrated significant effects on shock reversal with hydrocortisone.

• Patients in septic shock with a baseline cortisol level > 34 µg/dL are at high risk for death. Since their adrenal glands are capable of producing cortisol, it is unlikely that they will benefit from steroid replacement.

• The best evidence suggests that all patients with septic shock should undergo an ACTH stimulation test. Hydrocortisone (50 mg IV four times daily) should be administered until test results have returned.

• The following algorithm (Table 80-6) can serve as a guide for determining when to continue corticosteroid treatment.

• Ongoing multicenter trials should help to clarify the use of corticosteroids in the septic patient.

ACTIVATED PROTEIN C

• Sepsis is characterized by activation of procoagulant pathways, impaired fibrinolysis, and microvascular thrombosis. Activated protein C (APC) counteracts these abnormalities.

• At present, the only available form of recombinant human APC is drotrecogin alpha (Xigris).

• Clinical trials have demonstrated a significant survival benefit in patients with severe sepsis or septic shock who receive drotrecogin alpha within the first 48 hours of diagnosis. The benefit is more pronounced when therapy is started within 24 hours.

• Patients who are sicker benefit most.

○ Patients with only one organ failure do not benefit.

○ Patients with an APACHE II (Acute Physiology and Chronic Health Evaluation II) score < 25 do not benefit.

○ The APACHE II scoring system is a tool that predicts ICU mortality based on the patient's age, the presence of chronic disease, and physiologic and laboratory variables. Sicker patients have higher scores. The APACHE II score is most easily calculated by going to the Internet. APACHE calculators can be found at a number of sites including www.globalrph.com/xigris.htm and www.sfar.org/scores2/apache22.html

TABLE 80-7 Contraindications to the Use of Drotrecogin Alpha

CONTRAINDICATIONS	WARNINGS
Active internal bleeding	GI bleed within 6 weeks
Hemorrhagic stroke in last 3 months	Ischemic stroke in last 3 months
CNS trauma in last 2 months	Recent anticoagulation (subcutaneous heparin is ok)
Trauma with bleeding risk	Administration of aspirin > 650 mg or other platelet inhibitors within 7 days
Epidural catheter in place	
Intracranial mass lesion, arteriovenous malformation, or aneurysm	Thrombolytic therapy within 3 days
Known bleeding diathesis	Platelets < 30,000 per μL
Severe chronic liver disease	INR > 3.0
Pregnancy	Chronic renal failure requiring hemodialysis

Abbreviation: INR, international normalized ratio.

- Drotrecogin alpha is administered as a constant infusion for 96 hours at a rate of 24 μg/kg/hr.
- The major risk of drotrecogin alpha is bleeding.
  - In the largest trial evaluating drotrecogin alpha, 2.4% of patients experienced a serious bleeding event compared to 1% in the placebo group.
  - Bleeding risk is greatest during the infusion period. The infusion should be stopped 2 hours before surgery or invasive procedures. The drug can be started 12 hours after surgery or 2 hours after less invasive procedures (such as uncomplicated central line placement).
  - Bleeding risk is greatest in patients with a platelet count < 30,000 per μL. Interestingly, patients with DIC are the ones that benefit most. If platelet levels drop below 30,000 per μL during the course of infusion, platelets should be transfused.
- Contraindications and warnings for drotrecogin relate primarily to bleeding risk (see Table 80-7). Studies in children have shown no mortality benefit and demonstrate increased risk of intracranial hemorrhage.

CARE TRANSITIONS

- Patients who develop severe sepsis or septic shock should be transferred to the ICU. Intravenous fluids should be started immediately after the diagnosis of sepsis has been made. Fluid administration should not wait for transfer.
- It is safe to transfer patients from the ICU once sepsis has resolved, the patient has been weaned from vasopressors, and the primary infection has been controlled.
- If corticosteroids have been used to treat septic shock they should be continued for the full 7-day course, even if vasopressors have been successfully weaned.

There is the potential for rebound hypotension if steroids are discontinued too quickly.
- Many patients who survive sepsis have muscle weakness and deconditioning. Physical and occupational therapy should be consulted in these individuals. Speech and swallowing evaluation should be considered for individuals who required mechanical ventilation.
- If patient care is being transferred to a new medical team or physician, direct verbal communication is important. Key information includes
  - Any information that may not be readily apparent from progress notes
  - Results of family meetings, including any end-of-life discussions, family expectations, and unresolved issues
  - Incidental findings that require follow-up postdischarge
  - Identification of consultants who will see patient posthospitalization

BIBLIOGRAPHY

Absalom A, Pledger D, Kong A. Adrenocortical function in critically ill patients 24 h after a single dose of etomidate. *Anaesthesia.* 1999;54(9):861–867.

Annane D, Sebille V, Charpentier C, et al. Effect of treatment with low doses of hydrocortisone and fludrocortisone on mortality in patients with septic shock. *JAMA.* 2002;288(7):862–871.

Annane D, Sebille V, Troche G, et al. A 3-level prognostic classification in septic shock based on cortisol levels and cortisol response to corticotropin. *JAMA.* 2000;283(8):1038–1045.

Angus DC, Linde-Zwirble WT, Lidicker J, et al. Epidemiology of severe sepsis in the United States: analysis of incidence, outcome, and associated costs of care. *Crit Care Med.* 2001;29(7):1303–1310.

Bernard GR, Vincent JL, Laterre PF, et al. Efficacy and safety of recombinant human activated protein C for severe sepsis. *N Engl J Med.* 2001;344(10):699–709.

Brun-Buisson C, Doyon F, Carlet J. Bacteremia and severe sepsis in adults: a multicenter prospective survey in ICUs and wards of 24 hospitals. French Bacteremia-Sepsis Study Group. *Am J Respir Crit Care Med.* 1996;154(3 Pt 1):617–624.

Cooper MS, Stewart PM. Corticosteroid insufficiency in acutely ill patients. *N Engl J Med.* 2003;348(8):727–734.

Dellinger RP, Carlet JM, Masur H, et al. Surviving Sepsis Campaign guidelines for management of severe sepsis and septic shock. *Crit Care Med.* 2004;32(3):858–873.

Dunser MW, Mayr AJ, Ulmer H, et al. Arginine vasopressin in advanced vasodilatory shock: a prospective, randomized, controlled study. *Circulation.* 2003;107(18):2313–2319.

Kumar A, Roberts D, Wood KE, et al. Duration of hypotension before initiation of effective antimicrobial therapy is the critical determinant of survival in human septic shock. *Crit Care Med.* 2006;34(6):1589–1596.

Leibovici L, Paul M, Poznanski O, et al. Monotherapy versus beta-lactam-aminoglycoside combination treatment for gram-negative bacteremia: a prospective, observational study. *Antimicrob Agents Chemother.* 1997;41(5):1127–1133.

Levy MM, Fink MP, Marshall JC, et al. 2001 SCCM/ESICM/ACCP/ATS/SIS International Sepsis Definitions Conference. *Crit Care Med.* 2003;31(4):1250–1256.

Martin GS, Mannino DM, Eaton S, et al. The epidemiology of sepsis in the United States from 1979 through 2000. *N Engl J Med.* 2003;348(16):1546–1554.

Patel BM, Chittock DR, Russell JA, et al. Beneficial effects of short-term vasopressin infusion during severe septic shock. *Anesthesiology.* 2002;96(3):576–582.

Rackow EC, Falk JL, Fein IA, et al. Fluid resuscitation in circulatory shock: a comparison of the cardiorespiratory effects of albumin, hetastarch, and saline solutions in patients with hypovolemic and septic shock. *Crit Care Med.* 1983;11(11):839–850.

Rivers E, Nguyen B, Havstad S, et al. Early goal-directed therapy in the treatment of severe sepsis and septic shock. *N Engl J Med.* 2001;345(19):1368–1377.

Vincent JL, Bernard GR, Beale R, et al. Drotrecogin alfa (activated) treatment in severe sepsis from the global open-label trial ENHANCE: further evidence for survival and safety and implications for early treatment. *Crit Care Med.* 2005;33(10):2266–2277.

Vincent JL, Angus DC, Artigas A, et al. Effects of drotrecogin alfa (activated) on organ dysfunction in the PROWESS trial. *Crit Care Med.* 2003;31(3):834–840.

81 VENTILATORY SUPPORT

Joshua J. Solomon, Ryan McGhan, and William J. Janssen

EPIDEMIOLOGY/OVERVIEW

- Many patients with severe hypoxemia may be able to avoid invasive mechanical intubation with timely intervention.
- Hospitalists and respiratory therapists are often members of the rapid response team and also available as needed to patients in respiratory distress.
- Hospitalists can work with respiratory therapists and nurses to determine what the patient might need, such as noninvasive positive pressure ventilation (NIPPV) and/or oxygen and aerosol therapy before the oxygen requirements escalate to the point of intubation.

- Whenever a hypoxemic patient requires a high-flow nonrebreather mask or high-flow oxygen administration, hospitalists should assess the need for ventilatory support.
- Hospitalists should work with nurses and respiratory therapists to optimize oxygen delivery because invasive mechanical ventilation carries risks that can be avoided by utilizing noninvasive strategies for appropriate patients.
- Hospitalists can lead initiatives that ensure standardized procedures are in place for all inpatients requiring ventilatory support.

NONINVASIVE POSITIVE PRESSURE VENTILATION

DEFINITION

- NIPPV is positive pressure ventilation provided through a mask instead of an endotracheal tube.
- NIPPV can be delivered as continuous (also known as CPAP or continuous positive airway pressure, equivalent to positive end-expiratory pressure or PEEP) or bilevel (with set pressure support [PS] and PEEP).

GOALS OF NONINVASIVE POSITIVE PRESSURE VENTILATION
- NIPPV is used to provide short-term and nighttime ventilation to acutely hypoxemic patients who are able to cooperate and tolerate the mask.

COMMON INDICATIONS
- NIPPV is highly effective in patients with acute ventilatory failure from COPD and cardiogenic pulmonary edema.
- It may be used for other forms of acute ventilatory and respiratory failure, though the data supporting efficacy are less clear.
- Data are also unclear on the role of NIPPV for weaning from mechanical ventilation and postextubation respiratory failure.
- Chronic conditions that may benefit from NIPPV include neuromuscular disorders and obstructive sleep apnea.

RELATIVE CONTRAINDICATIONS
- NIPPV is not appropriate for patients who are unable to protect the airway caused by decreased level of consciousness (though it may reverse CO_2 narcosis in patients with ventilatory failure).
- NIPPV is not the treatment of choice for patients with shock or severe hemodynamic instability despite fluid resuscitation, patients with multiorgan system failure, or patients unable to clear copious secretions. See Table 81-1 for relative contraindications.

TABLE 81-1 Relative Contraindications to NIPPV

Facial burns, facial or head trauma, or surgery, esophageal surgery
Hemodynamic instability (shock, significant ventricular arrhythmias)
Inability to clear respiratory secretions and requirement for airway
  protection by intubation
Severely decreased mental status
Active upper GI bleeding
Inability to cooperate or tolerate mask
Pneumocephalus

INITIATION OF NIPPV

- Respiratory therapy will help select the appropriate interface and adjust for optimal settings that include inspiratory positive airway pressure (IPAP), expiratory airway pressure (EPAP), and FiO_2.
  - In general, avoid settings that create a peak IPAP > 20 cm which can increase the risk for aspiration.
- Patients need frequent evaluation to assess tolerance of the mask and need for subsequent intubation. When first initiated for respiratory failure, patient monitoring includes
  - Continuous electrocardiogram (ECG) and O_2 saturation
  - Vital signs every 15 minutes for the first hour, then every 30 minutes, followed by every 1–2 hours depending on stability
  - Mental status assessment
  - Presence of secretions and ability to clear them
- Emergent considerations for intubation include
  - Inability to cooperate or tolerate mask or need for restraints
  - Deterioration of PO_2 < 80 mm Hg or respiratory rate > 35
  - Further cognitive decline
  - Development of arrhythmias, myocardial ischemia (chest pain), hemodynamic instability, or deteriorating vital signs

MECHANICAL VENTILATION

INITIATING MECHANICAL VENTILATION

- Mechanical ventilators are used in patients with (1) *respiratory failure* or (2) *an inability to maintain a patent and safe airway.*
  1. Respiratory failure encompasses both ventilatory and hypoxemic failure
     - *Ventilatory respiratory failure* refers to an inability to adequately maintain alveolar ventilation and is characterized by a PCO_2 > 50 mm Hg on arterial blood gas sampling.
     - Causes of ventilatory respiratory failure include central respiratory depression, neuromuscular

disorders, medication overdoses (see Chap. 69), thoracic cage deformities, and airway obstruction.
  - *Hypoxemic respiratory failure* refers to an inability to maintain a PO_2 > 60 mm Hg on arterial blood gas measurement.
  - Causes of hypoxemic respiratory failure include pulmonary edema (see Chaps. 29 and 30), pneumonia, ARDS, atelectasis, pulmonary contusion, and pulmonary embolism (see Chap. 89).
  2. Patients with altered sensorium or mechanical obstruction of the upper airway may require endotracheal intubation and mechanical ventilation to secure a safe and patent airway.
     - Ultimately, the decision to initiate mechanical ventilation is a clinical decision that takes into account both the established criteria as well as the provider's judgment of the severity of the patient's illness and the ability to sustain the work of breathing necessary to match respiratory demand (see Table 81-2).

TYPES OF MECHANICAL VENTILATION DELIVERED BY ENDOTRACHEAL TUBE

- Mechanical ventilation modes are classified based on the preset variable for breath termination.
- *Volume cycling* is the most common mode of mechanical ventilation. The ventilator delivers flow until a preset volume is reached. In this mode, airway pressures during inspiration are variable and are dependent on the compliance of the lungs. Lungs with low compliance will have higher pressures at a given inspiratory volume than lungs with high compliance.
  - *Controlled mechanical ventilation (CMV)*—In CMV, the clinician sets the V_t, f, PEEP, and FiO_2. The ventilator also has a set V_e and delivers the predetermined number of breaths per minute. Patient-initiated breaths are not sensed by the ventilator and do not contribute to the overall minute ventilation (in other words, the patient is unable to "overbreathe" the ventilator).
  - *Assist-control (A/C)*—In A/C, the clinician sets the V_t, f, PEEP, and FiO_2. Each time the ventilator senses an inspiratory effort, a full V_t is delivered. If a patient does not initiate spontaneous breaths, the ventilator delivers breaths at the preset f. The ventilator therefore has a minimum V_e ($V_t \times f$) based on the set parameters. A higher V_e can be achieved if the patient "over-breathes" the set f. A/C is the most commonly used ventilator mode and minimizes the patient's work of breathing during spontaneous breathing.

TABLE 81-2   Ventilator Definitions

- Ventilator settings that the operator enters into the ventilator are defined as follows:
  - **Tidal Volume (V_t)** is volume of a delivered ventilator breath in milliliters.
  - **Respiratory rate (f)** is the number of breaths delivered by the ventilator in 1 minute.
  - **PEEP** refers to the positive pressure maintained in a patient's airways by the ventilator at the end of expiration.
  - **PS** is the pressure sustained by the ventilator once a patient initiates a breath. This pressure is sustained until inspiratory flow tapers to a preset level. In a PS mode, V_t is determined by patient effort.
  - **Fraction of inspired oxygen (FiO_2)** is the percentage of oxygen present in inspired gas. Room air has an FiO_2 of 21%.

Important physiologic parameters that can be measured from the ventilator include
- **Plateau pressure (P_{plat})** is the pressure at the end of inspiration.
  - It is measured during a manual breath hold on the ventilator at the end of inhalation.
  - Because there is no air movement at the time of measurement, this is also known as "static pressure."
  - Plateau pressure represents the force exerted on inflated lungs by the relaxation of the respiratory muscles and the elastic recoil of the lung tissue.
  - Normal values range from 10 to 25 cm H_2O.
  - Causes of elevated plateau pressures are listed in Table 81-1. Patient effort can affect the ventilator reading of plateau pressure.
- **Peak pressure (P_{pk})** is the highest recorded pressure during inspiratory flow on volume control ventilation (see below).
  - It represents the resistance to airflow in the ventilatory circuit including the endotracheal tube and conducting airways.
  - Because air is moving at the time of measurement, peak pressure is a "dynamic pressure."
  - Normal values range from 10 to 30 cm H_2O.
  - Causes of elevated peak pressures are listed in Table 81-2. Patient effort can affect the ventilator reading of a peak pressure.
- **MAP** is the mean pressure throughout the respiratory cycle measured in cm H_2O.
- **Minute ventilation (V_e)** is the total volume of air that a patient breathes in 1 minute.
  - It is the product of the tidal volume and the respiratory rate ($V_t \times f$) and is expressed in liters/minute.
  - Normal V_e during spontaneous respiration is <10 L/min.
- **Compliance** refers to the relationship between lung volume and pressure.
  - It is represented by the equation $\Delta v/\Delta p$ (change in volume over change in pressure, expressed in mL/cm H_2O).
  - Normal compliance is 50–170 mL/cm H_2O.
  - Anything that restricts expansion of the chest wall or increases the "stiffness" of the lung parenchyma will lower lung compliance. Poorly compliant lungs will have a small change in volume for a given applied pressure.
  - Examples of processes that decrease measured lung compliance include pulmonary edema, ARDS, pneumonia, and obesity.
  - When the alveolar septa are lost in a disease such as emphysema, the lungs have a high compliance. Emphysematous lungs have a large change in volume for a given pressure.
- **I:E ratio** is the ratio of time spent in inspiration vs. the time spent in expiration during a ventilator-delivered breath.
  - An I:E ratio of 1:2 means one-third of the time is inspiration and two-thirds of the time is expiration.
  - The amount of time that a patient spends in each part of the respiratory cycle depends on the respiratory rate. For example, if the respiratory rate is 10 breaths/min, each breath must take 6 seconds. An I:E ratio of 1:2 implies that the inspiratory time is 2 seconds and expiratory time is 4 seconds.

- *Intermittent mandatory ventilation (IMV)*—In IMV, the clinician sets the V_t, f, PEEP, and FiO_2. The ventilator delivers a mandatory breath at regular intervals based on the set f and V_t. A minimum V_e is therefore established. In addition, the patient is allowed to breathe spontaneously through the ventilator circuit. The volume of the spontaneous breath is determined entirely by the patient. The total V_e that the patient receives is the sum of the set V_t and the spontaneous V_t. This mode increases the patient's work of breathing during a spontaneous breath but may improve patient comfort.
- *Synchronized intermittent mandatory ventilation (SIMV)*—SIMV is a special form of IMV. Like IMV, the clinician sets the V_t, f, PEEP, and FiO_2. PS is also set. Most present day ventilators have the ability to sense a patient-initiated breath. When this occurs, the ventilator delivers airflow at the set PS. As with IMV, the total V_e is the sum of the set V_t and the spontaneous V_t, the spontaneous work of breathing is less than that of IMV, provided that enough PS is provided.

- *Pressure cycling* is a mode of ventilation where the ventilator delivers flow until a preset pressure is reached. In this mode, the V_t is variable and depends on the compliance of the lung. Lungs with low compliance will have a smaller V_t at a given inflation pressure than lungs with a high compliance.
  - *Pressure control ventilation (PCV)*—In PCV, the clinician sets the driving pressure, PEEP, f, and FiO_2. The delivered V_t is determined by the pressure difference between the driving pressure and PEEP, as well as by the compliance of the lung. Minute ventilation is variable and cannot be controlled in this mode. This mode is used for its potential to limit airway pressures as well as its potential to improve oxygenation by sustaining the MAP for longer intervals than are generally achieved with volume-cycled modes.
- *Flow cycling* is a mode of ventilation where the ventilator delivers a breath at a set pressure until a predetermined reduction in flow is reached. In this mode, the V_t as well as V_e is variable and dependent on patient effort.

○ *Pressure support ventilation (PSV)*—In PSV, the clinician sets the pressure of the delivered breath (millimeters of mercury). When a patient initiates a breath, the air is delivered at the set pressure until flow falls to a predetermined level (usually 25% of the maximum airflow). Minute ventilation is variable and depends on the patient's respiratory frequency and the volume of each breath. The patient's work of breathing is inversely proportional to the set PS.

INITIAL MODES AND SETTINGS

- The initial mode and settings are variable and depend on the patient's underlying illness and reason for endotracheal intubation.
- Both IMV and A/C provide full support while allowing some diaphragmatic activity, which may prevent atrophy of the respiratory musculature.
- A/C is the most commonly used ventilatory mode in the medical intensive care unit and is appropriate as the initial mode for most causes of respiratory failure.
- *Tidal volume*—Recent studies have shown that large tidal volumes with consequent alveolar over distention (termed "volutrauma") can lead to the development of lung injury.
  ○ In patients with no underlying lung pathology, an initial V_t of 8–10 mL/kg of *ideal* body weight is acceptable. Note: actual body weight should not be used. See Table 81-3 to calculate ideal body weight.
  ○ In a patient with underlying acute lung injury (ALI) or ARDS, it has been shown that a V_t of 6 mL/kg confers a survival advantage over the conventional 12 mL/kg of ideal body weight (see ALI/ARDS below).
- *Respiratory rate*—Initial respiratory rates can be set from 12 to 16 bpm. In patients on a "low" V_t strategy (eg, 6 mL/kg for ARDS) or patients with a significant acidosis as a cause of intubation and mechanical ventilation, initial respiratory rates may range from 20 to 30.
- *PEEP*—Initial PEEP should be set at 5 cm H_2O in all patients, except for those with increased intracranial pressure and possibly those with shock and known volume depletion. PEEP can then be increased to improve oxygenation in patients with hypoxemic respiratory failure. PEEP should not exceed 20 cm H_2O. PEEP can be particularly helpful in cases

TABLE 81-3   Calculating Ideal Body Weight (kg)

Males = 50 + (2.3 × [height (inches) − 60])
Females = 45.5 + (2.3 × [height (inches) − 60])

TABLE 81-4   Causes of Increased Plateau Pressure

Intrapulmonary
  Pulmonary edema
  Atelectasis
  ARDS
  Pulmonary fibrosis
  Pneumonia
  Air trapping/hyperinflation
Extrapulmonary
  Pneumothorax
  Hemothorax
  Pleural effusion
  Flail chest
  Pneumomediastinum
Extrathoracic
  Ascites
  Abdominal compartment syndrome
  Obesity
  Chest wall disorders
    Scoliosis
    Kyphosis
  Patient effort ("fighting the vent")

where edema is present in the lungs (such as CHF and ARDS).
- *FiO₂*—Initial FiO_2 should be set at 100%. FiO_2 can then be titrated downward to a goal of ≤ 60% while maintaining an oxygen saturation ≥ 90%.

PHYSIOLOGIC GOALS

- The goals of mechanical ventilation are to meet the metabolic needs of the patient with the least amount of ventilatory support.
- *Plateau pressures*—Elevated plateau pressures can cause barotrauma and pneumothorax. The target plateau pressure should be ≤ 30 cm H_2O (see Table 81-4).
- *Peak pressures*—Elevated peak pressures have *not* been associated with an increased risk of lung injury or pneumothorax. There is no target peak pressure and this measurement can be used to monitor response to therapy in treatment of bronchoconstriction (see Table 81-5).

TABLE 81-5   Causes of Increased Peak Pressure

Bronchoconstriction
  Asthma
  COPD
Mechanical airway obstruction
  Mucous plug
  Endobronchial lesion
Extracorporeal obstruction
  Kinked ventilator circuit
  Obstructed endotracheal tube
    Patient biting
    Mucous plug
Patient-ventilator interaction
  "Fighting the vent"
  Coughing
Any cause of increased plateau pressure (see Table 81-1)

- *FiO$_2$*—The FiO$_2$ should be titrated to a goal of ≤ 60% while maintaining an oxygen saturation ≥ 90%. Prolonged administration of high concentrations of oxygen (> 60%) can lead to lung injury.
- *PEEP*—PEEP and FiO$_2$ are the main contributors to the PO$_2$ in a well-ventilated patient. FiO$_2$ can be titrated easily with a quick response in oxygenation. The effects of a change in PEEP are realized much more slowly. For this reason and the risk of oxygen toxicity, FiO$_2$ should be titrated before PEEP. Once a patient is stable and oxygenating well, PEEP should be titrated downward to a goal of 5 cm H$_2$O.

SEDATION IN MECHANICALLY VENTILATED PATIENTS

- Most patients will require both sedation (eg, benzodiazepines, propofol) and analgesia (eg, fentanyl, morphine) in order to tolerate mechanical ventilation.
  - Options include bolus administration or continuous infusion
  - Continuous infusion and use of longer-acting agents may prolong duration of ventilation
- Consider short-acting agents such as propofol for patients who need frequent neurologic assessment or patients who will only require a brief period of ventilation.
- Agitated patients may "fight" the ventilator; ventilator-patient dyssynchrony may interfere with effective gas exchange
  - Dyssynchrony should be first addressed by determining why the patient is agitated. This may be pain, a problem with the ventilator circuit, an inappropriate or uncomfortable ventilator strategy, and so on.
  - Dyssynchrony may be treated by increasing sedation once underlying causes for agitation have been ruled out.
  - Paralysis should be avoided unless there are life-threatening problems with gas exchange. Paralytics are a major risk factor for critical illness polymyopathy/polyneuropathy.
  - If paralytics are used, adequate sedation must also be ensured.
- Continuous sedation should be interrupted daily to assess the patient's neurologic status.
  - This has been shown to reduce the time on mechanical ventilation, time in the ICU, and need for diagnostic testing of the central nervous system (CNS).
  - The best approach is provided by nurses in a protocol-driven fashion.

- Nurses must coordinate with respiratory therapists for weaning trials and with physician assessment for decisions regarding extubation.
- Patients should be watched for signs of withdrawal after cessation of sedation and analgesia.

VENTILATOR MANAGEMENT FOR SPECIFIC CONDITIONS

ACUTE LUNG INJURY AND ACUTE RESPIRATORY DISTRESS SYNDROME
- ARDS is defined as
  1. PaO$_2$/FiO$_2$ < 200
  2. Bilateral radiographic infiltrates consistent with pulmonary edema
  3. No clinical evidence of left atrial hypertension (ie, no cardiogenic pulmonary edema)
- ALI is defined by the same criteria except PaO$_2$/FiO$_2$ < 300.
- Specific criteria have been set forth for mechanical ventilation in patients with ALI or ARDS. These criteria are available at www.ardsnet.org. See Table 81- 6 for ventilator management of these and other common conditions.

INTRINSIC POSITIVE END-EXPIRATORY PRESSURE
- Expiratory flow is limited in patients with obstructive lung disease so they are at risk for air-trapping and intrinsic PEEP. As airway obstruction worsens during an exacerbation, they have dynamic hyperinflation. This increase in lung volume increases the work of breathing and leads to residual positive pressure in the airway at end-exhalation. The increase in residual positive pressure is referred to as auto PEEP or intrinsic PEEP (iPEEP). In pressure-triggered ventilation, the patient must overcome the iPEEP and then generate enough pressure to trigger a ventilator-delivered breath.
- iPEEP can be detected in the following ways:
  - Documenting persistent expiratory flow at the initiation of the next breath on the flow-time graph of the ventilator.
  - Performing an end-expiratory breath hold. This allows equalization of pressures between the alveoli and the airway opening. The recorded pressure is the iPEEP.
  - Wheezing audible with auscultation persisting until the onset of the next inspiration.
- iPEEP can be minimized by three strategies:
  - Decreasing the respiratory rate (f). This allows more time for exhalation.
  - Decreasing the V$_t$. When a patient gets smaller breaths, less air needs to be exhaled to empty the lungs.
  - Lowering the I:E ratio (goal should be 1:3 to 1:5). This results in shorter inspiratory times (increased

TABLE 81-6   Ventilator Management for ALI or ARDS, COPD, Asthma

	ALI OR ARDS	COPD	ASTHMA
Goals of ventilation	• Meet physiologic requirements while minimizing plateau pressures and volutrauma	• Correct life-threatening acid-base abnormalities • Provide support during pharmacologic treatment of bronchospasm, infection, and airway edema • Rest muscles of respiration • Prevent hyperinflation	• Avoid excessive airway pressure • Minimize lung hyperinflation
Initial ventilator settings	• Set the mode to A/C • Set initial tidal volume to 8 mL/kg of predicted body weight (Table 81-3) and titrate down by 1 mL/kg every 2 hours until a target tidal volume of 6 mL/kg is reached • Set initial respiratory rate to approximate the baseline V_e (to keep $\leq$ 35 L) • Set the initial FiO_2 to 100% and PEEP to 5 cm H_2O	• Initial mode should be A/C to facilitate respiratory muscle rest • V_t can be set at 8–10 mL/kg of ideal body weight • Respiratory rate should be set to target the patient's estimated $PaCO_2$ and decreased if there is evidence of dynamic hyperinflation (see below in iPEEP) • I:E ratio should be set to favor a long expiratory time (I:E ratio of 1:3 to 1:5) • PEEP should be set initially at 5 cm H_2O and adjusted to < 75% below the iPEEP	• Initial mode should be A/C • V_t can be set at 6–10 mL/kg of ideal body weight • Respiratory rate can be set at 10–14 bpm • I:E ratio should be set to favor a long expiratory time (I:E ratios of 1:3 to 1:5) • PEEP should initially be set at 0 cm H_2O in sedated patients because the work of breathing is usually minimal and the area of obstruction in acute attacks is the large noncollapsable airways • As the attack resolves, the patient actively triggers the ventilator and the predominant area of obstruction becomes the small airways. Applied PEEP is likely beneficial at this stage and should be initiated at low levels ($\leq$ 8 cm H_2O)
Oxygenation goal	• Target a goal PaO_2 of 55–80 mm Hg and a target SpO_2 of 88%–95% • The FiO_2 should be titrated downward from the initial setting of 100% to the lowest possible value that maintains oxygenation goals • Once FiO_2 has been minimized, PEEP should be titrated upward from 5 cm H_2O to the level indicated in Table 81-4 Increasing PEEP should permit a further drop in FiO_2	• Target a goal PaO_2 of 55–80 mm Hg and a target SpO_2 of 88%–95% • The FiO_2 should be titrated downward from the initial setting of 100% to the lowest possible value that maintains oxygenation goals	• Target a goal PaO_2 of 55–80 mm Hg and a target SpO_2 of 88%–95% • The FiO_2 should be titrated downward from the initial setting of 100% to the lowest possible value that maintains oxygenation goals
Plateau pressure goal	• Target a plateau pressure $\leq$ 30 cm H_2O. Check plateau pressures every 4 hours and after a V_t or PEEP change • If P_{plat} > 30 cm H_2O, decrease the V_t by 1 mL/kg/hr to a minimum of 4 mL/kg • If P_{plat} < 25 cm H_2O and V_t < 6 mL/kg, increase V_t by 1 mL/kg until P_{plat} > 25 cm H_2O or V_t = 6 mL/kg • If severe dyspnea occurs, increase the V_t by 1 mL/kg to a maximum of 8 mL/kg as long as P_{plat} < 30 mL/kg	• Target a plateau pressure $\leq$ 30 cm H_2O. Check plateau pressures every 4 hours and after a V_t or PEEP change • If plateau pressure > 30 cm H_2O, the focus must be on determining and correcting underlying etiology (Table 81-2). Patients with COPD are at high risk for air trapping and pneumothorax	• Target a plateau pressure $\leq$ 30 cm H_2O. Check plateau pressures every 4 hours and after a V_t or PEEP change • If plateau pressure > 30 cm H_2O, the focus must be on determining and correcting underlying etiology (Table 81-2). Consider air trapping and pneumothorax as most likely
pH Goal	• If arterial pH < 7.15, increase f to maximum of 35. If pH remains < 7.15, may consider HCO_3 infusion or increasing V_t in 1 mL/kg increments and exceeding the target P_{plat} • If arterial pH 7.15–7.30, increase f until pH > 7.30 or $PaCO_2$ < 25 (up to a maximum f of 35). If pH remains 7.15–7.30, may consider HCO_3 infusion • If pH >7.45, decrease f if possible		

(Continued)

TABLE 81-6   Ventilator Management for ALI or ARDS, COPD, Asthma (*Continued*)

	ALI OR ARDS	COPD	ASTHMA
iPEEP		iPEEP can be minimized by three strategies • Decreasing the respiratory rate (f) This allows more time for exhalation. • Decreasing the V_t. When a patient gets smaller breaths, less air needs to be exhaled to empty the lungs • Lowering the I:E ratio (goal should be 1:3 to 1:5). This results in shorter inspiratory times (increased inspiratory flow rate) and longer expiratory times	• As in COPD, expiratory flow limitation in acute asthma can cause hyperinflation and intrinsic PEEP. Strategies to limit this hyperinflation are similar to those used for COPD and include increasing the expiratory time and decreasing the tidal volume
Permissive hypercapnia			In asthma, strategies to minimize dynamic hyperinflation can reduce the V_e to levels that lead to the development of an acute respiratory acidosis with elevated $PaCO_2$ levels and reduced pH. Excluding patients with increased intracranial pressure and myocardial depression, this is usually well tolerated. Our experience recommends consideration of a bicarbonate infusion for a pH of ≤ 7.20

inspiratory flow rate) and longer expiratory times. See Table 81-7 for arterial oxygenation and PEEP in ARDS.

WEANING AND EXTUBATION

• There is no single clinical variable or test that determines a patient's readiness and ability to wean from mechanical ventilation. Instead, a constellation of clinical parameters and an overall assessment best determines the appropriate time and type of wean.
• It is difficult to recommend a level of "aggressiveness" in weaning and extubating patients. There are risks with delayed extubation as well as with early extubation and reintubation. Though there is no good clinical study, the accepted appropriate reintubation rate is somewhere between 5% and 10%.

TABLE 81-7   Arterial Oxygenation and PEEP in ARDS

FiO_2	0.3	0.4	0.4	0.5	0.5	0.6	0.7	0.7
PEEP	5	5	8	8	10	10	10	12
FiO_2	0.7	0.8	0.9	0.9	0.9	1.0	1.0	1.0
PEEP	14	14	14	16	18	20	22	24

SOURCE: Adapted from the NIH NHLBI ARDS Clinical Network Mechanical Ventilation Summary.

• A respiratory care practitioner and nurse-driven ventilator management protocol for weaning readiness reduces the duration of mechanical ventilation.
• *Readiness for spontaneous breathing*—The following criteria should be used to determine whether a patient receiving ventilatory support should be considered for a spontaneous breathing trial (SBT):
  ○ Reversal of the primary process that led to intubation and ventilation
  ○ Adequate oxygenation ($FiO_2 \leq 0.4$–0.5, PEEP ≤ 5–8 cm H_2O)
  ○ Adequate arterial pH (pH ≥ 7.25)
  ○ Hemodynamic stability with no active MI or vasopressor dependence
  ○ The ability to initiate an inspiratory effort
  ○ Absence of significant fever, acidosis, or anemia
  ○ Absence of significant electrolyte abnormalities such as hypophosphatemia and hypomagnesemia
  ○ Adequate mentation
• *Types of SBTs*—Once the determination has been made that a patient is ready to breathe on his/her own, an SBT should be performed. The two different protocols for SBTs include
  1. About 30–120 minutes on a T-piece—the patient is disconnected from the ventilator and oxygen flows past the endotracheal tube.
  2. About 30–120 minutes on PS—the ventilator is set at 5 cm H_2O of PEEP and 5–7 cm H_2O of PS (smaller diameter endotracheal tubes may need higher levels of PS).

- *Tolerance of the SBT*—Many criteria have been used to determine tolerance of an SBT and likelihood of successful extubation. If a patient meets these criteria after 30–120 minutes on an SBT, extubation should be considered.
  - Gas exchange
    - $SaO_2 \geq$ 85% to 90%
    - $PaO_2 \geq$ 50–60 mm Hg
    - Arterial pH $\geq$ 7.32
    - Increase in $PaCO_2 \leq$ 10 mm Hg compared to when patient was managed prior to the SBT
  - Hemodynamic stability
    - HR < 120–140 beats/min
    - HR not changed > 20% compared with pre-SBT HR
    - SBP < 180–200 and > 90 mm Hg
    - BP changed < 20% compared with pre-SBT BP, no vasopressors
  - Stable ventilation
    - RR $\leq$ 30–35 breaths/min
    - RR not changed > 50% compared with pre-SBT RR
  - Stable mentation—no somnolence, coma, agitation, or anxiety
  - No evidence of respiratory distress or excessive work of breathing
  - Presence of a cuff leak (rules out laryngeal edema)
    - Defined as > 110 mL tidal volume lost with cuff deflated on the endotracheal tube

BIBLIOGRAPHY

ARDSnet. Ventilation with lower tidal volumes as compared with traditional tidal volumes for acute lung injury and the acute respiratory distress syndrome. The Acute Respiratory Distress Syndrome Network [see comment]. *N Engl Med.* 2000;342(18):1301–1308.

Aubier M, Murciano D, Lecocguic Y, et al. Effect of hypophosphatemia on diaphragmatic contractility in patients with acute respiratory failure. *N Engl Med.* 1985;313(7): 420–424.

Dhingra S, Solven F, Wilson A, et al. Hypomagnesemia and respiratory muscle power. *Am Rev Resp Dis.* 1984;129(3): 497–498.

Ely EW, Baker AM, Evans GW, et al. The prognostic significance of passing a daily screen of weaning parameters. *Int Care Med.* 1999;25(6):581–587.

Esteban A, Alia I, Gordo F, et al. Extubation outcome after spontaneous breathing trials with T-tube or pressure support ventilation. The Spanish Lung Failure Collaborative Group [erratum appears in *Am J Resp Crit Care Med.* 1997 Dec;156(6):2028]. *Am J Resp Crit Care Med.* 1997;156(2 Pt 1): 459–465.

Keenan SP, Sinuff T, Cook DJ, et al. Does noninvasive positive pressure ventilation improve outcome in acute hypoxemic respiratory failure? A systematic review [see comment]. *Crit Care Med.* 2004;32(12):2516–2523.

MacIntyre NR, Cook DJ, Ely EW, Jr., et al. Evidence-based guidelines for weaning and discontinuing ventilatory support: a collective task force facilitated by the American College of Chest Physicians; the American Association for Respiratory Care; and the American College of Critical Care Medicine. *Chest.* 2001;120(6 suppl):375S–395S.

MacIntyre NR. Current issues in mechanical ventilation for respiratory failure. *Chest.* 2005;128(5 suppl 2):561S–567S.

Marelich GP, Murin S, Battistella F, et al. Protocol weaning of mechanical ventilation in medical and surgical patients by respiratory care practitioners and nurses: effect on weaning time and incidence of ventilator-associated pneumonia. *Chest.* 2000;118(2):459–467.

Miller RL, Cole RP. Association between reduced cuff leak volume and postextubation stridor. *Chest.* 1996;110(4): 1035–1040.

Moonsie I, Davidson C. Weaning from mechanical ventilation. *Clin Med.* 2005;5(5):445–448.

Oddo M, Feihl F, Schaller MD, et al. Management of mechanical ventilation in acute severe asthma: practical aspects. *Int Care Med.* 2006;32(4):501–510.

Park JE, Griffiths MJ. Recent advances in mechanical ventilation. *Clin Med.* 2005;5(5):441–444.

Parrillo J, Phillip R. *Critical Care Medicine: Principles of Diagnosis and Management in the Adult*, Vol 1. 2nd ed. St. Louis, MO: Mosby; 2001.

Peter JV, Moran JL, Phillips-Hughes J, et al. Effect of noninvasive positive pressure ventilation (NIPPV) on mortality in patients with acute cardiogenic pulmonary edema: a meta-analysis. *Lancet* 2006;367(9517):1155–1163.

Pilbeam SP. CJM. *Mechanical Ventilation.* 4th ed. St Louis, MO: Mosby; 2006.

Ram FS, Wellington S, Rowe B, et al. Noninvasive positive pressure ventilation for treatment of respiratory failure due to severe acute exacerbations of asthma [update of *Cochrane Database Syst Rev.* 2005;1:CD004360; PMID: 15674944]. *Cochrane Database Syst Rev.* 2005;3:CD004360.

Schweickert WD, Gehlbach BK, Pohlman AS, et al. Daily interruption of sedative infusions and complications of critical illness in mechanically ventilated patients [see comment]. *Crit Care Med.* 2004;32(6):1272–1276.

Sethi JM, Siegel MD. Mechanical ventilation in chronic obstructive lung disease. *Clin Chest Med.* 2000;21(4): 799–818.

Vassilakopoulos T, Zakynthinos S, Roussos C. The tension-time index and the frequency/tidal volume ratio are the major pathophysiologic determinants of weaning failure and success. *Am J Resp Crit Care Med.* 1998;158(2):378–385.

Yang KL, Tobin MJ. A prospective study of indexes predicting the outcome of trials of weaning from mechanical ventilation [see comment]. *N Engl Med.* 1991;324(21): 1445–1450.

82 PREVENTION OF ACUTE RENAL FAILURE IN THE HOSPITAL

Glen M. Kim

EPIDEMIOLOGY/OVERVIEW

- The prevention of in-hospital acute renal failure (ARF) is important because of the burden of associated morbidity, mortality, and healthcare costs.
- The incidence of ARF is estimated to be 5% to 7% in tertiary care medical and surgical hospitals; although a lack of a standard definition of ARF limits epidemiologic estimates.
- The development of in-hospital ARF is associated with increased LOS and poor clinical outcomes. Mortality rates range from 5% to 10% in uncomplicated ARF to 50% to 70% in the ICU setting.
- Up to 80% of episodes of in-hospital ARF have been attributed to the following causes:
  - Decreased renal perfusion (volume depletion, CHF, cardiogenic and septic shock)
  - Major surgery (coronary artery bypass, valve replacement, vascular procedures)
  - Aminoglycosides and radiocontrast administration
- With the exception of contrast-induced nephropathy (CIN), few preventive strategies exist beyond the avoidance of nephrotoxins and states predisposing to renal ischemia.

PATHOPHYSIOLOGY

- While the pathophysiology of ARF is an expansive topic, *decreased renal perfusion* and *nephrotoxicity* are two important mechanisms relevant to preventive strategies in the hospital.
- *Medications and other exogenous drugs* that may cause ARF by decreased renal perfusion or nephrotoxicity are shown in Table 82-1.
- The risk of *postischemic acute tubular necrosis (ATN)* is increased in states of decreased renal perfusion including volume depletion, bleeding, acute pancreatitis, CHF, cardiogenic and septic shock, arrhythmias with hypotension, and major surgeries.
- In *surgical patients*, preoperative volume deficits, anesthesia, intra-operative fluid losses and hypotension, arterial clamping, and cardiopulmonary bypass may decrease renal perfusion and increase the risk of ATN.
- Angiotensin-converting enzyme *(ACE) inhibitors* may decrease glomerular filtration rate (GFR) in settings of renal hypoperfusion such as low cardiac output, renal artery stenosis, volume depletion, and concurrent use of vasoconstrictor agents (eg, nonsteroidal anti-inflammatory drugs [NSAIDs]). Clinical settings in which ACE inhibitors may cause ARF are shown in Table 82-2.
- *NSAIDs* inhibit preglomerular vasodilation by prostaglandins which may result in renal ischemia, especially under conditions of low effective circulating volume. Other mechanisms for NSAID-induced ARF include acute interstitial nephritis (AIN) and nephrotic syndrome.
- *Nephrotoxins* may be exogenous or endogenous.
  - Common exogenous nephrotoxins associated with in-hospital ARF include aminoglycosides, radiocontrast, and various chemotherapeutics (see Table 82-1).

TABLE 82-1 Drug and Other Exogenous Causes of ARF

COMMON MEDICATIONS	ANTIMICROBIALS	CHEMOTHERAPY AND IMMUNOSUPPRESSANTS	OTHERS
Loop diuretics	Aminoglycosides	Cisplatin	Heroin
ACE inhibitors	Protease inhibitors	Carboplatin	Cocaine
ARBs	Acyclovir	Cyclosporine	Dextrans
NSAIDs	Amphotericin B	Tacrolimus	Bisphosphonates
	Foscarnet	Ifosfamide	Aristolochic acid (Chinese herb)
	Pentamidine	Methotrexate	Oral sodium phosphates (e.g., Fleet Phospho-soda)
			Ethylene glycol
			Bacterial toxins

Abbreviations: ACE, angiotensin-converting enzyme; ARBs, angiotensin receptor blockers; NSAIDs, nonsteroidal anti-inflammatory drugs.

TABLE 82-2 Clinical Settings in which ACE Inhibitors may Cause ARF

Preexisting renal impairment
Effective volume depletion
Volume depletion/diuretic use
CHF
Cirrhosis
Concurrent vasoconstrictor agents (NSAIDs, cyclosporine)
Advanced age
Renovascular disease
Bilateral renal artery stenosis/stenosis of single kidney

- *Aminoglycoside*-induced nephrotoxicity is thought to involve binding of cationic aminoglycosides to anionic phospholipids in the luminal membrane of the proximal tubule, leading to uptake in the proximal tubule, accumulation, and subsequent tubular injury. In theory, once-a-day dosing saturates binding sites and limits the amount of aminoglycoside taken into the tubules.
- *CIN* is thought to involve vasoconstrictive ischemia and direct cytotoxicity. This topic is discussed separately in this chapter.
  - Clinical settings of endogenous nephrotoxins include hyperuricemia in tumor lysis syndrome (TLS), myoglobinuria from crush injuries or rhabdomyolysis, and hemoglobinuria secondary to intravascular hemolysis.
    - In heme pigment-associated ARF (myoglobin and hemoglobin), obstruction of tubules by pigment casts, direct tubular injury, and renal ischemia secondary to third spacing may contribute to ATN.
    - In *TLS*, spontaneous or chemotherapeutic-induced cell turnover may result in ARF secondary to precipitation of urate and calcium phosphate in renal tubules.

PREVENTIVE STRATEGIES

- A first step to preventive strategies is identifying patients at risk for hospital-acquired ARF. Risk factors include sepsis, shock, major surgery, underlying renal insufficiency, heart failure, and exposure to nephrotoxins.
- In general, the *maintenance of adequate renal perfusion* and the *avoidance of nephrotoxic agents* are the mainstays of prevention of in-hospital ARF. Specific prophylactic strategies for CIN are discussed separately.
  - *Optimizing renal perfusion* includes achieving and maintaining intravascular volume, optimizing cardiac output, and avoiding insults such as significant hypotension.

- *Maintaining intravascular volume and stable hemodynamics* is particularly important in perioperative management of surgical patients who are at higher risk for ATN.
- Patients at risk for *NSAID-induced renal failure* include elderly patients, those with underlying renal insufficiency, and states of decreased effective circulating volume such as heart failure, cirrhosis, and volume depletion. Similar risks apply to the administration of *ACE inhibitors*, particularly in CHF patients undergoing aggressive diuresis.
  - Patients with underlying renal or hepatic impairment are at increased risk for *aminoglycoside-induced nephrotoxicity*. In these patients, alternative antibiotics should be considered.
    - When administered, aminoglycosides should be dosed carefully by creatinine clearance and monitoring of serum drug levels. Aminoglycosides may cause ARF even if levels are therapeutic.
    - Although once-a-day dosing has a theoretical benefit of decreased tubular toxicity, no definitive data support this practice in adults.
  - In *heme pigment-induced ARF*, aggressive volume repletion and diuresis help to prevent intratubular cast formation.
    - Massive amounts of IV fluids may be needed: 1–2 L/hr for initial volume repletion and then 200–300 mL/hr to maintain diuresis.
    - Once diuresis is established, urine alkalinization to pH > 6.5 may theoretically decrease renal toxicity of myoglobin and hemoglobin and intratubular pigment cast formation. The metabolic alkalosis may also help protect against hyperkalemia in rhabdomyolysis. Urinary alkalinization requires monitoring, however, and there are little data favoring this therapy over NS.
  - Prevention of ARF from TLS involves initiating allopurinol at least 3 days before initiation of chemotherapy. In patients with baseline hyperuricemia, serum uric acid concentration should be normalized prior to chemotherapy. Rasburicase, a urate oxidase, reduces serum uric acid levels more effectively than allopurinol and should be considered as an alternative to allopurinol for prevention and treatment of hyperuricemia in high-risk patients.
    - Aggressive IV hydration in high-risk patients should begin 24–48 hours prior to chemotherapy and then continued for 48–72 hours after chemotherapy. Target UO should be at least 3 L/d as volume status tolerates.
    - Urine alkalinization increases the solubility of uric acid. IV isotonic sodium bicarbonate and/or acetazolamide may be titrated to increase urinary pH to 7.0–8.0. As in prevention of ARF in rhabdomyolysis,

urine alkalinization, however, is controversial and carries risks of hypocalcemia and calcium phosphate precipitation in renal tubules.

○ The prevention of ARF secondary to *cisplatin* also requires aggressive hydration and diuresis. Amifostine may be considered if high dose cisplatin is administered.

○ Likewise, prehydration with NS decreases the incidence of ARF secondary to *amphotericin B*. Lipid formulations of amphotericin B may be less nephrotoxic than nonlipid formulations and are recommended for patients at high risk for nephrotoxicity.

○ Data do not support the prophylactic use of *mannitol* or *low-dose dopamine* (< 5 µg/kg/min) for the prevention or reduction in severity of ATN. Renal-dose dopamine infusion may increase GFR and UO, but has not been demonstrated to benefit mortality, need for dialysis, or LOS.

○ *Loop diuretics* may be used for volume management in patients with ATN who have become oliguric, but this is neither a preventive measure or to reverse ATN.

CONTRAST-INDUCED NEPHROPATHY

EPIDEMIOLOGY/OVERVIEW

• With advances in radiographic and interventional procedures, increasing numbers of hospitalized patients are receiving radiocontrast agents. In 2000, approximately 1,318,000 diagnostic cardiac catheterizations and 561,000 interventions were performed; these numbers do not include other procedures such as contrast-enhanced CT scans.

• CIN is a recognized complication of radiologic procedures using iodinated radiocontrast media and is an important cause of hospital-required renal failure.

• CIN has no standard definition, but is generally characterized as an acute decline in renal function following administration of radiocontrast media. In clinical trials, the most commonly used definition has been an *absolute increase in SCr of 0.5 mg/dL or a relative increase of 25% from baseline within 48 hours of administration of contrast.*

○ Increases in SCr of as little as 0.25 mg/dL or 25% within 3 days of contrast exposure have been associated with increased 30-day in-hospital mortality and length of hospital stay. It is unclear, however, whether CIN contributes directly to this mortality or is a marker for underlying comorbidities.

• Although the incidence of CIN is low in patients with normal renal function, it can be much higher in patients with underlying renal disease.

○ Overall, the incidence of CIN is estimated to be 1% to 6% in the general population and < 2% in patients with normal baseline renal function.

○ Chronic kidney disease (CKD) increases the incidence to 12% to 27%.

○ In patients with both CKD and diabetes mellitus (DM), the incidence of CIN may be as high as 50%.

• Patients with acute MI undergoing angioplasty are at higher risk of CIN than patients undergoing elective interventions. Incidence rates of 15% have been reported in patients undergoing cardiac catheterization. An estimated 0.3% to 4% of cases of CIN among cardiac catheterization patients require hemodialysis (usually temporary) and over 7000 deaths are attributed to contrast nephropathy annually.

PATHOPHYSIOLOGY

• The pathogenesis of acute renal insufficiency induced by radiocontrast agents is not fully understood. Two major theories are *medullary renal ischemia* and *direct nephrotoxicity.*

○ At baseline, the renal medulla is a hypoxic environment susceptible to ischemic insult. Contrast agents may cause vasoconstrictive ischemia by altering the balance of local nitric oxide, prostaglandins, adenosine, and endothelin.

○ The osmotic load and viscosity of contrast may also increase the work of active transport and oxygen demand, increase tubular hydrostatic pressure, and further reduce medullary blood flow.

○ Ischemia may result in oxidative stress and potentiate direct *cytotoxicity*. Cytotoxic effects include vacuolization, interstitial inflammation, cellular necrosis, and enzymuria.

○ Comorbid medical conditions such as underlying renal disease, states of decreased effective circulating volume, and exogenous nephrotoxins may exacerbate these pathologic mechanisms.

○ In patients with MI undergoing percutaneous coronary intervention (PCI), factors contributing to CIN may include decreased systemic perfusion secondary to left ventricular (LV) dysfunction, large volume of contrast medium, and limited time to administer renal prophylactic therapies.

CLINICAL PRESENTATION/DIFFERENTIAL DIAGNOSIS

• CIN is typically self-limited and transient, manifesting within the first 24–48 hours after contrast exposure, with recovery of renal function beginning within

3–5 days, and resolution within 7–10 days. Renal failure is typically *nonoliguric and reversible.*

- Small persistent increases in creatinine levels are associated with increased mortality. In severe cases, oliguric renal failure may ensue with SCr peaking 5–10 days after contrast exposure. Some patients may require dialysis.
- Urinalysis demonstrates ATN: coarse granular casts, renal tubular epithelial cells, and amorphous debris.
- Differential diagnosis for a rise in SCr following radiocontrast administration includes CIN and other causes of postischemic ATN. Additionally, in patients with atherosclerosis undergoing arteriography, the differential should include *renal atheroemboli.* Embolic lesions, livedo reticularis, hypocomplementemia, and delayed onset ARF with little or no recovery of renal function are consistent with renal atheroemboli.

PREVENTIVE STRATEGIES

- Optimal therapy to prevent CIN remains uncertain.
- Existing clinical studies have been limited by a lack of a uniform definition of CIN, variations in contrast and hydration regimens, the use of creatinine as a surrogate for GFR, and inadequate power to evaluate clinical outcomes.
- An important first step to preventing CIN is identifying associated *risk factors for CIN.* The most important risk factor is preexisting renal insufficiency, particularly when secondary to diabetic nephropathy.
  - SCr >1.5 mg/dL has been reported to predict increased risk of CIN, but there is no consensus cutpoint, particularly because SCr varies with age, muscle mass, gender, and ethnicity.
  - Consider estimated glomerular filtration rate (eGFR) < 60 mL/min/1.73 m^2 to identify patients at increased risk, although higher thresholds may be needed if other CIN risk factors are present.
  - Other potential risk factors include diabetes alone, concurrent use of nephrotoxic medications, dehydration, age > 70 years, female gender, and states of reduced perfusion such as hypovolemia and CHF. See Table 82-3.
- When clinically possible, the risk of contrast nephropathy may be obviated by *the use of alternative imaging techniques* such as ultrasound, noncontrast CT, or magnetic resonance imaging (MRI).
  - While there are reports of ARF after gadolinium administration in patients with significant underlying renal dysfunction, contrast-enhanced MRI using gadolinium poses little risk of nephrotoxicity when used in small doses (< 0.3 mmol/kg).

TABLE 82-3   Risk Factors for CIN

Preexisting renal impairment
DM (with renal disease)
Urgent procedures
Intra-aortic balloon pump
Age > 70 years
Female gender
Effective volume depletion
LVEF < 40%
Hypotension
Concurrent use of vasoconstrictive (NSAIDs) or nephrotoxic medications
Radiocontrast
High osmolarity
High-volume/multiple CM studies

Abbreviation: LVEF, left ventricular ejection fraction.

  - Of note, however, recent data suggest increased risk of *nephrogenic systemic fibrosis* in patients with end-stage renal disease (ESRD) who receive gadolinium. Pending further clarification, consider avoiding gadolinium in patients with ARF and CKD (stage 4/5).
- *Nephrotoxic and vasoconstrictive medications should be avoided for at least 24 hours* prior to the administration of contrast media, particularly in high-risk patients or those with eGFR < 60 mL/min. See Table 82-1.
- *Volume repletion and maintenance of adequate intravascular volume* optimizes renal blood flow and GFR. While RCTs have not studied hydration alone vs. placebo, volume expansion is generally recognized as an important prophylactic measure. The optimal type and duration of IV fluid, however, is unknown.
  - Administration of *periprocedure isotonic NS* is associated with a lower incidence of CIN compared with half-NS and with uncontrolled oral intake.
    - Various NS regimens have been studied. See Table 82-4 for recommendations.
    - Volume status must be carefully monitored with the administration of periprocedure NS.
    - The potential mechanism of NS includes increased delivery of sodium to the distal nephron, reduced activation of the renin-angiotensin system, and maintenance of renal perfusion.
  - *Alkalinizing renal tubular fluid* may reduce free radical formation and decrease viscosity of contrast agents within the vasa recta.
    - In one study, periprocedure administration of isotonic sodium bicarbonate was associated with a lower incidence of CIN (1.7%) compared with isotonic sodium chloride (13.6%).
    - Of note, the comparison involved a small bolus of IV sodium chloride or bicarbonate *1 hour preprocedure* followed by continuous infusion for

TABLE 82-4   Prophylactic Strategies for CIN

	INTERVENTION	DOSING	COMMENTS
Volume expansion	Isotonic sodium chloride	NS 1–1.5 mL/kg/hr for 6–12 hours preprocedure and continued 6–24 hours postprocedure	• IV volume expansion with periprocedure NS is superior to 0.45 NS or oral fluids. NS infusion requires monitoring of volume status
Antioxidant	Isotonic sodium bicarbonate	D5 w/3 amps bicarbonate (150 mEq). Initial IV bolus of 3 mL/kg/hr × 1 hour immediately before procedure, followed by 1 mL/kg/hr during and 6 hours post-procedure	• In one study, isotonic sodium bicarbonate was superior to isotonic sodium chloride bolus and drip beginning *1 hour preprocedure*. This bicarbonate regimen, however, has not been compared with longer duration, periprocedure NS regimens • Consider alkalinization when there is short notice for a contrast procedure and little time for prophylactic measures. This therapy requires monitoring for metabolic alkalosis and volume overload • Further studies of bicarbonate therapy are needed to determine optimal duration and effectiveness compared with volume expansion with NS
	NAC	600–1200 mg po bid beginning the day before procedure	• Research protocols testing NAC have been heterogeneous and few have been powered to assess clinical outcomes. Despite over 20 RCTS and 11 meta-analyses, the benefits of NAC are sill inconclusive. Further studies are needed to clarify the role of NAC in CIN prevention • One study suggests that attenuation of increased SCr is artifactual while other data suggest extra renal protective effects
Contrast agent	Low osmolarity, low volume	Use minimum volume of low-osmolar or iso-osmolar contrast	• Low-osmolar agents are widely used as the default contrast agent for CT and cardiac catheterization • Iso-osmolar agents are more expensive but should be considered in high-risk patients

Abbreviation: NAC, N-acetylcysteine.

6 hours postprocedure. The alkalinization regimen was not tested against volume expansion using a more standard regimen of several hours of periprocedure NS.

- The question of whether to administer a shorter course of sodium bicarbonate infusion or longer periprocedure NS regimens remains unresolved. Although the alkalinization study was not used for patients undergoing emergent procedures, its applicability may be in situations where there is little time for prophylactic measures (~1 hour). Additional confirmatory trials with bicarbonate must be performed before conclusive recommendations can be made.
- Sodium bicarbonate infusion requires monitoring of volume status and alkalinization. See Table 82-4 for dosing.

• *Minimize total contrast volume.* Contrast volume is an independent predictor of CIN. While there is likely a dose-dependent risk of renal dysfunction, an optimal threshold dose is unknown.

○ Recommended doses of contrast: < 300–400 mL if SCr is normal, < 150 mL if SCr 1.5–3.4 mg/dL, and < 100 mL if SCr > 3.4 mg/dL. CIN is rare if contrast volume is < 100 mL. (A typical diagnostic catheter coronary catheterization procedure, for example, may involve 60 cc vs. an interventional procedure may require over 200 cc.)

○ If more than one contrast-requiring study is needed, the *studies should be spaced by at least 48 hours.* Some experts suggest the use of an iso-osmolar agent if a follow-up contrast study is needed; however, this practice has not been evaluated in trials. See below.

• *Minimize contrast osmolarity.*

○ Radiocontrast agents can be generally classified as hyper osmolar (1500–1800 mOsm/kg), "low-osmolar" (600–900 mOsm/kg), and iso-osmolar (290 mOsm/kg). Of note, "low-osmolar" is two to three times the plasma osmolality.

- Hyper osmolar agents have been demonstrated to lead to higher incidence of CIN compared with "low-osmolar" agents. "Low-osmolar" agents are thus commonly used, but increasing data support the use of iso-osmolar contrast agents in high-risk patients. Despite the higher costs of iso-osmolar contrast media, the use of the agents may be cost-effective.

- The use of *prophylactic hemodialysis or hemofiltration* is not recommended based upon available data. While dialysis can remove contrast media, randomized trials have not demonstrated a decrease in CIN or clinical benefit with prophylactic *hemodialysis*. A few trials have suggested benefit with *hemofiltration*, but the intervention itself removes creatinine and may have affected outcomes in these studies. Moreover, these therapies are expensive, complicated, and carry additional risk.

- The antioxidant properties of *ascorbic acid* may help mitigate oxidative stress and free radical production in CIN.
  ○ In animals, ascorbic acid has been shown to attenuate renal damage from cisplatin, aminoglycosides, and postischemic stress.
  ○ In a double-blind RCT of ascorbic acid vs. placebo among 231 patients undergoing nonemergent cardiac catheterization (mean baseline SCr 1.36–1.46), the incidence of CIN was 9% after ascorbic acid vs. 20% in the placebo group. Ascorbic acid is inexpensive and safe in humans and has potential as a prophylactic measure for CIN. Further data and confirmation in other centers are needed to clarify the role of ascorbic acid in CIN prevention.

- Over the past 5 years, the use of *N-acetylcysteine (NAC)* has been the most widely studied prophylaxis strategy. Over 20 trials and 11 meta-analyses have yielded conflicting results and no clear strategy for the use of NAC. NAC may reduce the incidence of CIN, but this effect is not reported consistently across currently available trials. Differences in contrast media osmolarity and volume, definitions of CIN, patient populations, hydration protocols, timing of procedures, and NAC regimens, have lead to significant heterogeneity of trials. Of 11 meta-analyses, 7 concluded the effect of NAC was beneficial while 4 found the data inconclusive.
  ○ The purported nephroprotective mechanism of NAC is unclear.
    ■ NAC is a thiol-containing antioxidant that may confer renal protection by scavenging oxygen-derived free radicals or by enhancing the vasodilatory effects of nitric oxide.
    ■ Additionally, the reported nephro-protective effects of NAC may reflect extrarenal mechanisms.

  In patients with acute MI, NAC has been associated with increased coronary reperfusion, reduced infarct size, and preservation of LV function.
    ■ Alternatively, some data suggest that the effects of NAC on SCr are artifactual, reflecting altered tubular secretion and metabolism of creatinine rather than changes in GFR or renal injury.
  ○ Given the low cost and side effects of NAC, some favor the use of *600–1200 mg po bid for 2 days*, beginning the day before the procedure for patients at risk for CIN. Studies comparing 600 and 1200 mg po bid regimens suggest greater benefit with the higher dose. Data from the available clinical trials, however, do not definitively support the use of these regimens.
  ○ Several studies have reported a dose-dependent effect at NAC suggesting that a higher dose is needed when a greater amount of contrast is required.
    ■ In a recent study of 354 patients with acute MI undergoing primary angioplasty (median creatinine 1.02–1.06), administration of a total dose of 6000 mg of NAC plus periprocedure NS resulted in lower incidence of CIN (8%) compared with 3000 mg NAC plus hydration (15%) or hydration alone (33%). Additionally, mortality was significantly lower in groups receiving NAC (3% to 5%) compared with hydration alone (13%), perhaps reflecting cardio protective effects of NAC. Limitations of this study, however, included high complication rates in the control group and the administration of larger than average contrast volumes. Further studies are needed to clarify the use of high-dose NAC in emergent coronary angiography.

BIBLIOGRAPHY

Bellomo R, Chapman M, Finfer S, et al. Low-dose dopamine in patients with early renal dysfunction: a placebo-controlled randomised trial. Australian and New Zealand Intensive Care Society (ANZICS) Clinical Trials Group. *Lancet.* 2000;356: 2139–2143.

Gami AS, Garovic ED. Contrast nephropathy after coronary angiography. *Mayo Clinic Proc.* 2004;79:211–219.

Griffin MR, Yared A, Wayne AR. Nonsteroidal anti-inflammatory drugs and acute renal failure in elderly persons. *Am J Epidemiol.* 2000;151:488–496.

Hoffman U, Fischereder M, Kruger B, et al. The value of N-acetylcysteine in the prevention of radiocontrast agent-induced nephropathy seems questionable. *J Am Soc Nephrol.* 2004; 15:407–410.

Humes HD. Aminoglycoside nephrotoxicity. *Kidney Int.* 1988; 33:900–911.

Jo S, Youn T, Koo B, et al. Renal toxicity evaluation and comparison between visipaque (iodixanol) and hexabrix (ioxaglate) in patients with renal insufficiency undergoing coronary angiography: the RECOVER study: a randomized controlled trial. *J Am Coll Cardiol.* 2006; 48:924–930.

Marenzi G, Assanelli E, Marana I, et al. N-acetylcysteine and contrast-induced nephropathy in primary angioplasty. *N Engl J Med.* 2006;354:2773–2782.

Marenzi G, Lauri G, Campodonico J, et al. Comparison of two hemofiltration protocols for prevention of contrast-induced nephropathy in high-risk patients. *Am J Med.* 2006;119: 155–162.

McCullough PA, Bertrand ME, Brinker JA, et al. A meta-analysis of the renal safety of isosmolar iodixanol compared with low-osmolar contrast media. *J Am Coll Cardiol.* 2006;48: 692–699.

Mehta RL, Chertow GM. Acute renal failure definitions and classification: time for change? *J Am Soc Nephrol.* 2003;14: 2178–2187.

Morcos SK, Thomsen HS, Webb JA. Contrast-media-induced nephrotoxicity: a consensus report. Contrast Media Safety Committee, European Society of Urogenital Radiology (ESUR). *Eur Radiol.* 1999;9:1602–1613.

Pannu N, Wiebe N, Tonelli M. Prophylaxis strategies for contrast-induced nephropathy. *JAMA.* 2006;295: 2765–2779.

Parfrey P. The clinical epidemiology of contrast-induced nephropathy. *Cardiovasc Intervent Radiol.* 2005;28 (suppl 2):S3–S11.

Rudnick MR, Kesselheim A, Goldfarb S. Contrast-induced nephropathy: how it develops, how to prevent it. *Cleve Clin J Med.* 2006;73:75–87.

Rudnick MR, Berns, JS, Cohen RM, et al. Nephrotoxic risks of renal angiography: contrast-media associated nephrotoxicity and atheroembolism—A critical review. *Am J Kidney Dis.* 1994;24:713.

Stacul F. Reducing the risks for contrast-induced nephropathy. *Cardiovasc Intervent Radiol.* 2005;28 (suppl 2): S12–S128.

Spargias K, Alexopoulos E, Kyrzopoulos S, et al. Ascorbic acid prevents contrast-mediated nephropathy in patients with renal dysfunction undergoing coronary angiography or intervention. *Circulation.* 2004;110:2837–2842.

Stacul F, Adam A, Becker CR, et al, CIN Consensus Working Panel. Strategies to reduce the risk of contrast-induced nephropathy. *Am J Cardiol.* 2006;98: 59K–77K.

Townsend RR, Cohen DL, Katholi R, et al. Safety of intravenous gadolinium (Gd-BOPTA) infusion in patients with renal insufficiency. *Am J Kidney Dis.* 2000;36:1207–1212.

Weisbord SD, Chen H, Stone RA, et al. Associations of increases in serum creatinine with mortality and length of hospital stay after coronary angiography. *J Am Soc Nephrol.* 2006;17: 2871–2877.

83 ACUTE RENAL FAILURE

Prabhdeep Sandhu and Adam C. Schaffer

EPIDEMIOLOGY/OVERVIEW

- ARF is an important issue in hospital medicine, given the increase in LOS and mortality associated with ARF. ARF may be the presenting complaint, a consequence of the underlying illness (eg, sepsis), or the result of medications received in the hospital or other iatrogenic factors.
- Previously there had been many different definitions of ARF. An emerging consensus definition uses the term acute kidney injury, which is defined by Levin et al. as: "an abrupt (within 48 hours) reduction in kidney function currently defined as an absolute increase in SCr of either ≥ 0.3 mg/dL or a percentage increase of $\geq 50\%$ (1.5-fold from baseline) or a reduction in UO (documented oliguria of < 0.5 mL/kg/hr for > 6 hours)."
- A complementary system categorizes renal failure across a spectrum of severity, according to the RIFLE criteria (*r*isk, *i*njury, *f*ailure, *l*oss, *E*SKD—see Table 83-1). This classification scheme uses both GFR criteria and UO criteria.
- Typically, a diagnosis of ARF is also categorized according to the accompanying UO.
  - Nonoliguric (> 400 mL/24 hr)
  - Oliguric (< 400 mL/24 hr)
  - Anuric (< 100 mL/24 hr)
- Whether ARF is nonoliguric, oliguric, or anuric is significant for both diagnosis and prognosis.
- Estimates of the incidence of ARF in hospitalized patients vary considerably, depending on the ARF definition used and the population studied.
  - An analysis of the 2001 National Hospital Discharge Survey by Liangos et al. showed that the frequency of ARF, defined by ICD-9 codes, was 1.9%. In patients with ARF, LOS was increased by an average of 2 days, the adjusted odds ratio (OR) for in-hospital mortality was 4.1, and the adjusted OR for discharge to a short- or long-term care facility was 2.0.
  - A prospective study by Nash et al. of 4622 consecutive patients admitted to a tertiary care hospital revealed that ARF (defined as an increase in SCr of at least 0.5 mg/dL, depending on baseline SCr) occurred in 7.2% of patients. The most common causes of ARF were decreased renal perfusion (most

TABLE 83-1   RIFLE Criteria

	GFR CRITERIA	UO CRITERIA
Risk	Increased SCr × 1.5 or GFR decrease > 25%	UO < 0.5 mL/kg/hr × 6 hr
Injury	Increased serum SCr × 2 or GFR decrease > 50%	UO < 0.5 mL/kg/hr × 12 hr
Failure	Increased SCr × 3 or GFR decrease > 75% or a SCr > 4 mg/dL	UO < 0.3 mL/kg/hr × 24 hr or anuria × 12 hr
Loss	Complete loss of kidney function > 4 weeks	
ESKD	Complete loss of kidney function > 3 months	

SOURCE: Adapted from Bellomo R, Ronco C, Kellum JA, et al. Acute dialysis quality initiative workgroup. Acute renal failure—definition, outcome measures, animal models, fluid therapy and information technology needs: the Second International Consensus Conference of the Acute Dialysis Quality Initiative (ADQI) Group. *Crit Care* (London, England). Aug 2004;8(4):R204-R212,UI: 15312219; Bellomo R, Kellum JA, Ronco C. Defining and classifying acute renal failure: from advocacy to consensus and validation of the RIFLE criteria. *Int Care Med.* Mar 2007;33(3):409–413,UI:17165018.

often from volume contraction and hypotension), medications (most often aminoglycosides and NSAIDs), radiographic contrast media, postoperative conditions, and sepsis. The overall mortality rate among the ARF patients was 19.4%, with a mortality rate of 37.8% among those patients with an increase in SCr of >3 mg/dL.

○ An observational cohort study by Mehta et al. of 618 ICU patients with ARF found that the leading causes of ARF were ischemic ATN (primarily because of unknown precipitants, hypotension, and sepsis), followed by nephrotoxic ATN (primarily because of radiocontrast, rhabdomyolysis, antibiotics, and calcineurin inhibitors). In this cohort, the in-hospital mortality rate was 37%.

• ARF is also associated with significantly increased hospital costs. A study by Chertow et al. of almost 20,000 consecutive adults admitted to an urban academic medical center demonstrated a mean adjusted increase in total hospital costs of $7499 with a SCr increase of at least 0.5 mg/dL, and $22,023 with a SCr increase of at least 2.0 mg/dL.

PATHOPHYSIOLOGY

• A common, useful approach to ARF is to categorize it into prerenal, intrarenal (also referred to as intrinsic renal), and postrenal etiologies. This scheme is helpful in approaching both the pathophysiology and diagnosis of ARF (Table 83-2).

• Two of the most common causes of ARF in hospitalized patients, prerenal hypovolemia and ischemic ATN, should be thought of as a continuum, with prolonged

TABLE 83-2   Classification of the Major Causes of ARF

CAUSE	EXAMPLES
Prerenal	
Hypovolemia	Hemorrhage (eg, GI bleed), vomiting, overdiuresis
Hypotension	Cardiogenic shock, sepsis
Pharmacologic	NSAIDs, ACEI/ARBs
Vascular, large-vessel	Stenosis, thrombosis, dissection
Intrarenal	
ATN (ischemic)	Hypotension, sepsis
ATN (toxic)	Aminoglycosides, IV contrast, amphotericin B, cisplatin, myoglobin
AIN glomerular	Glomerulonephritis (eg, postinfectious GN, cryoglobulinemia, lupus nephritis)
Vascular, small-vessel	Vasculitis, atheroemboli, thrombotic microangiopathy, DIC
Postrenal	
Ureteral obstruction	Calculi, tumor, clot, lymphadenopathy, retroperitoneal fibrosis
Bladder outlet obstruction	Neurogenic, tumor
Urethral obstruction	BPH, malpositioned or obstructed Foley catheter, stricture

Abbreviation: ACEI, angiotensin-converting enzyme inhibitor; BPH, benign prostatic hyperplasia.
SOURCE: Adapted from Singri N, Ahya SN, Levin ML. Acute renal failure. *JAMA.* Feb 12 2003;289(6):747–751, UI: 12585954; Hilton R. Acute renal failure. *BMJ.* Oct 14 2006;333(7572):786–790, UI: 17038736; and Lameire N, Van Biesen W, Vanholder R. Acute renal failure. *Lancet.* Jan 29-Feb 4 2005;365(9457):417–430,UI: 15680458.

hypovolemia leading to renal hypoperfusion, resulting in damage to the renal tubules and ATN.

- In prenal cases, the kidney adaptively tries to conserve sodium (and hence water), and so the tubules will reabsorb a large proportion of the filtered sodium. The degree of renal sodium avidity can be quantitatively assessed using the fractional excretion of sodium (FE_{Na}). The FE_{Na} (as a percent) is calculated as

$$(\text{urine sodium} \times \text{plasma creatinine} \times 100)/$$
$$(\text{plasma sodium} \times \text{urine creatinine}).$$

- The FE_{Na} has a number of limitations.
  ○ It is not reliable in the setting of diuretic treatment, as diuretics effect increased urine sodium losses.
  ○ It is not reliable in the setting of a normal or near-normal GFR.
  ○ It is not reliable in the setting of an increased bicarbonaturia, such as may occur with severe vomiting. In these cases, the increased sodium excretion (and increased FE_{Na}) may be caused by its excretion as sodium bicarbonate, in order to compensate for the alkalosis.
- In cases where the FE_{Na} may be unreliable because of diuretic use, an alternative is to use the fractional excretion of urea (FE_{urea}), which is less influenced by diuretic use than is the FE_{Na}. FE_{urea} suggests a prerenal etiology when < 35% (analogous to FE_{Na} < 1%) and supports ATN when > 50% (analogous to FE_{Na} > 2%).
- These indices can prove useful in helping diagnose the cause of ARF, when considered in the larger clinical context, as will be discussed in the next section.

CLINICAL PRSENTATION, DIFFERENTIAL, MAKING THE DIAGNOSIS

- ARF is often detected based on elevations in serum BUN and creatinine values measured as part of routine laboratory tests, and may be asymptomatic.

- The use of SCr to assess renal function has a number of limitations.
  ○ If a patient initially has a normal GFR, this GFR can fall significantly with only a modest increase in the creatinine.
  ○ SCr may inaccurately represent GFR in nonsteady state conditions, such as ARF.
- Alternative serum markers of renal function, such as cystatin C, are currently under investigation, though they are not yet in wide clinical use.
- The history and physical examination should be geared to assisting in categorizing the patient into one of the three major categories of ARF (prerenal, intrarenal, and postrenal).
  ○ A history of vomiting, deceased oral intake, or bleeding—and examination findings suggestive of hypovolemia—support a diagnosis of prerenal ARF.
  ○ A history of receiving nephrotoxic drugs or undergoing radiographic studies that involved IV contrast support a diagnosis on intrarenal ARF.
  ○ A history of anuria or the passage of large blood clots in the urine—and examination findings, such as suprapubic fullness from a distended bladder—support a diagnosis of postrenal ARF.
- Initial testing should include, in addition to serum electrolytes: urinalysis (both dipstick and urine sediment analysis) and urine electrolytes (urine sodium, urine creatinine, and, if on a diuretic, urine urea). These tests can suggest what type of ARF is present (Table 83-3).
- Further laboratory testing will be guided by the history and physical examination, and initial laboratory results.
  ○ Urine eosinophils can be obtained to assess for AIN.
  ○ SCr kinase should be obtained if there is a suspicion for rhabdomyolysis. A urine dipstick positive for blood (which cross-reacts with myoglobin) in the absence of any red blood cells (RBCs) in the urine sediment should raise the possibility of rhabdomyolysis.
  ○ If there is a suspicion for glomerulonephritis (GN), such as might result from the finding of red cell casts and proteinuria on initial urinalysis, then

TABLE 83-3 Urine Chemistry and Urinalysis Findings in ARF

ETIOLOGY OF ARF	$URINE_{Na}$	FE_{Na}	FEU_{Urea}	PROTEINURIA	URINE SEDIMENT
Prerenal	< 20	< 1%	< 35%	Minimal	Bland
Intrarenal					
ATN	> 30	> 2%	> 50%	Minimal	Granular casts
AIN	Variable	Variable	Variable	Minimal	Eosinophils
GN	< 20	< 1%	< 35%	> 250 mg/d	RBC casts
Postrenal	Variable	Variable	Variable	Minimal	Bland or RBCs

SOURCE: Adapted from: Weisbord SD, Palevsky PM. Acute renal failure in the intensive care unit. *Sem Resp Crit Care Med*. Jun 2006;27(3):262–273, UI: 16791759; Singri N, Ahya SN, Levin ML. Acute renal failure. *JAMA*. Feb 12 2003;289(6):747–51, UI: 12585954; and Albright RC Jr. Acute renal failure: a practical update. Mayo *Clin Proc*. Jan 2001;76(1):67–74, UI: 1115541.

serologic tests to help with the diagnosis of GN can be sent.

- C3 and C4, which are decreased in postinfectious GN, lupus nephritis, cryoglobulinemia, membranoproliferative GN, and atheroembolic disease
- C-ANCA (circulating-antineutrophil cytoplasmic antibody; proteinase 3-ANCA), which is elevated in Wegener's granulomatosis
- P-ANCA (perinuclear-antineutrophil cytoplasmic antibody; myeloperoxidase-ANCA), which is elevated in microscopic polyangiitis and Churg-Strauss syndrome
- Antinuclear antibody (ANA), which is elevated in lupus nephritis
- Antiglomerular basement membrane (anti-GBM) antibody, which is positive in Goodpasture's syndrome
- Cryoglobulins, which are positive in cryglobulinemia
- Hepatitis B and C serologies, which can be associated with membranous, membranoproliferative, and cryoglobulinemic GN
- Serum protein electrophoresis (SPEP)/urine protein electrophoresis (UPEP), which will be abnormal in multiple myeloma
- HIV antibody test, which if positive could suggest HIV-associated nephropathy (a collapsing focal segmental glomerulosclerosis)

◦ If the patient has a cancer—especially a hematologic malignancy and/or a large tumor burden—with rapid malignant cell turnover, then the possibility of TLS should be considered. Serum uric acid and phosphate should be checked, both of which are elevated in TLS.

◦ If there is an anion gap metabolic acidosis and the possibility of methanol or ethylene glycol ingestion, then serum osmolality should be obtained, with a osmolal gap (measured plasma osmolality calculated plasma osmolality) > 10 mOsm/kg supporting the diagnosis of the ingestion.

- Renal ultrasound examination should be obtained early in the workup of ARF unless the etiology of the ARF is readily apparent. Renal ultrasound should be obtained immediately if there is a suspicion for obstruction or a structural abnormality. The duplex Doppler component of the ultrasound can show renal vein thrombosis, and may indicate renal artery stenosis. Other imaging modalities may also have a role in specific situations.

◦ CT scan (noncontrast) can be useful if a mass is suspected of contributing to the ARF.

◦ MRI is also useful in imaging renal masses. MR angiography can help diagnose renovascular disease. However, the recent recognition of nephrogenic systemic fibrosis and its association with MR gadolinium contrast given to patients with renal insufficiency must be considered before MR studies are performed, especially MR angiography, which uses higher doses of gadolinium.

◦ Nuclear renal scanning may be useful when assessment of the split kidney function will aid in the diagnosis. Gallium scanning may have a role in distinguishing ATN from AIN. The inflammatory state of AIN will demonstrate increased renal uptake on the gallium scan, whereas in ATN, in which inflammation in the kidney is minimal, very little renal uptake will be seen.

- Renal biopsies are infrequently performed in the workup of ARF, on the assumption that the results of the biopsy are unlikely to alter management. This assumption has been challenged by Richards et al. in a study reporting that in 22 of 31 (71%) cases in which biopsies were performed for ARF, the results did alter management.

- In patients admitted for reasons unrelated to their kidneys, who then go on to develop nonoliguric ARF while in the hospital, the most common causes are ischemia (from causes such as sepsis and hypotension), hypovolemia, radiocontrast-induced nephropathy, and nephrotoxic insults from drugs, such as aminoglycosides and NSAIDs. Therefore, the initial evaluation of these patients should focus on looking for episodes of hypotension, the administration of potentially nephrotoxic drugs, and whether any IV contrast has been given to the patient.

- Though less common, three causes of ARF that inpatient clinicians should be aware of, which are sometimes overlooked, are atheroembolic renal disease, rhabdomyolysis, and acute phosphate nephropathy from phosphate-based bowel cleansing preparations.

◦ Atheroembolic disease refers to embolization of cholesterol plaques from the walls of large arteries that then obstruct the renal microvasculature. Atheroembolic disease typically occurs after intravascular instrumentation or anticoagulation, though it can occur spontaneously. A renal biopsy is required to confirm the diagnosis, though supporting laboratory findings include peripheral eosinophilia and hypocomplementemia, and livedo reticularis may be seen on physical examination.

◦ Release of myoglobin during rhabdomyolysis can lead to ARF. Rhabdomyolysis has many causes, including compression from immobility and drugs (including cocaine, statins, and daptomycin). Supporting laboratory findings include an elevated SCr kinase, dark urine, and a urine dipstick positive for blood with no RBCs seen on urine microscopy.

◦ Acute phosphate nephropathy refers to renal failure from deposition of calcium phosphate in the kidney, which can occur after use of an oral sodium phosphate bowel cleansing preparation, such as Fleet Phospho-soda. In a study by Markowitz et al., the mean time to presentation with renal failure because of acute phosphate nephropathy was 1 month, though patients presented as soon as 3 days after the bowel cleansing. Diagnosis is made by renal biopsy.

TRIAGE AND INITIAL MANAGEMENT

- The initial assessment of the patient with renal failure must determine whether the ARF is severe enough to require hemodialysis or other renal replacement therapy.
- Indications for hemodialysis in ARF include the following, when refractory to medical therapy (described below)
  - Hyperkalemia (K > 6.5 mEq/L)
  - Volume overload that is clinically significant (eg, resulting in respiratory compromise)
  - Acidemia (pH < 7.1)
  - Uremia that is symptomatic (eg, causing pericarditis, vomiting, change in mental status)
- Although a discussion of the optimal modality and dose of renal replacement therapy is beyond the scope of this outline, there are data that suggest that, when renal replacement therapy is indicated, more intensive therapy (eg, daily intermittent hemodialysis) is beneficial in ARF.
- Indications for admission to the ICU include hemodynamic instability accompanying the ARF that requires continuous renal replacement therapy (eg, continuous venovenous hemofiltration). Another possible indication for ICU admission is severe volume overload causing respiratory distress.
- Hyperkalemia can be managed medically using a number of treatments.
  - IV calcium mitigates the electrophysiologic effect of hyperkalemia on the heart. Calcium exerts its effect within minutes, though the effect is short-lived.
  - Dextrose 50% and IV insulin shift potassium from the serum compartment to the intracellular compartment. The insulin is responsible for the potassium compartment shift, and the glucose prevents hypoglycemia.
  - Beta-2-agonists also shift potassium intracellularly. Terbutaline may be used, though albuterol is often more readily available and is also an option.
  - Sodium bicarbonate leads to alkalinization, which results in hydrogen ion shifts from the intracellular compartment to the serum compartment, accompanied by potassium shifts from the serum compartment to the intracellular compartment, in order to maintain electroneutrality.

  - IV insulin, beta-2-agonists, and alkalinization do not remove potassium from the body; they merely temporarily shift potassium out of the serum compartment. Therefore, more definitive therapy that removes potassium from the body is also required.
  - Besides dialysis, the main medical therapy to remove potassium from the body is the orally administered potassium exchange resin sodium polystyrene sulfonate (Kayexalate), at an initial dose of 15–30 g.
  - Loop diuretics may be tried to achieve potassium loss in the urine. However, in the setting of severe ARF, diuretics may be ineffective.
  - Urine flow to the distal portion of the nephron is required for aldosterone-mediated potassium secretion. Therefore, in the setting of severe volume depletion, hyperkalemia may result from inadequate flow to the distal nephron. In these cases, volume resuscitation may be helpful in restoring normokalemia.
- Diuretics may be tried to manage hypervolemia in ARF. However, if the ARF is severe, patients may not respond. Escalating doses of a loop diuretic, addition of a thiazide diuretic, and a loop diuretic drip can be tried, especially if the hypervolemia is severe and there will be a delay in initiating hemodialysis. Though diuretics can be used for management of hypervolemia in the setting of ARF, they are not indicated merely to increase UO in ARF in the absence of hypervolemia (see below).
- An acidosis can be managed medically with the use of IV sodium bicarbonate. IV sodium bicarbonate is only indicated in severe acidosis, such as when the serum bicarbonate falls to approximately 15 mEq/L or below. An arterial blood gas should be obtained to assess the magnitude of the acidemia. Sodium bicarbonate provides a large amount of sodium, which can worsen hypervolemia. The 1 mEq/mL sodium bicarbonate contained in prefilled 50-mL syringes has the sodium equivalent to 5.9% saline.
- Once the initial metabolic or volume disturbances from the ARF are addressed, management consists of supportive care and correcting the underlying cause of the ARF. The treatment will depend on the most likely etiology of the ARF.
- In cases of prerenal, hypovolemic ARF, the treatment is IV hydration, generally with NS. Careful documentation of fluid inputs and UO are important, so that the increase in UO that would be expected when hypovolemic ARF is treated with IV hydration can be documented.
- For ATN, it is crucial to make sure the kidneys are not subjected to any further nephrotoxic insults, to give

them an opportunity to recover. Nephrotoxic medications, such as NSAIDs, angiotensin-converting enzyme inhibitor (ACEI)/angiotensin receptor blockers (ARBs), aminoglycosides, as well as IV contrast, must be assiduously avoided. Preventing hypotension is also important and so holding or altering the doses of any antihypertensive medications should be considered.

- The treatment of postrenal ARF depends on the level of obstruction. If the obstruction is caused by benign prostatic hyperplasia (BPH), then simply inserting a Foley catheter may be adequate initial treatment. If the obstruction is higher up in the urinary tract, then urgent urologic consultation should be obtained, and insertion of a ureteral stent or percutaneous nephrostomy tubes may be required.
- Various pharmacologic therapies have been used to treat ARF from ATN, though there is little clear evidence demonstrating their efficacy.
  - Loop diuretics are sometimes used with the goal of "converting" oliguric ARF to nonoliguric ARF. A RCT ($n = 338$) by Cantarovich et al. concluded that using either IV or po furosemide did not provide a mortality benefit or hasten renal recovery.
  - Dopamine, given in low "renal" doses, with the objective of ameliorating ARF by increasing renal blood flow, does not appear to provide a benefit. Bellomo et al. (2000), conducted an RCT ($n = 328$) of ICU patients with SCr > 1.7 mg/dL or increases in creatinine > 1.0 mg/dL and did not find any beneficial effect from low-dose dopamine in terms of peak SCr or need for renal replacement therapy.
  - Atrial natriuretic peptide (ANP), which increases GFR, did not show a benefit (in terms of dialysis-free survival) in an RCT ($n = 504$) by Allgren et al. of patients with ARF and SCr increases of at least 1 mg/dL.

DISEASE MANAGEMENT STRATEGIES

- Given the lack of effective medical therapies for ARF because of ATN, the most effective approach is prevention.
- Three of the most important steps to prevent ARF are avoiding nephrotoxins, avoiding hypotension, and maintaining normal intravascular volume.
- Given that patients with preexisting renal insufficiency are at especially high risk for ARF from nephrotoxins, potentially nephrotoxic medications must be dosed appropriately for a patient's GFR.
  - Automatically calculating the GFR based on the daily labs and making this calculated GFR prominently available to the clinical team, and the active

involvement of the pharmacy department in scrutinizing whether a given medication is dosed appropriately, are both potentially useful steps.
- Specific measures exist to prevent CIN. These measures are discussed in detail in Chap. 82.

CASE TRANSITIONS

- Document and communicate all drug allergies.
- Communicate all complications of the hospitalization to the receiving physician.
- For patients who require hemodialysis in the hospital because of ARF, if they are otherwise clinically stable, they can be discharged to the care of a nephrologist at an outpatient hemodialysis facility, who can care for the patient and monitor the patient for signs of renal recovery.
- Ensure appropriate follow-up with a nephrologist for all patients with renal insufficiency.

BIBLIOGRAPHY

Allgren RL, Marbury TC, Rahman SN, et al. Anaritide in acute tubular necrosis. Auriculin Anaritide Acute Renal Failure Study Group. *N Engl J Med.* Mar 20 1997;336(12): 828–834, UI:9062091.

Bellomo R, Chapman M, Finfer S, et al. Low-dose dopamine in patients with early renal dysfunction: a placebo-controlled randomised trial. Australian and New Zealand Intensive Care Society (ANZICS) Clinical Trials Group. *Lancet.* Dec 23–30 2000;356(9248):2139–2143, UI:11191541.

Bellomo R, Kellum JA, Ronco C. Defining and classifying acute renal failure: from advocacy to consensus and validation of the RIFLE criteria. *Int Care Med.* Mar 2007;33(3):409–413, UI:17165018.

Cantarovich F, Rangoonwala B, Lorenz H, et al. High-Dose Furosemide in Acute Renal Failure Study Group. High-dose furosemide for established ARF: a prospective, randomized, double-blind, placebo-controlled, multicenter trial. *Am J Kid Dis.* Sep 2004;44(3):402–409, UI:15332212.

Chertow GM, Burdick E, Honour M, et al. Acute kidney injury, mortality, length of stay, and costs in hospitalized patients. *J Am Soc Nephrol.* Nov 2005;16(11):3365–3370, UI:16177006.

Guo X, Nzerue C. How to prevent, recognize, and treat drug-induced nephrotoxicity. *Clev Clin J Med.* Apr 2002;69(4): 289–290, 293–294, 296–297 passim,UI: 11996200.

Kellum J, Leblanc M, Venkataraman R. Renal failure (acute) [update of *Clin Evid.* Jun 2005;(13):1070–1092;PMID:16135288]. *Clin Evid.* Jun 2006;(15):1191–1212, UI: 16973048.

Lameire N, Van Biesen W, Vanholder R. Acute renal failure. *Lancet.* Jan 29-Feb 4 2005;365(9457):417–430, UI:15680458.

Levin A, Warnock DG, Mehta RL, et al. Acute Kidney Injury Network Working Group. Improving outcomes from acute kidney injury: report of an initiative. *Am J Kid Dis.* Jul 2007;50(1):1–4, UI:17591518.

Liangos O, Wald R, O'Bell JW. et al. Epidemiology and outcomes of acute renal failure in hospitalized patients: a national survey. *Clin J Am Soc Nephrol.* Jan 1 2006;1(1):43–51.

Marenzi G, Assanelli E, Marana I, et al. N-acetylcysteine and contrast-induced nephropathy in primary angioplasty. *N Engl J Med.* Jun 29 2006;354(26):2773–2782, UI: 16807414.

Markowitz GS, Stokes MB, Radhakrishnan J. et al. Acute phosphate nephropathy following oral sodium phosphate bowel purgative: an underrecognized cause of chronic renal failure. *J Am Soc Nephrol.* Nov 2005;16(11):3389–3396, UI: 16192415.

Mehta RL, Pascual MT, Soroko S. et al. Program to improve care in acute renal disease. Spectrum of acute renal failure in the intensive care unit: the PICARD experience. *Kid Int.* 66(4): Oct 2004;1613–1621, UI:15458458.

Nash K, Hafeez A, Hou S. Hospital-acquired renal insufficiency. *Am J Kid Dis.* May 2002;39(5):930–936, UI:11979336.

Richards NT, Darby S, Howie AJ, et al. Knowledge of renal histology alters patient management in over 40% of cases. *Nephrol Dial Transplant.* 1994;9(9):1255–1259, UI:7816285.

Singri N, Ahya SN, Levin ML. Acute renal failure. *JAMA.* Feb 12 2003;289(6):747–751, UI: 12585954.

84 CHRONIC KIDNEY DISEASE

Li-Li Hsiao and Valerie Luyckx

EPIDEMIOLOGY/OVERVIEW

- Chronic kidney disease (CKD) is a worldwide public health problem affecting 50 million people.
- CKD is defined using either of the two criteria (National Kidney Foundation, International Society of Nephrology)
  - Kidney damage for ≥ 3 months as defined by structural or functional abnormalities of the kidney, with or without decreased glomerular filtration rate (GFR). Kidney damage is manifest either by pathologic abnormalities, abnormalities in the composition of the blood or urine, or abnormalities on imaging tests.
  - CKD should be suspected when the GFR < 60 mL/min/1.73 m^2 for > 3 months, with or without kidney damage.
- According to GFR and presence of proteinuria and/or hematuria, CKD is classified into five stages. (See Table 84-1.)
- About 11% of the US population is affected by CKD and the prevalence and incidence are rising.
  - The incidence of "new-onset" kidney disease (defined as the estimated glomerular filtration rate, eGFR, < 64 mL/min/1.73 m^2 in men and < 59 mL/min/1.73 m^2 in women) is approximately 0.5% per year.
  - According to the Third National Health and Nutrition Examination Survey (NHANES III), the prevalence of stage 3 and 4 CKD (eGFR 15–59 mL/min/1.73 m^2) among US adults age 20 and over was 4.5%.
  - The number of individuals with kidney failure requiring treatment with dialysis or transplantation in the United States is projected to increase from 450,000 in 2003 to 650,000 in 2010.
- The total costs for management of kidney disease is approaching 24% of Medicare expenditures; about double that of 10 years ago.
- CKD is "under-diagnosed" and "under-treated" in the United States resulting in poor outcomes and high cost.
- The associated adverse outcomes of CKD, such as end-stage renal disease (ESRD), cardiovascular disease (CVD), and premature death are preventable if detected early.
- Hospitalists are positioned to identify and screen individuals at increased risk of CKD, and initiate management strategies designed to prevent or lessen the progression of CKD.

PATHOPHYSIOLOGY

- The primary functions of the kidneys are to maintain near constancy of the volume and composition of the extracellular fluid. These functions are usually remarkably well-preserved until late in the course of chronic renal disease.
- When nephrons are lost through disease or surgical resection, the least affected remaining nephrons undergo adaptive physiologic responses. Nephron hypertrophy and hyperfunction combine to compensate for the acquired renal functional deficits.
- Over time, and in the presence of ongoing renal risk factors, the nephron adaptation becomes maladaptive perpetuating an ongoing cycle of injury and compensation, accompanied by progressive loss of renal function. (See Table 84-2.)

TABLE 84-1 Stages of CKD and Surveillance Recommendations

STAGE DESCRIPTION	GFR (mL/min/1.73 m²)	RELATED TERMS AND SURVEILLANCE FREQUENCY
1 Kidney damage with normal or increased GFR	> 90	Albuminuria, proteinuria, hematuria 12 monthly
2 Kidney damage with mild decreased GFR	60–89	Albuminuria, proteinuria, hematuria 12 monthly
3 Moderate decreased GFR	30–59	Chronic renal insufficiency Early renal insufficiency 6 monthly (12 monthly if stable)
4 Severe decreased GFR	15–29	Chronic renal insufficiency Late renal insufficiency Pre-ESRD 3 monthly (6 monthly if stable)
5 Kidney failure	< 15 (or dialysis)	Renal failure, uremia, ESRD 3 monthly

Source: Modified from American Society of Nephrology. Chronic kidney disease and progression. *Nephrology Self-Assessment Program (NephSAP)*. Vol 5, No 3. ASN Offices: Washington, DC; May 2006 and Sheffield Kidney Institutes.

• CKD is usually a consequence of systemic diseases that are treatable.
  ○ Diabetes Type II is the leading cause of CKD and ESRD worldwide. Type I diabetes is associated with a greater risk of CKD compared to Type II, but the number of patients is smaller. The incidence of diabetes-associated renal disease is constantly increasing as the world wide epidemic of Type II diabetes is emerging.
  ○ Systemic hypertension is the second major cause of ESRD world wide.
  ○ Other major causes of CKD include chronic glomerular diseases (eg, IgA nephropathy), CKD in the transplant, and other diseases such as vasculitis, renovascular, tubulointerstitial, and cystic diseases. (See Table 84-3.)
• Early initiation of management strategies titrated to treatment goals is imperative to interrupt the cycle of ongoing renal injury and nephron loss, and attenuate renal disease progression.
• Adverse consequences of CKD, which deteriorate as renal disease progresses, include anemia, volume overload, metabolic acidosis, hyperparathyroidism, and malnutrition.

TABLE 84-2 Traditional and Nontraditional Risk Factors for CVD in CKD Patients

TRADITIONAL RISK FACTORS	NONTRADITIONAL RISK FACTORS
High blood pressure	Anemia
Left ventricular hypertrophy	C-reactive protein
Dyslipidemia	Lipoprotein
Diabetes	Fibrinogen
Smoking	Factor VIII
Low physical activity	Interleukin-6
Alcohol use	

Source: Modified from Shlipak, et al. Cardiovascular mortality risk in chronic kidney disease: comparison of traditional and novel risk factors *JAMA*. 2005;293:1737–1745.

CLINICAL PRESENTATION AND DIAGNOSIS

• Symptoms and signs of CKD develop late, therefore it is critical to maintain a high index of suspicion for patients at increased risk, in order to make an early diagnosis and initiate therapeutic strategies. Suggested surveillance times are outlined in Table 84-4.

TABLE 84-3 Potential Risk Factors for Susceptibility to and Initiation of CKD

CLINICAL FACTORS	SOCIODEMOGRAPHIC FACTORS
Diabetes	Old age
Hypertension	Ethnic minority status: African American, American Indian, Hispanic, Asian, or Pacific Islander
Autoimmune diseases	
Systemic infections	
Urinary tract infections	
Urinary stones	Low income/education
Lower urinary tract obstruction	
Neoplasm	
Family history of CKDs	
Recovery from acute kidney failure	
Reduction in kidney mass	
Exposure to certain drugs such as	
• Radiographic contrast	
• Selected antimicrobial agents (eg, aminoglycosides and amphotericin B)	
• Nonsteroidal anti-inflammatory agents, including cyclooxygenase type 2 inhibitors	
• Angiotensin-converting enzyme inhibition and angiotensin-2 receptor blockers	
• Cyclosporine and tacrolimus Low birth weight	

Source: With permission from National Kidney Foundation: Clinical practice guidelines for managing dyslipidemias in chronic kidney disease. *Am J Kidney Dis*. Apr 2003;41(4 Suppl 3):S1–S91.

TABLE 84-4   Uremic Symptoms and Signs of CKD

SYMPTOMS	SIGNS
Volume overload	Volume overload
Secondary to reduced sodium excretion	Hypertension
Hypertension	Lethargy
Secondary to reduced filtration surface	Pallor
area, sodium retention, renovascular	Pericardial rub
disease, etc.	Evidence of scratching
Pruritis	Uremic frost
Secondary to uremia, calcium-phosphate	Uremic fetor
deposition, high PTH	Bruises
Bruising and bleeding	Asterixis
Secondary to uremic platelet dysfunction	
Lack of appetite	
Secondary to uremia, metabolic acidosis,	
metallic taste	
Bone pain and fracture	
Secondary to hyperparathyroidism	
Nocturnal leg cramps	
Poor concentration and sleep	
Secondary to uremia	
Fatigue	
Secondary to uremia, anemia, metabolic acidosis	
Hiccups	

Abbreviation: PTH, parathyroid hormone.

- Serum creatinine (SCr) alone is an inaccurate marker of renal function as it is dependent of patient age, gender, ethnicity, and muscle mass.
  - Because of lack of standardization, calibration differences of SCr can be up to 0.3 mg/mL from one laboratory to another. Ideally, repeated tests in an individual patient, therefore, should be done in the same laboratory.
- Given the lack of overt signs and symptoms in the majority of patients with CKD, and the low sensitivity of SCr, formulae have been developed to estimate GFR, allowing for
  - Detection and diagnosis of CKD
  - Estimation of prognosis depending on stage of CKD (Table 84-1)
  - Guidance of appropriate dosing of medications to avoid drug toxicity
  - Monitoring the rate of progression of CKD over time
  - Identification of patients with reduced GFR despite "normal" SCr, who may be at increased risk of acute renal failure (eg, postcardiac surgery, radiocontrast administration, etc.)
- Two equations are most commonly used by nephrologists to estimate GFR for patients 18 years of age or older.
  1. The *Cockcroft-Gault equation* estimates creatinine clearance (CrCl)

  $$(mL/min) = (140 - age) \times weight\ (0.85\ weight\ if\ female) \div 72 \times SCr$$

  2. The *Modification of Diet in Renal Disease equation* estimates GFR

  $$(mL/min/1.73\ m^2) = 175 \times (SCr)^{-1.154} \times (age)^{-0.203} \times (0.742\ if\ female).$$

  If patient is black, multiply by 1.21.

- Screen all patients at increased risk for CKD by checking a urinary dipstick and sediment.
  - The presence of hematuria together with proteinuria on dipstick strongly suggests a renal source of the abnormalities, which may necessitate further investigations, serologic testing, renal biopsy, and so on.
  - The presence of urinary casts is suggestive of the pathologic process
    - Red cell casts suggest glomerulonephritis
    - White cell casts suggest pyelonephritis or interstitial nephritis
    - Granular or muddy brown casts suggest acute tubular necrosis
    - Broad waxy casts suggest advanced CKD
  - Urine microscopy also detects presence of cells, casts, crystals, lipid droplets, bacteria.
- All patients at increased risk for CKD should be screened for proteinuria—defined as: normoalbuminuria: < 30 mg/d; microalbuminuria: 30–300 mg/d; proteinuria: > 300 mg/d.
  - Early morning samples are most sensitive for detection of microalbuminuria.
  - Two of three samples should fall within the microalbuminuric or macroalbuminuric range to confirm classification.
  - Spot urine samples correlate well with 24-hour urine protein collections and are acceptable surrogates especially for follow-up monitoring.
  - Standard urine dipsticks detect total protein above a concentration of 10–20 mg/dL, which is insensitive in detecting microalbuminuria or positively charged serum proteins such as immunoglobulin light chains and Bence-Jones protein.
    - If the routine dipstick is positive, PCR is cheaper for quantitative proteinuria detection and follow-up.
    - If dipstick is negative but renal disease is suspected, albumin-to-creatinine ratio (ACR) is recommended.
  - Factors causing false positive results include dehydration, hematuria, exercise, urinary tract infection, drugs that alkalinize urine pH.
  - Factors causing false negative results include excessive hydration, urine proteins other than albumin, positively charged serum proteins such as some immunoglobulin light chains.
  - The albumin-specific dipstick, which detects urine albumin above a concentration of 3–4 mg/dL, is useful for detecting microalbuminuria, but is expensive.
- 24-hour urine collections allow for the measurement of GFR and of 24-hour urine protein excretion. Radio-isotope scans are another possible method for measuring GFR.
  - When measuring CrCl to estimate GFR, it is important to assess completeness of the urine collection.

This may be estimated for patients based on the daily creatinine excretion.

- Under age 50, creatinine excretion should be 20–25 mg/kg lean body weight for men and 15–20 mg/kg for women.
- Over age 50, there is a progressive decline in creatinine excretion to ~ 50% by age 90.

○ CrCl (mL/min) =
$$\frac{[(Ucr \text{ in mg/dL} \times \text{urine volume in L/d}) \div SCr \text{ in mg/dL}] \times 1000}{1400}$$

○ CrCl should ideally be adjusted for body surface area (BSA).
  - BSA = the square root of [(height in cm × weight in kg) ÷ 3600]
  - Adjusted CrCl (mL/min per 1.72 m²) = (CrCl × 1.73) ÷ BSA

- Specific tests for etiology of renal dysfunction, if indicated, may include antinuclear antibody (ANA), C3, C4, hepatitis C, hepatitis B, rapid plasma reagin (RPR), cryoglobulins, serum protein electrophoresis (SPEP), urine protein electrophoresis (UPEP), antistreptolysin O titre (ASOT), blood cultures, renal biopsy.
- Renal imaging of the kidney with ultrasound is easy, safe, and may identify
  ○ A reversible process (hydronephrosis, stones)
  ○ The cause of CKD (multiple cysts; discrepancy in renal size consistent with renal artery stenosis)
  ○ The chronicity of CKD (as reflected by small kidneys bilaterally, atrophy, absence of a kidney)

DISEASE MANAGEMENT STRATEGIES

See Table 84-5.
- Once CKD is established, it is usually irreversible.
- The major focus of management is to minimize further renal injury and halt renal disease progression.
- A multidisciplinary approach is often needed to optimize all renal risk factors in an individual patient to meet established treatment goals
  ○ Control blood pressure (BP)
  ○ Manage diabetes
  ○ Reduce proteinuria
  ○ Optimize nutrition
  ○ Identify and treat cardiovascular risk factors
  ○ Manage complications of CKD
  ○ Prepare for renal replacement therapy (see Table 84-6)

CONTROL OF BLOOD PRESSURE IN PATIENTS WITH CKD

- Hypertension is both a cause and a complication of CKD.
- Uncontrolled hypertension is associated with rapid decline of GFR and development of CVD complications.

TABLE 84-5 Precautions for Hospitalists in Managing Patients with CKD

- Be aware of CKD as a risk factor for acute renal dysfunction
- Avoid nephrotoxins
- Appropriately dose all drugs as renal function changes
- Maintain euvolemia
- Caution with intravenous contrast because of risk of contrast-induced nephropathy
  ○ Prescribe preventative measures for patients with the highest risk of developing contrast-induced renal insufficiency, especially those patients with a combination of CKD and diabetes (see Chap. 82).
- Avoid gadolinium in patients with CKD because of risk of nephrogenic fibrosing dermopathy (NSF) (see Chap. 85 for more information on NSF)
- Have heightened awareness of subtle changes in GFR reflecting loss of renal function
- Anticipate the eventual need for dialysis and obtain early renal consultation
- Save nondominant arm from blood draws, IVs
- Avoid "iatrogenic" need for urgent dialysis
  ○ Cautious use of hydration if patients have poor urine output
  ○ Treat hyperkalemia early, before potassium rises significantly
  ○ Avoid potassium supplements in patients with CKD or acute renal failure

- Systolic blood pressure (SBP) is more important than diastolic blood pressure (DBP) in predicting progression of CKD.
- BP reduction is renoprotective in diabetic and nondiabetic patients with CKD.
- All antihypertensive agents have a role in reducing progression of renal disease if they allow achievement of targets.
  ○ A target BP of < 130/80 mm Hg for all CKD patients; < 120/80 mm Hg for CKD patients with proteinuria.
  ○ A low sodium diet is imperative (see Table 84-7).

TABLE 84-6 Renal Remission Clinic Targets for Multidrug Approach to CKD

BP	
No proteinuria	< 130/80 mm Hg
Proteinuria > 1 g/d	< 120/80 mm Hg
Proteinuria	< 0.5 g/d
Glycemic control (HbA1c)	< 7%
LDL cholesterol	< 100 mg /dL
Control anemia	Hb 11–12 g/dL or Hct 33%–36%
Lifestyle changes	Stop smoking
	Moderate physical activity
	Keep ideal body weight
	Low salt diet
	Limit protein intake to 0.8 g/kg/bw
	Avoid nephrotoxic drugs (ie, NSAID)
	Caution with herbal remedies

Abbreviations: LDL, low-density lipoprotein; Hb, hemoglobin; Hct, hematocrit; NSAID, nonsteroidal anti-inflammatory drug.
SOURCE: Modified from American Society of Nephrology. Chronic kidney disease and progression. *Nephrology Self-Assessment Program (NephSAP)*. Vol 5, No 3. ASN Offices: Washington DC; May 2006.

TABLE 84-7 Pharmacologic Therapy of Hypertension in CKD

- ACEI or ARB are first line
  - Combination ACEI + ARB at submaximal doses is better than either alone at maximal doses
  - ACEI and/or ARB should be titrated as high as tolerated
- Diuretics may be necessary as second line for better BP and volume control especially in African American patients. Loop diuretics are more effective than Thiazides at lower GFRs and are useful in controlling potassium in late stages of CKD
- Beta-blockers have been shown to reduce proteinuria and may be first line in patients with CVD
- Calcium channel blockers
  - Nondihydropyridine-calcium channel blockers, for example, diltiazem and verapamil, have been shown to reduce proteinuria and are more powerful than beta-blockers
  - Dihydropyridine-calcium channel blockers, for example, amlodipine, are effective in reducing BP but may exacerbate edema and worsen proteinuria. They should be reserved as later agents necessary to get SBP below 120–130 mm Hg.

DIABETES MANAGEMENT

- Intensive treatment of hyperglycemia prevents CKD, slows progression of established CKD, and may prevent diabetic renal disease.
  - Aim for a target HbA1C < 7%, irrespective of the presence or absence of CKD for individuals with diabetes.
  - Most oral hypoglycemic agents and insulin have increased half-lives in CKD and doses may need to be adjusted or medications changed as CKD progresses.
    - Rosiglitazone is largely hepatically excreted and may be the best first-line oral hypoglycemic agent in CKD.
    - Exercise caution prescribing metformin and remember to discontinue this drug if the patient has any deterioration of renal function or undergoes a procedure.

REDUCTION OF PROTEINURIA

- The magnitude and the duration of proteinuria has a strong and direct association with the rate of progression of kidney disease.
- The target is to reduce proteinuria < 0.5 g/d or less, regardless of the specific nature of the underlying renal disease.
- Therapeutic options include angiotensin-converting enzyme inhibitors (ACEI) and angiotensin receptor blocker (ARB). See Table 84-8.
- Other drugs shown to reduce proteinuria include beta-blockers, nondihydropyridines, statin, and possible spironolactone.

OPTIMIZATION OF NUTRITION

- Dietary modifications may reduce the progression of CKD but care must be taken to avoid hypoalbuminemia.
- Target dietary protein intake for patients with CKD, stage 1–4: 0.8–1 g/kg body weight/day has been associated with attenuation of progression of CKD.

TABLE 84-8 ACEI and ARB for Renal Protection and Reduction of Proteinuria

ACEI have been shown to reduce renal disease progression and delay need for dialysis in Type I diabetic nephropathy and nondiabetic nephropathy. ARBs have been shown to reduce renal disease progression, development of ESRD, and Type II diabetic nephropathy

- The combination of ACEI + ARB is more effective than each drug alone in reduction of proteinuria and attenuating progression of kidney disease in nondiabetic nephropathy (COOPERATIVE Study)
- The effects of ACEI and ARBs are likely class effects and benefits are likely not restricted by cause of CKD
- Renoprotective and antiproteinuric benefits of ACEI and ARB are over and above benefits of BP control in patients with CKD
- ACEI and ARB should be titrated to maximal dose tolerated, irrespective of whether the patient has hypertension or not

Potential adverse effects of ACEI and ARB require monitoring

- SCr and potassium should be measured 1–2 weeks after initiation and each dose increase, and repeated weekly if creatinine rises
- Acute increase SCr by 30%–35% after initiation of ACEI/ARB therapy is often observed. This association is predominantly present in patients with a baseline SCr of < 3 mg/dL. A 30% increase of SCr is acceptable if SCr remains stable after regular follow-up for 2–3 months. Only withdraw ACEI in patients with acute increasing SCr exceeding above threshold over a shorter period of time
- Hyperkalemia (K^+ > 5.1 mEq/L) develops in ±10% of patients with advanced stages of CKD and diabetic nephropathy treated with ACEI. The incidence may be lower with ARB. See the section on hyperkalemia under Management of Complications of CKD in this chapter
- Persistent dry cough is more common with ACEI than ARB, usually beginning within weeks to months of initiation of therapy
- Angioedema is more common with ACEI (0.1% to 0.7% patients) than ARB and may present at any time during therapy
- ACEI and ARB are contraindicated in pregnancy, women of reproductive age should be counseled to take contraceptive precautions and notify their physician as soon as pregnancy is planned or discovered

- Patients with nephrotic syndrome should receive supplementary dietary protein to replace urinary protein losses.

IDENTIFICATION AND TREATMENT OF CARDIOVASCULAR RISK FACTORS

- The risk of CVD is significantly increased in patents with *any* reduction of GFR.
- Target LDL < 100 mg/dL in patients with stages 1–4 CKD.
- Cholesterol-lowering agents such as a statins may also have antiproteinuric effects in synergy with ACEI.

MANAGEMENT OF COMPLICATIONS OF CKD

- *Hyperkalemia* is a common complication of CKD and acute hyperkalemia must be managed as an emergency.
  - Low potassium diet should be routinely prescribed.
  - Avoid over-the-counter (OTC) anti-inflammatory drugs, which enhance the risk of hyperkalemia, and herbal remedies.
  - Consider loop-diuretics to mitigate the increases in serum potassium, especially in patients with volume-dependent hypertension and edema.

TABLE 84-9 Therapeutic Options for Anemia of CKD

- Iron levels should be monitored every 3 months and oral or intravenous iron used as necessary to maintain transferrin saturation ≥ 20% with a ferritin between 100 and 500 ng/mL
- Renal production of erythropoietin, which stimulates bone marrow to produce red blood cells, declines with advancing CKD
- ESA include epoetin alpha and beta, which closely resemble the endogenous molecule and have similar pharmacokinetics
  - Erythropoietin: 50–100 U/Kg subcutaneously or intravenously three times a week
  - Darbepoetin, a second-generation molecule with a prolonged half-life: 0.45 µg/kg/week dosed q 2–4 weeks
  - Hb should be monitored monthly on ESA. The target of initial ESA therapy is to increase Hb levels by 1–2 g/dL/month. The minimum interval between ESA dose adjustments is 2 weeks.
- In patients who are seemingly refractory to ESA, consider iron deficiency, chronic or occult infection, occult gastrointestinal bleeding, and concurrent B_{12} or folate deficiency.

Abbreviation: ESA, erythropoiesis-stimulating agents.

- Potassium-binding resins are well tolerated and effective in reducing the serum potassium.
- Use oral sodium bicarbonate for patients with moderate-to-severe CKD and persistent metabolic acidosis.
- Lower or withdraw ACEI or ARB when serum potassium is persistently > 5.5 mEq/L.
- *Anemia* is defined as a hemoglobin (Hg) level < 13.5 g/dL in adult males and < 12 g/dL in adult females. Hg is the preferred method for assessing anemia, because the hematocrit (Hct) is a derived value that may be affected by plasma volume (see Table 84-9).
  - Patients with eGFR < 60 mL/min/1.73 m² should be evaluated by measuring Hb, Hct, serum iron, ferritin, transferrin saturation levels, percentage of hypochromic red blood cells, or reticulocytes at least yearly.
    - The erythropoietin measurement is not useful in assessing anemia.
    - Other causes of anemia should be ruled out. (See Chap. 49.)
  - Anemia in CKD is associated with adverse patient outcomes, including increased hospitalizations, CVD, cognitive impairment, and mortality.
  - Treatment of anemia may regress left ventricular hypertrophy (LVH), delay progression of renal failure, improve survival and quality of life in patients with CKD.

- Treatment goals are Hb of 11–12 g/dL or Hct of 33% to 36%.
- Overcorrection of anemia is associated with increased CVD mortality.
- *Calcium/phosphorus/vitamin D/parathyroid hormone (PTH) metabolism* derangements should be anticipated in *CKD*. See Table 84-10
  - Hypocalcemia, hyperphosphatemia, and deficiency of 1,25-vitamin D lead to hyperparathyroidism, bone disease (renal osteodystrophy), soft tissue and vascular calcification.
  - Levels of calcium, phosphorus, intact plasma parathyroid hormone (iPTH) should be measured in all patients with eGFR < 60 mL/min/1.73 m² (see Tables 84-11 and 84-12).
- *Malnutrition* should be identified and addressed at the time of diagnosis of CKD.
  - Protein malnutrition is a common finding as a result of inadequate protein intake, impaired digestion and absorption, concomitant inflammation, increased protein losses.
  - Hypoalbuminemia at initiation of dialysis is a poor prognostic factor.

CARE TRANSITIONS

- The hospitalist can play a key role in early diagnosis of CKD and initiation of renoprotective strategies, which need to be continued and monitored over the long term.
- Patients should be referred to nephrology early, ideally at or before Stage 3.
- Patients who have advanced uremia when first present to nephrologists have less favorable outcomes after the onset of ESRD.
- Advantages associated with early referral include
  - Patient education about CKD and its implications
  - Concentrated efforts to reach therapeutic targets
  - Preservation of access by choosing an arm early and save for arteriovenous fistula (AVF) creation
    - Avoid blood drawing, intravenous, peripherally inserted central catheter (PICC), or subclavian line placements on the chosen, usually nondominant, side

TABLE 84-10 Target Ranges for Therapy of Calcium, Phosphorus, and PTH

CKD STAGE	eGFR RANGE (mL/min/1.73 m²)	TARGET PTH (pg/mL)	SERUM PHOSPHORUS (mg/dL)	SERUM Ca (mg/dL)	CAXPHOS PRODUCT
3	30–59	35–70	2.7–4.6	Normal range	< 55
4	15–29	70–110	2.7–4.6	Normal range	< 55
5	< 15 or dialysis	15–300	3.5–5.5	8.4–9.5	< 55

SOURCE: Adapted with permission from National Kidney Foundation. Clinical practice guidelines for bone metabolism and disease in chronic kidney disease. *Am J Kidney Dis.* 2003;42(Suppl 3):57–5200.

TABLE 84-11 Therapeutic Strategies to Manage Hyperphosphatemia

Hyperphosphatemia is defined as a serum phosphorus > 4.6 mg/dL in Stage 3 and 4 CKD. Management includes
- Restrict dietary phosphorus to 800–1000 mg/d
- Oral phosphate binders should be added with each meal when dietary therapy is not sufficient
  - Calcium binders are first line in forms of $CaCO_3$, TUMS, calcium acetate. Elemental calcium provided by calcium-containing phosphate binders should not exceed 1500 mg/d. Total elemental calcium intake including dietary calcium should not exceed 2000 mg/d.
  - Non-calcium-binders, for example, aluminum, magnesium-containing phosphate binders may also be used with caution for up to 2 weeks at a time. Aluminum is the most effective calcium binder, but can accumulate and cause long-tern toxicity. It is used to rapidly reduce severely elevated phosphorus level.
  - Sevelamer can cause nongap metabolic acidosis in CKD patients, and is only indicated for hyperphosphatemia treatment in ESRD.

- Preemptive creation of AVF or peritoneal dialysis (PD) catheter insertion
- Earlier referral for transplant evaluation
- Better management of the nutritional and metabolic consequences of advances in CKD
- Assessment of the risk of CVD in patients identified with CKD should be performed once a patient is stabilized, likely postdischarge (see Table 84-2).
  - Patients with CKD are among the "highest risk" group for CVD; even mild-to-moderate renal dysfunction is associated with increased rate of death from coronary artery disease, congestive heart failure (CHF), cerebrovascular disease, peripheral vascular disease.

TABLE 84-12 THERAPEUTIC STRATEGIES TO MANAGE HYPERPARATHYROIDISM

Target PTH levels in CKD are 2–3 times normal
- First-line therapy is correction of serum calcium and phosphate
- If iPTH levels are above the target range, measure 25. hydroxyvitamin D
  - If 25-hydroxyvitamin D < 30 ng/mL, initiate oral ergocalciferol (vitamin D_2) for 6 months to replete stores
  - If 25-hydroxyvitamin D > 30 ng/mL, start active oral vitamin D sterols, for example, calcitriol, alfacalcidol, paricalcitol, or doxercalciferol when serum calcium is < 9.5 mg/dL and phosphorus is < 4.6 mg/dL
  - Active 1,25-hydroxyvitamin D suppresses PTH synthesis but can raise serum calcium and serum phosphate
  - Therapy should be withheld if calcium × phosphorous product is > 55
- At present there are no data to support the use of calcium-receptor agonists (Cinacalcet) to suppress PTH synthesis in CKD. Calcium-receptor agonists, however, have been shown to reduce the iPTH in ESRD
- In more severe cases of renal osteodystrophy (typically seen in ESRD patients on dialysis), when medical therapies are ineffective in controlling hyperparathyroidism, surgical parathyroidectomy may be warranted

BIBLIOGRAPHY

Anavekar NS, et al. Relation between renal dysfunction and cardiovascular outcomes after myocardial infarction. *N Engl J Med.* 2004;351:1285–1295.

Bakris GL, et al. Preserving renal function in adults with hypertension and diabetes: a consensus approach. National Kidney Foundation Hypertension and Diabetes Executive Committees Working Group. *Am J Kidney Dis.* 2000;36: 646–661.

Go AS, Chertow GM, Fan D, et al. Chronic kidney disease and the risks of death, cardiovascular events, and hospitalization. *N Engl J Med.* 2004;351:1296–1305.

KDOQI. KDOQI clinical practice guidelines and clinical practice recommendations for diabetes and chronic kidney disease. *Am J Kidney Dis.* 2007;49:S12–S154.

Levey AS, et al. National Kidney Foundation practice guidelines for chronic kidney disease: evaluation, classification, and stratification. *Ann Intern Med.* 2003;139:137–147.

Masoudi FA, Plomondon ME, Magid DJ, et al. Renal insufficiency and mortality from acute coronary syndromes. *Am Heart J.* 2004;147:623–629.

National Kidney Foundation. K/DOQI clinical practice guidelines for chronic kidney disease: evaluation, classification, and stratification. *Am J Kidney Dis.* 2002;39:S1–S266.

Shlipak MG, Fried LF, Stehman-Breen C, et al. Chronic renal insufficiency and cardiovascular events in the elderly: findings from the Cardiovascular Health Study. *Am J Geriatr Cardiol.* 2004;13:81–90.

Shlipak MG, et al. Cardiovascular mortality risk in chronic kidney disease: comparison of traditional and novel risk factors. *JAMA.* 2005;293:1737–1745.

USRDS. The United States Renal Data System. *Am J Kidney Dis.* 2003;42:1–230.

85 CARE OF THE HOSPITALIZED DIALYSIS PATIENT

J. Kevin Tucker

EPIDEMIOLOGY/OVERVIEW

- In 2002, there were approximately 309,000 patients with ESRD on dialysis in the United States, and that number is projected to exceed 600,000 by 2010. The leading cause of ESRD in the United States is diabetes mellitus, followed by hypertension.
  - African Americans are more likely to develop ESRD from hypertension than are Caucasians, and

this propensity to develop ESRD among African Americans with hypertension accounts for much of the overrepresentation of minority populations in American dialysis facilities.

- The optimal care of ESRD patients requires coordinated care among the hospitalist, consulting nephrologist, medical nurse, and the dialysis nurse.
- Many of the common complications of ESRD are also seen in advancing CKD, including malnutrition, anemia, and hyperparathyroidism, and their management is covered in Chap. 84. Other medical complications causing ESRD patients to present to the hospital are reviewed below.

DISEASE MANAGEMENT STRATEGIES

Complications of hemodialysis (HD) vascular access are a major cause of morbidity among dialysis patients. About 20% of all hospitalizations in ESRD patients are due to problems with vascular HD access.

- General considerations
  - The extremity in which there is a vascular HD access should not be used for venipuncture nor for BP measurements.
  - The preferred HD access is an AVF. The AV graft is used when a native fistula cannot be successfully created. Catheters are used when neither a fistula nor a graft can be created or as a "bridge" until the fistula is mature.
- *Fever, bacteremia, and dialysis graft/catheter infection*
  - ESRD patients are relatively immunocompromised, with decreased cellular and humoral immunity and are more likely to develop community-acquired and healthcare-associated pneumonias and tuberculosis. However, the HD patient who presents with fever should be assumed to be bacteremic until proven otherwise.
  - The HD procedure in which two needles are introduced through the skin into an AVF or an AV graft may allow for the inadvertent introduction of bacteria into the blood stream, despite the use of aseptic technique.
    - Because it contains no synthetic materials, an AVF rarely becomes infected.
    - An AV graft, which contains a synthetic material such as polytetrafluoroethylene (PTFE) interposed between an artery and a vein, is more likely than an AVF to become infected. An infected AV graft will typically present with warmth, erythema, and induration. A healthy-looking graft should be considered a likely focus of infection in the patient who has persistently positive blood cultures despite treatment with appropriate antibiotics

and warrants examination of the graft by the surgical team. An infected AV graft may appear completely normal externally but upon surgical exploration may be found to be grossly purulent. An infected AV graft should be surgically excised and the wound irrigated. Systemic antibiotics should be administered for 3–4 weeks.

- The HD catheter, which is an indwelling foreign body, may be the primary focus of infection or may become secondarily infected when bacteremia originates at another site. If blood cultures are positive and the patient has an indwelling HD catheter, the catheter should be removed and replaced at an alternative site when follow-up blood cultures have been documented to be negative (see Fig. 85-1).
  - If there is no appropriate alternative site for placement of a HD catheter and there is no evidence of a tunnel infection, the catheter may be exchanged over a guidewire with continued systemic antibiotic therapy for 3–4 weeks.
  - If blood cultures remain positive despite removal of the infected catheter and administration of appropriate antibiotics, and there is no other obvious source of infection, the workup should then focus on looking for metastatic foci of infection. Transthoracic and/or transesophageal echocardiography should be considered to look for signs of endocarditis if blood cultures remain persistently positive. The patient who develops new-onset back pain or neurologic signs in the setting of HD catheter-associated bacteremia should have a magnetic resonance imaging (MRI) to look for an epidural abscess.
- A complete blood count, chest x-ray, blood cultures, and careful physical examination with particular

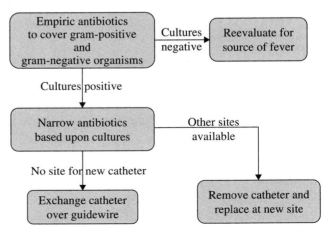

FIG. 85-1 Management of fever in a HD patient with a catheter.

attention to the vascular access should lead to diagnosis of the usual most common causes of fever in dialysis patients.

- When the dialysis patient is hospitalized for fever, it is important to follow-up on any blood cultures that were drawn in the outpatient dialysis facility. If antibiotics were given in the outpatient dialysis unit before the patient came to the hospital, blood cultures drawn in the hospital may be negative.
○ Initial management of the HD patient who presents with fever should include empiric treatment with broad-spectrum antibiotics, covering both gram-positive and gram-negative organisms.
  - Antibiotic therapy should be narrowed once cultures and sensitivities of the causative organism are available.
  - Antibiotic therapy for bacteremia is usually continued for a total of 3–4 weeks and may be continued as an outpatient with the antibiotics administered in the outpatient dialysis facility.
○ Choosing appropriate antibiotic therapy
  - Vancomycin is an appropriate empiric antibiotic choice in most situations for gram-positive coverage; however, its long-term use for treatment of methicillin-sensitive organisms should be avoided

to prevent the emergence of vancomycin-resistant organisms. (See Table 85-1.) Cefazolin can be used as an alternative to treat methicillin-sensitive organisms, and it can be dosed at dialysis.
  - Gentamycin is an appropriate empiric antibiotic choice in most situations for gram-negative coverage.
- *Malfunctioning fistulas, grafts, and dialysis catheters*, often because of clotting, are also frequent vascular HD access issues.
○ The HD procedure often requires heparin anticoagulation to prevent the extracorporeal circuit from clotting. In the hospitalized dialysis patient, the dialysis procedure may be performed without heparin, particularly if the patient is going for a procedure or has a bleeding diathesis. The dialyzer is frequently rinsed with saline to prevent clotting within the extracorporeal circuit when the dialysis procedure is done heparin-free.
○ Heparin is the standard anticoagulant used to "lock" HD catheters to prevent them from clotting. In patients who are intolerant of heparin, most commonly because of heparin-induced thrombocytopenia (HIT), an alternative anticoagulant solution such as citrate is used to lock the HD catheter.

TABLE 85-1 Drug Dosing in ESRD

Selected antibiotics

Vancomycin should be administered as a loading dose of 15–20 mg/kg ideal body weight. Most patients who are dialyzing with large surface area/high-flux dialyzers will require a supplemental dose after each HD treatment to maintain a therapeutic trough blood level of 15–20 µg/mL. The supplemental dose should be based upon an individual center's experience with their dialyzers. For most patients, a 500-mg dose of vancomycin given during the last hour of dialysis will maintain therapeutic predialysis vancomycin concentrations
Gentamicin should be administered as an initial loading dose of 1–2 mg/kg followed by a supplemental dose after each dialysis treatment of half of the loading dose. Dosing of gentamicin in the obese patient should be based upon adjusted body weight rather than actual total body weight. Use of the actual total body weight may lead to doses that are too high and increase the risk of otovestibular toxicity
Cefazolin 0.5–1.5 g q 24–48 hours, supplemental dose after HD 0.5–1.0 g
Ceftazidim 1–2 g q 48 hours, supplemental dose after HD 1.0 g
Nafcillin and clindamycin do not require dose adjustment in ESRD
Levofloxacin should be administered at an initial dose of 500 mg, with subsequent doses of 250 mg given every other day rather than daily in ESRD
Metronidazole should be given as 50% of the usual dose and given after HD
Imipenem should be given as 25% of the usual dose. ESRD patients are at higher risk of imipenem-induced seizures

Selected oral hypoglycemic agents

Glyburide should be avoided in ESRD patients because of its prolonged half-life
Glipizide is the preferred sulfonylurea for ESRD patients
Metformin should not be used in ESRD patients because of the risk of lactic acidosis

Selected miscellaneous drugs

Gabapentin is commonly over dosed in ESRD patients. The ESRD patient with gabapentin toxicity will typically present with tremors, extrapyramidal symptoms, or mental status changes. Gabapentin should be given in a dose of 200–300 mg after HD and only on HD days

Anticoagulants

Low molecular weight heparins, such as enoxaparin, should be avoided in dialysis patients because their half-lives are unpredictable and may be associated with excessive bleeding
Warfarin may be used in ESRD patients for the usual indications such as atrial fibrillation. However, there is no evidence that anticoagulation with warfarin prevents graft or fistula thrombosis. A carefully coordinated plan for anticoagulation management needs to be in place when a dialysis patient is placed on warfarin. It should not be assumed that the INR will be monitored by the nephrologist or the dialysis facility

- Among HD patients with HIT antibodies, thrombocytopenia and thrombotic events are rare. See Chap. 90 for more information on HIT.
  - There is no evidence that anticoagulation with warfarin prevents graft or fistula thrombosis.
  - Consultation with surgery and/or interventional radiology may be required to assess the dialysis access device patency, to administer lytic therapy if clotting is a problem, and to revise or replace the device when necessary.

EMERGENT DIALYSIS

The dialysis patient who presents with respiratory compromise from volume overload or severe metabolic abnormalities (hyperkalemia with electrocardiogram [ECG] changes, metabolic acidosis) should be considered for emergent dialysis. Usual treatment strategies should also be applied to these patients since the mobilization of an after-hours dialysis team may take up to 4 hours in some institutions.

- In many hospitals, after-hours dialysis may be performed in a remote part of the hospital, where other personnel are not readily available to help in case of an acute deterioration in the patient's condition. In those circumstances, the patient who requires emergent dialysis should preferentially be triaged to an intensive care unit, where the HD procedure can be performed with continuous monitoring.
- Dietary noncompliance and/or missed dialysis treatments are the most common causes of the need for emergent dialysis, and these issues need to be addressed prior to discharge.
- *Hyperkalemia* management is also addressed in Chap. 87A and B and Chap. 84. Two additional points of note, specific to ESRD patients:
  - Fasting for procedures is a common cause of hyperkalemia in the hospitalized HD patient even when no exogenous potassium is given. This fasting hyperkalemia may be prevented by the administration of dextrose, for example, D10W at 20–30 mL/hr, to prevent shifting of potassium from the intracellular compartment to the extracellular compartment.
  - ESRD patients are more sensitive to the effects of beta-adrenergic blockage on serum potassium concentration. Nonselective beta-blockers, for example, propranolol, labetalol, and carvedilol, reduce beta-adrenergic stimulation of potassium uptake by cells, thus raising the serum potassium.
- *Volume overload* caused by dietary fluid and/or sodium excess is the leading cause of dyspnea in HD patients. Dialysis patients are most vulnerable to this problem during their long 2-day weekend interval between dialysis treatments.
  - Review of the flowsheets from the outpatient dialysis facility will reveal how much fluid has been removed during recent treatments and whether or not the target dry weight has been achieved (see Table 85-2).
  - Poorly controlled hypertension in the setting of a stiff, noncompliant, hypertrophied left ventricle may lead to the development of pulmonary edema despite normal total body volume.

CHEST PAIN

- *CVD* is the leading cause of death in patients with ESRD; hence acute coronary syndromes must be considered in the differential diagnosis of dialysis patients presenting with chest pain (see Chaps. 21, 22, and 23).
  - In HD patients who have no signs of chronic inflammation (eg, low serum albumin, high serum ferritin, or high C-reactive protein), serum cholesterol is a predictor of cardiovascular events.
  - Coronary vascular calcification is a major risk factor for atherosclerotic CVD and occurs very early in the course of dialysis, even in young patients. A chronically elevated calcium $\times$ phosphorous product is a good marker for the likelihood of coronary vascular calcification.
  - Hypertension and chronic volume overload predispose HD patients to develop LVH. Acute drops in BP in the presence of LVH may lead to the development of subendocardial ischemia in the absence of obstructive atherosclerotic coronary lesions.

TABLE 85-2   Assessing Dry Weight

The "dry weight" is the weight at which the patient has no signs or symptoms of volume overload. Some patients at dry weight will not require antihypertensive medications. In other patients, however, volume status and BP do not correlate well.
- When a dialysis patient is admitted to the hospital in a volume overloaded state, the dry weight should be reassessed
  - If the patient has been achieving his target dry weight at outpatient dialysis and is still clinically volume overloaded at that weight, then the dry weight needs to be lowered
  - Whenever the patient loses body mass as a result of an illness, the dry weight should be lowered to reflect the loss of body mass
  - If the patient is becoming hypotensive during dialysis in reaching the target dry weight and has no signs or symptoms of fluid excess, he/she may have gained body mass, and the dry weight needs to be increased. There are also a number of strategies that may help to stabilize the BP during the HD procedure
    - Limit interdialytic weight gain to 2 kg
    - Hold antihypertensive medications on dialysis days
    - Cool temperature dialysate (induces vasoconstriction)
    - Sodium modeling (reduces the change in plasma osmolality)

- *Uremic pericarditis*, which typically occurs in patients who are inadequately dialyzed, may also present with chest pain.
  - Patients with uremic pericarditis will often describe relief of the pain with sitting upright.
  - Physical examination findings may include hypotension, pulsus paradoxus, elevated jugular venous pressure, and/or a pericardial friction rub.
  - An echocardiogram should be performed to look for wall motion abnormalities and for a pericardial effusion.
    - If there are echocardiographic signs of cardiac tamponade, the pericardial effusion should be percutaneously drained.
    - Uremic pericarditis with a pericardial effusion is generally treated with intensive, that is, daily dialysis. Heparin should not be given to the patient with a uremic pericardial effusion because of the risk of bleeding into the pericardial space. The dialysis procedure in such cases is usually done without heparin anticoagulation.

SKIN DISORDERS ASSOCIATED WITH END-STAGE RENAL DISEASE

- *Calciphylaxis* results from medial calcification of small vessels, resulting in tissue necrosis. It is most commonly seen in ESRD patients on dialysis but has been described in several other disorders.
  - Risk factors for calciphylaxis include obesity, hyperparathyroidism, diabetes mellitus, rapid or dramatic weight loss, warfarin use, and protein C or protein S deficiency. Calciphylaxis occurs more commonly in women than men in a ratio of about 3:1.
  - The lesions of calciphylaxis (early stages may resemble cellulitis, advancing to purpuric plaques, and necrotic ulcers) occur most commonly on the lower extremities and tissues with high adipose content, such as the abdominal pannus or the breast. Onset is often correlated with local trauma.
  - The diagnosis is best made by tissue biopsy. However, the lesions sometimes worsen after a biopsy; so in the right clinical setting, treatment may be initiated without histologic confirmation of the diagnosis.
  - The initial management of the patient with calciphylaxis should focus on control of the serum phosphorous and the calcium × phosphorous product.
  - Calciphylaxis has a high mortality rate resulting from concomitant wound infection and sepsis. Local wound care by specialized wound care nurses and the administration of broad-spectrum systemic antibiotics is warranted. Consultation with a burn specialist or plastic surgeon is also advisable.

- Hyperbaric oxygen and sodium thiosulfate have also been used as adjunctive therapies in the treatment of calciphylaxis.
- *Nephrogenic systemic fibrosis (NSF)/nephrogenic fibrosing dermopathy* is a new disease seen in ESRD patients, characterized by symmetric bilateral thickening of the skin, beginning in the distal extremities and migrating proximally, and may be confused with scleroderma (the absence of Raynaud's and ANA antibodies in NSF helps distinguish the two). It may be associated with fibrosis of muscle tissue, heart, and lungs. It causes significant disability due to loss of joint mobility and in it's more fulminant form results in death.
  - Epidemiological studies have linked this new disorder to the use of gadolinium for contrast-enhanced MRI.
  - Diagnosis is made by deep incisional or punch biopsy of affected skin.
  - There is no clearly beneficial treatment available. Patients who have recovered renal function and no longer require dialysis have experienced remission of NSF.
- Prevention is by avoidance of gadolinium in patients with advanced CKD.

DRUG DOSING IN END-STAGE RENAL DISEASE PATIENTS ON DIALYSIS

Although antibiotics are the group of medications most frequently given to HD patients that require dose adjustment, many different categories of commonly prescribed drugs and other pharmacotherapeutic agents require dose adjustment in ESRD (see Table 85-1).

- The clearance of a given drug by dialysis is dependent upon its molecular weight, water solubility, and degree of protein binding. Drugs that are highly water soluble with little protein binding, for example, lithium, are very efficiently removed by HD, while more lipid-soluble compounds and those that are highly protein bound, for example, phenytoin, are not efficiently removed by HD.

CARE TRANSITIONS

- At the time of discharge from an acute hospitalization, the care plan should be communicated to the outpatient dialysis facility and the nephrologist who takes care of the patient in the community. The following information should be given to the outpatient dialysis facility:
  - Dry weight.
  - Changes in the dialysis prescription.
  - Changes in erythropoietin dose.
  - If the patient is to be discharged to home to complete a course of antibiotics given at dialysis, the

nephrologist should be involved in the discharge planning process. Dialysis units typically have a limited choice of antibiotics on their formularies.

- PICC lines should be avoided in ESRD patients. The PICC line may ruin a potential site for future dialysis access. An antibiotic regimen that can be given at dialysis will preclude the need for a PICC line.
- Disease management by nurse case managers, who follow patients in the outpatient dialysis facility may improve outcomes by supporting patients in the management of
  ○ Anemia (Hb, iron, transferrin saturation)
  ○ Bone disease (calcium, phosphorous, PTH)
  ○ Nutrition (serum albumin)
  ○ Vascular access
  ○ Adequacy of dialysis (urea reduction ratio, Kt/V)
  ○ BP control
  ○ Volume status (dry weight assessment)
  ○ Patient compliance with dietary restrictions and dialysis

BIBLIOGRAPHY

Ariano RE, Fine A, Sitar DS, et al. Adequacy of a vancomycin dosing regimen in patients receiving high-flux hemodialysis. *Am J Kidney Dis.* 2005;46:681–687.

Aronoff G, et al. *Drug Prescribing in Renal Failure.* 4th ed. Philadelphia, PA: American College of Physicians; 1999.

Allon M. Medical and dialytic management of hyperkalemia in hemodialysis patients. *Int J Artif Organs.* 1996; 19:697–699.

Besarab A, Bolton WK, Browne JK, et al. The effects of normal as compared with low hematocrit values in patients with cardiac disease who are receiving hemodialysis and epoetin. *N Engl J Med.* 1998;339:584–590.

Brucculeri M, Cheigh J, Bauer G, et al. Long-term intravenous sodium thiosulfate in the treatment of a patient with calciphylaxis. *Semin Dial.* 2005;18:431–434.

Dheenan S, Henrich WL. Preventing dialysis hypotension: a comparison of usual protective maneuvers. *Kidney Int.* 2001;59: 1175–1181.

Ifudu O. Care of patients undergoing hemodialysis. *N Engl J Med.* 1998;339:1054–1062.

Owen WF, Lew NL, Liu Y, et al. The urea reduction ratio and serum albumin concentration as predictors of mortality in patients undergoing hemodialysis *N Engl J Med.* 1993;329: 1001–1006.

Pastan S, Bailey J. Dialysis therapy. *N Engl J Med.* 1998;338:1428–1437.

Robinson D. Suchocki P, Schwab S. Treatment of infected tunneled venous access hemodialysis catheters with guidewire exchange. *Kidney Int.* 1998;53:1792–1794.

Robinson D, Suhocki P, Schwab SJ. Treatment of infected tunneled venous access hemodialysis catheters with guidewire exchange. *Kidney Int.* 1998;53:1792–1794.

Singh AK, Szczech L, Tang KL, et al. for the Choir Investigators. Correction of anemia with epoetin alfa in chronic kidney disease. *N Engl J Med.* 2006;355:2085–2098.

86 ACID-BASE DISORDERS
David V. Gugliotti

EPIDEMIOLOGY/OVERVIEW

- Acid-base disturbances occur frequently in acutely ill hospitalized patients.
- Blood pH is maintained by acid-base homeostasis mechanisms in the kidneys and the lungs and by buffer systems present in the body.
- Acid-base abnormalities are classified as acute or chronic in nature.
- Simple acid-base disorders have one primary abnormality, while mixed disorders have more than one abnormality.
- Timely and accurate interpretation of abnormalities and prompt intervention to treat their underlying cause(s) is necessary to avoid consequences from severe acid-base disturbances.

PATHOPHYSIOLOGY

Normal diet generates endogenous volatile acids (CO_2) from carbohydrate metabolism and nonvolatile acids (H^+) from protein metabolism. An average 1 mEq/kg/d of endogenous acid is generated by the typical western diet.

- A variety of medical conditions cause derangement of intrinsic acid-base balance, and the introduction of exogenous acids disrupts this balance as well.
- Endogenous and exogenous acids or bases must be neutralized to maintain optimal pH for normal metabolic processes.
  ○ Alveolar ventilation is responsible for excretion of CO_2 produced by normal or abnormal metabolism.
  ○ The kidney is responsible for reclaiming filtered bicarbonate and generating new bicarbonate to match the loss of bicarbonate, resulting from buffering of hydrogen ion introduced by metabolism.
- Blood pH ($-\log [H^+]$) is determined by the ratio of HCO_3^- (serum bicarbonate) and $PaCO_2$ (partial

pressure of CO_2 in arterial blood). A primary alteration in [H^+], bicarbonate, or PCO_2 will result in an abnormal pH.

- The Henderson equation, adapted from the Henderson-Hasselbach equation, represents the body system relationship between the HCO_3^- and $PaCO_2$ ratio and hydrogen ion concentration [H^+]

$$[H^+] = 24 \times \frac{PaCO_2}{HCO_3^-}$$

- Acidemia is defined as blood pH < 7.36. An acidosis is a pathologic process that decreases the serum bicarbonate (metabolic acidosis), or raises the $PaCO_2$ (respiratory acidosis).
  - Metabolic acidosis may be either normal anion gap or wide anion gap. Some patients also have "hybrid metabolic acidosis" or a combination of the two.
    - Anion gap metabolic acidosis is caused by the addition of acids to the body system, resulting in effective loss of bicarbonate by buffering of acid and elevation of the anion gap.
    - A nonanion gap acidosis (hyperchloremic metabolic acidosis) is caused by loss of bicarbonate from the body system coupled with chloride retention and preservation of the normal anion gap.
  - Respiratory acidosis is caused by impaired CO_2 release due to impaired ventilation, and may occur acutely or chronically.
- Alkalemia is defined as blood pH > 7.44. An alkalosis is a pathologic process that raises the serum bicarbonate (metabolic alkalosis) or decreases the $PaCO_2$ (respiratory alkalosis).
  - Metabolic alkalosis is caused by addition of alkali to the body system, losses of acid from the gastrointestinal system or the kidneys, or concentration of bicarbonate in the extracellular fluid.
  - Respiratory alkalosis is caused by excess excretion of CO_2 from the lungs, and can occur acutely or chronically.
- All acid-base challenges are buffered—in the early phases of an acid-base disturbance, extracellular and intracellular buffers minimize pH changes. Each of the four primary acid-base abnormalities then results in relatively predictable compensation responses to impede deviations from normal pH.
  - Respiratory disorders evoke a compensatory renal response correcting the pH back toward normal.
  - Metabolic disorders evoke a respiratory compensatory response.
  - The longer-term correction of an acid-base derangement is accomplished by alteration of the lung or kidney handling of acids or bases.

CLINICAL PRESENTATION, DIFFERENTIAL, MAKING THE DIAGNOSIS

- Diagnosis of acid-base disorders is based on clinical suspicion and the finding of abnormal laboratory values (pH, $PaCO_2$, HCO_3^-).
- pH and $PaCO_2$ are measured directly in arterial blood gases (ABG), while the bicarbonate from blood gases is calculated using the Henderson-Hasselbach equation.
- Bicarbonate is directly measured in plasma chemistries—at normal body pH total venous carbon dioxide exists in the form of bicarbonate.
- Acidemia may result in hypotension, decreased cardiac output, decreased peripheral vascular resistance, hyperkalemia, altered mental status, and Kussmal's respirations (rapid, deep, and labored).
- Alkalemia causes cardiac dysrhythmias, hypoventilation, neuromuscular irritability (fasciculations, tetani, muscle cramping), encephalopathy, and hypokalemia.

DIAGNOSTIC APPROACH ACID-BASE DISORDERS

- A stepwise approach to the diagnosis of acid-base disorders insures accurate and consistent interpretation of abnormalities.
- The use of acid-base nomograms may be helpful for diagnosis of simple acid-base disturbances. Shaded areas on typical acid-base nomograms define 95% confidence limits for simple acid-base disorders. Values outside shaded areas imply the presence of mixed disorders, but nomograms limit further specific interpretation.
- Table 86-1 summarizes a general, stepwise approach to the diagnosis of acid-base disorders.
- Urine electrolyte and osmolality measurements can be used to identify disorders of acid-base metabolism as well as fluid and electrolytes.
  - To examine the renal response to an abnormal condition such as acidosis, it is important to realize that there are "expected" ranges rather than "normal" results.
    - Patients with abnormal renal and adrenal function and patients who use diuretics will have a different expected response.
    - Patients with a low "effective" intravascular volume usually conserve Na^+ and Cl^- in the urine whereas euvolemic patients will excrete all excess Na^+ and Cl^- of dietary origin.
    - During oliguria, however, the expected range will change and there is overlap in the concentration of Na^+ in the urine in these two situations.
  - The concentration of Na^+ in the urine is used diagnostically to determine the cause of normal AG metabolic acidosis.

TABLE 86-1   General Approach to the Diagnosis of Acid-Base Disorders

1. History and physical examination
   - Perform a detailed medical history, including previous medical illnesses, acute changes in health status, medication changes, fevers/infections, vomiting or diarrhea, and ingestion
   - The physical examination should include vital signs, noting the respiratory pattern, assessing perfusion and neurologic status, and reflexes
2. Simultaneous measurement of ABG and plasma chemistries to determine any abnormality of pH, $PaCO_2$, and bicarbonate
   - Use the measured values of pH and $PaCO_2$ (from the ABG) plugged into the Henderson equation to calculate the HCO_3^- and compare to the measured value from plasma chemistries

   $[H^+] = 24 \times (PaCO_2/HCO_3^-)$ $[H^+]$ estimate = 80–last 2 digits of pH (7.40)

   - The two values should agree within 2–3 mEq/L (if agreement is not present, suspect laboratory error or samples not obtained simultaneously, thus the ABG is unreliable)
3. Identification of the primary acid-base disorder
   - Look at the pH. Is acidemia or alkalemia present?
   - The direction of the pH relative to 7.40 defines the primary process
   - Whichever side of 7.40 the pH is on, the process that caused it to shift to that side is the primary abnormality
     ○ Primary metabolic acidosis decreases HCO_3^- and pH
     ○ Primary metabolic alkalosis increases HCO_3^- and pH
     ○ Primary respiratory acidosis increases $PaCO_2$ and decreases pH
     ○ Primary respiratory alkalosis decreases $PaCO_2$ and increases pH
4. Calculations
   - Plasma anion gap = $Na^+ - (Cl^- + HCO_3^-)$, normal is 12 ± 2 mEq/L
   - The normal anion gap reflects unmeasured anions—mostly the negative charge on albumin, but also minor negative charges (SO_4^{2-}, PO_4^{3-})
   - The addition of unmeasured anions (lactate, salicylate, B-hydroxybutyrate, etc.) will increase the anion gap
   - An elevated AG indicates a metabolic acidosis by definition
   - Decreased anion gap (< 8) may be caused by decreased albumin or increased cations (Mg^{2+}, Ca^+, K^+, Li^+)
   - For each 1 g/dL decline in plasma albumin, 2.5 should be added to the anion gap
   - For an anion gap between 12 and 20, a specific cause for increased anion gap may be difficult to find, but the greater the anion gap (usually > 20) the more likely a specific metabolic acidosis will be found[4]
   - Exogenous or endogenous acids (H^+A^-) are buffered by HCO_3^- and an unmeasured anion (A^-) is introduced in the system and represents the increased anion gap, as noted in the following equations:

   $H^+A^- + HCO_3^- \leftrightarrow H_2CO_3$ (carbonic acid) $+ A^-$

   $H_2CO_3^- \rightarrow H_2O + CO_2$ (removed by alveolar ventilation)

   - Each unit increase in AG should result in equivalent decrease in HCO_3^- in a pure anion gap acidosis
   - **Delta gap defined as the change in AG relative to the change in HCO_3^-** (calculated when AG present)
   - Differences in change of AG and HCO_3^- means the presence of mixed metabolic disorder (difference greater than 2–3 mEq/L)

   Δ **AG > Δ HCO_3^- = AG acidosis + metabolic alkalosis** (HCO_3^- level > expected for the addition of the unmeasured ion)

   Δ **AG < Δ HCO_3^- = AG acidosis + non-AG acidosis** (HCO_3^- level < predicted based on the change in anion gap from the unmeasured ion)
   - **Osmolar Gap defined as measured serum osmolality—calculated osmolality**

   - Suspicion for ingestion of toxins as the cause of anion gap acidosis should prompt calculation of OG (↑methanol, ethylene glycol)
   - **Urine AG defined as UNa + UK + – UCl–**
   - Nonanion gap acidosis is further evaluated by checking the UAG to characterize renal vs. GI losses of bicarbonate (see urine anion gap).
   - Renal losses of bicarbonate from RTA may be further characterized by measurement of urine pH, serum potassium, and fractional excretion of bicarbonate depending on suspicion of the RTA type
   - Plasma renin activity, serum aldosterone concentration, and serum cortisol concentration may be needed to confirm type 4 RTA
5. Compensation formulas
   - Use compensation formulas to determine expected findings
     ○ Metabolic acidosis: $PaCO_2 = 1.5 (HCO_3^-) + 8 (\pm 2)$ Winter's Formula
     ○ Metabolic alkalosis: $PaCO2 = 0.9 (HCO_3^-) + 9 (\pm 2)$
     ○ Acute respiratory acidosis: plasma HCO_3^- concentration should rise by about 1 mmol/L for each 10 mm Hg increase in $PaCO_2$ (± 3 mmol/L)
     ○ Chronic respiratory acidosis: plasma HCO_3^- concentration should rise by about 4 mmol/L for each 10 mm Hg increase in $PaCO_2$ (±4 mmol/L)
     ○ Acute respiratory alkalosis: plasma HCO_3^- concentration should fall by about 1–3 mmol/L for each 10 mm Hg decrease in $PaCO_2$ (usually not < 18 mmol/L)
     ○ Chronic respiratory alkalosis: plasma HCO_3^- concentration should fall by about 2–5 mmol/L/10 mm Hg decrease in $PaCO_2$ (usually not < 14 mmol/L)
   - Compensation generally does not correct the pH to normal, and does not overshoot
   - If compensation is not in the expected range (or if the pH is normal when an acid-base disorder is present), then there is another acid-base disorder present

Use the characterization of acid-base disorder to diagnose specific causes based on clinical suspicion
   - Metabolic acidosis—any condition resulting in retention of acid (primary event) or increased ventilation with decrease in PCO_2 (secondary event) with signs and symptoms of metabolic acidosis: fatigue, dyspnea, abdominal pain, vomiting, Kussmaul's respiration, hyperkalemia, leukemoid reaction, insulin resistance, arteriolar dilation, hypotension, myocardial depression (pH < 7.2)
   - Metabolic alkalosis—any condition resulting in increased bicarbonate (primary event) or decreased ventilation with increase in PCO_2 (secondary event) with signs and symptoms of metabolic alkalosis: weakness, muscle cramps, hyperreflexia, alveolar hypoventilation, dysrhythmias
   - Mixed disturbances: most common respiratory acidosis and metabolic acidosis caused by cardiopulmonary arrest, lung disease with severe hypoxemia, shock with respiratory failure
     ○ Respiratory acidosis and metabolic acidosis caused by cardiopulmonary arrest, lung disease with severe hypoxemia, shock with respiratory failure (most common).
     ○ Respiratory alkalosis and metabolic acidosis caused by salicylate intoxication, gram-negative sepsis, liver failure
     ○ Respiratory acidosis and metabolic alkalosis caused by cor pulmonale treated with diuretics
     ○ Respiratory alkalosis and metabolic alkalosis caused by cirrhosis treated with diuretics
     ○ Metabolic alkalosis and metabolic acidosis caused by vomiting with severe volume depletion leading to lactic acidosis

Abbreviation: RTA, renal tubular acidosis.

○ The concentration of Cl^- in the urine is helpful in determining the cause of metabolic alkalosis.
○ The fractional excretion of Na^+ (FE_{Na}^+) is more sensitive and specific in distinguishing prerenal from renal azotemia.

$$FE_{Na}\% = \frac{Urine\,[Na] \times Plasma\,[Creatinine]}{Plasma\,[Na] \times Urine\,[Creatinine]} \times 100$$

FE_{Na} reflects the amount of sodium excreted by the body relative to the amount filtered by the kidney. In the setting of acute oliguric renal failure, the following may be observed:

- $FE_{Na} < 1\%$ usually, but not invariably, indicates prerenal azotemia.
- A $FE_{Na} < 1\%$ has also been seen in chronic prerenal failure, such as cirrhosis, and severe CHF, acute renal failure superimposed on chronic renal failure, rhabdomyolysis, and radiocontrast-induced renal failure.
- $FE_{Na} > 1\%$ (usually > 3%) indicates renal damage.
- The urine osmolality may be helpful, although again there can be overlap between prerenal and renal causes.

• Urine anion gap or urine net charge (UAG) is used for characterization of hyperchloremic (nonanion gap) acidosis to determine if HCO_3^- losses are coming from the urine or the GI tract.

$$UAG = UNa^+ + UK^+ - UCl^- \quad (Normal\; -10\;to\;+10\;mEq/L)$$

○ UAG is a reflection of the kidney's ability or inability to acidify the urine by secretion of NH_4^+ (ammonium ion).
○ Electroneutrality must be maintained in the urine, therefore elevated urine NH_4^+ will be matched by increased urine chloride and alter the gap between charges of the urine electrolytes.
○ If acidosis is caused by impaired renal tubular function, the kidney has impaired ability to produce NH_4^+ resulting in $Cl^- < Na^+ + K^+$.
  - UAG > 10 ("positive") indicates impaired renal tubular function.
○ If losses of HCO_3^- are occurring because of an extrarenal disorder, the kidney would compensate by increasing production of NH_4^+ resulting in $Cl^- > Na^+ + K^+$.
  - UAG < −10 ("negative") indicates extrarenal losses of HCO_3^-
• Osmolar gap (OG) is the difference between the measured serum osmolality and the calculated serum osmolality.
○ Determination of the freezing point of serum is how the serum osmolality is directly measured.

○ The calculated osmolality ($mOsm/H_2O$) is

$$2(Na) + \frac{glucose}{18} + \frac{blood\;urea\;nitrogen\;(BUN)}{2.8}$$

- This equation will not accurately estimate extracellular fluid osmolality if other solutes are present in sufficient amounts.
- Hence a difference or "gap" between measured and calculated osmolality of more than 10 mOsm/kg suggests the presence of another solute, such as lactate, ethanol, mannitol, or ethanol.
- The osmotic contribution of alcohol can be calculated as ethanol mg/dL ÷ 4.6.
- If an OG persists despite factoring in the alcohol contribution, other unmeasured osmolytes are present in the body as seen with methanol, ethylene glycol, isopropyl alcohol ingestion as well as mannitol administration, or if Na^+ is falsely low as seen with hyperlipidemia and hyperproteinemia.
- Uremia, lactic acidosis, ketoacidosis, and salicylate intoxication will be associated with an OG < 25 Osm/kg.
- Isopropyl alcohol increases the OG but not the anion gap because acetone is not an anion.
○ An OG > 50 mOsm/L is associated with a high mortality.

TRIAGE AND INITIAL MANAGEMENT

• The hospitalist can take a systematic approach to analyze acid-base disturbances in the acutely ill hospitalized patient by measuring serum electrolytes and ABG pH and PCO_2, as outlined above and in Table 86-1.
○ Is the patient acidemic or alkalemic?
○ Is the acid-base derangement primary respiratory or metabolic?
○ If respiratory, is it acute or chronic?
○ If metabolic, is it a normal or wide anion gap acidosis and is the respiratory system adequately compensating?
○ If a wide anion gap acidosis, are there any additional metabolic disturbances?
• Once a specific primary or mixed acid-base disturbance is diagnosed, along with assessment of compensation, the specific etiology should be investigated in order to initiate treatment and correction of the underlying disorder.
• Management of a specific acidosis or alkalosis process may depend on the acuity of onset of the disorder and requires frequent reassessment to judge progress toward normalization of acid-base status.
• Table 86-2 categorizes major types of acid-base disorders, including differential diagnosis, clinical features, and specific treatments.

TABLE 86-2   Major Types of Acid-Base Disorders and Management Considerations

PRIMARY ACID-BASE DISORDER	CLINICAL FEATURES AND DIAGNOSIS	MANAGEMENT CONSIDERATIONS
• **METABOLIC ACIDOSIS— ELEVATED ANION GAP**	• pH < 7.36 and HCO_3^- < 20–22 • Anion gap elevation indicates the presence of unmeasured anions resulting from buffering and loss of HCO_3^- by an acid	

• Lactic acidosis	• Most cases of lactic acidosis from tissue hypoxia arise from circulatory failure
	
	• Check lactic acid level if clinical suspicion is present along with anion gap acidosis
	• Lactic acid concentration > 4 mmol/L indicates that metabolic acidosis is at least in part related to net lactic acid accumulation (normal lactate is approx. 1 mmol/L)
	• Type A—evidence of impaired tissue oxygenation
	  ○ Cardiogenic, hemorrhagic, or septic shock
	  ○ Acute hypoxemia
	  ○ Carbon monoxide
	• Type B—no impaired tissue oxygenation
	  ○ Liver disease (reduces lactate metabolism), renal failure, thiamine deficiency, malignancy, ETOH ingestion in malnourished patients
	  ○ Metformin (cause unknown—risk increased with volume depletion and contrast agents)
	  ○ Nucleoside reverse transcriptase inhibitors for HIV infection (eg, zidovudine, stavudine)
		• Anion gap elevation, at ICU admission, is a useful predictor of hyperlactemia (> 5 mmol/L) (Kamel et al., 1990)
		• Lactate may be a useful indicator of illness severity and help predict mortality
		• Therapy is focused on insuring adequate tissue oxygenation, and treating underlying causes
		• Provide high inspired O_2 fraction, volume repletion, inotropes if needed
		• Minimize vasoconstrictors
		• Consider surgical intervention for trauma or ischemic tissue
		• Prescribe empiric antibiotics for sepsis
		• Discontinue metformin in high-risk patients
		• Consider dialysis for lactate or toxin removal
		• Alkali therapy may be an option for acute, severe acidemia (pH < 7.1), but administration may be problematic and the use of alkali is controversial

• D-Lactic acidosis	• D-Lactate is formed as a byproduct of metabolism by bacteria • D-Lactic acidosis can accumulate in human GI tract with jejunal bypass or short bowel syndrome	• Low carbohydrate diet and antibiotics for bacterial overgrowth
• KETOACIDOSIS		
• Diabetic ketoacidosis (DKA)	• DKA is usually associated with hyperglycemia • Fatty acids are metabolized to ketoacids (acetoacetate and B-hydroxybutyrate) • See Chap. 34	• It is important to replete fluid losses, administer insulin, and identify and treat infection or associated triggers for DKA • Correction of electrolyte deficits • Small amounts of bicarbonate may be needed with severe acidemia (pH < 7.0) • pH 6.90–7.00 give 50 mEq (1 ampule) and 10 mEq KCl in 200 mL water IV over 2 hours • pH < 6.90 give 100 mEq (2 ampules) and 20 mEq KCl in 400 mL water IV over 4 hours
• Alcoholic ketoacidosis	• This is typically seen with chronic ETOH use with low food intake and abrupt ETOH withdrawal • Mostly B-hydroxybutyrate is found in the serum • The blood glucose is usually low or normal	• Treat dehydration, usually with glucose in isotonic saline • Hypophosphatemia is common and may be severe (risk for rhabdomyolysis) • Correct K^+, Mg^+, and vitamin supplementation (especially thiamine and folate)
• Starvation ketosis	• This usually occurs 24–48 hours after fasting and may become more severe with exercise and pregnancy	• Administration of glucose and insulin
• INGESTIONS (DRUGS AND TOXINS)		
• Ethylene glycol (antifreeze)	• This ingestion is colorless, odorless, sweet • Ethylene glycol is metabolized to glycolic acid and oxalate by alcohol dehydrogenase (CNS, cardiopulmonary, and renal toxicity) • OG may be elevated (usually only early) • Check blood ethylene glycol levels • Look for oxalate crystals in urine or fundoscopic examination • Fluorecein (chemical added to antifreeze) may be seen with Wood's lamp but has limited diagnostic utility	• Treat with supportive measures *and* competitive inhibition of alcohol dehydrogenase: Fomepizole 15 mg/kg IV followed by 10 mg/kg every 12 hours *or* IV Ethanol (10% in D5W) 600 mg/kg initially followed by 154 mg/kg/hr (target serum ETOH level 100–200 mg/dL) • Treatment continued until ethylene glycol level < 20 mg/dL • Consider HD, particularly if severe acidosis
• Methanol	• Methanol raises plasma osmolality (early) and is metabolized to formaldehyde and formic acid (CNS toxins) by alcohol dehydrogenase	• Treat similar to ethylene glycol-induced metabolic acidosis until methanol level < 20 mg/dL

(Continued)

TABLE 86-2   Major Types of Acid-Base Disorders and Management Considerations (*Continued*)

PRIMARY ACID-BASE DISORDER	CLINICAL FEATURES AND DIAGNOSIS	MANAGEMENT CONSIDERATIONS
	• Optic nerve hyperemia may occur • Check blood methanol leve	
• Salicylates	• Salicylate ingestion causes predominantly a respiratory alkalosis, but AG acidosis in mixed disorder • Check salicylate level • Salicylate level is part of AG elevation, along with ketones and lactate	• Perform gastric lavage • Charcoal is administered via nasogastric tube • Cautiously consider use of alkali to lower blood pH 7.45–7.50 with resultant urinary alkalization
• Paraldehyde	• Very rarely occurs now	• Intravenous saline is supportive
• Toluene exposure	Toluene from glue sniffing produces benzoic and hippuric acid metabolites • OG may be elevated • UAG can also be positive with toluene poisoning when a large amount of the anion hippurate is excreted in the urine and results in ($Cl^- \ll Na^+ + K^+$).	
• Renal failure/uremia	• Acute, acute superimposed on chronic renal failure or chronic in nature, renal disease does not typically cause uremic symptoms until severe	• See Chaps. 83 and 84
METABOLIC ACIDOSIS—NORMAL ANION GAP	• This is notable for pH < 7.36 and HCO_3^- < 20–22 • Bicarbonate is lost with retention of chloride, thus anion gap in the normal range	
• Renal tubular acidosis (RTA)	• Hyperchloremic acidosis, normal anion gap, UAG > 10 (positive) is seen with RTA If urine pH < 5.5, check serum K^+ to distinguish between type 2 and type 4 RTA	
• Proximal RTA (type 2)	The proximal defect is in reclaiming HCO_3^- mainly in proximal tubule. Associated laboratory findings include: • Plasma K^+ usually low • Urine pH < 5.3 in steady state • Acidosis which is milder than type 1 due to intact HCO_3^- reabsorption distally • Plasma HCO_3^- usually 14–20 mmol/L The possible etiologies include • Multiple myeloma, Fanconi syndrome, ifosfamide therapy cause damage to proximal tubule epithelium • Acetazolamide, cystinosis inhibit carbonic anhydrase Diagnostic test results are • Urine pH > 5.3 if above absorption threshold (alkali administration will increase pH) • Baseline $FE_{HCO_3^-}$ is low (calculated similarly to FE_{Na}) • HCO_3^- is given to raise plasma HCO_3^- to near normal then urine pH measured (pH < 5.5 for Dx) along with $FE_{HCO_3^-}$ ($FE_{HCO_3^-}$ should be > 10–15% for Dx)	• Treat with oral bicarbonate 10–30 mEq/kg/d (sodium bicarbonate tablets: 650 mg = 7.6 mEq) • K^+ supplementation is often necessary
• Distal RTA (type 1)	Defect of H^+ secretion is in the distal tubule. Associated laboratory findings include • K^+ low or normal • Urine pH > 5.3 • Plasma HCO_3^- low (often < 14 mmol/L) • Inability to acidify urine in the setting of systemic acidosis The possible etiologies • Sjögren's syndrome, amphotericin B, lithium, volume depletion, urinary obstruction, sickle cell disease, HIV infection	• Treat with oral bicarbonate 1–3 mEq/kg/d • K^+ replacement often not needed because acidosis correction reduces K^+ excretion • Abnormal Ca^+ metabolism with hypercalciuria, nephrolithiasis, and nephrocalcinosis
• Type 4 RTA (low renin, low aldosterone)	This is notable for inadequate aldosterone support of renal acidification (aldosterone promotes Na^+ reabsorption, along with K^+ and H^+ secretion distally). Associated laboratory findings include • Hyperkalemia • Low plasma renin activity, low serum aldosterone • Decreased cortisol level with primary adrenal insufficiency	• Treat with kayexalate for elevated potassium • Withdrawal of offending medications if indicated • Treat underlying medical conditions

(Continued)

TABLE 86-2   Major Types of Acid-Base Disorders and Management Considerations (*Continued*)

PRIMARY ACID-BASE DISORDER	CLINICAL FEATURES AND DIAGNOSIS	MANAGEMENT CONSIDERATIONS
	The possible etiologies include • Heparin, NSAIDs, ACE inhibitors, HIV infection (decreased aldosterone production), cyclosporin B, K^+-sparing diuretics, trimethoprim (aldosterone resistance) Adrenal insufficiency, TB • Diabetic nephropathy, chronic interstitial nephritis (decreased renin-angiotensin system activity), obstructive uropathy, sickle nephropathy	
• GI loss of bicarbonate	This is notable for • Hyperchloremic acidosis, normal anion gap, UAG < −10 (negative) • Usually accompanied by volume depletion due to large quantities of HCO_3^- loss • Fractional excretion of sodium is often low (< 1–2%) • Hypokalemia due to large quantities of K^+ loss in stool, and increased renin/aldosterone The possible etiologies include: • Diarrhea, external pancreatic or small bowel drainage, and ureteral to bowel diversions; also drug-related diarrhea from magnesium sulfate or cholestyramine (bile acid diarrhea)	• Infuse saline to restore euvolemia and renal perfusion • Correct potassium and magnesium deficits • Identify and correct underlying cause of GI losses
• Dilutional acidosis	This occurs commonly during recovery from ketoacidosis when rapid saline infusion causes chloride retention with loss of HCO_3^- • Sodium salts of ketoacids are excreted, and potential HCO_3^- buffered and lost • Usually in the setting of some renal functional impairment	• Expect nonanion gap acidosis after treatment of significant ketosis
METABOLIC ALKALOSIS	pH > 7.44 and HCO_3^- > 26–28 Important diagnostic tests include • Assessment of volume status, BP, and K^+ • Urine chloride measurement to differentiate chloride responsive from chloride unresponsive	
• Chloride responsive	This occurs commonly in hospitalized patients Important diagnostic tests include • Urine chloride < 10 Possible etiologies include • GI acid loss from vomiting, nasogastric suction (HCl loss) • Renal acid loss from thiazide or loop diuretics (urinary excretion of ammonium chloride [NH_4Cl] without alteration in total body HCO_3^-) • Hypovolemia (contracted volume of extracellular fluid) • Posthypercapneic state (enhanced renal HCO_3^- absorption and generation)	• Treat dehydration with intravenous normal saline • Discontinue diuretics • If continued gastric drainage required, H_2 blockers or proton pump inhibitors can reduce gastric acid loss • Acetazolamide can accelerate renal HCO_3^- loss • Administer HCl or initiate HD in severe cases
• Chloride unresponsive	• Urine chloride > 20 Possible etiologies include • Hyperaldosteronism (aldosteronoma or Conn's syndrome), Cushing's syndrome (increased net acid excretion from mineralocorticoids) • High renin states with HTN (renal artery stenosis) • Hypokalemia (activation of renal H^+/K^+ ATPase) • Refeeding alkalosis • Bartter's and Gitelman's syndrome (genetic disorders)	• Remove underlying stimulus for HCO_3^- generation • Prescribe spironolactone for increased mineralocorticoid states • Consider surgery for adrenal adenomas • Correct hypokalemia

(Continued)

TABLE 86-2   Major Types of Acid-Base Disorders and Management Considerations (*Continued*)

PRIMARY ACID-BASE DISORDER	CLINICAL FEATURES AND DIAGNOSIS	MANAGEMENT CONSIDERATIONS
RESPIRATORY ACIDOSIS	• pH < 7.36 and $PCO_2 \geq 45$ Possible etiologies include • Inhibition of respiratory drive due to opiates, anesthetics, sedatives, central sleep apnea, obesity, CNS lesions/trauma, excessive oxygen in a patient with chronic compensated hypercarbia • Respiratory muscle disorders or chest wall restriction due to myasthenia gravis, Guillain-Barré syndrome, spinal cord injury, multiple sclerosis, ALS, kyphoscoliosis, chest wall deformity • Upper airway obstruction due to obstructive sleep apnea, laryngospasm, aspiration • Intrinsic lung disease due to pneumonia, severe asthma, pneumothorax, acute respiratory distress, COPD, interstitial lung disease	• Provide ventilatory support if severe or acute • This can be via noninvasive ventilation with CPAP or BiPAP • Eliminate medications that depress respiratory drive • Lung expansion maneuvers may be employed to maximize ventilation
RESPIRATORY ALKALOSIS	• pH > 7.44 and $PCO_2 \leq 35$ Possible etiologies include • Hypoxemia from CHF, anemia, or pulmonary disease (pneumonia, pulmonary embolism, pulmonary edema, fibrosis) • Central stimulation from primary hyperventilation, hepatic failure, salicylate toxicity, pregnancy, sepsis, or neurologic disorders • Anxiety or pain • Mechanical ventilation	• Correct underlying disorder • Provide oxygen supplementation for hypoxia • Adjust ventilator settings in patients on mechanical ventilation

Abbreviations: ETOH, ethanol; DKA, diabetes ketoacidosis; CNS, central nervous system; ALS, amytrophic lateral sclerosis; COPD, chronic obstructive pulmonary disease; CPAP, continuous positive airway pressure; BiPAP, bi-level positive airway pressure.

DISEASE MANAGEMENT STRATEGIES

• Hospitalists should refine their abilities to assess volume status in ill hospitalized patients and be familiar with intravenous fluid management, including the types of intravenous fluids and electrolyte replacement options.
• Prevention of acid-base problems in the hospital may include specific protocols, such as for the prevention of metformin-induced lactic acidosis related to intravenous contrast dye administration. (See Chap. 82.)
• Intensive diabetes management strategies can prevent iatrogenic diabetic ketoacidosis (DKA), a common preventable complication of in-hospital diabetes treatment. (See Chap. 36.)
• Patients with ongoing fluid losses, such as nasogastric suction, diarrhea, aggressive diuresis, and postsurgical patients need careful and attentive evaluation of fluid shifts and electrolytes for effective prevention and management of acid-base disturbances.

CARE TRANSITIONS

• Once an acid-base disorder has been appropriately diagnosed and treated, care should be taken to prevent recurrence—particularly, timely communication of information with the patient's primary care physician regarding details of the hospital course, possible complications, and follow-up needs.
• Intensive diabetes education and referral to endocrinology can improve compliance with insulin therapy and prevent frequent DKA, especially with complex insulin regimens.
• Psychiatry, substance abuse, or social work services may be needed for ingestion and toxin exposures, particularly for suicide attempts or alcohol abuse.
• Make sure to give specific instructions to patients regarding reinstitution of medications, particularly in cases of acute renal failure or medication-related disorders.

BIBLIOGRAPHY

Adrogué HJ, Madias ND. Management of life threatening acid-base disorders, first of two parts. *N Engl J Med.* 1998; 338(1):26–34.
Adrogué HJ, Madias ND. Management of life threatening acid-base disorders, second of two parts. *N Engl J Med.* 1998; 338(2):107–111.
Du Bose TD. Acid-base disorders. In: Brenner BM, ed. *Brenner and Rector's The Kidney.* 7th ed. Philadelphia, PA: W.B. Saunders; 2004:921–996.

Haber RJ. A practical approach to acid-base disorders. *West J Med.* 1991;155(2):146–151.

Kamel KS, Ethier JH, Richardson R, et al. Urine electrolytes and osmolality: when and how to use them. *Am J Nephrol.* 1990;10:89–102.

Rocktaeschel J, Morimatsu H, Uchino S, et al. Unmeasured anions in critically ill patients: can they predict mortality? *Crit Care Med.* 2003;31(8):2131–2136.

Sterns RH. Fluid, electrolyte and acid-base disturbances. *J Am Soc Nephrol.* 2003;2(1):1–33.

Wiseman AC, Linas S. Core curriculum in nephrology, disorders of potassium and acid-base balance. *Am J Kidney Dis.* 2005; 45(5):941–949.

Whittier WL, Rutecki GW. Primer on clinical acid-base problem solving. *Dis Mon.* 2004;50(3):122–162.

87A DISORDERS OF SODIUM AND WATER

Kambiz Zandi-Nejad and Chin C. Tang

EPIDEMIOLOGY/OVERVIEW

- Hyponatremia is the most commonly encountered electrolyte abnormality with an estimated prevalence of 2.5% to 42.6% in hospitalized patients.
  - Although two-thirds of cases of hyponatremia in hospitalized patients develop after admission, hyponatremia is common in outpatients as well with a prevalence of about 7%.
  - Many cases of hyponatremia are incidental to the reason for admission, but do have prognostic importance.
  - The prevalence of hyponatremia increases with advancing age. By the eighth decade, the odds ratio for hyponatremia is 5.8, and for severe hyponatremia (serum sodium < 116 mmol/L), it is almost 13.
- Hypernatremia is much less common than hyponatremia, with an estimated prevalence of 6.9% in hospitalized patients and 0.7% in clinic patients.
  - Although not the direct cause in many cases, hypernatremia is associated with a high mortality rate in hospitalized patients, particularly if the presence of hypernatremia has been of longer duration.
  - The development of hypernatremia in hospitalized patients is usually iatrogenic or preventable and may be a measure of quality care in the intensive care unit (ICU).

PATHOPHYSIOLOGY

- Disorders of sodium balance, unlike that of other electrolytes measured, is a reflection more of water homeostasis and less of the electrolyte being measured. Hyponatremia and hypernatremia reflect an increased or decreased water-to-sodium ratio, respectively. In either case, the total body sodium can be normal, less than normal, or greater than normal.
- Total body water (TBW) is controlled by the interplay between baroreceptors that regulate antidiuretic hormone (ADH, also known as arginine vasopressin [AVP]) and osmoreceptors that regulate thirst in addition to ADH release; in cases of conflicting input, the signal from baroreceptors will prevail (Fig. 87A-1).
- ADH enhances water absorption by the kidneys via insertion of preformed water channels into the luminal surface of the renal collecting tubules. Urine concentration should, therefore, increase and urine volume should decrease.
  - The maximum urine osmolality achieved in ADH presence is ~ 1200 mOsm/kg, while the maximally dilute urine has an osmolality of ~ 50–80 mOsm/kg.
- Plasma osmolality, of which sodium is the overwhelming determinant, is tightly maintained between 285 and 295 mOsm/kg. Osmoreceptors respond to a change of plasma osmolality of as little as 1% through its effects on ADH and help keep the plasma osmolality and serum sodium in its narrow ranges despite wide variations in daily intake of water.
- Decreased effective arterial volume is also a strong stimulus for ADH release through its effects on baroreceptors; congestive heart failure (CHF), cirrhosis, and nephrotic syndrome are common examples.
- ADH release and thirst are suppressed by hypo-osmolality and volume overload.

CLINICAL PRESENTATION, DIFFERENTIAL, MAKING THE DIAGNOSIS

- The key to diagnosing the etiology of, and treatment for, both hyponatremia and hypernatremia is the determination of the patient's volume status, both total and effective circulatory volume. Proper measurement of orthostasis may be invaluable in assessing the volume status and should be done by the physician.
  - Hypovolemic patients may present with orthostasis, dry oral mucosa, tachycardia, hypotension, or syncope.
  - Hypervolemic patients present with pulmonary congestion, peripheral edema, and/or ascites but may

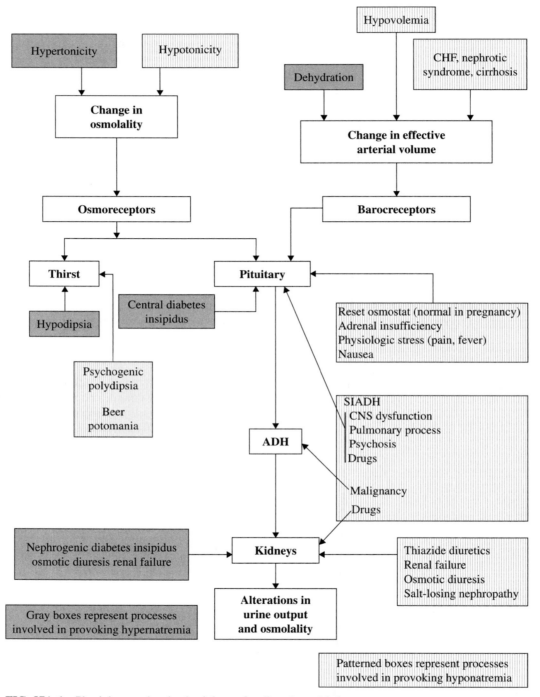

FIG. 87A-1   Physiology and pathophysiology of sodium (water) balance.

also have symptoms and signs of a low effective circulatory volume.

• The symptoms of hyponatremia and hypernatremia result from fluid shifts into (hyponatremia) or out of (hypernatremia) central nervous system (CNS) cells.

The presence and severity of the symptoms depend on the rapidity of development, magnitude, and duration of serum sodium change. The faster or more severe the degree of sodium level changes, the more apparent the symptoms.

MANAGEMENT STRATEGIES

- The formulae presented in this section serve as guides for the selection and rate of fluid administration. Serum sodium must be monitored closely and adjustments made during treatment.
- Since serum sodium concentration is a measure of body water and not sodium balance, management strategies consists of manipulation of TBW.
- TBW is 60% of lean body weight in men and 50% of lean body weight in women. That fraction may decrease to 50% and 45% in elderly men and women, respectively.
- The treatment of hyponatremia revolves around hypertonic or isotonic saline administration or fluid restriction, depending on the severity and etiology of the hyponatremia. (See Table 87A-1.)
- The treatment of hypernatremia always requires the administration of water.
- The rate of correction of hyponatremia and hypernatremia can generally be done at the same rate at which it occurred; unfortunately, this rate is often unknown.
  - Rapid correction of serum sodium level is usually not necessary and is potentially dangerous.
  - The exception is when there are severe neurologic symptoms present.
- The effect of 1 L of IV fluid on serum sodium can be estimated as follows for either hypo- or hypernatremia:
  - Change in serum sodium = (infusate Na + infusate K) − serum Na/(TBW + 1 L)
  - TBW = lean body weight × (0.6 for men, 0.5 for women and elderly men, 0.45 for elderly women)

HYPONATREMIA

CLINICAL PRESENTATION
- Many cases of hyponatremia are discovered incidentally and symptoms are nonspecific. More sophisticated testing may, however, detect disorders of attention and gait.
- Symptoms of hyponatremia become more apparent in patients who have a lower sodium level (< 125 mmol/L), experience a more rapid decline in sodium level, or have preexisting CNS disease such as a seizure disorder.
- As hyponatremia becomes more severe (progressively < 125 mmol/L), patients may develop nausea, malaise, ataxia, headache, lethargy, confusion, seizure, coma, and finally, brain herniation and death.

DIFFERENTIAL DIAGNOSIS
- Hyponatremia usually occurs when there is an increase, appropriate or inappropriate, in ADH.
- Hyponatremia can rarely occur with excessive water ingestion, which can overcome the kidney's ability to

TABLE 87A-1 Sodium and Potassium Content of Commonly Used Intravenous Fluids

IV SOLUTIONS COMMONLY USED IN ADULTS WITHOUT ADDITIVES	INFUSATE NA+ (mmol/L)	INFUSATE K+ (mmol/L)
D5W	0	0
0.2% NS	34	0
Each ampule of sodium bicarbonate (often diluted into 11 L of D5W)	50	0
0.45% NS	77	0
Lactated ringers	130	5.4
0.9% NS	154	0
3% NS	513	0

excrete water. However, even in these cases, there is often a concomitant defect in ADH regulation or function.
- Hypovolemic hyponatremia occurs when there is
  - True hypovolemia (eg, shock), as evidenced by extracellular and intravascular volume contraction that leads to appropriate ADH secretion.
  - Cerebral and renal salt wasting, adrenal insufficiency, vomiting and diarrhea, and diuretic use, particularly thiazide-like diuretics.
- Euvolemic hyponatremia occurs when there is
  - Physiologic stress, including pain and fever, nausea with or without vomiting, and hypothyroidism through an increase in ADH secretion or a failure to suppress ADH.
  - Adrenal insufficiency, which removes the negative feedback of cortisol on ADH-CRH release so that ADH together with corticotropin-releasing hormone (CRH) continues to be secreted by the pituitary.
  - The syndrome of inappropriate antidiuretic hormone (SIADH), a term used to describe the nonphysiologic, inappropriate secretion or effect of ADH (Table 87A-2).

TABLE 87A-2 Causes of SIADH

CNS INFECTIONS, SURGERY, MASSES, VASCULAR EVENT	MEDICATIONS
Pulmonary infections, illnesses, and masses	Tricyclic antidepressants
Malignancy	Serotonin-reuptake inhibitors
Psychosis	Opiate derivatives
HIV infection	Cyclophosphamide
Positive pressure ventilation	Phenothiazines
Guillain-Barreé syndrome	Carbamazepine
	Monoamine-oxidase inhibitors
	Sulfonylureas
	Vasopressin
	Oxytocin
	Nicotine
	Clofibrate
	Vincristine
	NSAIDs

Abbreviations: HIV, human immunodeficiency virus; NSAIDs, nonsteroidal antiinflammatory drugs.

- The pathophysiology of SIADH includes the inappropriate secretion of ADH by the pituitary, enhancement of the action of ADH on the kidneys, and the ectopic production of ADH.
  - Several illnesses, including malignancies, CNS or pulmonary diseases, psychiatric illnesses, medications, or infection can cause SIADH.
- Hypervolemic hyponatremia is characterized by a decreased effective arterial volume with increased TBW and volume; patients usually have edema and/or ascites on physical examination.
  - Although sodium absorption is also increased due to the activation of the renin-angiotensin-aldosterone cascade, water absorption exceeds that of sodium, hence, causing hyponatremia.
  - CHF, nephrotic syndrome, and cirrhosis are the classic examples in which the decreased effective intravascular volume sensed by the baroreceptors

results in increased ADH secretion and hyponatremia (see Fig. 87A-2).

MAKING THE DIAGNOSIS

- First, true hyponatremia must be distinguished from pseudohyponatremia.
  - A normal or elevated plasma osmolality together with hyponatremia characterizes pseudohyponatremia.
  - Pseudohyponatremia is usually associated with the presence of excessive amounts of lipids or proteins in the serum or in association with high concentration of effective solutes in the serum.
  - It may occur even with newer methodologies (ion-specific electrodes) commonly used in most laboratories; this appears to be primarily due to pre-analysis dilution of the sample. Checking a plasma osmolality will uncover this situation.

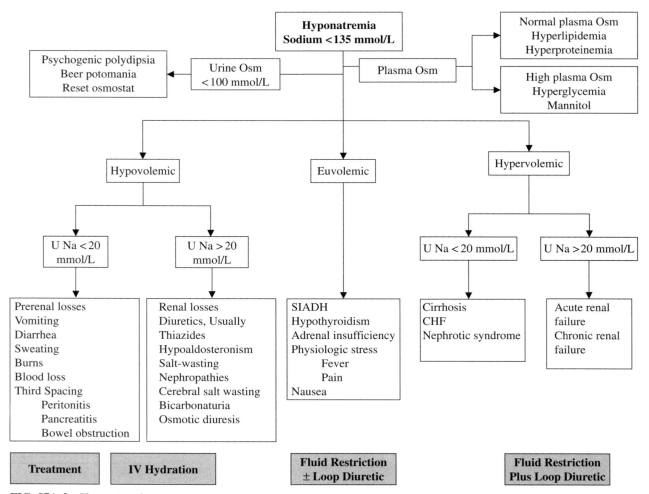

FIG. 87A-2 Hyponatremia.
SOURCE: Modified with permission from Kumar S, Berl T. Sodium. *Lancet.* 1998,352:220–228.

- If hyperglycemia is present, sodium is corrected by adding 1.6 mmol/L for every 100 mmol/L glucose > 100 mmol/L.
- Other solutes that can decrease the measured serum sodium include sorbitol, mannitol, and IV contrast.
- Alcohol and urea readily cross cell membranes, are not effective osmoles, and thus do not affect serum sodium.
- Secondly, the hospitalist should determine the patient's volume status using the physical examination and complimentary laboratory tests to determine total and effective circulatory volume.
  - The urine sodium should be < 20 mmol/L in hypovolemic patients.
  - The fractional excretion of sodium (FE_{Na}) and the fractional excretion of urea (FE_{Urea}), often used in the workup of acute renal failure to distinguish between prerenal azotemia and ATN, may also be helpful in assessing the effective circulatory volume in patients with hyponatremia.
    - A FE_{Na} < 1% and a FE_{Urea} < 35% may be suggestive of a low effective circulatory volume.
    - Whereas recent loop and distal diuretic use may confound the results of the urine sodium and FE_{Na}, it does not appear to have a significant effect on FE_{Urea}.
  - However, these tests should only be used in combination with other measures (eg, clinical examination) to determine the effective circulatory volume and with close attention to their limitations and shortcomings.
    - For example, in patients with normal renal function and euvolemia, the FE_{Na} may be as low as 0.1%.
    - Hypervolemic patients with pulmonary congestion, peripheral edema, and/or ascites may also have a low effective circulatory volume despite an increased total volume; hence, their urine sodium and FE_{Na} are often low as well.
  - Be sure to also check the patient's weight in the assessment of volume status.
- Third, the following tests are required to confirm the cause of hyponatremia: blood urea nitrogen (BUN), creatinine, glucose, total protein, albumin, and plasma osmolality; urinalysis; and urine sodium, creatinine, osmolality, and if diuretics were recently used, urea.
- The following criteria should be met before a diagnosis of SIADH is made:
  - No recent diuretic use
  - Euvolemia
  - Hypotonic hyponatremia
  - Urine osmolality > 100 mOsm/kg
  - Urine sodium > 40 mmol/L
  - Normal renal, cardiac, hepatic, adrenal, and thyroid function
  - Normal acid-base status
  - Normal serum potassium level

TRIAGE AND INITIAL MANAGEMENT

- Rapid correction of hyponatremia is indicated in cases of hyponatremia accompanied by seizures or obtundation.
  - Hypertonic saline should be administered with the goal of raising the serum sodium 1–2 mmol/L/hr until symptoms have resolved.
  - A ceiling of 8 mmol/L increase in serum sodium over the first 24 hours should be observed. Serum sodium should be measured every 1–2 hours and the patient should be monitored in the ICU or ED.
  - Furosemide can be given as adjunctive therapy.
- Most cases of hyponatremia that are not being treated with hypertonic saline can be managed on a general medical floor.
- To get a very rough estimate of the negative fluid balance necessary to achieve a target sodium for euvolemic and hypervolemic patients:

$$\text{Excess fluid (in liters)} = \text{TBW} - (\text{actual Na/target Na}) \times \text{TBW}$$

- Central pontine myelinolysis (ie, osmotic demyelination syndrome) can occur when hyponatremia is corrected too rapidly. Hyponatremia should not be corrected at a rate > 1 mmol/L/hr and not > 8 mmol/L over 24 hours. This significantly reduces the risk for central pontine myelinolysis.
  - The development of symptoms such as dysarthria, dysphagia, or extremity weakness after initial improvement of neurologic symptoms should raise the suspicion of central pontine myelinolysis.
  - Magnetic resonance imaging (MRI) is the neurodiagnostic modality of choice, although most lesions can be seen on computed tomography (CT) scan. The diagnosis is often made clinically since radiologic findings may take up to 4 weeks to develop.
- Hypovolemic hyponatremia should be treated with fluid resuscitation with 0.9% saline (normal saline [NS]).
  - This should be done cautiously as volume correction leads to shutdown of ADH secretion. Once ADH secretion is inhibited, the serum sodium can correct very rapidly. This may clinically reveal itself as a rapid increase in the output of dilute urine.
  - If too rapid a rate of correction occurs, free water or even desmopressin may be administered to slow the rate of sodium level correction.

- Euvolemic hyponatremia should be treated with fluid restriction. Fluid intake should be less than urine output.
  - Loop diuretics can be given to augment negative fluid balance and to hamper the concentrating ability of the kidney.
  - If adrenal or thyroid insufficiency is the cause of hyponatremia, cortisol, or thyroid hormone replacement therapy, respectively, is often sufficient.
  - If in vitro fertilization (IVF) is given to a patient with SIADH, and the osmolality of the IVF is less than the urine osmolality, hyponatremia will worsen.
- Hypervolemic hyponatremia should be treated with fluid restriction. Loop diuretics are frequently necessary.

DISEASE MANAGEMENT STRATEGIES
- Once patients with hypovolemic hyponatremia are volume-repleted with NS, maintaining euvolemia is essential, either by treating the underlying disease, or matching fluid losses.
- Patients with SIADH should be kept on fluid restriction. Obviously, any underlying, reversible cause should be identified and treated.
  - If the urine osmolality is < 400 mOsm/kg, fluid restriction should be adequate.
  - If the urine osmolality is > 600 mOsm/kg, furosemide 20 mg po daily to bid or demeclocycline 300–600 po bid will likely be necessary. Lithium is an alternative but is rarely used due to its narrow therapeutic index.
  - A high-salt, high-protein diet may be instituted in order to facilitate urinary free water excretion.
  - Patients with hypervolemic hyponatremia should be managed with salt and fluid restriction plus diuretics and be monitored by daily weights.
- AVP V_2-receptor antagonists are emerging as promising treatment options. These drugs promote the excretion of dilute urine.
- Tolvaptan (initial dose of 15 mg po daily) has been shown to be effective in the treatment of hyponatremia due to CHF, cirrhosis, and SIADH, and its use has been initiated at several medical centers for these indications.

HYPERNATREMIA

CLINICAL PRESENTATION
- The signs of volume depletion that may variably be seen with hypernatremia are orthostasis, tachycardia, decreased skin turgor, dry oral mucosa, and altered mental status.

- Hypernatremia will develop only if the patient does not drink enough water (either because of lack of access to water or, very rarely, hypodipsia) or iatrogenically if the patient receives rapid hypertonic sodium infusions (eg, total parenteral nutrition [TPN] or sodium bicarbonate infusions).
- Profuse perspiration, vomiting, diarrhea, or osmotic diuresis results in hypotonic fluid loses, dehydration, and ultimately hypernatremia.
  - Dehydration denotes loss of both extracellular and intracellular water.
  - This is unlike hypovolemic hyponatremia, where there is extracellular volume depletion, but maintenance of the overall intracellular volume.

DIFFERENTIAL DIAGNOSIS
- Central diabetes insipidus (CDI) and nephrogenic diabetes insipidus (NDI) predispose to hypernatremia, but manifest with hypernatremia only when the thirst mechanism is impaired or the patient has inadequate access to water.
  - The usual presenting sign of diabetes insipidus is not hypernatremia, but rather polyuria and polydipsia.
  - However, patients with otherwise undiagnosed diabetes insipidus may develop hypernatremia as their presenting symptom during a hospitalization since this may be the first time their access to water is limited.
  - Most patients with diabetes insipidus have an incomplete, or partial, defect in secreting or responding to ADH.
- The defect in CDI is failure to produce/secrete ADH.
  - Alterations in the anatomy of the hypothalamus from trauma, neurosurgery, malignancy, or infiltrative disease can cause CDI.
- The defect in NDI is the kidney's failure to respond to ADH.
  - Lithium use, hypercalcemia, and persistent glycosuria can result in NDI.

MAKING THE DIAGNOSIS
- Check serum potassium, glucose, calcium, albumin, ADH level (in selected cases), and urine osmolality (see Fig. 87A-3).
- The underlying reason for inadequate access to water should also be investigated. This may involve a workup for infection, stroke, overdose, or other reasons.
- A urine osmolality < 300 mOsm/kg in a hypernatremic patient suggests complete NDI or CDI.
  - Patients with partial CDI and NDI have a higher urine osmolality (300–800 mOsm/kg) when hypernatremia develops.

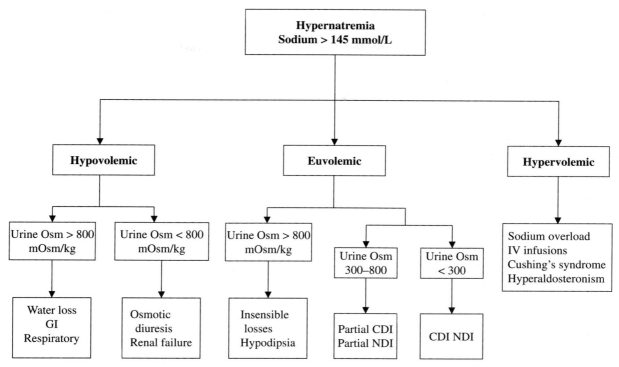

FIG. 87A-3 Causes of hypernatremia.
SOURCE: Modified with permission from Kumar S, Berl T. Sodium. *Lancet.* 1998,352:220–228.

- These two conditions can also be distinguished from each other by the response to desmopressin.
- The water deprivation test is used to determine the etiology of patients with polyuria, of which diabetes insipidus is often a diagnostic consideration.
  ○ Patients with hypernatremia are already hyperosmolar by definition. If diabetes insipidus is suspected, the response to desmopressin can be measured without water restriction as long as they remain hypernatremic and hyperosmolar (plasma osmolality > 295 mOsm/kg).
  ○ If these conditions are met, a baseline ADH and urine osmolality can be drawn. dDAVP 1 μg IV is given and the urine osmolality is rechecked at 30 and 60 minutes.
  ○ The urine osmolality will increase by more than 50% in CDI and less then 50% in NDI. ADH should be low in CDI and high in NDI.

TRIAGE AND INITIAL MANAGEMENT

- Overly rapid correction of hypernatremia can cause cerebral edema, which is marked by seizures and coma. This should be evident on CT scan.
  ○ Hypernatremia should not be corrected at a rate > 0.5 mmol/L/hr or 12 mmol/L over 24 hours.

  ○ The TBW deficit = TBW [(plasma Na/140) − 1)]
- Free water can be administered as tap water enterally or 5% dextrose in water (D5W) parenterally.
- If there are signs of hemodynamic instability in a patient with hypernatremia, isotonic saline should be infused first.
  ○ Once stability has been achieved, the hypernatremia can be addressed with hypotonic fluids.

DISEASE MANAGEMENT STRATEGIES

- Patients with hypernatremia must have ready access to water.
- Most patients with diabetes insipidus will maintain normal serum sodium as long as they have ready access to water. However, the polyuria, particularly nocturia, may be troubling to the patient.
- Patients with CDI can be treated with dDAVP 10 mcg QHS. It can be given intramuscularly, intranasally, or orally. Other therapies include chlorpropramide, carbamazepine, clofibrate, and thiazide diuretics.
- Treatment for NDI is more problematic and consultation with nephrology is advised. Thiazide diuretics and salt restriction can be tried. Amiloride may help in patients with lithium-induced NDI.

CARE TRANSITIONS

- Hyponatremia and hypernatremia are often not the primary reason for the patient's admission and disposition is usually dictated by his/her primary diagnosis.
- If thiazide diuretics are the culprit of a patient's hyponatremia, resumption of these medications is not recommended prior to discharge and an alternative agent should be considered.
- Patients should have their electrolytes checked 3–5 days after discharge.
- Emphasis must be placed on maintaining treatment for their water imbalance, whether it is fluid restriction and diuretics for hyponatremic patients or free access to water for patients with diabetes insipidus.
- It is especially important for patients with hyponatremia, because of the risk of heart failure or cirrhosis, to follow a strict regimen of fluid and salt restriction and medication adherence.

BIBLIOGRAPHY

Abbott R, Silber E, Felber J, et al. Osmotic demyelination syndrome. *BMJ*. 2005;331:829–830.

Adrioge J, Madias N. Hyponatremia. *N Engl J Med*. 2000;342:1581–1589.

Andersson B. Regulation of water intake. *Physiol Rev*. 1978;58:582–603.

Asadollahi K, Beeching N, Gill G. Hyponatremia as a risk factor for hospital mortality. *QJM*. 2006;99:877–880.

Carvounis C, Nisar S, Guro-Razuman S. Significance of the fractional excretion of urea in the differential diagnosis of acute renal failure. *Kidney Int*. 2002;62:2223–2229.

Chassagne P, Druesne L, Capet C, et al. Clinical presentation of hypernatremia in elderly patients: a case control study. *J Am Geriatr Soc*. 2006,54:1225–1230.

Decaux G. Is asymptomatic hyponatremia really asymptomatic? *Am J Med*. 2006;119(7A):S79–S82.

Kumar S, Berl T. Sodium. *Lancet*. 1998,352:220–228.

Makaryus A, McFarlane S. Diabetes insipidus: diagnosis and treatment of a complex disease. *Cleve Clin J Med*. 2006;73(1):65–71.

Pirzada N, Ali I. Central pontine myelinolysis. *Mayo Clin Proc*. 2001;76:559–562.

Reynolds R, Padfield P, Seckl J. Disorders of sodium balance. *BMJ*. 2006;332:702–705.

Rose B, Post T. *Clinical Physiology of Acid-Base and Electrolyte Disorders*. 5th ed. New York, NY: McGraw-Hill; 2001.

Schrier R, Gross P, Gheorghiade M, et al. Tolvaptan, a selective oral vasopressin V2-receptor antagonist, for hyponatremia. *N Engl J Med*. 2006;355:2099–2112.

Turchin A, Seifter J, Seely E. Mind the gap. *N Engl J Med*. 2003;349:1465–1469.

Upadhyay A, Jaber B, Madias M. Incidence and prevalence of hyponatremia. *Am J Med*. 2006;119(7A):S30–S35.

Zarich S, Fang LS, Diamond JR. Fractional excretion of sodium. Exceptions to its diagnostic value. *Arch Intern Med*. 1985;1415:108–112.

87B DISORDERS OF POTASSIUM

Kambiz Zandi-Nejad and Chin C. Tang

EPIDEMIOLOGY/OVERVIEW

- Hypokalemia, is defined as serum $K^+ < 3.5$ mmol/L.
  - Hypokalemia is a common finding in both outpatients (average 15% to 30%) and inpatients (up to 20%) with mild hypokalemia (serum K^+ of 3–3.5 mmol/L) constituting the majority (~75%) of cases.
- Hyperkalemia is defined as serum $K^+ \geq 5.5$ mmol/L.
  - Hyperkalemia is reported in 1% to 10% of hospitalized patients of which ~10% have significant hyperkalemia ($K^+ \geq 6.0$ mmol/L).
- Major consequences of both hypokalemia and hyperkalemia manifest primarily in the following systems:
  - Cardiovascular
  - Muscles
  - Kidneys
- An excess of cardiac death primarily accounts for the mortality increase.
  - Hypokalemia may increase mortality of inpatients by tenfold.
  - Hyperkalemia is associated with a higher mortality rate of 14% to 41%
- Hospitalists play an important role in preventing, diagnosing, and treating electrolyte disturbances, many of which are iatrogenic.

PATHOPHYSIOLOGY

- The serum potassium level is tightly kept at 3.5–5.0 mmol/L, despite wide variation in daily potassium intake, through *internal* and *external* potassium balance.
- The total body potassium content is estimated at ~3500 mmol or ~50 mmol/kg of which ~98% is intracellular, resulting in intracellular and extracellular fluid potassium concentrations of ~150 and ~4 mmol/L, respectively.

- Internal potassium balance, the movement of potassium between intracellular and extracellular spaces, occurs in minutes. This transfer plays a critical role in maintaining a tight serum potassium level, particularly when large amounts of potassium enter the circulation over a short period.
  - The Na^+-K^+-ATPase pump is the major route for potassium entrance into the cells and maintains the high intracellular-extracellular potassium concentration gradient. Potassium passively exits the cells primarily through potassium channels.
  - Insulin and beta-2-catecholamines enhance cellular potassium uptake, whereas hyperosmolality and alpha-catecholamines enhance potassium efflux.
- External potassium balance, the excretion of potassium through urine (~90% to 95%) and stool (~5% to 10%), requires several hours to eliminate the total daily potassium intake of ~70–140 mmol/L for a healthy person at steady state.
  - Potassium excretion by the kidney is mainly regulated at the distal part of the nephron, namely the cortical collecting duct (CCD) and the connecting segment (CNT), primarily by principal cells. See Fig. 87B-1.
  - Factors affecting renal potassium excretion include urine flow rate; distal sodium delivery; intraluminal charge; aldosterone, vasopressin, and serum potassium concentration
  - Of note, potassium excretion in the stool can significantly increase in certain conditions such as chronic kidney disease (CKD) and diarrhea.
- Acid-base disorders can affect the serum K^+ concentration through both internal and external potassium balance.
  - For any given change in pH, acidemia has a stronger effect on internal potassium balance than alkalemia. This effect is limited mainly to nonorganic acidoses.

Unlike nonorganic anions such as chloride, organic anions such as lactate follow hydrogen ion into the cells, thereby precluding potassium efflux.
  - In chronic acid-base disorders, the effect on external potassium balance is dominant.
- The transtubular potassium gradient (TTKG) is used to estimate the potassium concentration at the end of CCD. It is valid only if the urine osmolality exceeds that of the plasma and if the sodium concentration in urine is at least 25 mmol/L. TTKG is calculated using the following equation: [urine K^+/plasma K^+]/[urine osmolality/plasma osmolality]. Normal values for TTKG vary and depend on the serum potassium levels.
  - In patients with hypokalemia TTKG " 2–3 is considered normal.
  - In patients with hyperkalemia TTKG > 6–7 is considered normal.

HYPOKALEMIA

CLINICAL PRESENTATION
- Hypokalemia may reduce tissue metabolism and oxygen consumption, thereby promoting vasoconstriction.
- Arrhythmias and vascular constriction can result.
- Skeletal muscle weakness may present as diaphragmatic weakness and respiratory distress or even diaphragmatic paralysis and respiratory arrest.
  - Rhabomyolysis, weakness, and paralysis may in fact be the first manifestation of severe hypokalemia ($K^+ < 3.0$ mmol/L)
- Smooth muscle weakness may also occur and present as ileus or urinary retention.
- Changes affecting the kidneys include increased ammoniogenesis, acute renal failure, end-stage renal disease (ESRD), and salt retention.

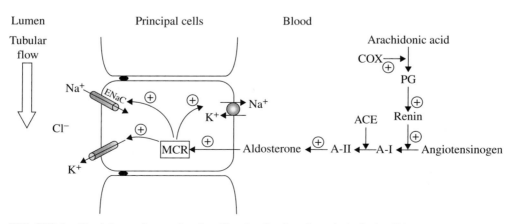

FIG. 87B-1 Physiology of potassium handling by distal nephron (principal cells).

○ Hypokalemia may be a major contributing factor for hepatic encephalopathy in patients with advanced liver disease. This is mainly due to increased ammoniogenesis by renal proximal tubule cells in the setting of hypokalemia.

○ NDI may be a manifestation of severe hypokalemia.

DIFFERENTIAL DIAGNOSIS

• Hypokalemia can be associated with normal body potassium content due to potassium shift into cells or as a result of a true deficit of total body potassium.

• The major causes of potassium redistribution into cells are listed in Table 87B-1.
  ○ Although the majority of causes under this category are due to increased cellular potassium uptake, inhibition of potassium efflux (eg, barium intoxication) from cells can also occur.
  ○ Importantly, endogenous sources of excess beta-2-catecholamines may be seen with stressful conditions such as head injury, alcohol withdrawal, and acute myocardial infarction and should not be overlooked.

• Total body potassium deficit due to increased potassium loss can be through renal or nonrenal routes.

• Increased potassium loss by the kidneys involves several mechanisms.
  ○ Total body potassium deficit due to obligatory renal potassium loss is very rare because most foods have potassium content that exceeds the level of obligatory renal potassium loss.

TABLE 87B-1 Major Causes of Potassium Redistribution into Cells

Insulin excess
Exogenous beta-2-adrenergic excess
  • Decongestants
  • Bronchodilators
  • Tocolytic agents
Endogenous beta-2-adrenergic excess
  • Head injury
  • Acute myocardial infarction
  • Alcohol withdrawal
Hyperthyroidism
Theophylline
Caffeine
Barium ingestion
Chloroquine intoxication
Verapamil intoxication
Familial hypokalemic periodic paralysis
Rapid and significant production of blood cells

○ The main pathophysiologic mechanisms underlying excessive renal potassium excretion are increased distal potassium secretion or increased tubular flow. See Fig. 87B-2.

• The major nonrenal source of potassium loss is the gastrointestinal (GI) tract due to infectious (eg, infectious diarrhea) or noninfectious etiologies (eg, celiac disease, ileostomy, GI fistulas, chronic laxative abuse).
  ○ Hypokalemia associated with vomiting or nasogastric suctioning is primarily because of increased

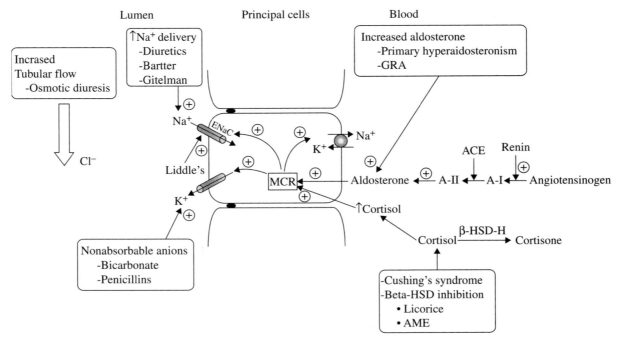

FIG. 87B-2 Pathophysiology of hypokalemia due to increased renal potassium excretion.

renal potassium loss secondary to hypochloremic metabolic alkalosis and volume contraction associated with these conditions. Gastric fluid per se only contains ~6–8 mmol/L of potassium.

○ Profuse sweating may cause hypokalemia, especially if the patient has other conditions that predispose to hypokalemia. Sweat only contains ~5–10 mmol/L of potassium.

MAKING THE DIAGNOSIS

- Diagnosis is based on a serum potassium level of ≤ 3.5 mmol/L.
- Very rarely a low serum potassium level can be spurious; it is usually seen in leukemic patients with a high white blood cell count and is due to postvenipuncture potassium uptake by these cells.
- However, the diagnosis is neither complete nor acceptable unless the cause of hypokalemia is identified. This is usually achievable by following a systematic approach (Fig. 87B-3).
- Inquire about:
  ○ Medications (particularly diuretics, laxatives, antibiotics such as amphotericin B, chemotherapeutic agents such as cisplatin, and beta-2-agonists)
  ○ Diet (eg, potassium intake), dietary supplements (eg, licorice)
  ○ Associated symptoms (eg, diarrhea and vomiting)
  ○ Medical history and concomitant medical conditions (eg, head injury)
  ○ Family history
  ○ The timing and evolution of hypokalemia, especially helpful in determining the cause in hospitalized patients.
    ▪ Hypokalemia due to potassium loss takes days to develop
    ▪ Transcellular shift can precipitate a significant drop in the potassium level within hours.
- Physical examination should be directed at blood pressure, volume status, and signs of specific disorders associated with hypokalemia (eg, Cushing's syndrome).
- Initial laboratory investigation should include kidney function tests; electrolyte profile, including calcium and magnesium; arterial blood gas (ABG); complete blood count (CBC); osmolality; and urinary pH, osmolality, creatinine, Na^+, K^+, and Cl^-.
- Further laboratory studies such as plasma renin and aldosterone levels may be required to make the diagnosis (Fig. 87B-3).

TRIAGE AND INITIAL MANAGEMENT

- Once the diagnosis of hypokalemia is made, the first goal is to prevent, diagnose, and manage life-threatening conditions particularly in high-risk patients.

- All patients with potassium disorder should have a 12-lead electrocardiogram (ECG) as part of their initial workup.
- Hypokalemia can be associated with the following ECG changes:
  ○ A flattened T wave
  ○ A prominent U wave (U wave with amplitude more than T wave)
  ○ Ventricular arrhythmias (see Fig. 87B-4)
- Promptly identify and treat high-risk patients.
  ○ Patients who have electrocardiographic changes, muscle weakness, and respiratory distress require urgent treatment and close observation in the emergency room or ICU until they are stable.
  ○ Elderly patients (age > 65 years), patients with organic heart disease, or those receiving digitalis or antiarrhythmic medications, and patients with liver failure also have an increased risk of dysrhythmia with even mild degrees of hypokalemia (K^+ of 3.0–3.5 mmol/L).
  ○ Patients who experience a rapid decline of potassium level to < 2.5 mmol/L may suddenly develop dysrhythmias.
- Although potassium replacement is usually reserved for patients with a true deficit, it should be considered in patients with hypokalemia due to transcellular shift when serious complications are present or imminent.
  ○ The potassium replacement in these patients, however, should be done cautiously and with close follow-up and frequent monitoring of potassium level, given the high risk of overcorrection or rebound hyperkalemia.
- Dietary potassium may be used as the first line of therapy in mild cases.
  ○ However, it may not be effective in patients with concomitant chloride deficiency (eg, diuretic use) because dietary potassium is primarily present in the form of potassium phosphate and potassium citrate.
  ○ Both of these forms of potassium may accentuate metabolic alkalosis associated with chloride deficiency and volume contraction, thereby, increasing renal potassium excretion.
- In patients with hypokalemia and chloride-responsive metabolic alkalosis, volume replacement may increase bicarbonaturia and renal potassium excretion.
  ○ Therefore it should be done with caution, along with potassium replacement, and with frequent monitoring of serum potassium level.
- The choice of potassium salt depends on the clinical situation.
  ○ Potassium chloride is the default salt of choice because it can help correcting chloride-responsive metabolic alkalosis and may raise serum potassium

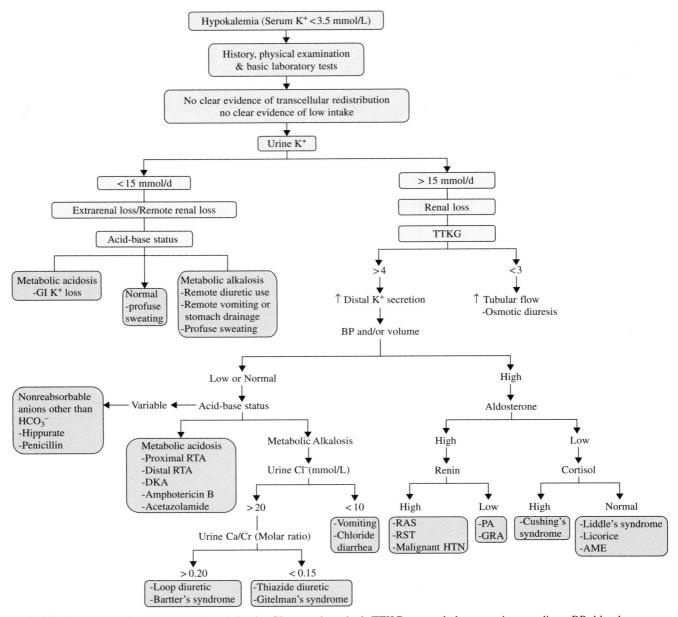

FIG. 87B-3 Diagnostic approach to hypokalemia. GI: gastrointestinal; TTKG: transtubular potassium gradient; BP: blood pressure; RTA: renal tubular acidosis; DKA: diabetic ketoacidosis; RAS: renal artery stenosis; RST: renin secreting tumor; HTN: hypertension; PA: primary aldosteronism; GRA: glucocorticoid remediable aldosteronism; AME: apparent mineralocorticoid excess.
SOURCE: Adapted from Mount DB, Zandi-Nejad K. Disorders of potassium balance. In: Brenner BM, ed. *Brenner and Rector's The Kidney.* 8th ed. Philadelphia, PA: W.B. Saunders; 2008.

level faster, since chloride is mainly an extracellular anion.

○ Potassium bicarbonate is primarily indicated for patients with concomitant hypokalemia and metabolic acidosis (eg, patients with diarrhea, renal tubular acidosis [RTA]).

○ Potassium phosphate should be reserved for patients with both phosphate and potassium deficiencies (eg, patients

with diabetic ketoacidosis). If administered intravenously, the dose should be limited to 50 mmol over 8 hours to prevent hypocalcemia and metastatic calcification. In cases of moderate-to-severe hypokalemia it should be given along with another potassium salt.

• Intravenous (IV) potassium should be limited to patients with signs and symptoms of hypokalemia, high-risk patients (initially), and patients unable to

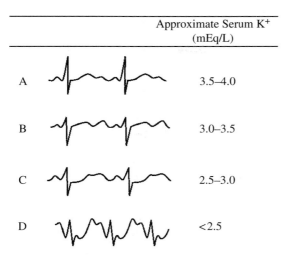

Approximate Serum K⁺ (mEq/L)

A   3.5–4.0

B   3.0–3.5

C   2.5–3.0

D   <2.5

FIG. 87B-4 ECG changes associated with hypokalemia. (A) U waves may be normal finding; (B) U waves with amplitude more than T waves may be a sign of hypokalemia; (C) QU interval should not be mistaken as prolonged QT interval; (D) The PR interval is prolonged and QRS duration may increase. Supraventricular and ventricular ectopic rhythm may occur in high-risk patients.
SOURCE: From Osorio FV, Linas SL. Disorders of potassium metabolism. In: Schrier RW, ed. *Atlas of The Diseases of The Kidney,* Vol. 1. 3.1–3.18.

use the enteral route. The following recommendations are based on potassium chloride as the salt of choice.
○ Usual concentration is 20–40 mmol of potassium chloride in 1 L of dextrose-free vehicle solution.
○ Higher concentration of up to 400 mmol/L (eg, 40 mmol in 100 mL of NS) may be used with extreme caution and only in an ICU setting.
○ The usual rate of administration is 10–20 mmol/hr. Higher infusion rates of up to 80 mmol/hr have been used in life-threatening conditions and may be associated with transient hyperkalemia.
○ ECG monitoring is recommended for infusion rates of more than 10 mmol/hr.
○ IV potassium should be administered preferably through a large central vein; femoral is usually preferred to internal jugular and subclavian.
• Several forms of oral potassium chloride are available (Table 87B-2).
○ A dose of 40–100 mmol of potassium chloride per day, divided in 2–3 doses, is effective in maintaining serum potassium level in desirable range in more than 90% of patients on diuretic therapy. In some patients, larger doses or the addition of a potassium-sparing diuretic may be necessary.
○ Potassium chloride may be toxic in doses of ≥ 2 mmol/kg.

TABLE 87B-2 Major Causes of Potassium Redistribution Out of Cells

Hypertonicity
• Hyperglycemia
• Mannitol
Beta-blockers (nonselective)
Insulin deficiency
Metabolic acidosis (nonorganic)
Digoxin toxicity
Exercise
Succinylcholine
Hyperkalemic periodic paralysis
Arginine hydrochloride infusion
ε-Aminocaproic acid

DISEASE MANAGEMENT STRATEGIES
• The management strategy should focus on the following three elements:
○ Diagnosis and prevention of life-threatening conditions
○ Replacement of the potassium deficit (if any)
○ Diagnosis and correction of the underlying cause
• Replacing potassium is the cornerstone of the treatment.
○ Replacement is necessary for any patient with potassium level < 3.0 mmol/L, high-risk patients with potassium level < 4.0 mmol/L, and asymptomatic patients with mild to moderate hypertension and potassium level of < 4.0 mmol/L.
○ Replacement should be done cautiously to prevent overcorrection and rebound hyperkalemia, particularly for patients with hypokalemia due to redistribution and for patients with kidney function impairment.
○ In the absence of an abnormal transcellular shift, it is estimated that serum potassium level drops by ~0.3 mmol/L for every 100 mmol reduction in total body potassium content.
○ The potassium level should be raised to a safe range rapidly (eg, via IV administration) with the remainder of the deficit replaced at a slower rate over days.
○ Whenever possible and appropriate, repletion through the enteral route is preferable to IV route. In fact, an oral dose of 75 mmol of potassium chloride may increase serum potassium level by 1–1.4 mmol/L.
• In addition to potassium supplementation, strategies to reduce potassium loss through the use of potassium-sparing diuretics (eg, spironolactone, triamterene, amiloride) or medications (eg, ACE-I) should be considered.
• Mg^{2+} deficiency enhances renal potassium excretion through mechanism(s) yet to be fully understood and is one of the common causes of refractory

hypokalemia. Mg^{2+} levels should be measured in all patients with hypokalemia and corrected accordingly.
- Nephrology consultation should be considered for patients with renal potassium loss and no readily identifiable cause. Psychiatric consult should be considered in some patients (eg, laxative abuse)

HYPERKALEMIA

CLINICAL PRESENTATION
- Major consequences of hyperkalemia are also cardiac (rhythm disturbances), muscular (weakness, paralysis), and renal (affecting kidney acidifying capability).
- Skeletal muscle weakness and paralysis may be secondary to hyperkalemia itself or as part of the familial hyperkalemic periodic paralysis.

DIFFERENTIAL DIAGNOSIS
- Hyperkalemia may be due to an increase in total body potassium or a result of transcellular shift. In most cases, however, the cause is multifactorial.
- The major causes of hyperkalemia due to transcellular potassium redistribution are listed in Table 87B-3.
- Increased potassium intake is a rare cause of hyperkalemia in the setting of normal kidney function. In the majority of cases not associated with transcellular shift, some degree of impaired urinary potassium excretion usually does exist. This impairment is usually due to either reduced tubular flow or reduced distal potassium secretion (Fig. 87B-5).
- Principal cells and the effect of aldosterone on these cells play a major role on the ability of kidneys to excrete potassium. In the absence of reduced tubular flow, the usual culprits are (1) conditions associated with low aldosterone level or (2) an impaired response to it by principal cells. See Figs. 87B-1, 87B-3.
- In patients with advanced CKD, intestinal potassium excretion plays a more significant role; constipation may be a significant contributory factor in the development of hyperkalemia among these patients.
- The spurious causes of hyperkalemia (pseudohyperkalemia) should be considered in the differential diagnosis.
  ○ The most common causes are fist clenching, tourniquet use, hemolysis, severe thrombocytosis (usually

TABLE 87B-3   Oral Preparations of Potassium Chloride

SUPPLEMENT	ATTRIBUTES
Controlled-release micro-encapsulated tablets	Disintegrate better in stomach than encapsulated microparticles; less adherent and less cohesive
Encapsulated controlled-release microencapsulated particles	Fewer erosions than wax-matrix tablets
Potassium chloride elixir	Inexpensive, tastes bad, poor compliance; few erosions; immediate effect
Potassium chloride (effervescent tablets) for solution	Convenient, but more expensive than elixir; immediate effect
Wax-matrix extended-release tablets	Easier to swallow; more GI tract erosions compared with microencapsulated formulations

SOURCE: Adapted from Cohn JN, Kowey PR, Whelton PK, et al. New guidelines for potassium replacement in clinical practice: a contemporary review by the National Council on Potassium in Clinical Practice. *Arch Intern Med.* 2000;160:2429–2436.

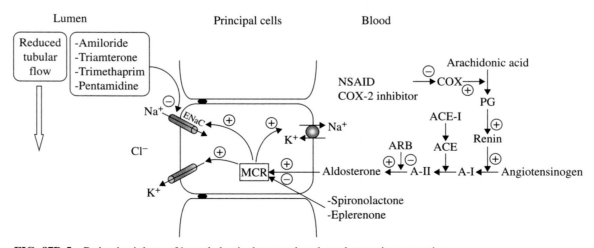

FIG. 87B-5 Pathophysiology of hyperkalemia due to reduced renal potassium excretion.

platelet count of more than 1 million), and severe leukocytosis.
- ○ In patients with severe leukocytosis or thrombocytosis plasma potassium level can be used to differentiate pseudohyperkalemia.

MAKING THE DIAGNOSIS
- A systematic approach can usually identify the cause of hyperkalemia. (See Fig. 87B-6.)
- The history and physical examination should focus on risk factors for impaired kidney function, urine output, medications, diet and dietary supplements, blood pressure, and volume status.

- Basic laboratory testing should include kidney function tests; electrolyte profile; blood glucose level; osmolality; ABG; CBC; and urinary pH, osmolality, creatinine, and electrolyte profile, including 24-hour urine K^+.
- Several medications can cause hyperkalemia by altering internal potassium balance favoring potassium exit from cells.
- An increased potassium load may be endogenous or exogenous; in the absence of impaired renal potassium excretion, increased potassium load is an uncommon cause of hyperkalemia.
  - ○ The common sources for *exogenous* potassium are foods and food supplements rich in potassium,

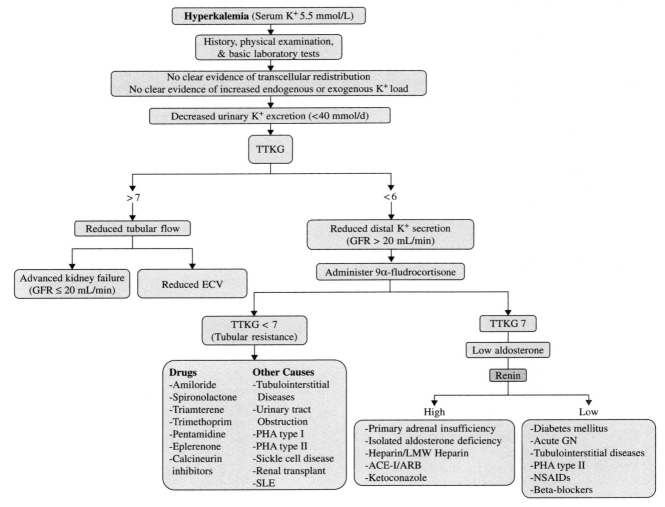

FIG. 87B-6 Diagnostic approach to hyperkalemia. TTKG: transtubular potassium gradient; GFR: glomerular filtration rate; ECV: effective circulatory volume; acute GN: acute glomerulonephritis; HIV: human immunodeficiency virus; NSAIDs: nonsteroidal anti-inflammatory drugs; LMW H: low molecular weight heparin; ACE-I: angiotensin-converting enzyme inhibitor; ARB: angiotensin II receptor blocker; PHA: pseudohypoaldosteronism; SLE: systemic lupus erythematosus.
SOURCE: Adapted from Mount DB, Zandi-Nejad K. Disorders of potassium balance. In: Brenner BM, ed. *Brenner and Rector's The Kidney.* 8th ed. Philadelphia, PA: W.B. Saunders; 2008.

massive red blood cell transfusion, and use of potassium salts of medications (eg, penicillin K or potassium phosphate).

○ The common sources of endogenous potassium are GI bleeding, hematomas, tissue necrosis (eg, rhabdomyolysis), and tumor lysis syndrome.

• In the absence of advanced kidney failure and low urine flow, a TTKG value of < 6 is reflective of decreased potassium secretion in CCD, which may be due to either aldosterone deficiency or resistance.

○ An increase in TTKG value ≥ 7 in response to 9α-fludrocortisone (a mineralocorticoid) is suggestive of aldosterone deficiency, whereas a lesser or no response is indicative of aldosterone resistance.

• Hyporeninemic hypoaldosteronism is the most common form of aldosterone deficiency in adults.

○ The usual presentation is in a patient with mild degree of kidney function impairment and tubulointerstitial involvement.

○ The level of hyperkalemia is usually disproportionate to the degree of kidney function impairment.

○ Commonly, it is associated with mild nonanion gap metabolic acidosis (a condition also known as type IV RTA).

• Several medications are frequent contributors. Among them potassium-sparing diuretics, nonsteroidal anti-inflammatory drugs (NSAIDs including COX-2 inhibitors), angiotensin-converting enzyme (ACE) inhibitors, angiotensin II receptor blockers (ARB), heparin and low molecular weight heparin (LMWH), and beta-blockers are the more common offenders.

Triage and Initial Management

• The criteria for admission in hyperkalemia are not well defined. This is in part due to the lack of a universally accepted definition for mild, moderate, or severe hyperkalemia and in part because clinical consequences of hyperkalemia depend on other variables such as calcium level, acid-base status, and chronicity.

• All patients with hyperkalemia should have a 12-lead ECG as part of their initial workup.

• The ECG changes and cardiac arrhythmias associated with hyperkalemia are true medical emergencies.

○ These ECG changes may be progressive and include tall, peaked, narrow-base T waves, prolonged PR interval, flattening of P waves, and widening of the QRS complex with eventual blending with T waves also known as sine waves.

○ However, it is important to remember that the ECG changes may progress from normal to ventricular fibrillation and asystole precipitously. See Fig. 87B-7.

○ The ECG changes have a low sensitivity of about 50%, especially in patients with CKD.

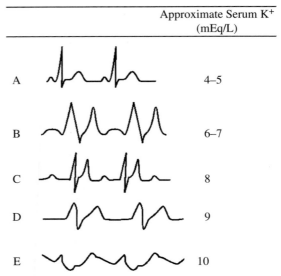

	Approximate Serum K⁺ (mEq/L)
A	4–5
B	6–7
C	8
D	9
E	10

FIG. 87B-7 ECG changes associated with hyperkalemia. (A) Normal ECG; (B) Peaked narrow-based T waves and are best seen in leads II, III, and precordial leads V2-V4; (C) Peaked T waves, PR prolongation, and QRS widening; (D) and (E) Absence of P waves, progressive widening of the QRS eventually blending with T waves (also known as a "sine-wave pattern"), and ultimately ventricular fibrillation and asystole.
SOURCE: From Osorio FV, Linas SL. Disorders of potassium metabolism. In: Schrier RW, ed. *Atlas of The Diseases of The Kidney*, Vol. 1. 3.1–3.18.

• Nevertheless, given the limitations of ECG, we recommend the following patients to be admitted and treated emergently:

○ Any patient with hyperkalemia and any ECG changes consistent with hyperkalemia, including peaked T waves.

○ Any patient with severe hyperkalemia (K⁺ ≥ 6.0 mmol/L), irrespective of ECG findings.

• Emergency treatment of hyperkalemia involves antagonizing the effects of hyperkalemia on membrane potential, rapid reduction of potassium level by shifting of potassium into cells, and ultimately removing potassium from the body. Serum potassium level should be repeated in 1–3 hours and frequently thereafter as needed.

• Administration of calcium antagonizes the effects of hyperkalemia on membrane potential.

○ Calcium gluconate and calcium chloride are equally effective if used at equivalent millimolar doses of elemental calcium. They are effective even in normocalcemic patients.

○ Each milliliter of 10% calcium gluconate and calcium chloride has 8.9 mg (0.22 mmol) and 27.2 mg (0.68 mmol) of elemental calcium, respectively.

○ The usual dose is 10 mL of 10% calcium gluconate or 3–4 mL of 10% calcium chloride infused IV

slowly over 2–3 minutes (calcium chloride should be administered through a central vein). The effect starts in 1–3 minutes and lasts 30–60 minutes. The dose can be repeated every 5 minutes if ECG changes persist as necessary.
  ○ In patients treated with digoxin, 10 mL of 10% calcium gluconate should be added to 100 mL of D5W and infused IV over 20–30 minutes; avoid giving in solutions containing bicarbonate.
- Administration of insulin and glucose shifts potassium into the cells.
  ○ Treatment with insulin and glucose is the most consistent and reliable method and is effective in almost all patients, including patients with CKD and ESRD.
  ○ Its potassium-lowering effect starts in 10–20 minutes, peaks at 30–60 minutes, and lasts for 4–6 hours. At its peak, it can drop the potassium level by 0.5–1.2 mmol/L.
  ○ The recommended dose is 10 units of regular insulin given as an IV bolus and immediately followed by 50 mL of 50% dextrose. This should be followed by 10% dextrose in water infusion at 50 mL/hr. Monitor blood glucose level on an hourly basis.
  ○ Insulin without glucose may be administered to diabetic patients with blood glucose level ≥ 200–250 mg/dL with frequent monitoring of blood glucose level. Administration of glucose without insulin is strongly discouraged.
- Beta-2-adrenergic agonists should not be used as a single agent, particularly in ESRD patients in whom up to 40% are resistant to its potassium-lowering effect.
  ○ The recommended dose is 10–20 mg of albuterol in 4 mL of NS, nebulized over 10 minutes. Its potassium-lowering effect begins in 30 minutes, peaks at 90 minutes, and lasts for 2–6 hours. At its peak, it can lower the potassium level by 0.5–1.0 mmol/L. The IV form is currently not available in the United States.
  ○ There is an average increase of ~10 beats per minute in heart rate and no significant change in systolic or diastolic blood pressure. Nevertheless, they should be used with extreme caution in high-risk patients (eg, patients with ischemic heart disease).
- The effects of beta-2-adrenergic agonists and insulin are synergistic. The combination therapy may drop the potassium level by ~1.2–1.5 mmol/L.
- The role of sodium bicarbonate in the acute treatment of hyperkalemia has been questioned, particularly in patients with CKD and ESRD. It is primarily recommended in patients with hyperkalemia and concomitant acidosis.
- Potassium removal from the body is the definitive initial treatment for acute hyperkalemia. Although diuretics may be helpful in this regard, the main modalities are dialysis, particularly hemodialysis, and cation exchange resins (sodium polystyrene sulfonate [SPS, Kayexalate]).
  ○ It is prudent that these measures only be used with other treatment options aimed at acutely lowering potassium level because of the usual logistic delay in the initiation of hemodialysis and the rather slow effect of Kayexalate on serum potassium level of at least several hours.
  ○ Each gram of SPS binds 0.5–1.0 mmol of potassium in exchange for 2–3 mmol of sodium. The recommended oral dose is 15–30 g of SPS in 70% sorbitol (usually 30–60 mL) 2–4 times a day. Its full potassium-lowering effect may take up to 24 hours or even longer to develop. The efficacy of single-dose SPS has been recently challenged and repeated doses are usually necessary.
  ○ SPS can be administered rectally as a retention edema (without sorbitol).
  ○ Ischemic colitis and colonic necrosis are the most serious complications of SPS and much less common with the oral form. The incidence of these complications is higher in postoperative period particularly following abdominal surgery (eg, kidney transplant).
- Low-risk patients with potassium level of ≤ 5.8–6.0 mmol/L and no ECG changes may be treated with potassium removal strategies and frequent monitoring of the potassium level and ECG; diagnostic evaluation to identify and treat the cause of hyperkalemia should be initiated at the same time.

DISEASE MANAGEMENT STRATEGIES
- The management strategy should focus on three elements:
  ○ Diagnosis and treatment of life-threatening conditions.
  ○ Removal of excessive potassium.
  ○ Diagnosis and correction of the underlying cause (Fig. 87B-6).
- Do not overlook hidden causes of hyperkalemia such as potassium salt of certain medications (eg, penicillins) and salt substitute (each gram contains 10–13 mmol of potassium chloride).

CARE TRANSITIONS

- Check the potassium level 3–5 days following discharge from the hospital, particularly if the underlying cause has not been identified or corrected by the time of discharge. The process of identifying and correcting the underlying cause should be initiated before discharge.
- Closely monitor patients initiated on medications known to be associated with potassium balance disturbances

during their hospital admission. For example, check the potassium level 3–5 days following initiation or any dose increment of an ACE-I or an ARB.

BIBLIOGRAPHY

Cohn JN, Kowey PR, Whelton PK, et al. New guidelines for potassium replacement in clinical practice: a contemporary review by the National Council on Potassium in Clinical Practice. *Arch Intern Med.* 2000;160:2429–2436.

Gennari FJ. Hypokalemia. *N Engl J Med.* 1998;339:451–458.

Mount DB, Zandi-Nejad K. Disorders of potassium balance. In: Brenner BM, ed. *Brenner and Rector's The Kidney.* 7th ed. Philadelphia, PA: W.B. Saunders; 2004:997–1040.

Mount DB, Zandi-Nejad K. Disorders of potassium balance. In: Brenner BM, ed. *Brenner and Rector's The Kidney,* 8th ed. Philadelphia, PA: W.B. Saunders; in press.

Osorio FV, Linas SL. Disorders of potassium metabolism. In: Schrier RW, ed. *Atlas of the Diseases of the Kidney,* Vol. 1. 3.1–3.18.

Parham WA, Mehdirad AA, Biermann KM, et al. Hyperkalemia revisited. *Tex Heart Inst J.* 2006;33:40–47.

VENOUS THROMBOEMBOLISM

88 PREVENTION OF VENOUS THROMBOEMBOLISM IN MEDICAL AND SURGICAL PATIENTS

Sylvia C. McKean

EPIDEMIOLOGY/OVERVIEW

The term *venous thromboembolism* (VTE) refers to pathologic venous thrombosis.
• Deep venous thrombosis (DVT) of the lower extremities is the most common.
• DVT may lead to pulmonary embolism (PE).
• PE can occur suddenly without warning.
• More than 7.7 million medical service inpatients and 3.4 million surgical service inpatients are at risk for developing VTE and the number is likely to rise as the population ages.
• About two-thirds of VTE cases and deaths are hospital acquired.
• Fatal PE may be the most common preventable cause of hospital death and may account for up to 10% of hospital deaths.
• VTE contributes to > 250,000 hospitalizations annually, and the mortality rate associated with the complications of PE can reach 17.5% at 90 days.
• Three factors, previously identified by the German pathologist Rudolph Virchow in 1856—venous stasis,

vessel wall damage, and hypercoagulability—are still responsible for VTE today. (See Table 88-1.)
• Although risk factors can help identify patients who are at risk for VTE and the subpopulations which are at greater risk, it is not possible to identify in advance specifically which individuals will develop a PE.
• Classic signs and symptoms of DVT only occur in approximately one-third of individuals, and PE often occurs without warning or chance to resuscitate the patient.
• On an international scale, VTE prophylaxis is underutilized.
• Given the scope of VTE and effective evidence-based prophylaxis regimens, hospitals should undertake a strategy of VTE prevention as a "universal precaution" for hospitalized patients. Hospitalists can play a pivotal role in helping their hospitals meet target VTE prevention goals.

SCOPE OF THE PROBLEM IN HOSPITALIZED PATIENTS

• Every year, an estimated 200,000 to 600,000 Americans will suffer from either DVT or PE.
• Public agencies are educating the public about VTE as a major but under recognized problem in acutely ill hospitalized medical patients, and it is the number one cause of unexpected hospital deaths. (See Table 88-2.)
• Performance measures for VTE prevention have been developed for general surgical patients. (See Table 88-3.)

TABLE 88-1   Virchow's Triad

Venous stasis when blood pools due to impaired venous return thereby allowing clotting factors to reach levels high enough to initiate clotting
- Venous stasis can develop in any immobilized limb, but it occurs most frequently in the legs
- Patients with varicose veins are at increased risk due to venous stasis and because varicose veins may be a marker for prior DVT

Vessel wall damage when platelets are exposed to collagen in the subendothelium, triggering the release of a substance that causes platelets to collect at the injured site and initiate the clotting mechanism
- Elderly patients are more likely to have atherosclerosis and venous valvular insufficiency, both of which may be associated with decreased endothelial anticoagulant activity, reduced blood flow, and increased fibrinogen turnover along with reduced levels of antithrombin III, and fibrinolytic activity. Age, therefore, is an important predictor of risk

Hypercoagulability, or the increased tendency for blood to clot, may be congenital or acquired
- Lifelong, genetic predeterminants for thrombosis cannot be measured routinely and may become manifest with certain settings such as hospitalization and the development of comorbid disease
- This risk increases with age, pregnancy beginning in the first trimester, and with cancer
- Tumor cells can interact with platelets, clotting, and fibrinolytic proteins
- Chemotherapeutic agents and drugs, such as hormonal replacement therapy or birth control pills, can increase the risk of VTE, especially in patients genetically predisposed
- Hypercoagulability can be triggered when bleeding, shock, heparin-induced platelet 4 immune complex formation (HIT), and hypothermia cause changes in coagulation that lead to thrombin formation and development of a clot

Abbreviation: HIT, heparin-induced thrombocytopenia.

- Targeted VTE performance measures across the continuum of care may include, but are not limited to, risk assessment/stratification, prophylaxis/prevention, therapy, and patient education (www.JointCommission.org).

TABLE 88-2   Public Agency Initiatives Related to VTE

VTE prevention has been identified as the number one priority by the AHRQ in a report entitled "Making Health Care Safer: A Critical Analysis of Patient Safety Practices."

The AHRQ systematic review ranks 79 patient-safety interventions based on the strength of the evidence supporting more widespread implementation of these procedures. This recommendation was based on "overwhelming evidence that thromboprophylaxis reduces adverse patient outcomes while, at the same time, decreasing overall costs."

The AHRQ, through its Evidence-based Practice Centers, sponsors the development of evidence reports and technology assessments that provide comprehensive, science-based information on common, costly medical conditions and new healthcare technologies to assist healthcare organizations in their efforts to improve the quality of healthcare in the United States. (The AHRQ Evidence Report/ Technology Assessment, Number 31: Prevention of VTE).

NQF and JCAHO recently announced a project to standardize performance measures for the prevention of DVT.

Abbreviations: AHRQ, Agency for Health Care Research and Quality; NQF, National Quality Forum; JCAHO, Joint Commission on Accreditation of Healthcare Organizations.

TABLE 88-3   VTE Prevention in Surgical Patients

Leapfrog Group Practice # 17 specifies that each patient should be evaluated regularly for risk and that appropriate methods should be used to prevent VTE.

The NQF performance measures are the percent of surgery patients with documented VTE risk assessment, the percent of patients with recommended VTE prophylaxis ordered, and the percent of patients who have received appropriate VTE prophylaxis.

The Surgical Care improvement Project measures are the percent of surgery patients with recommended VTE prophylaxis, the percent of patients with ordered prophylaxis, and the percent of patients with appropriate prophylaxis. Additional measures are the percent of patients with postoperative PE and the percent of patients with DVT during the index hospitalization or within 30 days of surgery.

RISK FACTORS FOR DEVELOPING VENOUS THROMBOEMBOLISM

- A patient's risk of VTE varies depending on multiple factors including age, specific medical conditions, severity of illness, medical treatment, type of surgery, duration of immobilization, and the presence of underlying hypercoagulable states such as malignancy.
- The five most frequent comorbidities in patients who developed DVT were hypertension, surgery within 3 months, immobility within 30 days, cancer, and obesity (DVT-Free prospective registry).
  - Hypertension is associated with a high prevalence of atherosclerotic blood vessel changes and surgery is associated with endothelial damage.
  - The presence of cancer in hospitalized patients causes a two- to four-fold increase in the incidence of VTE in both medical and surgical patients.
  - For the obese patient, a continuous weight scale, body mass index (BMI) range of 28.5–30, there is an increased risk of PE at autopsy, not just for the morbidly obese (Framingham data). A retrospective review of patients with PE—data from more than 100,000 nurses at Brigham and Women's Hospital, based on self-reported weight—obesity was identified as the number one risk factor—not just the morbidly obese (NursesHealth Study).
- Elaborate blood tests that look for genetic and biochemical abnormalities do not increase our ability to predict whether someone will have another blood clot.
- Whatever the risk factors for VTE, it is the immediate situation—hospitalization for acute medical illness and/or surgery—that greatly increases the risk.

RISK ASSESSMENT TOOLS

- While there are many tools for determining risk of VTE in hospitalized patients, it is important to have a low threshold for using VTE prophylaxis.

- A simple risk assessment tool for physicians to be able to apply to their setting on admission and at regular intervals may enhance compliance with evidence-based VTE performance measures.
- One example of a simple VTE risk assessment tool designed for use in medical patients is The DVT-Free Consensus Panel algorithm, which recommends that all patients should be screened for VTE prophylaxis.
  - Note that in patients with reduced mobility and only one other listed risk factor, VTE prophylaxis is recommended. The "old, sick, or surgical" patient should be considered of sufficient risk to initiate pharmacologic prophylaxis unless there is a contraindication.
  - Patients who do not initially meet criteria for VTE prophylaxis should be reassessed daily, and VTE prophylaxis initiated if indicated (Table 88-5).
  - See risk assessment tools and a downloadable quality improvement workbook available on the Society of Hospital Medicine Web site at: http://www.hospitalmedicine.org

MODALITIES OF VENOUS THROMBOEMBOLISM PROPHYLAXIS

- Modalities for VTE prevention include mechanical and pharmacologic prophylaxis.
- Graduated compression stockings (GCS) increase venous blood flow, while intermittent pneumatic compression increases venous blood flow and endogenous fibrinolysis.
  - Both require virtually continuous use.
  - Evidence of efficacy of mechanical prophylaxis is limited in medical patients due to differences in equipment design, frequency of use, use in combination with antiplatelet or anticoagulant drugs, and lack of blinding in randomized controlled trials (RCTs).
- Inferior vena caval (IVC) filter is a mechanical barrier which prevents PE, but does not halt the thrombotic process and in fact increases the risk of further DVT below and sometimes through the filter.
  - IVC filter insertion is recommended for patients with proven proximal DVT, and either an absolute contraindication to full-dose anticoagulation therapy or planned major surgery in the near future.
  - Removable IVC filters may be a safer alternative to permanent devices.
- Pharmacologic prophylaxis includes the use of "mini-dose" unfractionated heparin (UFH), LMWH, a pentasaccharide fondaparinux, and warfarin. Although it is effective for the prevention of heart attack and stroke, aspirin and/or other antiplatelet agents when used alone is not the standard of care for prevention of VTE. (See Chap. 90.)

THE EVIDENCE FOR MEDICAL PATIENTS

- Before the development of LMWH, "mini-dose" UFH 5000 units administered subcutaneously (SC) bid or tid was the standard pharmacologic preventive regimen for medical patients in the United States despite lack of evidence.
- In the multicenter European Thromboembolism-Prevention in Cardiac or Respiratory Disease with Enoxaparin (THE-PRINCE) trial, 665 patients were enrolled in the randomized study to receive VTE prophylaxis with either enoxaparin 40 mg daily ($n = 239$) or heparin 5000 units tid ($n = 212$).
  - The primary efficacy endpoint was the occurrence of thromboembolic events as confirmed by DVT-bilateral venography, ventilation perfusion lung scan, chest x-ray/perfusion lung scan, and pulmonary angiography.
  - The efficacy endpoint occurred in 8.4% of patients in the enoxaparin group vs. 10.4% in the UFH group (P = NS).
  - Bleeding events were less frequent in the enoxaparin group, but the difference compared with the UFH group was not statistically significant. Other adverse events were significantly less common in the enoxaparin group.
- Results of a recent meta-analysis of earlier trials showed that prophylactic low-dose UFH and LMWH were associated with a lower incidence of DVT and PE (56% to 58% risk reduction [RR]) relative to no prophylaxis, and there was no significant difference in effectiveness between the agents.
  - However, LMWH was associated with a reduced risk of major hemorrhage by 52% (P = 0.049) compared with UFH.
- Compared with data for UFH 5000 units tid, the data for UFH 5000 units bid are less convincing.
  - Studies evaluating doses of UFH of 5000 units bid were small, not randomized, and there were variations in the endpoints measured.
  - A recent meta-analysis of 12 studies—1664 patients in the tid arm and 6314 patients in the bid arm—found that bid dosing of UFH had fewer major bleeds and tid dosing of UFH had somewhat better efficacy.
- There have been three rigorously conducted, randomized, double-blinded, placebo-controlled trials evaluating the efficacy and safety of LMWHs, enoxaparin (*MEDENOX*), and dalteparin (*PREVENT*), and a synthetic and specific inhibitor of activated Factor X (Xa), fondaparinux (*ARTEMIS*), to placebo for the prophylaxis of VTE in medical patients.
  1. *MEDENOX* (Prophylaxis in *Med*ical Patients with *Enox*aparin). The MEDENOX trial, a double-blind, multicenter, placebo-controlled study, randomized

866 medical patients to receive pharmacologic pro-phylaxis with enoxaparin 40 mg/d SC or enoxa-parin 20 mg/d SC compared with placebo.

- The primary efficacy endpoint of VTE (ie, DVT or PE) between days 1 and 14 occurred in 5.5% of the enoxaparin 40-mg group, 15% of the 20-mg group, and 14.9% of the placebo group (63% RR, enoxaparin 40 mg vs. placebo; $P < 0.001$).
- The significant reduction in the incidence of all VTE and proximal and distal DVT in the 40-mg group was maintained during the 3-month follow-up period.
- The frequency of hemorrhage, thrombocytopenia, and death was not statistically significantly different between the groups.

2. *PREVENT* (*Pro*spective *Ev*aluation of Dalteparin *E*fficacy for Preven*t*ion of VTE in Immobilized Patients Trial). The PREVENT trial, a randomized, double- blind, placebo-controlled, multicenter study, randomized 3706 medical patients to receive phar-macologic prophylaxis with dalteparin 5000 units per day SC compared with placebo.

- The primary efficacy endpoint of the incidence of VTE by day 21 occurred in 2.77% in the dalteparin group and 4.96% in the placebo group (55% RR; $P = 0.0015$).
- The frequency of bleeding rates and other adverse events was not significantly different between the groups at day 21.

3. *ARTEMIS* (*Ar*ixtra for *T*hrombo*e*mbolism Prevention in a *M*edical *I*ndications *S*tudy). The ARTEMIS trial randomized 849 patients > 60 years of age admitted with acute cardiac, respiratory, infectious, or inflam-matory conditions to receive pharmacologic prophy-laxis with fondaparinux 2.5 mg/d SC compared with placebo.

- The primary endpoint of venogram-confirmed or symptomatically observed DVT between days 6 and 15 occurred in 5.6% of patients in the fon-daparinux group and 10.5% in the placebo group (49.5% RR; $P = 0.029$).
- There was no difference in the incidence of major bleeding between the groups.
- Fondaparinux showed a trend toward reducing overall mortality from 6.0% in the placebo group to 3.3% in the fondaparinux group.

THE IMPLEMENTATION GAP FOR MEDICAL PATIENTS

- Although there are effective evidence-based prophy-lactic strategies to prevent VTE in medical patients, there is an implementation gap in applying what we

know about VTE prophylaxis in clinical practice (DVT-Free).

- A significant number of patients (71%) who devel-oped DVT did not receive VTE prophylaxis.
- Of the 29% of patients ($n = 1557$) who did receive prophylaxis, 410 had DVT diagnosed while they were outpatients and 1147 were diagnosed while they were inpatients.
- Medical patients were much less likely to receive prophylaxis compared with surgical patients.

- Physicians may underestimate the incidence of hospital-acquired VTE, because clinical symptoms of VTE in the prospective DVT-Free Registry did not become manifest until posthospital discharge for many patients.

- All medical patients who are discharged should be edu-cated about the signs and symptoms of VTE and the importance of seeking treatment quickly if they occur.

THE EVIDENCE FOR SURGICAL PATIENTS

- Just as for medical inpatients, the higher the risk, the more clinicians rely on pharmacologic therapy and the more the risk extends beyond discharge. The rec-ommended duration depends on the type of surgery.

MECHANICAL PROPHYLAXIS IN GENERAL SURGERY

- In GCS-alone method, 13% of patients (81/624) developed DVT compared to placebo 27% (154/581) based on pooled results from 9 RCTs.
- In GCS plus another method, 2% (10/501) developed DVT compared to placebo 15% based on pooled results from 7 RCTs.
- Odds ratio of 0.24 suggests GCS plus another method is more effective than GCS alone (Amaragiri and Lees, 2003.

PHARMACOLOGIC PROPHYLAXIS IN GENERAL SURGERY

- Administration of low-dose UFH results in a 68% reduction in DVT and a 67% reduction in PE fol-lowing surgery and a 21% reduction in total mortality ($P < 0.02$) (Collins et al., 1988).
- In a prospective, double-blind, randomized multicenter trial with prophylaxis started 2 hours prior to abdomi-nal or pelvic surgery for cancer, a 10-day regimen of enoxaparin reduced the observed rate from 29% to 15%. Following a 25- to 31-day regimen of enoxa-parin, the observed rate was 5%. The safety results showed no significant difference between the two drugs. (ENOXACAN Study Group, 1997).

- A meta-analysis comparing LMWH and UFH was notable for a RR of 0.68 for DVT, 0.43 for PE, and 0.75 for bleeding in favor of LMWH.

PHARMACOLOGIC PROPHYLAXIS IN ORTHOPEDIC PATIENTS

- Aspirin has no clear benefit for hip or knee arthroplasty.
- LMWH has superior efficacy to vitamin K antagonists for major orthopaedic surgery (proximal, total DVT) with no difference in bleeding or prevention of clinical PE.
- Fondaparinux has been found to be superior in hip fracture and knee arthroplasty, but may be associated with more bleeding than LMWH. Superiority of efficacy in PENTHIFRA trial may be related to early dosing of fondaparinux and relatively late dosing of enoxaparin.
- American College of Chest Physicians (ACCP) recommends pharmacologic prophylaxis.
  - Enoxaparin 40 mg SQ up to 12 hours preoperation, resuming 12–24 hours postoperatively. Dose of enoxaparin can be adjusted to 30 mg once daily in patients with CrCl < 30 mL/min. LMWH has superior efficacy to vitamin K antagonists for major orthopedic surgery (proximal and total DVT) with no difference in bleeding or prevention of clinical PE.
  - Fondaparinux 2.5 mg SQ daily. Fondaparinux has a longer half-life of 17–21 hours, and there is no antedote for reversal; it is contraindicated in patients < 50 kg or with CrCl < 30 mL/min.
  - Despite required monitoring, warfarin is a drug with unpredictable dosing, drug interactions, and usually takes 3–5 days to become therapeutic. LMWH or fondaparinux should be prescribed along withcoumadin for about 4–5 days until a maintenance target INR (international normalized ratio) of 2–3 reached.

PHARMACOLOGIC PROPHYLAXIS IN TRAUMA PATIENTS

- The Seventh ACCP Consensus Conference for the Prevention of VTE recommends the use of LMWH for the majority of moderate-risk and high-risk trauma patients.
  - LMWH should be started once primary hemostasis has been achieved usually within 36 hours.
  - LMWH can be safely used in patients with head injury without frank hemorrhage, lacerations or contusions of internal organs, the presence of a retroperitoneal hematoma associated with pelvic fracture, or complete spinal injuries if no evidence of ongoing bleeding.
  - LMWH superior to low-dose UFH for VTE prevention.
  - Continuous mechanical prophylaxis preferable to no prophylaxis in patients with contraindications to LMWH in prophylactic doses.

PHARMACOLOGIC PROPHYLAXIS IN SURGICAL PATIENTS WITH MALIGNANCY

- Numerous RCTs have reported improved overall survival in patients who have received LMWH (compared with UFH or coumadin) given to postoperative patients and for the treatment of DVT in medical patients with cancer.
- For patients undergoing gynecologic surgery for cancer, even a brief prophylactic period achieved enhanced survival with LMWH compared with UFH.
- LMWH may have antineoplastic properties (ie, direct antitumor, antiangiogenic, and immune system modulary action).

THE IMPLEMENTATION GAP FOR SURGICAL PATIENTS

- Overall, a higher proportion of surgical inpatients with DVT had received prophylaxis compared with medical patients, but the rate was still too low (DVT-Free) 57.5% vs. 38.1% respectively; $P < 0.0001$.
- The prevalence of VTE risk in patients without VTE prophylaxis is 10% to 40% among general surgical patients and 40% to 60% in patients following major orthopaedic surgery.
  - One-quarter to one-third of these thrombi are proximal.
  - Proximal thrombi are much more likely to produce symptoms and result in PE.
  - Asymptomatic thrombi are also associated with the chronic postphlebitic syndrome in 24% of cases.
- The incidence of VTE in surgical patients is related to patient-specific, anesthetic, and surgical risk factors (see Table 88-4).
  - About one-half of perioperative DVTs begin in the operating room and the risk of perioperative DVTs is greatest within 2 weeks of the surgical procedure.
  - The risk of fatal PE is greatest 3–7 days postoperatively.
- In the absence of prophylaxis, rates of postoperative VTE are high, particularly for orthopedic procedures, and vary with the type of procedure: knee (65%), hip (50%).
- Hip fracture surgery has the highest rate of fatal PE (5%) and VTE risk persists postdischarge.
- After orthopedic surgery, fatal PE correlates with overall mortality and acute PE is the second most common cause of death following cardiac causes.
- Clinicians should weigh the risk of clotting against the risk of bleeding. Around 40 out of every 10,000 total hip replacement (THR) patients will die from fatal PE compared with 1–2 fatal bleeds.
- The scope of the problem is significant because approximately 500,000 total joint arthroplasties,

TABLE 88-4   VTE Risk Factors in Surgical Patients

PATIENT RISK FACTORS

Age; malignant disease (the risk of VTE and fatal PE is two- to fourfold higher in cancer surgeries); history of previous VTE; extent of traumatic injury (patients with multisystem or major trauma have a DVT risk > 50%. PE is the third leading cause of death in this group); spinal cord injury; lower extremity or pelvic fractures; prolonged immobility, including prolonged preoperative hospital stay; femoral venous line insertion or major venous repair

In one study of 2070 patients undergoing elective abdominal surgery (Flordal et al., 1996), preoperatiom hospitalization ≥ 6 days, preoperative transfusion > 1 unit, and leg ulcers were also identified as independently associated with major postoperative VTE

ANESTHESIA-RELATED RISK FACTORS

General anesthesia carries a greater risk of VTE than spinal or epidural anesthesia and the duration of anesthesia matters
- Procedures lasting more than 30 minutes increase the risk of VTE
- Duration more than 3.5 hours regardless of the type of surgery confers a marked increase risk

SURGICAL RISK FACTORS

Even low-risk procedures carry some risk of DVT (2%) and PE (0.2%) (Geerts et al., 2004)
- Outpatient surgery is relatively low risk
- Minor surgery such as inguinal hernia repair, appendectomy is associated with 0.1%–0.6% risk of developing VTE
- Major abdominal surgery such as liver, pancreatic, gastric, and bowel surgery up to 25% of patients develop DVT and 0.8%–1.7% PE
- VTE rates without prophylaxis are high for many surgical procedures: neurosurgery (29%), general surgery (20%), gynecologic surgery (11%)
- Orthopedics procedures carry the greatest risk (see text)

TABLE 88-5   VTE Prophylaxis in Hospitalized Patients

Of 100 general surgery patients without VTE prophylaxis, anticipate that 25% will develop DVT, decreased to approximately 6% with LMWH prophylaxis, an RRR of 76%

Of 100 patients undergoing hip fracture, anticipate that 48% will develop DVT, decreased to approximately 27% with LMWH, an RRR of 44%

Of 100 patients undergoing neurosurgery, anticipate that 22% will develop DVT, decreased to approximately 18% with LMWH plus elastic stocking, an RRR of 18%

Of 100 patients on the general medical service, anticipate that 15% will develop DVT, decreased by approximately 50% with pharmacologic prophylaxis

Data from Geerts W et al.

either hip or knee, are performed annually in the United States.
- Complications postoperatively, such as infection, immobilization, and dehydration also increase the risk.
- When balancing the risk of clotting vs. the risk of bleeding, surgeons and consultants may overestimate the risk of bleeding with pharmacologic prophylaxis and underestimate the risk of clotting. Physicians are unable to reliably identify individual patients who do not require prophylaxis and recommendations should be based on the evidence from RCTs, reflecting the type of operation, age of patient, and presence of additional risk factors such as cancer. (See Table 88-5.)

PHARMACOLOGIC PROPHYLAXIS INPATIENTS EXCLUDED FROM RCTS

- Many surgical patients receive postoperative analgesia through indwelling epidural catheters inserted just before surgery. Epidural hematoma is a devastating, preventable complication that causes permanent neurologic compromise in more than half of the patients. Factors to consider include the following:
  - There may be some short-term pain-control benefits but morbidity and mortality benefits less clear.
  - The risk of postoperative DVT is decreased by approximately 40% to 80% with LMWH if started no later than 24 hours after surgery.
  - Once daily LMWH dosing for VTE prophylaxis can be safely prescribed for patients with indwelling epidural catheters as long as there is adherence to the following principles:
    - Avoid LMWH in patients with coagulopathy and/or receiving drugs that affect hemostasis, and in patients who had a traumatic insertion of the epidural catheter
    - Insertion of preoperative needle occurs > 12 hours after last LMWH dose
    - Administration of the first dose of LMWH occurs 6–8 hours after surgery
    - Epidural removal occurs 20 hours after preceding dose of LMWH and subsequent administration of LMWH occurs > 2 hours after removal
  - Once-daily LMWH dosing does not apply to fondaparinux, which is a pentasaccharide with a long (17-hour) elimination half-life. Fondaparinux should not be prescribed in this setting.
- For patients with renal insufficiency, there may be an increased risk of bleeding from prophylactic doses of heparin due to renal clearance.
  - Patients with renal insufficiency in the ICU, however, have a fourfold increased risk of VTE compared with those without renal failure (odds ratio, 3.7; 95% confidence interval, 1.3–11.2).
  - The evidence is that likely low-dose LMWH is safe in patients with CrCl 30–99 mL/min based on studies that assessed higher, therapeutic doses of LMWH for VTE treatment or ACS, including ESSENCE (Efficacy and Safety of Subcutaneous Enoxaparin in Non-Q Wave Coronary Events) and TIMI (Thrombolysis in Myocardial Infarction) IIB.
- Lack of clinical trials requires individualized assessment of balance of risk of bleeding vs. benefit in these special populations.

- For patients with contraindications to initial pharmacologic prophylaxis, mechanical devices should be placed on the patient prior to anesthesia primarily for neurosurgery, spine, and plastic surgery. This includes elastic stockings and sequential compression devices.

SYSTEMS IMPROVEMENT

- Although education can increase physician awareness of the need to treat predictable complications of hospitalization, the implementation gap between the evidence provided by RCTs and practice followed by hospital mandates (Leapfrog, National Quality Forum [NQF], Joint Commission on Accreditation of Healthcare Organizations [JCAHO]) requires system-level changes that are multidisciplinary, making it easy for clinicians to practice evidence-based care.
- Hospitalists should critically review prophylaxis, provide hospital-specific data to clinicians, identify and lower barriers, devise strategies to bridge the gap between knowledge and practice, develop automated reminder systems and participate in clinical research.
- An example of a successful quality improvement/research initiative from the Brigham and Women's Hospital utilized a computer alert in the hospital order entry system to improve VTE prophylaxis in patients at highest risk of VTE, reducing the incidence of DVT and PE in hospitalized patients (Kucher et al. are: 2005). Key lessons from this project
  ○ A preexisting wealth of educational information on hospital Web sites was ineffective, and multiple seminars and lectures on VTE prophylaxis had little impact on practice.
  ○ The most important result of this study is that clinical alerts had an effect on both the approach to care and outcomes during the 3-year study period.
- Although a computerized decision support system linked to the patient database and a computer order entry system were used in this case, these two key features of the intervention—use of a simple point-based risk assessment tool and a reminder to physicians about the need for VTE prophylaxis, can be implemented at any healthcare institution. The risk assessment tool can be incorporated into daily patient assessments that are routinely performed, and a reminder can be placed on the chart of appropriate patients (DVT-Free Algorithm). Although physicians often underestimate the risk, the percentage of hospitalized patients who will develop VTE without prophylaxis can be predicted from RCTs. (See Table 88-5.)
- There are several resources available to guide hospitalists through the key steps of implementing a quality improvement initiative for VTE prophylaxis. (See Table 88-6.)

TABLE 88-6   Web-Based Resources for DVT Prevention Initiatives

DVT Consensus Panel Guidelines and Recommendations available at: http://www.thrombosisconsult.com/ThrombosisPosters/VTEDPathway.pdf

Key steps in the redesign process are outlined in detail, along with example quality improvement tools, in the Society of Hospital Medicine Workbook for Improvement: Optimize Prevention of Venous Thromboembolism at your Medical Center http://www.hospitalmedicine.org/AM/Template.cfm?Section=Search_Advanced_Search&Template=/Search/SearchDisplay.cfm

There is additional information on implementing quality improvement projects, specifically on rapid cycle improvement, available on the Institute for Health Care Improvement (IHI) Web site, at www.ihi.org

Example guidelines for VTE prophylaxis are available at the National Guideline Clearing House: http://www.guideline.gov/search/searchresults.aspx?Type=3&txtSearch=venous+thromboembolism&num=20

BIBLIOGRAPHY

Akkar AK, Davidson BL, Haas SK. Investigators Against Thromboembolism (INATE) Core Group. Compliance with recommended prophylaxis for venous thromboembolism: improving the use and rate of uptake of clinical practice guidelines. *J Thromb Haemost.* 2004;2:221–227.

Amaragiri SV, Lees TA. Elastic compression stockings for prevention of deep vein thrombosis. *Cochrane Database Syst Rev.* 2000;3:CD001484. Review

American Public Health Association (APHA). White Paper: Deep-Vein Thrombosis: Advancing Awareness to Protect Patient Lives. Public Health Leadership Conference on Deep-Vein Thrombosis. Washington, DC; Feb. 26, 2003. Available at: www.apha.org/ppp/DVT_White_Paper.pdf. Accessed Dec 2005.

Anderson FA, Jr, Zayaruzny M, Heit JA, et al. Estimated annual numbers of US acute-care hospital patients at risk for venous thromboembolism. *Am J Hematol* 2007;82(9):777–782.

Burris HA. Low-molecular-weight heparins in the treatment of cancer-associated thrombosis: a new standard of care? *Semin Oncol.* 2006:33(2 suppl 4):S3–S16.

Cohen AT, Gallus AS, Lassen MR, et al. Fondaparinux vs. placebo for the prevention of venous thromboembolism in acutely ill medical patients (ARTEMIS). *J Thromb Haemost.* 2003;1(suppl 1):P2046. Abstract.

Collins R, Scrimgeour A, Yusuf S, et al. Reduction in fatal pulmonary embolism and venous thrombosis by perioperative administration of subcutaneous heparin. Overview of results of randomized trials in general, orthopedic, and urologic surgery. *N Engl J Med.* 1988;318(18):1162–1173.

Dentali F, Douketis JD, Gianni M, et al. Meta-analysis: anticoagulant prophylaxis to prevent symptomatic venous thromboembolism in hospitalized medical patients. *Ann Intern Med.* 2007; 146(4):278–288.

Durieux P. Electronic medical alerts—so simple, so complex. *N Engl J Med.* 2005;352:1034–1036.

ENOXACAN Study Group. Efficacy and safety of enoxaparin versus unfractionated heparin for prevention of deep vein thrombosis in elective cancer surgery: a double-bline randomized multicentre trial with venographic assessment. *Br J Surg.* 1977;84(8):1099–1103.

Flordal PA, Berggvist D, Burmark US, et al. Risk factors for major thromboembolism and bleeding tendency after elective general surgical operations. The Fragmin Multicentre Study Group. *Eur J Surg* 1996;162(10):783–789.

Geerts W, Pineo G, Heit J, et al. Prevention of venous thromboembolism: the Seventh ACCP Conference on Antithrombotic and Thrombolytic Therapy. *Chest.* 2004;126(3 suppl): 338S–400S.

Goldhaber SZ. Venous thromboembolism: an ounce of prevention (editorial). *Mayo Clin Proc.* 2005;80:725–726. Available at: http://www.mayoclinicproceedings.com/inside.asp? AID= 927&UID=. Accessed Dec 3, 2005.

Goldhaber SZ, Tapson VF, for the DVT FREE Steering Committee. A prospective registry of 5,451 patients with ultrasound-confirmed deep vein thrombosis. *Am J Cardiol.* 2004;93:259–262.

Goldhaber SZ, Grodstein F, Stampfer MJ. A prospective study of risk factors for pulmonary embolism in women. *JAMA.* 1997 25;277(24):1933.

Goldhaber SZ, Turpie AGG. Prevention of venous thromboembolism among hospitalized medical patients. *Circulation.* 2005;111:e1–e3.

Hull RD, Pineo GF, Francis C, et al. LMWH prophylaxis using dalteparin in close proximity to surgery vs warfarin in hip arthorplasty patients. *Arch Intern Med.* 2000;160:2199–2207.

Hull RD, Pineo GF, Francis C, et al. LMWH prophylaxis using salteparin extended out-of-hospital vs in-hospital warfarin/out-of-hospital placebo in hip arthroplasty patients. *Arch Intern Med.* 2000;160:2208–2215.

JCAHO/National Quality Forum: Call for thromboembolism (VTE-DVT/PE) performance measures. Available at: http://www.jcaho.org/pms/core+measures/request+for+core+measures.htm.

King CS, Holley AB, Jackson JL, et al. 2-3 times daily heparin dsing for thromboembolism prophylaxis in the general medical population: a meta-analysis. *Chest.* 2007;131:507–516.

Kleber FX, Witt C, Vogel G, et al. for THE-PRINCE Study Group. Randomized comparison of enoxaparin with unfractionated heparin for the prevention of venous thromboembolism in medical patients with heart failure or severe respiratory disease. *Am Heart J.* 2003;145:614–621.

Kleinbart J, Williams WV, Rask K. AHRQ Evidence Report/Technology Assessment, Number 31: Prevention of Venous Thromboembolism. Available at: http://www.ncbi.nlm.nih.gov/books/bv.fcgi?rid=hstat1.section.61086. Accessed Dec 3, 2005.

Kucher N, Koo S, Quiroz R, et al. Electronic alerts to prevent venous thromboembolism among hospitalized patients. *N Engl J Med.* 2005;352:969–977.

Leizorovicz A, Cohen AT, Turpie AGG, et al. for the PREVENT Medical Thromboprophylaxis Study Group. Randomized, placebo-controlled trial of dalteparin for the prevention of venous thromboembolism in acutely ill medical patients. *Circulation.* 2004;110:874–879.

Making Health Care Safer: A Critical Analysis of Patient Safety Practice. AHRQ Publication No. 01-E058. Available at: http://www.ncbi.nlm.nih.gov/books/bv.fcgi?rid=hstat1.chapter.59276. Accessed Dec 2005.

Mismetti P, Laporte-Simitsidis S, Tardy B, et al. Prevention of venous thromboembolism in internal medicine with unfractionated or low-molecular-weight heparins: a meta-analysis of randomised clinical trials. *Thromb Haemost.* 2000;83:14–19.

Prandoni P. Acquired risk factors for venous thromboembolism in medical patients. *Hematology.* 2005. Available at: http://www.asheducationbook.org/cgi/content/abstract/2005/1/458. Accessed Dec 2005.

Samama MM, Cohen AT, Darmon JY, et al. for the Prophylaxis in Medical Patients with Enoxaparin Study Group. A comparison of enoxaparin with placebo for the prevention of venous thromboembolism in acutely ill medical patients. *N Engl J Med.* 1999;341:793–800.

Thrombotic disorders. Merck Manual. 17th ed. Available at: http://www.merck.com/mrkshared/mmanual/section11/chapter132/132a.jsp. Accessed Dec 3, 2005.

89 VENOUS THROMBOEMBOLISM

Amir Jaffer and Franklin Michota

EPIDEMIOLOGY/OVERVIEW

- DVT and PE are a continuum of the same disease process termed VTE.
- VTE is the third leading cause of cardiovascular death in the United States after myocardial infarction and stroke with an estimated 200,000 deaths annually related to PE.
- VTE is a common disease requiring hospitalization with an average annual incidence of 117 cases per 100,000.
- Autopsy studies demonstrate large numbers of silent events leading to widely reported estimates of 2 million DVT cases annually.
- Studies utilizing ventilation perfusion scanning demonstrate almost 50% of patients with DVT have silent PE as well.
- Population studies confirm that over 60% of community patients with a first lifetime DVT are nursing home residents or patients recently discharged from the hospital.

PATHOPHYSIOLOGY

- DVT is usually a clot that forms in the deep veins of the lower extremities.
- DVT occurring in the upper extremities represents 10% of all VTE, particularly axillosubclavian vein thrombosis in the context of central venous catheters.

- Spontaneous upper extremity DVT, also known as Paget-Schroetter syndrome, occurs in healthy young people, often associated with compressive anomalies of the thoracic outlet, such as a cervical rib.
- PE occurs when a portion or all of a DVT breaks loose and travels to the lungs occluding one or more of the pulmonary arteries. Acute PE increases pulmonary vascular resistance, which causes an increase in right ventricular (RV) pressure. Consequently, RV microinfarction causes troponins to leak, and RV shear stress may be associated with elevated B-natriuretic peptides.
- The development of DVT is influenced by the presence of VTE risk factors and three underlying etiologic factors for thrombosis: venous stasis, endothelial injury, and hypercoagulability.
- It is not known how the various factors interact to determine a single patient's individual VTE risk, yet there is evidence that overall VTE risk increases in proportion to the number of VTE risk factors present.

CLINICAL PRESENTATION, DIFFERENTIAL, MAKING THE DIAGNOSIS

- Patients with DVT can present with symptoms of lower extremity swelling, calf pain, redness, dilated superficial veins, and warmth. Physical examination can show unilateral edema, palpable cords, erythema, tenderness along the deep venous distribution, calf pain on dorsiflexion of the foot (positive Homan's sign), and fever.
- DVT signs and symptoms are neither sensitive nor specific, and approximately 80% of patients will not have the disease and instead have one of the following: leg trauma, internal derangement of the knee, ruptured Baker's cyst, cellulitis, obstructive lymphadenopathy, lymphedema, drug-induced edema, calf muscle pull or tear, superficial thrombophlebitis, or the postphlebitic syndrome.
- Quantifying the patient's VTE risk factors will help create a clinical pretest probability for the presence of DVT that should lead to diagnostic testing. (See Table 89-1.)
- Signs and symptoms of PE, including chest pain (70% of patients), tachypnea (70%), cough (40%), tachycardia (33%), shortness of breath (25%), syncope (5%), and signs of DVT (10%) are similarly nonspecific. Patients may also have coexisting conditions such as pneumonia, CHF, or COPD which produce similar symptoms.
- The differential diagnosis for PE is broad and ranges from lethal causes of chest pain, such as myocardial

TABLE 89-1   Clinical Model for Predicting Pretest Probability for DVT

Active cancer (ongoing treatment or within 6 months)	1 point
Paralysis, paresis, or recent plaster immobilization of lower extremities	1 point
Bedridden > 3 days or major surgery within 4 weeks	1 point
Localized tenderness along the distribution of the deep venous system	1 point
Entire leg swollen	1 point
Calf swelling by more than 3 cm than asymptomatic leg	1 point
Pitting edema	1 point
Collateral superficial veins	1 point
Alternative diagnosis as likely or greater than the possibility of DVT	−2 points

Score (points)	Clinical probability of DVT
0	Low
1 or 2	Moderate
> 3	High

SOURCE: Reproduced from Wells PS, et al. Value of assessment of pretest probability of deep-vein thrombosis in clinical management. *Lancet.* 1997;350(9):1795–1798.

infarction or aortic dissection, to more benign conditions such as viral pleurisy, chest wall muscle inflammation, or bronchitis.
- Tests clinically available today to assist in DVT diagnosis include: D-dimer testing, compression duplex ultrasound, contrast CT venous imaging, contrast venography, and MRI.
- Compression ultrasonography is the preferred diagnostic test because it is noninvasive, relatively inexpensive, and readily available.
- D-Dimer (a fibrin split product) assays are useful adjuncts to noninvasive testing because they have high negative predictive values and can help in ruling out disease. However, due to their low positive predictive value, D-dimer assays are insufficient to diagnose VTE in the inpatient setting. (See Table 89-2.)
- Tests available today to assist in PE diagnosis include the same tests used for DVT diagnosis as well as chest CT, time-resolved MR angiography, ventilation perfusion scanning, and pulmonary angiography.
- Chest CT PE protocol is preferred to ventilation perfusion scanning, which is often indeterminate for the majority of patients.
- For patients with contraindications to the administration of iodinated contrast material, MR imaging provides high temporal resolution of arterial phase-only images of the main pulmonary artery through the segmental branches with excellent interobserver agreement.

TABLE 89-2 Approach to the Diagnosis of DVT

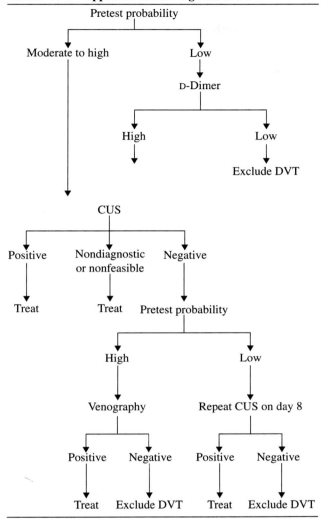

SOURCE: Reproduced from Kyrle PA, Eichinger S. Deep-vein thrombosis. *Lancet*. 2005;365:1163–1174.

- Chest radiography and ECGs may rapidly suggest alternative diagnoses.
- ABG measurements have little diagnostic value. (See Table 89-3.)

TRIAGE AND INITIAL MANAGEMENT

RISK STRATIFICATION

- Optimal management of acute PE requires patient risk stratification. PE patients with RV dysfunction, with or without normal blood pressure, have a poorer prognosis than PE patients with preserved RF function.
- Physical signs of RV dysfunction include distended neck veins, a parasternal heave, an accentuated P2, and a tricuspid regurgitation murmur.

TABLE 89-3 Approach to the Diagnosis of PE

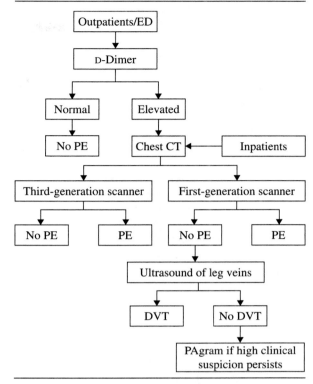

SOURCE: Reproduced from Goldhaber SZ, Elliott G. Acute pulmonary embolism: part II; risk stratification, treatment, and prevention. *Circulation*. 2003:108:2726–2729.

- Depending on the presentation of the patient and size of the embolism, risk stratification includes
  ○ Assessment of vital signs
  ○ Measurement of troponin and B-type natriuretic peptides (BNPs)
  ○ Echocardiography to estimate RV function and pulmonary artery pressure
  ○ Chest CT scan to estimate RV and PE size
- RV hypokinesis has been shown to double the 30-day mortality, and RV enlargement by chest CT has a significantly higher 30-day mortality than patients with normal RVs.
- Despite normal blood pressure on admission, patients with an elevated cTNI (cardiac troponin I) ≥ 0.07 µg/L and BNP ≥ 600 ng/L have a high mortality risk, whereas a normal cTNI and BNP < 600 ng/L is associated with an excellent prognosis.

THERAPY

- Risk stratification is used to guide therapy—thrombolysis vs. anticoagulant therapy.
- PE patients with hypotension (< 90 mm Hg or a drop in systolic arterial pressure of at least 40 mm Hg for at least 15 minutes) are termed "massive" PE and

require critical care. Therapy for massive PE in many instances is considered lifesaving and includes anticoagulation as well as fibrinolysis or embolectomy.

- Thrombolysis with tissue-plasminogen activator is effective in patients with hemodynamic compromise, but routine use in patients with normal vital signs and RV compromise is controversial due to concerns about safety (increased risk of intracranial hemorrhage compared with heparin).
  - The intracranial bleeding rate is approximately 3% to 5%.
  - The Food and Drug Administration (FDA) has approved PE thrombolysis for patients with massive PE. An analysis of the International Cooperative Pulmonary Embolism Registry (ICOPER) found, however, no reduction in 90-day mortality rate of patients with massive PE.
  - Catheter-directed thrombolysis into the pulmonary vasculature is under study.
- Surgical removal of an embolism may be performed either with a catheter or during open-heart surgery for patients with massive bleeding, preventing anticoagulation.
- IVC filters are indicated prior to surgical removal of embolism or when there is failure of anticoagulation resulting in recurrent PE. Although there is a higher incidence of DVT in association with IVC filters. ICOPER data suggest that patients with massive PE may fare better than the nonfilter group.
- Prompt initiation of anticoagulant therapy (see Chap. 90) is essential in the acute management of VTE for the majority of patients, except those who are actively bleeding or in whom the risk of bleeding clearly outweighs benefits.
- Currently, several groups of drugs are available for acute-phase anticoagulation for VTE. The preferred initial agent for uncomplicated VTE treatment is LMWH. (See Table 89-4.)
- Once patients are therapeutic with acute-phase anticoagulation, patients should begin chronic oral anticoagulation (OAC) with vitamin K antagonists. Acute-phase anticoagulation should continue for a minimum of 4–5 days (7–10 days for symptomatic PE) overlapping with OAC. Long-term anticoagulation with LMWH instead of warfarin has been shown to have a survival benefit in cancer patients.
- Patients with uncomplicated VTE may be triaged to out-of-hospital treatment. (See Table 89-5.)
- Catheter-directed fibrinolytic therapy for DVT should generally be reserved for patients with severe iliofemoral DVT, where there is risk of limb ischemia and/or high risk for subsequent postphlebitic syndrome.
  - Catheter-directed fibrinolytic therapy, with subsequent surgical correction of underlying anatomic

TABLE 89-4   FDA-Approved Initial Therapy for VTE

UFH
  Use normogram—80 U/kg IV bolus followed by continuous IV drip 18 U/kg/hr
  Goal aPTT = 60–80 (may vary from institution to institution; therapeutic range should correspond to heparin levels of 0.3–0.7 U/mL)
LMWH
  Enoxaparin 1 mg/kg SC q 12 hour
  Enoxaparin 1.5 mg/kg SC q 24 hour
  Dalteparin 200 IU/kg SC q 24 hour
  Tinzaparin 175 IU/kg SC q 24 hour
Fondaparinux
  5 mg SC daily if weight < 50 kg
  7.5 mg SC daily if weight 50–100 kg
  10 mg SC daily if weight > 100 kg

Abbreviation: aPTT, activated partial thromboplastin time.

anomalies, may be the treatment of choice in Paget-Schroetter syndrome, reducing the risk of significant long-term morbidity from postphlebitic syndromes in the upper extremity of these typically young patients.
  - Catheter-directed thrombolysis may reduce the incidence of the postthrombotic syndrome, increase venous patency and valvular function. However, major bleeding can occur in 11% of cases.
- Other options to restore patency of thrombosed veins include open surgical thrombectomy and percutaneous mechanical thrombectomy. These modalities are not considered standard of care but may have benefit depending upon clinical setting. (See Table 89-6.)

SUBSEQUENT THERAPY

- Duration of OAC therapy requires balancing the risks of recurrent and fatal VTE off warfarin therapy against the risks of recurrent and fatal bleeding on OAC.
- Anticoagulation should be continued indefinitely for patients with idiopathic VTE. (See Table 89-7.)
- Jobst or equivalent compression stockings (30–40 mm Hg) should be prescribed to all patients with DVT unless they have severe arterial insufficiency.

DISCHARGE FOLLOW-UP

- Risk stratification can assist in decision-making regarding the timing of discharge. Low-risk patients with PE may be potential candidates for outpatient treatment.
- Recurrent embolism may occur in a small percentage (3%) of patients treated for acute PE, and the majority of these were fatal. Risk factors for recurrent VTE, bleeding, and mortality are immobilization, hospitalization, advanced age, the presence of COPD, and cancer. These patients may benefit from continued hospitalization for the duration of their treatment.

TABLE 89-5 Management of DVT

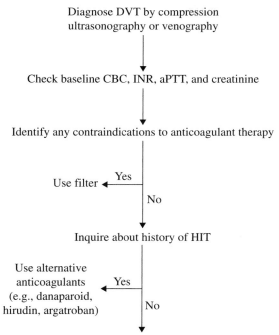

Diagnose DVT by compression ultrasonography or venography

↓

Check baseline CBC, INR, aPTT, and creatinine

↓

Identify any contraindications to anticoagulant therapy

↓

Use filter ◄—— Yes

No

↓

Inquire about history of HIT

Use alternative anticoagulants (e.g., danaparoid, hirudin, argatroban) ◄—— Yes

No

↓

Assess the need for hospitalization by identifying any of the following:

An extensive iliofemoral DVT with circulatory compromise

An increased risk of bleeding, which requires close monitoring of therapy

A limited cardiorespiratory reserve

A risk of poor compliance with home therapy or inadequate support (i.e., community, social, or medical)

A contraindication to LMWH, which would necessitate IV heparin therapy

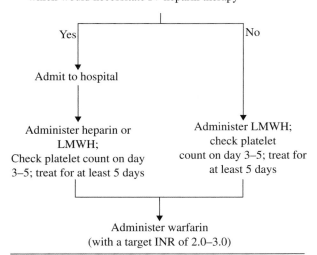

Yes | No

Admit to hospital

↓

Administer heparin or LMWH; Check platelet count on day 3–5; treat for at least 5 days | Administer LMWH; check platelet count on day 3–5; treat for at least 5 days

↓

Administer warfarin (with a target INR of 2.0–3.0)

SOURCE: Reproduced from Bates SM, Ginsberg JS. Clinical practice: treatment of deep-vein thrombosis. *N Engl J Med.* 2004;351:268–277.

TABLE 89-6 Approach to Risk Stratification of Patients with Acute PE

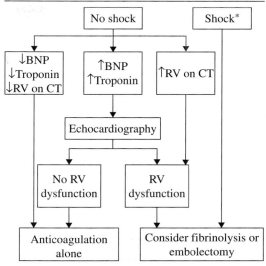

No shock | Shock*

↓

↓BNP ↓Troponin ↓RV on CT | ↑BNP ↑Troponin | ↑RV on CT

↓

Echocardiography

↓

No RV dysfunction | RV dysfunction

↓

Anticoagulation alone | Consider fibrinolysis or embolectomy

*Shock = hypotension (< 90 mm Hg or a drop in systolic arterial pressure of at least 40 mm Hg for at least 15 minutes). (with permission?)

SOURCE: Reproduced from Piazza G, Goldhaber SZ. Acute pulmonary embolism. *Circulation.* 2006;114:e42–e47.

TABLE 89-7 Guidelines for Duration of Anticoagulant Therapy for VTE

RISK FACTOR FOR VTE	DURATION OF TREATMENT (TARGET INR 2.0–3.0)
Major transient risk factor	3 months
Minor risk factor	3–6 months
Unprovoked	Indefinite

Unprovoked but also
    Isolated calf DVT
    Moderate to high risk
    of bleeding
	6 months

Uncontrolled malignancy	Indefinite (preferable with LMWH)

Uncontrolled malignancy but also
    Very high risk of bleeding
    Additional reversible provoking
    risk factor
	6 months

Major transient risk factor = surgery within 3 months, hospitalization, plaster cast immobilization

Minor transient risk factor = estrogen therapy within 6 weeks, prolonged air travel (> 10 hours), pregnancy, less marked leg injury or immobilization

Bleeding risk factors = age > 65, previous stroke, previous GI bleeding, peptic ulcer disease, renal impairment, thrombocytopenia, liver disease, diabetes mellitus, use of antiplatelet therapy, poor patient adherence, structural lesion associated with bleeding (including tumor)

SOURCE: Reproduced from Kearon C. Long-term management of patients after venous thromboembolism. *Circulation.* 2004;110(9 suppl 1):110–118.

TABLE 89-8   Patient Education for Outpatient LMWH Therapy

The pharmacist or nurse and the supervising physician need to coordinate the clinical, nonclinical, and educational aspects of the outpatient treatment of VTE. A case manager or coordinator can help verify that the patient's prescription provider covers the cost of LMWH.

The nurse or pharmacist must educate the patient and/or caregiver about the following:

1. How to perform LMWH injections, including technique, sites for injection, and proper disposal of syringes
2. Understanding the condition of acute VTE and the associated risks and complications
3. Understanding the treatment regimen of LMWH and warfarin (what the drugs do, dosing schedule, potential side effects, and drug and food interactions)
4. Education about the signs of bleeding and other adverse events and how to respond to them
5. An explanation of laboratory tests and subsequent dose changes
6. How to access emergency assistance
7. Period and time of next follow-up appointments

- Patients hospitalized on anticoagulant therapy require a platelet count at least every other day for monitoring the development of heparin induced thrombocytopenia.
- For those patients being discharged home on outpatient LMWH therapy, a CBC should be checked on day 3 and day 7 of therapy. Patients will need patient education and prescriptions for both the LMWH and warfarin. (See Table 89-8.)
- Patients need their INR checked at least every other day until the INR is consistently 2.0–3.0.
- Communication with the outpatient provider, who will be responsible for monitoring newly initiated anticoagulant therapy after discharge, is essential to ensure a safe transition of care.
- In fact, patients, especially the elderly, are at highest risk of bleeding during the first month of initiation of warfarin therapy.
- Medication errors related to anticoagulants can be a significant source of patient morbidity/mortality. Referral to an anticoagulation clinic, when available, is often the safest strategy.

BIBLIOGRAPHY

Augustinos P, Ouriel K. Invasive approaches to treatment of venous thromboembolism. *Circulation* 2004;110(9 suppl 1):I27–I34.
Aujesky D, Roy P-M, Monach CP, et al. Validation of a model to predict adverse outcomes in patients with pulmonary embolism. *Eur Heart J.* 2006;27:476–481.
Bates SM, Ginsberg JS. Clinical practice: treatment of deep-vein thrombosis. *N Engl J Med.* 2004;351(3):268–277.
Buller HR, et al. Antithrombotic therapy for venous thromboembolic disease: the seventh ACCP conference on antithrombotic and thombolytic therapy. *Chest.* 2004;126(3 suppl):410S–428S.
Goldhaber SZ, Elliott CG. Acute pulmonary embolism: part II; risk stratification, treatment, and prevention. *Circulation.* 2003;108:2834–2838.
Kearon C. Long-term management of patients after venous thromboembolism. *Circulation* 2004;110 (9 suppl 1):110–118.
Kyrle PA, Eichinger S. Deep-vein thrombosis. *Lancet.* 2005;365:1163–1174.
Kucher N, Goldhaber SZ. Management of massive pulmonary embolism. *Circulation.* 2005;112:e28–e32.
Nijkeuter M, Sohne M, Tick L, et al. The natural course of hemodynamically stable pulmonary embolism. Clinal outcome and risk factors in a large prospective cohort study. *Chest.* 2007;131(2):517.
Piazza G, Goldhaber SZ. Acute pulmonary embolism. *Circulation.* 2006;114:e42–e47.
Stein PD, Hull PD, Patel KC, et al. D-Dimer for the exclusion of acute venous thrombosis and pulmonary embolism: a systematic review. *Ann Intern Med.* 2004;140(8):589–602.
Wells PS, Anderson DR, Rodger M, et al. Evaluation of D-dimer in the diagnosis of suspected deep-vein thrombosis. *N Engl J Med.* 2003;349(13):1227–1235.
Wells PS, et al. Value of assessment of pretest probability of deep-vein thrombosis in clinical management. *Lancet.* 1997;350(9):1795–1798.

90 ANTICOAGULANT THERAPIES

Rosalynn M. Nazaria and Michael Laposata*

EPIDEMIOLOGY/OVERVIEW

- Hospitalized patients often have multiple factors contributing to a high risk for the development of a blood clot.
- The major principle guiding the use of anticoagulant therapies for the prevention and treatment of thrombosis in these patients involves striking the appropriate balance between bleeding and clotting.
- An understanding of the physiologic processes involved in clot formation and the pharmacologic mechanism of action, cost, risk, and benefit profile of the various anticoagulant therapies is necessary for safe and effective clinical management of hospitalized patients.

*Disclosure: Dr. Michael Laposata is a member of the GlaxoSmithKline Speaker's Bureau.

PATHOPHYSIOLOGY

CLOT FORMATION

- Clot formation begins with a contraction of the blood vessel wall and a narrowing of the vessel lumen.
- Platelets within the circulation then adhere to subendothelial proteins, such as collagen, which become exposed as a result of vascular injury, and become activated.
- Once activated, platelets release the contents of their granules and other substances to activate circulating platelets and form a platelet aggregate.
- After initiation of platelet plug formation, the coagulation cascade is activated, with the end product being fibrin, which strengthens the platelet plug.
- When clot formation becomes excessive, the lumen of the blood vessel can become partially or completely obstructed by the clot, producing thrombosis.
- Thrombosis can occur in veins to produce DVT or PE or in arteries to produce arterial thrombosis, myocardial infarction, or stroke.
- There are many *acquired* risk factors that predispose to thrombosis. The most commonly encountered ones include: surgery, trauma, immobilization, malignancy, a high estrogen state from pregnancy or estrogen supplementation, obesity, smoking, and the presence of antiphospholipid antibodies.
- In addition, a number of *hereditary* risk factors for thrombosis have been identified including the factor V Leiden mutation, the prothrombin 20210 mutation, deficiency of protein C, protein S, or antithrombin, and many other rare inherited disorders.
- The accumulation of multiple risk factors, either congenital, acquired, or a combination of both, that exceeds the threshold for clot formation is responsible for the development of thrombosis.

PRIMARY AND SECONDARY PROPHYLAXIS OF VENOUS THROMBOEMBOLISM

- Prior to the use of pharmaceutical compounds, thrombosis prophylaxis was commonly achieved by physical methods such as early ambulation, external compression of the leg by active or passive leg exercises, the use of graduated pressure stockings, and the use of electrical or pneumatic calf compression devices.
- Options for prevention of clot formation include inhibition of platelets or inhibition of the coagulation cascade.
- Primary prophylaxis is an attempt to prevent the first thrombotic event.
- Indications for primary prophylaxis include: post-surgery, trauma, a medical condition that predisposes

to thrombosis, and multiple genetic or acquired risk factors for thrombosis.
- Secondary prophylaxis refers to the prevention of recurrent thrombosis in a patient who has already suffered one thrombotic event.
- Medications useful for thrombosis prophylaxis can be divided into: antiplatelet drugs that impair platelet function and anticoagulant drugs that inhibit clot formation and limit further clot extension.
- Thrombolytic agents dissolve existing thrombi and are not considered anticoagulants.
- Bleeding is an important adverse effect of all pharmacologic agents used for thrombosis prophylaxis. (See Table 90-1.)

TABLE 90-1 Potential Adverse Effects of Anticoagulant Therapies*

DRUG	POTENTIAL ADVERSE EFFECT
Warfarin	• Hemorrhage • Cholesterol embolization syndrome ("purple toe" syndrome) • *General:* hypersensitivity reaction, hematoma, priapism • *Dermatologic:* skin necrosis • *Hepatic:* hepatitis
UFH	• Hemorrhage • HIT and thrombosis syndrome ("white clot" syndrome) • *General:* hematoma, osteoporosis (with long-term, high-dose use) • *Dermatologic:* injection site erythema, ulceration, tissue necrosis • *Hepatic:* elevated hepatic aminotransferase levels
LMWH -Enoxaparin -Dalteparin	• Hemorrhage • HIT • *General:* hypersensitivity, confusion • *Cardiac:* atrial fibrillation, CHF • *Dermatologic:* injection site rash, tissue necrosis • *GI:* nausea, diarrhea • *Hematologic:* anemia • *Hepatic:* elevated liver function studies • *Pulmonary:* dyspnea
Fondaparinux	• Hemorrhage • *General:* fever • *Dermatologic:* injection site hemorrhage, pruritus • *Hematologic:* anemia • *Hepatic:* elevated hepatic aminotransferase levels
Lepirudin	• Hemorrhage • *General:* anaphylaxis, fever • *Cardiac:* CHF • *Hepatic:* elevated liver function studies • *Pulmonary:* cough, bronchospasm, dyspnea
Argatroban	• Hemorrhage • *General:* hypotension, fever, infections • *Cardiac:* atrial fibrillation, ventricular tachycardia • *GI:* abdominal pain, nausea, vomiting, diarrhea • *Renal:* abnormal renal function

*Data from product prescribing information packets—see reference section for a complete listing.

ANTIPLATELET AGENTS

- Aspirin has long been used for both prophylaxis and treatment of thrombosis particularly in the arterial circulation, where platelets play a major role in clot formation.
- RCT have shown that aspirin alone is ineffective for the prevention of venous thrombosis and PE when compared with other prophylactic regimens in hospitalized patients with multiple risk factors.
- Clopidogrel (Plavix) is also commonly used as a platelet inhibitor.
- There are a number of NSAIDs that inhibit platelet function reversibly.
- Among the intravenously administered antiplatelet drugs are the glycoprotein IIb/IIIa inhibitors, utilized largely for interventional cardiology.
- Aspirin exerts its effect by irreversibly inhibiting the enzyme cyclooxygenase, resulting in decreased thromboxane A_2 production.
- Clopidogrel inhibits platelets by blocking the ADP receptor for platelet activation.
- NSAIDs produce platelet dysfunction by reversibly inhibiting cyclooxygenase.
- The glycoprotein IIb/IIIa receptor antagonists (Reopro, Integrilin, Aggrastat) all work by inhibiting platelets by binding to the glycoprotein IIb/IIIa receptor binding site.
- Aspirin resistance is growing in recognition and there may be a significant number of patients who are poorly responsive to aspirin, clopidogrel, or both.

ANTICOAGULANT AGENTS

The remainder of this chapter will focus on the anticoagulants: warfarin, UFH, LMWH, fondaparinux, argatroban, and lepirudin.

WARFARIN

Drug Action

- The original oral anticoagulant that resembles warfarin (coumadin) is dicoumarol, which is no longer utilized due to slow and erratic GI tract absorption.
- Phenprocoumon and acenocoumarol are in clinical use but not in the United States.
- There are a number of potent rodenticides that resemble warfarin structurally and have the same mechanism of action.
- Warfarin acts by inhibiting the enzyme vitamin K epoxide reductase, thereby increasing the level of inactive vitamin K epoxide and decreasing the level of active vitamin K.
- This impairs the complete synthesis of the four vitamin K-dependent coagulation factors (factors II, VII, IX, and X), as well as protein C and protein S.
- Warfarin does not eliminate the presence of these factors. Therefore, it takes a typical patient 5 days or longer to generate stable depletion of these four coagulation factors.
- Patients are usually maintained at a target INR ranging from 2.0 to 3.0, or 2.5 to 3.5.
- Warfarin overdose may result in elevations of the INR above the target range.
- If the INR is only slightly elevated, warfarin can be discontinued for 1 or 2 days followed by resumption of therapy at the same dose.
- For significant elevations of the INR in the range of 5.0–9.0, vitamin K can be administered to reduce the risk of lethal bleeding. As little as 1 mg of vitamin K orally may be sufficient for reducing the INR into the therapeutic range.
- If life-threatening bleeding occurs, warfarin should be discontinued and fresh-frozen plasma administered to stop the bleeding and increase the concentration of the vitamin K-dependent coagulation factors.

Use in Prophylaxis

- The conditions in which warfarin is used for prophylaxis (INR target range of 2.0–3.0) include: valvular heart disease, atrial fibrillation, and tissue heart valves. For mechanical heart valves an INR target range of 2.5–3.5 is recommended.
- Some practitioners have recommended an INR of 1.5–2.0 lifelong, after a treatment period of at least 6 months at an INR of 2.0–3.0, for patients who have had a single spontaneous thrombotic event. However, it has also been shown that maintaining an INR of 2.0–3.0 lifelong further reduces the incidence of recurrent venous thrombosis.

Use in Treatment

- The four vitamin K-dependent factors affected by warfarin have different half-lives: factor VII has a very short half-life of 4–7 hours; factor IX has a half-life of 12–24 hours; the half-life for factor X is 40–45 hours; and factor II has the longest half-life of the four factors at 60–70 hours.
- Initially, treatment must be monitored daily with the INR to determine whether a dose adjustment is necessary. This is achieved by measuring the time it takes for a clot to form (prothrombin time [PT]) using the patient's plasma and a source of calcium and thromboplastin.

- The thromboplastin reagent, especially if it is obtained from rabbit brain, has variable sensitivity to coagulation factor deficiencies, even if made by the same manufacturer. Use of recombinant thromboplastin for measurement of the PT and subsequent calculation of the INR is associated with greater reproducibility of the PT and INR.
- The INR utilizes the international sensitivity index (ISI) for a given thromboplastin reagent to "normalize" the measured PT value. The formula for the international normalized ratio is: *INR = (patient PT/mean of normal PT range)^{ISI}*.
- Reagents with a low ISI have a high sensitivity to coagulation factor deficiencies, while reagents with a high ISI have a low sensitivity to factor deficiencies.
- In clinical practice, the anticoagulant effects of warfarin can be altered by other medications resulting in a significantly increased or decreased INR.
- Certain drugs may compete for warfarin metabolism via the hepatic cytochrome P450 enzyme pathway or inhibit vitamin K-producing intestinal flora resulting in an increased INR.
- Pharmacologic agents known to potentiate the effect of warfarin include bactrim, ciprofloxacin, erythromycin, isoniazid, omeprazole, dilantin, cimetidine, quinine, and tamoxifen among others.
- Pharmacologic agents that can inhibit the effect of warfarin include penicillin, sucralfate, phenobarbital, trazodone, and oral contraceptive pills.
- Herbal medications and certain components of the diet may also interact with warfarin.
- The combination of warfarin with aspirin or NSAID medications should generally be avoided due to an increased risk of bleeding.
- Warfarin is contraindicated in women who are pregnant or who may become pregnant. (See Table 90-2.)

UNFRACTIONATED HEPARIN
Drug Action

- UFH, or heparin, is a polysaccharide of variable chain length with repeating units of glucosamine and uronic acid.
- Heparin does not work independently as an anticoagulant but produces its anticoagulant effect by interacting with antithrombin and forming a trimolecular complex with heparin, antithrombin, and the activated coagulation factor to be inhibited.
- UFH treatment results in the inhibition of all coagulation factors in their activated form, including factor IIa (thrombin) and factor Xa.

Use in Prophylaxis

- The use of UFH in prophylaxis has little merit, with the possible exceptions being treatment of patients

TABLE 90-2 US FDA Pregnancy Risk Categories Defined

CATEGORY	PREGNANCY RISK
A	RCT fail to show a risk to the fetus (all trimesters)
B	*Either* no controlled trials in pregnant women, but animal studies failed to show a risk to the fetus, *or* adverse effect demonstrated in animal studies but controlled trials in pregnant women failed to show a risk to the fetus
C	*Either* adverse effect demonstrated in animal studies but no controlled trials in pregnant women have been performed, *or* no animal or human data are available
D	Evidence-based risk to fetus has been shown in pregnant females. (Benefit may outweigh the risk of use if limited to life-threatening.) situations with no available alternate treatments)
X	The drug is contraindicated in women who are or may become pregnant. (Evidence-based risk of use of the drug outweighs any potential benefit.)

SOURCE: Adapted from http://www.fda.gov/fdac/features/2001/301_preg.html#categories. Used with permission.

with renal failure who cannot clear LMWH or fondaparinux effectively, and those patients anticipating an epidural because of the longer half-life of LMWH and fondaparinux relative to UFH.

Use in Treatment

- Heparin is formulated for administration via subcutaneous injection or IV delivery. Heparin treatment results in rapid inactivation of coagulation factors. For that reason, heparin is effectively used to initiate anticoagulation until oral anticoagulation with warfarin reaches a therapeutic level.
- The minimum heparin and warfarin treatment overlap is 5 days. The two anticoagulants are used concurrently for at least 5 days until an INR within the desired therapeutic range is demonstrated on 2 consecutive days, at which time discontinuation of heparin is possible.
- When heparin or LMWH is given for prophylaxis, there is no monitoring requirement. However, for patients who are obese, have abnormal renal function, or in children, there is a need to monitor LMWH. (See section Low Molecular Weight Heparin.)
- Full-dose UFH is monitored by measuring the partial thromboplastin time (PTT). The target range for PTT is at least 1.5 times the mean of the normal range. Therefore, for a normal range of 26–34 seconds, the mean is 30 seconds, and the target range is at least 45 seconds. Commonly, a therapeutic range of 60–80 seconds is used. (See Table 90-4.)

TABLE 90-3   Anticoagulant Drug Dosing: Special Considerations*

DRUG	PREGNANCY RISK CATEGORY[†]	RENAL INSUFFICIENCY[‡]
Warfarin	X	• No dosage adjustment is necessary
UFH	C	• No dosage adjustment is necessary
LMWH	B	• For creatinine clearance < 30 mL/min: the recommended dosage adjustment for Enoxaparin in prophylaxis is 30 mg SQ × 1 daily and 1 mg/kg SQ × 1 daily for treatment of VTE • Sufficient data for evidence-based renal dose adjustments for Enoxaparin and Dalteparin are not available, but reduced doses are recommended in patients with impaired renal function
Fondaparinux	B	• Evidence-based guidelines are not available, but use in patients with creatinine clearance < 30 mL/min is contraindicated
Lepirudin	B	• In patients with renal impairment, the bolus dose is to be reduced to 0.2 mg/kg body weight. The maintenance dose is to be reduced as follows[§]:

Creatinine clearance (mL/min)	Adjusted dose (% of original dose)
45–60	0.075 mg/kg/hr (50%)
30–44	0.045 mg/kg/hr (30%)
15–29	0.022 mg/kg/hr (15%)
< 15	Stop infusion

DRUG	PREGNANCY RISK CATEGORY	RENAL INSUFFICIENCY
Argatroban	B	• No dosage adjustment is necessary

*Data from product prescribing information packets—see reference section for a complete listing.
[†]See Table 90-2 for Pregnancy risk category definitions.
[‡]Defined as creatinine clearance < 30 mL/min; see Table 90-5 for calculation of creatinine clearance.
[§]Guidelines derived from Refludan (Lepirudin) product information packet.
Abbreviations: UFH, unfractionated heparin; LMWH, low molecular weight heparin (eg, Enoxaparin, Dalteparin); VTE, venous thromboembolism.
Note: Renal dosing is of particular importance for geriatric patients (esp. Fondaparinux and Lepirudin).

• In the event of a heparin overdose without any evidence of bleeding, heparin should be discontinued and the patient watched carefully for at least 2 hours. If

TABLE 90-4   Weight-Based UFH Nomogram

PTT	HEPARIN IV INFUSION RATE (body weight in kg)
Initial "loading" dose	80 units/kg bolus dose, then 18 units/kg hourly
PTT < 35 seconds	80 units/kg bolus dose, increase drip 4 units/kg hourly
35–45 seconds	40 units/kg bolus dose, increase drip 2 units/kg hourly
46–70 seconds	No change
71–90 seconds	Decrease drip 2 units/kg hourly
> 90 seconds	Decrease drip 4 units/kg hourly

Derived from Raschke RA, Reilly BM, Guidry JR, et al. The weight-based heparin dosing nomogram compared with a "standard care" nomogram. *Ann Intern Med.* 1993;119:874–881. Used with permission.
Note: Recommended laboratory testing algorithm for patients on UFH:
• Obtain PTT, PT, and CBC at time of initial dose.
• Obtain CBC with platelet count at least every 3 days throughout the duration of therapy.
• Obtain a "STAT" PTT 6 hours after bolus dose and after any change in the infusion rate.
• After two consecutive PTTs within the therapeutic range (46–70 seconds), the frequency of monitoring can be reduced to once daily if no dosage changes are made.

there are no signs and symptoms of bleeding, heparin can then be reinitiated, but at a lower dose.
• For significant heparin-associated bleeding, heparin is promptly discontinued and protamine sulfate, a heparin antagonist, is administered to neutralize the heparin.
• Heparin can produce markedly different PTT values, even at a single concentration of heparin in vivo, depending upon the reagent used to measure the PTT. There is no INR equivalent for the PTT, as there is for the PT.
• There is insufficient data to support the use of UFH in pregnant women. (See Table 90-3.)

LOW MOLECULAR WEIGHT HEPARIN
Drug Action

• There are four FDA-approved LMWH preparations: Enoxaparin, Dalteparin, Ardeparin, and Tinzaparin; by trade names these are Lovenox, Fragmin, Normiflo, and Innohep, respectively.
• When LMWH is injected SC, its bioavailability is > 90%, and is independent of dose, whereas UFH injected SC for prophylaxis has a bioavailability that ranges from 10% to 90%, and it is not independent of the dose.
• Unlike standard heparin, LMWH preferentially inhibits factor Xa due to its shorter chain length,

which prevents the binding of the LMWH molecule to the coagulation factor directly.

Use in Prophylaxis

- LMWH and UFH have similar efficacy, although LMWH trends to better efficacy for prevention of thrombosis.
- There is essentially no bleeding risk with prophylactic doses of either LMWH or UFH, with spinal puncture being a noteworthy exception.
- There is approximate dose equivalence between the two major LMWHs in use for prophylaxis, enoxaparin, and dalteparin. One approach is 40 mg of enoxaparin daily, which is approximately equivalent to 2500 units of dalteparin daily; 30 mg of enoxaparin twice daily is approximately equivalent to 5000 units of dalteparin daily.

Use in Treatment

- The half-life of UFH (1–2 hours) is shorter than the half-life for LMWH (3–5 hours). In the hospital setting, it is not uncommon to use UFH instead of LMWH because it permits brief interruptions of anticoagulation for invasive procedures.
- Laboratory monitoring of LMWH is not required, but it is recommended for patients with renal dysfunction, an elevated BMI or a very low BMI, those undergoing long-term treatment, in pregnancy, and in children (especially neonates). (See Table 90-3.)
- Unlike standard heparin, LMWH only marginally elevates the PTT. However, due to its relative selectivity for factor Xa, the anticoagulant effect of LMWH can be monitored using the antifactor Xa assay. The target range is 0.5–1.0 units/mL.
- The approximate dose equivalence between the two major LMWHs used for treatment is as follows: 1 mg/kg of enoxaparin twice daily is approximately equivalent to 100 units/kg of dalteparin twice daily, and 1.5 mg/kg of enoxaparin daily is approximately equivalent to 200 units/kg of dalteparin daily.
- Protamine sulfate in a 1% solution cannot completely reverse antifactor Xa activity, but it is recommended for reversal of anticoagulation with LMWH because it neutralizes a significant percentage of its activity.

Heparin-Induced Thrombocytopenia

- UFH and LMWH can both induce bleeding, heparin-induced thrombocytopenia (HIT), and osteoporosis. However, LMWH has a much lower incidence of HIT and osteoporosis compared to UFH. In addition, many clinical trials have reported similar or decreased bleeding with LMWH in comparison to UFH.

- To monitor for HIT, it is advisable to follow the platelet count in patients receiving UFH or LMWH at a minimum of every 3 days. Often platelet counts are obtained daily in hospitalized patients, and this is reasonable.
- HIT is mediated by the development of antibodies to the heparin-platelet factor 4 (PF4) complex. Only a fraction of patients who develop these antibodies will develop thrombocytopenia, and only a fraction of these will activate enough platelets to induce venous or arterial thrombosis.
- Enzyme-linked immunosorbent assay (ELISA)-based laboratory testing can confirm the presence of heparin-PF4 antibodies for the diagnosis of HIT, but it may take several days to obtain results.
- If there is a high pretest probability for HIT, heparin should be promptly discontinued and appropriate alternative anticoagulant therapy begun prior to laboratory confirmation of heparin-PF4 antibodies.
- Clinical parameters that raise the pretest probability for HIT include a decrease in the platelet count from baseline by > 50% within a 48-hour period, or thrombocytopenia occurring approximately 4–14 days following the induction of heparin therapy in the absence of other etiologies.
- It is important to consider the temporal relationship between exposure to heparin and the variation in absolute platelet count, as HIT is an immune-mediated condition.
- Other clues to the development of HIT include the occurrence of a thrombotic event during treatment with heparin, an acute systemic reaction to IV heparin administration, and/or the development of skin lesions at the site of heparin injection.
- In patients who develop HIT from UFH, use of LMWH is not an acceptable alternative due to its ability to cross-react with the HIT-related antibody.
- LMWH is significantly more expensive than UFH, but despite the higher cost per dose, LMWH may actually be more cost-effective than UFH in the total patient encounter.
- One appropriate alternative to heparin is treatment with a direct thrombin inhibitor, such as lepirudin or argatroban (see below for further discussion of these agents) and warfarin. Once a therapeutic INR is achieved, the direct thrombin inhibitor can be discontinued and the patient maintained on warfarin alone.
- In patients with HIT, the platelet count should rise following the discontinuation of heparin.
- A platelet count of at least 100,000 per μL in the absence of any heparin for at least 3–5 days is advised prior to the initiation of warfarin, as this can exacerbate the thrombosis syndrome.

FONDAPARINUX

Drug Action

- Fondaparinux is a synthetic five-sugar compound that interacts with the active site of antithrombin, which binds to heparin-related compounds.
- The binding of fondaparinux results in a conformational change in the antithrombin molecule allowing it to bind factor Xa, and subsequently, inhibit its procoagulant effect. However, fondaparinux does not produce a prolongation of the PT or the PTT.
- Fondaparinux undergoes renal clearance. Its use is contraindicated in patients with a creatinine clearance of < 30 mL/min. (See Table 90-5.)
- There is no known effective reversal agent for fondaparinux, but factor VIIa and fresh-frozen plasma have been used.
- Fondaparinux reaches a maximum plasma concentration 1–3 hours following administration. It is formulated for administration via subcutaneous injection only.
- Fondaparinux has a long plasma half-life of 17–21 hours with once daily dosing at 2.5 mg, which requires attention to renal function because of the inability to reverse the anticoagulant.

Use in Prophylaxis

- Randomized trials have shown that fondaparinux given 6 hours following wound closure is effective for postoperative venous thrombosis in patients undergoing hip or knee surgery. A delay of 6–12 hours from the time of wound closure to the initiation of therapy with fondaparinux is recommended to reduce the risk of clinically significant postoperative bleeding.

Use in Treatment

- Fondaparinux is available for use in treatment of thrombosis. For patients weighing > 50 kg, the appropriate treatment dose is 5 mg daily by subcutaneous injection; for patients weighing 50–100 kg, the dose is 7.5 mg daily; and for patients weighing > 100 kg, the dose is 10 mg daily.

TABLE 90-5 Cockcroft-Gault Creatinine Clearance Approximation Formula

$$\text{Creatinine clearance (mL/min)} = \frac{(140 - \text{age}) \times \text{mass (in kg)}}{72 \times \text{serum creatinine (mg/dL)}}$$

Multiply result by 0.85 in females
Normal reference range: > 90 mL/min

SOURCE: Derived from http://www.nephron.com. Copyright 2007, Stephen Z. Fadem, MD, FACP, FASN. All rights reserved. Used with permission.

LEPIRUDIN

Drug Action

- Lepirudin is a direct thrombin inhibitor, and thereby, inhibits the action of factor IIa in the coagulation cascade.
- Lepirudin is biotechnologically manufactured as a recombinant protein and has been proven to be a safe and effective anticoagulant for patients with HIT.

Use in Prophylaxis

- Desirudin, which differs from lepirudin only in the first two N-terminal amino acids of the molecule, has been licensed for the prevention of DVT.

Use in Treatment

- Similar to fondaparinux, lepirudin has no reversal agent, is renally cleared, and is recommended for use in patients with HIT who have adequate renal function.
- The plasma half-life of lepirudin is approximately 1 hour in patients with normal renal function, but can exceed 50 hours in patients with ESRD. Dose adjustment is necessary for patient with renal dysfunction. For patients with severe renal insufficiency, use of lepirudin is contraindicated. (See Table 90-3.)
- Approximately 40% of patients receiving lepirudin develop antibodies that paradoxically potentiate its anticoagulant properties.
- The anticoagulant effect of lepirudin is monitored by measuring the PTT with a target range of 1.5–2.5 times the mean of the normal range.
- Lepirudin is formulated for IV administration at a concentration of 5 mg/mL. The use of a bolus at the initiation of treatment was initially recommended at a dose of 0.4 mg/kg for patients weighing 50–110 kg. The bolus dose should not be administered to patients with a baseline PTT > 2.5 times normal.
- Many practitioners now suggest the use of lepirudin as a continuous IV infusion of 0.15 mg/kg without administration of a bolus dose.
- More frequent monitoring with adjustment of the infusion rate is recommended for patients with a body weight < 50 kg or > 110 kg for which standard weight-based dosage guidelines cannot readily be applied.
- The first PTT should be measured 4 hours after the initiation of lepirudin therapy.
- If the PTT is > 2.5 times baseline, the infusion should be stopped for 2 hours and then restarted at 50% of the original infusion rate.
- If the PTT is < 1.5 times baseline, the infusion rate should be increased by 20% over the original infusion rate.
- For long-term management of patients with HIT, lepirudin therapy should be overlapped with warfarin.

The overlap between lepirudin and warfarin should mimic that between heparin or LMWH and warfarin.
- Since lepirudin can interfere with the measurement of the INR used to monitor the anticoagulant effect of warfarin, the lepirudin dose should be adjusted to maintain the PTT at the lower end of the therapeutic range (approximately 1.5 times the baseline PTT) in an effort to reduce the interference of lepirudin and permit proper interpretation of the INR value.

ARGATROBAN

Drug Action

- Argatroban is a synthetic direct thrombin inhibitor derived from arginine.
- Argatroban is formulated for IV administration and undergoes hepatic clearance. Therefore, it is useful for the prophylaxis or treatment of thrombosis in patients with HIT who have impaired renal function.
- Argatroban may still be utilized in patients with liver disease, although dose adjustment may be necessary to prevent plasma accumulation of the drug due to delayed hepatic clearance.
- A standard infusion rate of 2 μg/kg/min is recommended for the treatment of patients with HIT weighing between 50 and 140 kg that have normal hepatic function.
- Argatroban is monitored by measuring the PTT, with a target range of 1.5–2.5 times the mean of the normal range.
- While there is no known reversal agent for argatroban, it has a short plasma half-life of only 20–30 minutes.

Use in Prophylaxis

- There is currently no role for argatroban in the prophylaxis of thrombosis.

Use in Treatment

- The anticoagulant effects of argatroban are produced immediately upon infusion, but 1–3 hours are required to attain a steady-state plasma level.
- The guidelines for overlap between argatroban and warfarin for long-term anticoagulation of patients with HIT are similar to that of heparin, LMWH, fondaparinux, and lepirudin in combination with warfarin.
- However, argatroban significantly interferes with calculation of the INR. Thus, the INR result cannot be interpreted to determine whether therapeutic levels of warfarin have been achieved prior to the discontinuation of argatroban.
- Manufacturer produced nomograms to extrapolate the INR for warfarin alone, from the INR value calculated for warfarin in the presence of argatroban, show much scatter of the data, and therefore, show little concordance between the extrapolated INR value and the actual INR.
- Other options for monitoring the anticoagulant effect of warfarin when coadministered with argatroban include discontinuing the argatroban for 3 hours and then performing the INR, or using the chromogenic factor X assay as an alternative to the INR, since factor X is among the coagulation factors inhibited by warfarin.

SUMMARY

- Reviewed in this chapter are the mechanism of action, indications, and assays for laboratory monitoring of anticoagulants used in the prophylaxis and treatment of thromboses including warfarin, UFH, LMWH, fondaparinux, lepirudin, and argatroban. (See Table 90-6.)

TABLE 90-6 Summary of Anticoagulant Therapies*

DRUG	INDICATIONS FOR USE	ROUTE OF ADMINISTRATION	LAB TEST FOR MONITORING
Warfarin	Treatment of arterial and venous thrombosis and prophylaxis in patients with atrial fibrillation, prosthetic heart valves, peripheral vascular disease, and following hip or knee replacement surgery	Oral	INR
UFH	Treatment of arterial and venous thrombosis; can also be used as prophylaxis	SQ, IV	PTT
LMWH	Prophylaxis and treatment of thrombosis	SQ	Antifactor Xa assay if indicated
Fondaparinux	Prophylaxis and treatment of thrombosis	SQ	Antifactor Xa assay if indicated
Lepirudin	Anticoagulation in patients with HIT	IV	PTT
Argatroban	Anticoagulation in patients with HIT	IV	PTT

*Data from product prescribing information packets—see reference section for a complete listing.

- For hospitalists, understanding these principles for the use of anticoagulant therapies is critical for the prevention, diagnosis, and treatment of thromboembolic disorders (including HIT), while minimizing the risk of clinically significant bleeding in hospitalized patients.
- Recommendations for the administration of anticoagulant therapies offered in this chapter are intended to be used as a guideline. Appropriate clinical correlation is suggested prior to the application of these principles in clinical practice.

BIBLIOGRAPHY

Argatroban Prescribing Information. http://us.gsk.com/products/assets/us_argatroban.pdf. Accessed June 4, 2007.

Clagett G, Anderson F, Heit J, et al. Prevention of venous thromboembolism. *Chest.* 1995;108:312S–334S.

Di Nisio M, Middeldorp S, Buller H. Direct thrombin inhibitors. *N Engl J Med.* 2005;353:1028.

Enoxaparin Prescribing Information. Available at: http://products.sanofi-aventis.us/lovenox/lovenox.html. Accessed June 4, 2007.

Fadem SZ. The nephron information center. Cockcroft-Gault calculator. Copyright © 2007. All rights reserved. Available at: http://www.nephron.com/cgi-bin/CGSIdefault.cgi. Accessed May 5, 2007.

Fondaparinux Prescribing Information. Available at: http://us.gsk.com/products/assets/us_arixtra.pdf. Accessed June 4, 2007.

Greinacher A, Volpel H, Janssens U, et al. Recombinant hirudin (lepirudin) provides safe and effective anticoagulation in patients with heparin-induced thrombocytopenia: a prospective study. *Circulation.* 1999;99:73.

Heparin Prescribing Information. Available at: www.pfizer.com/pfizer/download/uspi_PI.pdf. Accessed June 4, 2007.

Hirsh J, Fuster V, Ansell J, et al. American Heart Association/American College of Cardiology Foundation guide to Warfarin therapy. *Circulation.* 2003;107:1692.

Hirsh J, Raschke R. The seventh ACCP conference on antithrombotic and thrombolytic therapy. Heparin and low molecular weight heparin. *Chest.* 2004;126:188S.

Laposata M, Green D, Van Cott EM, et al. College of American Pathologists conference XXXI on laboratory monitoring of anticoagulant therapy. The clinical use and laboratory monitoring of low molecular weight heparin, danaparoid, hirudin and related compounds, and argatroban. *Arch Pathol Lab Med.* 1998;122:799.

Lepirudin Prescribing Information. Available at: http://www.refludan.com.au/corporateweb/refludanau/home.nsf/AttachmentsByTitle/RefludanProductInformation/$FILE/RefludanProductInformation.pdf. Accessed June 4, 2007.

Meadows M. Pregnancy and the drug dilemma FDA consumer magazine. 2001;35(3). Available at: http://www.fda.gov/fdac/features/2001/301_preg. html#categories. Accessed May 5, 2007.

Raksob G, Hirsh J. Controversies in timing of the first dose of anticoagulant prophylaxis against venous thromboembolism after major orthopedic surgery. *Chest.* 2003;124(6):379S–385S.

Raschke RA, Reilly BM, Guidry JR, et al. The weight-based heparin dosing nomogram compared with a "standard care" nomogram. *Ann Intern Med.* 1993;119(9):874.

Warfarin Prescribing Information. Available at: www.malwarfarin.com/MALWarfarin_PI.pdf. Accessed June 4, 2007.

Warkentin T. Heparin-induced thrombocytopenia: pathogenesis and management. *Br J Haematol* 2003;121:535.

Warkentin T, Greinacher A. Heparin-induced thrombocytopenia: recognition, treatment and prevention. *Chest.* 2004;126:311S–337S.

White CM. Thrombin-directed inhibitors: pharmacology and clinical use. *Am Heart J.* 2005;149:S54.

Section 8
HOSPITALISTS AS EXPERTS

91 DECONDITIONING
Joanne Borg-Stein and Claudia Wheeler

EPIDEMIOLOGY/OVERVIEW

- Deconditioning is the constellation of deteriorating changes in organ system physiology that are induced by inactivity and reversed by activity.
- It occurs as early as the second day of hospital admission; it is iatrogenic and preventable.
- Patients experience a new burden of functional impairment in the hospital that improves at a much slower rate than the acute illness.
- The effects of deconditioning influence disposition and increase length of stay (LOS).
- The hospitalist should understand the physiologic effects of immobility and the factors that contribute to functional decline. Appropriate steps should be implemented to prevent and treat deconditioning in the hospitalized patient, including promotion of early mobility and an appropriate exercise program.
- Contributing factors (see Table 91-1).
  - Routine bed rest orders are often implemented without medical justification. In one study, bed rest was ordered in 33% of 498 patients and 60% had no medical justification. Lack of an activity order is also a problem. In a study of a major academic teaching center, no-activity order was in effect on 13% of the 3500 patient days reviewed.
  - Inconsistency among staff in regard to implementing the order desired by the physician contributes significantly. In one study, when activity was ordered, actual patient activity differed from that ordered by the physician on 41% of the days.
  - In the above study, patients who remained in bed or in a chair rarely received physical therapy (PT),

never had physician orders for exercise, and never performed exercises with nursing staff. What does bed rest mean for the patient?

PATHOPHYSIOLOGY AND CLINICAL PRESENTATION

Deconditioning because of prolonged bed rest affects every organ system in the body, with profound effects on patient health and well being.

1. Musculoskeletal: In addition to decreased mobility, the effects of deconditioning on the musculoskeletal system result in loss of endurance as well as pain and stiffness.
   - Immobilization in a shortened position promotes more rapid degeneration of the muscles. Functionally, the typical flexed neck, flexed hip, and flexed knee hospital bed position is not ideal (Fig. 91-1).
     - Atrophy is a normal response to decreased activity as the body does not support redundant tissues. Atrophy resulting in muscle wasting and weakness results in a loss of strength. There is a 1% to 1.5% loss of initial strength per day on strict bed rest, with a 10% to 20% loss of strength per week, which plateaus at approximately 25% to 40%.
     - Loss of strength varies by muscle group: elbow flexors experience a 6.6% overall loss of strength, shoulder flexors 8.7%, dorsiflexors 13.3%, and plantar flexors 20.8%.
     - Antigravity muscles (gastrocnemius-soleus and back muscles) lose strength disproportionately, approximately twice as fast as small muscles. Functionally, this results in impaired ambulation.
     - Recovery of muscle strength after immobilization can be two or more times longer than the period of immobilization.

515

TABLE 91-1   Factors Contributing to Functional Decline in Hospitalized Patients

FACTOR	IMPLICATION
Modern hospital design and services	• Small rooms • Noisy floors • Obstacles in the room lead to falls
Activity order	• Lack of an activity order • Ordering appropriate level of activity • Inconsistency among staff following activity order • Lack of medical justification for bed rest

Age	• Age >70
	  ○ 1/3 will experience a decline in ADLs
	• Age >85
	  ○ Increased risk for new walking dependence
	  ○ Associated with discharge to nursing home
	  ○ Higher post discharge mortality

Functional impairment prior to admission	• Preadmission impairment with at least one ADL • Use of walker or wheel chair prior to admission • Lower mental status on admission
Comorbidities	• More than four comorbid conditions • Cancer diagnosis • Rehospitalization

ADL, activities of daily living.

- Bones are affected by deconditioning, including:
  ○ Immobilization osteoporosis results from the lack of stress on bones which promotes osteoclastic activity. It occurs as early as 30 hours after immobilization in animal studies. There is a 1% loss of vertebral mineral content per week.
  ○ In addition to generalized osteoporosis, local bone loss in areas of partial immobilization (such as casting) or paralysis can fracture with relatively nontraumatic activities such as transferring.
  ○ Heterotopic ossification is bone growth in abnormal locations, especially around joints,

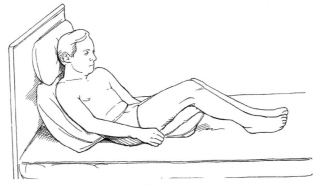

FIG. 91-1 Common hospital bed position.
(SOURCE: From Buschbacher RM, Porter CG. Deconditioning, conditioning, and the benefit of exercise. In: Braddom R, ed. *Physical Medicine and Rehabilitation*. 2nd ed. W.B. Saunders; 2000: 702–726, Figure 34-3, Chap. 34, pg 707.) (Used with permission from W.B. Saunders Company)

and may cause pain and limited range of motion (ROM). It is indirectly caused by immobility, although the mechanism is not well understood. On plain films, it appears as calcification in the soft tissues around a joint, and is most often seen in people status post-trauma.
- The tendons and ligaments also become weaker, primarily at the myotendinous junction and at the insertion at bone.
- Joints are affected by deconditioning in several ways:
  ○ There is cartilage degeneration. Joint surfaces in contact with each other develop pressure necrosis and erosion. Joint surfaces that are not in contact with each other develop fissures and loss of smoothness. Cartilage becomes stiffer; there is osteophyte proliferation, fibrofatty tissue infiltration, synovial atrophy, deterioration of subchondral bone, and ankylosis.
  ○ Joint effusions secondary to immobility are often seen in paralyzed patients (spinal cord injury, Guillain-Barre syndrome, and other neuromuscular diseases). The effusions are hypothesized to be secondary to inadequate muscular control of intra-articular joint structures.
- Contractures are abnormal limitation of passive joint ROM that, if not treated, results in bony ankylosis of the joint.
- Contractures can arise from the musculature, skin and soft tissue, or joints.
- Common contractures and their sequelae can result in permanent impairment (Table 91-2).
  ○ Hip flexion contracture results in compensatory lordosis (back pain), knee flexion, and shortened step length.
  ○ Hip external rotation contracture causes a stiff-legged gait pattern and excess stress on medial knee ligaments.
  ○ Knee flexion contractures result in plantar flexion (toe walking) and crouched gait.
  ○ Ankle plantar flexion contracture causes genu recurvatum and an absence of heel strike.
  ○ Shoulder flexion, adduction, and internal rotation results in inability to reach a back pocket, comb hair, or reach above shoulder level.
  ○ Elbow flexion contracture if mild, results in little functional loss. If severe, it interferes with dressing and weakens triceps position.
  ○ Wrist flexion contracture weakens grip.
  ○ Finger flexion contracture results in inability to open hand to grasp.
2. Integument
- The typical hospital bed position puts pressure on bony prominences such as the sacrum and

TABLE 91-2   Common Joint Contractures and Their Sequelae

JOINT CONTRACTURE	SEQUELAE
Hip flexion	Compensatory lordosis (back pain), knee flexion, shortened step length
Hip external rotation	Stiff-legged gait pattern, excess stress on medial knee ligaments
Knee flexion	Plantar flexion (toe walking), crouch gait
Ankle plantar flexion	Genu recurvatum, absence of heel strike
Shoulder flexion, adduction, and IR	Cannot reach back pocket, comb hair, or reach above shoulder level
Elbow flexion	If mild, little functional loss; if severe, interferes with dressing and weakens triceps position
Wrist flexion	Weakens grip
Finger flexion	Cannot open hand to grasp

IR, internal rotation.

SOURCE: From Buschbacher RM, Porter CG. Deconditioning, conditioning, and the benefit of exercise. In: Braddom R, ed. *Physical Medicine and Rehabilitation.* 2nd ed. W.B. Saunders; 2000:702–726, Figure 34-3, Chap. 34, pg 707. (Used with permission from W.B. Saunders Company)

ischial tuberosities, resulting in skin breakdown and ulceration.
- Hospitalized patients are often unable to change their position in bed secondary to weakness or mental status changes, or may remain relatively immobile because of lines and tubes.
- Edema develops in dependent areas such as the lower extremities and sacrum.
- Subcutaneous bursitis also occurs over bony prominences and can be painful.

3. Cardiovascular
- At rest, there is an increased heart rate (HR) and decreased stroke volume. Cardiac output (CO) is unchanged or slightly decreased. Rate of oxygen consumption (Vo_2) is unchanged. There is decreased cardiac size and volume, decreased left ventricular end-diastolic (LVED) volume. Systolic and diastolic blood pressures are unchanged. Arteriovenous oxygen differences are unchanged or slightly increased.
- With prolonged bed rest, redistribution of body fluids results in decreased plasma volume, decreased total blood volume, decreased RBC mass, as well as mineral and plasma protein loss.
- Prolonged bed rest may also result in orthostatic intolerance, the loss of the appropriate reflexive vasoconstriction in response to blood pooling in the venous system upon standing. This may be secondary to altered carotid baroreflex or a change in autonomic balance. It is accompanied by signs and symptoms of orthostatic hypotension; light-headedness, dizziness, nausea, sweating, pallor, tachycardia, and drop in systolic blood pressure.

4. Hematologic
- Immobility tips the scale in Virchow triad toward thrombosis.
  ◦ Decreased calf blood flow secondary to stasis increases the risk of deep vein thrombosis (see Chaps. 88 and 89).
  ◦ There is also increased blood fibrinogen.
  ◦ Patients who have suffered a stroke, are status post-trauma, or have cancer are particularly at risk of thrombus formation.

5. Respiratory
- Deconditioning affects the respiratory system by increasing the respiratory rate, forced vital capacity, and slightly increasing total lung capacity, while residual volume, functional residual capacity, maximal minute ventilation, and vital capacity remain unchanged.
- Vital capacity may actually decrease in time because of chest wall contracture.
- These changes in respiratory physiology may
  ◦ Cause V/Q mismatch.
  ◦ Increase the risk of pulmonary embolism (PE).
  ◦ Promote a lack of deep breathing, resulting in atelectasis and increased risk of pneumonia.

6. Gastrointestinal
- Decreased gut motility results in constipation and decreased appetite.
- Hospitalized patients often do not drink enough fluids, which may be secondary to lack of thirst, fear of excessive urination, or decreased mental status.

7. Genitourinary
- Immobility causes diuresis resulting in electrolyte loss, increased calculus formation, decreased glomerular filtration rate (GFR), and decreased ability to concentrate urine.
- Foley catheters:
  ◦ Result in many patients having difficulty voiding once they are removed, resulting in increased postvoid residual volumes and overflow incontinence.
  ◦ Increase the incidence of urinary tract infection (UTI). In patients who are elderly, immunocompramised, acutely ill or malnourished, UTI may have an occult presentation. These patients may not experience the typical dysuria of a UTI, but will rather develop mental status changes or will

quickly progress to sepsis, with further impairment of their mobility.

8. Endocrine
   - Alterations in hormone levels (including parathyroid, thyroid, adrenal, pituitary, growth, androgen, renin, and angiotensin) secondary to immobility have vast effects on the body.
   - Some of the more common effects include
     - Impaired glucose tolerance—finger stick blood sugars can help to keep tabs on glucose tolerance, and diet changes and insulin can be used to manage hyperglycemia until it normalizes.
     - Altered circadian rhythm—respecting hours of sleep by avoiding overnight blood draws and medication administration will help with sleep hygiene in the hospital.
     - Altered temperature and sweating responses.
9. Metabolic
   - Atrophy results in decreased lean muscle mass and increased body fat.
   - Electrolyte loss is commonly observed, including nitrogen, calcium, phosphorus, potassium, and sulfur.
   - Immobilization hypercalcemia and hypercalciuria can result from increased osteoclastic activity.
   - It is associated with immobilization osteoporosis. It frequently occurs in young males' status post-trauma.
     - As bone is resorbed, calcium levels rise. Symptoms include nausea, vomiting, abdominal pain, lethargy, muscle weakness, and anorexia. If not treated, it can be fatal.
     - It is treated with intravenous (IV) furosemide and hydration. IV pamidronate and calcitonin can be used in refractory cases.
10. Neurologic/Behavioral
    - The neurologic system is affected by immobility both peripherally and centrally.

- Peripherally, compression neuropathies can occur over areas of bony prominence. Commonly fibular head pressure causes peroneal nerve compression in the hospital bed resulting in foot drop.
- Centrally, the decreased balance, decreased coordination, sleep disturbance, increased auditory threshold, and decreased visual acuity that occur secondary to immobilization put hospitalized patients at risk for falls.
- Sensory deprivation can cause decreased attention span, altered time awareness, and decreased hand-to-eye coordination.
- Depression and anxiety can be obstacles for motivating patients to get out of bed and participate in therapy.

MANAGEMENT STRATEGIES

The best treatment for deconditioning is prevention (Table 91-3) and requires a multidisciplinary team approach
- Education:
  - Detecting patients at risk for deconditioning is essential to the prevention of its deleterious effects.
  - The entire team (physicians, nurses, care assistants, and rehabilitation staff) and, most importantly, the patient and family need to be educated about the dangers of prolonged bed rest.
- Exercise:
  - Mobility has a major influence on disposition. Addressing level of activity is an essential part of the admission orders, and it should be frequently reevaluated. It is quite easy and time efficient to evaluate bed mobility and ambulation on morning rounds.
  - Consult physical and occupational therapists early for patients in whom prolonged bed rest is predictable.

TABLE 91-3   Prevention of Deconditioning

PREVENTION MEASURE	EXPLANATION
Education	Physicians, nurses, care assistants, rehabilitation staff, patient, and family should be aware of dangers of prolonged bed rest and benefits of early mobility
Exercise	Activity order on patient should be justified and frequently reevaluated, to include strengthening, stretching, ROM, and mobility training
ADLs	Encourage independence with toileting, bathing, and dressing
Decrease barriers to mobility	Remove tubes and lines as early as possible. Reduce use of physical and chemical restraints
Positioning	Scheduled position changes, pressure relieving boots, and a pressure-relieving mattress. Lie in prone position to stretch hip and knee flexors
DVT prophylaxis	For the duration of immobilization (see Chap. 88)
Nutrition	Monitor nutritional status, intake, and obtain nutrition consultation for supplements if necessary
Pain control	Find the balance between adequate pain control for participation in therapies and prevention of excess sedation (see Chap. 93)
Pharmacologic	Reduce polypharmacy and the use of psychotropics and sedatives that increase the risk of falls
Depression	Treat depression aggressively as it prevents participation in therapies. Consider short-term use of stimulant until antidepressant is effective
Discharge planning	Early consideration to the safest and most appropriate level of care on discharge. The ability to stand and walk in the hospital can significantly impact disposition

ADLs, activities of daily living; DVT, deep vein thrombosis; ROM, range of motion.

○ Sitting up in the chair or bed with the legs dangling reduces orthostatic intolerance.

○ The optimal type and amount of exercise in hospitalized patients is not known. Most likely a combination of strengthening, stretching, ROM, and mobility training would be the best approach.

○ Isometric muscle strength can be maintained by performing daily isometric contractions of 10% to 20% maximal tension for 10 seconds in duration. Maintenance of knee extensor strength with five sets of leg presses performed at 80% to 85% of 1 repetition maximum (RM), the weight a person can lift one time only, every other day.

○ Stretching seems to delay atrophy in animal studies and may even cause growth. Staff must take care not to be overly aggressive stretching a contracture, as this may cause dislocation or damage.

○ In regards ROM exercises, it is not clear how frequently soft tissues should be passed through a full ROM to prevent contracture. More studies need to be done in this area.

• Encourage independence with activities of daily living (ADLs).

○ Toileting, bathing, and dressing should be performed in a safe manner, while focusing on maximizing independence.

○ Some patients may benefit from adaptive equipment.

• Decreasing barriers to mobility during acute hospitalization is imperative.

○ Tubes and lines are obstacles that inhibit ambulation. Remove Foley catheters and IV lines as soon as possible.

○ Low bed positions help to prevent falls.

○ Reduce the use of restraints, both physical and chemical.

○ Community areas for socialization encourage patients to leave their rooms and spend time out of bed.

○ Dedicated walking paths for ambulatory patients demonstrate the importance of ambulation during acute hospitalization and provide a safe area free of obstacles.

• Positioning prevents contractures and pressure ulcers in immobilized patients.

○ Hip and knee flexion contractures can be prevented by spending time in the prone position, which stretches the hip and knee flexors.

○ Prevent skin breakdown by ordering scheduled position changes, pressure-relieving boots, and a pressure-relieving mattress.

○ Once an area of skin breakdown has developed, be aggressive with treatment (consider consulting a wound care nurse specialist for appropriate dressings and therapies).

• Deep venous thrombosis (DVT) prophylaxis (see Chap. 88).

• Nutrition (see Chap. 92):

○ Low serum albumin, reflecting protein malnutrition, is one of the best predictors of mortality in postsurgical and severely ill patients.

○ Malnutrition is present in 30% to 40% of hospitalized elderly.

○ Nutritional status should be monitored carefully as it directly impacts healing.

○ Nutrition consultation may be helpful in the selection of appropriate supplementation.

• It is important to find the optimal balance of pain control (see Chap. 93).

○ Too much sedation will lead to prolonged bed rest and may increase the risk of falls.

○ Inadequate pain control prevents full participation in therapies.

• Pharmacologic:

○ Reduce polypharmacy and limit the use of psychotropics.

○ Avoid medications that increase risk of falls and sedation (benzodiazepines, anticholinergics).

• Depression hinders participation in therapy. A short course of stimulant may help alleviate symptoms until an antidepressant takes effect.

CARE TRANSITIONS

• Disposition greatly depends on functional status. Early consideration of the safest and most appropriate level of care on discharge is imperative.

○ Home discharge requires independence with mobility and self-care.

○ Home with services discharge is appropriate for patients who are able to care for themselves, but still require rehabilitation or nursing services for wound care or mobility, for example.

○ Acute rehabilitation is appropriate for patients who need medical supervision, but can participate in > 3 hours of therapy daily.

○ A skilled nursing facility (SNF) may be more appropriate for patients who need some medical supervision, but are only able to engage in 3 hours or less of therapy daily. Nursing home placement may be most appropriate for patients who are unable to care for themselves and need intermittent medical supervision.

○ Hospice services allow patients with terminal conditions to manage their pain and end-of-life needs with dignity.

BIBLIOGRAPHY

Bamman M, Clarke M, Feeback D, et al. Impact of resistance exercise during bed rest on skeletal muscle sarcopenia and myosin isoform distribution. *J Appl Physiol.* 1998;84(1):157–163.

Bamman M, Hunter G, Stevens B, et al. Resistance exercise prevents plantar flexor deconditioning during bed rest. *Med Sci Sports Exerc.* 1997;29(11):1462–1468.

Belin de Chantemèle E, Pascaud L, Custaud M, et al. Calf venous volume during stand-test after a 90-day bed-rest study with or without exercise countermeasure. *J Physiol.* 2004;561(2): 611–622.

Bleeker M, DeGroot P, Pawelczyk J, et al. Effects of 18 days of bed rest on leg and arm venous properties. *J Appl Physiol.* 2004;96:840–847.

Bleeker M, DeGroot P, Poelkens F, et al. Vascular adaptation to 4 wk of deconditioning by unilateral lower limb suspension. *Am J Physiol Heart Circ Physiol.* 2005;288:1747–1755.

Bleeker M, DeGroot P, Rongen G, et al. Vascular adaptation to deconditioning and the effect of an exercise countermeasure: results of the Berlin Bed Rest study. *J Appl Physiol.* 2005;99: 1293–1300.

Bonner CD. Rehabilitation instead of bed rest? *Geriatrics.* 1969;24(6):109–118.

Brown C, Friedkin R, Inouye S. Prevalence and outcomes of low mobility in hospitalized older patients. *JAGS.* 2204;52(8): 1263–1270.

Buschbacher RM, Porter CG. Deconditioning, conditioning, and the benefit of exercise. In: Braddom R, ed. *Physical Medicine and Rehabilitation.* 2nd ed. W.B. Saunders; 2000:702–726.

Cao P, Kimura S, Macias B, et al. Exercise within lower body negative partially counteracts lumbar spine deconditioning associated with 28-day bed rest. *J Appl Physiol.* 2005;99:39–44.

Fisher N, Pendergast D, Calkins E. Muscle rehabilitation in impaired elderly nursing home residents. *Arch Phys Med Rehab.* 1991;72:181–185.

Gillis A, MacDonald B. Deconditioning in the hospitalized elderly. *Can Nurse.* 2005;101:16–20.

Halar EM, Bell KR. Immobility and inactivity: physiological and functional changes, prevention, and treatment. In: DeLisa J, ed. *Physical Medicine and Rehabilitation: Principles and Practices.* 4th ed. Lippincott, Williams and Wilkins; 2004:1447–1467.

Hirsch C, Sommer L, Olsen A, et al. The natural history of functional morbidity in hospitalized older patients. *JAGS.* 1990;38:1296–1303.

Lazarus B, Murphy J, Coletta E, et al. The provision of physical activity to hospitalized elderly patients. *Arch Intern Med.* 1991;151(12):2452–2456.

Mahoney J, Sager M, Jalaluddin M. New walking dependence associated with hospitalization for acute medical illness: incidence and significance. *J Gerontology.* 1998;53A(4): M307–M312.

Mallery L, MacDonald E, Hubley-Kozey C, et al. The feasibility of performing resistance exercise with acutely ill hospitalized older adults. *BMC Geriat.* 2003;3:1–8.

McVey L, Becker P, Saltz C, et al. Effect of a geriatric consultation team on functional status of elderly hospitalized patients. *Ann Intern Med.* 1989;110(1):79–84.

Palmer R, Bolla L. When your patient is hospitalized: tips for primary care physicians. *Geriatrics.* 1997;52(9):36–42, 47.

Pawelczyk J, Zuckerman J, Blomqvist CG, et al. Regulation of muscle sympathetic nerve activity after bed rest deconditioning. *Am J Physiol Heart Circ Physiol.* 2001;280:2230–2239.

Sager M, Franke T, Inouye S, et al. Functional outcomes of acute medical illness and hospitalizations in older persons. *Arch Intern Med.* 1996;156(6):645–652.

Siebens H, Aronow H, Edwards D, et al. A randomized controlled trial of exercise to improve outcomes of acute hospitalization in older adults. *J Am Geriat Soc.* 2000;48:1545–1552.

Spaak J, Montmerle S, Sundblad P, et al. Long-term bed rest–induced reductions in stroke volume during rest and exercise: cardiac dysfunction vs. volume depletion. *J Appl Physiol.* 2005;98:648–654.

Warshaw G, Moore J, Friedman W, et al. Functional disability in the hospitalized elderly. *JAMA.* 1982;248(7):847–850.

92 NUTRITION AND THE HOSPITALIZED PATIENT

Vihas Patel and Malcolm K. Robinson

EPIDEMIOLOGY/OVERVIEW

- Malnutrition is common in hospitalized patients, ranging from 30% to 55% of inpatients.
- Malnutrition is associated with increased complications, lengths of stay, and healthcare costs.
- For hospitalists, nutrition care may be a challenging, but ultimately rewarding, endeavor, helping to improve wound healing and reducing morbidity, mortality, and rehospitalization rates.
  - For patients, hospitalization may be the first time their nutrition status is being evaluated, and presents us with an opportunity to intervene to improve their nutrition health.
  - Hospitalists, who are frequently called upon to consult on a variety of patients on medical and surgical subspecialty services, may be ideally suited to coordinate a hospital-wide nutrition intervention program where staffing demands allow for only cursory nutrition screening via nurse interviews and patient questionnaires.
  - These hospitalist-led nutrition rounds in community hospitals may help to identify the patient particularly susceptible to malnutrition earlier, and trigger more aggressive intervention.
- A nutrition care plan should be made for all hospitalized patients to improve overall outcome and should consist of screening, assessment, and development of an action plan.

○ Once implemented, the plan should be monitored and reformulated as indicated.

○ The plan may be as simple as providing foods from the hospital menu or as complex as total parenteral nutrition (TPN) supplemented with anabolic agents.

PATHOPHYSIOLOGY

• Illness stimulates release of a number of hormones which inhibit insulin release from the pancreas, blunt peripheral tissue responsiveness to insulin, and stimulate gluconeogenesis, proteolysis, and the hypermetabolic state.

○ Epinephrine, norepinephrine, cortisol, and various cytokines, notably interleukin-6 (IL-6), prevent the adaptive response of ketone body production and reduced metabolic rate seen in simple starvation.

• As a result, critically ill individuals depend on amino acids from lean tissue as building blocks for gluconeogenic pathways in the liver.

• There are increases in both protein synthesis and protein catabolism, with proteolysis overwhelming protein synthetic rates.

• The net result is rapid degradation of lean body mass, leading to decreased ability for the host to repair damaged tissue, fight infection, and recover from critical illness.

• Significant disability develops without nutritional support for those patients who cannot eat adequate calories and protein by mouth.

• Nutrition support may consist of oral supplements, tube feedings, TPN, or a combination thereof. Such support slows degradation of lean body mass in the sick by increasing protein synthesis to approach, but not equal, the increase in catabolism.

TRIAGE AND INITIAL MANAGEMENT

• A previously healthy person who is admitted to the hospital and is anticipated to fast for 1 or 2 days does not need nutritional support. However, if inadequate nutrition persists for weeks, weight loss will ensue.

○ This loss will accelerate if there is added critical illness.

○ When loss of body weight exceeds 30%, there is an increased likelihood of death.

○ Consensus and expert opinion mandate nutrition support well before such a critical state is reached.

• Nutrition screening should be the first step in developing an overall nutrition care plan. Ideally, a nutrition expert should evaluate all patients on hospital admission.

○ However, limited staff and resource availability often make this infeasible.

○ Consequently, many hospitals use a patient questionnaire administered by a nurse as their primary nutrition-screening tool.

• Alternatively, some healthcare facilities use a laboratory-based nutrition screening process in which plasma proteins indicative of nutritional status are evaluated in all patients on admission.

○ Such proteins include albumin, retinol-binding protein, and prealbumin.

○ Prealbumin may be the best of these three but more studies are needed to validate this possible finding.

• Factors indicative of malnutrition include:

○ Involuntary loss or gain of > 10% of usual body weight within 6 months or > 5% of usual body weight in 1 month.

○ Body weight of 20% more or less than ideal body weight, especially in the presence of chronic disease or increased metabolic requirements.

○ Inadequate nutrition intake including an impaired ability to ingest or absorb food adequately for at least 7–10 days. This would include severely ill patients with pancreatitis, peritonitis, major injury, or extensive burns.

○ Patients who do not meet one of these three general indications should be reassessed after 7 days.

• If nutrition screening identifies an individual who is malnourished or at risk for malnourishment, one should then determine energy (calorie) and protein needs.

ENERGY

• Both overfeeding and underfeeding calories in the hospital setting are associated with a variety of complications. Hence, calories should be administered in an amount sufficient to meet basal energy expenditure (BEE), hypercatabolism related to disease stress, and provide for physical activity without overfeeding calories.

• BEE can be estimated from predictive equations with reasonable accuracy. The most common predictive equations are the Harris-Benedict equations for men and women, where weight (W) in kg, height (H) in cm, and age (A) in years:

$$BEE_{men} \text{ kcal/d} = 66.5 + (13.8 \times W) + (5 \times H) - (6.8 \times A)$$

$$BEE_{women} \text{ kcal/d} = 655 + (9.5 \times W) + (1.8 \times H) - (4.7 \times A)$$

○ The Harris-Benedict equation has to be multiplied by a disease stress factor to account for hypercatabolism of disease and an activity factor.

◦ The disease stress factor can vary from 1.1 for mild illnesses up to 2.0 for burns covering a large proportion of the body surface area.

◦ The activity factor ranges from 1.0 for the heavily sedated, vented patient to 1.3 for the fully ambulatory patient. This estimated amount generally falls within a range of 30–35 kcal/kg/d for most individuals but can be inaccurate for those who are at the extremes, eg, those who are thin, obese, old, or the sickest, such as burn patients.

• In those for whom predictive equations are less accurate, indirect calorimetry using a metabolic cart is considered the gold standard for calorie determination in the clinical setting.

◦ The metabolic cart measures oxygen consumption and carbon dioxide production and calculates resting energy expenditure (REE) using the Weir equation. REE is then multiplied by an activity factor to account for how physically active the patient is.

◦ In contrast to the Harris-Benedict equation, the metabolic cart reading does not need to be multiplied by a stress factor because it already accounts for illness-related hypercatabolism.

• Obesity can be considered a form of malnutrition, which may affect the outcome of hospitalized patients. Although seemingly counterintuitive, it should be noted that obese individuals can be undernourished when there is significant acute weight loss.

◦ Hence they are prone to complications of nutritional deficiency similar to "normal"-weight individuals. Even if adequately fed, obese patients have a higher incidence of wound infections and hernias and may have a higher incidence of respiratory, cardiac, and thromboembolic complications.

◦ Nutrition support should be initiated expeditiously in obese patients with illnesses that produce significant catabolism. Starvation places these patients at risk for loss of lean body mass.

◦ Nutritional requirements in obese patients may be predicted using an "adjusted" body weight [((actual body weight − ideal body weight) × 0.25) + IBW] in the Harris-Benedict equation. This is an attempt to account for the increase in lean body mass seen in the obese patient. Alternatively, calorie intake can be estimated at 18–20 cal/kg actual body weight.

PROTEIN, CARBOHYDRATES, AND LIPIDS

• Protein demands in most hospitalized patients fall in the range of 1.2–1.5 g/kg/d. Protein should be included as part of the overall calorie calculations above.

• When calculating protein needs for an obese individual, the adjusted body weight should be used. The remaining calories are provided as lipid or fat and carbohydrate.

• Lipid should be provided to meet 20% to 25% of total calorie administration to prevent essential fatty acid deficiency. Lipid infusions above these levels are thought to cause immunosuppression and should be avoided.

• Carbohydrate is provided to make up the remaining calories not met through protein and fat administration. In general, carbohydrate should not be administered at an intravenous infusion rate > 5–7 mg/kg/min to avoid excessive carbon dioxide production that may compromise those with poor respiratory function, and to help maintain glucose control.

WATER AND ELECTROLYTES

• Water requirements are individualized to fluid balance and solute load. Alterations in fluid and electrolyte needs are managed in a patient-specific manner, taking into account disturbances of volume, concentration, and/or composition.

• The fluid requirement for adults is generally met with volumes of 30–40 mL/kg/d, or at 1–1.5 mL/kcal expended.

• Enteral electrolyte doses follow recommended dietary allowance (RDA) reference values. The standard dosing ranges for parenteral electrolytes assumes normal organ function, without abnormal losses.

VITAMINS AND TRACE ELEMENTS

• Vitamins and trace elements are essential nutrients that act as coenzymes and cofactors involved in metabolism.

• For patients with severe hyperbilirubinemia (eg, total bilirubin > 5.0), the copper and manganese should be removed from TPN to avoid toxicity, as these elements are not excreted normally.

INITIATING NUTRITION SUPPORT

• The third step in designing a nutrition plan is determining if the patient is meeting his or her estimated protein and calorie needs.

• If the patient is malnourished and not meeting their needs, the nutrition support is implemented. This usually consists of tube feeds or TPN. A vital decision in the nutrition care algorithm is the route of administration (see Fig. 92-1).

• Enteral nutrition is indicated for patients with a functional gastrointestinal tract whose oral nutrient intake is insufficient to meet estimated needs.

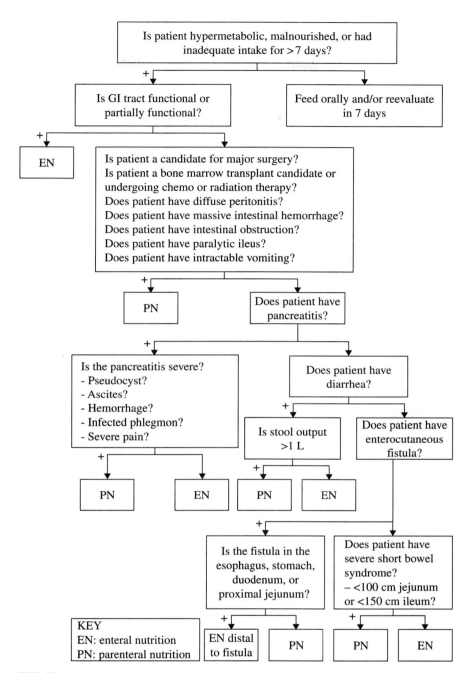

FIG. 92-1 Initiating nutrition support.

- Enteral nutrition is contraindicated in diffuse peritonitis, intestinal obstruction, intractable vomiting, paralytic ileus, intractable diarrhea, and gastrointestinal ischemia.
- Enteral nutrition should not be initiated until the patient is hemodynamically stable. Although commonly used as indicators of intestinal function, bowel sounds and passage of flatus are unreliable predictors of the eventual tolerance of enteral nutrition.

- Advantages of enteral nutrition over parenteral nutrition include reduced cost, better maintenance of gut integrity, reduced infection, and decreased hospital length of stay.
- Disadvantages are tube-feed intolerance as indicated by nausea, vomiting, and diarrhea which may make it difficult to meet nutrient goals. In addition, there is a risk of tube-feed aspiration.

ENTERAL ACCESS

- When selecting an enteral access device, the hospitalist must consider the patient's gastrointestinal anatomy and function, anticipated duration of enteral nutrition, and the potential for aspiration.
  - The nasoenteric tube is the most commonly used method for temporary enteral access because it has low complication rates, is relatively inexpensive, and easy to place.
  - Conversion to a tube enterostomy is indicated when long-term (eg, > 2–3 weeks) feeding is anticipated. Complications associated with tube enterostomies include perforation, hemorrhage, wound infection, bowel obstruction, bowel necrosis, and stomal leakage.
  - All feeding tubes are subject to mechanical complications, especially clogging. When water fails to declog feedings tubes, use of combinations of activated pancreatic enzymes and sodium bicarbonate mixed with water has been successful.
- Tube feeding may be administered into the stomach or small intestine.
  - The advantages of gastrostomy tubes are that they may be easier to place and allow for bolus, rather than continuous feedings. The disadvantages are that gastric feedings require intact gag and cough reflexes and adequate gastric emptying.
  - Small bowel access is indicated in clinical conditions in which tracheal aspiration, reflux esophagitis, gastroparesis, gastric outlet obstruction, or previous gastric surgery precludes gastric feedings, or when early postoperative feeding after major abdominal procedures is planned.
- Prevention of aspiration entails identification of high-risk patients, elevation of the head of the bed, careful monitoring of tube feeding delivery and patient tolerance, and adequate airway management.
  - Studies have not consistently demonstrated a benefit of small bowel feedings over gastric feedings to prevent aspiration. However, lack of an accepted definition of clinically significant aspiration makes interpretation of these studies difficult.
  - The physical presence of a nasogastric tube across the lower esophageal sphincter probably impairs sphincter function and promotes reflux of gastric contents.

INITIATING AND ADVANCING TUBE FEEDS

- Once the decision has been made to institute enteral feeding, and access has been obtained, the next decision is type of tube feed.
- Tube feeds may be classified as "polymeric" or "elemental."

- Polymeric diets contain carbohydrates; fats; and proteins in complex, undigested forms.
  - Carbohydrates are present as oligosaccharides, polysaccharides, or maltodextrins. Fats consist of medium- or long-chain triglycerides. The protein may be either intact or partially hydrolyzed.
  - Polymeric diets are usually isotonic, lactose free, and available in ready-to-use liquid form. Polymeric diets are suitable for most hospitalized patients.
- Elemental diets contain carbohydrate in the form of dextrose or oligosaccharides, protein as crystalline amino acids, or short peptides and fats as medium-chain triglycerides or essential fatty acids.
  - Because they are not palatable, elemental diets are rarely used as oral supplements.
  - Elemental diets may be appropriate in patients who have not had enteral nourishment for prolonged periods and/or have pathology of the intestinal mucosa which limits the ability to digest the macronutrient composition of polymeric formulas. Of note, however, elemental formulas are hypertonic and therefore may exacerbate diarrhea.
- After selecting the appropriate formula, it is started at a continuous delivery rate of 30 mL/h for 24 hours.
  - The patient's head should be elevated during enteral feeding to reduce the risk of regurgitation.
  - The presence of a tracheostomy or endotracheal tube does not ensure that regurgitated gastric contents will not be aspirated.
- Feeding intolerance is assessed continually until the tube feeding has been advanced to goal and the patient has remained stable on a regimen for several days.
  - Emesis, diarrhea, abdominal bloating, or a high gastric residual may indicate poor tolerance.
  - Although controversial, "high" gastric residual is generally defined as > 150–250 mL.
  - Blue food coloring is no longer used to monitor patients for microaspiration as there have been several case reports of death with this practice related to mitochondrial toxicity.
- If the patient tolerates the initial trial of enteral feeding, then the regimen may be advanced by 10–25 mL/h every 4–6 hours until the goal rate is achieved.
- If the risk of aspiration is minimal, intragastric feedings are preferred as they are better tolerated physiologically, easier to administer, and less restrictive for the patient than continuous feeding into the small intestine. Gastric feeds are less restrictive because they can be administered as boluses of 250–500 mL over 20–60 minutes.
- Patients fed into the small bowel should receive isotonic formulas delivered at an initial rate of 30 mL/h with the aid of a peristaltic pump. Hypertonic formulations have been associated with small bowel injury and necrosis.

- The most frequent complication is diarrhea. There are many causes of diarrhea in hospitalized patients receiving enteral nutrition, including antibiotic therapy and toxin-producing Clostridium difficile, fat or carbohydrate malabsorption, bacterial overgrowth as well as gastric acidity.
  - If all the other causes have been ruled out, the desired therapeutic approach is to adjust the enteral nutrition regimen as necessary rather than to discontinue it completely.
  - Only one variable of the feeding regimen (osmolality, volume, rate, or type of diet) should be altered at a time. Diluting formulas with water ("1/2" strength) is generally not recommended as a therapy for diarrhea as this just reduces the caloric value of the formula with little impact on the volume of diarrhea.
- Although enteral feeding is the preferred route of feeding, TPN is better than no or inadequate feeding for prolonged periods (eg, >7–10 days) and should be initiated in those who cannot tolerate enteral feeding.
- If the decision to administer TPN is made, a dedicated central access must be obtained.
  - The osmolarity of TPN is > 900 mOsm/L, compared to blood, which is typically 200–300 mOsm/L. The hyperosmolarity of TPN requires infusion into a central vein where it can be rapidly diluted upon infusion into the bloodstream, preventing phlebitis and thrombosis.

PARENTERAL ACCESS

- Parenteral nutrition administration requires central venous access in order to provide nutrients at greater concentrations than is possible through peripheral veins.
- For hospitalized patients, temporary central venous catheters inserted through the subclavian vein or peripheral arm veins (ie, peripherally inserted central catheter or PICC) are often most appropriate.
- Catheters inserted through the femoral vein are associated with higher risk of venous thrombosis and catheter-related sepsis and are not recommended for parenteral nutrition.
- For long-term therapy in a nonhospital setting, subcutaneously tunneled catheters (eg, Hickman catheters) or implanted subcutaneous infusion ports (eg, port-a-cath) are most commonly used.
- The management of catheter-related sepsis should involve catheter removal and appropriate antibiotic coverage.
  - Prophylactic catheter exchange over a guidewire has not been shown to decrease the risk of catheter-associated infection.[6]
  - Central venous catheters impregnated with chlorhexidine and silver sulfadiazine or with minocycline and rifampin are associated with a lower rate of blood stream infection than untreated catheters. Because of the higher cost of these catheters it is probably reasonable to restrict their use to units with particularly high infection rates.

  - No one device has been shown to provide the lowest rate of complications with the greatest therapeutic benefit and ease of maintenance for all patients.

TOTAL PARENTERAL NUTRITION PRESCRIPTION

- The TPN prescription is determined by the nutritional assessment. The patient's energy, protein, and fluid requirements should be calculated and the patient's need for specialized nutrients and other additives should be considered. See Table 92-1.

TABLE 92-1   TPN Worksheet and Sample Calculation

You are caring for a 55-year-old woman with gastric outlet obstruction from adenocarcinoma. She vomits everything taken by mouth. While she is undergoing cardiac workup for surgery, a central line is inserted with a dedicated port for TPN. Her height is 66 in (168 cm) and weight is 60 kg. She ambulates without difficulty.

1. Estimate BEE, where W in kg, H in cm, and A in years based on Harris-Benedict equation:

$$BEE_{women} \text{ kcal/d} = 655 + (9.5 \times 60 \text{ kg}) + (1.8 \times 168 \text{ cm}) - (4.7 \times 55 \text{ years}) = 1268$$

and
disease stress factor: 1.1 for mild
activity factor: 1.3 for the ambulatory patient

$$BEE \times 1.1 \times 1.3 = 1813 \text{ kcal/d}$$

or simply,

kcal/kg/d	clinical situation
20–25	elderly, debilitated, bedridden, nonstressed
25	ventilated and sedated
25–30	maintenance, mild stress, minimal activity
30–35	significant activity, weight gain

$$30 \times 60 \text{ kg} = 1800 \text{ kcal/d}$$

2. Calculate daily protein requirement:

Protein (g/kg/d)	clinical situation
0.8–1.0	elderly, minimal stress, maintenance
1.0–1.3	mild to moderate stress, repletion
1.3–1.5	severe stress, aggressive repletion

$$\text{dry weight} \times 1.2 = 72 \text{ g/d}$$

3. Calculate fluid needs:

$$60 \text{ kg} \times 30 \text{ mL/kg} = 1800 \text{ mL}$$

4. Final calorie breakdown:

Protein:	72 g × 4 kcal/g = 288 kcal
25% fat:	1800 kcal × 0.25 = 450 kcal
Dextrose:	1800 – 288 – 450 = 1062 kcal
	1062 kcal/3.4 kcal/g = 312 g

5. Most institutions require macronutrient orders per liter bag of TPN:

Fluid:	1.8 L/d
Protein:	72 g/1.8 L = 40 g/L (or 4.0% amino acid)
Dextrose:	312 g/1.8 L = 173 g/L (or 17% dextrose)
Fat:	450 kcal/d
Goal TPN:	1.8 L D17, AA4.0% with 450 calories additional fat

6. Day 1, order TPN containing 50% of goal needs, baseline labs including electrolytes, liver enzymes, renal parameters, triglyceride level, and fingerstick glucose checks with insulin coverage

7. Day 2, advance TPN to goal if patient tolerates above

TPN, total parenteral nutrition.

- Always start with half of the estimated needs on the first day and increase to full estimated needs on the second to allow for assessment of tolerance (hyperglycemia, hypertriglyceridemia, hypophosphatemia).
- Parenteral amino acids provide 4 kcal/g. Carbohydrate in parenteral nutrition is in the form of dextrose monohydrate and provides 3.4 kcal/g and *not* 4 kcal/g as the nonhydrated form of dextrose dose.
- The maximum oxidative rate (maximum glucose infusion rate) is 5 mg/kg/min to maintain glucose control and minimize carbon dioxide production which may compromise the individual with respiratory dysfunction.
- Fat provides 9.3 kcal/g. Lipids in TPN are also an important source of essential fatty acids. Lipid infusion should not exceed 2.5 g/kg since excessive fat infusion can cause immunosuppression.
- Lipid infusion may also be limited by hypertriglyceridemia > 400 mg/dL and the associated risk of pancreatitis. Lastly, lipid infusion may be impossible in patients with egg or soy allergies.
- Although there are many ways to estimate fluid needs, the fluid requirement for adults is generally met with volumes of 30–40 mL/kg/d, or at 1–1.5 mL/kcal expended.
- Other TPN additives, such as electrolytes, vitamins, and trace elements, will also need to be prescribed with consideration of the patient's renal and hepatic function.

DISEASE MANAGEMENT STRATEGIES

MONITORING NUTRITION

- Monitoring patients maintained on nutrition support is necessary to determine efficacy, detect and prevent complications, evaluate changes in clinical condition, and document clinical outcomes.
- Changes in clinical condition and activity level may require periodic recalculation of energy requirements. If the patient is not responding appropriately, indirect calorimetry may be used to guide changes and reassess needs periodically. As oral feeding improves, TPN and tube feeds should be weaned or discontinued.
- It should be noted that no amount of nutritional support can help a malnourished individual until the primary disease process is controlled. Devitalized tissue must be removed, infection must be controlled, and organ failure must be optimized for nutrition support to have an impact. "Inadequate response to nutrition"

may in fact represent inability to control the primary disease process and not inadequate nutrition.
- Studies have shown that hypoalbuminemia is associated with poor clinical outcome.[4]
  - Although albumin levels may have prognostic value, they have been found to be poor indicators of the adequacy of nutrition support in the hospital setting.
  - Serum transferrin has a short half-life (8.8 days) and may more accurately reflect acute protein depletion and replenishment.
  - Frequent measurements of prealbumin (half-life of 2–3 days) may help assess nutrition status changes in response to therapy. It is important to note that prealbumin levels may be raised or lowered by factors other than nutritional status. This includes patient hydration status, liver or renal dysfunction, the presence of inflammatory conditions, and use of drugs such as corticosteroids.
- Patients should also be monitored for complications associated with nutrition support.
  - The life-threatening refeeding syndrome is a complication that may arise during aggressive administration of both enteral and parenteral nutrition support.
  - Rapid reintroduction of large amounts of carbohydrate feedings can result in metabolic abnormalities, including hypophosphatemia, hypokalemia, and hypomagnesemia.
  - At greatest risk for the syndrome are chronically starved marasmic patients whose bodies have adapted largely to use of free fatty acids and ketone bodies as energy sources.
- Both hyperglycemia and hypoglycemia are potential complications of nutrition support. Efforts to monitor and control blood glucose during nutrition support are prudent, given the association of hyperglycemia with decreased immune function and increased risk of infectious complications.
  - Data from a large controlled trial in intensive care unit patients showed that keeping blood glucose levels below 127 mg/dL (7 mmol/L) significantly reduced mortality from sepsis-related multisystem organ failure.[5]
  - The challenge for hospitalists when providing nutrition support to patients with diabetes is to achieve and maintain euglycemia. Blood glucose control should be optimized *before* nutrition support begins.
  - There is increasing evidence that glucose control is important in hospitalized patients because hyperglycemia can adversely affect immune function and fluid balance as well as contribute to gastroparesis and impaired small bowel motility.

- For insulin-dependent patients who are receiving TPN, the same amount of insulin that would normally be taken is added to the parenteral nutrition solution and titrated to blood glucose concentrations.
- Abrupt discontinuation of parenteral nutrition is not recommended in patients with diabetes because of the potential for hypoglycemia.
- "Ramping" down is not necessary in patients without diabetes and the infusion can be discontinued all at once as these patients do not typically become hypoglycemic.
- Gastroparesis in and of itself is not an indication for parenteral nutrition. Gastroparesis may be managed with pharmacologic agents and low-fat and fiber-free enteral formulas. Alternatively, feeding into the small bowel via nasojejunal or jejunostomy tubes may allow enteral nourishment in the patient with gastroparesis.
- Other complications include hypertriglyceridemia, which may occur in some patients receiving intravenous fat emulsion. This may lead to the development of pancreatitis.
- Overfeeding with dextrose calories may result in the production of excess carbon dioxide. This may lead to difficulty with ventilatory support and weaning.
- Hepatobiliary complications, ranging from steatosis to cholestasis, as well as metabolic bone disease may arise during administration of parenteral nutrition.

CARE TRANSITIONS

- Malnutrition affects many hospitalized patients, impacting their morbidity, mortality, length of stay, and healthcare cost. For these reasons, nutrition support of the hospitalized patient can be a challenging yet rewarding endeavor.
- Hospitalists can collaborate with nutrition experts to design comprehensive nutrition care plans consisting of screening, assessment, prescription, and monitoring for efficacy and complications.
- This nutrition care plan may have to be reformulated for care transition to home or extended care facility.

BIBLIOGRAPHY

ASPEN Board of Directors and the Clinical Guidelines Task Force. Guidelines for the use of parenteral and enteral nutrition in adult and pediatric patients. *JPEN J Parenter Enteral Nutr.* 2002;26(1 Suppl):1SA–138SA.

McGee DC, Gould MK. Preventing complications of central venous catheterization. *N Engl J Med.* 2003;348(12): 1123–1133.

Robinson MK, Trujillo EB, Mogensen KM, et al. Improving nutritional screening of hospitalized patients: the role of prealbumin. *JPEN J Parenter Enteral Nutr.* 2003;27(6):389–95.

Rolandelli RH, Gupta D, Wilmore DW. Nutritional support. In: Souba WW, et al, eds. *ACS Surgery: Principles and Practice.* WebMD Inc.; New York: 2005:1566–1587.

van der Berghe G, Wouters P, Weekers F, et al. Intensive insulin therapy in critically ill patients. *N Engl J Med.* 2001;345(19): 1359–1367.

The Veterans Affairs Total Parenteral Nutrition Cooperative Study Group. Perioperative total parenteral nutrition in surgical patients. *N Engl J Med.* 1991;325(8):525–532.

93 PAIN MANAGEMENT
Darin J. Correll

BACKGROUND

- Pain can be defined as an unpleasant sensory and emotional experience associated with actual or potential tissue damage. It is probably the most common presenting or associated symptom in patients in the hospital.
- The Joint Commission on Accreditation of Healthcare Organizations (JCAHO) mandates that all patients have the right to adequate assessment and management of pain and that they must be informed that this is a part of their treatment (Table 93-1).
- In studies of postoperative patients, better pain control leads to possible benefits in terms of fewer cardiovascular and respiratory complications; probable benefits in terms of endocrine and immunologic outcomes and definite benefits in terms of gastrointestinal and hematologic outcomes. Table 93-2 lists the possible negative physiologic consequences, by system, of uncontrolled pain.
- Other reasons to control pain in the acute setting are that patients are often more concerned about being in pain than they are about the primary reason for being in the hospital, quality of recovery is improved, and acute pain can become persistent if not treated properly.

DEFINITIONS

- Acute pain is relatively brief in duration. It is most commonly experienced following injury to the body from some defined source and ends when the injury has healed.

TABLE 93-1   JCAHO Pain Assessment and Management Standards for Hospitals

STANDARD	INTENT
1. Patients have the right to appropriate assessment and management of pain	a. Initial assessment and regular reassessment of pain
	b. Education of all relevant providers in pain assessment and management
	c. Education of patients, and families when appropriate, regarding their roles in managing pain as well as the potential limitations and side effects of pain treatments
	d. After taking into account personal, cultural, spiritual, and/or ethnic beliefs, communicating to patients and families that pain management is an important part of care
2. Pain is assessed in all patients	a. The organization identifies patients with pain
	b. The assessment and a measure of pain intensity and quality (e.g., pain character, frequency, location, and duration), appropriate to the patient's age, are recorded in a way that facilitates regular reassessment and follow-up according to criteria developed by the organization
3. Patients are educated about pain and managing pain as part of treatment, as appropriate	a. Patients and families are instructed about understanding pain, the risk for pain, the importance of effective pain management, the pain assessment process, and methods for pain management, when identified as part of treatment

JCAHO = Joint Commission on Accreditation of Healthcare Organizations.

- Persistent (or chronic) pain is of relatively long duration, often lasting months to years. It is generally considered pain that lasts beyond the time at which an injury has healed or is excessive for the level of injury. It may be associated with ongoing and/or progressive illness or have no clear etiology at all.
- Hyperalgesia is the experience of a significant amount of pain from a mildly noxious stimulus.
- Allodynia is the experience of pain from a nonnoxious stimulus.

PAIN MANAGEMENT GUIDELINES

- Listen to and believe the patient; pain is always subjective and the provider must accept the patient's report of pain.
- Pain is the consequence of the filtering, modulating, and distorting of the afferent nerve activity (nociceptive input) through the affective (limbic system) and cognitive processes unique to each individual.
- One positive thing from the fact that pain is an affective and cognitive experience is that the placebo response to analgesics is real and can be helpful. Using a placebo should never include lying to patients or giving them an inactive substance to determine if

TABLE 93-2   Physiologic Consequences of Uncontrolled Pain

Cardiovascular	Tachycardia, hypertension, increased cardiac workload
Pulmonary	Hypoxia, hypercarbia, atelectasis, decreased cough
Gastrointestinal	Decreased gastric emptying, nausea/vomiting, ileus
Renal	Urinary retention
Endocrine	Increased adrenergic activity, catabolic state, sodium/water retention
Immunologic	Impairment, slowed wound healing
Musculoskeletal	Splinting, contractures, decreased mobility (DVT)
Hematologic	Increased coagulability
Neurologic	Anxiety, fear, anger, fatigue, delirium

DVT, deep vein thrombosis.

they are lying or to punish them. Instead, the benefit of the placebo effect is that if a patient believes that a particular therapy is going to work, it is more likely to work. Therefore, truthfully "talk up" genuine attempts at analgesia. This also works in reverse; if a patient tells you a particular therapy "never works for them," then more than likely it isn't going to work.
- Assess the patient's level of pain and degree of pain relief appropriately and regularly.
- Diagnose and treat the nonpain aspects of the patient's disease appropriately.
- Treat pain quickly; do not withhold therapy while seeking a diagnosis; pain treatment will not impair the ability to diagnosis a disease.
- Use a comprehensive plan that addresses the multidimensional aspects of pain. This may require an interdisciplinary team approach (eg, hospitalist, pain specialist, anesthesiologist, surgeon, psychiatrist/ psychologist, physical therapist), especially for patients with persistent pain.
- Always discuss the analgesic plan with the patient and family, understand the patient's expectations for pain management, and offer reasonable goals for the therapy.
- A multimodal approach for managing pain is always better than using a single modality to its "limit"; this may include both pharmacologic and nonpharmacologic measures. This approach allows for the best possible analgesia with the lowest incidence of side effects.
- Understand the use of several agents within each class of analgesics, including side effects expected, because individual responses vary greatly.
- If pain is present most of the time or expected to last for an extended period of time (eg, greater than a few weeks), dose around the clock or with long-acting agents. As-needed (prn) dosing of immediate-release agents is also needed for breakthrough pain. If pain is intermittent or expected to last a short time (eg, less than a couple weeks), prn dosing of immediate release agents can be used.

- Communication with the patient's primary care provider regarding the discharge analgesic plan is essential, especially if there has been an alteration to a prior analgesic regimen. Ensure that the patient has adequate follow-up to monitor for the effectiveness of the analgesic regimen and development of possible side effects on discharge from the hospital. There should also be a follow-up plan for a taper off of analgesics—if the patient was not on chronic analgesics prior to admission.

PAIN ASSESSMENT

- Location—where the patient is experiencing pain and any radiation from the primary location.
- Intensity—using scales appropriate to the patient and situation.
- Character—have the patient describe the pain using adjectives.
- Pattern—is the pain constant, intermittent, worse at certain times of day?
- Aggravating and alleviating factors—is there anything that makes the pain worse or better?
- Impact on functional ability—does the pain affect the patient's activities of daily living as an outpatient, but also is it affecting the ability to cough, get out of bed, ambulate, and so on while in the hospital?
- Prior analgesic history—what therapies have either worked or not worked in the past?
- Ongoing analgesics—is the patient taking any analgesic agents presently, and if so, the exact doses?

- Concomitant health history—medical and psychologic comorbidities, social and family history.
- Physical examination—a directed examination of the location of the pain as well as a generalized physical examination of the patient, as appropriate.
- Diagnostic tests—the use of tests to diagnose the etiology of pain may be useful in some situations (eg, x-rays to diagnose a fracture, magnetic resonance imaging (MRI) to diagnose nerve impingement in the spinal cord, or electromyogram (EMG) to diagnose a neuropathy). However, absence of an abnormality on a test should not be used to discount a patient's report of pain.

PAIN INTENSITY

- The most commonly used measurement tools for intensity of pain in the inpatient acute setting are the single-dimension scales (Table 93-3).
- A numerical rating scale is a written scale with the numbers 0 to 10 spaced evenly across a page where 0 is "no pain at all" and 10 is "the worst pain imaginable." Patients are instructed to circle the number that represents the amount of pain they are experiencing at the time of evaluation. A more common variation of this scale is the verbal numeric scale where patients are asked to verbally state a number between 0 and 10 to correspond to their present pain intensity.
- Some people prefer to use words to describe the intensity of their pain; these are termed verbal descriptor scales.
- Variations of the single-dimension scales that may be of benefit in the elderly or cognitively impaired are scales

TABLE 93-3   Single-Dimension Scales

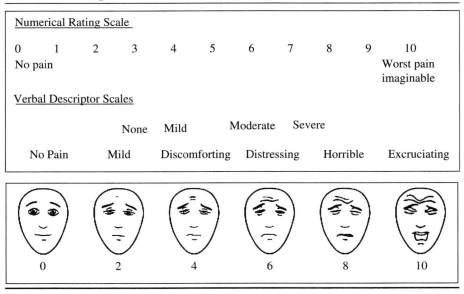

Numerical Rating Scale

0	1	2	3	4	5	6	7	8	9	10
No pain										Worst pain imaginable

Verbal Descriptor Scales

	None	Mild	Moderate	Severe	
No Pain	Mild	Discomforting	Distressing	Horrible	Excruciating

| 0 | 2 | 4 | 6 | 8 | 10 |

The Faces Pain Scale.
Source: Revised from *PAIN*. 2001;93:173–183. Used with permission from IASP.
For administration instructions see www.painsourcebook.ca

that use drawn faces ranging from a content-looking, smiling face to a distressed-looking face (eg, Faces Pain Scale or Wong-Baker Faces Scale) instead of relying on the patient choosing a number or word for their pain.

- The benefits of single-dimension scales are that they are quick and easy to use; this is important in the acute setting when repeated measures are needed over a brief period of time.
- One disadvantage of single-dimension scales is that they attempt to assign a single value to a complex, multidimensional experience. Another disadvantage is that patients can never know if the present experience is the "worst." A final disadvantage is that these scales have a ceiling at the upper-most end in that if a value of "10" is chosen and the pain worsens, the patient officially has no way to express this change.
- Several multidimensional scales exist that attempt to assess various aspects of the patient's pain experience (eg, McGill Pain Questionnaire, Brief Pain Inventory, Multidimensional Affect, and Pain Survey).
- The major benefit of multidimensional scales is that they take into account the complex nature of the pain experience.
- The major disadvantage of using these scales in the acute setting is that they are too long for rapid or repeated use.
- One compromise is to attempt to address a limited multidimensional aspect of pain, possibly using a few single-dimension scales to address the issues that appear to be important to hospitalized patients—pain, anxiety, depression, anger, fear, and interference with physical activity.

DETERMINE MECHANISM OF PAIN

- In order to choose the correct therapy for treating pain, the underlying mechanism or generator of the pain needs to be determined (Table 93-4).

- One of the best ways to determine this is to have the patient use adjectives to describe the character of the pain (eg, aching, burning, dull, electric-like, sharp, shooting, stabbing, tender, throbbing).

CONCOMITANT HEALTH HISTORY

- Medical conditions that may lead to or contribute to pain include cancer, diabetes, osteoarthritis, rheumatoid arthritis, herpes zoster infection, or spinal cord injury.
- Psychologic conditions that have been shown to adversely affect a patient's pain experience, therefore needing appropriate diagnosis and therapy, are anxiety (most prevalent in acute pain states), depression (most prevalent in persistent pain states), fear, catastrophizing, and certain personality disorders.
- A family history may reveal the presence of substance abuse in others related to the patient, which is a risk factor for addiction in the patient.
- A social history is important to determine the use of alcohol or tobacco, to use appropriate agents to prevent the development of withdrawal (ie, benzodiazepines or nicotine patches). Also, elicitation of substance abuse is important to guide therapy and prevent withdrawal by proper selection of agent and dose.

PHYSICAL EXAMINATION

- Pain (especially acute) may be associated with tachycardia, hypertension, diaphoresis, and tachypnea.
- However, since measures of sympathetic activation are common and nonspecific, physical findings in hospitalized patients offer little help in the diagnosis and treatment of pain in an awake, competent patient.

TABLE 93-4 Determine Mechanism of Pain

PAIN MECHANISM	CHARACTER	EXAMPLES	TREATMENT OPTIONS
Somatic	Usually well localized and constant; aching, sharp, stabbing	• Laceration • Fracture • Burn • Abrasion • Localized infection or inflammation	• Heat/Cold • Acetaminophen • NSAIDs • Opioids • Local anesthetics (topical or infiltrate)
Visceral	Not well localized; can be constant or intermittent; generalized ache, pressure, or cramping, can be sharp	• Muscles/Spasm • Colic or obstruction (GI or renal) • Sickle cell • Internal organ infection or inflammation	• NSAIDs • Opioids • Muscle relaxants • Local anesthetics (nerve blocks)
Neuropathic	Can be localized (i.e., dermatomal) or radiating, can also be generalized and not well localized; burning, tingling, electric shock, lancinating	• Trigeminal • Postherpetic • Postamputation • Peripheral neuropathy • Nerve infiltration	• Anticonvulsants • Tricyclic antidepressants • Muscle relaxants • NMDA antagonists • Neural/Neuraxial blockade

- They can be used as surrogate measures in someone who cannot verbalize their pain experience.
- Patients may not exhibit any alterations in vital signs despite significant levels of pain, especially persons who have persistent pain.

ANALGESIC MODALITIES

- Nonpharmacologic measures: In general, the scientific data on the use of these measures are limited; however, most of them have little risk and if the patient believes that the therapies are going to help then they are likely to be of at least some benefit, because of the cognitive and affective nature of pain.
- Pharmacologic measures: there are many different agents available for use that fall into three basic categories:
  - Nonopioid analgesics
  - Opioids
  - Adjuvant analgesics
- There is no one correct way to treat a patient in pain. It is best to individualize therapy for each patient. There are some schemes that can be used to guide the development of a regimen (Table 93-5). These schemes encompass the concepts of using a multimodal approach, the addition or alteration of agents when pain control is inadequate, and the need to alter or diminish agents as pain resolves.

NONPHARMACOLOGIC MEASURES

- Application of cold (to reduce inflammation) or heat (to reduce spasms) to muscles or joints are commonly employed techniques, but the evidence for a benefit is mixed.
- Hypnosis has been shown to reduce pain specifically associated with medical procedures; however it requires specific training and time to administer.
- Transcutaneous electrical nerve stimulation (TENS) has shown conflicting results in terms of an analgesic benefit in the acute setting, but has relatively good evidence to show it reduces the need for pharmacologic analgesics.
- Relaxation and guided imagery have shown little evidence for any benefit in the acute setting.
- Attentional techniques can be complicated in that one needs to determine which approach is better for a particular patient. Some patients will do better when

TABLE 93-5 Suggested Pain Management

The World Health Organization has devised the following "Analgesic Ladder" to use for the treatment of cancer pain. The concepts behind it are useful in the management of all types of pain, both persistent and acute.

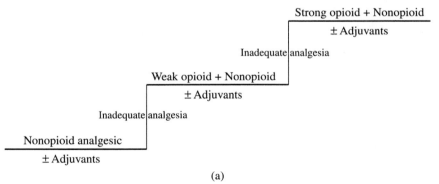

(a)

The World Federation of Societies of Anaesthesiologists has devised the following "Analgesic Ladder" to use for the treatment of acute/postoperative pain.

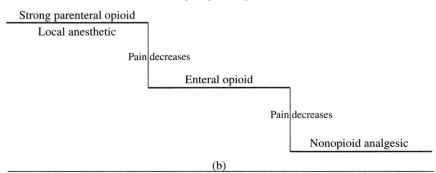

(b)

TABLE 93-6   Select Nonopioid Analgesics

AGENT	ADULT DOSING	MAXIMUM DOSE	COMMENTS
Acetaminophen	650–1000 mg q 6 hours	4000 mg	Single doses above 1000 mg do not improve analgesia
Choline magnesium trisalicylate	1000–1500 mg bid	3000 mg	Caution in liver disease, avoid in severe liver disease
Diclofenac	50 mg bid-qid	200 mg	Low GI effect incidence, but possible increased renal effects, recent data suggest increased negative CV effects
Etodalac	200–400 mg q 6–8 hours	1000 mg	Low GI and renal effect incidence, safest NSAID in liver disease
Ibuprofen	400–600 mg q 4–6 hours	3000 mg	<1500 mg qd has low risk of GI effects, possible increased renal effects, inhibits CV benefits of aspirin when given concomitantly
Ketorolac	30 mg q 6 hours	120 mg	High risk of renal and GI complications; use for no more than 5 days; 15 mg q 6 hours in renal impairment, age >65 years, weight <50 kg
Nabumetone	750–1500 mg qd or bid	1500 mg	Low GI effect incidence
Naproxen	250–500 mg q 6–12 hours	1500 mg	Possible increased liver and renal effects, probably least negative CV effects
Celecoxib	100–200 mg qd	200 mg	Use 100 mg dose if possible; long-term use has increased negative CV effects

GI, gastrointestinal; CV, cardiovascular

instructed to shift attention away from the pain, whereas others will do better if they are instructed to attend to a particular "part" of the pain experience (ie, the sensory component as opposed to the emotional component).

- Acupuncture and electroacupuncture have been shown to be of benefit in the acute setting both to improve pain and to reduce common side effects of opioid analgesics; however it requires specific training and time to administer.

NONOPIOID ANALGESICS (TABLE 93-6)

- Nonacetylated salicylates (choline magnesium trisalicylate and salsalate) have a low incidence of gastrointestinal disturbance probably because of no effect on platelets and bleeding.
- Acetaminophen is not an anti-inflammatory agent and is not associated with gastrointestinal disturbances or platelet effects. Acetaminophen, however, can be hepatotoxic.
- Nonselective nonsteroidal anti-inflammatory drugs (NSAIDs) have negative effects on platelets, gastrointestinal, and renal systems. Recent data suggest that there may be increased risk of major cardiovascular events with certain NSAIDs. No one NSAID appears to be more effective as an analgesic than any other, but there is great inter patient variability in response; thus changing agents may be of benefit if one does not seem to be effective.
- COX-2 selective NSAIDs have no affect on platelet aggregation, less effect on the GI mucosa, but equal chance of renal toxicity compared to nonselective NSAIDs. Should not be considered as first-line agents, given high cost and should not be used long term at high doses, given the data that they increase the risk of major cardiovascular events.

OPIOIDS: TERMINOLOGY

- Tolerance—a physiologic phenomenon in which an individual's response to a drug's effect diminishes over time, or in order to maintain the same effect the drug dose needs to be increased. Tolerance development is the result of a down-regulation of the agonist's receptors.
- Dependence—a state of physiologic adaptation that develops with continued use of a drug that manifests as a withdrawal syndrome if the drug is abruptly stopped, the dose is dramatically reduced, or an antagonist is given.
- Addiction—a primary, chronic, neurobiologic disease with many factors influencing its development. It manifests as drug-seeking behaviors, impaired control over the drug, and continued use despite negative effects. *Tolerance to and/or dependence on opioids do not equal addiction*!
- Pseudoaddiction—a term used to describe iatrogenically induced patient behaviors that mimic "drug seeking" and "craving" that occur solely because of the undertreatment of pain. When the pain is adequately managed the behaviors resolve.

OPIOID THERAPY BASICS

- Generally it is recommended to use pure opioid agonists, especially with moderate to severe pain, as opposed to the agonist/antagonists.
- The commonly used agonists can be classified as in Table 93-7.

TABLE 93-7   Opioid Classification

NOT RECOMMENDED	WEAK	STRONG
Meperidine	Codeine	Fentanyl
Propoxyphene	Hydrocodone	Hydromorphone
	Tramadol	Methadone
		Morphine
		Oxycodone
		Oxymorphone

- Efficacy relates to the proportion of available receptors an agonist needs to bind in order to exhibit its full effect. This may become relevant in the opioid tolerant (ie, because of the presence of down-regulated receptors)—low-efficacy opioids (eg, codeine, hydrocodone, propoxyphene, meperidine, morphine) often cannot provide adequate analgesia; when there are not enough receptors available, they effectively become partial agonists. In these cases, high-efficacy opioids (eg, hydromorphone, oxycodone, methadone) are more likely to result in better analgesia.
- Be familiar with the characteristics of several opioid agonists (Table 93-8).

- The optimal analgesic dose varies widely among patients, even the opioid naïve.
- The analgesic effect and side effects from opioids varies widely between patients. Ask the patient which opioids have either worked or not worked in the past and/or have given them intolerable side effects. There are at least 10 different mu receptor subtypes, the expression of which differs between individuals, and the various opioids have different levels of effect at each. This may explain the inter-patient variation in opioid effectiveness and side effects.
- Monitor patients closely for effectiveness and side-effects whenever there is a change of agent and/or

TABLE 93-8   Opioid Characteristics

AGONIST	ROUTE	EQUIANALGESIC DOSE (MG)	ONSET (MIN)	PEAK EFFECT (MIN)	DURATION OF EFFECT (H)
Morphine	IV	10	5–10	10–30	3–5
	Oral	30	15–60	60–120	4–6
	Oral CR	–	30–120	180–240	8–12
	Oral SR	–	30–120	480–600	8–24
Codeine	IM	120	10–30	90–120	4–6
	Oral	200	30–45	60	3–4
Hydromorphone	IV	1.5	5–20	15–30	3–4
	Oral	7.5	15–30	90–120	4–6
Oxycodone	Oral	20	15–30	30–60	4–6
	Oral CR	–	30–60	90–180	8–12
Methadone	IV	10*	10–20	60–120	4–6
	Oral	20*	30–60	90–120	4–12
Fentanyl	IV	0.1	<1	5–7	0.75–2+
	TD	(See Table 93-11)	720–1080	1440–4320	48–72
Oxymorphone	IV	1	5–10	30–60	3–6
	Oral†	10	meaningful relief = 60		4–6

IV, intravenous; CR, controlled release; SR, sustained release; IM, intramuscular; TD, transdermal.

†Recent FDA approval of oral form, therefore limited clinical experience; also available as a 12 hour extended release form.

*These doses are based on single administration and should only be used to convert between po and IV methadone. If converting a patient who has been on a different opioid use, the following table that takes into account the dose-dependent potency changes seen with methadone:

Equianalgesic Conversion to Methadone‡

ORAL MORPHINE EQUIVALENT THAT PATIENT IS TAKING	ORAL METHADONE (MG)	ORAL MORPHINE (MG)
<100 mg/d	1	4
101–300 mg/d	1	8
301–600 mg/d	1	10
601–800 mg/d	1	12
801–1000 mg/d	1	15
>1000 mg/d	1	20

To determine the starting dose of oral methadone
- Convert the patient's daily opioid dose into oral morphine equivalents.
- Convert the daily oral morphine equivalents to a daily oral methadone dose using the table.
- Reduce the calculated daily oral methadone dose by 30% to 50%.
- Divide the resulting reduced daily dose by 3.
- Prescribe this dose of oral methadone (in mg) every 8 hours.

‡This chart is not meant to be used to convert from methadone to other opioids. There is limited data on the conversion from methadone to other agents and often inadequate analgesia results. Thus if it is necessary to convert from methadone to another opioid agonist, it is best performed in stages with close monitoring of the patient for effectiveness (e.g., over a 3-day period introduce the new agent as the methadone dose is tapered by 1/3 each day).

route or if there is the addition of another analgesic to the regimen.

OPIOID CHOICES

- Codeine is not a good first choice because of the fact that maybe around 30% of the population does not have an active form of the enzyme (ie, cytochrome P450 2D6) necessary to convert codeine into an active drug in the body (ie, morphine).
- All opioids should be used with caution in patients with renal or hepatic insufficiency, where lower doses or longer dosing intervals may be necessary. Morphine is relatively contraindicated in patients with severe renal insufficiency because of the accumulation of the metabolite, morphine-6-glucuronide, which can lead to sedation and respiratory depression.
- *Meperidine is not recommended for pain management.* Its active metabolite, normeperidine, can accumulate in a day or two to levels that cause nervous system excitation (tremors, muscle twitching, convulsions). It causes a strong euphoric feeling especially when given IV push. It is a weak agonist as well as having low efficacy. It usually causes more nausea than other agents.
- *Proproxyphene is not recommended for pain management.* Its active metabolite, norpropoxyphene, can accumulate with high doses, renal or hepatic insufficiency, or in the elderly, leading to nervous system toxicity. It is a weak agonist as well as having low efficacy.
- Hydrocodone use needs to be monitored closely because of the acetaminophen component in all the available preparations. Also, the most frequent nonmedical use of a pharmaceutical agent leading to an emergency department visit is hydrocodone combination preparations.

OPIOID ADMINISTRATION

- Whenever possible, the enteral route of administration is best as it is the easiest route and offers the most stable pharmacokinetics.
- If not able to use the enteral route or if unable to attain adequate analgesia in a timely manner, use intravenous (IV) administration.
- Intramuscular administration is not recommended (*it hurts* and has unpredictable pharmacokinetics).
- With a competent patient, the use of an intravenous patient-controlled analgesia (PCA) has been demonstrated

to offer the best overall pain management option (see section: PCA Basics).

OPIOID DOSING

- Recommended starting doses for moderate to severe pain in the opioid naïve are found in Table 93-9.
- If a patient is not receiving enough pain relief at a given dose, increase the dose by 25% to 50%.
- If a patient is having pain before the next dose is due, reduce the interval and/or increase the dose.
- Rotation from one opioid to another may be necessary in several circumstances
  ○ If a few attempts have been made at increasing the dose of an opioid, such that a patient is receiving a "reasonable" dose and still not receiving any pain relief, rotation to a different opioid may provide better analgesia. The patient may not have the "correct" receptor population to bind a particular opioid.
  ○ If a patient is having intolerable side effects not treated with appropriate agents, rotation to a different opioid may provide a better side effect profile. The patient may have a high receptor population that binds a particular opioid in regions that cause side effects.
  ○ If a particular opioid is not available by the route of administration required in a given patient, rotation to a different opioid is a reasonable option.
  ○ If a patient has been on an opioid for an extended period of time and is demonstrating signs of tolerance to the analgesic effects, rotation to a different opioid may provide better analgesia; usually at less than the expected equianalgesic dose (see section: Equianalgesic-Dosing Charts). Better analgesia may also occur by switching opioids in patients, who have been on an opioid for extended periods, when they have an acutely painful insult in addition to their chronic pain state.

TABLE 93-9 Recommended Starting Doses of Opioids for Adults More Than 50 kg

AGONIST	ORAL	IV
Codeine	15–60 mg q 3–4 hours	n/a
Hydrocodone	5–10 mg q 3–6 hours*	n/a
Tramadol	50–100 mg q 4–6 hours†	n/a
Oxycodone	5–10 mg q 3–4 hours	n/a
Morphine	10–30 mg q 3–4 hours	5–10 mg q 2–4 hours
Hydromorphone	2–6 mg q 3–4 hours	1–1.5 mg q 3–4 hours
Oxymorphone	10–20 mg q 4–6 hours‡	1 mg q 3–4 hours

*Daily dose limited by acetaminophen component in available preparations.
†Maximum recommended 24-hour dose: 400 mg in adults <75 years old; 300 mg in adults >75 years old.
‡Recent FDA approval of oral form, therefore limited clinical experience.

EQUIANALGESIC-DOSING CHARTS

- See Table 93-8.
- These are based on the relative potency of the various opioid agonists as determined by single-dose clinical studies and experience.
- Several different versions exist, thus the calculations are estimates only and clinical judgment is always required.
- Incomplete cross-tolerance exists between the various opioids. This means that patients will not be "as tolerant" to a new opioid agonist as they were to the one they were on previously. Thus, when converting between opioids (for any of the reasons mentioned in section: Opioid Dosing), the calculated equianalgesic dose of the new agent must be reduced by 25% to 75% in order to prevent over-sedation and/or respiratory depression.
- Table 93-10 shows how to switch from parenteral hydromorphone to oral oxycodone as an example of opioid rotation/conversion.

SUSTAINED-RELEASE OR LONG-ACTING OPIOIDS

- Sustained-release formulations should generally only be initiated in the acute setting if pain is present most of the time and it is assumed that the pain generator will last for an extended period of time (eg, > 2 weeks). If the pain is more incident related or expected to be of a brief duration, then immediate-release agents should be employed.
- If initiating or increasing a sustained-release opioid (eg, if > 4 rescue doses are needed in 24 hours while on a sustained-release agent as well), start or go up on the sustained-release agent by 50% to 100% of the total 24-hour breakthrough dose used.
- When using a sustained-release opioid, also provide doses of an immediate release opioid equivalent to 10% to 15% of the 24-hour total, to be used every few hours on a prn basis.
- Transdermal fentanyl is not appropriate for acute pain, especially in the opioid naïve. There is a black box warning against its use in the acute setting because of the risk of severe respiratory depression from the delayed peak effect of the drug as the pain level decreases. It is intended for use in patients who are already tolerant to opioids of comparable potency. Table 93-11 gives recommendations for conversion from other opioids to transdermal fentanyl.
- Methadone is not appropriate as the first-line agent in the acute setting, especially in the opioid naïve. Its use requires an understanding of the unique pharmacology of the drug; especially its extended duration of action and its dose-dependent potency (see Table 93-8). Also, as it takes a few days to reach a stable plasma concentration, patients will need to be followed closely to monitor for effectiveness and side effects. It must also be realized that methadone is a racemic mixture of a mu agonist and an NMDA antagonist (see section: Adjuvant Analgesics), which makes patients have a lesser degree of analgesic-tolerance development. Recent FDA precautions state that patients must be made aware of the long duration of action of methadone, instructed not to take extra doses nor mix it with other medications, and to be familiar with signs of overdose.

TABLE 93-10   Example of Opioid Conversion

1. Patient used 15 mg of IV hydromorphone in the past 24 hours.
2. According to the equianalgesic table:

   1.5 mg of IV hydromorphone = 20 mg of oral oxycodone

   $$\frac{1.5 \text{ mg of IV hydromorphone}}{20 \text{ mg of oral oxycodone}} = \frac{15 \text{ mg of IV hydromorphone}}{X}$$

   $$X = 200 \text{ mg of oral oxycodone per day}$$

3. Taking into account incomplete cross-tolerance, decrease the total daily opioid dose by 25% to 75%:

   $$200 - (0.25 \times 200) = 150 \text{ mg of oral oxycodone per day}$$
   $$200 - (0.75 \times 200) = 50 \text{ mg of oral oxycodone per day}$$

4. Dose initially every 4 hours:

   $$150/6 \cong 25 \text{ mg oxycodone every 4 hours}$$
   $$50/6 \cong 8 \text{ mg oxycodone every 4 hours}$$

Therefore, order oxycodone 10–25 mg every 4 hours as needed for pain.

TABLE 93-11   Dose Conversion Guidelines from Another Opioid to Transdermal Fentanyl

24-HOUR ORAL MORPHINE EQUIVALENT DOSE (MG/D)*	TRANSDERMAL FENTANYL INITIAL DOSE (MCG/H)
60–134	25
135–224	50
225–314	75
315–404	100
405–494	125
495–584	150
585–674	175
675–764	200
765–854	225
855–944	250
945–1034	275
1035–1124	300

*Convert other opioid to oral morphine equivalents using an equianalgesic dose table. This table should not be used to convert from transdermal fentanyl to another opioid because the conversion to transdermal fentanyl in this table is conservative. Therefore use of this table to convert from transdermal fentanyl to another opioid can overestimate the amount of the new agent resulting in overdosage/respiratory depression.

WEANING OPIOIDS

- If the cause of pain is effectively eliminated, patients will require the discontinuation of opioids while preventing the occurrence of physical withdrawal.
- When weaning a patient from long-acting agents, decrease the dose of the long-acting agent by 25% to 50% every 2 days. Once the patient is off the sustained-release form, the immediate-release agent can be weaned.
- When weaning a patient from immediate-release agents, reduce the opioid dose by 50% for 2 days and then reduce the daily dose by 25% every 2 days thereafter until the total dose (in oral morphine equivalents) is 30 mg/d. The drug may be discontinued after 2 days on the 30 mg/d dose.

PCA BASICS

A patient-controlled analgesia (PCA) is meant to be used by patients as a maintenance therapy. If the patient is in moderate to severe pain when it is initiated, IV loading doses must be used to achieve comfort because the incremental dosing of the PCA will not achieve comfort in a reasonable period of time. This method of administration helps overcome the wide inter-patient variation in opioid requirements by allowing the patient to control the dosing regimen.

- PCA—opioid choice, dose, and lockout interval
  - Morphine: most common first-choice agent.
  - Fentanyl: quicker onset and shorter duration than morphine. This is good if one is concerned about accumulating effects, but it is bad in that patient must "constantly" activate the PCA—can be difficult for some patients to get sleep at night.
  - Hydromorphone: generally more effective in patients who are opioid tolerant, because of its high efficacy.
  - In the opioid-naïve patient, Table 93-12 indicates the recommended starting doses and suggestions for how to change the dose if the patient does not receive adequate pain relief.
  - Commonly used lockout intervals range from 5 to 10 minutes. Even though time to peak effect may be longer than this, in practice no major differences are seen with longer lockouts for specific opioids. There have also been no good studies to suggest that a particular lockout interval is better than any other.

- PCA—basal rates
  - May be needed in opioid-tolerant patients or if fentanyl is used.
  - Not recommended in opioid-naïve, elderly, obstructive sleep apnea, or morbidly obese patients.
  - Decrease or discontinue the basal rate if a patient is not activating the PCA (ie, they do not need to self-administer a dose) or if side effects increase, in order to maintain the inherent safety of this method of pain management.

OPIOID-INDUCED SIDE EFFECTS

Nausea, vomiting, pruritus, constipation, sedation, and respiratory depression are the most common opioid-related side effects. The opioid-naïve patient is more likely to develop these effects. Tolerance eventually develops to all these effects, except constipation. Many of these side effects are discussed in greater detail, particularly regarding management strategies for patients requiring long-term use of opioids for persistent pain and terminal illness, in Chap. 94.

- Treatment of these side effects can be accomplished by
  - Changing the dose or schedule of the agent
  - Rotation to a different agent (side effects vary widely among patients to the different opioid agonists)
  - Specific therapy to counteract the side effect
  - Addition of another analgesic and/or adjuvant to decrease the needed dose of the opioid (ie, opioid-sparing effect)
- Constipation should be expected with the use of opioids and the prophylactic use of stool softeners (eg, docusate) and stimulant laxatives (eg, senna preparations) is recommended.
- Nausea/vomiting can be treated with any of the various agents available (eg, prochlorperazine, ondansetron, metoclopramide, promethazine) as none has proven more or less effective.
  - Metoclopramide is a promotility agent, thus it has limited antinausea effects and is most effective if there is vomiting.
  - Promethazine or possibly prophylactic use of a scopolamine patch may be more effective if the patient has a history of motion sickness or if nausea comes on with movement, as opioids sensitize the inner ear labyrinthine system.

TABLE 93-12   Suggested Starting PCA Dose and Dose Changes

	MORPHINE	HYDROMORPHONE	FENTANYL
Staring PCA dose	1.0–1.5 mg	0.2 mg	20–25 mcg
PCA dose change	0.5 mg	0.1 mg	5–10 mcg

- Pruritus is a very commonly experienced side effect and in the absence of a rash/allergic reaction it is a central mu-related phenomenon.
  - Diphenhydramine is only effective if the etiology is definitely because of histamine release, which is usually only the case for large doses of morphine given quickly or a true allergic reaction.
  - Nalbuphine 5 mg IV q 4 h prn is more effective in that it treats the cause, by antagonism of the central mu receptors.
- Sedation may be a troublesome side effect, particularly when using opiates to alleviate persistent pain in terminal illness—see the section on sedation in Chap. 94 for management strategies in this population.
- The proper treatment of respiratory depression from opioid agonists is given in Table 93-13.

ADJUVANT ANALGESICS

- See Table 93-14.
- Antiepileptics: Effective for treatment of neuropathic pain. May have analgesic effects in the acute setting as well.

TABLE 93-13   Treatment of Suspected Opioid-Induced Respiratory Depression

Suggested definition of respiratory depression
- Oxygen saturation below 90% or decrease of more than 5% from baseline in patients with baseline oxygen saturation of < 90%.

and

- Respiratory rate < 8 breaths/min.

Primary, nonpharmacologic treatments of respiratory depression
- If patient is taking effective breaths but at a rate of < 8 per minute
  - Tactile and verbal stimulation, naloxone administration may not be essential
- If patient is taking ineffective breaths and/or with a respiratory rate < 4 per minute
  - May require ventilatory assist with bag-valve mask and supplemental oxygen. This should be instituted while diluting and administering naloxone

Naloxone should only be considered in the following situations:
- Patient is unarousable or minimally arousable to tactile/verbal stimulation
- Patient is requiring ventilatory assistance

Proper naloxone dilution and dosing
- 1 ampule (0.4 mg) of naloxone must be diluted with 9 mL of saline to yield 0.04 mg/mL.
- Administer to patient in 1–2 mL increments (0.04–0.08 mg) at 2–3-minute intervals until response.
- If no change in respiratory depression after 0.4 mg naloxone has been titrated, consider another etiology other than opioid induced.
- If there is some, but not enough, improvement after 0.4 mg of naloxone has been titrated, continue titration.
- Naloxone's half-life is less than most of the opioid agonists so be aware that respiratory depression may recur. Therefore, be prepared for the need to readminister naloxone boluses or consider use of a naloxone infusion.

- Tricyclic antidepressants: Effective for treatment of neuropathic pain. Doses used are lower than for depression and onset of analgesia is faster (ie, days) than antidepressant effects (ie, weeks).
- Local anesthetics: Topical application of a cream can be useful for brief topical dermal anesthesia or a patch can be used for treatment in various neuropathic pain syndromes.
- Glucocorticoids: Used in cancer pain management to reduce inflammation from tumor invasion of nerves.
- Skeletal muscle relaxants: Useful for relief of muscle injury/spasms.
- Antispasmodics: Treatment of pain with a spastic component or in neuropathic pain states.
- NMDA antagonists: Have no primary analgesic effects but do have opioid-sparing, opioid tolerance-reversing and anti-hyperalgesic effects.
- Alpha-2 agonist: analgesic and opioid-sparing effects.
- Benzodiazepines: Treatment of anxiety or insomnia. Be aware of the development of dependence with long-term use.
  - These agents do not have any analgesic properties.
  - May be useful to help patients fall asleep, making it easier to "deal" with pain.
  - Anxiety can play a role in pain states especially acute pain; when this is added to persistent pain an antianxiety medication may be useful.
  - Use with caution in acute pain, especially when high doses of opioids are required, as significant sedation and respiratory depression can occur in the benzodiazepine-naïve patient.
  - In anxious patients with pain, adequate titration with analgesics should occur before the addition of a benzodiazepine.

ACUTE PAIN IN THE OPIOID TOLERANT

- If the patient has experienced some event that has increased their pain, opioid use can be expected to be higher than just replacement of what the patient was on before coming in to the hospital and it can be *significantly* higher than in opioid-naïve patients.
- More pain complaints and higher pain scores should be expected.
- Discussion of reasonable goals and expectations of analgesic therapy with the patient is crucial.
- Start with the higher efficacy opioids but always be prepared to change the regimen if needed as variance in response to the various opioids exists in this population as well.
- The use of multimodal therapy in this patient population is especially important.

TABLE 93-14   Select Adjuvant Analgesics

CLASS	AGENT	ADULT DOSING	SIDE EFFECTS/COMMENTS
Antiepileptics	Gabapentin	Start with 300 mg po q 8 hours, increase by 300 mg qd after a few days to a max of 3600 mg/d in divided doses	Dizziness and somnolence; do not stop abruptly
	Pregabalin	Start with 50 mg po q 8 hours or 75 mg po q 12 hours; in 1 week increase to max of 300 mg/d in divided doses	
Tricyclic antidepressants	Amitriptyline Nortriptyline	25 mg po qhs; increase to max of 150 mg/d in a single or divided doses	Anticholinergic symptoms (e.g., dry mouth, confusion), sedation, and hypotension
Local anesthetics	Lidocaine 2.5% and prilocaine 2.5% cream	2–2.5 gm/10–25 cm² skin for 1–2 hours before procedure	Localized skin reactions; rare cardiovascular and/or CNS toxicity; prilocaine may contribute to methemoglobinemia in patients treated with other agents known to cause this
	Lidocaine patch 5%	Up to three patches for up to 12 hours within a 24 hour period	Localized skin reactions; rare cardiovascular and/or CNS toxicity; only FDA indication is for treatment of post-herpetic neuralgia
Glucocorticoids	Dexamethasone	4–8 mg po q 8–12 hours	Typical steroid-induced side effects from long-term use (> 2–3 months) usually outweigh benefits; concomitant use with NSAIDs is not recommended
Skeletal muscle relaxants	Cyclobenzaprine Tizanidine Orphenadrine	5–10 mg po q 8 hours 4–8 mg po q 6–24 hours 100 mg po q 12 hours 60 mg IV q 12 hours	Long-term use can lead to the development of dependence
Antispasmotic	Baclofen	10 mg po q 8 hours, titrate slowly to max of 80 mg/d in divided doses	Drowsiness; may impair renal function; abrupt D/C may cause seizures
NMDA antagonists	Ketamine	0.1–0.2 mg/kg/hour IV	Sedation, dreams, and hallucinations possible but infrequent at analgesic (low) dose, treat with the addition of benzodiazepine or dose reduction
	Dextromethorphan	Start with 30–90 mg po q 8 hours, increase to max of 360 mg/d in divided dose	Best dose and regimen not well defined
Alpha-2 agonist	Clonidine	0.2 mg/d via a transdermal patch, left on for 1 week	Hypotension & sedation; monitor for rebound hypertension on D/C if used for > 1 week

WHEN TO CONSULT

- Severe pain that remains uncontrolled after multiple attempts at escalating drug doses and use of multiple classes of agents.
- Severe concomitant psychiatric illness (eg, anxiety, depression, substance abuse).
- Need for performance of certain diagnostic tests (eg, diagnostic epidural injections).
- Need for help with specific treatment modalities that the provider cannot administer, such as physical therapy, surgery, complementary therapies, or invasive treatment modalities (eg, epidural injections, intrathecal pumps, spinal cord stimulators).

BIBLIOGRAPHY

American Pain Society. *Principles of Analgesic Use in the Treatment of Acute Pain and Cancer Pain.* 5th ed. Glenview, IL: American Pain Society; 2003.

Carr DB, Goudas LC. Acute pain. *Lancet.* 1999;353:2051.

Galvagno SM, Correll DJ, Narang S. Safe oral equianalgesic opioid dosing for patients with moderate-to-severe pain. *Res Staff Phys.* 2007;53:17.

Gordon DB, Dahl JL, Miaskowski C, et al. American Pain Society recommendations for improving the quality of acute and cancer pain management. *Arch Intern Med.* 2005;165:1574.

Gruener D, Lande SD, eds. *Pain Control in the Primary Care Setting.* Glenview, IL: American Pain Society; 2006.

Morrison RS, Meier DE, Fischberg D, et al. Improving the management of pain in hospitalized adults. *Arch Intern Med.* 2006;166:1033.

Pereira J, Lawlor P, Vigano A, et al. Equianalgesic dose ratios for opioids: a critical review and proposals for long-term dosing. *J Pain Symptom Manage.* 2001;22:672.

United States Food and Drug Administration/Center for Drug Evaluation and Research Web site; http://www.accessdata.fda.gov/scripts/cder/drugsatfda/index.cfm. Accessed 5/30/2007.

Whelan CT, Jin L, Meltzer D. Pain and satisfaction with pain control in hospitalized medical patients. *Arch Intern Med.* 2004;164:175.

94 PALLIATIVE CARE: OVERVIEW AND SYMPTOM MANAGEMENT

Jane deLima Thomas and David F. Giansiracusa

INTRODUCTION

- During the second half of the twentieth century, improvements in healthcare resulted in a decrease in sudden and premature deaths and an increase in the population of patients living with chronic illness.
- More than 90% of Americans will experience a protracted, life-threatening illness, whereas less than 10% will die suddenly of a myocardial infarction, an accident, or another unexpected event.
- The evolution of our healthcare system—as well as our system of Medicare reimbursement which addresses Hospice as a separate benefit requiring patients to forego many life-prolonging treatments—has caused a dichotomous approach to patients with chronic or life-threatening illness: either trying to cure disease and prolong life or to provide comfort care.
- One consequence is that many patients die in institutions receiving aggressive treatment, with supportive, symptom-oriented treatment minimized or overlooked. Despite a 1996 Gallup poll showing that 90% of respondents expressed a wish to die at home, nearly 80% of patients currently die in hospitals or nursing homes.
- It is crucial, therefore, that physicians caring for hospitalized patients become familiar and comfortable with dealing with the complex symptom and psychosocial issues that face patients at the end of life.

OVERVIEW OF PALLIATIVE CARE

- Palliative care is an approach to care which improves quality of life for patients and families facing life-threatening illness, through the prevention and relief of suffering by means of early identification and impeccable assessment and treatment of pain and other problems, physical, psychosocial, and spiritual.
- Important characteristics of palliative care include the following:
  - It is multidisciplinary, and often includes physicians, nurses, social workers, chaplains, pharmacists, and complementary medicine practitioners.
  - The goals of care are tailored to, and reflective of, the particular situation, aims, and priorities of the patient and family.

- Aggressive symptom management is a key tenet, with an eye toward relieving suffering in all its manifestations: physical, emotional, social, and spiritual.
- Good communication is paramount for the tasks performed by palliative care clinicians: coordinating care across specialties, addressing goals of care and advanced directives, establishing a comprehensive discharge plan, and providing psychosocial and spiritual support to the patient and family, see Chap. 96.
- Palliative care can and should be offered *simultaneously* with other medical treatment.

EVALUATION AND MANAGEMENT OF PAIN

- As noted above, aggressive symptom management is a key component of good palliative care. Many patients with life-limiting illnesses have poorly managed pain; it has been estimated that 25% of cancer patients die without good pain management. For a detailed overview of pain management, please see Chap. 93. What follows is an approach to the evaluation of pain and pain management that focuses on aspects related to the care of the terminally ill patient.

EVALUATION OF PAIN/PALLIATIVE CARE APPROACH

- An important philosophy in the palliative care approach is that pain is subjective and therefore *the patient's self-report is the gold standard*. When the patient cannot communicate, clinicians must rely on family/caregiver report, observation, and previous experience with the patient.
- After eliciting a thorough history and performing a physical examination, the clinician should form a differential diagnosis of the etiology of the pain: is it progression of disease, a complication of therapy, or another process such as bladder distension, neuropathy, rheumatic disorder, or peptic ulcer disease?
- A more sophisticated assessment includes evaluation of what the pain *means* to the patient: does the patient associate increased pain with worsening disease? With impending death? With treatment failure?
- Concomitant with a determination of the etiology of pain is an assessment of the type of pain the patient is experiencing, since different types of pain—somatic, visceral, and neuropathic—require different treatment approaches.
  - Neuropathic pain is often less responsive to opioids alone and requires the use of adjuvant medications such as gabapentin and other anticonvulsants, steroids, tricyclic antidepressants, and Lidoderm patches.

◦ Bony pain because of metastatic disease responds to a combination of treatments including opioids (often methadone is helpful), nonsteroidal anti-inflammatory medications, bisphosphonates, calcitonin, steroids, radiation therapy, and even radiopharmaceuticals.

The WHO ladder was developed for the treatment of cancer pain and can be used as a guideline for the selection of analgesics (see Table 93-5 in Chap. 93). Some points worth emphasizing when treating pain as part of palliative care

- There is rarely cause for a patient to be on more than one long-acting and one short-acting opioid at a time with one exception: sometimes having both oral and intravenous short-acting opioids available can be helpful for patients who are nauseated or dysphagic.
- When a patient is admitted with significant pain, it is important to make sufficient pain medication available, often continuing the patient's long-acting opioid as at home (if he's taking one) and making a short-acting opioid available frequently.
- The rule of thumb is that a short-acting ("breakthrough") dose should be equivalent to 10% to 20% of the total opioid dose the patient takes in 24 hours (see Table 94-1).
- For patients presenting with severe pain, use of a PCA or patient-controlled analgesia should be considered, often with a continuous infusion of medication as well as a demand dose (see section on PCA in Chap. 93).

Patients can have highly individual and variable responses to different pain medications, with specific medications proving either more or less efficacious than anticipated depending on the patient's own idiosyncratic response. When a patient is experiencing intolerable side effects or inadequate pain relief despite aggressive up-titration of medication, consider changing to another opioid (see section on rotating opiates in Chap. 93 and also Table 94-2).

- Three cautionary notes regarding commonly used opioids follow:
  ◦ Have care when using fentanyl patches.
    ▪ Use with caution in an opioid-naïve patient. A low-dose 25 mcg fentanyl patch is equivalent of 1 mg of morphine intravenously per hour or 72 mg oral morphine daily.

TABLE 94-1 Example of Calculating a Breakthrough Dose

Q. What is the appropriate breakthrough dose of morphine for a patient taking MS Contin 120 mg orally bid and 4 doses of MSIR 15 mg in the day prior to admission?

A. The total morphine dose in 24 hours is 300 mg, so the appropriate oral short-acting morphine dose is 10% to 20% of 300 mg, or 30–60 mg. It should be made available every 3–4 hours.

TABLE 94-2 Example of Opioid Rotation

Q. A patient with metastatic breast cancer is on a 50 mcg fentanyl patch with MSIR (short-acting po morphine) for breakthrough pain. She has been taking 15 mg MSIR at least four times on most days and still has pain much of the time. She wishes to switch to an all-oral regimen because the fentanyl patches irritate her skin. How do we switch her from a fentanyl patch to long-acting morphine (MS Contin)?

A. Her 50 mcg fentanyl patch is the equivalent of approximately 100–144 mg po morphine daily. Reduce that by 25% to 50%, which yields about 50–100 mg po morphine daily. Add the breakthrough doses of po morphine, totaling 60 mg daily, which does not have to be reduced by 25% to 50%, since it is the same medication we are switching her to and therefore not subject to incomplete cross-tolerance. The daily total is 110–160 mg po morphine daily. Since the patient is still having pain much of the time, she could be started on MS Contin 60–75 mg po bid with MSIR 15–30 mg po q 3–4 hours prn pain. If there is reason to be more conservative in the conversion, for example, the patient is cachectic and we are unsure how much fentanyl is being absorbed in the first place, a more cautious approach would be to start her on 45 mg MS Contin bid with MSIR 15 mg po q 3–4 hours prn pain. Either way, active, careful monitoring of her pain and her response to the new regimen is warranted, especially in the first few days after the change.

- Fentanyl patches should be placed above the waist on ambulatory patients (above or below the waist on nonambulatory patients), and should be placed on intact skin overlying an area with some subcutaneous fat; a good site on most patients is the underside of the upper arm.
- Fentanyl patches should not be used in febrile patients since the uptake of medication is increased, or in patients with rapidly changing opioid needs since fentanyl patches are relatively cumbersome to change dosing.
- After application of a fentanyl patch, little medication is provided for hours 1–6, about half the dose for hours 6–12, then the full dose 12 hours after application. Likewise, the full dose, or almost that, will persist for the first 12 hours after removing a fentanyl patch, then about half the dose for 12–18 hours after removal.

◦ Have care when using methadone, which can be a highly effective analgesic especially for patients with mixed nociceptive/neuropathic pain syndromes.
  ▪ Methadone requires some experience to use; it has a long half-life and doses should not be changed more frequently than every 72 hours.
  ▪ Also rotating to methadone from another opioid or vice versa can be complicated and requires some expertise.

◦ Have care when using opioid infusions. The protocol should be to use bolus doses (equivalent to 50% to 100% of the hourly infusion dose) for episodes of pain instead of merely increasing the infusion rate, even for dying patients.
  ▪ Increase the infusion rate only if the patient requires regular boluses.

■ Remember that increasing the infusion rate will not relieve pain immediately, but rather take an hour or more to have an effect.

TOLERANCE AND SIDE EFFECTS OF OPIOIDS

• Concerns about side effects of opioids often cause clinicians to undertreat pain. Most patients will develop tolerance to the side effects of opioids within 2–7 days of starting or increasing the dose of medication (except for constipation, which persists as discussed below), without developing tolerance to the analgesia of opioids. A list of potential side effects follows, with suggestions for management

• Sedation
  ○ Sedation is a bothersome side effect for many patients taking opioids, but it usually wanes in the first few days after opioid initiation or dose escalation.
  ○ Many patients starting a new opioid regimen have had significant pain and impaired sleep; these patients can sleep a great deal in the first days in part because they are more comfortable and able to sleep for first time in a while.
  ○ On the other hand, sedation can be a warning of potential respiratory depression; patients will pass through a somnolent phase before respiratory function is impaired (addressed below).
  ○ If a patient complains of somnolence after a week of taking a new opioid or increased dose of opioid, look for other causes of sedation. The differential diagnosis includes a new intracranial process (eg, tumor, bleed), metabolic disturbance such as hypercalcemia or hyponatremia, uremia, hepatic failure, infection, or other medications such as H2 blockers, benzodiazepines, other sleep aids, and anticholinergics. It is important to evaluate for the possible contribution of alcohol.
  ○ If these potential causes are eliminated, consider opioid rotation or dose reduction; a reasonable start is to reduce the dose by 25% and observe the patient both for pain relief as well as sedation.
  ○ If there is a strong reason to continue the patient on his current opioid regimen despite persistent sedation, consider adding a psychostimulant. Methylphenidate, modafinil, and dextroamphetamine have been used to help patients feel more awake and cognitively sharp when taking opioids, and they often have the added benefits of mood enhancement and appetite stimulation as well.
    ■ Methylphenidate can be started at 2.5 mg orally bid and titrated up to a maximum of 60 mg daily (given in divided doses at 8 AM and noon to avoid keeping the patient awake at night, although another dose can be given at 4 PM if warranted); it should be avoided in patients with arrhythmias, delirium, or psychosis.
    ■ Modafinil is used less often and can be started at 100 mg orally daily and titrated up to 400 mg orally daily.
    ■ More recently, some palliative care clinicians have started to use donepezil to enhance cognitive function especially in patients who have not only opioid-induced sedation but underlying brain disease as well. Donepezil can be tried at 2.5 mg orally at bedtime, increased to 2.5 mg bid if effective, and should have a discernible impact within a day or two.

• Respiratory depression
  ○ An important fact to remember is that patients will become somnolent before their respiratory function is affected. Clinicians will not compromise even a tenuous patient's respiratory status with opioids if that patient remains awake.
  ○ Management of opioid-induced respiratory depression includes decreasing or holding the opioid, providing stimulation, providing oxygen therapy, and in severe cases giving naloxone.
  ○ Since naloxone reverses analgesia, an incremental dosing approach is recommended: see Table 93-13, Chap. 93.

• Constipation
  ○ Constipation is another symptom (like pain) for which the patient's definition provides useful information; important questions to ask when assessing constipation are, "How frequently did you move your bowels before you started the pain medication?" "What frequency of moving your bowels would you consider normal?"
  ○ Constipation can present simply, with the patient complaining of hard or infrequent bowel movements, or more subtly with abdominal pain, nausea, or even mental status changes, especially in the elderly. Constipation can even happen concurrently with diarrhea, with liquid material bypassing hardened, immobile stool.
  ○ Constipation is one opioid side effect that does not wane with time, in part because opiate receptors in the gut continue to be stimulated as long as the patient is taking the medication.
  ○ Nonpharmacologic measures, such as exercise and increased fluid and soluble fiber intake, should be encouraged when appropriate.
  ○ Virtually all patients on opioids should also be treated with a scheduled bowel regimen to prophylax against constipation. The combination of a stool softener (eg, docusate sodium) with a laxative

(eg, senna) often proves sufficient but escalating the regimen may be warranted, as noted below.

○ Avoid bulk-forming, insoluble fiber laxatives such as Metamucil and Citrucel, which will often exacerbate the problem, potentially leading to ileus.

○ For patents with opioid-related constipation, a stepwise approach is recommended (see Table 94-3).

○ If early measures are ineffectual, a rectal examination can be helpful to rule out distal impaction, especially since opioids can cause anorectal sphincter tightening and desensitization.

○ Constipation despite aggressive measures warrants evaluation for the presence of small bowel obstruction or ileus, especially when no stool or gas is passed or the patient has significant nausea and vomiting (please see the section on nausea and vomiting below for a discussion on bowel obstruction).

○ It is important to evaluate for the use of other medications that may contribute to constipation: antacids, anticholinergics, calcium channel blockers, iron, and ondansetron, all of which are medications used often in patients with chronic progressive illness.

• Nausea and vomiting
○ Many patients complain of nausea when starting opioids; fortunately, this side effect frequently resolves within a few days. Nausea in response to taking an opioid does *not* constitute an allergy to that medication!

○ Opioid-induced nausea is multifactorial in etiology, with likely contributors including stimulation of the chemoreceptor trigger zone in the fourth ventricle, intracerebral histamine release leading to stimulation of the vomiting center in the medulla, and decreased gut motility leading to constipation and stimulation of vagal mechanoreceptors.

TABLE 94-3   Stepwise Approach to Opioid-Related Constipation

(1) Docusate sodium 100 mg orally bid and senna two tablets orally at bedtime

(2) Docusate sodium 100 mg orally tid and senna 2–4 tablets bid

(3) Add lactulose 30–60 mg orally bid or polyethylene glycol (Miralax) 17–34 g orally daily (realize that lactulose is less expensive but can cause gas and cramps, especially in patients with abnormal gut architecture, strictures, tumors, etc.)

(4) Add a bisacodyl suppository bid until bowel movement or a daily enema until bowel movement. Mineral oil enemas are helpful in lubricating hard stool whereas tap water enemas and soap suds enemas can be helpful for stimulation of the bowel to move softer stool. Sometimes a mineral oil enema for lubrication followed by a soap suds enema for bowel stimulation is the most effective approach.

(5) In extreme cases, consider oral naloxone (Narcan) 1–4 mg bid-tid, which can address opioid-related constipation without reversing systemic analgesia

○ Patients often benefit from prochlorperazine 10 mg orally tid-qid, either regularly scheduled or as needed when opioid therapy is initiated, with the understanding that the prochlorperazine will likely be discontinued after a few days once the patient becomes tolerant to the opioid.

○ Other neuroleptics, such as haloperidol and olanzapine, are also reasonable choices.

○ If nausea persists beyond the first week of starting an opioid, consider other causes of nausea, including other medications (eg, iron sulfate), oral or esophageal thrush, peptic ulcer disease, gastritis (especially in patients on NSAIDs in combination with their opioid), delayed gastric emptying, constipation, bowel obstruction, chemotherapy/radiation therapy, hypercalcemia, hyponatremia, hepatic or renal failure, CNS disease, and vertigo.

○ Identifying the likely etiology of a patient's nausea will guide treatment, as illustrated in Table 94-4.

○ One cause of nausea and vomiting, which is particularly distressing and merits specific discussion, is malignant bowel obstruction, a common complication of patients with advanced abdominal and pelvic malignancies.

■ Patients generally present with nausea, vomiting, and continuous or colicky pain.

■ Although the treatment of choice is surgery, contraindications to surgery include previous surgery revealing inoperable disease, reobstruction, intra-abdominal carcinomatosis, diffuse intra-abdominal tumors or multiple masses, extensive ascites, poor nutritional status, poor performance status, and patient refusal to have surgery.

■ For patients with recent symptoms and potentially reversible bowel obstruction and without colicky or cramping abdominal pain, the following medication regimen is recommended: metoclopramide 60–120 mg intravenously or subcutaneously daily (divided into q 4–6-hour doses), octreotide 0.3–0.6 mg daily as either a constant intravenous infusion or 0.1–0.2 mg boluses subcutaneously every 8 hours, dexamethasone 4 mg tid intravenously or subcutaneously daily, and parenteral opioids for pain control.

■ If metoclopramide increases the abdominal pain, it should be discontinued and haloperidol or another neuroleptic agent used to treat the nausea and vomiting.

■ If the patient's obstruction and symptoms persist and the patient is not a surgical candidate, metoclopramide should be discontinued and haloperidol 2–5 mg in divided doses daily given intravenously or subcutaneously. In this case, the octreotide should be continued and if partially effective, increased up to 0.9 mg a day, the opioids should

TABLE 94-4   Treatment of Nausea and Vomiting by Etiology

ETIOLOGY	TREATMENT
Initiation or escalation of opioid therapy	Prochlorperazine 10 mg po tid-qid, haloperidol 0.5–1 mg po/IV q 4–12 hours or olanzapine 2.5–5 mg po/SL daily-qid
Oropharyngeal thrush	Fluconazole 200 mg IV on the first day then 100 mg IV daily for 5 days
Gastritis/peptic ulcer disease	Proton pump inhibitor, e.g., omeprazole 20–40 mg po daily-bid
Delayed gastric emptying	Metoclopramide 10–20 mg po/IV q 4–12 hours or 1–5 mg/hr IV/SC
Constipation	Docusate with senna. Also lactulose, polyethylene glycol, bisacodyl, enemas, oral naloxone (see section on constipation)
Bowel obstruction	Octreotide, metoclopramide, dexamethasone, and parenteral opioids (see paragraph on bowel obstruction)
Chemotherapy/radiation therapy	Ondansetron 4–8 mg po/IV bid-tid and/or lorazepam 0.5–2 mg po q 4–12 hours
Liver/renal failure	Haloperidol 0.5–1 mg po/IV q 4–12 hours or olanzapine 2.5–5 mg daily-qid
CNS disease	Dexamethasone 2–10 mg po/IV bid
Vertigo	Scopolamine transdermal patch

SOURCE: Modified from Abrahm J. *A Physician's Guide to Pain and Symptom Management in Cancer Patients*. 2nd ed. Baltimore, MD: Johns Hopkins University Press; 2005.

be continued for pain control, and a venting gastrostomy should be considered.

○ Two further notes about the treatment of nausea and vomiting

  ▪ Remember that ondansetron, often thought to be a particularly effective antiemetic, can cause constipation and actually worsen nausea. Ondansetron is most helpful for chemotherapy and radiation therapy-induced nausea and vomiting, but is not as effective for nausea and vomiting from other etiologies.

  ▪ Lorazepam is often used in oncology settings for the treatment of nausea and vomiting, and is particularly effective for anticipatory nausea associated with recurrent chemotherapy or radiation therapy treatments. Lorazepam can be very helpful for situations in which a patient's nausea and vomiting have a strong anxiety or anticipatory component, but is not as effective for nausea and vomiting from other etiologies.

• Delirium

  ○ Many patients experience delirium at the end of life (please see the section on care of the imminently dying patient in Chap. 95), and many clinicians either do not recognize delirium or they accept it as part of the dying process and do not treat it aggressively.

  ○ Delirium can be particularly distressing since it can compromise the patient's ability to be himself, something most patients and families find quite frightening and which enhances their sense of loss.

  ○ Delirium may also lead to injury, such as falls and unintended removal of tubes and lines, it can complicate the evaluation and treatment of the underlying illness or other symptoms, and it can delay discharge.

  ○ Delirium can manifest overtly with hallucinations, agitation, delusions, paranoia, and disordered thinking, or it can manifest subtly as a "hypoactive delirium" with withdrawal, sleepiness, and more subtle inattention and disordered thinking.

○ Assessment of delirium can be difficult, especially since one of the hallmarks is that symptoms can wax and wane, so that one clinician may visit the patient and find him thinking clearly whereas another clinician may find the patient very confused and inattentive.

○ Opioids can cause delirium and are often blamed for causing delirium, but a rigorous and sophisticated approach is warranted in these often complex patients.

○ Patients on a stable dose of opioids who develop delirium warrant a careful workup for the underlying etiology, including evaluation for progression of disease, new infection, CNS disease, hepatic or renal insufficiency, metabolic derangements like hypercalcemia or hyponatremia, hypoxia, constipation, urinary retention, and other medications like benzodiazepines, H2 blockers, anticholinergics, and steroids.

○ If a patient is thought to be delirious, it is often helpful to consult psychiatry. Nonpharmacologic interventions can be effective: be sure the patient has glasses and hearing aids as needed, try to maintain distinct differences between night and day, post a calendar, clock, and other orienting materials clearly in the room, and frequently orient the patient to time, place, and situation.

○ Having friends and family present, whom the patient trusts, may help orient and calm the patient and help him feel safe. Conversation in the room should be soothing and the television should be turned off.

○ Pharmacologic treatment largely rests on the use of antipsychotic medications.

  ▪ One reasonable regimen is to use Haldol 0.5–1 mg IV or 1–2 mg orally q 4–12 hours (depending on the severity) with another 0.5–1 mg IV or 1–2 mg orally available q 2 hours as needed for agitation or confusion.

  ▪ Olanzapine is another medication used very frequently; usually starting with 2.5–5 mg orally or sublingually daily tid titrated up to a maximum of 20 mg daily.

- Quetiapine (Seroquel) is another helpful agent, especially for patients who are having a more active delirium since it causes sedation; it can be given from 25 mg orally daily to 300 mg orally daily.
- For refractory cases, especially in bed-bound patients, consider using chlorpromazine (Thorazine), which again is very sedating as well as calming.

○ One last note about the treatment of delirium: benzodiazepines are used frequently in the hospital setting to calm agitated patients, but these medications often exacerbate delirium, especially in elderly patients or patients with underlying brain disease. Benzodiazepines may appear to calm the agitation because they are sedating, but they often worsen the disorientation and confusion making it more difficult for patients to think clearly. For agitated delirium, consider using a sedating antipsychotic like quetiapine rather then using a benzodiazepine.
- Other opioid side effects

Other less common opioid side effects include pruritis, urinary retention, and myoclonus.

○ Pruritis occurs especially in opioid-naïve patients with opioids delivered intraspinally and often involves the face, neck, and upper thorax. Treatment includes changing or stopping the opioid and administering an antihistamine (although there is some question whether this type of pruritis is always histamine mediated). Ondansetron, paroxetine, nalmefene, and nalbuphine have also been shown to help.

○ Urinary retention: Urinary retention is another less-readily recognized opioid side effect that can cause discomfort and distress; it is caused by opioid stimulation of bladder smooth muscle. Like constipation, it can cause a cycle of increasing pain leading to increasing pain medication leading to increasing retention, and so on. Discontinuing anticholinergic medications can be helpful, as can adding bethanechol 10 mg orally tid to a maximum of 50 mg orally tid. In elderly patients who may already have an element of bladder outlet obstruction, adding finasteride 5 mg by mouth daily may help.

○ Myoclonus: Spasmodic muscle jerks are a sign of opioid neurotoxicity. They are associated with an accumulation of metabolites and are seen especially in settings with high opioid doses, dehydration, and renal failure. Meperidine is a particular culprit in causing myoclonus and should not be used for pain control (its sole indication is for the treatment of rigors). Treatment can include dose reduction,

opioid rotation, and the use of baclofen or dantrolene. In more severe cases, where there is a good reason to continue the patient on his current opioid regimen, the use of benzodiazepines like clonazepam, lorazepam, or midazolam can be effective. Lastly, for benzodiazepine-resistant patients a barbiturate infusion can be effective.

BIBLIOGRAPHY

Abrahm JL. *A Physician's Guide to Pain and Symptom Management in Cancer Patients.* 2nd ed. Baltimore, MD: The Johns Hopkins University Press; 2005.

Berger AM, Portenoy RK, Weissman DE (eds). *Principles and Practice of Palliative Care and Supportive Oncology.* 2nd ed. Philadelphia, PA: Lippincott Williams and Wilkins; 2002.

Doyle D, Hanks G, Cherny N, Calman K (eds). *Oxford Textbook of Palliative Medicine.* 3rd ed. New York: Oxford University Press; 2004.

Field MJ, Cassel CK (eds). *Approaching Death: Improving Care at the End of Life.* Washington, DC: National Academy Press; 1997.

Lynch M. Pain as the fifth vial sign. *J Intraven Nurs.* 2001;24: 85–94.

Morrison RS, Meier DE. Palliative care. *N Engl J Med.* 2004;350(25):2582–2590.

Ripamonti C, Mercadante S. How to use octreotide for malignant bowel obstruction. *J Support Oncol.* 2004;2:357–364.

Waller A, Caroline NL. *Palliative Care in Cancer.* 2nd ed. Boston, MA: Butterworth Heinemann; 2000.

WEB SITES

Cancer Pain Guidelines. The National Comprehensive Cancer Network. Guidelines for supportive care. http://www.nccn.org/physician_g/s/f_guidelines.html

Advanced Chronic Illness Guidelines. The National Census Project for Quality Palliative Care (NCP) home page. http://www.nationalconsensusproject.org

Center for Palliative Care, Harvard Medical School. pallcare@partners.org.

Center to Advance Palliative Care. http://capc.org/

The EPEC Project. Education in Palliative and End-of-Life Care, info@epec.net

EPERC-End of Life/Palliative Education Resource Center. Advancing End of Life Care Through an Online Community of Educational Scholars, http://www.eperc.mcw.edu/

Growth House. www.growthhouse.org/palliative. Excellent Web site for information on palliative and end-of-life care with links to other Web sites

95 PALLIATIVE CARE: CARING FOR THE DYING PATIENT

David F. Giansiracusa and Jane deLima Thomas

INTRODUCTION

- This chapter addresses the evaluation and management of dyspnea, anxiety, depression, spiritual/existential suffering, and care of the imminently dying patient.
- Several studies indicate that most patients with life-threatening illness experience multiple physical symptoms; in one study of patients with cancer, inpatients averaged 13.5 symptoms while outpatients averaged 9.7 symptoms.
- For information on symptoms not addressed in this chapter, please see the references and Web site listing at the end of the chapter for further resources.

DYSPNEA

- Dyspnea, the sense of difficulty in breathing or air hunger, is one of the most frightening and frequently experienced symptoms of patients with progressive, life-limiting illness.
- Approximately 40% of cancer patients experience significant dyspnea, and approximately 70% of those in hospice experience dyspnea at some time during their last 6 weeks of life.
- In patients with other life-limiting illnesses such as heart failure, chronic lung disease, renal and liver failure, advanced AIDS, and progressive neuromuscular disease, dyspnea can be even more common and distressing.
- Etiologies of dyspnea include:
  - Dyspnea is the result of the following:
    - Breathing requiring excessive work, as in pleural effusions, ascites, interstitial pulmonary disease, and neuromuscular disease.
    - Less ventilation for the effort of breathing, as in reactive airway disease and pulmonary embolism.
    - Hypercapnea caused by excessively deep breathing, as in metabolic acidosis or CNS disease.
  - Dyspnea is pathophysiologically mediated by the following:
    - Mechanoreceptor response to stretch in the lungs, airways, and chest wall.
    - Peripheral chemoreceptor response to hypoxemia in the aorta and carotid bodies.
    - Central chemoreceptor response to carbon dioxide.
    - Alveolar J-receptor response to fluid and microemboli.
- Evaluation of dyspnea includes:
  - Evaluation with medical interview, physical examination, and simple laboratory studies including chest radiographs, complete blood counts, electrolytes, and pulse oximetry can reveal the etiology of the dyspnea in more than 75% of patients.
  - Common causes include pulmonary and cardiac disorders, anemia, ascites, and in cancer patients with lung cancer or disease involving the mediastinum (eg, lymphoma), superior vena cava syndrome and pericardial disease. Evaluation in such patients may require, in addition to chest radiographs, an MRI of the chest and an echocardiogram.
- Treatment of dyspnea includes
  - Addressing the specific etiology and providing symptomatic relief of both the sense of air hunger as well as the anxiety that so often accompanies dyspnea.
    - Dyspnea because of superior vena cava syndrome generally responds to radiation therapy, usually given in combination with high doses of corticosteroids.
    - Dyspnea because of malignant obstruction of bronchi, blood vessels, and lymphatics can also respond to radiation therapy with high-dose steroids. In some cases, obstructed or stenotic bronchi can be stented.
    - Pleural effusions can be drained, but in the setting of cancer may require sclerotherapy or placement of a Pleurx pleural catheter. Consider using diuretics and reducing artificial feeding and IV hydration.
    - Pericardial disease may require pericardiocentesis and pericardial stripping or placement of a pericardial window.
    - Dyspnea because of abdominal ascites may respond to paracentesis and/or shunting. Again, consider reducing artificial feeding and IV hydration.
    - Blood transfusions can be helpful for dyspnea because of anemia.
    - If bronchospasm is present, consider adding nebulized albuterol and/or oral steroids. If bronchospasm is absent, consider using reduced doses of theophylline and adrenergic agents to minimize tremor and anxiety.
    - Supplemental oxygen for hypoxia of any etiology should be provided to maintain an oxygen saturation of 88% to 90% or partial pressure of oxygen of 55–60 mm Hg.

◦ Symptomatic treatment of dyspnea is very important, even when the underlying etiology has been identified and treated. Nonpharmacologic measures such as blowing air gently across the face of a dyspneic patient with a fan or open window may provide relief.

◦ Opioids are the mainstay of symptomatic pharmacologic therapy since they decrease the sense of air hunger. For opioid-naïve patients, starting with 2.5–5 mg of oral morphine every 2–4 hours or its equivalent is reasonable. For patients on opioids, an increase in dose by about 25% may relieve symptoms. Doses of opioids should be increased as needed to control the sense of respiratory distress while monitoring for symptomatic effectiveness and side effects.

◦ Anxiety, which so commonly accompanies dyspnea, may be treated with lorazepam 0.5–2 mg every 4–6 hours po/SL/IV. Clonazepam 0.5–1 mg by mouth at bedtime to tid may be used as an alternative. For patients with severe anxiety and panic caused by dyspnea, midazolam 0.2–2.0 mg IV slowly every 1–4 hours (or midazolam 0.5 mg IV every 15 minutes until acute anxiety is relieved) and possibly a midazolam constant IV infusion at 0.5–1.25 mg/hr, or morphine 5–10 mg IV or by nebulizer every 2–4 hours, or chlorpromazine 25 mg orally or 12.5–25 mg IV every 4–12 hours can be given. Relaxation techniques have also been shown to be very helpful for some patients.

ANXIETY AND DEPRESSION

• Patients with progressive, life-limiting illness frequently experience anxiety and/or depression.
• Anxiety and depression are important to recognize since they often:
  ◦ Intensify the distress of other symptoms, particularly pain and dyspnea
  ◦ Impact negatively the quality of life for patients and family members
  ◦ Respond to appropriate treatment
• Anxiety
  ◦ Evaluation of anxiety includes recognizing its manifestations and evaluating for medical conditions that could be contributing factors.
  ◦ Anxiety may be manifested as panic disorder with restlessness, a sense of doom, autonomic hyperactivity (palpitations, sweating, mouth dryness, chest tightness), irritability, as well as difficulty concentrating, relaxing, and sleeping. Nausea, vomiting, and diarrhea may also be experienced. Other patients experience anxiety with specific events; in

such patients, exploring the source(s), aggravators, and relievers of their anxiety can be very helpful.
  ◦ For patients who experience chronic, generalized anxiety, a thorough psychiatry history including episodes of panic, depression, phobias, post-traumatic stress disorder, and obsessive-compulsive disorder is required as well as consideration of possible contributing medical conditions, which may include the following:
    ▪ Cardiac disease: ischemia, arrhythmia, heart failure
    ▪ Hypovolemia
    ▪ Pulmonary disease: obstructive airway disease, PE, pneumonia, pneumothorax
    ▪ Metabolic derangements: hypoglycemia, hypoxia, fever, hyperthyroidism, hyper- and hypocalcemia, hyponatremia, hyperkalemia
    ▪ Neurologic disorders: akasthesia, encephalopathy, partial complex seizures
    ▪ Medications: corticosteroids, bronchodilators and other beta-adrenergic agents, psychostimulants (eg, caffeine), antidepressants, rebound from very short-acting benzodiazepines (eg, alprazolam), and withdrawal from alcohol, benzodiazepines, and opioids
  ◦ Treatment of anxiety includes nonpharmacological and pharmacological approaches (Table 95-1).
• Depression
  ◦ Identifying depression in patients with progressive, life-limiting illness may be difficult because of the somatic symptoms of anorexia, weightloss, sleep disturbances, and fatigue that so commonly accompany these illnesses. Key indicators of depression in patients with advanced disease are:
    ▪ The expression of being depressed
    ▪ Feeling sad
    ▪ Crying
    ▪ Being unable to derive pleasure from anything (anhedonia)
    ▪ Feeling worthless, guilty, hopeless, helpless, or suicidal
  ◦ Questions such as, "What brings you pleasure?", "Are there things you used to enjoy that no longer give you pleasure?", "What are you looking forward to?", "What do you see as your future?", "What are your worries?", "What is most difficult or troubling?", or, "What is hardest for you?" may facilitate conversation helpful in assessing a patient's mood.
  ◦ Assessing for depression should include awareness and evaluation of medical, social, and spiritual problems that may contribute to depression. Hyponatremia, hypercalcemia, malignancies of the central nervous system, interferon therapy, corticosteroids, and

TABLE 95-1   Treatment Approaches for Anxiety

NONPHARMACOLOGIC	
Counseling, relaxation techniques, hypnosis, behavioral training	

PHARMACOLOGIC	
Mild to moderate anxiety: benzodiazepines	Lorazepam 0.5–1 mg po, SL or IV q 1–4 hours Clonazepam 0.5–1 mg po q HS to tid Diazepam 5–10 mg PR for those unable to take oral medication
For moderate to severe anxiety: selective serotonin reuptake inhibitors (SSRIs) or mirtazapine	Example SSRI (many others available as well): sertraline 50 mg in the morning, double dose every 2–3 days to a maximum of 200 mg; in the elderly start with 25 mg; no adjustment needed with renal impairment, use with caution in hepatic impairment Mirtazapine 15 mg at bedtime, double dose every 1–2 weeks, maximum 45 mg; in the elderly start with 7.5 mg; dose must be adjusted in renal failure
In patients with anxiety and paranoia or hallucinations: antipsychotics	Haloperidol 0.5–1 mg po/IV bid-qid regularly or prn olanzapine 2.5–5 mg po or 5 mg wafers sublingually at bedtime

opioids may all affect mood as may physical symptoms (pain, nausea, shortness of breath), financial and family concerns, lack of sleep, and spiritual distress.

○ The choice of pharmacologic treatment of depression in palliative care is influenced by the prognosis of the patient (since various antidepressant medications have varying periods of time to reach effectiveness), and by the other potential benefits of specific medications.

▪ The antidepressants with most rapid onset of action, often within a day or two, are the psychostimulants, for example, methylphenidate, generally started at 2.5–5 mg at 8 AM and 12 noon (in order to minimize the chance of inhibiting sleep at night) with another possible dose as needed at 4 PM, titrated up to a maximum daily dose of 60 mg. Other commonly used psychostimulants are modafinil, generally started at 100 mg each morning and increased, if needed to 200 mg twice daily, and dextroamphetamine started at 2.5–5 mg each morning and repeated at noon as needed and titrated to a maximum daily dose of 60 mg.

▪ For patients with a prognosis of more than weeks to months, an SSRI is the drug of first choice, often started in conjunction with a psychostimulant. The dose of SSRI should be started low for 3–7 days then increased every week or two.

○ Other antidepressants may be considered depending on the need to treat additional symptoms.

▪ Mirtazapine is helpful in treating insomnia and anorexia as well as depression.

▪ Trazadone, a mild antidepressant, is sedating and can help with insomnia.

▪ Tricyclic antidepressants may be helpful for neuropathic pain, but often their anticholinergic side effects limit usefulness in patients with advanced disease. When a tricyclic antidepressant is desired, desipramine and nortriptyline (tricyclics with the mildest anticholinergic side effects) should be chosen and started at low doses, such as 10 mg at bedtime.

○ Although most physicians have some familiarity with identifying and treating depression, patients with life-limiting illness often benefit from a consultation with a psychiatrist, social worker, or psychologist, who can be helpful with the following issues:

▪ Providing emotional and psychosocial support
▪ Educating patients and their families
▪ Teaching coping skills
▪ Recognizing and treating adjustment disorders, anxiety, and depression
▪ Facilitating discussion among patients, families, and healthcare providers
▪ Other indications for requesting a psychiatric consultation are listed in the Table 95-2

SPIRITUAL DISTRESS

• Spiritual distress may manifest in a variety of ways. Patients may experience any or all of the following:
  ○ Loss of personhood or of meaning of life
  ○ Changes in their relationships with God

TABLE 95-2   Reasons to Request Psychiatric Consultation in the Care of a Dying Patient with Depression

• As the physician, being unsure of the diagnosis of depression
• Patient's lack of response to first-line antidepressant medication
• Patient is psychotic, confused, or delirious
• Patient has a history of a major psychiatric disorder
• Dysfunctional family dynamics are present
• Patient is suicidal or requesting hastened death (euthanasia or assisted suicide)

- ○ Fear of being punished by God
- ○ Fear of death and/or afterlife
- ○ A profound sense of guilt or of burdening loved ones
- These situations, as well as a patient's need for spiritual/religious rituals, are very appropriate reasons to request assistance of a chaplain, pastoral counselor, or member of the clergy. These spiritual counselors may help patients address their sense of guilt, feelings of abandonment or punishment by God, fears of death and afterlife, and need for sacraments and rituals.

CARE OF THE IMMINENTLY DYING PATIENT

- This section focuses on symptom management during the last hours and days of life; communication skills helpful in the care of these patients are discussed in the next chapter.
- Evidence suggests that the factors most important to patients as they are dying are the following:
  - ○ Optimizing physical comfort
  - ○ Maintaining a sense of continuity of self
  - ○ Maintaining and enhancing relationships
  - ○ Making meaning of both life and death
  - ○ Achieving a sense of control
  - ○ Confronting and preparing for death
- Signs of imminent death include the following: pain, noisy breathing, incontinence, restlessness, agitation, delirium, nausea and vomiting, anorexia, dysphagia, xerostomia, fatigue, dyspnea, cough, existential/ spiritual distress.
- Generally, these symptoms may be controlled with treatment. For patients with intractable distress after appropriate assessment and treatment, palliative sedation should be considered.
- *Pain*: The treatment of pain is discussed in Chap. 93. One frequent obstacle to adequate pain control in dying patients is the loss of the ability to take pain medication by mouth. Pain medications may need to be given by sublingual, buccal, transdermal, rectal, subcutaneous, or intravenous routes.
  - ○ Morphine or oxycodone concentrates (20–40 mg/mL) may be given buccally or sublingually every 2 hours.
  - ○ A transdermal fentanyl patch or sustained-release morphine preparation given rectally every 12 hours, together with the sublingual opioid concentrate for breakthrough pain every 1–2 hours, often provides good pain control.
  - ○ In the case of bone pain in which nonsteroidal anti-inflammatory agents and corticosteroids are being used, indomethacin can be given rectally and dexamethasone subcutaneously.
  - ○ For neuropathic pain, methadone and doxepin can be given rectally.

- ○ For patients requiring high doses of opioids, hydromorphone (Dilaudid) can be given intravenously or subcutaneously as a constant infusion with bolus doses for breakthrough pain.
- ○ Concentrated hydromorphone (hydromorphone HP) can be given in a 10 mg/mL concentration, allowing as much as 30 mg of subcutaneous hydromorphone to be subcutaneously infused each hour.
- ○ An opioid infusion can be useful for patients who have pain or dyspnea, but *not every dying patient needs to have one.* Many patients can have their symptoms managed using the above transdermal, rectal, and sublingual medications. If a patient does need an opioid infusion, it is important to also order opioid boluses for episodic pain or dyspnea; the bolus dose should be equivalent to 50% to 100% of the hourly infusion dose. The infusion rate should be increased only if the patient has needed regular boluses to remain comfortable.
- *Noisy breathing*: Sometimes referred to as a "death rattle," noisy breathing is often caused by retained upper airway secretions, occurs commonly as a patient nears death, and may be very distressing to family members and to staff caring for the patient. Repositioning the patient in a lateral recumbent position may be helpful, but often a drying agent is needed (Table 95-3).
  - ○ Atropine with morphine and dexamethasone given by nebulizer have also been used to dry out upper airway secretions.
  - ○ All of these agents cause mouth dryness, which can be treated using sips of water, ice chips, fruit-flavored ice pops, or artificial saliva.
  - ○ Good lip care is also important and can be achieved with applications of lip balm every few hours.
- *Terminal restlessness/agitation*: Nearly half of all actively dying patients will display restlessness or agitation, which may manifest with turning and moving in bed, nonpurposeful picking at sheets and other objects, moaning, muscle twitching, or intermittent wakefulness. Once patients have been evaluated and treated for possible reversible causes such as pain, urinary bladder distention, fecal impaction, nausea, and difficulty breathing, treatment possibilities include opioid dose adjustment, psychosocial and spiritual support, and treatment with a neuroleptic agent (Table 95-4).

TABLE 95-3 Drying Agents for Moist, Noisy Breathing

DRYING AGENT	DOSE/ROUTE/FREQUENCY
Hyoscyamine	0.125 mg sublingually tid to qid
Glycopyrrolate	0.1–0.2 mg IV tid to qid
Scopolamine	1–3 patches every 3 days; 0.2–0.6 mg every 2–4 hours IV or SQ

TABLE 95-4   Neuroleptic Therapy for Terminal Restlessness

Haloperidol	1–2 mg po, SQ, and IV every 6–12 hours with prn doses every 2 hours to maximum of 20 mg in 24 hours (intramuscular delivery is avoided because of pain)
Olanzapine	2.5–5 mg po or wafer sublingually q HS to bid plus prn every 4 hours
Chlorpromazine	25–50 mg po or IV q 4–8 hours or 25 mg prn q 4–12 hours

- *Shortness of breath*: Dyspnea should be treated with opioids, as noted above.
  - The anxiety often accompanying dyspnea may be treated with lorazepam 1 mg orally, sublingually, or intravenously every 2 hours.
  - In cases of dyspnea with severe anxiety/panic, continuing the opioids and adding midazolam 0.5–1 mg IV slowly then 0.1–1.25 mg/h SQ or IV or chlorpromazine 25 mg orally or rectally q 4–12 hours or 12.5 mg IV q 4–8 hours, may be very helpful.
- *Intractable suffering*: For patients who are actively dying and experiencing intractable physical, psychological, and/or spiritual/existential suffering, palliative sedation is available. Consultation should be obtained from experts in palliative care, pastoral care, and psychiatry.
- *Use of parenteral hydration*: The issue of parenteral hydration comes up frequently in the care of dying patients, often because of family concerns that their dying loved one will suffer and "die of thirst." After assessing how worried the patient and family are about this issue, it can be helpful to explain to family members that as people die, they often lose the sense of thirst but suffer from mouth dryness, which needs be meticulously addressed. Also, the burdens of artificial hydration, including the distress accompanying increased urine output, increased oropharyngeal secretions, nausea/vomiting, and increased edema of extremities, abdomen, and lungs, need to be explained to patients and family members. If hydration is to be given, it generally should be limited to a liter or a-liter-and-a-half a day while monitoring for signs of overhydration.
- *Hemorrhage*: Massive hemoptysis or exsanguinating bleeding, though occurring relatively rarely, are such distressing events for patients, family members, and care providers, that recognition of patients at risk, preparation, and emergent treatments merit discussion.
  - Patients most at risk are those with head and neck tumors, which may erode into the carotid arteries, and patients with lung lesions, which may erode into major vessels. Those caring for the patient should do the following:
    - Have ready dark-colored towels, sheets, and blankets to mask the blood
    - Have good intravenous access (a PICC line)
    - Have medications available and someone to administer rectal diazepam 10 mg; rectal, SQ or IV lorazepam 2 mg or IV midazolam 1–5 mg in pre-drawn syringes; morphine IV or SQ (for opioid-naïve patients 10 mg, and for patient on opioids the equivalent of a rescue/breakthrough dose, again in pre-drawn syringes)
    - Place the patient with bleeding side down in the Trendelenburg position

BIBLIOGRAPHY

See also Chap. 94—Palliative Care: Overview and Symptom Management.

Block SD. Assessing and managing depression in the terminally ill patient. *Ann Intern Med.* 2000;132:209–218.

Block SD. Psychological considerations, growth, and transcendence at the end of life. *JAMA.* 2001;285(22):2898–2905.

Byock I. *Dying Well: Peace and Possibilities at the End of Life.* New York: Riverhead Books; 1997.

Ferris FD, von Gunten CF, Emmanuel LL. Competency in end-of-life care: the last hours of life. *J Palliat Med.* 2003;6:605–613.

Steinhauser KE, Christakis NA, Clipp EC, et al. Factors considered important at the end of life by patients, family, physicians, and other care providers. *JAMA.* 2001;286:3007–3014.

WEB SITES

See Chap. 94—Palliative Care: Overview and Symptom Management.

96   PALLIATIVE CARE: COMMUNICATION

David F. Giansiracusa and Jane deLima Thomas

INTRODUCTION

- Communication is a fundamental clinical skill in palliative care.
- Patients at the end of life value comfort, a sense of control and dignity, relief of burden on loved ones, strengthening of relationships with significant others, and avoidance of prolonging the dying process, all of

which require excellent communication between the patient, family, and healthcare team.

- This chapter will address the following communication skills:
  - Overcoming barriers to good communication
  - Identifying patients' goals and preferences for care
  - Addressing psychosocial and spiritual issues
  - Giving bad news
  - Redirecting care to focus on comfort (including withholding or withdrawing medical interventions used to prolong life)
  - Confronting fears of patients and families
  - Communicating as death approaches and after the patient dies
  - Using the structured family meeting in the care of patients with life-limiting illness and their families
- Communication in palliative care begins by establishing goals of care which become the foundation for medical decision making.
  - Patients and family members cannot have meaningful discussions about preferences for treatment and specifically about advanced care planning (including resuscitation and mechanical life support) until they have a realistic understanding of their prognosis and treatment options. Discussions of the benefits and burdens of various options in realistic and understandable terms and in the context of obtainable goals are critically important.
  - In spite of the importance of sharing realistic prognoses with patients, often such conversations do not occur, or when they do prognoses are portrayed in overly optimistic terms.

BARRIERS TO GOOD COMMUNICATION

- Problems in communication can occur between the physician and patient, between physician and family, between patient, family and friends, and between healthcare providers.
- Reasons for communication problems in palliative care are multiple (see Table 96-1) and include the following:

TABLE 96-1　Barriers to Good Communication

- Closed questions
- Leading questions
- Discussing only neutral issues, for example, physical symptoms
- Ignoring cues
- Giving only selected attention to cues
- Providing premature and/or inappropriate advice
- Giving false assurances
- Switching the topic
- Passing the buck
- Premature problem solving
- Avoiding the patient

- Each of us—the physician, patient, family, friends, and other healthcare providers—often has a different view of the stage of the patient's illness and remaining options for care.
- Patients, family members, physicians, and other healthcare providers often withhold information in the spirit of protecting one another from upsetting news.
- True sources of distress may not be clearly communicated.
- Physicians sometimes use language which is upsetting and engenders a sense of abandonment (eg, "There is nothing more that I can do for you.") rather than saying, "There is much that we can do to care for you and relieve your symptoms, even though we do not have effective treatment against your cancer (or other medical condition)."

- Communicating with a patient-centered approach can facilitate learning about the patient as a whole person:
  - His expectations, values, goals and preferences for care
  - His symptoms and sources of suffering, needs, fears
  - His sources of support and methods of coping
  - His wishes for the remaining time

Important relationships which he may want to strengthen, enjoy, or bring closure.

- Approaching patients with genuine curiosity about their life stories, families, work, values, concerns, hopes, and important relationships not only provides the clinician with valuable information to assist with making medical recommendations and decisions, but also serves to establish a trusting, caring, supportive relationship between clinicians, patients, and family members. Further benefits of good communication are listed in the Table 96-2.
- To help patients and families disclose what is important to them, it is crucial for clinicians to create a safe and comfortable environment for sharing information.
  - Sit with patients and their families at the patient's eyelevel with a relaxed, open posture in a quiet area free of interruptions.

TABLE 96-2　Good Communication Helps Clinicians

- Understand who the patient is as a person
- Perform comprehensive assessments of physical and psychologic symptoms and sources of distress
- Determine what the patient and family know about the patient's condition
- Determine how much the patient wishes to be told, and with whom the patient wishes information to be shared
- Facilitate patient and family understanding of what they have been told
- Clarify wishes for advanced directives, surrogates, goals, and preferences for care
- Achieve closure at the end of life
- Support patients and family members through the illness and family members through bereavement
- Provide clinician peace of mind

- Arrange people so that everyone can make eye contact.
- Ask permission to pose sensitive and/or probing questions.
- Use open-ended questions (see Table 96-3).
- Encourage each person to participate.
- Provide a safe atmosphere for people to express emotions, fears, values, feelings, and spiritual concerns.
- Be observant and respectful.
- Be ready to respond to the patient's and family members' affect.
- Convey a caring and accepting attitude, provide presence, and actively listen while using silence, summaries, and attempts to clarify issues.
- Assess for understanding and respond to emotions.
- Minimize interruptions, and avoid changing the subject or moving in a new direction of conversation until the patient and family are done: "Before we move on, is there anything else on this topic you wish to ask me or tell me about?"

- The approach of "ask-tell-ask," in contrast to "tell-ask-tell," begins by inquiring what a patient or family member is thinking and feeling (patient-centered) rather than focusing on the clinician's agenda.
  - Begin with a question: "What is your understanding of how you are doing?" followed by active listening.
  - Then share some information: "These are some things we can do to help you be more comfortable."
  - Ask the patient, "What do you think about these options?" then attentively listen to the response.
- Demonstration of respect for the patient, the patient's experience, and the patient's emotions supports the patient and reduces the sense of isolation that so often accompanies having advanced illness. For example, "You have shared a lot of information with me... I appreciate this and feel that I now have a better understanding of you."
- Addressing patients' and family members' emotions may be difficult, particularly when those emotions include anger.

TABLE 96-3   Open-Ended Questions/Empathetic Comments

- "Would you be willing to share with me how are you doing?"
- "Could you tell me about yourself?"
- "Can you tell me more? Please help me understand how you are doing, how you feel, and what is important to you."
- "How were you hoping we could help you?"
- "I am interested in what you are feeling. What do you believe is happening? What are you experiencing?"
- "When you think about the future, what do you hope for?"
- "It seems that things have been difficult for you. May I ask, what is hardest for you?"

TABLE 96-4   Responding to Emotion with the *"Nurse"* Technique

- N-name the emotion: "It appears to me that you are upset/sad/angry."
- U-understand: "I would think that what you are going through is very difficult."
- R-respect: "You seem to be working very hard to care for your family even though you are dealing with so much yourself."
- S-support: "We will be here and do everything to ensure your comfort."
- E-explore: "What concerns you the most?" "If things do not go as well as we hope they will, what is most important to you?"

- It can be challenging but healing to receive an angry comment and *not take it personally*, even if it sounds like an attack.
- A response that supportively addresses the anger is, "It sounds like you and I have been thinking about the situation differently. Would you please share with me what your understanding is?"
- The "nurse" technique may also be useful in addressing intense emotions (see Table 96-4).

PSYCHOSOCIAL AND SPIRITUAL ISSUES

- Attention to psychosocial and spiritual/existential issues is a particularly important aspect of communication in palliative care.
  - Patients experiencing psychosocial and spiritual/existential distress are more likely to desire hastened death, and their family members more likely to experience extended or complicated grief and bereavement.
  - Specific questions may be helpful to explore psychosocial aspects of having advanced illness (see Table 96-5).

TABLE 96-5   Questions to Elicit Psychosocial Concerns

- **Meaning of illness:** "How have you made sense of why this is happening to you?" "What do you think is ahead?"
- **Coping style:** "How have you coped with hard times in the past?" "What have been major challenges you have confronted in your life?"
- **Social support:** "Who are the important people in your life now?" "How are they coping with your illness?"
- **Stressors:** "What is most difficult for you, for your family?" "What is most stressful?" "Do you have concerns/worries/fears about pain or other physical suffering?"
- **Spiritual resources:** "What role does faith or spirituality play in your life?" "What role has it played during difficult times in your past?"
- **Psychiatric vulnerabilities:** "Have you been anxious, depressed, frightened?" "Have you used/abused drugs or alcohol to cope?"
- **Economics:** "How much concern are financial issues for you, for your family?"
- **Patient-clinician relationship:** "How would you like me to help you in this situation?" "How may we best work together?" "How may I be of greatest help to your family?"

SOURCE: Modified from Block SD. Psychological considerations, growth, and transcendence at the end of life. *JAMA.* 2001;285(22): 2898–2905.

TABLE 96-6 Assessing the Role of Spirituality as it Impacts Patient Care

The "FICA" system*
- *F*aith and beliefs
- The *i*mportance and *i*nfluence of spirituality in the patient's life
- The spiritual *c*ommunity
- The manner in which the patient wishes the clinician to *a*ddress spiritual beliefs

The "SPIRIT" model†
- *S*piritual belief system
- *P*ersonal spirituality
- *I*ntegration with a spiritual community
- *R*itualized practices and restrictions
- *I*mplications for medical care
- Planning for a *t*erminal event

SOURCE: *Pulchalski CM, Romer AL. Taking a spiritual history allows clinicians to understand patients more fully. *J Palliat Med.* 2000;3:129–137.
†Maugans TA. The spiritual history. *Arch Fam Med.* 1996;5:11–16.

- Discussing a patient's spirituality and religious beliefs is important for a number of reasons.
  - A large majority of patients with advanced illness in the United States want their physicians to ask about spirituality.
  - Doing so allows clinicians to show interest in the patient as a person and helps the clinician get to know the patient's beliefs and values.
  - Spiritual and/or religious beliefs may have profound effects on the medical decisions patients make, from choices about taking medications for pain to decisions about cardiopulmonary resuscitation and life-prolonging interventions.
  - Spiritual and religious beliefs may help patients cope with their illness and impending death or, conversely, may cause patients increased fear and anxiety about dying and the afterlife, thereby preventing them from being able to accept the realities of their medical conditions.
  - Unresolved existential and spiritual concerns may be a great source of suffering and distress for patients and families.
- A number of mnemonic techniques have been developed as tools to help clinicians ask questions to elicit spiritual histories including the acronyms FICA and SPIRIT (see Table 96-6).
- Lastly, a simple, open-ended question that addresses patients' spirituality is, "What role does spirituality or religion play in your life?"

GIVING BAD NEWS

- Giving bad news is a communication challenge that can occur early in the care of patients with life-threatening illnesses as well as at multiple times during the course of illness.

TABLE 96-7 Suggestions for Giving Bad News

- Inform patients of the conversation in advance so they can invite others to the meeting.
- Invite other health care professionals whom you feel would be helpful to you, to the patient, and to the family.
- Make yourself, the patient, family members, and all others comfortable in a quiet room. Seat everyone so that they are able to make eye contact with each other.
- Begin the discussion by asking what the patient knows. "Before I share information with you, it would be very helpful if you tell me/us what you think is going on with you and what others have told you." Also, inquire as to what the family understands.
- Establish how much information the patient wishes to know and is able to comprehend. "Some patients wish to know all the details of their illness and treatment whereas others prefer to know the 'big picture' and then ask specific questions later. What do you prefer?"
- Give a "warning" comment such as, "I wish I had more positive information to share with you." or "I wish things were different."
- Give information in words patients and families can understand and in small amounts.
- After giving bad news, stop talking and be silent and present while the patient and family process the information.
- Elicit and respond to feelings. This may involve some encouragement such as, "I have shared some very unfortunate information with you. How may I be helpful at this time?"
- Ask the patient to summarize what you have told him.
- Clarify points of misunderstanding and misconception.
- Address feelings and reactions of patients and their families.
- Explain that this is just one of many conversations.
- Ask for questions.
- Provide psychological support, which may include the assistance of a colleague and assessment for patient self-harm.
- Make a specific plan for the next meeting/conversation and give the patient and family the means to contact you in the interim.

- Robert Buckman, in his helpful book *How to Break Bad News: A Guide for Health Care Professions*, as well as other authors have articulated how to convey distressing news to patients and respond to their reactions (see Table 96-7).
- When giving bad news, clinicians should explore for any feelings of guilt or responsibility in the patient for being ill, such as shame in a long-time smoker who is diagnosed with lung cancer.
- Assess the impact of the illness on the patient overall, including the effect on relationships, work, social life, hobbies, interests, sleep, and mood.
- Address issues such as the uncertainty of the future, the search for meaning, the loss of control, and the sense of isolation.
- Providing open communication may help reduce the anxiety and depression that often occur after learning bad news.

ADVANCED CARE PLANNING AND ADVANCED DIRECTIVES

- Realistic sharing of information and prognosis is an essential foundation for discussions about advanced care planning.

- Although clinicians expect patients and family members to ask about the patient's prognosis if they want to know it, evidence suggests that this frequently does not happen.
- For patients and families to have discussions and make rational choices about advanced care planning, they need to have accurate and realistic information about their prognoses as well as about the outcomes of resuscitation given their particular clinical conditions.
  - Sharing with a patient and family the evidence that patients with metastatic cancer, who have a cardiac arrest in the hospital, do not survive to be discharged home may help them in the decision-making process.
  - Describing what life may be like on mechanical life support after resuscitation in terms of potential neurologic injury, inability to talk and eat, and potential need for sedation may also allow patients and families to make more informed decisions.
  - Using the words "death" and "dying," for example, "Once you have died, do you want us to try to resuscitate you?" may bring a clearer sense of reality to the discussion.
  - Conversely, discussion of intubation and mechanical ventilation may be framed in the context of preventing death, as a treatment intervention used to allow time for a patient to recover from a reversible process. In such a discussion, the reality of the patient's condition, reasons for possible respiratory failure, and the desired duration of mechanical respiratory support become key issues.
- Regardless of the context, discussions about advanced care planning offer another opportunity to ask the question, "What is important to you if things do not go as well as we hope they will?"
- Discussions of advanced care planning should not be purely task focused, for example, "Do you want cardiopulmonary resuscitation if you die, if your heart stops, or if you cannot breathe?"
- Advanced care planning discussions most appropriately focus on clarifying what defines an acceptable quality of life for a patient and establishing goals of care under different clinical situations, rather than describing a "buffet" or "menu" of potential medical interventions.
- Advanced care planning is not an isolated task but a *process* that requires exploration of what is important to patients, what makes their lives worth living, what their hopes and goals are, what activities/events/relationships are important, what elements enhance their quality of life, and what eventualities would be unacceptable.
- The question, "Can you imagine any kind of existence which would be worse than death?" may help explore these issues and facilitate discussions and decisions about advanced care planning and advance directives.

- Once a patient has made decisions, it is critically important to document those decisions, to identify and inform a healthcare agent, to share wishes and preferences for treatment with those close to the patient and with those involved in the patient's care, and to document the dissemination of this information.
- When patients are unable to speak for themselves and no advanced directives are available, the focus should be clarifying what the patient would have wanted under these circumstances.
- A meeting of family and healthcare providers involved in the patient's care including the primary care physician as well as social workers, nurses, and chaplains who know the patient is often critically important.

REDIRECTING CARE TO FOCUS ON COMFORT

- Discussions about redirecting care or withholding or withdrawing life-prolonging medical interventions involve a review of the patient's values, preferences, and goals of care, changes in the patient's clinical course, clarification of the patient's current condition, and discussion of specific treatments in the context of goals and of alternative treatments the patient may receive if he declines more aggressive or life-prolonging therapy. Note: *Care* for the patient is never to be withdrawn or withheld.
- After such discussions, the plans to withhold or to withdraw aggressive treatment should be documented and that documentation given to the patient, family, and healthcare team as well as communicated to consultants.
- When talking with patients facing life-limiting illness, the request that "everything be done" may best be thought of as an expression of fear and grief and a sign of a need for support.
  - It is critical to maintain open communication and to clarify just what "doing everything" actually means.
  - Families should often be involved in assessments and plans for care, consistent with the patients' wishes, values, and preferences.
  - Families often need additional support to deal with their sense of loss and to deal with the possible need for resolution of relationships and for closure.

CONFRONTING FEARS OF PATIENTS AND FAMILY MEMBERS

- Patients with advanced, progressive, life-limiting illness are often concerned that their medical team will "give up" and abandon them.

○ It is valuable to be clear about the intent of interventions, and to use language that focuses on what can be done rather than what treatments are not going to be utilized.

- For example, patients and families often associate opioids, especially morphine, with death and dying. When opioids are discussed, it is important to explain that they may be very helpful to relieve pain and shortness of breath while also asking the patient and family if they have any concerns about opioid therapy.
- Another example is to explain that patients with very advanced illness often lose interest in eating and drinking. Discussing the burden and risks, as well as the potential benefits, of artificial hydration at the same time as benefits may help patients and family members feel that their loved ones will not suffer the sense of thirst or hunger that less ill people would.
- Explaining what will be done to provide relief (such as meticulous mouth care for dry mouth) also helps relieve a concern that family members may have that the patient is being ignored and allowed to suffer.

• Specific choice of words is likewise very important.

○ Using the term "intensive comfort measures" rather than "comfort measures only" or "allow a natural death" rather than "do not resuscitate" may help to unload emotionally heavy situations for patients and their families.

• When caring for patients with life-limiting illness, clinicians should explore for potential differences between the patient's priorities for symptom management and those of family members. These can differ for multiple reasons, one of which is that family members may be afraid of the underlying motivation of the patient.

○ A patient may not be concerned about not eating, whereas family members may feel distressed about the patient's lack of appetite because they interpret this as the patient "giving up."

○ Exploring with family members their feelings of distress and attending to these concerns can help clinicians facilitate optimal patient and family interactions and relieve the family members' anxiety and emotional distress when the patient dies and through the bereavement process.

• Requests for hastened death should be viewed as a plea for open dialogue about dying, a wish to discuss concerns about suffering and/or loss of control, and a possible indication of depression.

○ Patients may request physician-assisted suicide (PAS) or euthanasia for a variety of reasons.

- Patients may lack technical expertise; they view their physicians as the ones who will guide them through the end of suffering.

- Patients worry about anticipated symptoms.
- Patients may feel that their families are too burdened to care for them.
- Patients may be suffering intolerable physical, psychological, spiritual, or existential distress (see Chap. 94).

○ Exploring patients' and family members' fears, concerns, and wishes for end-of-life care may relieve the angst leading to a request for hastened death.

- Involving the assistance of other clinical colleagues such as social workers, psychologists, chaplains, and/or psychiatrists is often appropriate and helpful.
- With such help, many patients are able to experience growth and new meaning.

• After having explored with the patient and family the origin of the request and provided compassionate presence and listening, the physician should make it clear what he/she will or will not do.

○ The patient may need to be referred to another clinician if acceding to his persistent wish runs contrary to the ethics of the initial clinician. Laws about PAS vary from state to state, with Oregon being the only state that permits PAS, and only in selected cases.

COMMUNICATION AS DEATH APPROACHES

• As illness progresses, communicating with patients and families about approaching death is extremely important.

• As this is often a very emotionally charged and difficult subject for most people to consider and discuss, the conversation needs to be approached with great respect and delicacy.

○ Asking permission of the patient and family to talk with them about how things are going may help introduce the discussion.

○ Asking patients and families what *their* sense of things is and helping them process and reflect on their situation allows them to share their own concerns and awareness (again, the ask-tell-ask approach). Often, patients have a real sense of their condition and welcome the opportunity to talk openly. Asking the question, "What is your body telling you?" may facilitate such discussion.

○ The following questions can help address a patient's hopes, "Given that time is short, what is most important to you?" "What do you hope for now?"

○ Breaking the collusion of silence which patients, family members, and even healthcare provides often participate in, often in an attempt to "protect one another," may help facilitate needed dialogue and sharing.

- Encouraging or even coaching patients and families to express affection, appreciation, gratitude, forgiveness, and farewell may be particularly helpful.
  - Ira Byock, in his book *The Four Things that Matter Most*, suggests patients and family members may find it helpful to use the following phrases: "Please forgive me."; "I forgive you."; "I love you."; "Thank you"; and "Good-bye."
- Identifying resources, such as a social worker, to help patients and families create a legacy can likewise be very helpful.
- Collections of writings, photographs, drawings, scrapbooks, audio and/or videotapes, notes, and prewritten cards (particularly for children's and grandchildren's future special events such as birthdays, graduations, and weddings) may help patients and families engage in sharing activities and life reviews which honor and respect the life of the patient.
- Such legacy work may also help support patients and families through the terminal phases of illness and families through bereavement.
- As death becomes imminent, explaining to the family the anticipated signs and providing ongoing attention to the patient and to the grief of the family members may help ease the emotional pain.
- It can be helpful to explain to family members that even when their loved ones appear to be asleep and unresponsive, they may be able to hear and be aware of touch.
- Encourage family members to speak, read, share patient/family stories, and play favorite music. This provides families with ways to continue to express their affection and care for their dying loved one.
- Sharing with family members the signs that death may be very close, hours to days, may help prepare them for their loved one's death.
- Provide support to family members by attending to the patient's symptoms (see section on care of the imminently dying patient), as well as to the family members' distress.
- Encourage family members to give permission to their loved ones to die, for example, "We will miss you terribly, but we will take care of each other and we will be okay."
- Explaining to families that some patients die only when alone may relieve a sense of guilt if a family member is not present when the patient dies. To assist with a sense of closure, suggest to family members that they say "good-bye," if not out loud then to themselves, whenever they leave the patient's room.
- Referring a patient to hospice may facilitate the patient's and family members' comfort and quality of life, including best addressing values and preferences for care (see Table 96-8).

TABLE 96-8   Benefits of Hospice Care

- The emphasis is on quality of life for patients with terminal illness.
- Care is focused on the goals and values of patients and their families.
- A multidisciplinary team of nurses, social workers, nursing aids, chaplains, volunteers and physician, including referring physician, usually care for patients in their homes.
- Care is provided to relieve physical, psychological, social, financial, spiritual, and existential suffering.
- Medications, durable medical equipment (e.g., hospital bed, walker, wheelchair), and supplies required for patients' comfort are provided.
- 24 h/d home nursing care or hospitalization is available, if needed, for patients whose symptoms that cannot be controlled at home.
- Respite care is available to the family.
- Support for the bereaved is provided.
- Patients qualify for Medicare hospice benefit if they are expected to live for six months or less.

SOURCE: Modified from Abrahm J. *A Physician's Guide to Pain and Symptom Management in Cancer Patients.* 2nd ed. Baltimore, MD: Johns Hopkins University Press; 2005.

CARE OF THE FAMILY, STAFF, AND ONESELF AFTER A PATIENT DIES

- Communication with family members after a patient's death shows respect and caring and may help with bereavement and closure for family and clinicians alike.
  - Such communication can include spending time in the patient's room with the family after the patient has died, making telephone contact with family members in the weeks and months afterward, and sending condolence cards.
  - Continued contact with bereaved family members after the death also allows clinicians to assess the need for bereavement support groups and/or referral to professional counselors or psychiatrists.
  - Communicating with other involved staff and caring for oneself, such as by sharing feelings with a colleague or other members of your healthcare team, are also important facets of communication in end-of-life care.

THE STRUCTURED FAMILY MEETING

- A structured family meeting may be particularly helpful to address a number of communication tasks including establishing goals of care, sharing bad news, discussing advanced care planning and advanced directives, and discussing redirecting care or withholding/withdrawing certain medical interventions.
- Situations in which a family meeting may be particularly helpful are those in which no consensus or decisions have been reached, or those in which conflict exists within a family, between healthcare providers and patient/family, and/or among healthcare providers.

TABLE 96-9   Structure for a Family Meeting

(1) Premeet with healthcare providers (may include family) to clarify goals such as discussion of patient's condition, prognosis, advanced care planning, discharge planning; plan who is going to run the meeting and how others will contribute; establish which family members, friends, and care providers the patient wishes to attend.

(2) Introductions
  (a) Introduce self and others.
  (b) Review goals.
  (c) Establish rules: everyone will be given the opportunity to speak and ask questions; only one person speaks at a time while all others listen with respect, no interruptions are permitted.

(3) Review the patient's medical status.
  (a) What do the patient and family know?
  (b) What do they want to know?
  (c) Share information about the patient's current status, prognosis, and plan.
  (d) Ask for questions.

(4) For patients with decision-making ability: what decisions is the patient making? Also ask each family member about questions or concerns about treatment and how we as clinicians may help the patient.

(5) For nondecisional patients, ask family, "What do you believe the patient would want done?" "What do you think should be done?"

(6) Address conflict: "What leads you to your decisions?" "What causes you to feel the way you express?" If conflict persists, you may need to schedule a subsequent meeting.

(7) Identify other sources of support: chaplain, physicians, nurses, social workers, other family members, and/or friends.

(8) Wrap up: summarize the following.
  (a) Points of consensus
  (b) Points of disagreement
  (c) Decisions
  (d) Plans
  Also, support the patient and family with hope but caution against unrealistic expectations. Lastly, identify family spokesperson.

(9) Document the following in the medical record:
  (a) Who attended the family meeting
  (b) What decisions were made
  (c) What remains to be addressed
  (d) Plans for follow-up

(10) Establish a plan for future contact: scheduled telephone call, follow-up meeting, or office visit.

- These may also be situations in which ethics consultation may be very helpful. A proposed structure for family meetings is outlined in Table 96-9.

BIBLIOGRAPHY

See also Chap. 94—Palliative Care: Overview and Symptom Management.

Abrahm J. *A Physician's Guide to Pain and Symptom Management in Cancer Patients.* 2nd ed. Baltimore, MD: Johns Hopkins University Press; 2005.

Block SD. Assessing and managing depression in the terminally ill patient. *Ann Intern Med.* 2000;132:209–218.

Block SD. Psychological considerations, growth, and transcendence at the end of life. *JAMA.* 2001;285(22):2898–2905.

Block SD, Billings JA. Patient requests to hasten death: evaluation and management in terminal care. *Arch Intern Med.* 1994;154:2039–2047.

Buckman R. *How to Break Bad News: A Guide for Health Care Professionals.* Baltimore, MD: Johns Hopkins University Press; 1992.

Byock I. *Dying Well: Peace and Possibilities at the End of Life.* New York: Riverhead Books, 1997.

Byock I. *The Four Things That Matter Most: A Book about Living.* New York: Free Press; 2004.

Epstein RM, Alper BS, Quill TE. Communicating evidence for participatory decision making. *JAMA.* 2004;291(19):2359–2366.

Faulkner A, Maguire P. *Talking to Cancer Patients and Their Relatives.* Oxford: Oxford University Press; 2002.

Larson DG, Tobin DR. End-of-life conversations: evolving practice and theory. *JAMA.* 2000;284(12):1573–1578.

Meier DE, Back AL, Morrison RS. The inner life of physicians and care of the seriously ill. *JAMA.* 2001;286:3007–3014.

Steinhauser KE, Christakis NA, Clipp EC, et al. Factors considered important at the end of life by patients, family, physicians, and other care providers. *JAMA.* 2001;286:3007–3014.

Quill TE. Perspectives on care at the close of life: initiating end-of-life discussions with seriously ill patients: addressing the 'elephant in the room'. *JAMA.* 2000;284:2502–2507.

Quill TE, Arnold RM, Platt F. "I wish things were different": expressing wishes in response to loss, futility, and unrealistic hopes. *Ann Intern Med.* 2001;135(7):553–555.

Teno JM, Clarridge BR, Casey V, et al. Family perspectives on end-of-life care at the last place of care. *JAMA.* 2004;291:88–93.

von Gunten CF. Discussing hospice care. *J Clin Onc.* 2002;20:1419–1424.

von Gunten CF. Ferris FD, Emanuel LL. Ensuring competency in end-of-life care: communication and relational skills. *JAMA.* 2000;284(23):3051–3057.

WEB SITES

See Chap. 94—Palliative Care: Overview and Symptom Management.

HOSPITALISTS CARING FOR SPECIAL POPULATIONS

97 CARE OF VULNERABLE POPULATIONS

Cheryl Clark

OVERVIEW/DEFINITIONS

Vulnerable populations are groups that experience disparities in healthcare utilization, delivery, or health outcomes because of a mismatch between patients' resources and healthcare system resources such that patients' needs are unmet.

- The US Department of Health and Human Services (DHHS) and the Agency for Healthcare Research and Quality (AHRQ) highlight several groups that may be vulnerable in healthcare settings. As indicated by the DHHS, groups to whom hospitalists should pay particular attention include those who are vulnerable because of
  - Financial circumstances
  - Place of residence (eg, urban, rural)
  - Demographic characteristics (eg, age, race, ethnicity, sex, sexual orientation)
  - Functional disability or developmental status
  - Ability to communicate
- Hospitalists are best able to deliver quality in-patient care when deficits are defined as properties of systems that can be adapted to meet patients' needs.

WHERE DO VULNERABILITIES EXIST?

HOSPITALIZATION

Hospitalists should understand the interplay between patient factors and systems factors that contribute to risks for hospitalization and vulnerability in hospital settings.

- Hospitalization because of ambulatory care sensitive (ACS) conditions is thought to reflect the adequacy of primary healthcare, as well as the influence of social and environmental processes. National data from the Health Care Utilization Project (HCUP) and regional analyses show that several vulnerable priority populations have high risks for hospital admission.
  - Elders aged 65 and older are the largest group at risk for hospitalization. Data from HCUP show the most common diagnoses, and highest age-associated risks in 2000, are for
    - Congestive heart failure (CHF) with 2321 admissions per 100,000 population aged 65 and older versus 355 admissions per 100,000 population aged 45–64 years.
    - Bacterial pneumonia with 1815 admissions per 100,000 population aged 65 and older versus 323 admissions per 100,000 population aged 45–64 years.
    - Chronic obstructive pulmonary disease (COPD) with 1138 admissions per 100,000 population aged 65 and older versus 272 admissions per 100,000 population aged 45–64 years.
  - HCUP data indicate gender differences in risks for hospitalization are condition specific.
    - Women are more frequently hospitalized because of hypertension, asthma, and urinary tract infections.
    - Men are more vulnerable to admission for complications because of diabetes, namely, lower extremity amputation, as well as CHF and bacterial pneumonia.
  - Most available data regarding socioeconomic risks use the median income of the patient's community of residence to estimate personal resources. HCUP data show those residing in an area with a low median income are at highest risk for admissions for uncontrolled diabetes and chronic complications because of diabetes, asthma, and hypertension.

- In 2003, the rate of hospitalization for uncontrolled diabetes in areas with a median income less than $25,000 was 63.8 admissions per 100,000 population compared to 12.9 admissions per 100,000 population in areas with median incomes above $45,000.
- For certain racial groups, historical and contemporary social conditions in the United States lead to the intersection of multiple vulnerabilities, including an average lower socioeconomic status, lower rate of health insurance, and fewer community resources.
  - Nationwide Inpatient Survey (NIS) data from the 1990s show rates of hospitalization for chronic ACS conditions among African Americans and Hispanic groups are up to twice that of non-Hispanic whites.
  - HCUP data tracking hospitalizations for uncontrolled diabetes among those aged 65 and older show high admissions rates for Hispanic groups (130 admissions per 100,000 population), non-Hispanic African Americans (109 admissions per 100,000 population), and Native American/Alaskan Native populations admitted to Indian Health Service and Tribal hospitals (50 admissions per 100,000 populations) compared to non-Hispanic whites (31.6 admissions per 100,000 populations) and Asian/Pacific Islander groups (30.9 admissions per 100,000 populations).
- Low-functional health literacy has been suggested as an independent determinant of hospitalization because of a reduced ability to participate in outpatient self-care.
  - A study of Medicare enrollees with low literacy reported up to 30% higher risk-adjusted rates of admission compared to those with adequate literacy, assessed by Test of Functional Health Literacy in Adult Scores.
- HCUP data compare hospital admission rates between urban and rural residents for ACS conditions.
  - Where differences are found, rural residents have higher risks of hospitalization. Increased risks for rural residents are seen for uncontrolled diabetes without complications, hypertension, bacterial pneumonia, and COPD.
- Few data review the risks of hospitalization among homeless patients.
  - Data from the 1996 National Survey of Homeless Assistance Providers and Clients, collected by the US Census, showed 23% of 2974 homeless clients had been hospitalized for all causes within the past year, four times the US norms during that period.
- Reduced access to healthcare financing is a leading hypothesis explaining excess ACS admissions among the poor.
- An analysis of the 1997 NIS and census data showed Medicaid recipients had risks of ACS hospitalization that exceeded their excess prevalence of disease, compared to those with private insurance.

PROCESSES OF CARE

In keeping with national and local quality assurance initiatives to improve care in hospital settings, hospitalists should know the extent to which processes of care in their institutions are uniformly of high quality for all patients, particularly vulnerable subgroups. Specific vulnerable groups are at risk for low-quality processes of care.

- Elders in hospital settings are known to be vulnerable to polypharmacy, poor medication choices, improper medication dosing, and poor medical reconciliation at discharge (see Chap. 98).
- Recent data from the NIS and the CRUSADE cohort suggest gender differences in the use of catheterization, angioplasty, and stents in the treatment of acute coronary syndromes are decreasing over time, while gaps in surgical revascularization persist.
  - In the context of unstable angina therapy, women appear less likely to receive glycoprotein IIb/IIIa inhibitors in the acute setting, and appear somewhat less likely to receive statins acutely, and aspirin at discharge.
- Racial disparities in treatment patterns between African Americans and whites appear to persist for newer therapies for acute myocardial infarction.
  - Among African Americans, data from CRUSADE indicate lower use of glycoprotein IIb/IIIa inhibitors in the acute setting, low use of clopidogrel and statin therapy at discharge compared to whites.
  - A recent review of cardiac procedure utilization for acute coronary syndromes shows persistent gaps in invasive procedure use between African Americans and whites, and suggests disparities among Hispanic and Asian American groups.
  - Data from the National Healthcare Disparities Report (NHDR) suggest gaps in quality treatment for acute coronary syndromes among Hispanic, and Native American/Alaska Native groups as well.

OUTCOMES

The relationship between the quality of inpatient care and health outcomes is difficult to ascertain with current available research. Further study is required to understand the relationships between inpatient care systems and individual or social factors.

- Though an optimal rate of readmission has not been determined, early rehospitalization is thought, in part, to reflect inpatient processes of care.
  - A recent review of the literature shows up to twofold risks of 30-day readmission among geriatric populations (12%–16% of admissions readmitted) compared to the general population (5%–14% of admissions readmitted), and up to sixfold risks among ill geriatric patients initially hospitalized with CHF or COPD (35% readmitted).
  - Regional analyses show no consistent gender differences in risks for rehospitalization because of cardiac conditions.
  - Observational cohort studies in the mid-1990s to early 2000s investigate rehospitalization because of CHF. No consistent age and risk-adjusted gender differences in readmissions were found in regional studies including the Epidemiology, Practice, Outcomes, and Cost of Heart Failure (EPOCH) study in California, administrative data from the New York Statewide Planning and Research Cooperative System (SPARCS) database, and administrative data from Connecticut state hospitals.
- Further research is required to determine specific processes of care that consistently reduce mortality risks in vulnerable groups.
  - Condition-specific mortality benefits to quality-driven care have been monitored through the Assessing Care of Vulnerable Elders (ACOVE) project, a quality measurement initiative sponsored by the American College of Physicians-American Society of Internal Medicine Task Force on Aging.
    - The ACOVE project developed more than 200 measures of quality care for the elderly, many of which are relevant to hospital-based medical care.
    - Emerging data validating ACOVE measures of quality care among elders tie poor performance to increased longer term mortality at 500 days.
  - Other observational data have found reduced mortality associated with adherence to clinical guidelines for pneumonia.
  - Gender differences in early mortality (inpatient and 30-day mortality) have been inconsistently reported by condition or procedure.
    - In the context of acute myocardial infarction, data from Medicare's Cooperative Cardiovascular Project showed no 30-day mortality differences between men and women of all ages, despite differences in procedure utilization. However, gender differences in hospital mortality among younger populations, less than age 60, have been reported after coronary artery bypass grafting. Higher mortality has been reported among younger women compared to younger men.

- Early mortality outcomes by race/ethnicity have been studied in the context of CHF and acute myocardial infarction.
  - Observational studies of African Americans, Hispanics, and whites have found increased risks for rehospitalization, yet, survival *advantages* for African Americans and Hispanics in early mortality posthospitalization. Care in interpreting these findings is warranted. It is unclear whether outcomes reflect processes of care, use of hospitals to treat less severe disease among populations without access to care, or population-based factors.
  - Small risks of 1-year mortality were higher among lower income groups.
- The NHDR indicates Asian and Pacific Islanders are particularly at risk for low satisfaction with care. Data indicate these groups may not perceive their physicians listen or communicate well with them. The extent to which this occurs in inpatient settings should be investigated.

WHY DO DISPARITIES EXIST AMONG VULNERABLE GROUPS? EXPLANATORY DEBATES

Though further research is needed to understand the roots of disparities, hospitalists should be familiar with several frameworks and debates in the literature that attempt to explain disparities, and underlie intervention strategies.

- Differences in outcomes may reflect "fundamental vulnerabilities," or "disparities."
  - "Fundamental vulnerabilities" are individualized risks for poor outcomes that, despite quality care, may not be amenable to intervention with current knowledge. An example may include the relationship between advanced age and mortality in inpatient settings.
  - In contrast, "disparities" are poor outcomes thought to arise from inadequate processes of care, or inequitable social processes that result in poor outcomes for specific groups.
  - In teasing out these issues, performance should be studied with careful risk adjustment to compare similar individuals, but with attention to assessing the quality of care and outcomes for vulnerable groups.
    - For example, hospitalists or administrators may wish to design interventions for health plans or hospital services such that low-income patients receive the same quality of care, or achieve outcomes similar to higher income patients.
    - Institutions may wish to measure poor performance in caring for these groups, rather than "adjusting out" income disparities in processes or outcomes.

- *Patient preferences versus physician biases* are particularly relevant to procedure utilization.
  - It is difficult to untangle the extent to which disparities in processes of care or utilization result from patient-driven preferences and refusals versus physician management styles that have discriminatory effects.
    - Overt intent toward discrimination is difficult to uncover and may not be required to produce disparities in management and outcomes. Moreover, physicians may play a role in shaping patient preferences for treatment.
- "Diffusion of technology" effects may shape patterns of discrimination, such that disparities are greater where technology or practices are new, and standards of care are unclear.
  - Intervention studies may illuminate the impact of physician biases by observing the effect of adhering to structured protocols and guidelines, where standards of care are identified.
- *Intrainstitutional versus between-hospital (geography)* explanations for disparities posit vulnerable populations are at risk because of inequitable treatment within a given institution or because their care is provided disproportionately in places where quality is uniformly poor.
  - Complicating this debate, it is not clear whether current measures of quality for the majority are good indicators of quality for vulnerable groups.
  - Future efforts to collect institutional-level data on socioeconomic and demographic characteristics, and efforts to stratify performance by characteristics of vulnerable groups (eg, age, race, income, gender, language preference), may improve our ability to address inequalities at the institutional level and suggest broader strategies to improve quality of care at ailing institutions.
- The extent to which disparate health outcomes result from *poor access to quality medical care versus disproportionate exposure to injurious social and environmental conditions* is a continued policy debate. Interventions that create linkages between medical care and social and environmental services have promise for bridging this divide to provide comprehensive healthcare and health promotion for vulnerable groups (see Table 97-1).
  - The American Hospital Association reports a case example of a hospital-based effort to integrate medical care and population-based approaches to health promotion. A 330-bed medical center in Birmingham, Alabama, has created community partnerships to reduce crime in the area of the hospital, and has worked with beauty salon owners to disseminate health promotion materials to prevent cancer, heart disease, and diabetes.

TABLE 97-1 What Should I Know about Vulnerable Populations in Hospital Settings?

Vulnerabilities arise from interactions between social environments, healthcare systems, and individual characteristics that lead to
- Increased risk for preventable hospitalization
- Poor quality in process of care
- Poor outcomes posthospitalization

Though more research is needed to understand why disparities exist, the hospitalist should understand the basic explanatory debates that direct strategies to provide quality care to vulnerable groups

  - Additionally, hospital-based benefit programs have contributed to successful community-level improvements. Efforts to provide frameworks and strategies for coordinated activities may be needed to maximize results.

SKILLS AND PRACTICES

- An essential challenge for the hospitalist is to develop skills and practices that provide appropriate social and nonmedical services as well as appropriate medical care to vulnerable populations. Evidence-based best practices to ensure the quality of care for vulnerable populations are not uniformly recognized.
- However, emerging data from regional practices, clinical trials, interventions, and observational studies suggest practices that hold promise to improve hospital-based healthcare provision for vulnerable populations. Hospitalists should adopt best practices for assessing the needs of vulnerable populations.
  - Identify patients' vulnerabilities on admission, particularly those with potentially hidden vulnerabilities (low literacy, subtle language barriers, lack of insurance or ability to pay for prescriptions, or inadequate housing). The importance of this key skill must be highlighted as physicians may be unaware of disparities in processes or outcomes of care within their institutions or among the patients they serve.
  - Identify systems level underperformance in caring for vulnerable groups through improved data collection. Improved data collection for vulnerable groups in hospital settings is an important step toward developing system solutions.
- Hospitalists should adopt best practices for ensuring effectiveness, safety, timeliness, and patient-centered care provision. The Department of Health and Human Services reports successful practices for reducing health disparities through the NHDR. The NHDR highlights areas toward which hospital-based practitioners should expand their skill base by improving:

- ◦ Hospital treatment for pneumonia, and pneumococcal vaccination for African Americans
- ◦ Pneumococcal vaccination rates for Asian Americans
- ◦ Hospital-based treatment for myocardial infarction among Native Americans and Alaska Natives
- ◦ Smoking cessation, pneumococcal vaccination, and myocardial infarction treatment among Hispanic populations
- ◦ Hospital-based smoking cessation advice, timeliness of care, and patient-provider communication among the poor
- ◦ Vaccination among older and younger Medicare beneficiaries with disabilities
- • Some effective practices among subgroups that are not incorporated into commonly used quality measures include improving
  - ◦ Access to interpreter services and bilingual providers.
    - ▪ Observational research suggests improved outcomes from professional interpreters, and increased satisfaction for subgroups who received translation from bilingual providers.
    - ▪ In order to receive funding from Medicare and Medicaid, hospitals must provide language interpretation per a memorandum issued in 1998 by the Office for Civil Rights out of the Department of Health and Human Services.
- • Smoking cessation among gay and bisexual men.
  - ◦ A particularly high prevalence of smoking has been reported among bisexual and gay men.
  - ◦ A community-based group intervention piloted for gay men in the United Kingdom demonstrated a 76% quit rate after 7 weeks, suggesting a role for referrals to community-based services.
- • Hospitalist should become skilled at delivering comprehensive healthcare by providing timely referrals and adopting multidisciplinary approaches to caring for vulnerable groups (see Table 97-2). Hospitalists should be alert to best practices for referrals within their institutions and during transitions of care. A survey of emerging good practices suggests hospitalists should:
  - ◦ Provide respite care for the homeless.
    - ▪ New evidence from a county-hospital based intervention in Illinois demonstrates discharging patient to respite facilities providing interim housing, food, acute care health services by volunteer

TABLE 97-2   What Skills Should I Practice to Care for Vulnerable Populations?

- • To promote effectiveness, safety, timeliness, and patient-centered care, hospitalists should ensure that nonmedical and social services as well as appropriate medical care are provided to vulnerable groups
- • Hospitalists should provide referrals and use multidisciplinary services where indicated

health providers, facilities to organize medications, substance abuse counseling, case management, and referrals to permanent housing reduced hospitalization length of stay by 5 days, and reduced readmissions within 1 year by 49%.

- ◦ Employ multidisciplinary or case management approaches for chronic CHF management among elders.
- ◦ Utilize discharge checklists for the elderly.
- ◦ Provide patients with access to community-based health promotion programs.
  - ▪ A sustained community health promotion intervention in East Baltimore, integrated with access to inpatient services, was able to reduce mortality from hypertension among African American men by 57%.

ATTITUDES THAT PROMOTE EFFECTIVE CARE

Attitudes are the subjective, qualitative, and often unarticulated aspects of one's orientation to providing care. Attitudes and values that foster respect and trust are essential to cultivate quality and dignity in healthcare (see Table 97-3). This is particularly important for hospitalists who must establish rapport quickly, during times of crises, among populations who may feel socially marginalized. Though each patient-provider encounter is in some ways a unique experience, there are themes and principles that help hospitalists bridge mismatches between the resources of vulnerable groups and the health systems they encounter.

- • Literature reviews on communicating with vulnerable populations emphasize commitment to three concepts
  - ◦ *Self-reflection:* Reflected in self-awareness of the personal beliefs and assumptions the provider brings to the encounter.
  - ◦ *Listening:* Reflected in the ability to demonstrate a thorough comprehension of patient beliefs, needs, and expectations for care.

TABLE 97-3   What Attitudes Should I Cultivate to Care for Vulnerable Populations?

Hospitalists should develop
- • Rapport during fast-paced encounters, during times of crisis with patients who may feel socially marginalized
- • Attitudes that promote trust and impart dignity to vulnerable groups in order to facilitate providing quality care

Helpful attitudes include
- • Making a commitment to excel in *communicating*
- • Providing *informed consent* and *identity-centered care*
- • Promoting *advocacy* and promoting *accessibility*,
- • *Carefully planning transitions* from hospital settings to other sites of care

○ *Expressive skill:* Reflected in successful educational exchanges and negotiation with patients. One should consider using multiple modes of communication, including oral and visual aids for those with low health literacy or language barriers.

• Respect for a person's autonomy is a fundamental principle in providing care for vulnerable populations. The essential attitudes to ensure consent include:
  ○ Accurate description of therapies and alternatives.
  ○ Communication of the risks of receiving and refusing care.
  ○ Self-reflection to identify potentially inappropriate provider biases in presenting therapeutic options (such somatization by an elderly female as the cause of symptoms).

• Incorporating principles of cultural competence and patient-centered care is essential and often requires
  ○ An awareness of the culture, mores, and traditions of the populations served by the provider
  ○ Recognition and guarantee that cultural beliefs one ascribes to a group are pertinent for the individual
  ○ Provision of care tailored to patient's resources (eg, finances, insurance, housing) and beliefs
  ○ Inclusion of relevant others in healthcare decision-making (eg, same-sex partners)

• Hospitalists should help patients achieve quality in processes of care, and optimal health outcomes. Strategies may include
  ○ Timely utilization of consultants.
  ○ Helping patients access inpatient procedures.
  ○ Facilitating communication between inpatient services.
  ○ Facilitating interinstitutional transfer as appropriate.
  ○ Helping patients articulate and obtain their preferences for care.
  ○ Helping patients maximize access to healthcare financing.
  ○ Providing referrals for social and legal services as appropriate.

• Hospitalists should demonstrate a commitment to the principle of accessibility to help those with disabilities maximize their participation in care. Examples include
  ○ Adherence to architectural principles of universal design (including access ramps, proper lighting, removing clutter, audible and visual alarm systems).
  ○ Facilitation of communication through clear enunciation of spoken word, utilization of sign language interpreters, and hearing aids.
  ○ Requests for clarification when speech impediments impair comprehension.
  ○ Provision of adequate time for conversation so that patients and families can express their wishes.

• Ensuring strong connections to outpatient medical and social services may prevent adverse events after hospitalization.

• Effective communication with primary care physicians about social and nonmedical issues identified during the hospitalization is essential to providing smooth transitions in care.

• Discharge planning in vulnerable groups requires working with primary care physicians, and consulting social workers, nurses, care coordinators, specialists, or lay advocates early in the hospitalization to arrange appropriate disposition and services. Examples of services may include arranging or providing referrals to
  ○ Hospital-based/community-based financial safety nets.
  ○ Regular source of primary care.
  ○ Visiting nurse associations.
  ○ Elder services.
  ○ Hospice.
  ○ Medical respite care, housing authorities, shelters.
  ○ Substance abuse rehabilitation.
  ○ Legal services for immigrant groups.
  ○ Psychological or psychiatric services for torture victims.
  ○ Domestic violence advocates.

CONCLUSIONS

• Our understanding of the knowledge base, skill sets, and helpful attitudes for providing quality care to vulnerable populations is evolving.

• This review endeavors to empower hospitalists by surveying the evidence that exists to guide care as we continue to investigate best practices to reduce and eliminate disparate outcomes for these groups.

BIBLIOGRAPHY

Agency for Healthcare Research and Quality. *The National Healthcare Disparities Report.* Rockville, MD: AHRQ Publication No. 06–0017; 2005.

American Institutes for Research. Effective physician-patient communication. In: *Teaching Cultural Competence in Health Care: A Review of Current Concepts, Policies and Practices.* Washington, DC: Report prepared for the Office of Minority Health; 2002.

American Hospital Association 2006. Web resource: http://www.aha.org/aha/content/2004/pdf/case-al1-0408-princetonbap.pdf Last accessed January 19, 2007.

Annas G. A national bill of patients' rights. *New Engl J Med.* 1998;338:695–700.

Barnett PB. Rapport and the hospitalist. *Am J Med.* 2001;111(9B):31S–35S.

Benbassat J, Taragin M. Hospital readmissions as a measure of quality of healthcare: advantages and limitations. *Arch Intern Med.* 2000;160:1074–1081.

King TE, Wheeler M, Bindman A, et al., eds. *Medical Management of Vulnerable and Underserved Patients: Principles, Practice, Population.* New York: McGraw Hill; 2006.

Kruzikas DT, Jiang HJ, Remus D, et al. *Preventable Hospitalizations. Window into Primary and Preventive Care, 2000.* Rockville, MD: HCUP Fact Book No. 5. AHRQ Publication No. 04-0056, Agency for Healthcare Research and Quality; September 2004. Web resource: http://www.ahrq.gov/data/hcup/factbk5/ Accessed January 21, 2007.

Laditka JN, Laditka SB. Insurance status and access to primary healthcare: disparate outcomes for potentially preventable hospitalization. *J Health Soc Policy.* 2004;19:81–100.

Laditka JN, Laditka SB, Mastanduno MP. Hospital utilization for ambulatory care sensitive conditions: health outcome disparities associated with race and ethnicity. *Soc Sci Med.* 2003;57:1429–1441.

Chapter 5: Priorty populations. *National Healthcare Disparities Report, 2003.* Rockville, MD: Agency for Healthcare Research and Quality. Web resource http://www.ahrq.gov/qual/nhdr03/nhdr03.htm Last accessed: January 26, 2007.

Mace RL. Removing barriers to care: a guide for health professionals. The Center for Universal Design and The North Carolina Office on Disability and Health; 1998. Web resource: http://www.cdc.gov/ncbddd/dh/accessibilityguides.htm Last accessed January 20, 2007.

National Healthcare Disparities Report: Appendix D, Data Tables. Rockville, MD: Agency for Healthcare Research and Quality; 2006. Web resource: http://www.ahrq.gov/qual/nhdr06/. Last accessed: January 22, 2007.

Smedley BD, Stith AY, Nelson AR, eds. *Unequal Treatment: Confronting Racial and Ethnic Disparities in Health Care.* Washington DC: National Academies Press; 2003.

Youdelman M, Perkins J, Brooks JD, et al. Providing language services in state and local health-related benefits offices: examples from the field. The Commonwealth Fund, January 2007. Web resource: http://www.cmwf.org/publications/publications_show.htm?doc_id=444660 Last accessed January 15, 2007.

98 INPATIENT CARE OF THE FRAIL OLDER ADULT

Anne Fabiny

EPIDEMIOLOGY/OVERVIEW

- Older adults are at high risk of developing complications during a hospitalization because of the physiologic changes that accompany normal aging combined with disease-specific pathologic changes.
- Hospitalization can result in complications unrelated to the problem that caused admission or to its specific treatment. The following age-related factors create significant vulnerability to stresses experienced by older hospitalized adults:
  ○ Decline in muscle strength and aerobic capacity
  ○ Vasomotor instability
  ○ Reduced bone density
  ○ Diminished pulmonary ventilation
  ○ Impaired vision and hearing
  ○ Diminished thirst perception
  ○ Loss of skin integrity
- These complications can occur rapidly, are predictable, and can be minimized or prevented irrespective of admitting diagnosis and disease burden.
- Frail older adults are particularly vulnerable to complications during hospitalization. Although as of yet there is no one commonly accepted definition of frailty, one hypothesis is that frailty is a clinical syndrome.
  ○ Differing syndrome definitions have included various combinations of the following: weakness, fatigue, weight loss, decreased balance, low levels of physical activity, slowed motor processing and performance, social withdrawal, mild cognitive changes, and increased vulnerability to stressors.
  ○ None of the many definitions of frailty include advanced age; however, older adults are well represented within the population of frail hospitalized patients.
- Older patients will consume more and more of the hospitalist's time and hospital resources between now and 2050.
  ○ In 2002, the rate of hospital discharge for persons aged 65 and older was more than three times the comparable rate for person aged 45–64.
  ○ By 2030, there will be about 71.5 million older persons in the United States, more than twice their number in 2000; they will comprise 20% of the total population.
- It is the growth in the number of the oldest old, those 85 years of age and older that is of greatest public concern.
  ○ From 1995 to 2010, this population is expected to grow by 56%, as compared with 13% for the population 65–84. And while the expected increase from 2010 to 2030 is less than 50%, the increase from 2030 to 2050 is 116%.
  ○ The cumulative growth in the 85 and above population from 1995 to 2050 is anticipated to be more than 400%.
- For many older adults, hospitalization results in complications and functional decline despite cure or repair of the condition for which they were admitted.

TRIAGE AND INITIAL MANAGEMENT

Several elements of care need to be considered at the time of admission of a frail elder.

- The geriatric history should include the following:
  ○ Baseline functional status, see Table 98-1
  ○ Baseline cognitive function

TABLE 98-1   A Sample Baseline Functional Status Tool

FUNCTIONAL REVIEW OF SYSTEMS (INFORMATION FROM PATIENT AND/OR FAMILY)			
SELF-CARE	ADLs	IADLs	HOME SUPPORTS
Scoring for ADLs/ **IADLs** 0 = independent 1 = supervision 2 = partial assistance 3 = total assistance	____bathing ____dressing ____transfers ____toileting ____feeding	____telephone ____transportation ____cooking ____shopping ____housework ____finances	____VNA (____hrs/wk) ____HHA (____hrs/wk) ____PT (____hrs/wk) ____OT (____hrs/wk) ____speech therapy ____meals on wheels ____hospice ____social worker

Ambulation: ____across room   **Assist devices:**
____one block   **History of falls:** If yes, injury? (describe)
____one flight stairs

Mental Health:

	Cognitive	Depression	Behavior
	____difficulty remembering ____gets disoriented ____unsafe behavior ____forgets names ____poor judgment	____sleep ____interest ____guilt ____energy ____concentration ____appetite ____psychomotor retardation agitation ____suicidal	____delusions ____hallucinations ____wandering ____resistance to care ____socially inappropriate ____Other:

ROS:
Vision ____glasses ____cataracts ____glaucoma ____mac degen ____other
Hearing ____aid
Nutrition ____10 lb wt. loss in last 6 months ____5 lb wt. loss in last 1 month
____dentures ____special diet, specify:
Bladder ____lost of urine
Bowel ____recent change in bowel habits, specify:

Home situation: ____house/apartment ____nursing home ____senior housing
Home environment: ____stairs to enter ____stairs within ____throw rugs ____other, specify:
Lives With: ____spouse ____children ____other family, specify: ____other, specify:
General level of physical activity:
Other local social supports:

Family interview:
Spokesperson:_____ Local phone #:
Principal caregiver:_____ Local phone #:
____permission to talk to family denied
____family education on goals of hospitalization
____family involvement in D/C plan
Additional relevant information:

Scoring for Other Questions
1 = Yes
0 = No

○ Identification of the primary caregiver
○ Medications
  ▪ Who manages them?
  ▪ Who procures them?
  ▪ How are they paid for?
  ▪ Are they taken as prescribed? Trust and verify!
  ▪ Does each medication have an indication?
  ▪ Are the doses and scheduling appropriate?
  ▪ Could one or a combination of drugs cause the presenting illness?
  ▪ Ask about over-the-counter and herbal preparations, particularly sleep aids.

○ Immunizations—make sure pneumococcal and influenza vaccines are up-to-date (see vaccination guidelines in Table 77-3 in Chap. 77).
  ▪ A tetanus booster is only effective if the person had the original series of tetanus immunizations as a child and has been getting the booster every 10 years.
  ▪ Because World War II soldiers were the first people in this country to receive the DPT series of shots, very elderly patients who were teenagers or older in the 1940s did not receive the original series of immunizations. This patient population will not benefit from a booster.

○ Social history
  ▪ Where does the patient live?
  ▪ With whom?
  ▪ Are there family members or caregivers nearby?
  ▪ Does the patient already have an established relationship with a visiting nurse or home health agency?
○ Goals of care
  ▪ Identify the healthcare proxy.
  ▪ Advance care planning—includes code status, advanced directives.
  ▪ What is the goal of this admission? Treatment for cure, palliation of symptoms, placement in long-term care?
○ Anticipate discharge planning—involve case managers and/or social workers soon after admission to help with needs assessment and planning for discharge
  ▪ Will patient be able to return to home setting?
  ▪ If not, what setting will most likely be required?
  ▪ Talk to family/caregiver about likely options and transitions of care.
• The geriatric physical examination should be comprehensive, and pay special attention to the following:
○ Functional vision examination, that is, can you see me? Can you read this?
○ Functional hearing examination, that is, whisper or turn head so that examiner's face is not visible and speak to patient.
○ Skin—inspect pressure points over back, buttocks, sacrum, hips, malleoli, and heels.
○ Mental status.
  ▪ Mood
  ▪ Must first assess attention—days of the week or months of year backwards (performance is not dependent on education level or literacy)
  ▪ If inattentive, continue with delirium evaluation (see Chap. 62)
  ▪ If attentive, assess cognition with Mini-Cog Dementia Screen, which has been validated in ethnolinguistically diverse populations (Table 98-2)
  ▪ Neuromuscular examination
  ▪ Joints—rigidity or deformities
  ▪ Bed mobility—independent or needs assistance to go from lying to sitting to standing position
  ▪ Balance—quiet stand, Romberg, sternal nudge, and shoulder taps
  ▪ Gait—base, stride height and stride length, speed, stance time on each leg, use of assistive device

MANAGEMENT STRATEGIES

Several elements that need to be considered irrespective of diagnosis, and many need to be reevaluated daily include:
• Sleep
○ Sleep deprivation can cause delirium and an altered sleep-wake cycle is a feature of delirium.

○ A change in the architecture of sleep is a normal part of aging. Older adults spend more time in stage 1 and stage 2 sleep and less time in rapid eye movement (REM) stage 3, and stage 4 sleep. This predisposes them to easy arousal and disrupted sleep in a noisy, unfamiliar environment.
○ Do not order around-the-clock vital signs unless absolutely necessary.
○ Do not order nighttime medication administration unless absolutely necessary.
○ Anticipate difficulty sleeping, or altered sleep-wake cycle if delirious, and provide hypnotic medications such as trazodone.
• Mobility
○ Assess patient's mobility on rounds every day. See Chap. 91.
○ If there is a change in functional status at time of admission, order physical therapy consult at admission.
○ Assess for pain and manage aggressively.
○ As soon as patient is physically able
  ▪ Minimize immobility and order up in chair three times daily.
  ▪ Ambulating with patient does not always require physical therapy consult or physical therapist! Order "ambulate with assistance three times daily" and encourage visiting family members to assist with ambulation.
• Bowels
○ Anticipate constipation and maintain adequate hydration, order stimulant laxatives, and osmotic cathartics as needed.
○ Stool softeners are not particularly effective, but you can use them.
• Mental status
○ If not delirious at time of admission, confusion can develop at any point during hospitalization.
○ For elderly surgical patients, postoperation day 2 is when delirium most commonly presents. See Chap. 62.
• Dementia
○ Chronic cognitive impairment because of vascular dementia or Alzheimer disease (AD) is a common problem among adults aged 85 and older and is associated with prolonged average length of stay (LOS).
○ These patients have increased risk of functional decline and delirium during hospitalization.
○ Although the prevalence of AD and other dementias is only about 5% in adults aged 65 to 84, the range jumps to 30% to 50% of adults aged 85 and older.
  ▪ However, in one recent study, primary care physicians were unaware of cognitive impairment in more than 40% of their cognitively impaired patients.
  ▪ And there is poor concordance between the clinical diagnoses of cognitive impairment or dementia and a family informant's recognition of memory loss. A study in 2004 found that when

TABLE 98-2   Mini-Cog Dementia Screen

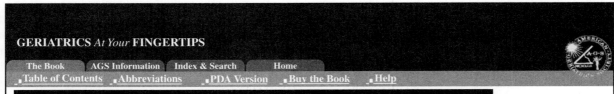

GERIATRICS *At Your* **FINGERTIPS**

| The Book | AGS Information | Index & Search | Home |
| Table of Contents | Abbreviations | PDA Version | Buy the Book | Help |

———————ASSESSMENT INSTRUMENTS

MINI-COG ASSESS MENT INSTRUMENT FOR DEMENTIA
PHYSICAL SELF-MAINTENANCE SCALE (ACTIVITIES OF DAILY LIVING, OR ADLs) ▼
INSTRUMENTAL ACTIVITIES OF DAILY LIVING SCALE (IADLs) ▼ GERI ATRIC DEPRESSION SCALE
(GDS, SHORT FORM) ▼ BRIEF HEARING LOSS SCREENER ▼ PERFORMANCE-ORIENTED MOBILITY
ASSESS MENT (POMA) ▼ ABNORMAL INVOLUNTARY MOVEMENT SCALE (AIMS) ▼ PAIN SCALES
FOR ASSESSING PAIN INTENSITY ▼ 10-MINUTE SCREENER FOR GERIATRIC CONDITIONS ▼ AUA
SYMPTOM INDEX FOR BPH ▼

The Mini-Cog Assessment Instrument for Dementia

The Mini-Cog assessment instrument combines an uncued 3-item recall test with a clock-drawing
test (CDT). The Mini-Cog can be administered in about 3 minutes, requires no special equipment,
and is relatively uninfluenced by level of education or language variations.

Administration

The test is administered as follows:

1. Instruct the patient to listen carefully to and remember 3 unrelated words and then to repeat the
   words.

2. Instruct the patient to draw the face of a clock, either on a blank sheet of paper, or on a sheet
with the clock circle already drawn on the page. After the patient puts the numbers on the clock
face, ask him or her to draw the hands of the clock to read a specific time, such as 11:20. These
instructions can be repeated, but no additional instructions should be given. Give the patient as
much time as needed to complete the task. The CDT serves as the recall distractor.

3. Ask the patient to repeat the 3 previously presented words.

Scoring

Give 1 point for each recalled word after the CDT distractor. score 1–3.

A score of 0 indicates positive screen for dementia.

A score of 1 or 2 with an abnormal cdt indicates positive screen for dementia.

A score of 1 or 2 with a normal cdt indicates negative screen for dementia.

A score of 3 indicates negative screen for dementia.

The CDT is considered normal if all numbers are present in the correct sequence and position,
and the hands readably display the requested time.
SOURCE: Borson S, Scanlan J, Brush M, Vitaliano P, Dokmak A. The mini-cog: a cognitive "vital signs"
measure for dementia screening in multi-lingual elderly. *Int J Geriatr Psychiatry.*
2000;15(11):1021–1027.

Borson S, et al. The Mini-Cog as a screen for dementia: validation in a population-based sample. *J Am Geriatr Soc.* 2003;51:1451-1454.

family informants reported memory loss, 30% of older adults were found not to have a cognitive loss. Among participants in whom family informants reported no memory loss, 75% were diagnosed with dementia or cognitive impairment.

- Therefore, just because there is no documentation of cognitive impairment or dementia in an older adult's medical record, and family members deny any cognitive problems, does not mean it does not exist!

○ Keep in mind that you cannot diagnose dementia or executive dysfunction in a delirious patient.

- If a patient is *not* delirious and you suspect cognitive impairment, use the Mini-Cog Screening Tool at the bedside, or refer for further evaluation as an outpatient.
- If the patient is delirious with no documented cognitive impairment, have a high suspicion for it and refer for further neuropsychologic testing as an outpatient after the delirium has cleared.

• Depression

○ This mood disorder is no more common in older adults than younger adults.

○ Its clinical features, however, can be different, with fewer neurovegetative signs and more anxiety.

○ Older adults may more often present with somatic complaints.

○ Because many symptoms of chronic medical problems can mimic some neurovegetative signs, the Geriatric Depression Scale Short Form is a useful diagnostic tool. See Table 98-3.

• Nutrition

○ Frail older adults are at particular risk for inadequate nutritional intake for a variety of reasons, including

- Loss of smell, taste, and thirst as a normal part of aging
- Poor dentition and/or loss of teeth
- Ill-fitting dentures
- Inability to obtain adequate food supplies secondary to poor mobility or lack of financial resources
- Cognitive impairment
- Underlying depression

○ An inpatient nutrition consult may be less useful than a home-based assessment through a visiting nurse association or licensed home care agency.

○ A change in weight is the best indicator of nutritional compromise rather than any laboratory findings. See Chap. 92 and Table 98-4.

• Medications

○ If an admission medication does not have an indication, investigate its use and either find the indication or discontinue the medication.

TABLE 98-3   Geriatric Depression Scale (GDS, Short Form)

Choose the best answer for how you felt over the past week.	
1. Are you basically satisfied with your life?	yes/**no**
2. Have you dropped many of your activities and interests?	**yes**/no
3. Do you feel that your life is empty?	**yes**/no
4. Do you often get bored?	**yes**/no
5. Are you in good spirits most of the time?	yes/**no**
6. Are you afraid that something bad is going to happen to you?	**yes**/no
7. Do you feel happy most of the time?	yes/**no**
8. Do you often feel helpless?	**yes**/no
9. Do you prefer to stay at home, rather than going out and doing new things?	**yes**/no
10. Do you feel you have more problems with memory than most?	**yes**/no
11. Do you think it is wonderful to be alive now?	yes/**no**
12. Do you feel pretty worthless the way you are now?	**yes**/no
13. Do you feel full of energy?	yes/**no**
14. Do you feel that your situation is hopeless?	**yes**/no
15. Do you think that most people are better off than you are?	**yes**/no
Score 1 point for each bolded answer. Cutoff: normal (0–5), above 5 suggests depression.	

SOURCE: Jerome A, Yesavage MD. For 30 translations of the GDS, see http://www.stanford.edu/~yesavage/GDS.html

For additional information on administration and scoring refer to the following references:

1. Sheikh JI, Yesavage JA. Geriatric Depression Scale: recent evidence and development of a shorter version. *Clin Gerontol*. 1986;5:165-172.

2. Feher EP, Larrabee GJ, Crook TH, 3rd. Factors attenuating the validity of the Geriatric Depression Scale in a dementia population. *J Am Geriatr Soc*. 1992;40:906-909.

3. Yesavage JA, Brink TL, Rose TL, et al. Development and validation of a geriatric depression rating scale: a preliminary report. *J Psychiatr Res*. 1983;17:27.

Mini-cog Assessment Instrument for Dementia Δ Physical Self-Maintenance Scale (Activities of Daily living, or Adls) Δ Instrumental Activities of Daily Living Scale (Iadls) Δ Brief Hearing Loss Screener ∇ Performance-Oriented Mobility Assessment (Poma) ∇ Abnormal Involuntary Movement Scale (Aims) ∇ Pain Scales for Assessing Pain Intensity ∇ 10-minute Screener for Geriatric Conditions ∇ Aua Symptom Index for bph ∇

TABLE 98-4   An Example of a Daily Assessment Tool

PATIENT NAME:

MOBILITY							
Hospital day	1	2	3	4	5	6	7
Bed rest							
Bed to chair							
Ambulating with assistance							
Ambulating independently							

MENTATION							
Hospital day	1	2	3	4	5	6	7
Alert, awake, oriented							
Alert w/cognitive memory/deficits							
Not alert							
Comatose							

NUTRITION							
Hospital day	1	2	3	4	5	6	7
Eating regular diet							
Eating regular diet poorly							
Liquid diet							
Not eating (NPO)							

BOWEL							
Hospital day	1	2	3	4	5	6	7
Normal elimination habits							
Constipation/diarrhea							
Obstipation							

BLADDER							
Hospital day	1	2	3	4	5	6	7
Normal							
Incontinence/retention							
Foley							

SENSORY/COMMUNICATION							
Hospital day	1	2	3	4	5	6	7
Glasses							
Hearing aid							
Able to follow instructions							
Able to communicate							

PAIN							
Hospital day	1	2	3	4	5	6	7
No pain							
Well-controlled pain w/meds							
Uncontrolled/poorly controlled							

MOOD							
Hospital day	1	2	3	4	5	6	7
Normal							
Depressed affect							
Severely depressed							

○ Does the patient have a medical problem for which he/she should be on a medication and is not? Older adults are just as often not on a medication that is indicated for a particular disease as they are on medications that are not indicated.

○ Calculate creatinine clearance (normal serum creatinine and blood urea nitrogen do not necessarily indicate normal renal function in older adults) and adjust medication dosing appropriately

- ClCr = (140 − age in years) × weight in kg/72 × serum creatinine in mg/dL
  For women, multiply × 0.85
- Creatinine clearance calculator available free at www.intmed.mcw.edu/clincalc/creatinine.html

• The role of the geriatrician—when to consult

○ All hospitalists should be competent in the care of older adults. A geriatrician can be helpful, however, when the following conditions or situations exist

- The patient does not respond to interventions as anticipated.
- Goals of care are difficult to determine.
- Multiple medications and question of inappropriate prescribing are noted.
- Delirium becomes difficult to manage.
- An unanticipated complication arises.
○ A posthospital discharge outpatient geriatric assessment can be extremely helpful when a patient has multiple problems (ie, falls, question of cognitive impairment, unsafe living situation, complex medication regimen) that cannot be adequately addressed during the inpatient stay.

SYSTEM-BASED APPROACHES TO IMPROVING THE CARE OF HOSPITALIZED OLDER ADULTS

- Individual physicians can improve the medical care they provide to frail, older adult hospitalized patients, but it is clear that the systems of care in the hospital are not devised to best meet the complex needs of those patients. Two well-developed and highly sophisticated programs exist for hospitals and healthcare systems that want to improve the care they provide to this growing segment of the population.
- The Hospital Elder Live Program, HELP, this patient-care program, developed by Dr Sharon Inouye and clinicians at Yale School of Medicine, is designed to prevent delirium in hospitalized older adults. Resources are available at www.elderlife.med.yale.edu/public/for-clinicians.php
- The New York University College of Nursing, Nurses Improving Care for Health System Elders, NICHE Program. It is a national geriatric nursing program designed to achieve systematic nursing change that will benefit older hospitalized patients. Information and resources are available at www.hartfordign.org/programs/niche/index.html

CARE TRANSITIONS

- Discharge planning
  ○ Assess cognitive and functional status daily; will this patient be able to return to previous site of care/home?
  ○ Multidisciplinary team rounding with nursing, case management, and physical therapy may help anticipate and mitigate barriers to discharge.
  ○ Active involvement of the family/caregiver in discharge planning is essential, including communication regarding anticipated care needs at time of discharge and the goals of care at next site of care.
  ○ Refer to outpatient geriatric assessment clinic when issues such as questions of patient safety, ability to

follow through with recommendations, concern about driving, recurrent falls, or complex medication or medical regimens exist. A geriatrician can then make the appropriate referrals to community resources such as home-based services, driving assessment, geriatric case managers.
  ○ The Care Transitions Project at the University of Colorado, Denver Health Sciences Center, www.caretransitions.org, is an excellent resource for healthcare organizations that wants to improve their discharge planning systems and transitions of care. They have multiple validated tools for self-assessment and program improvement.

BIBLIOGRAPHY

Coleman EA, Berenson RA. Lost in transition: challenges and opportunities for improving the quality of transitional care. *Ann Int Med.* 2004;141:533–536.
Creditor MC. Hazards of hospitalization of the elderly. *Ann Int Med.* 1993;118:219–223.
Resnick NM, Marcantonio ER. How should clinical care of aged differ? *Lancet.* 1997;350:1157–1159.
Watson LC, Lewis CL, Fillenbaum GG. Asking family members about memory loss. Is it helpful? *J Gen Int Med.* 2005;20:28–32.
www.geriatricsatyourfingertips.org This resource can be downloaded to your handheld device at no charge at: www.geriatricsatyourfingertips.org/front-back/pda.asp

99 ONCOLOGIC EMERGENCIES FOR THE HOSPITALIST
Rundsarah Tahboub

This chapter will deal with three of the most common oncologic emergencies treated by hospitalists: hypercalcemia of malignancy, neutropenic fever, and epidural spinal cord compression.

HYPERCALCEMIA OF MALIGNANCY

OVERVIEW

- Hypercalcemia of malignancy is one of the most common life-threatening metabolic emergencies in cancer patients, occurring in up to 20% of cases.
- Hypercalcemia predicts very poor prognosis in a cancer patient. About 50% of patients die within 30 days of this diagnosis.

- While hypercalcemia may occur in both solid tumors and leukemia
  - The most common cancers associated with hypercalcemia are breast cancer and multiple myeloma.
  - Less common are nonsmall cell lung cancer and renal cell carcinoma.

PATHOPHYSIOLOGY

Hypercalcemia of malignancy is secondary to increased bone resorption and this may happen by four different mechanisms (by decreasing frequency of occurrence)

- Humoral hypercalcemia of malignancy (80%) because of tumor secretion of parathyroid hormone-related peptide (PTH-rp).
  - This is the most common cause of hypercalcemia in malignancy, and should be suspected as the etiology of hypercalcemia in solid tumors (squamous cell cancer, renal cell, breast, ovarian cancer) without evidence of bony metastases and in some non-Hodgkin lymphoma patients.
  - PTH-rp also increases renal retention of calcium.
- Local osteolytic hypercalcemia (20%): osteolytic metastases with local release of prostaglandins and cytokines such as TGF-beta, interleukin-6, and tumor necrosis factor. Common in breast cancer, nonsmall cell lung cancer, and multiple myeloma

- Tumor production of calcitriol (Hodgkin's disease)
- Rarely by ectopic production of PTH (<1%)

CLINICAL PRESENTATION, DIFFERENTIAL, MAKING THE DIAGNOSIS

- Signs and symptoms may be vague and nonspecific especially if calcium levels are <12 mg/dL. Remember "stones, bones, moans and groans."
- Presentation varies depending on levels of hypercalcemia and the acuity of rise of calcium levels.
  - Mild-to-moderate hypercalcemia
    - Fatigue, nausea, vomiting, anorexia, constipation, polydipsia, poyluria, and bone pain
  - As levels rise, more neuropsychiatric symptoms develop
    - Lethargy, muscle weakness, confusion, psychosis, delirium, and coma
    - Hypotension and ECG changes such as shortening of the QT interval, bradycardia and first-degree AV block
    - Volume depletion can be quite severe and is secondary to central diabetes insipidus, and isosthenuria
- There are many potential causes of hypercalcemia in the hospitalized patient (see Table 99-1), but the most common are malignancy (65%) and hyperparathyroidism (25%).

TABLE 99-1   Differential Diagnosis of Hypercalcemia in Hospitalized Patients

65% hypercalcemia of malignancy
25% hyperparathyroidism
- Primary—most often from parathyroid adenomas, typically mild hypercalcemia (≤ 11, levels more than 13 would be exceedingly rare)
- Secondary—such as in end-stage renal disease
Milk-alkali syndrome (high intake of calcium carbonate associated with hypercalcemia, metabolic alkalosis, and renal insufficiency)
Paget disease of the bone
Immobilization
Medications
- Estrogens
- Tamoxifen
- Hypervitaminosis A
- Hypervitaminosis D
- Lithium
- Thiazide diuretics
- Theophylline
Granulomatous diseases, particularly sarcoidosis
Rhabdomyolysis
Endocrine
- Hyperthyroidism
- Pheochromocytoma
- Adrenal insufficiency
Genetic
- Familial hypocalciuric hypercalcemia
- Metaphyseal chondrodysplasia
- Congenital lactase deficiency
Pseudohypercalcemia
- Patients with hypoalbuminemia and dehydration
- Patients with multiple myeloma that secretes a calcium-binding paraprotein

- Most patients who present to the hospital with hypercalcemia of malignancy have a known history of cancer.
- In patients with no known diagnosis of their hypercalcemia, a thorough history and physical examination should be preformed to elicit the cause of hypercalcemia.
  - Initial studies should include complete blood count, differential, BUN, creatinine, urine analysis, serum protein electrophoresis, and chest x-ray.
  - An intact PTH should always be measured.
    - There is higher incidence of primary hyperparathyroidism in patients with malignancy.
  - Measuring PTH-rp is not routinely necessary as the etiology of hypercalcemia is usually evident clinically from the initial evaluation outlined above.
  - Measuring ionized calcium levels may be of value especially in patients with hypoalbuminemia.
- Factors that may trigger hypercalcemia in patients with malignancy include
  - Thiazide diuretics
  - Immobilization
  - Administration of hormonal therapy in breast cancer patients

TRIAGE AND INITIAL MANAGEMENT

- Reasons to hospitalize
  - Severe (calcium level >12) or symptomatic hypercalcemia, especially when altered mental status is present with its associated risks of aspiration and falls.
  - Acute renal insufficiency regardless of degree of hypercalcemia.
  - Dehydration, particularly if there is an inability to maintain/increase fluid intake at home.
- Initial therapy
  - Remove all exogenous calcium and discontinue any potential causative medications (lithium, thiazide diuretics, vitamin D, calcitriol).
  - Minimize use of sedative medications and encourage ambulation if possible.
  - Intravenous hydration with normal saline is the most critical initial therapy in patients with hypercalcemia, as the majority have moderate to severe volume depletion and hydration will also stimulate calciuresis.
    - Start with normal saline at an initial rate of 200–300 mL/h to achieve urine output of 100–150 mL/h, with careful monitoring of Ins and Outs and clinical examination to avoid volume overload. Volume repletion is still important in patients with heart disease and renal disease but with close monitoring.
  - Loop diuretics may be used if volume overload develops. Routine use of loop diuretics is no longer

recommended. If loop diuretics must be used, vigilance is required to minimize the possible adverse consequences of hypokalemia and volume depletion which may worsen hypercalcemia.
  - Consider starting calcitonin and a bisphosphonate (see below).
  - Close monitoring of neurologic status, urine output and renal function, calcium, phosphorus, and potassium levels is essential, and depending on the severity of the patient's condition may need to be done in a step-down unit or critical care setting.
  - Hypophosphatemia frequently occurs with hypercalcemia of malignancy and should be treated concomitantly as it may make lowering calcium levels difficult.
    - Replace orally or through a nasogastric tube.
    - Intravenous administration should be avoided as it may cause severe hypocalcemia, seizures, or renal failure.
    - The goal for the phosphate serum level should be 2.5–3.0 mg/dL.
- Immediate consultation for hemodialysis should be considered in the following settings:
  - Serum calcium >15 mg/dL
  - Severe renal failure
  - Coma
  - Contraindications exist to aggressive hydration

DISEASE MANAGEMENT STRATEGIES

Please refer to Table 99-2.
- Bisphosphonates are the safest, most widely studied, and most potent treatment for hypercalcemia of malignancy when compared to other therapies. Zoledronic acid is the bisphosphonate of choice for hypercalcemia of malignancy because of its increased potency and ease of administration.
  - Bisphosphonates work by inhibiting osteoclastic bone resorption.
  - Most are poorly absorbed orally (the exception is clodronate, available in Canada but not the United States).
  - They should be started immediately
    - Initial response occurs in 2–4 days
    - About 60%–90% of patients will have normal calcium levels in 4–7 days
    - The effect lasts 1–3 weeks, and varies by the specific agent used
  - There is concern of worsening renal function when using bisphosphonates.
  - They may also cause transient flu-like symptoms; the most common side effects are mild nausea, constipation, or diarrhea.

TABLE 99-2   Medications for the Treatment of Hypercalcemia of Malignancy

DRUG	DOSE	COMMENTS
FIRST LINE: IV BISPHOSPHONATES (AGENTS AVAILABLE IN THE UNITED STATES)		
Zoledronic acid	4 mg IV over 15 minutes although 8 mg dose can be used, it is associated with more renal toxicity	88% of patients have normalization of their calcium level with a single 4 mg dose. Longer duration of action (4–6 weeks) Use with creatinine up to 4.5 Use with caution in patients with multiple myeloma on thalidomide
Pamidronate	60–90 mg IV over 2–4 hours Use 60 mg for calcium levels up to 13.5 Use 90 mg for calcium levels above 13.5	70% of patients have normalization of their calcium level with a single 90 mg dose Less expensive than zoledronic acid Duration of action 2–4 weeks Use in creatinine up to 3.0
Etidronate	7.5 mg/kg IV in 250 mL saline over 4 hours on at least 3 consecutive days (5 days for optimal response) 20 mg/kg po daily to maintain normocalcemia	Relatively weak agent compared to zoledronic acid and pamidronate Duration of action 1–7 weeks
Ibandronate	2–4 mg IV	Decreases serum levels of PTH-rp Side effects include fever, hypophosphatemia, and GI distress
SECOND LINE THERAPY		
Calcitonin	4–8 units/kg IM or SC every 6–12 hours Intranasal route ineffective in treating hypercalcemia	Tachyphylaxis occurs within 48–72 hours
Glucocorticoids		May be used in patients with lymphomas or other underlying steroid-responsive diseases
Gallium nitrate	200 mg/m^2 continuous infusion over 5 days	Advantage—effective for both PTH-rp-mediated and non-PTH-rp-mediated hypercalcemia Disadvantages—nephrotoxicity and method of administration

◦ Osteonecrosis/avascular necrosis of the jaw has been associated with the use of IV bisphosphonates. Variables that predispose to osteonecrosis of the jaw include
  ▪ Underlying dental problems, dental extraction/local infection, or trauma
  ▪ Sequential therapy, particularly with high-potency bisphosphonates
  ▪ Longer duration of bisphosphonate use
• Second-line agents are to be used if bisphosphonates are ineffective or contraindicated, or in cases of severe hypercalcemia when their earlier onset of action may be beneficial.
  ◦ Calcitonin inhibits osteoclast maturation and bone resorption, and also promotes renal calcium excretion.
    ▪ Onset of action is within 4–6 hours, although tachyphylaxis occurs within ~48 hours.
    ▪ Side effects include mild nausea (common) and anaphylaxis/hypersensitivity reactions (rare).
    ▪ Typically initiated at a dose of 4 units/kg IM or SC every 12 hours, may be given 4–8 units/kg every 6 hours.

CARE TRANSITIONS

Recurrence of hypercalcemia should be avoided through appropriate followup
• When possible, treat the underlying malignancy.
• Ongoing outpatient bisphosphonate therapy and maintaining adequate hydration are essential.

NEUTROPENIC FEVER

OVERVIEW

• Fever is defined as a single oral temperature of >38.3°C or (101°F) or a temperature of >38°C (100.4°F) for more than 1 hour.
• Neutropenia is defined as an absolute neutrophil count (ANC) of <500 cells/mL.
• Serious infections developing in patients with neutropenia are a major cause of morbidity and mortality.

PATHOPHYSIOLOGY

- Neutropenia may develop in cancer patients receiving myelosuppressive chemotherapeutic agents.
- Factors that increase risk of infection in neutropenic patients include
  - The degree of neutropenia. Highest risk associated with ANC <100 cells/mL
  - Rapid rate of decline of the ANC
  - Longer duration of neutropenia

CLINICAL PRESENTATION, DIFFERENTIAL, MAKING THE DIAGNOSIS

- Signs and symptoms may be diminished or absent in patients with severe neutropenia. For example, the chest x-ray may not show an infiltrate in a patient with pneumonia, or a patient may have a UTI but no pyuria secondary to the decreased neutrophil count.
- A thorough history and physical examination should be performed on any neutropenic patient with fever with special focus on the most commonly infected organs in this situation, including the peridontum, pharynx, lungs, lower esophagus, perineum/anus (rectal examinations should not be performed in neutropenic patients), eyes/fundus, skin, especially vascular access sites.
- Fever may sometimes be absent in a neutropenic patient despite the presence of infection. Other signs should be looked for such as hypotension, altered mental status, tachypnea, tachycardia, or hypothermia.
- Other sources of fever in neutropenic patients include: drug fevers, transfusion reactions, thromboembolic disease, and the underlying malignancy itself.
- Initial immediate tests should include
  - Cultures
    - Two sets of blood cultures, including a set from any indwelling line or port, before any antibiotics are given.
    - Urine analysis and culture.
    - Consider stool for *Clostridium difficile* in patients with abdominal pain or diarrhea and who have received antibiotics recently.
    - Cerebrospinal fluid studies if neurologic symptoms exist (not recommended to be obtained routinely).
  - Radiologic
    - Chest x-ray
    - Abdominal films upright and supine in patients with gastrointestinal symptoms
    - Consider CT scans of chest, abdomen, pelvis if clear localizing symptoms are present and plain x-rays show no abnormalities
  - Other labs: CBC, BUN, creatinine, liver enzymes should be followed during the course of treatment to ensure that the patient is not developing toxicity

from treatments and/or evidence of organ failure from sepsis.

TRIAGE AND INITIAL MANAGEMENT

OUTPATIENT MANAGEMENT

- Low-risk neutropenic patients with fever may be managed as outpatients with oral or intravenous antibiotics.
- These patients must be selected carefully and should have lower risk of complications or mortality.
  - Age <60 years
  - No localizing signs or symptoms of infection or systemic toxicity
    - Normal chest x-ray
    - No hypotension, respiratory rate <24, peak temperature <39°C
  - Absence of chronic pulmonary disease, diabetes mellitus (DM), confusion, blood loss, dehydration, history of fungal infection, or receiving antifungals in past 6 months.
  - They must have immediate access to medical care in case of change in their condition.
  - See Table 99-3 for factors associated with low risk of serious infection in patients with neutropenia and infection for further detail.
- See Fig. 99-1 for initial empiric drug therapy in the outpatient setting.

INPATIENT MANAGEMENT

- If the patient is high risk (does not meet the above criteria for outpatient management), then they should be admitted to the hospital.
- Initial empiric intravenous drug therapy for the neutropenic patient with fever may follow three different pathways based on the 2002 recommendations of the Infectious Disease Society of America (IDSA). See Fig. 99-1 for an overview.

TABLE 99-3 Factors Associated with Low Risk of Serious Infection in Patients with Neutropenia and Infection

Absence of neurologic deficits or mental status changes
Absence of abdominal pain
Absence of comorbidities (shock, hypoxia, pneumonia, deep organ infection)
Absolute monocyte count >100
Normal chest x-ray
Normal or mild abnormalities in hepatic or renal function tests
Duration of neutropenia <7 days and resolution expected in 10 days
No IV catheter site infection
Malignancy in remission
Peak temperature <39°C

From 2002 Guidelines for use of Antimicrobial Agents in Neutropenic Patients with Cancer.

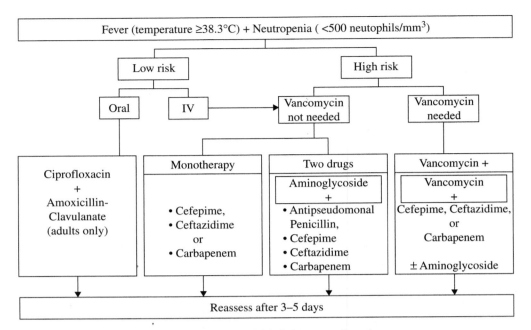

FIG. 99-1 Algorithm for initial management of febrile neutropenic patients. From 2002 Guidelines for use of Antimicrobial Agents in Neutropenic Patients with Cancer.

- The course of therapy chosen depends on many factors specific to the patient, such as prior history, suspected site of infection, severity of illness, patients' allergies, and possible drug interactions and local drug susceptibilities.
- The need for vancomycin should be determined initially. See Table 99-4. Vancomycin should not be used routinely in all patients as this may increase the emergence of vancomycin-resistant organisms.
  - Vancomycin has not been shown to reduce the overall mortality because of gram-positive cocci as a group but may affect mortality specifically in patients with viridans streptococci.
  - If no organisms requiring vancomycin have been isolated in first 24–48 hours, it should be discontinued.
- Therapy options when vancomycin is not indicated
  - Single drug therapy: use a third- or fourth-generation cephalosporin or a carbapenem.
  - Two-drug therapy, vancomycin not indicated: Most common combination includes aminoglycoside plus antipseudomonal carboxy penicillin.

TABLE 99-4 Indications for Vancomycin

Vascular catheter-associated infection
Known or suspected MRSA infection
High institutional risk for MRSA
Initial cultures positive for gram-positive cocci
Evidence of sepsis
Severe beta-lactam allergy
Severe mucositis

MRSA, methicillin-resistant *Staphylococcus aureus*.

DISEASE MANAGEMENT STRATEGIES

- The initial drug regimen should be followed for 3–5 days and the patient's need for further antimicrobials be reassessed based on their response to the initial therapy on available culture data.
- If the patient is afebrile after the first 3–5 days and the organism is known
  - The antibiotic regimen should be tailored to treat the specific organism with the least toxicity and cost.
  - The duration of therapy should at least be of the same duration for that infection in a normal host but may need to be prolonged based on the severity of the initial presentation.
  - The ANC should be >500 cells/mL before discontinuing antibiotics.
- If the patient is afebrile after the first 3–5 days but no organism was identified
  - Low-risk patients: (no sepsis, rapid defervescence, ANC >100 cells/mL) will probably do well on oral antibiotics and outpatient therapy. May stop therapy when ANC >500 cells/mL.
  - High-risk patients
    - ANC <100 cells/mL, unstable or has mucositits: continue empiric antibiotics, until
    - ANC >100 cells/mL, stable, intact skin and mucous membranes: then continue antibiotics until afebrile for 5–7 days.
- If a neutropenic patient has persistent fevers after the first 3–5 days, nonbacterial infection, a resistant

organism, emergence of a second infection, abscess or drug fever should be suspected.

- The patient should be reevaluated and this should include review of all culture results, a thorough reexamination, chest x-ray, and imaging of any organs suspected of infection.
- If patient remains febrile after 5 days and no clear cause is evident, one of the following approaches may be taken
  - Continue with initial antibiotics especially if patient appears stable and neutropenia is expected to resolve quickly.
  - Change or add antibiotics such as adding aminoglycoside or vancomycin as indicated, and depending on the initial drug regimen chosen.
  - Initiate empirical antifungal therapy: it may be difficult to diagnose a fungal infection (candida or aspergillus) in neutropenic patients and delaying therapy until clinical evidence of fungal infection emerges, is associated with high mortality.
    - Aspergillus should be suspected in patients with prolonged neutropenia, history of respiratory tract colonization with aspergillus, or cutaneous, pulmonary, or central nervous system signs of aspergillus.
    - Neutropenic patients with oral, esophageal candidiasis or colitis are at risk for candidemia.
    - See Table 99-5.
- Empiric antiviral therapy is not recommended.
  - Treat with acyclovir or valacyclovir or famciclovir if there is clinical evidence of viral disease such as varicella zoster or herpes simplex.

TABLE 99-5 Antifungal Therapy Options

- Amphotericin B is a broad-spectrum antifungal agent and should be dosed at 0.5–0.6 mg/kg/d for suspected candidal infections and 1.0–1.5 mg/kg/d for aspergillus
- Liposomal amphotericin B has less toxicity than amphotericin deoxycholate; however it is significantly more expensive
- Voriconazole is an appropriate alternative to amphotericin B for empiric therapy and has less toxicity
- Fluconazole is an appropriate option in institutions where incidence of aspergillus and drug-resistant candida is low but should not be used if there is a high suspicion of aspergillus such as patients with sinus or pulmonary lesions or patients on fluconazole prophylaxis
- Caspofungin is as effective and associated with less toxicity when compared with liposomal amphotericin B and may be used for empiric therapy
- Every effort should be made to determine whether a fungal infection exists in order to determine if continued antifungal therapy is necessary (repeat CT scans of sinuses, brain, lungs, abdomen, biopsy of any suspicious lesions . . . etc)
- Candidemia can be treated with fluconazole or amphotericin or caspofungin if sensitive
- Pulmonary aspergillus can be treated with voriconazole or amphotericin alone
- If CNS or systemic aspergillus infection is suspected, combination therapy with voriconazole plus caspofungin with or without high-dose amphotericin B

CNS, central nervous system; CT, computed tomography.

- Cytomegalovirus infections are uncommon in neutropenic patients except those in post–bone marrow transplant patients and should be treated with ganciclovir or foscarnet.
- Colony-stimulating factors are not recommended for routine use in treatment of febrile or afebrile neutropenic patients especially in uncomplicated cases. They may be considered in patients with prolonged neutropenia, multiorgan dysfunction, or patients not responding to appropriate antimicrobial therapy.

CARE TRANSITIONS

- Duration of treatment: the most important factor in determining duration of therapy is the ANC.
- See Fig. 99-2 for a suggested approach.

EPIDURAL SPINAL CORD COMPRESSION

OVERVIEW

- Spinal cord compression most commonly occurs in association with the following cancers: breast cancer, prostate cancer, and lung cancer.
- The most commonly affected area is the thoracic spine (~60%), followed by the lumbar spine (30%).
- About 98% of cancer patients who present with back pain will have bone or epidural metastases.
- Spinal cord compression will occur in 20% of patients with known vertebral metastases.
- Around half the patients with spinal metastases have multiple levels involved.
- Spinal metastasis and cord compression may be the first sign of metastasis or may even be the first sign of cancer and, therefore, further staging of the cancer may be necessary to make treatment decisions.
- Cauda equina syndrome occurs when compression occurs below the level of the distal end of the spinal cord at L1 and the compression in this case occurs to the lumbosacral nerve roots.

PATHOPHYSIOLOGY

- The thecal sac which contains the spinal cord is enclosed by the vertebral body anteriorly and the lamina, pedicles, and spinous process posteriorly. The outer layer of the thecal sac is the dura. The space between the dura and the bone is the epidural space.
- Spinal cord compression occurs when tumor invades the epidural space and compresses the thecal sac.

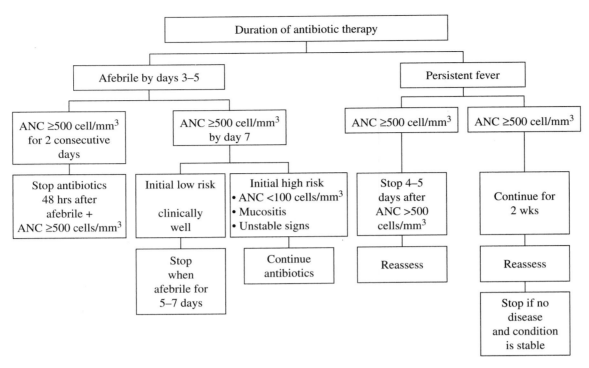

FIG. 99-2   Duration of antibiotic therapy in neutropenic patients.
From 2002 Guidelines for use of Antimicrobial Agents in Neutropenic Patients with Cancer.

- Tumor invading the epidural space will usually incase the thecal sac and can obstruct the epidural venous plexus causing vasogenic edema, which if not treated can lead to spinal infarct.
- The degree of compression and the resultant presentation can vary from asymptomatic/minor compression to severe strangulation of the thecal sac resulting in paralysis.

CLINICAL PRESENTATION, DIFFERENTIAL, MAKING THE DIAGNOSIS

- Unfortunately there often exist significant delays in the diagnosis of spinal cord compression, and as a result roughly half of patients will initially present in a nonambulatory state.
- Symptoms of spinal cord compression
  - Pain: spinal cord compression should be suspected in any patient with known metastatic cancer and new onset back pain.
    - Pain is present in >80% of patients on initial presentation and may precede any neurologic symptoms by several weeks.
    - Pain initially may be localized but then can develop a radicular pattern, especially in case of lumbosacral lesions.
    - Pain may be worse in the supine position.
    - Pain usually worsens in intensity with time.

- High cervical metastases may present as an occipital headache.
- Patients with T12 or L1 lesions may present with flank pain, iliac crest, or sacroiliac joint pain.
- Lesions in C7 to T1 may cause interscapular pain.
- Abrupt worsening of pain may be secondary to compression fractures.
  - Myelopathy: motor or sensory deficits below a specific spinal level, bowel and bladder dysfunction, or change in tendon reflexes
    - More than half the patients present with weakness at diagnosis.
    - Weakness is most severe in cases of thoracic compression.
    - Weakness progresses to loss of ability to walk and then leads to paralysis.
    - Weakness of the lower extremities is usually symmetrical but patients may also have a motor radiculopathy.
    also secondary to unilateral nerve root compression.
    - Sensory loss is less common. Patients may have parasthesias and this may present in a radicular fashion and more commonly occurs in lumbar rather than thoracic lesions.
    - Compression of the cauda equine will result in saddle sensory loss.
    - Bladder or bowel dysfunction is a late finding and usually manifests as urinary retention.

- The initial evaluation
  - ○ Stable back pain: Patient's pain is not severe or new and there are no neurologic deficits.
    - ▪ Workup can be done as an outpatient. Initial workup should include spinal x-rays and bone scan.
    - ▪ X-rays will detect 70% of vertebral metastases and is helpful in detecting compression fractures. False-negative results remain unacceptably high as 50% of the vertebral bone must be destroyed before an x-ray is abnormal and, therefore, further imaging is usually needed.
    - ▪ Bone scans will visualize the entire spine. Its positive predictive value is 40% for metastases as there are other conditions that may lead to a positive scan. A bone scan will not visualize the thecal sac.
    - ▪ If x-rays or bone scan are abnormal, an MRI should be done to confirm the presence of tumor and determine the extent of disease.
  - ○ Unstable back pain: If pain rapidly worsens or any neurologic symptoms exist, immediate evaluation (within 24 hours) with MRI of the entire spine to evaluate for multiple areas of metastasis and degree of compression is warranted. MRI is the gold standard for evaluating patients with spinal cord compression
    - ▪ MRI can visualize the entire spine and is more sensitive than bone scan for the diagnosis of metastasis.
    - ▪ MRI is more convenient than a CT myelogram (an alternative for patients in whom MRI is contraindicated).
    - ▪ MRI imaging is important for staging, and in preparation for radiation therapy (RT).

- ○ Urgent neurosurgical evaluation should also be requested.
- Differential diagnosis (see Table 99-6).

TRIAGE AND INITIAL MANAGEMENT

- Reasons to hospitalize: Frequently cancer patients will present initially to the emergency room with complaints of back pain and no outpatient work has been done. These patients should be hospitalized for
  - ○ Severe pain
  - ○ Inability to care for self
  - ○ High suspicion of impending cord compression even if neurologic deficits have not developed
  - ○ Neurologic deficits/myelopathy
- Any patient with proven spinal cord compression on MRI or otherwise should be immediately hospitalized for emergent care.
- Initial management
  - ○ Bed rest until further evaluation of spinal stability has been done.
  - ○ Frequent evaluation of neurologic examination by nursing staff (neurochecks)
  - ○ Preventative care (deep vein thrombosis prophylaxis, decubitus ulcer prevention, prevention of constipation, watching for urinary retention).
  - ○ Physical and occupational therapy consultation.
  - ○ Pain control.
  - ○ Steroids (see below).
  - ○ Neurosurgery and radiation oncology consultation should be obtained early in all patients suspected of

TABLE 99-6 Differential Diagnosis of Back Pain in Patients with Underlying Malignancy

Musculoskeletal causes (spinal stenosis, disc disease, muscle spasms, etc) Spinal epidural abscess	• Usually occur in lumbar or cervical regions not thoracic • Pain is not usually worse in supine position • Suspect in cases of IV drug abuse, vertebral osteomyelitis, bacteremia • May be very similar in presentation and even on imaging • Biopsy may be needed to make the diagnosis
Leptomeningeal carcinomatosis	• May present similar to cauda equina syndrome along with headache, mental status changes, cranial nerve palsies • Usually not associated with back pain • MRI will not show thecal compression, may show leptomeningeal enhancement • CSF is needed to make the diagnosis
Radiation myelopathy	• May occur 9–15 months after radiation • Ascending numbness and upper motor neuron findings • MRI usually will differentiate
Spontaneous spinal epidural hematomas	• In anticoagulated patients, those with AV malformations, or bleeding disorders

AV, atrioventricular; CSF, cerebrospinal fluid; IV, intravenous; MRI, magnetic resonance imaging.

cord compression and immediately in any patient with neurologic deficits.

DISEASE MANAGEMENT STRATEGIES

- The goal for therapy of spinal cord compression is relief of pain, preserving, and improving neurologic function as is appropriate based on the patient's overall condition and prognosis.
- Corticosteroids
  - Corticosteroids may improve pain within a few hours of administration.
  - High-dose steroids have been shown to improve neurologic function, but may be associated with significant side effects (hyperglycemia, adrenal axis suppression, increased risk of infection, and many others).
    - A typical high-dose regimen would be dexamethasone (100 mg IV followed by 24 mg 4 times a day for 3 days then tapered over 10 days) and should be considered for patients with paraparesis or paraplegia.
  - Low-dose regimens have not been demonstrated to be of neurologic benefit in randomized controlled trials, but are frequently used in patients with pain and minimal neurologic deficits.
    - A typical low-dose regimen would be dexamethasone (10 mg IV followed by 16 mg a day in divided doses).
  - Patients with pain and small epidural lesions and no deficits may not require corticosteroids and may proceed to RT directly.
- RT
  - Was the initial treatment of choice before radical surgery became available. It is also used for pure palliative reasons.
  - Should be used in patients who are not surgical candidates.
  - Poor response to RT occurs in the following situations
    - Nonambulatory
    - Greater that 14 days between start of motor deficits and initiation of therapy
    - Presence of solid organ or other bony metastases
  - RT leads to resolution of pain in most patients and is usually well tolerated. Patients who receive doses of radiation to large areas of the spine may develop gastrointestinal symptoms such as esophagitis, diarrhea, and mucositis.
  - Response to RT is dependent on
    - Preradiation function is the most important predictor to the response to RT.
    - Sensitivity of the tumor to radiation: Lymphoma, multiple myeloma, prostate cancer, and breast

cancer are the most responsive and less likely to develop local recurrence after radiation.

- Radical resection plus RT: aggressive anterior tumor resection, along with spinal reconstruction and stabilization (with methacrylate), followed by RT 1 week postoperatively, is the optimal choice for restoration/preservation of neurologic functioning in selected patients.
  - Patients must be selected carefully depending on the overall medical condition and prognosis from cancer.
  - This approach is best suited for patients with minimal disease burden and may be necessary in cases of vertebral instability or bone impinging on the thecal sac or in tumors that are not likely to respond to RT.
  - Studies show that this approach is associated with higher incidence of regaining ability to walk than RT alone.
- Systemic chemotherapy: Some tumors causing spinal cord compression may respond to chemotherapy such as Hodgkin disease, non-Hodgkin lymphoma, neuroblastoma, germ cell neoplasms, and breast cancer.
- Hormonal therapy: May be useful in cases of breast and prostate cancer.
  - Orchiectomy and high-dose ketoconazole may have a rapid effect on patients with prostate cancer and be beneficial in acute cord compression.

CARE TRANSITIONS

- Prognosis and recurrence
  - Median survival after diagnosis of spinal cord compression is 6 months.
  - The single most important prognostic factor is neurologic status on presentation. Those who present ambulatory usually remain so.
  - Prognosis is better in ambulatory patients with single site of metastasis and in patients with newly diagnosed breast cancer, prostate cancer, Hodgkin and non-Hodgkin lymphoma.
  - Lung cancer carries a worse prognosis.
  - Poorer prognosis for patients with multiple vertebral metastases, solid organ metastases, paraplegia, and incontinence.
- Discharge planning
  - Patients may be discharged home if they have stable neurologic examination.
  - Patients discharged home may require home physical therapy, occupational therapy, and visiting nurse/home health aides to assist in care.
  - Ensure adequate ongoing pain control at discharge.
  - Consider referral to hospice care as appropriate based on expected prognosis.

BIBLIOGRAPHY

Abraham JL. Management of pain and spinal cord compression in patients with advanced cancer. *Ann Intern Med.* 1999:131:37–46.

Basgoz N. Neutropenia. In: *Hospital Medicine.* 2nd ed. Lippincott Williams & Wilkins; 2005:615–619.

Hughes WT, Armstrong D, Bodey GP, et al. Guidelines for use of Antimicrobial Agents in Neutropenic Patients with Cancer. IDSA Guidelines;2002.

Luce JA. Hypercalcemia. In: *Hospital Medicine.* 2nd ed. Lippincott Williams & Wilkins; 2005:924–927.

Luce JA. Neurologic emergencies. In: *Hospital Medicine.* 2nd ed. Lippincott Williams & Wilkins; 2005:917–921.

Schiff D. Clinical features and diagnosis of epidural spinal cord compression, including cauda equine syndrome. 2007 Uptodate.

Schiff D. Treatment and prognosis of epidural spinal cord compression, including cauda equine syndrome. 2007 Uptodate.

Stewart AF. Hypercalcemia associated with cancer. *NEJM.* 2005;352:4.

Walsh TJ. Caspofungin versus liposomal amphotericin B for empirical antifungal therapy in patients with persistent fever and neutropenia. *NEJM.* 2004;1812(9):1391–1402.

Walsh TJ. Voriconazole compared with liposomal amphotericin B for empirical antifungal therapy in patients with neutropenia and persistent fever. *NEJM.* 2002;346(1):225–234.

100 SKILLED NURSING FACILITY CARE

Darrell W. Craig

OVERVIEW

- Approximately 1.5 million Americans reside in more than 16,000 skilled nursing facilities in the United States. In 1 year, more than 3 million Americans will receive services provided by a skilled nursing facility.
- Skilled nursing facilities are becoming more focused on short-term subacute stays and less on long-term care, with lengths of stay <90 days increasing from 46.1% in 1977 to 91.7% in 1999.
- Three different types of care may be occurring in the same physical setting in skilled nursing facilities
  - *Long-term care* has focused on the care of individuals with debilities related to chronic illnesses, especially dementia.
  - *Subacute care* focuses on rehabilitation and skilled nursing for individuals who in years past were treated in the acute-care hospital setting.
  - *Hospice care* has expanded in the nursing home setting recently.
- Nursing homes increasingly are the site of death for those Americans dying of chronic illnesses: almost one-quarter of nontraumatic deaths occur in nursing homes.
- Responsibilities of the physician are outlined in detail in Part 483.40 of the Code of Federal Regulations (see Table 100-1).

TRANSITIONAL CARE

- During care transitions, such as hospital to subacute rehabilitation facility or from the facility back to the hospital, the following requirements are ideal:
  - Uniformity in the care plan, allowing for communication across care settings.
  - Availability of highly relevant medical information including current problem lists, medications, allergies, advanced directives, cognitive and physical status, and contact information of the patient's advocates.
- Knowledge of the types and levels of service provided at a skilled nursing facility is necessary to plan for an appropriate transition. Skilled nursing facilities vary in the types of services that they provide. Some facilities are unable to provide for IV therapies, while others may handle long-term ventilators or left ventricular assist pumps.

INTERDISCIPLINARY CARE

- Skilled nursing facility provides an opportunity to practice in an interdisciplinary manner. Mandatory physician visits may be as infrequent as every 60 days in some situations (Table 100-1). Frequency of nonregulatory physician visits is based on medical necessity. With high-acuity subacute patients, this may be as frequent as daily. The need for a physician visit is often guided by information conveyed to the attending physician by facility staff.
- Physicians are assisted in maximizing the quality of care at the facility by
  - *Registered nurses and licensed practical nurses,* overseen by a director of nursing, perform daily assessments, administer medications, and provide treatments. They are responsible for the development of nursing care plans that should coordinate with the overall plan of care that the physician is responsible for approving. Infection control at the facility is overseen by the director of nursing or designee.

TABLE 100-1   Responsibilities of the Physician in a Skilled Nursing Facility

§ 483.40 Physician services.

A physician must personally approve in writing a recommendation that an individual be admitted to a facility. Each resident must remain under the care of a physician

(a) *Physician supervision.* The facility must ensure that
  (1) The medical care of each resident is supervised by a physician
  (2) Another physician supervises the medical care of residents when their attending physician is unavailable
(b) *Physician visits.* The physician must
  (1) Review the resident's total program of care, including medications and treatments, at each visit required by paragraph (c) of this section
  (2) Write, sign, and date progress notes at each visit
  (3) Sign and date all orders with the exception of influenza and pneumococcal polysaccharide vaccines, which may be administered per physician-approved facility policy after an assessment for contraindications
(c) *Frequency of physician visits.*
  (1) The resident must be seen by a physician at least once every 30 days for the first 90 days after admission, and at least once every 60 days thereafter
  (2) A physician visit is considered timely if it occurs not later than 10 days after the date the visit was required
  (3) Except as provided in paragraphs (c)(4) and (f) of this section, all required physician visits must be made by the physician personally
  (4) At the option of the physician, required visits in SNFs after the initial visit may alternate between personal visits by the physician and visits by a physician assistant, nurse practitioner, or clinical nurse specialist in accordance with paragraph (e) of this section
(d) *Availability of physicians for emergency care.* The facility must provide or arrange for the provision of physician services 24 hours a day, in case of an emergency
(e) *Physician delegation of tasks in SNFs.*
  (1) Except as specified in paragraph (e)(2) of this section, a physician may delegate tasks to a physician assistant, nurse practitioner, or clinical nurse specialist who meets the following criteria:
    (i) Meets the applicable definition in §491.2 of this chapter or, in the case of a clinical nurse specialist, is licensed as such by the State
    (ii) Is acting within the scope of practice as defined by State law
    (iii) Is under the supervision of the physician
  (2) A physician may not delegate a task when the regulations specify that the physician must perform it personally, or when the delegation is prohibited under State law or by the facility's own policies
(f) *Performance of physician tasks in NFs.* At the option of the State, any required physician task in an NF (including tasks which the regulations specify must be performed personally by the physician) may also be satisfied when performed by a nurse practitioner, clinical nurse specialist, or physician assistant who is not an employee of the facility but who is working in collaboration with a physician

56 FR 48875, Sept. 26, 1991, as amended at 67 FR 61814, Oct. 2, 2002.

○ *Certified nursing assistants* provide the bulk of the individual care provided in nursing homes. They are often the most knowledgeable about changes in a patient's mental status or changes in functional abilities.

○ *Physical therapists, occupational therapists, and speech and language pathologists* are responsible for establishing rehabilitation goals and directing therapies to achieve these goals. They often determine when an individual has reached a level of independence with therapies that would afford a transition to a less restrictive environment than the skilled nursing facility. Speech pathologists often provide dysphagia and cognitive rehabilitation services in addition to their work with improving communication.

○ *Registered dieticians* are responsible for ensuring the proper diet for residents and monitoring of adequate nutrition and hydration.

○ *Social workers* often serve as a liaison to family members and assist in planned care transitions.

○ *Consulting pharmacists* are required by regulations to review medications on a monthly basis and assist in compliance with federal and state regulations.

○ *Mental health professionals* are generally available as consultants on contractual arrangements with the facilities.

• Physician visits, in addition to allowing for a medical assessment including reviews of medications and laboratory data, provide an opportunity to review documentation of other interdisciplinary team members. Medication review should follow guidelines in Table 100-2.

• Details of financing of skilled nursing facility visits under Medicare are presented in Table 100-3.

ADVANCED CARE PLANNING

• Most recent available data suggests that only about 35% of nursing home residents have advance directives.

• Portability of advanced directives is poor—information regarding discussions of goals of treatment or limitations of treatment unfortunately does not often pass from the hospital to the nursing facility, or vice versa.

• To aid in their decision-making, patients and their surrogates may be informed that only 2% of individuals

---

TABLE 100-2   Regulations and Guidelines Regarding Unnecessary Medications

Regulations

- Each resident's medication regimen must be free from unnecessary medications
- An unnecessary medication is any medication when used
  - In excessive doses (including duplicate therapy)
  - Without adequate monitoring
  - Without adequate indications for its use
  - In the presence of adverse consequences which indicate the dose should be reduced or discontinued
  - Any combinations of the reasons above
- Antipsychotics—based on a comprehensive assessment of a resident, the facility must ensure that
  - Residents who have not used antipsychotic drugs are not given these drugs unless antipsychotic drug therapy is necessary to treat a specific condition as diagnosed and documented in the clinical record
  - Residents who use antipsychotic drugs receive gradual dose reductions and behavioral interventions, unless clinically contraindicated, in an effort to discontinue these drugs

Interpretive guidelines

- Previously, individuals with known chronic psychiatric illnesses were exempt from gradual dose reductions. Attempts at gradual dose reduction are required twice in the first year and then yearly unless clinically contraindicated. Documentation by the physician is required if dose reduction is clinically contraindicated by stating that target symptoms have returned or worsened after the last dose reduction and that attempted dose reductions would impair a resident's function or increase distressful behaviors
- Before sedatives and hypnotics are prescribed, documentation is required that an assessment of potential causes of insomnia has occurred and indicated interventions have failed. Attempts to taper hypnotics must occur quarterly and all medications, no matter what pharmacologic class, used for induction or maintenance of sleep fall under this regulation
- All psychopharmacologic medications, including antidepressants and mood stabilizers require the same attempts at dose reduction as antipsychotics
- Documentation requirements required to avoid citations under the unnecessary medication use guidelines include
  - Evaluation of the continued need for proton pump inhibitors or H2 antagonists beyond 12 weeks of therapy
  - Adequate GFR for the safe use of certain medications such as nitrofurantoin
  - Adequate laboratory monitoring for anticonvulsants, diuretics, lipid-lowering agents, and so on
  - Appropriate evaluation is performed before medication is prescribed, such as the need to document that an anemia is because of iron deficiency before iron sulfate is prescribed
  - The need for medications with known anticholinergic properties, and the lack of alternative therapies, must be clearly stated

---

who had cardiopulmonary arrest in nursing homes survived 1 year.

- Detailed discussions regarding transfer from skilled nursing facilities to the hospital setting should take place.

A request for DNR should not be interpreted as a preference for less aggressive care. In addition to discussions of desire for resuscitation, patients and their surrogates should be queried regarding desire for hospitalization.

TABLE 100-3   Skilled Nursing Facility Benefit Under Medicare Part A

- Requirements
  - Acute-care hospitalization for 3 consecutive days, not counting the day of discharge
  - Admission to the skilled nursing facility within 30 days of hospital discharge
  - Services required in the skilled nursing facility are related to the condition treated during the hospitalization
  - Skilled nursing services or rehabilitation services are required on a daily basis
  - A physician must certify at the time of admission, at 14 days, and every 30 days thereafter that skilled care services are needed on a daily basis
  - Skilled nursing facility care is covered for up to 100 days per benefit period
  - The skilled nursing facility benefit is renewable for another benefit period if
    - The individual has not been in a skilled nursing facility or a hospital for at least 60 days in a row
    - The individual remains confined to a skilled nursing facility, skilled care (as defined by level of service provided) has not been received for at least 60 days in a row
- Benefits
  - A semiprivate room
  - All meals, including special diets
  - Nursing care
  - Rehabilitative therapies
  - Medications prescribed by a physician
  - Medical supplies
  - Use of appliances and equipment

- Decisions regarding artificial nutrition and hydration should be addressed early on and in the context of the individual's present debilities, prognosis, and overall goals of care. Families may be informed that in patients with dysphagia the use of enteral feedings with gastrostomy feeding tubes does not decrease the risk of developing aspiration pneumonia.
- A study of the sites of death in nursing home residents indicated that younger skilled nursing facility residents and those with less severe cognitive impairment were likely to die in hospital rather than in the facility. One-quarter of those patients who died after transfer to an acute hospital died in the first 24 hours and only 50% survived beyond day 5.
- Nursing home residents are eligible for hospice benefits at the end of life; quality of pain and symptom control can improve with the addition of hospice care. For those individuals in the skilled nursing facility under their Medicare Part A benefit for posthospitalization rehabilitation, election of hospice care will eliminate Medicare coverage of room and board costs which would then need to be covered by other resources.

INFECTION CONTROL

- Colonization with antibiotic-resistant bacteria is common in long-term care facilities.
  - Individuals who are colonized with antimicrobial-resistant pathogens should not be denied admission to long-term care facilities and decolonization should not be required.
  - Individuals colonized with antimicrobial-resistant organisms should not be restricted in their participation in social or group activities unless there is reason to believe that they are shedding large numbers of bacteria.
- Physicians practicing in the skilled nursing facility setting should avoid contributing to the development of antibiotic-resistant bacteria through the use of appropriate antibiotics and avoiding antibiotic treatment of viral illnesses and asymptomatic bacteriuria.
- Use of indwelling Foley catheters for the management of urinary incontinence is discouraged. State surveyors require documentation of the medical necessity for the use of urinary catheters (eg, urinary retention from a neurogenic bladder).
- Guidelines for use of influenza and pneumococcal vaccines should be followed.

COMMON CLINICAL ISSUES

- Infectious diseases
  - *Clostridium difficile* diarrhea: Debilitated patients that have been treated with broad-spectrum antibiotics are highly susceptible. Universal and enteric precautions should be utilized. Since about one-quarter of the antibiotics used in skilled nursing facilities cannot be justified, antibiotics should be used only when clearly indicated and targeted to a specific pathogen whenever possible.
  - *Pneumonia*: Leading cause of death in the nursing home population. Risk factors include swallowing difficulties, advanced dementia, Parkinson disease or other neurologic conditions, and poor oral hygiene. Pathogens causing pneumonia in long-term care residents are comparable to those of community-acquired pneumonia. Nosocomial pathogens need to be considered. Pneumonia can often be treated in the skilled nursing facility. Criteria for hospitalization are listed in Table 100-4.
  - *Norwalk and Norwalk-like viral gastroenteritis*: Outbreaks of this common, generally self-limited, illness are common in skilled nursing facilities. Because of the frailty of the population, dehydration is common. Strict adherence to universal and enteric precautions by staff is a must and employees should not be allowed to work if they have signs and symptoms of illness during an outbreak.
- Behavioral disorders common in patients with dementia
  - *Psychotic symptoms and aggressive behaviors*: Effects of atypical antipsychotics are modest and are complicated by increased somnolence, extrapyramidal side effects, abnormal gait and increased risk of falls, and increased risk of stroke.
  - *Wandering and pacing behaviors*: There is no pharmacologic therapy for treatment of these common symptoms of dementia. Providing an appropriate physical environment to accommodate these behaviors is essential. Physical restraints and the use of medications as chemical restraints must be avoided.
  - *Inappropriate sexual behavior*: Sexual activity continues throughout the life span. With dementia, however, inappropriate sexual activity is not uncommon and is best dealt with through behavioral therapy. It is incumbent on the facility and facility staff to

TABLE 100-4   Criteria for Transfer to Hospital for Treatment of Pneumonia

Hospitalization for treatment of pneumonia is recommended when two or more of the following symptoms exist:
- Oxygen saturation <90%
- Systolic BP <90 or 20 mm Hg lower than baseline
- Respiratory rate of >30
- Oxygen requirements above 3 L/min
- Uncontrolled COPD, CHF, or DM
- Unarousable, if previously conscious
- New or increased agitation

BP, blood pressure; CHF, coronary heart failure; COPD, chronic obstructive pulmonary disease; DM, diabetes mellitus.

protect other residents and staff from undesired sexual advances.

- Falls
  - *Risk assessment on admission and proper care planning* is required. The use of an interdisciplinary care team for fall prevention assessments has been shown to be effective in reducing falls and injuries. The physician and clinical pharmacist have responsibility for identifying medications that may be contributing to falls.
  - *Vitamin D deficiency* is common in the elderly and especially in those who are institutionalized. Replacement with 700–800 IU of vitamin D daily has been associated with a reduction in falls and hip fractures.
  - *Assessment for the presence and severity of osteoporosis* should not be overlooked. Consideration should be given to the use of antiresorptive agents or teriparatide injections.
  - *The use of hip padding* ("hipsters") is an inexpensive way to provide some reduction in the incidence of hip fractures in the nursing home population.
- Dehydration
  - Aging associated with impaired thirst mechanism and increased renal excretion of salt and water because of the age-related reduction in renin and aldosterone production.
  - Fluids need to be regularly offered to residents of nursing facilities who often have disabilities that limit their ability to access water.
  - Ongoing need for diuretic therapy needs to be part of medication review at each visit.
  - Though not widely used, hypodermoclysis is an option for rehydration when IV access is not readily available for those patients for whom it is appropriate to provide artificial hydration.
- Pressure ulcers
  - *Prevention*: Understanding the risk factors of poor nutrition, moisture, pressure, and immobility is the primary approach to pressure ulcers in the modern nursing home.
  - Wound care protocols should be utilized for the proper treatment based on size, location, and stage.
- Weight loss
  - *Depression and adverse drug reactions* are most common reversible causes.
  - *Calorie-dense oral supplements* frequently prescribed when inadequate nutritional intake is identified. Inadequate nursing staff time to deliver and assist with between meal supplements may be a barrier to effectiveness. Supplements may be used at time of medication administration to enhance caloric intake.
  - *Megestrol acetate* is often used as an appetite stimulant to promote weight gain. Studies of its use in nursing home residents are limited and evidence of benefit is unclear.

101 PREOPERATIVE EVALUATION OF THE PATIENT UNDERGOING NONCARDIAC SURGERY

Satyen S. Nichani and Steven L. Cohn

OVERVIEW

- Thirty million people undergo major noncardiac surgery in the United States each year.
- The goal of the preoperative medical encounter is to assess the patient's current medical status, perform diagnostic tests if required, grade the severity of medical problems associated with adverse surgical outcomes, weigh the risks and benefits of the proposed procedure in the individual patient, and optimize all medical conditions, including medications, during the perioperative period.
- The preoperative evaluation begins with a thorough history and physical examination of the patient, with an emphasis on current symptoms, cardiopulmonary status, past medical illnesses, and previous surgical outcomes. It also includes a comprehensive review of all current medications including the use of tobacco, alcohol, other drug use, and herbal medications. The patient's exercise capacity is also determined, which serves as a marker of the patient's functional reserve.
- The preoperative consultant should communicate all recommendations to the referring physician directly in a timely manner and provide follow-up as needed. Additional tests should be ordered only if they have the potential to add significantly to the existing information, assist decision-making, and alter patient management.[1]

- This chapter will provide an overview of preoperative evaluation of the most common comorbid conditions.

CARDIOVASCULAR EVALUATION

- Overview
  - Coronary artery disease is the leading cause of postoperative mortality because of a medical illness. Every year, more than 50,000 people suffer perioperative myocardial infarctions (MIs).[2]
    - Only half of these patients with an MI present with some sign or symptom that triggers the suspicion of the treating clinician. Perioperative cardiac events may be missed because of postoperative analgesia, lack of patient communication secondary to sedation and/or intubation, and the attribution of potential signs and symptoms of an MI to alternative diagnoses.
  - Cardiac complications include cardiac death, MI, unstable angina, heart failure (HF), and life-threatening dysrhythmias, primarily ventricular tachycardia and ventricular fibrillation. Various pathophysiologic changes occur during surgery, which may precipitate myocardial ischemia and infarction.
    - Surgical trauma, anesthetic agents, pain, bleeding, and fasting state induce a stress response which increases levels of circulating catecholamines and cortisol, with resultant increases in heart rate, blood pressure, and myocardial oxygen demand.
    - Hypothermia and bleeding may compromise myocardial oxygen delivery.
    - Surgical trauma and anesthetic agents also induce an inflammatory and procoagulant state, which facilitates coronary plaque fissuring and acute coronary thrombosis.
  - Perioperative cardiac events occur in 1% to 5% of unselected patients undergoing noncardiac surgery.[3]

They increase the average length of hospital stay significantly and contribute to substantially higher costs, making them the most common reasons for preoperative evaluations.

- Preoperative evaluation
  - The goal of the preoperative cardiac evaluation is to assess and stratify the patient's clinical risk for cardiac morbidity and mortality, decide whether further cardiac testing is indicated, and recommend interventions to reduce perioperative cardiac complications.
  - A number of cardiac risk indices have been developed to estimate individual risk and assist the physician and the patient in clinical decision-making. These include the American Society of Anesthesiologists (ASA) Physical Status, Canadian Cardiovascular Society index, Goldman Original Cardiac Risk index (1977), Cooperman (1979), Detsky Modified Cardiac Risk index (1986), Larsen (1987), Eagle (1989), Pedersen (1990), Vanzetto (1996), American College of Physicians (ACP, 1997), Lee Revised Cardiac Risk index (1999), and American College of Cardiology/American Heart Association (1996; Updated 2002 and 2007).
  - The Lee Revised Cardiac Risk index[4] identified six independent clinical predictors of adverse cardiac outcomes: high-risk type of surgery, history of ischemic heart disease, history of congestive heart failure (CHF), history of cerebrovascular disease, preoperative treatment with insulin, and preoperative serum creatinine > 2.0 mg/dL. Major cardiac complications included MI, pulmonary edema, ventricular fibrillation or primary cardiac arrest, and complete heart block. This simple index is easy to perform and quantifies risk numerically to assist the physician and the patient in weighing cardiac risks associated with surgery: the low-risk group with 0–1 risk factors had a 0.4% to 1.3% rate of major cardiac complications, whereas those with 2 risk factors had a 4% to 7% rate of complications, and a high-risk group with 3 or more risk factors had a 9% to 11% rate of complications. However, the Regulatory & Clinical Research Institute, Inc. (RCRI) does not suggest whether or not to do further testing prior to elective surgery.
  - The American College of Cardiology/American Heart Association (ACC/AHA) Updated Guidelines for Perioperative Cardiac Evaluation[5] (Fig. 101-1) utilizes a strategy based on clinical predictors, surgery-specific risk, and exercise capacity. Patient self-reported ability to participate in an activity equivalent to at least four metabolic equivalents of task (METs) is considered to indicate adequate functional reserve.
    - High-risk surgical procedures (> 5% complications) include aortic and major vascular surgery, emergent major operations, and anticipated prolonged surgical procedures associated with large fluid shifts and/or blood loss.
    - Intermediate risk surgeries (complication rate 1% to 5%) include carotid endarterectomy surgery, major head and neck surgery, intraperitoneal and intrathoracic surgery, and major orthopedic surgery.
    - Low risk (<1% complications) include most other procedures, such as cataract surgery and superficial procedures.
    - Patients undergoing emergent procedures have a two to four fold increased risk of perioperative cardiac complications.
  - Noninvasive testing has excellent negative predictive value (> 95%) but poor positive predictive value (15% to 20%). Assuming no contraindications to either test, the choice between dobutamine stress echocardiography (DSE) and dipyridamole thallium nuclear imaging (DTI) should depend on availability and local expertise. Results are generally comparable although DSE has fewer false positive. A notable exception is in the presence of a bundle branch block where DTI is preferred over DSE or standard exercise testing. DSE should be avoided in patients with significant arrhythmias, marked hypertension or hypotension, and suspected critical aortic stenosis, whereas bronchospasm and chronic obstructive pulmonary disease (COPD) are relative contraindications to intravenous dipyridamole or adenosine testing.
- Risk reduction strategies
  - Prophylactic medical therapy
    - Beta-blockers prescribed perioperatively blunt the sympathetic response associated with surgery and seem to reduce adverse cardiac outcomes.
    - Atenolol given immediately preoperatively and continued postoperatively until hospital discharge reduced perioperative ischemia and overall mortality following hospital discharge at 6–24 months.
    - Bisoprolol given to high-risk patients (with positive results on DSE) undergoing vascular surgery significantly reduced the perioperative incidence of cardiac death and nonfatal MI.
    - Subsequent investigators (DIPOM, MaVS, and POBBLE), however, failed to show similar benefit, and results from larger ongoing trials (POISE, DECREASE IV) are awaited to better answer this question. Preliminary results from POISE showed a decrease in nonfatal perioperative MIs and cardiac death but an increase in strokes and total mortality as well as significant hypotension and bradycardia requiring treatment. Some of these adverse effects may be because of the study protocol using a high dose of extended release metoprolol that was started just before surgery.
      - Currently, the ACC recommends continuing the use of beta-blockers perioperatively in all patients already on beta-blockers undergoing major surgery, prescribing beta-blockers perioperatively

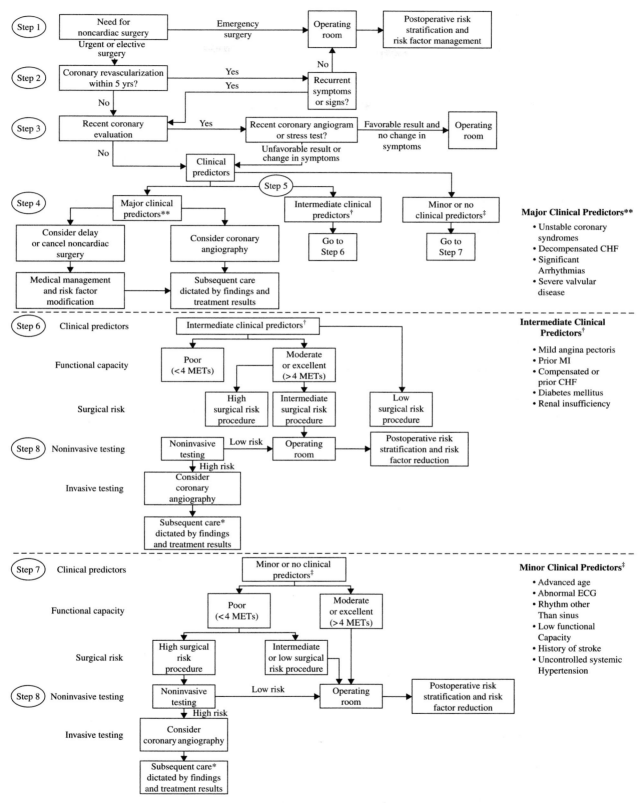

FIG. 101-1   The ACC/AHA approach to preoperative cardiac assessment.

for patients who have or are at high cardiac risk for coronary artery disease undergoing vascular, high, or intermediate-risk surgery.

- When possible, prophylactic beta-blockers should be started well before surgery and the dose titrated to achieve a resting heart rate of 55–65 beats per minute (bpm). Tight heart rate control has been correlated with reduced perioperative cardiac complications, but caution should be exercised in using protocols to adjust the dose– clinical evaluation is necessary to assess the reason for heart rate or blood pressure changes. Beta-blockers should be continued for at least 7 (and preferably 30) days postoperatively.
  - Alpha-2-agonists (clonidine), a possible alternative for patients with contraindications to beta-blockade, have limited evidence showing benefit in reducing perioperative ischemia and cardiovascular (CV) events.
  - Lipid-lowering agents (statins) have been reported to be beneficial in multiple observational studies; however, there has only been one small randomized controlled trial so statins cannot yet be recommended as prophylaxis to prevent perioperative CV complications. They should probably be continued in patients already taking them.
- Coronary revascularization
  - Observational data suggested that patients who had previous coronary artery bypass grafting (CABG) or percutaneous coronary intervention (PCI) that later underwent noncardiac surgery had fewer perioperative deaths and nonfatal MIs. However, these observations did not take into account the morbidity/mortality of the cardiac intervention itself.
  - The coronary artery revascularization prophylaxis (CARP) trial failed to show that prophylactic revascularization improved outcomes (primarily long-term mortality) compared to intensive medical therapy in patients with stable cardiac symptoms undergoing elective vascular surgery.
  - At this time prophylactic revascularization in general should not be recommended just to get the patient through surgery.
  - Furthermore, patients receiving stents who then require noncardiac surgery are potentially at increased risk if they do not complete a 4–6 week course of dual antiplatelet therapy after placement of a bare metal stent.
  - The recommended duration of therapy for drug-eluting stents was at least 3–6 months, depending on the type of stent (paclitaxel or sirolimus), but there have been case reports of in-stent thrombosis and fatal MI after discontinuation of antiplatelet therapy beyond these intervals. The AHA recently recommended uninterrupted dual antiplatelet therapy for at least 12 months.
- Additional CV considerations
  - CHF is a major risk factor for perioperative complications and should be controlled prior to elective surgery.
  - Hemodynamically significant arrhythmias need to be treated and the heart rate controlled before the patient has surgery.
  - Significant valvular disease, primarily symptomatic aortic stenosis, should be evaluated before major surgery. Ideally the valve should be replaced; if the patient refuses, however, many of these patients can get through surgery successfully with careful hemodynamic monitoring and medical management.
  - Consider endocarditis prophylaxis for patients with prosthetic valves, previous endocarditis, or complex congenital heart disease undergoing invasive dental or upper respiratory procedures as per the AHA guidelines.
  - Hypertension in general is only a minor risk factor and should rarely lead to cancellation of surgery. Values frequently quoted as increasing perioperative risk are diastolic BP >110 mm Hg and systolic BP >200 mm Hg; however, there is little evidence to support this. Having antihypertensive medication on board may minimize intraoperative blood pressure lability.

PULMONARY EVALUATION

- Overview
  - Postoperative pulmonary complications (PPCs) include atelectasis, pneumonia, exacerbation of underlying chronic airway disease, respiratory failure requiring mechanical ventilation, aspiration pneumonia, acute respiratory distress syndrome, pneumothorax, and pulmonary embolism. These complications are common, occur in 5% to 10% of all surgical patients, and are an important cause of perioperative morbidity and mortality.
  - The ACP recently published a systematic review of preoperative risk assessment and risk reduction strategies.
- Preoperative evaluation
  - A number of risk factors have been shown to increase the incidence of PPCs. These can be divided into surgery-related and patient-related factors.
  - Surgery-related risk factors
    - The most important predictor of risk is the type of surgery and its proximity to the diaphragm. Thoracic, abdominal, aortic aneurysm repair, and

vascular surgery are associated with higher PPC risk. However, neurosurgery and major head and neck procedures are also high risk for PPCs. Limited evidence suggests that laparoscopic surgery, as opposed to open, may be associated with fewer complications.

- Emergency surgeries, duration > 3 hours, and use of general anesthesia are also associated with an increased incidence of complications. The use of longer-acting neuromuscular-blocking agents, such as pancuronium, should be avoided in patients at high risk of pulmonary complications, and shorter-acting agents such as vecuronium or atacurium are preferred
  - ○ Patient-related risk factors
    - These include COPD, advanced age, cigarette smoking, CHF, partial or total functional dependence, ASA class greater than II, impaired sensorium, alcohol use, and malnutrition (Table 101-1).[6] No significant increase in the risk of these complications has been observed in patients with morbid obesity or mild-to-moderate asthma.
    - Although a low serum albumin level (< 3.5 g/dL) is an important predictor of PPCs, nutritional

TABLE 101-1 Odds Ratios for Risk Factors for Developing PPCs

RISK FACTOR	ODDS RATIO
A. Procedure related	
Surgical site	
• Aortic	6.09
• Thoracic	4.24
• Any abdominal	3.01
• Upper abdominal	2.91
Emergency surgery	2.21
Prolonged surgery	2.26
General anesthesia	1.83
B. Patient related	
Age*	
60–69 years	2.09
70–79 years	3.04
COPD	1.79
Cigarette smoking	1.26
CHF	2.93
Functional dependence	
• Total	2.51
• Partial	1.65
ASA Class II or greater[†]	4.87
Impaired sensorium	1.39
Alcohol use	1.21

*Compared to patients < 60 years of age.
[†]Compared to patients with ASA Class less than II.
Abbreviations: ASA, American Society of Anesthesiologists; CHF, congestive heart failure; COPD, chronic obstructive pulmonary disease; PPCs, postoperative pulmonary complications.
SOURCE: Smetana GW, Lawrence VA, Cornell JE; American College of Physicians. Preoperative pulmonary risk stratification for noncardiothoracic surgery: systematic review for the American College of Physicians. *Ann Intern Med.* Apr 2006 18;144(8):581–595.

supplementation either in the form of total parenteral nutrition or total enteral nutrition has not been shown to improve postoperative outcomes.

- Cigarette smoking is associated with nearly a six-fold increase in the risk of PPC. However, whether smoking cessation is beneficial prior to surgery is controversial in view of conflicting study results. Several studies showed no benefit or an increased risk in patients who quit smoking within 1–2 months of surgery. It is therefore recommended that smokers be advised to stop smoking at least 2 months before surgery if possible.

- Risk reduction strategies
  - ○ A thorough history and careful physical examination may reveal clues to the presence of occult pulmonary pathology.
    - The presence of chronic cough, unexplained dyspnea, low exercise capacity, abnormal or decreased breath sounds, and a prolonged expiratory phase should prompt an investigation preoperatively.
    - Patients experiencing an acute exacerbation of their obstructive airway disease should have their surgery delayed and treated aggressively.
  - ○ All patients with COPD should be treated with inhaled ipratropium and short-acting inhaled beta-2-agonists used as needed for symptomatic relief.
    - If acute bacterial respiratory infection is suspected, a course of antibiotics is appropriate. However, routine use of perioperative antibiotics does not reduce the risk of postoperative pneumonia.
  - ○ In patients with asthma, a short course of perioperative corticosteroids does not increase the incidence of postoperative infections.
  - ○ Spirometry does not accurately predict the risk of PPCs, and routine preoperative spirometry is not recommended for assessing pulmonary risk in patients undergoing extrathoracic surgery. It is usually reserved for selected patients with obstructive airway disease to determine optimal reduction in airway resistance and for patients with unexplained pulmonary symptoms.
  - ○ Chest x-rays may have some value in patients undergoing high-risk procedures but are not usually helpful in patients without signs or symptoms of respiratory disease.
  - ○ Atelectasis is best prevented with adequate analgesia, lung expansion maneuvers, and early ambulation.
    - Postoperative epidural analgesia may provide effective analgesia.
    - Incentive spirometry, deep breathing, and continuous positive airway pressure are effective in preventing PPC. These strategies are more effective when patients are educated about these techniques prior to surgery.

○ Selective nasogastric suctioning of patients with postoperative nausea or vomiting, intolerance of oral feeds, or symptomatic abdominal distention following elective laparotomy resulted in a lower incidence of atelectasis and pneumonia.

ENDOCRINOLOGIC EVALUATION

• Diabetic patients undergoing surgery have increased postoperative mortality. They have higher rates of postoperative wound infections and suffer from impaired healing when glycemic control is poor perioperatively. Tight glucose control with intensive insulin therapy reduces complication rates and mortality in patients in surgical intensive care units.[8]
  ○ The goals of the preoperative evaluation of the diabetic patient are reducing perioperative morbidity and mortality, avoiding hyperglycemia, hypoglycemia, and ketosis. A preoperative hemoglobin A_{1c} level of <7% is optimal. Perioperative management must include frequent bedside glucose monitoring.
  ○ The preoperative clinical evaluation of the diabetic patient should include the examination of CV, renal, and autonomic systems.
    ▪ A 12-hour fasting period is recommended for patients suspected to have gastroparesis, which increases the risk of regurgitation and aspiration on induction of anesthesia. Breakfast is omitted on the day of surgery.
    ▪ Oral antidiabetic agents are held on the day of surgery and resumed with the patient's first meal postoperatively.
    ▪ Generally, insulin-dependent patients are given one-half to two-thirds of their daily insulin requirements as intermediate acting insulin subcutaneously on the morning of surgery. Tight glycemic control using a glucose insulin potassium continuous infusion is commonly used for critical care patients. Usual insulin therapy is restarted once the patient resumes eating and adjusted to the caloric intake.
    ▪ Use of short-acting insulin by sliding scale as the patient's only insulin treatment is discouraged because of the greater likelihood of fluctuations in blood glucose levels.
• Adrenal insufficiency. Perioperative adrenal insufficiency may result from inadequate cortisol production because of the suppression of the hypothalamic-pituitary-adrenal (HPA) axis in patients with prolonged use of exogenous corticosteroids. It may also occur in patients with primary adrenal insufficiency, or those who suffer an adrenal insult secondary to hemorrhage or sepsis in the postoperative period.

  ○ All patients on long-term corticosteroid therapy should have their HPA axis assessed prior to surgery or be given supplemental steroids perioperatively.
  ○ Adrenal insufficiency in patients undergoing major surgery should be treated with stress doses of corticosteroids with a rapid taper to outpatient doses.[9] Both corticosteroids and mineralocorticoids should be given.
  ○ Glycemic control should be monitored for all patients on glucocorticoids.
• Thyroid disease
  ○ Patients with mild-to-moderate hypothyroidism seem to do relatively well with minimal compensation. There is no reason to postpone surgery unless the patient is severely symptomatic or myxedematous.
  ○ On the other hand, elective surgery should be postponed for patients with hyperthyroidism until treated properly or euthyroid, because of the risk of development of thyroid storm perioperatively.
• Patients with pheochromocytoma need to be properly treated before surgery to prevent perioperative CV complications.

HEMATOLOGIC EVALUATION

• The preoperative hematologic evaluation of the surgical patient must include details about any abnormal bleeding, thromboembolic disease, malignancy, liver or kidney disease, family history of similar conditions, nutritional status, alcohol abuse, and medications. In the absence of a bleeding risk clinically, screening blood tests (platelet count, prothrombin time [PT], activated partial thromboplastin time) are rarely helpful.
  ○ Antiplatelet agents (aspirin, clopidogrel, ticlopidine) and nonsteroidal anti-inflammatory drugs (NSAIDs) can prolong bleeding time and are usually stopped prior to surgery depending on the half-life and indication for use.
  ○ All herbal medications should be stopped prior to surgery as they may interfere with adequate hemostasis.
• Perioperative anemia is common. Postoperative anemia is typically multifactorial, owing to surgical blood loss, dilution from intravenous fluids, marrow suppression secondary to drugs, inflammation, and repeated phlebotomy.
  ○ There is significant variation in transfusion practices among physicians.[10] The type of surgical procedure, patient age, and a history of cardiopulmonary disease are considerations in deciding the transfusion threshold.
  ○ There is little evidence to support the practice of keeping the hemoglobin above 10 g/dL, and the decision to transfuse should be based on physiologic rather than numeric transfusion triggers.
  ○ All strategies to prevent anemia in the perioperative period should be considered in an effort to minimize exposure of surgical patients to blood transfusion.

○ In adult patients with sickle cell disease, preoperative exchange transfusion not necessary, and there is no clear benefit of preoperative blood transfusion.
• For patients with thrombocytopenia, there is no clearly defined threshold platelet count for transfusions in the perioperative context, but expert consensus recommends platelet transfusion to achieve a platelet count above 50,000 per µL.

EVALUATION OF RENAL, HEPATIC, AND NEUROLOGIC SYSTEMS

• Renal
  ○ Postoperative renal dysfunction is an important cause of perioperative morbidity and mortality. The etiology is usually multifactorial. The commonest cause is hypoxic acute tubular necrosis secondary to hypotension, hypovolemia, and/or dehydration. Other risk factors include preexisting renal insufficiency, Type I diabetes mellitus, age more than 65 years, major vascular surgery, and recent exposure to nephrotoxic agents (such as radiocontrast dyes, aminoglycoside antibiotics, and NSAIDs.) Adequate hydration and maintenance of normovolemia is the most effective preventive strategy. Patients on renal replacement therapy should be dialyzed on the day before surgery, and arrangements must be made for ongoing dialysis postoperatively.
• Hepatic
  ○ Surgical risk in patients with chronic liver disease or cirrhosis is best evaluated using the modified Child-Pugh score or the Model of End-Stage Liver Disease (MELD) score.[13] In general, elective surgery is avoided in patients with Child-Pugh Class C, acute viral or alcoholic hepatitis, and severe coagulopathy. Elevated transaminase levels detected incidentally preoperatively may require further workup but usually do not uncover significant disease that alters perioperative management.
• Neurologic
  ○ The risk of a postoperative *stroke* in general surgery (excluding cardiac, neurologic, and carotid procedures) is < 1%. Although patients with a previous stroke or carotid disease may be at increased risk, further workup and prophylactic carotid endarterectomy is rarely indicated prior to noncardiac surgery except in symptomatic patients (transient ischemic attack [TIA]).[14]
  ○ Postoperative *delirium* occurs in approximately 10% of patients. Some risk factors include advanced age, alcohol abuse, preoperative cognitive impairment suggested by a Telephone Interview for Cognitive Status (TICS) score <30, poor functional status (Specific Activity Scale functional class IV), use of anticholinergic drugs, preoperative glucose and electrolyte

abnormalities, thoracic and aortic aneurysm surgery. Proactive geriatrics consultation and adequate control of postoperative pain can reduce the development of this serious complication.

REFERENCES

1. Cohn SL, Macpherson DS. Overview of the principles of medical consultation. In: Rose BD, ed. *UpToDate*. Waltham, MA: UpToDate; 2006.
2. Devereaux PJ, Goldman L, Yusuf S, et al. Surveillance and prevention of major perioperative ischemic cardiac events in patients undergoing noncardiac surgery: a review. *CMAJ*. 2005 Sep 27;173(7):779–788.
3. Auerbach AD, Goldman L. Beta-blockers and reduction of cardiac events in noncardiac surgery: scientific review. *JAMA*. 2002 Mar 20;287(11):1435–1444.
4. Lee TH, Marcantonio ER, Mangione CM, et al. Derivation and prospective validation of a simple index for prediction of cardiac risk of major noncardiac surgery. *Circulation*. 1999 Sep 7;100(10):1043–1049.
5. Fleisher LA, Beckman JA, Brown KA, et al. ACC/AHA 2007 guidelines on perioperative cardiovascular evaluation and care for noncardiac surgery: a report of the American College of Cardiology/American Heart Association Task Force on Practice Guidelines (Writing Committee to Revise the 2002 Guidelines on Perioperative Cardiovascular Evaluation for Noncardiac Surgery) developed in collaboration with the American Society of Echocardiography, American Society of Nuclear Cardiology, Heart Rhythm Society, Society of Cardiovascular Anesthesiologists, Society for Cardiovascular Angiography and Interventions, Society for Vascular Medicine and Biology, and Society for Vascular Surgery. *J Am Coll Cardiol*. 2007;50:e159–e241.
6. Smetana GW. Preoperative pulmonary evaluation. *N Engl J Med*. 1999 Mar 25;340(12):937–944.
7. Smetana GW, Lawrence VA, Cornell JE; American College of Physicians. Preoperative pulmonary risk stratification for noncardiothoracic surgery: systematic review for the American College of Physicians. *Ann Intern Med*. 2006 Apr 18;144(8):581–595.
8. van den Berghe G, Wouters P, Weekers F, et al. Intensive insulin therapy in the critically ill patients. *N Engl J Med*. 2001 Nov 8;345(19):1359–1367.
9. Coursin DB, Wood KE. Corticosteroid supplementation for adrenal insufficiency. *JAMA*. 2002 Jan 9;287(2):236–240.
10. Shander A, Knight K, Thurer R, et al. Prevalence and outcomes of anemia in surgery: a systematic review of the literature. *Am J Med*. 2004 Apr 5;116(suppl 7A):58S–69S.
11. Geerts WH, Heit JA, Clagett GP, et al. Prevention of venous thromboembolism. *Chest*. 2001;119:132S–175S.
12. Dajani AS, Taubert KA, Takahashi M, et al. Prevention of bacterial endocarditis. Recommendations by the American Heart Association. *Circulation*. 1997 Jul 1;96(1):358–366.
13. Farnsworth N, Fagan SP, Berger DF, et al. Child-Turcotte-Pugh versus MELD score as a predictor of outcome after

elective and emergent surgery in cirrhotic patients. *Am J Surg.* 2004 Nov;188(5):580–583.
14. Blacker DJ, Flemming KD, Link MJ, et al. The preoperative cerebrovascular consultation: common cerebrovascular questions before general or cardiac surgery. *Mayo Clin Proc.* 2004 Feb;79(2): 223–229.

ADDITIONAL READING

Cohn SL. Preoperative medical consultation. In: Goldman L, Ausiello D, eds. *Cecil's Textbook of Medicine.* 23rd ed. Elsevier Inc., 2008.

Grines CL, Bonow RO, Casey DE Jr. et al. Prevention of premature discontinuation of dual antiplatelet therapy in patients with coronary artery stents: a science advisory from the American Heart Association, American College of Cardiology, Society for Cardiovascular Angiography and Interventions, American College of Surgeons, and American Dental Association, with representation from the American College of Physicians. *Circulation.* 2007;115:813–818. Epub 2007 Jan 15.

Wilson W, Taubert KA, Gewitz M, et al. Prevention of infective endocarditis: guidelines from the American Heart Association: a guideline from the American Heart Association Rheumatic Fever, Endocarditis, and Kawasaki Disease Committee, Council on Cardiovascular Disease in the Young, and the Council on Clinical Cardiology, Council on Cardiovascular Surgery and Anesthesia, and the Quality of Care and Outcomes Research Interdisciplinary Working Group. *Circulation.* 2007;116:1736–1754. Epub 2007 Apr 19. Erratum in: Circulation. 2007;116:e376–e377.

102 PERIOPERATIVE MEDICATION MANAGEMENT

Vibhu Sharma and Steven L. Cohn

INTRODUCTION

- Perioperative medical management is challenging, given the increasing age and medical complexity of patients undergoing surgery. Hospitalists are uniquely positioned to impact the care of the surgical patient by being involved in their care in the perioperative period.
- The following outline of management of medications in the perioperative period is based on clinical experience and expert opinion, as well as the limited available published literature on the subject. See Table 102-1.

GENERAL PRINCIPLES

- Query the surgical patient about prescription as well as over-the-counter medications. Ideally, patients should bring in all their medications for review to the preoperative visit to avoid confusion about which medications to continue and which ones need to be stopped.
- Carefully evaluate the risks and benefits of each medication and decide whether to continue, discontinue, or modify the patient's current regimen. Consider
  - The potential benefits of beginning a drug prior to surgery for prevention of infection, thrombosis, infection, myocardial ischemia, aspiration, and/or stress ulceration.
  - The risks of discontinuing a drug prior to surgery, including: withdrawal symptoms, rebound effects, and clinical worsening intraoperatively or postoperatively.
  - The risks of continuing a drug perioperatively including: bleeding, hypoglycemia, drug interactions with anesthetic agents.
- Make clear recommendations about all medications in your report.
  - Oral medications that are continued in the perioperative period should be administered the morning of surgery, and the orders for NPO should clearly indicate "except for medications with a sip of water."
  - If the medication would not ordinarily be administered before 10 AM and surgery is scheduled earlier, be sure to specify to give "on call to the OR."

RECOMMENDATIONS BY DRUG CATEGORY

CARDIOVASCULAR MEDICATIONS/ ANTIHYPERTENSIVES

Stable preoperative blood pressures usually imply stable intraoperative pressures; uncontrolled blood pressure preoperatively increases the risk of intraoperative hypotension or hypertension and cardiac ischemia.
- Alpha-2-agonists (clonidine) may
  - Aid in diminishing the risk of perioperative cardiac ischemia and also in decreasing the amount of anesthesia required for maintenance.
  - Be associated with a classic withdrawal syndrome (hypertension, tachycardia, tremors, anxiety) if abruptly discontinued.
  - Decrease preoperative anxiety and BP lability as well as extreme blood pressure fluctuations.
  - Be used in high-risk patients where beta-blockers are contraindicated.
- *Recommendations*: continue usual dose perioperatively including dose on morning of the day of scheduled

TABLE 102-1   Summary of Perioperative Medication Management

MEDICATION CLASS	RECOMMENDATION
Anticoagulants and other drugs affecting hemostasis	• Continue for minor surgery • Discontinue at appropriate interval before major surgery • Consider bridging anticoagulation for patients at high risk of interim thrombosis
CV medications	• Continue most agents • Initiate beta-blockers in patients at high risk of perioperative cardiac morbidity • Withhold diuretics on the morning of surgery especially if signs of volume depletion
Gastrointestinal agents	• Continue • Substitute parenteral forms in patients who are NPO for prolonged periods or those at high risk for stress ulceration
Pulmonary agents	• Continue
Diabetic agents	• Withhold oral hypoglycemics on morning of surgery and resume when patient resumes eating • For Type I diabetics, continue some form of insulin (long acting or intravenous) at all times • For Type II diabetics, decrease dose of morning intermediate insulin depending on anticipated duration of NPO status and time of surgery
Thyroid agents	• Continue thyroid replacement. Parenteral substitution needed only if prolonged (days) NPO state • Postpone surgery until hyperthyroidism controlled
Oral contraceptives, hormone replacement, and SERMs	• Discontinue several weeks before surgery in patients at high risk for perioperative venous thromboembolism, otherwise continue
Lipid-lowering agents	• Continue "statins" • Discontinue other agents
Corticosteroids	• Continue chronic corticosteroids. Increase dosage to account for surgical stress
Psychotropic agents	• For most patients, continue SSRIs. Consider holding several weeks before surgery in patients in which perioperative hemorrhage could be catastrophic (CNS surgery) • Continue tricyclic antidepressants, benzodiazepines, lithium, and antipsychotics • For MAOs, continue or discontinue depending on anesthesiologist preference
Chronic opioids	• Continue. Substitute equianalgesic or higher doses to manage surgical pain
Rheumatologic agents	• Continue methotrexate • Discontinue other DMARDs and anticytokines • Continue hypouricemic agents
Neurologic agents	• Continue antiseizure medications • Hold anti-Parkinsonian agents briefly • Continue agents for myasthenia gravis
Herbal agents	• Discontinue all agents

Abbreviations: CNS, central nervous system; DMARD, disease-modifying antirheumatic drug; MAO, monoamine oxidase inhibitor; NPO, nil per os (nothing by mouth); SERM, selective estrogen receptor modulator; SSRI, selective serotonin reuptake inhibitor.
SOURCE: From Cohn SL, Macpherson DS. Perioperative medication management. In: Cohn SL, Smetana GW, Weed HG, eds. *Perioperative Medicine—Just the Facts*. New York, NY: McGraw-Hill; 2006.

surgery. If prolonged NPO status is expected, start transdermal preparation 24–48 hours preoperatively while oral dose is weaned.
  ○ Anticipate that hypotension and bradycardia may occur.
• Beta-blockers
  ○ Decrease heart rate and myocardial oxygen demand.
  ○ Can decrease perioperative ischemia (and possibly nonfatal MI and death) in high-risk cardiac patients; may be harmful for low-risk patients (increased incidence of symptomatic bradycardia and hypotension).
  ○ Abrupt discontinuation is associated with rebound ischemia, hypertension, and tachycardia.
• *Recommendations*: continue perioperatively
  ○ Start prophylactically before major vascular surgery or other intermediate-high risk surgery in patients

with ischemia on stress testing or those with coronary heart disease (angina, previous MI).
  ○ Consider prophylactic use for other patients undergoing vascular surgery or those at intermediate-high cardiac risk for intermediate-high risk surgery.
  ○ Start days or weeks (ideally at least 1 week) before surgery whenever possible.
  ○ Titrate to resting heart rate of 50–70 bpm and continue preoperatively (on morning of scheduled surgery) and through the perioperative period.
  ○ Administer intravenously if unable to take orally.
  ○ Avoid if significant bronchospasm, pulmonary edema, and high-grade AV block.
• Alpha- and alpha-beta blockers
  ○ The former are used to treat benign prostatic hypertrophy and pheochromocytoma. The latter are used to treat HF and hypertension.

- *Recommendations*: continue perioperatively
  - If treating pheochromocytoma, begin at least a week prior to surgery.
  - Intravenous labetalol is used commonly for intraoperative blood pressure control.
- Calcium channel blockers
  - Diltiazem may reduce perioperative ischemia and postoperative arrhythmias (based on limited studies).
- *Recommendations*: continue preoperatively if being used for management of hypertension or supraventricular tachycardias.
  - These agents may be substituted for beta-blockers in the presence of asthma and COPD.
- Diuretics
  - These agents may cause hypovolemia and hypokalemia acutely; however, if the patient has been on a diuretic for several weeks, a steady state has probably been reached.
- *Recommendations*: typically withhold dose on the morning of surgery to prevent intravascular volume depletion; however, if there is a history of stable CHF, diuretics should be continued through the perioperative period.
  - Stop diuretics if blood pressure is borderline the morning of surgery, the patient appears volume depleted, or the blood urea nitrogen (BUN)/creatinine ratio suggests a "prerenal picture." Restart once on a diet.
  - Monitor potassium levels closely.
  - These agents can be administered intravenously if necessary.
- Nitrates
  - Prophylactic use has not been shown to reduce perioperative coronary events.
- *Recommendations*: continue perioperatively
  - Can apply nitropaste 1–2 in the morning of surgery to substitute for oral long-acting nitrates.
- ACEI/ARB
  - Antihypertensive effect mediated by blockade of the rennin-angiotensin system.
  - These may be associated with increased incidence of hypotension with induction of anesthesia requiring fluid or pressor administration; however, they were not associated with an increase in perioperative MI.
- *Recommendations*: controversial; however they are usually continued as the potential benefit of the drug is thought to outweigh the possible development of hypotension. Consider withholding if baseline BP is low on the morning of surgery.

CARDIOVASCULAR MEDICATIONS/ ANTIARRHYTHMICS

- Common medications include digoxin, sotalol, amiodarone, and others.

- Consider cardiac consultation.
- *Recommendations*: continue perioperatively
  - Consider obtaining serum levels when indicated (digoxin).
  - Avoid hypercalcemia and hypokalemia, both of which predispose to digoxin toxicity.

CARDIOVASCULAR MEDICATIONS/ LIPID-LOWERING AGENTS

- Statins also appear to prevent acute coronary plaque rupture and have been associated with a mortality benefit in patients undergoing vascular surgery.
- Bile acid sequestrants and fibric acid derivatives have no demonstrable benefits in the immediate perioperative period and may be associated with erratic absorption of other medications.
- *Recommendations*: continue statins
  - Possibly consider starting prophylactically in high cardiac risk patients undergoing vascular or high-risk surgery, especially if the patient has an indication for statin therapy.
  - Stop niacin/clofibrate a day prior to surgery.
  - Discontinue colestipol, cholestyramine, and ezetimibe the day prior to surgery to allow for fat-soluble medications to be absorbed.

MEDICATIONS AFFECTING HEMOSTASIS/ ANTIPLATELET AGENTS

- Aspirin
  - This agent irreversibly inhibits cyclooxygenase; therefore 7–10 days required for repopulation by functional platelets.
  - Some studies noted increased perioperative bleeding and need for transfusions while others did not.
  - Case reports noted an increase in thromboembolic events within 30 days of discontinuing aspirin.
- *Recommendations*: although often discontinued 5–10 days before surgery, consider the indication for therapy and risk of bleeding. Discuss with the surgeon.
  - Continue perioperatively in cardiac or peripheral vascular surgery. Aspirin decreases mortality if begun within 48 hours after CABG.
- Clopidogrel (and ticlopidine)
  - These agents irreversibly inhibits adenosine diphosphate (ADP)-induced platelet aggregation and have been associated with increased bleeding.
- *Recommendations*: discontinue clopidogrel at least 5 days before cardiac surgery. Stop ticlopidine 10–14 days before surgery.
  - Postpone elective surgery at least 4–6 weeks after PCI with bare metal stent placement to continue dual antiplatelet therapy.

- ○ With drug-eluting stents, the latest recommendation is to continue dual antiplatelet therapy uninterrupted for at least 12 months. If surgery is necessary sooner, continue aspirin if possible and stop clopidogrel 5–7 days prior to surgery. Restart as soon as feasible thereafter.
  - ○ Consider cardiac consultation.
- Dipyridamole
  - ○ This drug inhibits activity of adenosine deaminase and phosphodiesterase leading to accumulation of adenosine and cyclic adenosine monophosphate (cAMP) and inhibiting platelet aggregation.
  - ○ It also allows for coronary vasodilation by the same mechanism.
  - ○ The effect is reversible with a half-life of 10 hours.
- *Recommendations*: no data to advise whether to stop or continue; if discontinuing, consider stopping 2–3 days before surgery (5 half-lives).
- Pentoxifylline
  - ○ This drug lowers blood viscosity and improves erythrocyte flexibility
  - ○ It is associated with increased risk for bleeding with or without other anticoagulants or antiplatelet agents
- *Recommendations*: stop 8 hours before surgery (on the morning of surgery)
- Cilostazol
  - ○ This drug is a reversible PDE3 inhibitor; half-life: 12 hours
- Recommendations: stop 48 hours before surgery.
- COX 2 inhibitors
  - ○ Celecoxib does not affect platelet aggregation at usual doses (up to 400 mg/d).
  - ○ It may reduce requirements for perioperative analgesics.
- *Recommendations*: stop 1–3 days before surgery in view of recent controversy over possible increased CV events.

MEDICATIONS AFFECTING HEMOSTASIS/ ANTICOAGULANTS

- Warfarin
  - ○ The risk of bleeding with continuation of the drug needs to be balanced with the risk of a thromboembolic event.
  - ○ Achieving a target international normalized ratio (INR) can be especially challenging in the hospital setting because of drug-drug interactions, dietary changes, and transiently stopping the drug in anticipation of procedures.
- *Recommendations*: warfarin can be continued for minor surgical procedures with low bleeding risk.
  - ○ You can safely discontinue 3–5 days before surgery and check INR preoperatively (should be subtherapeutic, preferably < 1.5) if bleeding risk is greater than risk of thromboembolism.
  - ○ Consider bridging therapy with heparin (unfractionated heparin [UFH] or low molecular weight heparin [LMWH]) if older metallic valve, mitral (vs. aortic) position, or at high risk for thromboembolism without anticoagulation. Bridging therapy requires weighing the risk of hemorrhage versus the risk of thromboembolism.
  - ○ For VTE prophylaxis of orthopedic surgical patients, some experts begin warfarin the evening before orthopedic surgery (hip or knee replacement, hip fracture) as an option for deep vein thrombosis (DVT) prophylaxis. Titrate to INR 2–3. See Chapter 88.
- Low molecular weight heparins (LMWHs)
  - ○ In general, no monitoring is necessary regarding the level of anticoagulation. Anti-Xa activity can be checked if it is of concern in special populations (morbidly obese, severely underweight, renal failure). When to check the anti-Xa activity level is controversial.
  - ○ Different LMWHs have different indications, half-lives, contraindications, and warnings. Consult the manufacturer's labeling.
  - ○ Anticoagulant effects are only partly reversible with protamine sulfate.
- *Recommendations*: stop full dose LMWH 24 hours before surgery and restart once deemed safe by the surgeon.
  - ○ The last dose of full dose LMWH should be given no less than 24 hours before planned neuraxial (spinal or epidural) anesthesia or lumbar puncture; prophylactic doses of LMWH need to be held 12 hours prior. Allow at least 2 hours from spinal needle/catheter removal before starting or restarting LMWH.
  - ○ Begin or continue if indicated for DVT prophylaxis. The dosing regimen varies based on the specific agent and whether the drug is started before or after surgery.
  - ○ Periodically monitor platelet counts (every 3 days with full anticoagulation dose).
- Unfractionated heparin (UFH)
- *Recommendations*: stop full dose anticoagulation 4–6 hours before surgery and begin postoperatively when deemed safe by the surgeon.
  - ○ Restart UFH as soon as 6 hours postoperatively provided there is adequate hemostasis and low risk of bleeding. Do not administer for at least 72 hours after a craniotomy and follow closely with the neurosurgeon.
  - ○ Start or continue low dose UFH (q 8–12 hours) for DVT prophylaxis depending on level of risk of bleeding in combination with mechanical prophylaxis.

○ Monitor platelet count (for heparin-induced thrombocytopenia, HIT).
- Synthetic pentasaccharides (fondaparinux)
  ○ Anticoagulation effect is mediated by antithrombin III-mediated Factor Xa inhibition. Although elevated PF4 antibodies have been associated with fondaparinux, antibody-mediated HIT has not been reported.
- *Recommendations*: begin 6 hours postoperatively in patients undergoing lower extremity orthopedic surgery.
  ○ Fondaparinux has a significantly longer half life of 17 hours and is generally avoided for spinal interventions.
  ○ Contraindicated with severe renal impairment.

PULMONARY

Optimization of pulmonary function in patients with known COPD or asthma is the major goal of preoperative pulmonary management, especially in patients undergoing thoracic or upper abdominal surgery.
- Inhaled agents include beta-agonists, ipatropium, steroids
- *Recommendations*: continue
- Systemic corticosteroids
  ○ Evaluate possibility of suppression of HPA axis.
  ○ If history of steroid use at a physiologic dose or greater for at least 3 weeks in the past 6 months, the patient may not be able to generate the appropriate adrenocortical response to the stress of surgery.
- *Recommendations*: continue or increase the dose of corticosteroids based on the history, usual dose, and duration of therapy, and anticipated stress of surgery.
  ○ You can give a bolus of 50–100 mg of hydrocortisone followed by 25–50 mg q 8 hours, adjusting dose and duration to ongoing stress of surgery. A maximum of 200 mg/d is adequate.
  ○ Consider giving mineralocorticoids as well.
- Theophylline
  ○ This drug may be associated with perioperative arrhythmias in supratherapeutic range.
- *Recommendation*: check drug level
  ○ Either continue on morning of surgery or stop it the night before.
- Leukotriene inhibitors
- *Recommendations*: continue perioperatively

ENDOCRINE/DIABETIC AGENTS

- Tight perioperative glucose control is important to reduce incidence of infections and possibly improve outcome in critically ill patients.
- Frequently sample blood glucose to determine insulin requirements and minimize hypoglycemia.
- Oral hypoglycemics

- *Recommendations*: depends on the agent
  ○ Sulfonylureas/glitazones: hold dose on the morning of surgery.
  ○ Metformin: usually stop the day prior to surgery. (Some experts recommend 48 hours before surgery; however, the risk of lactic acidosis does not appear to be different from other hypoglycemic agents).
  ○ Restart oral hypoglycemics when the patient is able to eat normally and renal function is stable.
- Insulins
- *Recommendations*:
  ○ Normal pressure hydrocephalus [NPH]: administer half (to two-thirds) of the usual dose on the morning of surgery.
    ▪ Follow fingersticks frequently while starting D5 one-half NS.
    ▪ For prolonged surgical procedures, cover with regular insulin boluses or an insulin drip at 1–2 units/h.
  ○ Mixed insulin (70/30): can give one-half to two-thirds of equivalent dose of the NPH portion. Fingerstick and give regular insulin on sliding scale basis.
  ○ Long-acting basal insulin (Lantus): depending on degree of glucose control and type of procedure one can continue usual dose or decrease it the night before surgery.

ENDOCRINE/THYROID DISORDERS

- Mild-to-moderate hypothyroidism is not associated with adverse perioperative events. However, elective procedures in patients who are clinically or chemically hyperthyroid need to be postponed, until adequate control achieved.
- *Recommendations*:
  ○ Continue replacement therapy with levothyroxine; however, intravenous use is not necessary if patient will not be eating for up to a week. For longer durations, administer 50% to 70% of usual oral dose intravenously daily.
  ○ Continue antithyroid medications in usual dosages perioperatively, and check thyroid function preoperatively if not done checked recently.

ENDOCRINE/ESTROGENS

- Oral contraceptives, selective estrogen receptor modulators (SERMs), hormone replacement therapy (HRT) are associated with an increased risk of venous thromboembolism.
- *Recommendations*: theoretically, elective surgery with a high risk for VTE should prompt discontinuation of

hormonal contraception 2–3 weeks prior to surgery, and alternative contraception should be instituted (if feasible). However, this is rarely done in actual clinical practice. A pregnancy test before surgery is mandatory if hormonal contraception is discontinued and patients need to be counseled to use barrier methods of contraception after discontinuation and through the first cycle after resumption of contraception.

- Patients undergoing elective surgery with low risk for VTE can continue hormonal contraception and should receive perioperative DVT prophylaxis.

NEUROLOGIC MEDICATIONS/ANTISEIZURE

- *Recommendations*: continue seizure medications and monitor drug level.
  - ○ Antiepileptics (except Valproate) induce metabolism of each other and other drugs.
  - ○ Valproate and phenytoin can be administered intravenously if necessary.

NEUROLOGIC MEDICATIONS/ ANTI-PARKINSONIAN

- Perioperative complications related to motor dysfunction are common (dysphagia, poor cough reflex), and the risk of delirium associated with surgery is high.
- Discontinuation of anti-Parkinson's medications can induce the neuroleptic malignant syndrome (NMS).
- *Recommendations*: give levodopa/carbidopa (LD/CD) the evening prior to surgery but withhold dose morning of surgery and until patient is able to take medicines orally.
  - ○ Hold LD/CD/entacapone preparations longer before surgery.
  - ○ Stop tolcapone 1 day before surgery.
  - ○ Administer pramipexole and ropinirole on the morning of surgery and restarted once oral intake is resumed.
  - ○ The last dose of bromocriptine and pergolide should be administered the morning of the day before surgery and resumed once oral intake has been reinstated, as long as hemodynamic stability is maintained.
  - ○ Selegiline needs to be discontinued several days before surgery. This is a "Type B" monoamine oxidase (MAO) inhibitor, and concerns about interactions with tyramine-like substances are minimal at doses below 10 mg; however, avoid concurrent use with selective serotonin reuptake inhibitors (SSRIs) and other medicines associated with the serotonin syndrome or NMS.
  - ○ Diphenhydramine and benztropine can be administered parenterally if necessary, and are useful in patients in whom an exacerbation of symptoms occurs because usual therapy has been withheld.

NEUROLOGIC MEDICATIONS/ MYASTHENIA GRAVIS

- Exacerbations can occur in the perioperative period, and myasthenic crisis may precipitate respiratory insufficiency.
- *Recommendations*: substitute short-acting pyridostigmine for the long-acting preparations the evening before the surgery.
  - ○ Pyridostigmine is optional on the morning of surgery.
  - ○ Pyridostigmine can be administered intramuscularly or intravenously for patients unable to resume oral intake for a prolonged period of time. Administer 1/10th of usual dose intramuscularly and 1/30th of the usual dose intravenously at the usual interval for oral dosing. Alternatively, a continuous infusion at 2 mg/h may be used.

ANTIPSYCHOTICS/ANTIDEPRESSANTS

- Lithium: can prolong the effect of muscle relaxants, can cause volume depletion secondary to nephrogenic diabetes insipidus, and can induce hypothyroidism.
- *Recommendations*: monitor levels and administer dose on morning of surgery.
  - ○ Monitor fluid and electrolyte status (especially sodium).
  - ○ Check thyroid function preoperatively if not done recently.
- MAO inhibitors: beware of serotonin syndrome. Avoid meperidine (Demerol), dextromethorphan, and vasoconstrictors, such as phenylephrine, during anesthesia.
- *Recommendations*: usually discontinue 2 weeks preoperatively.
  - ○ Consider psychiatry consultation preoperatively, in concert with anesthesia, to determine risks/benefits of continuing if decision is made to do so. Anesthesiologists may choose to continue MAO inhibitors if deemed an "MAO safe procedure."
  - ○ Avoid tyramine-containing foods (cheese, wine) if on MAO inhibitors and decision made to continue the drug in the perioperative period.
- SSRIs
  - ○ These drugs inhibit platelet aggregability.
    - ▪ There is an association with gastrointestinal (GI) bleeding in the perioperative period and also one study that suggested more transfusion requirements in patients on SSRIs undergoing orthopedic surgery.
  - ○ Abrupt discontinuation may result in a withdrawal syndrome.
- *Recommendations*: consider tapering and stopping 3 weeks before neurosurgical procedures; otherwise continue through the day of surgery.

- Tricyclics
  - These medications inhibit reuptake of norepinephrine and serotonin in the presynaptic membrane.
  - They can be proarrhythmic, however, there is sparse clinical data.
- *Recommendations*: usually continue perioperatively (but some suggest tapering and stopping before surgery).
- Anxiolytics
  - Benzodiazepines are commonly used in the perioperative period to reduce anxiety. Abrupt discontinuation can lead to a classic withdrawal syndrome that can closely mimic delirium tremens.
- *Recommendations*: continue benzodiazepines and buspirone in usual doses in the perioperative period.
  - Administer intravenously if patient will be "NPO" for a prolonged period.
- Antipsychotic agents
  - Haloperidol has been used for its sedative and antiemetic properties.
  - Perioperative experience with the newer antipsychotic agents (quetiapine, ziprasidone, olanzapine, risperidone) is limited.
- *Recommendations*: continue this class of medication perioperatively.
  - Haloperidol may be administered intramuscularly or intravenously. Olanzapine can be administered intramuscularly if necessary.

GASTROINTESTINAL MEDICATIONS

- H2 blockers and PPIs (proton pump inhibitors) are indicated for stress ulcer prophylaxis.
- *Recommendations*: continue acid-suppression drugs on day of surgery; some can be given intravenously if necessary.
  - Reglan: can be administered 1 hour prior to surgery in patients known to have (or at high risk for) gastroparesis (eg, diabetics).

OPIOID ANALGESICS

- Higher doses of opioid medication may be necessary perioperatively in patients on chronic opioid therapy.
- Withdrawal symptoms and exacerbation of chronic pain are to be expected if there is abrupt discontinuation. Symptoms can vary from a mild withdrawal syndrome to seizures, tremulousness, severe anxiety, agitation, confusion, and hypertension.
- *Recommendations*: continue opioids in the perioperative period.
  - Substantial escalation of dose from baseline may be necessary to achieve adequate analgesia.
  - Ensure equianalgesic doses of parenterally substituted opioids to allow for adequate analgesia.
  - Do not overlook prescribing an effective bowel regimen in the perioperative period for all patients receiving opioids.

RHEUMATOLOGIC MEDICATIONS/GOUT

- Surgical procedures can induce flares of gout, possibly because of abrupt changes in uric acid levels because of rapid fluid shifts.
- *Recommendations*: can continue probenecid, allopurinol, and colchicine.
  - Parenteral colchicine is discouraged because of the risk of skin necrosis with accidental subcutaneous infiltration.
- Flares of gout can be treated with NSAIDs or with corticosteroids.

RHEUMATOLOGIC MEDICATIONS/ DISEASE-MODIFYING ANTIRHEUMATIC DRUGS

- These include methotrexate, hydroxychloroquine, sulfasalazine, leflunomide, and azathioprine. Some may cause immunosuppression and may potentially increase risk of postoperative infections.
- A randomized trial in patients undergoing orthopedic surgery showed no increased rate of infection in patients who continued weekly methotrexate compared to those who discontinued it 2 weeks prior to surgery.
- Most disease-modifying antirheumatic drugs (DMARDs) are renally excreted and therefore may accumulate in the face of renal insufficiency inducing bone marrow suppression.
- *Recommendations*
  - Methotrexate can be continued through the perioperative period as long as renal function is normal.
  - Azathioprine and sulfasalazine can be continued.
  - Leflunomide needs to be discontinued 2 weeks prior to surgery given its long half-life.

RHEUMATOLOGIC MEDICATIONS/ ANTICYTOKINES

- Etanercept (tumor necrosis factor [TNF] receptor), Adalimumab, Infliximab (anti-TNF alpha antibodies), Rituximab (anti-CD20 antibody), and Anakinra (interleukin [IL]-1 receptor antagonist) are newer immune response modifying agents used primarily in the treatment of rheumatologic disease.

- *Recommendations*: infliximab has been shown to be safe if continued through surgery.
  - Consult rheumatology; consider stopping the others 1–2 weeks prior to surgery and resuming 1–2 weeks postoperatively.

VITAMINS AND HERBS

- Valerian and kava have been associated with excessive sedation.
- Garlic, gingko, and ginseng have been associated with bleeding complications.
- *Recommendations*: stop at least 7 days prior to surgery.

BIBLIOGRAPHY

Cohn SL. Perioperative Medication Management. http://pier. acponline.org/physicians/diseases/d835/d835.html [Accessed August 11, 2006.] In PIER [online database]. Philadelphia, PA: American College of Physicians; 2006.

Cohn SL, Macpherson DS. Perioperative medication management. In: Cohn SL, Smetana GW, Weed HG, eds. *Perioperative Medicine— Just the Facts.* New York: McGraw-Hill; 2006.

Cygan R, Waitzkin H. Stopping and restarting medications in the perioperative period. *J Gen Intern Med.* 1987; 2:270–283.

Muluk V, Macpherson DS. Perioperative medication management. In Rose BD, ed. *UpToDate.* Wellesley, MA: UpToDate; 2006.

Physicians' Desk Reference. Montvale, NJ: Thomson PDR; 2006.

103 PREOPERATIVE SCREENING TESTS

Ali Azarm and Steven L. Cohn

OVERVIEW

- Physicians often order a constellation of tests routinely prior to surgery. This process is an expensive practice in terms of the cost of each test and the need for the follow-up of an unexpected abnormal result. The aim of this chapter is to provide an evidence-based guide for utilization of screening tests for preoperative evaluation.
- Preoperative testing should be selective, not routine, based on the findings on history and physical examination. See Table 103-1.

- Current literature has consistently demonstrated that "routine" preoperative screening testing has little, if any, impact on perioperative outcomes, particularly in asymptomatic patients undergoing low-risk procedures.
  - Hospital guidelines should be updated to reflect the most recent evidence and recommendations from the medical literature.
- In order to prevent medico-legal problems, all abnormal findings should be addressed and documented in the patient's medical record.

CONCEPTS IN PREOPERATIVE TESTING

- Definition of abnormal test results
  - Test results are of three basic types: continuous, ordinal, and categorical.
  - Continuous test results, which contain most blood tests, theoretically are measured from 0 through infinity. Other tests may have ordinal (eg, degree of proteinuria detected by dipstick) or categorical results (eg, normal vs. abnormal chest x-ray).
  - For continuous test results, the "normal" value is defined by the reference range (95% of normal population) which is determined by the numbers falling within 2 standard deviations of the mean. Therefore, 5% of the population will have what is labeled as an "abnormal" test result.
  - The greater the number of tests that are ordered, the higher the probability that one or more will be abnormal. Therefore, the practice of ordering multiple "routine" blood tests preoperatively may result in substantially high false positive or false negative results.
- Rationale for preoperative testing
  - Physicians usually order routine preoperative tests for several reasons: to detect unsuspected abnormalities that may change management, to obtain a baseline value for monitoring and comparison during and after surgery, and for medico-legal purposes.
  - The main issue is whether ordering a test adds any incremental value to what is obtained from the clinical evaluation alone. Assuming an abnormal result is detected, does it affect surgical risk and does it need to be addressed before surgery? If the answers to these questions are no, then the test did not need to be ordered preoperatively. Furthermore, an abnormal result may create an additional medico-legal risk.
  - Clinicians usually ignore 30% to 60% of abnormalities detected in routine preoperative tests.[1] In a large study of 2000 patients undergoing elective surgery, investigators found that 60% of tests which had been ordered routinely should not have been performed if a reasonable indication was defined initially. Although 4.1%

TABLE 103-1 Recommendations for Laboratory Testing before Elective Surgery

TEST	ABNORMALITIES INFLUENCING MANAGEMENT (%)	LR(+)*	LR(−)	INDICATIONS
Hemoglobin	0.1	3.3	0.90	Anticipated major blood loss or symptoms or signs of anemia
White blood cell count	0.0	0.0	1.00	Symptoms of infection, myeloproliferative disorder, or myelotoxic medications
Platelet count	0.0	0.0	1.00	History or signs of bleeding disorder, myeloproliferative disorder, or myelotoxic medications
PT	0.0	0.0	1.01	History or signs of bleeding disorder, chronic liver disease, malnutrition, recent or long-term antibiotic use
PTT	0.1	1.7	0.86	History of bleeding disorder
Electrolytes	1.8	4.3	0.80	Renal insufficiency, CHF, medications that affect electrolytes
Renal function	2.6	3.3	0.81	Age > 50 years, hypertension, cardiac disease, major surgery, medications that may affect renal function
Glucose	0.5	1.6	0.85	Diabetes (or strong family history), obesity, symptoms of diabetes
Liver function tests	0.1	—	—	No indication for screening. Consider albumin measurement for major surgery or chronic illness
Urinalysis	1.4	1.7	0.97	No indication for screening
Electrocardiogram	2.6	1.6	0.96	Men > 45 years or women > 55 years with CAD or ≥ 2 risk factors for CAD, such as diabetes and hypertension
Chest radiograph	3.0	2.5	0.72	Age > 70 years, cardiac or pulmonary disease, symptoms or examination findings of cardiac or pulmonary disease

*LR(+) = positive likelihood ratio; LR(−) = negative likelihood ratio.
Abbreviations: PT, prothrombin time; PTT, partial prothrombin time.
SOURCE: Modified with permission from Smetana GW, Macpherson DS. The case against routine preoperative laboratory testing. *Med Clin North Am.* 2003;87:7.

of the results were abnormal, based on the reference range, only 0.4% of the results were both not indicated and abnormal; furthermore, only 0.15% of the not indicated tests had potentially significant abnormalities related to perioperative management.[2]

○ Characteristics associated with a good screening test include

- High prevalence of the disease being sought
- High sensitivity and specificity of the test
- Noninvasive and inexpensive
- Leads to detection of disease that is asymptomatic and would not have been diagnosed otherwise by clinical examination alone
- Detects a disease that is more important to be diagnosed preoperatively than postoperatively (eg, contributes to perioperative morbidity)

COMMONLY ORDERED PREOPERATIVE TESTS

HEMOGLOBIN

- The prevalence of an abnormal hemoglobin concentration perioperatively was found to be 1.8% in a review of eight studies.[3]
- Significant blood loss during surgery may lead to tissue hypoxia if anemia is not corrected perioperatively;

however, a patient with normal cardiopulmonary function should be able to compensate for a chronic anemia with a hemoglobin as low as 7 g/dL.

- Mild-to-moderate anemia rarely requires a blood transfusion, and few studies have correlated preoperative anemia with surgical risk.

Recommendations for preoperative hemoglobin

○ Patients undergoing a major surgery with expected significant blood loss and the need for further blood transfusion

○ History of anemia or diseases usually associated with it (malignancy, chronic kidney disease)

○ Signs or symptoms of anemia (pallor, tachycardia)

- Patients undergoing minor surgery or a procedure not anticipated to result in significant blood loss do not require preoperative hemoglobin measurement.

WHITE BLOOD CELL COUNT

- The prevalence of white blood cell WBC abnormalities preoperatively is low (1%). Furthermore, these abnormalities have not been found to correlate with perioperative morbidity and mortality.
- Recommendation for preoperative WBC
  ○ Not indicated routinely without signs and symptoms of infection, myeloproliferative disorders, or recent chemotherapy

PLATELET COUNT

- The incidence of unexpected abnormalities of platelet count is < 1% in patients undergoing surgery and rarely alters surgical management.
- Recommendation for preoperative platelet count
  - Not indicated routinely unless the history and physical examination suggest the possibility of abnormal hemostasis or the presence of known conditions or drugs that predispose patients to thrombocytopenia or thrombocytosis (eg, myeloproliferative disorders, heparin).

COAGULATION TESTS

- PT/INR and partial thromboplastin time (PTT) are often ordered by physicians to identify patients at risk for perioperative bleeding.
- However, these tests are rarely helpful in the absence of a history of bleeding or findings suggestive of a bleeding disorder. Furthermore, an abnormal test result did not usually alter the management nor result in perioperative bleeding.[3]
- Elevated *prothrombin time* is expected in conditions like chronic liver disease, malnutrition, and in patients taking warfarin or antibiotics that result in vitamin K deficiency.
- Recommendation for PT/INR
  - Routine measurement of prothrombin time is not recommended for patients undergoing surgery unless coagulopathy is suspected based on history and physical examination, or the patient is on warfarin, in which case the PT/INR is necessary to guide the perioperative anticoagulation treatment.
- Despite the fact that an elevated PTT is more common than an abnormal prothrombin time, it rarely influences management or affects surgical outcome.
  - The most common cause of an elevated PTT is insufficient blood filling of the specimen tube.
  - Hemophiliacs (Factor VIII or IX deficiency) have usually been diagnosed; Factor XI deficiency is often associated with Ashkenazi Jewish ancestry and a family history of bleeding; Factor XII deficiency is not associated with an increasd bleeding risk.
  - Lupus anticoagulant is more likely to cause thrombosis than bleeding.
- Recommendation for PTT
  - PTT should not be obtained as a routine screening test preoperatively.
- Although bleeding time may be abnormal in patients taking aspirin or other antiplatelet drugs (NSAIDs), its value in predicting an uneventful perioperative outcome is not clear, and an abnormal test result does not usually change management.
- Recommendation for bleeding time
  - Bleeding time should not be measured before surgery unless the history and physical examination suggest a bleeding tendency and other tests (PT, PTT, platelet count) are normal.

ELECTROLYTES

- The main objective of measuring serum electrolytes on a routine basis preoperatively is to prevent perioperative arrhythmias.
- Theoretically, alteration of serum levels of electrolytes, particularly *hypokalemia or hyperkalemia*, may predispose patients to potentially lethal arrhythmias. However, evidence does not show that unexpected abnormal electrolytes affect surgical management (only 1.8%).[3]
- Furthermore, a study of patients undergoing major cardiac or vascular surgery found no increase in ventricular arrhythmias in patients with mild hypokalemia (≥ 3.0 mEq) vs. those with normal potassium levels.[4]
- Recommendations for serum electrolytes
  - Screening electrolytes may be indicated if the patient's history suggests certain conditions likely to be associated with abnormalities.
  - These conditions include renal insufficiency, CHF, adrenal insufficiency, diarrhea, and the use of ACEIs, ARBs, diuretics, digoxin, and NSAIDs.

GLUCOSE

- Diabetes, particularly those patients requiring insulin treatment, is a risk factor for postoperative cardiac complications.
  - The revised cardiac risk index[5] and ACC/AHA guidelines[6] list diabetes as an risk predictor.
- However, the finding of an unexpected elevation of glucose usually carries no risk to patients undergoing elective surgery.
  - In a recent review, only 0.5% of all values were both abnormal and influenced preoperative management. The majority of abnormal values belong to patients with established diabetes mellitus.
- Recommendations for glucose measurement
  - Do not obtain serum glucose as a routine preoperative screening test in asymptomatic patients; however, it is reasonable to screen those with risk factors for diabetes, including obesity or glucocorticoid use, or symptoms of polyuria or polydipsia.

○ Obtain serum glucose in patients with known diabetes to assess control of the disease and guide perioperative management.

RENAL FUNCTION TESTS

- A growing body of evidence emphasizes the role of preoperative screening for renal insufficiency since an elevated serum creatinine is a predictor of postoperative complications.
  - ○ In the revised cardiac risk index,[5] preoperative serum creatinine > 2.0 mg/dL is one of six predictors of risk for postoperative cardiac complications.
  - ○ The revised ACC/AHA guidelines[6] on preoperative cardiac evaluation for noncardiac surgery classifies renal insufficiency as an "intermediate" clinical risk predictor.
  - ○ Goldman's original cardiac risk index[7] and Detsky's modified cardiac risk index,[8] used in the ACP guidelines, list serum creatinine > 3.0 as a risk predictor.
- The prevalence of an abnormal serum creatinine increases with age and in a recent review, was 2.6% preoperatively and tended to influence patient management.
  - ○ Dose adjustment of some medications (eg, muscle relaxants) requires knowledge about renal function.
- Recommendation for obatining a preoperative serum creatinine
  - ○ The elderly
  - ○ Patients with renal insufficiency, hypertension, diabetes mellitus or CV disease
  - ○ Patients undergoing major surgery
  - ○ Patients taking medications that may adversely affect renal function.

LIVER FUNCTION TESTS

- Liver cirrhosis has an unfavorable impact on the surgical outcome. This risk increases with disease severity that correlates with the Childs-Pugh criteria or MELD score.
- Conversely, asymptomatic elevation of liver enzymes, mainly transaminases, does not appear to influence the surgical outcome, and in only 0.1% of cases did detection of abnormal liver enzymes alter the management.
- Low serum albumin predicted perioperative complications in a large multivariate analysis, with the risk of mortality increasing with serum albumin concentrations < 3.5 g/dL,[9] and predicted PPCs in another study. Nevertheless, the results of a low serum albumin rarely affects management, and it is not clear that increasing a low serum albumen would improve the surgical outcome.

- Recommendations for liver function tests (LFTs)
  - ○ Do not routinely obtain screening liver enzymes for preoperative evaluation.
  - ○ Consider preoperative screening for a low serum albumin in patients who have predisposing conditions, including malnutrition, enteropathy, chronic liver disease, and nephropathy. Note, however, that it is not routinely obtained as the results are unlikely to change management.

URINALYSIS

- Potential reasons for obtaining a urinalysis preoperatively include identifying patients with asymptomatic bacteriuria, undetected renal disease, and asymptomatic diabetes.
  - ○ Although asymptomatic bacteriuria theoretically could increase the risk of prosthetic device infection, this is mainly anecdotal. Many abnormal results are not treated, and most prosthesis implant patients receive prophylactic antibiotics regardless of the results.
  - ○ Diabetes and undiagnosed renal disease are better detected by other tests or need not be identified preoperatively.
- Although the incidence of abnormal urinalysis may be significant, existing data do not support the rationale of obtaining urinalysis preoperatively because an abnormal result rarely influenced management or surgical outcome.
- Recommendation for urinalysis
  - ○ Do not obtain a routine urinalysis preoperatively unless the patient has urinary tract symptoms or will undergo urologic instrumentation.

ELECTROCARDIOGRAM

- The rationale to perform 12-lead electrocardiogram (ECG) preoperatively is to identify patients who are potentially at increased risk of CV complications and to obtain a baseline ECG for comparison in case of a further cardiac event.
- There are disparities in the literature and clinical practice in terms of obtaining routine preoperative ECG.[10]
- Despite the relatively high frequency of abnormal ECG findings, patient management was rarely affected.[3]
  - ○ The most useful finding would be that of a silent MI such as Q waves; however, even this abnormality rarely changes management unless the patient is undergoing major surgery.
  - ○ Arrhythmias, such as atrial fibrillation, atrial or ventricular ectopy, and tachy or bradyarrhythmias can usually be detected by physical examination, in

which case the ECG would only serve to confirm the diagnosis.

○ Other abnormalities, such as asymptomatic bundle branch block and left ventricular hypertrophy, are unlikely to change management.

○ Goldman's original cardiac risk index[7] included nonsinus rhythm and frequent atrial premature contractions (APCs) or premature ventricular contractions (PVCs) as markers of cardiac disease for risk prediction, but they are not part of the revised cardiac risk index.[5] History of an MI or Q waves on ECG were risk predictors in both indices.

• Although ECG abnormalities are more likely in older patients, age alone should probably not mandate obtaining a preoperative ECG.

○ A multicenter randomized controlled trial[11] in asymptomatic patients undergoing cataract surgery demonstrated that preoperative ECG did not result in improved risk stratification.

○ These findings were confirmed by a new multivariate analysis[12] which concluded that routine ECG is not necessary in asymptomatic patients undergoing low-risk or low-intermediate risk surgical procedures.

○ The new ACC/AHA guideline[6] updates indicate that "routine" ECG in the asymptomatic patients is not supported unless combined with two or more atherosclerotic risk factors.

• Recommendations for ECG testing, including

○ Preoperative ECG is indicated for patients who are at increased risk of postoperative cardiac complications

■ Known cardiac disease or suspicion of cardiac disease in the clinical evaluation

■ Men > 45 years of age and women > 55 years of age in the presence of two or more atherosclerotic risk factors (eg, hypertension, hypercholesterolemia, diabetes)

■ Conditions that predispose patients to electrolyte abnormalities such as diuretic use

■ Patients undergoing major intermediate- to high-risk surgeries

CHEST RADIOGRAPH

• Chest radiography is usually performed in order patients to identify abnormalities that could potentially predict increased risk of postoperative cardiopulmonary complications or be used as a baseline for comparison in the event of a postoperative event.

• Advanced age and the presence of cardiopulmonary disease are associated with an increased likelihood of an abnormal study.

• Although a significant proportion of screening preoperative chest x-rays are abnormal, these abnormal findings rarely lead to alteration in patient management.[3]

• A recent systematic review demonstrated that the prevalence of chest x-ray abnormalities is low in asymptomatic patients less than the age of 70, and there is insufficient evidence for or against routine CXR for patients more than the age of 70.[13]

• Recommendations for chest radiograph (CXR)

○ According to these studies, we suggest preoperative chest x-ray in patients with active preexisting or suspected cardiopulmonary disease (based on the history and findings on physical examination) and possibly in patients more than the age of 70 with other risk factors undergoing intermediate to high-risk surgery.

REFERENCES

1. Roizen MF. More preoperative assessment by physicians and less by laboratory tests. *N Engl J Med.* 2000;342: 204–205.
2. Kaplan EB, Sheiner LB, Boeckmann AJ, et al. The usefulness of preoperative laboratory screening. *JAMA.* 1985;253:3576.
3. Smetana GW, Macpherson DS. The case against routine preoperative laboratory testing. *Med Clin North Am.* 2003;87:7.
4. Hirsh IA, Tomlinson DL, Slogoff S, et al. The overstated risk of hypokalemia. *Anesth Analg.* 1988;67:131.
5. Lee TH, Marcantonio ER, Mangione CM, et al. Derivation and prospective validation of a simple index for prediction of cardiac risk of major noncardiac surgery. *Circulation.* 1999;100:1043.
6. Eagle KA, Berger PB, Calkins H, et al. ACC/AHA 2007 guidelines on perioperative cardiovascular evaluation and care for noncardiac surgery: a report of the American College of Cardiology/American Heart Association Task Force on Practice Guidelines (Writing Committee to Revise the 2002 Guidelines on Perioperative Cardiovascular Evaluation for Noncardiac Surgery) developed in collaboration with the American Society of Echocardiography, American Society of Nuclear Cardiology, Heart Rhythm Society, Society of Cardiovascular Anesthesiologists, Society for Cardiovascular Angiography and Interventions, Society for Vascular Medicine and Biology, and Society for Vascular Surgery. *J Am Coll Cardiol.* 2007;50:e159–e241.
7. Goldman L, Caldera DL, Nussbaum, SR, et al. Multifactorial index of cardiac risk in noncardiac surgical procedures. *N Engl J Med.* 1977;297:845–850.
8. Detsky AS, Abrams HB, McLaughlin JR, et al. Predicting cardiac complications in patients undergoing noncardiac surgery. *J Gen Intern Med.* 1986;1:211–219.
9. Gibbs J, Cull W, Henderson W, et al. Preoperative serum albumin level as a predictor of operative mortality and morbidity: results from the national VA Surgical Risk Study. *Arch Surg.* 1999;134:36.
10. Yuan H, Chung F, Wong D, et al. Current preoperative testing practices in ambulatory surgery are widely disparate: a survey of CAS members. *Can J Anaesth.* 2005;52:675–679.

11. Schein O, Katz J, Bass E, et al. The value of routine preoperative testing before cataract surgery. *N Engl J Med.* 2000;342:168.

12. Noordzij P, Boersma E, Bax JJ, et al. Prognostic value of routine preoperative electrocardiography in patients undergoing noncardiac surgery. *Am J Cardiol* 2006;97:1103–1106.

13. Joo H, Wong J, Naik V, et al. The value of screening preoperative chest x-rays: a systematic review. *Can J Anaesth.* 2005;52(6):568–574.

104 POSTOPERATIVE COMPLICATIONS

Danielle Scheurer and Cregg Ashcraft

OVERVIEW

- Hospitalists should play an active role in preventing and managing postoperative complications.
- The focus of preoperative risk assessment has shifted away from preoperative cardiac testing to optimizing the medical conditions of patients so that they can withstand the stress of surgery.
- In preoperative clinics and in the hospital setting, hospitalists have an opportunity to develop strategies for the prevention of postoperative complications. Using beta-blockers as an example
  - Instead of simply recommending perioperative beta-blockade for cardiac protection, hospitalists can develop a beta-blocker protocol to maintain heart rates between 55 and 70 bpm. (See Chaps. 101 and 102.)
  - During consultation for an individual patient, hospitalists can go beyond simply recommending beta-blockade, and make specific recommendations with dosages so that careful beta-blocker titration is more likely to occur and complications such as stroke, increased mortality, and renal failure are less likely.
- Hospitalists should actively communicate with surgeons to clarify perioperative goals.
  - Hospitalists have moved from the traditional consultation role of writing recommendations in the chart once daily to more active management, which requires a clear delineation of responsibilities.
  - Surgical services may differ in their assumptions about the role and responsibilities of the hospitalist.
  - Nurses and other members of the healthcare team need to know who is the primary contact for concerns

about wound infection, bleeding, delirium, VTE, and other postoperative complications (see Chaps. 11 and 105).

- Postoperative complications hospitalists frequently actively manage include
  - Persistent postoperative fever
  - Hospital-acquired infection
  - Respiratory distress (see Chap. 73)
  - Chest pain (see Chap. 21)
  - Hypertension or hypotension
  - Blood loss anemia (see Chap. 52)
  - Acute renal failure (see Chaps. 82 and 83)
  - Acid-base and fluid-electrolyte issues (see Chaps. 86, 87A, and 87B)
  - Hyperglycemia/hypoglycemia (see Chap. 36)
  - Delirium (see Chaps. 62 and 61)
  - Pain management (see Chap. 93)
  - VTE (see Chap. 89)
- This chapter will discuss postoperative fever, including surgical site infections (SSIs), PPCs, and postoperative CHF.

POSTOPERATIVE FEVER

- Postoperative fever is one of the most common reasons for postoperative medical consultation.
  - Postoperative fever may occur in up to 90% of patients, depending on type of surgery.
  - The majority of fevers that occur within the first 48 hours after surgery abate spontaneously without a definite cause ever being found.
  - Atelectasis, very common after surgery or prolonged bed rest, has often been implicated, but a causal relationship has been difficult to establish.
- As the differential for postoperative fever is broad, the evaluation should include
  - A comprehensive history, carefully assessing
    - Postoperative symptoms
    - Perioperative drug administration, particularly antibiotics
    - Perioperative transfusions and type of blood product
  - A comprehensive physical examination, including
    - The surgical site (may require surgical expertise)
    - Extremities for evidence of DVT or gout
    - Skin for rashes or other evidence of an allergic reaction
    - The presence of foreign bodies (intravascular catheters, urinary catheters, nasogastric tubes, etc.) that predispose to nosocomial infections
- The evaluation should take into account
  - Patient risk factors.

- • The presence of delirium
- • Immune status
- • Possible alcohol or other substance withdrawal
- ○ The type of surgery and possible intraoperative complications.
  - • Intra-abdominal procedures precipitating acute pancreatitis,
  - • Hematomas
  - • Infection of any materials implanted during the surgery
- ○ The timing of postoperative fever is an important diagnostic clue to determine the etiology (see Table 104-1).
- • The most common infectious causes of postoperative fever are
  - ○ Urinary tract infections, the frequency of which is related to the duration of use of the catheters (see Chap. 55).
  - ○ SSIs—discussed in more detail below.
  - ○ Hospital-acquired pneumonia (see Chap. 78).
  - ○ Intravenous catheter-associated infections (see Chap. 56).
  - ○ Antibiotic-associated diarrhea because of *Clostridium difficile* (see Chap. 41).

SURGICAL SITE INFECTIONS

- • SSIs account for 3.7 million excess hospital days, and carry relative risks of intensive care unit (ICU) admission and death of 2.2 and 1.6, respectively. Approximately, 500,000 surgical patients are affected annually.
  - ○ This occurrence rate is likely an underestimation since most SSIs occur after hospital discharge and are not captured by conventional surveillance.
- • In recognition of the magnitude of the problem, reducing the risk of healthcare-associated infections, including SSIs, is a national patient safety goal.
- • The rate of occurrence depends on the type of surgery and the patient risk category.
  - ○ The highest rates occur after abdominal and organ transplant surgeries.
  - ○ Genitourinary, gynecologic, orthopedic, vascular, and cardiothoracic surgeries are intermediate risk.
  - ○ The lowest rates occur after endocrine and eye surgeries.
- • Most infections occur at the time of surgery, and the microbiology reflects the skin, viscus, or mucosal flora that is surgically compromised.
- • The epidemiology of SSIs has not changed substantially in the past decade (the most common organisms being *Staphylococcus aureus*, Coagulase-negative Staphylococcus, *Escherichia. coli*, and *Enterococcal* species), but there has been an increase in fungal and resistant gram-positive organisms (methicillin-resistant *S. aureus* [MRSA] and vancomycin-resistant enterococci

[VRE] have increased 11% and 12% from 1998 to 2003).
- • Skin flora infections are usually monomicrobial.
- • Visceral and mucosal flora infections are usually polymicrobial.
- • Less commonly, inoculation of the surgical field can occur as a result of contact with healthcare workers (hand or nasal carriage), bandages, or irrigants. There are multiple patient and environmental factors associated with SSIs, only some of which are modifiable (Table 104-2).
- • According to National Nosocomial Infection Surveillance (NNIS), the risk category (0–3) depends on the ASA preoperative assessment score, the contamination of the wound, and the duration of the surgery.
- • The clinical presentation depends on the type of SSI. According to the Centers for Disease Control (CDC), these infections are classified into incision or organ/space, and incision infections are further divided into superficial (skin and subcutaneous tissue) and deep (deep soft tissue-muscle and fascia).
  - ○ Incision infections account for two-thirds of all cases, and organ/space infections account for one-third of all cases.
  - ○ Signs and symptoms of infection present within a week in 50% of patients and within 2 weeks in 90% of patients.
  - ○ The CDC definition, however, delineates any infection that occurs within 30 days of the operation (and up to a year if related to an implant) as an SSI.
  - ○ Signs and symptoms usually include localized pain, erythema, drainage, subcutaneous swelling, foul odor, fever, and elevated WBC (or other markers or inflammation such as erythromycin sedimentation rate [ESR] or C-reactive protein [CRP]).
- • Although empiric treatment of SSI, based on the site of infection and likely pathogen(s) is important, definitive treatment will often require surgical exploration and debridement.
- • Category I recommendations to reduce the incidence of SSIs from the Hospital Infection Control Practices Advisory Committee (HICPAC) include the following:
  - ○ Use appropriate prophylactic antibiotics: antibiotics within 1 hour of incision and up to 24 hours after surgery have been shown to markedly reduce the incidence of SSIs (Table 104-3).
  - ○ Control diabetes: blood sugars > 200 within 48 hours postoperatively increase the risk of SSIs. (See Chap. 36.)
  - ○ Provide smoking cessation counseling: multiple studies confirm recent smoking as an independent risk factor for the development of SSI.

TABLE 104-1 Causes of Postoperative Fever

FEVER PRESENTING DURING OR WITHIN A FEW HOURS OF SURGERY	FEVER PRESENTING WITHIN 1 WEEK OF SURGERY	FEVER PRESENTING FROM 1–4 WEEKS OF SURGERY	FEVER PRESENTING MORE THAN 1 MONTH AFTER SURGERY
Medication reactions (malignant hyperthermia from anesthetics, allergic reactions to antibiotics)	Medication reactions (allergic reactions to antibiotics)	Medication reactions (drug fever from antibiotics, histamine blockers, phenytoin, and carbamazepine used for postoperative neurosurgical seizure prophylaxis, among others)	
Transfusion reactions	Transfusion reactions		
Infection present prior to surgery (including dirty/infected surgical sites and preexisting infections unrelated to the surgical problem, such as urinary tract infection or pneumonia)	Infection present prior to surgery		
Fulminant surgical site infection (necrotizing fasciitis and fulminant myonecrosis because of *Clostridium* or beta-hemolytic Group A *Streptococcus*)	Surgical site infection (including toxic shock syndrome from colonization of wound dressings with beta-hemolytic Group A *Streptococcus* or *S. aureus*)	Surgical site infection	Surgical site infection (especially more indolent pathogens, or associated with implanted device or prosthesis)
	Nosocomial infections (hospital-acquired and ventilator-associated pneumonia, urinary catheter-associated urinary tract infection, central venous access catheter-associated infections)	Nosocomial infections; antibiotic-associated diarrhea (*C. difficile*)	Nosocomial infections; antibiotic-associated diarrhea (*C. difficile*)
			Other infections: • cellulitis (because of impaired lymphatic drainage such as in the leg following saphenous vein graft harvest) • bacterial endocarditis (s/p valve replacement or from perioperative bacteremia in a patient with valvular heart disease who did not receive appropriate prophylaxis) • viral (such as Cytomegalovirus [CMV] or Hepatitis B or C from postoperative transfusion, or CMV reactivation following transplant surgery)
Trauma Adrenal insufficiency	Noninfectious causes: MI; pulmonary embolism; thrombophlebitis; hematomas; alcohol withdrawal; gout/pseudogout; pancreatitis; acalculous cholecystitis	Noninfectious causes: pulmonary embolism; thrombophlebitis	Noninfectious causes: postpericardiotomy syndrome

TABLE 104-2 Factors Associated with SSI Risk (Mangrum)

PATIENT FACTORS	ENVIRONMENTAL FACTORS
Diabetes	OR personnel traffic
Smoking	OR ventilation
Immunosuppression	Foreign bodies (prostheses, drains)
Malnutrition	Duration of hospital stay before surgery
Age	Duration of surgery and surgical scrub
Remote focus of infection	Preoperative skin preparation
Obesity	Preoperative shaving
Colonization or nasal carriage of *S. aureus*	Surgical technique (electrocautery, hemostasis, tissue trauma, dead space)

OR, operating room.

○ Treat other foci of infection: according to HICPAC, elective surgery should be postponed until the remote infection is cleared. Discretion must be used to determine when the infection is "cleared."

○ Avoid shaving the surgical site: if hair removal is necessary, use electric clippers immediately before surgery, since shaving significantly increases the risk of SSIs.

○ Protect the postoperative site: use a sterile dressing for 24–48 hours and wash hands before and after each contact. There is no evidence that sterile technique needs to be continued past 48 hours with primary closure sites (should be continued in open wounds).

○ Use an infection surveillance and control program: this has been shown to decrease infection rates by 30%. It should include a trained physician and nurse (1 per 250 beds) and a system for reporting infection rates to surgeons (Haley).

TABLE 104-3 Antibiotics for Prevention of SSIs (Bratzler, ACOG)

TYPE OF SURGERY	FIRST-LINE TREATMENT	BETA-LACTAM ALLERGIC
CV and vascular	Cefazolin Cefuroxime Cefamandole	Vancomycin Clindamycin
Colorectal surgery*	Cefotetan Cefoxitin Cefazolin/Metronidazole	Clindamycin (with Gent, Cipro, or Aztreonam) Metronidazole (with Gent or Cipro)
Orthopedic surgery	Cefazolin Cefuroxime	Vancomycin Clindamycin
Gynecologic surgery	Cefazolin Cefotetan Cefoxitin	Clindamycin (with Gent, Cipro, or Aztreonam) Metronidazole (with Gent or Cipro)

*Should combine with bowel prep: neomycin/erythromycin or neomycin/IV metronidazole.

○ Preoperative measures that have not been proven to reduce the risk of SSIs include: weight loss, immunosuppressive medication reduction, nutritional repletion, eradication of staph nasal colonization, restrictive blood transfusion triggers, and bathing with an antiseptic agent.

PULMONARY COMPLICATIONS

• Pulmonary complications often result from a perioperative decrease in vital capacity, residual volume, *forced expiratory volume* in the first second of expiration (FEV_1), and functional residual capacity.
• These decreases
  ○ Start within 5 minutes of anesthesia induction
  ○ Tend to peak at postoperative day 2
  ○ Return to baseline by day 5
• Decreases in pulmonary volumes, diaphragmatic dysfunction, loss of sigh breaths, prolonged recumbency, and depression of respiratory drive contribute to V/Q mismatching and resultant hypoxia.
• Although preoperative evaluations focus more on the prevention of cardiac complications, pulmonary complications are more common in postoperative patients. In one study of veterans administration (VA) patients after elective abdominal surgery, PPCs occurred in 10% and cardiac complications occurred in 6%.
• The spectrum of PPCs is wide and includes
  ○ Atelectasis
    ▪ The clinical presentation of atelectasis varies depending on its severity, and can range from no symptoms to profound shortness of breath and hypoxia. The hypoxia is most pronounced on postoperative day 2, but can persist for up to 5 days. The physical examination is characterized by unilateral or bilateral crackles at the bases, and chest radiograph shows reduced expansion in the same area.
  ○ Pneumonia
    ▪ Postoperative (and aspiration) pneumonias present more insidiously with any combination of shortness of breath, hypoxia, tachypnea, cough, fever, or signs of consolidation on examination (egophony), and can also be accompanied by bronchospasm or pleural effusions. (See Chap. 78.)
  ○ COPD exacerbation
    ▪ Postoperative exacerbations of underlying pulmonary disease present similar to nonpostoperative exacerbations. (See Chaps. 74 and 75.)
  ○ Bronchospasm
    ▪ Postoperative bronchospasm usually presents more acutely with shortness of breath, hypoxia, tachypnea, and wheezing.

- Postoperative bronchospasm is usually a result of aspiration, allergic reaction (usually to medications), or exacerbation of underlying bronchospastic disease (asthma or COPD).
  ◦ Pulmonary embolism
    - Pulmonary embolism, including fatty embolism in orthopedics patients, should always be considered in the differential of a postoperative patient with respiratory compromise.
    - The postoperative incidence of these varies from 2% to 19%, depending on the patient population and definition used.
- Other PPCs include pleural effusions and aspiration events.
  ◦ Pleural effusion is very common, and occurs in up to 50% of patients after abdominal surgery, and usually resolves spontaneously. Postoperative pleural effusions are likely because of a decrease in pleural pressures with enhanced filtration across the microvascular barrier, as well as lymphatic disruption because of a change in respiratory motion.
  ◦ Aspiration at the time of intubation is rare and usually occurs either in emergency surgery or in patients with a high ASA class. Steps to decrease perioperative aspiration risk include control of postoperative vomiting and limiting the duration of nasogastric tube insertion.
- Initial management should include an assessment of the degree of hypoxia (by pulse oximetry or arterial blood gas) and maneuvers to resolve the hypoxia (by oxygen alone, or with the addition of continuous positive airway pressure [CPAP], bi-level positive airway pressure [BiPAP], or endotracheal intubation).
- The history should focus on preoperative diagnoses, onset and duration of symptoms, and exacerbating and alleviating interventions. Hypoxia is usually accompanied by tachypnea unless hypoventilation is the cause of the hypoxia, or respiratory depression is coexistent. (See Chap. 73.)
- Dyspnea (see Chap. 73) may also be related to nonpulmonary complications, including
  ◦ Postoperative ischemia (see Chap. 101)
  ◦ Arrhythmias (particularly atrial fibrillation, Chap. 25)
  ◦ Pulmonary embolism (see Chap. 88)
- Subsequent management depends on the etiology of the hypoxia and may include any combination of chest percussion, incentive spirometry, deep breathing, diuresis, antibiotics, mucolytics, steroids, bronchodilators, anticholinergics, or anticoagulation.
- Strategies to reduce the risk of PPCs include assessing preoperative risk in order to optimize care in the preoperative period.
  ◦ There are multiple published indices to estimate risk of postoperative pneumonia and respiratory failure.

- Prior to 2002, the Goldman-based Combined Cardiac Pulmonary Risk Index (CPRI) was the most commonly utilized risk index, but it is not well validated and requires pulmonary function tests and arterial blood gases on all patients.
- The Multifactorial Risk Index is well validated, easy to use, and more commonly utilized. The only limitation is that it assesses only the risk of pneumonia (not other pulmonary complications). The index risk factors are listed in Table 104-4. Patients in risk classes 1 through 5 have a risk of postoperative pneumonia of < 1%, 1%, 5%, 11%, and 16%, respectively, corresponding to points of 0–15, 16–25, 26–40, 41–55, and > 55.
- The ACP Clinical Guideline defines high-risk patients as those with COPD, age > 60, ASA class 2+, functional dependence, HF, and low albumin, as well as those undergoing procedures > 3 hours (abdominal, thoracic, neurosurgery, head/neck, vascular, emergency, and general anesthesia).
  ◦ Counsel smoking cessation
    - Smoking within 2 months of surgery carries a much higher risk of pulmonary postoperative complications than those with cessation of > 2 months.

TABLE 104-4 Pulmonary Complications—Multifactorial Risk Index

RISK FACTOR	POINT VALUE
Type of surgery	
Abdominal aortic aneurysm	15
Thoracic	14
Upper abdominal	10
Neck	8
Neurosurgical	8
Vascular	3
Age	
> 80	17
70–79	13
60–69	9
50–59	4
Functional status	
Totally dependent	10
Partially dependent	6
Weight loss > 10% in 6 months	7
History of COPD	5
General anesthesia	4
Impaired sensorium	4
History of CVA	4
BUN	
< 8 mg/dL	4
22–30 mg/dL	2
> 30 mg/dL	3
Transfusion > 4 units	3
Emergency surgery	3
Chronic steroid use	3
Smoker (within a year)	3
EtOH (> 2/day in last 2 weeks)	2

○ Aggressively treat asthma/COPD

▪ This includes ipratropium for COPD, beta-agonists for any bronchoconstriction, the addition of systemic steroids for those not well controlled, and the addition of antibiotics for those with evidence of lower respiratory tract infections.

▪ Peak flows should be optimized to 80% of the patients' personal best.

○ Limit the duration of surgery if possible

▪ Surgeries lasting < 1 hour, 1–2 hours, 2–4 hours, and > 4 hours have PPCs of 4%, 23%, 38%, and 73% respectively.

▪ This is ultimately a surgical decision, but for high-risk patients, the hospitalist should communicate this risk directly with the surgeon.

○ Attempt local or spinal vs. general anesthesia

▪ Neuroaxial anesthesia (vs. general) reduces pneumonia and respiratory depression by 39% and 59%, respectively.

▪ The type of anesthesia is decided by the anesthesiologist, but for high-risk patients, hospitalists should communicate this risk directly with the anesthesiologist.

○ Control pain

▪ Epidural pain control is associated with fewer pulmonary complications than parenteral opioids.

▪ Adequate pain control may reduce the risk of postoperative delirium which can predispose to aspiration.

○ Avoid prolonged duration of using nasogastric tubes

▪ NG tubes used temporarily for the relief of gastric distention, nausea, or vomiting can prevent aspiration of stomach contents. However, prolonged or unnecessary use increases the risk of pneumonia.

○ Lung expansion maneuvers

▪ Incentive spirometry or deep breathing exercises can reduce pulmonary complications by up to 50% after upper abdominal surgery.

▪ There are less data to support this routinely in other surgical populations.

▪ There are no data to support one modality over the other.

Postoperative Heart Failure

• HF is the most common postoperative cardiac complication in hospitalized patients, occurring in approximately 5%.

○ The highest risk (18%) occurs in patients with diabetes or previous cardiac disease (MI, valvular disease, or HF).

○ It carries a mortality of approximately 11% and is difficult to predict preoperatively.

○ Preoperative signs of active HF confer the highest risk of postoperative HF, but a past history of HF still confers significant risk. Both are included in most perioperative cardiac risk indices as an independent risk factor for perioperative CV events.

• The pathophysiology of perioperative HF is complex, given that HF is a heterogeneous diagnosis.

• It appears that both hypovolemia and hypervolemia can predispose to postoperative HF.

○ Lower intravenous volume during surgery can increase the risk of HF likely because of reduced preload and altered Starling physiology.

○ However, excessive fluid administration has also been linked to fatal pulmonary edema.

○ Another factor shown to contribute to postoperative HF is significant perioperative deviations of systolic blood pressure (> 40 mm Hg increase or decrease).

○ "Negative pressure pulmonary edema" can occur in patients after the relief of temporary laryngospasm (or other upper airway obstruction). It appears to be related to the negative intrathoracic pressure created with inspiration against a closed glottis, with subsequent pulmonary capillary transudation upon relief of the obstruction. This entity is rare and the prognosis is good with airway management and oxygenation.

• Strategies to reduce the incidence of postoperative HF include.

○ Preoperative assessment of exercise tolerance: this correlates significantly with the risk of perioperative CV events and should be assessed in all patients. Patients with "poor" functional status (defined as the inability to walk four blocks or climb two flights of stairs) are more likely to experience perioperative CV events (defined as MI, arrhythmia, hypotension, or CHF).

○ Assess for current signs or symptoms of HF: in patients with current signs or symptoms of HF (S_3, jugular venous distention (JVD), or pulmonary edema), it is prudent to defer surgery until these are resolved/medical management optimized.

○ Assess for past symptoms of HF: in patients with a past history of HF, perioperative ACE inhibitors and diuretics in appropriate doses are the most beneficial in reducing the risk of perioperative HF.

○ Preoperative assessment of ejection fraction (EF) should not be a routine part of the preoperative work up. Although EF appears to independently predict the risk of postoperative pulm edema, echocardiography information does not appear to change the risk when clinical variables are also assessed. Therefore, a thorough HF history and physical examination should suffice in most patients.

- Administer appropriate intraoperative volume: although excessive fluid administration has been linked to fatal pulmonary edema, hypovolemia has also been linked to postoperative pulmonary edema and should similarly be avoided.
- Avoid blood pressure fluctuations: significant fluctuations in mean SBP (< or > 40 mm Hg) has been shown to be an independent predictor of postoperative HF.
- Perioperative pulmonary artery (PA) catheters should not be routinely utilized: they have never proven to be beneficial, even in high-risk patients.

BIBLIOGRAPHY

Postoperative Fever

Bratzler DW, Houck PM. Antimicrobial prophylaxis for surgery: an advisory statement from the National Surgical Infection Prevention Project. *Clin Infect Dis*. 2004;38(12):1706–1715.

Classen DC, Evans RS, Pestotnik SL, et al. The timing of prophylactic administration of antibiotics and the risk of surgical-wound infection. *N Engl J Med*. 1992;326(5):281–286.

Culver DH, Horan TC, Gaynes RP, et al. Surgical wound infection rates by wound class, operative procedure, and patient risk index. National Nosocomial Infections Surveillance System. *Am J Med*. 1991;91(3B):152S–157S.

Gaynes RP, Culver DH, Horan TC, et al. Surgical site infection (SSI) rates in the United States, 1992–1998: the National Nosocomial Infections Surveillance System basic SSI risk index. *Clin Infect Dis*. 2001;33 (suppl 2):S69–S77.

Haley RW, Culver DH, White JW, et al. The efficacy of infection surveillance and control programs in preventing nosocomial infections in US hospitals. *Am J Epidemiol*. 1985;121(2):182–205.

Horan TC, Gaynes RP, Martone WJ, et al. CDC definitions of nosocomial surgical site infections 1992: a modification of CDC definitions of surgical wound infections. *Infect Control Hosp Epidemiol*. 1992;13:606–608.

Kirkland KB, Briggs JP, Trivette SL, et al. The impact of surgical-site infections in the 1990s: attributable mortality, excess length of hospitalization, and extra costs. *Infect Control Hosp Epidemiol*. 1999;20(11):725–730.

Latham R, Lancaster AD, Covington JF, et al. The association of diabetes and glucose control with surgical-site infections among cardiothoracic surgery patients. *Infect Control Hosp Epidemiol*. 2001;22(10):607–612.

Mangram AJ, Horan TC, Pearson ML, et al. The Hospital Infection Control Practices Advisory Committee Guideline for the Prevention of Surgical Site Infection 1999. Infection Control and Hospital Epidemiology 1999;20(4):247–278 (or *http://www.cdc.gov/ncidod/dhqp/pdf/guidelines/SSI.pdf*)

Sands K, Vineyard G, Platt R. Surgical site infections occurring after hospital discharge. *J Infect Dis*. 1996;173(4):963–970.

Prevention of Postoperative Pulmonary Complications

American College of Physicians. Preoperative pulmonary function testing. *Ann Intern Med*. 1990;112:793.

Arozullah AM, Khuri SF, Henderson WG, et al. Participants in the National Veterans Affairs Surgical Quality Improvement Program. Development and validation of a multifactorial risk index for predicting postoperative pneumonia after major noncardiac surgery. *Ann Intern Med*. 2001;135(10):847–857.

Cheatham ML, Chapman WC, Key SP, et al. A meta-analysis of selective versus routine nasogastric decompression after elective laparotomy. *Ann Surg*. 1995;221(5):469–476.

Fisher BW, Majumdar SR, McAlister FA. Predicting pulmonary complications after nonthoracic surgery: a systematic review of blinded studies. *Am J Med*. 2002;112(3):219–225.

http://www.nhlbi.nih.gov/guidelines/asthma/asthgdln.pdf, page 100–101.

Kroenke K, Lawrence VA, Theroux JF, et al. Operative risk in patients with severe obstructive pulmonary disease. *Arch Intern Med*. 1992;152(5):967–971.

Lawrence VA, Hilsenbeck SG, Mulrow CD, et al. Incidence and hospital stay for cardiac and pulmonary complications after abdominal surgery. *J Gen Intern Med*. 1995;10(12):671–678.

Qaseem A, Snow V, Fitterman N, et al. Risk assessment for and strategies to reduce perioperative pulmonary complications for patients undergoing noncardiothoracic surgery: a guideline from the American College of Physicians. *Ann Intern Med*. 2006;144:575–580.

Rodgers A, Walker N, Schug S, et al. Reduction of postoperative mortality and morbidity with epidural or spinal anaesthesia: results from overview of randomised trials. *BMJ*. 2000;321(7275):1493.

Rosenberg J, Ullstad T, Rasmussen J, Hjorne FP, Poulsen NJ, Goldman MD. Time course of postoperative hypoxaemia. *Eur J Surg*. 1994;160(3):137–143.

Thomas JA, McIntosh JM. Are incentive spirometry, intermittent positive pressure breathing, and deep breathing exercises effective in the prevention of postoperative pulmonary complications after upper abdominal surgery? A systematic overview and meta-analysis. *Phys Ther*. 1994;74:3–10.

Warner MA, Warner ME, Weber JG. Clinical significance of pulmonary aspiration during the perioperative period. *Anesthesiology*. 1993;78(1):56–62.

Prevention of Postoperative Congestive Heart Failure

Arieff AI. Fatal postoperative pulmonary edema: pathogenesis and literature review. *Chest*. 1999;115(5):1371–1377.

Halm EA, Browner WS, Tubau JF, et al. Echocardiography for assessing cardiac risk in patients having noncardiac surgery. Study of Perioperative Ischemia Research Group. *Ann Intern Med*. 1996;125(6):433–441.

Reilly DF, McNeely MJ, Doerner D, et al. Self-reported exercise tolerance and the risk of serious perioperative complications. *Arch Intern Med*. 1999;159(18):2185–2192.

Sandham JD, Hull RD, Brant RF, et al. A randomized, controlled trial of the use of pulmonary-artery catheters in high-risk surgical patients. *N Engl J Med*. 2003;348(1):5–14.

105 SURGICAL COMANAGEMENT

Shaun Frost

SCOPE OF THE PROBLEM

THE NEED FOR SURGICAL COMANAGEMENT

- A number of contemporary issues make today's hospitalized surgical patients increasingly vulnerable to perioperative complications and adverse events.
  - Compared to a decade ago, surgical patients today are older, have more chronic medical conditions, and are taking more medications.
  - Perioperative complications are common, with CV events most frequently causing death.
  - Hospital systems of care are complex and challenging to navigate under increasing financial and resource utilization pressures.
  - Some consultants feel that they are inadequately trained to perform preoperative evaluations.
  - Advances in technology and science are challenging historical models of perioperative care delivery. For example, some anesthesiologists question whether the current anesthesia training curriculum adequately prepares them to diagnose, optimize, and treat the complex medical illnesses common among today's surgical patients.
  - Surgeons are spending an increasing amount of time in the operating room, limiting their availability to attend to postsurgical hospitalized patients. This may be a factor accounting for studies suggesting that surgeons perform suboptimally in employing effective strategies for perioperative VTE prophylaxis, beta-blockade, and prevention of wound infection.
- Optimal care of the hospitalized surgical patient requires a team approach that coordinates the expertise of the medical specialist and the surgical team.

HOSPITALISTS AS SURGICAL COMANAGERS

- Hospitalists are uniquely positioned to best partner with surgery teams to provide medical comanagement.
  - Perioperative medicine is a "core competency" for hospitalists as defined by the Society of Hospital Medicine.
  - Hospitalists are experts in treating and preventing common perioperative conditions including MI, delirium, hyperglycemia, hypertension, hyponatremia, VTE, pneumonia, alcohol withdrawal, and pain.
  - Hospitalists can effectively guide surgical patients through complicated systems of hospital care by providing expertise in communication, information management, resource allocation, care team leadership, care coordination, transitions of care, risk management, patient safety, and quality improvement.
  - Hospitalists' specialized knowledge in the areas of palliative care, end-of-life care, and nutrition are frequently useful in caring for select surgical populations.
  - Hospitalists' ready availability allows for immediate response to the needs of nurses, patients, and family members.

COMANAGEMENT VS. CONSULTATION

- Surgical comanagement (SCM) is distinctly different than traditional consultation.
- Requests for consultation should be differentiated from patient referrals.
  - A consultation is a request for another physician to give medical advice regarding patient diagnosis or management.
  - A referral is a request for another physician to assume direct responsibility for a portion or all of a patient's care. As surgical comanagers typically assume direct responsibility for the care they provide, SCM is much more a referral arrangement vs. a consulting relationship between hospitalist and surgeon.
- Consulting relationships are sometimes rendered ineffective when the recommendations of the consultant are not acted on. This may occur because of gaps in communication or delays in execution of recommendations. Comanagement eliminates these problems by creating a referral arrangement in which the medical comanager is granted the ability to provide direct patient care, as opposed to being limited to providing advice.
- The comanagement care model represents a departure from the consultative model in that the hospitalist becomes a true member of the care team.
  - This role is a natural extension of the Hospital Medicine model of care in that surgeons, like primary care physicians, are often physically unable to see patients repeatedly throughout the day.
  - Hospitalist comanagers typically have the ability to independently order tests, consultations, medications, and other therapies.
  - Hospitalist comanagers may serve as physicians of first call for nurses, assume responsibility for communication to and education of patients and families, coordinate discharge planning, and ensure that the patient's primary care physician is informed.

○ There is no standard structure to SCM services. Such services may be broadly categorized into models that are service based (ie, all orthopedic patients), diagnosis based (ie, all joint arthroplasty patients), or dictated by severity of illness (ie, all orthopedic patients with specific concomitant medical illness).

EVIDENCE THAT COMANAGEMENT ADDS VALUE

• Some investigators have reported that adding a medical specialist to the surgery team improves outcomes and adds value.
  ○ Macpherson et al. (1994) described a comanagement model in which an internist made daily rounds with surgeons, participated in clinical problem solving, and performed specific duties such as preoperative assessment, order writing for medical issues, management of postoperative medical problems, and participation in discharge planning. Compared to a care model that did not include an internist, the comanagement model significantly decreased length of stay, mean number of radiology tests ordered, and number of medications patients were prescribed at discharge. Revenue generated by the internist offset the cost of adding this physician to the care team.
  ○ Huddleston et al. (2004) described a comanagement model in which hospitalists were added to a surgery team to manage hip and knee arthroplasty patients more than the age of 75 years, and those with predefined comorbidities. The hospitalists were responsible for all medical management and related order writing 24 hours a day. Compared to patients randomized to receive standard care without hospitalist team members, the comanagement model significantly decreased minor postoperative complications and adjusted length of stay without affecting total cost of care. Also, surgeons and nurses were more satisfied with the comanagement model compared to the historical standard manner of providing care. In a separate report, these investigators also determined that among patients with hip fracture, their comanagement model decreased time to surgery.

SYSTEMS IMPROVEMENTS: HOW TO BUILD A COMANAGEMENT SERVICE

• Although there are various forms and structures to SCM services, a number of issues should be universally considered when hospitalists develop comanagement arrangements with surgeons.

ETHICAL CONSIDERATIONS

• The American Medical Association (AMA) has stated that any medical practice that divides care responsibilities among various care givers creates a variety of ethical considerations. To avoid potential ethical pitfalls in providing SCM, the AMA's Council on Ethical and Judicial Affairs offers a number of recommendations (Table 105-1).
• The American College of Surgeons' (ACS) Statement on Principles Underlying Perioperative Responsibility outlines practical and ethical considerations for surgeons involved in comanagement arrangements (Table 105-2).
• Opinions of governing bodies and organizations such as the AMA and the ACS should be incorporated into agreements among care team members providing comanagement.
• Preemptively considering potential ethical pitfalls when dividing care responsibilities will highlight opportunities to avoid the perception of fraud when hospitalists bill and collect fees for services provided. To avoid the perception of billing fraud, hospitalist comanagers must ensure that they provide specialized knowledge or services that other care team members can not offer. Fraud is typically not a concern when hospitalists provide or perform
  ○ Care for conditions unrelated to the diagnosis for which surgery was performed.
  ○ Critical care services.
  ○ Diagnostic procedures.
• Consulting a billing and coding specialist prior to providing comanagement services will help ensure that the process of remuneration for care delivery is conducted according to rules and regulations set forth by the Centers for Medicare and Medicaid Services.

TABLE 105-1   The American Medical Association's Council on Ethical and Judicial Affairs Recommendations for Avoiding Ethical Pitfalls in SCM

• Engage in SCM only to assure the highest quality care.
• Delineate responsibilities according to physician expertise.
• Designate a single physician to supervise care coordination.
• Employ safeguards to ensure confidentiality.
• Ensure patient consent to all services provided.
• Inform patients of all elements of the SCM arrangement.
• Ensure SCM does not violate ethical or legal restrictions on self referral.
• Base referrals on patient needs and caregivers skills.

TABLE 105-2   The American College of Surgeons' Statement on Principles Underlying Perioperative Responsibility

- The surgeon is responsible for proper preoperative preparation of the patient, which may require consultation of other physicians.
- The surgeon is responsible for postoperative care of the patient including personal participation in and direction of care.
- The surgeon must maintain an essential coordinating role when delegating aspects of care to other physicians.
- The surgeon is responsible for determining when the patient should be discharged from the hospital.
- It is unethical to turn over the postoperative care of a patient completely to the referring physician.
- When a patient is ready for discharge from the surgeon's care, it may be appropriate to transfer care to another physician.
- The premise of referral to another physician must be quality of care.

CREATING AN AGREEMENT FOR COMANAGEMENT

- To avoid conflicts and guarantee that patient care is uncompromised, Sanderson advocates that "forthright and reasoned discussions" take place between medical specialists and surgeons, with these discussions resulting in "guidelines and policies based on principles agreed to by both groups."
- Hospitalists and surgeons participating in SCM should develop protocols that specify how they will work together to deliver high-quality, safe, efficient, and coordinated patient care. These protocols should specifically address the following (Table 105-3):
  - *Purpose of the comanagement arrangement.* A statement of purpose will help ensure that ethical and legal standards are upheld. Possible elements to include are
    - Maximize quality and patient safety
    - Optimize resource utilization
    - Maximize operating room efficiency
    - Improve hospital bed availability
    - Improve patient, nurse, physician, and staff satisfaction
  - *Role definitions for comanagement participants.* Roles should be clearly defined and agreed upon to avoid misunderstanding of responsibility.
    - One care team member should be designated as having ultimate responsibility for the overall care outcome. This person will ensure that communication between care team members occurs in an effective manner, and will be responsible for mediating in situations of disagreement or conflict.
    - Assign primary responsibility for specific aspects of care such as order writing for medications and tests, completion of paperwork, requests for subspecialty consultation, first call for nursing, care coordination (ie, with case management, physical therapy, etc.), discharge planning, and wound management.
  - *Expectations for care delivery.* Expectations of each care provider should be mutually discussed and agreed upon by all participants. Consider setting clear expectations for the following:
    - Level of medical comorbidity required to initiate referral for hospitalist comanagement
    - Time to complete initial evaluations
    - Duration of hospitalist participation in care
    - Timing and number of postoperative visits by the surgeon
  - *Mechanism and timing of communications between hospitalist and surgeon.* Inadequate and ineffective communication will surely lead to suboptimal patient care. Consider specifically defining
    - A standard process for initiating comanagement that outlines reliable contact information including after-hours contacts and mechanisms to reach team members in emergency situations. Surgeons should also be told what patient-specific information is required at the time of referral, and if referral requests can be made verbally or in writing.
    - Designated times for daily care update communications.
    - Reasonable timelines for returning messages regarding nonurgent issues.
    - Optimal time of day and mechanism for contacting surgeons.
    - Reliable methods to reach surgeons regarding urgent and emergent issues.
  - *Services offered by the hospitalist.* Consider specifically offering the following:
    - Preoperative evaluation
    - Posthospital discharge rehabilitative or transitional care
    - Discharge planning
    - Best practices pathway adherence
    - Family meeting coordination
    - Patient and family education
- Measure the performance of the SCM service to monitor its success. Outcomes data to measure are presented

TABLE 105-3   Subjects to Consider when Creating a Protocol for SCM

- Purpose of the comanagement arrangement.
- Role definitions for all care team participants.
- Clearly defined expectations for the delivery of care.
- Mechanism and timing of communications between care team members.
- Services offered by the hospitalist.

TABLE 105-4 Outcome Measures that Reflect Performance of a SCM Service

- Mortality
- Morbidity
  - CV complications
  - Pulmonary complications
  - VTE
  - Delirium
  - Ileus
  - Urinary tract infection
  - Fever
  - Electrolyte disturbances
- Quality
  - Beta-blocker utilization
  - VTE prophylaxis
  - Blood sugar control
  - Incentive spirometry utilization
  - Blood transfusion rate
  - Pain control
- Resource utilization
  - Length of stay
  - Time from admission to surgery
  - Time from surgery to discharge
  - Time to transfer from Post Anesthesia Care Unit to floor
  - Rate of hospital readmission
  - Rate of transfer to ICU
  - Rate of transfer from SCM service to regular medicine or surgical services
  - Average number of ancillary tests and labs ordered
  - Average number of consults ordered
- Satisfaction
  - Patient and family
  - Nurse
  - Surgeon
  - Hospitalist
  - Primary care physician
- Cost of care

in Table 105-4. Strongly consider meeting with key stakeholders to review this data on a recurrent and regular basis.

CONCLUSIONS

- Today's hospitalized surgical patients are sicker and more complex than in decades past. Caring for surgical patients requires a team approach that draws on specialized medical and surgical knowledge to shepherd patients through an increasingly complex care delivery system.
- Given their availability and expertise, hospitalists are uniquely positioned to partner with surgeons to comanage the medical problems of surgical patients.

- SCM is distinctly different than traditional consultation. Comanagement requires a high level of involvement by the participating hospitalist, as well as a clearly defined and mutually agreed upon working agreement between hospitalist and surgeon that considers potential ethical and legal pitfalls that may occur when patient care is divided among multiple providers.

BIBLIOGRAPHY

The American Medical Association Council on Ethical and Judicial Affairs Report 5–I99, 1999. Accessed at *www.ama-assn.org/ama1/pub/upload/mm/369/ceja_5i99.pdf*, October 10, 2006.

Bull Am Coll Surg. Sept 1996;81:(9):39.

Huddleston JM, Long KH, Naessens JM, et al. Hospitalist-orthopedic team trial investigators: medical and surgical comanagement after elective hip and knee arthroplasty: a randomized controlled trail. *Ann Intern Med.* 2004;141: 28–38.

Macpherson DS, Parenti C, Nee J, et al. An internist joins the surgery service: Does co-management make a difference? *J Gen Intern Med.* 1994;9:440–444.

McKean S, Auerbach A, Frost S. Role of the hospitalist in perioperative medicine. In: Cohen S, Smetana J, Weed H, eds. *Just the Facts in Perioperative Medicine.* New York, NY: McGraw-Hill; 2006.

Phy MP, Vannes DV, Melton J, et al. Effects of a hospitalist model on elderly patients with hip fracture. *Arch Intern Med.* 2005;165:796–801.

Sanderson R. Ethical and legal concerns in relationships with cardiologists. *Ann Thoracic Surg.* 2001;72:3–5.

Sarraille W. Spotlight on eye doctors puts co-management in gray area. Hospitalist and Inpatient Management Report. 2003;5(7):96–97.

Stratton MA, Anderson FA, Bussey HI, et al. Prevention of venous thromboembolism: adherence to the 1995 American College of Chest Physicians consensus guidelines for surgical patients. *Arch Intern Med.* 2000;160(3):334–340.

Taylor RC, Pagliarello G. Prophylactic B blockade to prevent myocardial infarction perioperatvely in high risk patients who undergo general surgical procedures. *Can J Surg.* 2003; 46(3):216–222.

Tetzlaff JE, Maurer WG, Parker BM, et al. New directions in perioperative medicine? *J Clin Anesth.* 1999;11(2):143–145.

Wasey N, Baughan J, de Gara CJ. Prophylaxis in elective colorectal surgery: the cost of ignoring the evidence. *Can J Surgery.* 2003;46(4):279–284.

106 ADULT LEARNING PRINCIPLES AND HOSPITAL MEDICINE

Grace Huang

INTRODUCTION

- In academic settings, hospitalists are uniquely positioned to integrate teaching into their daily work flow and activities for a variety of reasons:
  - They are available at the point of care; therefore, learning interactions can occur informally and in person.
  - Hospitalists can play a leadership role in mentoring trainees, developing peer review of teaching and faculty development, and working with the residency program at their institutions to define the specific knowledge, skills, and attitudes required by the Accreditation Council for Graduate Medical Education (ACGME) outcome project and provide educational experiences as needed.
  - Whether hospitalists are community-based or affiliated with a teaching hospital, the potential learners can be students, trainees, other health professionals, or peers.
  - Hospitalists and other general medicine physicians may possess inherent characteristics that have led trainees to rate them highly as teachers.
  - The ability to transmit knowledge and communicate thought processes behind clinical decisions may improve the cohesiveness of the healthcare team and, ultimately, the care of the patient.
- The key to being an effective teacher is to understand how adults learn and how to apply these principles in practice.

PRINCIPLES

- Adult learning theory is a major organizing framework for professional education. Malcolm Knowles, widely viewed as its originator, outlines the following characteristics of adult learners:
  - *They are self-directed in their learning.* They want to participate actively in the defining, planning, execution, and evaluation of their instruction.
  - *Their prior experiences have applicability to their learning.* They draw on a rich source of existing knowledge and life experiences as they learn; creating connections to prior experience allows them to elaborate and build upon this knowledge base meaningfully.
  - *They need to see the relevance of learning to actual practice.* They seek knowledge and skills that meet their educational needs, whether vocational or personal. As such, they should be exposed to authentic tasks.
  - *They focus on problem-centered learning rather than subject-centered learning.* They prize practicality and goal-oriented instruction rather than knowledge for its own sake.
  - *They are motivated by internal rather than external pressures to learn.* They are no longer driven to learn largely because of standardized tests and class assignments, but by factors such as the need to feel confident or the desire to provide excellent care.

PRACTICAL APPROACHES

- Principles that characterize adult learners can translate into practical points for the academic hospitalist as he or she interacts with learners.
- Foremost, however, one must recognize the primacy of the teacher-learner relationship itself in promoting learning.

- Students regard the personal attributes of teachers, such as communication ability, friendliness, and enthusiasm as more important than professional skills such as punctuality and organization.
- Thus, an educator mindful of adult learning theory and good interpersonal skills can become an effective clinical teacher (Table 106-1).
- *Create a safe learning environment* to allow the self-directed learner to feel confident taking charge of his or her learning.
  - Take advantage of the time spent in the hospital to become well-acquainted with the trainees rotating in the hospital over time.
  - Make an extra effort to recognize individual learners' interests, strengths, and sensitivities.
  - Show kindness and respect to encourage trainees to verbalize uncertainty. A brusque tone or harsh words will impede the climate for learning.
  - Listen actively. Rephrase what a learner says to you to indicate that you heard and understood. ("Let me share what I heard you say….") Do not interrupt the trainee.
  - Emphasize the collaborative nature of patient care by using "we" liberally. Encourage learners to actively participate and to help set the agenda. ("What should we do?")
  - Show enthusiasm for teaching and use appropriate nonverbal communication skills.
- *Elicit a needs assessment* plan to help the learner vocalize his or her specific needs. Use this information to provide learner-centered instruction.
  - When a learner asks you a close-ended question, try turning the question back on him or her. ("What do you think?")
  - Get a sense of the learner's prior experience with the situation. ("Have you managed this type of case before?")
  - Check in periodically for understanding. ("What aspect of this is giving you most trouble?")

- *Facilitate learner autonomy* to promote self-directed learning.
  - Suppress the impulse to answer a pointed question with your opinions and orders. (Respond to "Can I send this patient home now?" with "What are your endpoints for discharge?")
  - Provide adequate guidance for the learner to arrive at a solution, but avoid leading questions that ultimately ask, "What am I thinking?" Be willing to delegate when appropriate.
- *Promote understanding and retention* to advance the learner's knowledge.
  - Use higher order questions that activate complex cognitive skills such as analysis, synthesis, and evaluation ("How would you categorize the various types of glomerulonephritis?") (Table 106-2).
  - Draw connections between clinical manifestations and the basic science mechanisms that underlie them.
  - Use common teaching scripts to convey easy-to-remember general principles. ("Because blood cultures are positive in 20% of community-acquired pneumonias, always remember to order blood cultures.") At the end of the session, have the team summarize what was learned.
- *Build on prior knowledge* to allow learners to bring their previous experiences meaningfully into the learning process.
  - Ask learners about similar clinical situations. ("Does this situation remind you of previous patients?")
- *Give feedback* to allow learners to gauge their own progress and identify next steps for learning. (See also Chap. 109.)
  - Feedback should be timely but at the right time.
  - Feedback should be collaborative, with agreement on next steps to improve.

TABLE 106-1 Attributes of Effective Clinical Teachers

CLINICAL-TEACHING DOMAINS	SOME EXAMPLES
Interpersonal relationship	Communicates effectively, serves as role model, provides mentorship, collaborates as fellow learner
Personality characteristics	Displays enthusiasm, friendliness, approachability, nonjudgmental
Teaching ability	Makes learners feel comfortable, sets goals, motivates learners, provides feedback
Professional competence	Displays expertise, advocates for patients

TABLE 106-2 Sample Questions that Promote Adult Learning Principles

ADULT LEARNER CHARACTERISTIC	SAMPLE QUESTION
Self-directed	"What aspects of the knee examination do you have the hardest time performing?"
Drawing on prior experience	"How did you treat your last patient with GI bleed and hypotension?"
Relevance-oriented	"What will you remember as a result of this case that you will think about the next time you have a patient with this problem?"
Problem-oriented	"What clinical questions do you have now that you've seen this patient with a rash?"
Internally motivated	"Which resources did you use to learn about the clinical problem?"

- ○ Feedback should be genuine and specific to actions supported by examples, not to the person. ("I noticed that the needle went in at too shallow an angle.")
- • *Foster reflection* to promote the habit of self-assessment and extract maximal learning out of experience.
  - ○ Use untoward events as opportunities for informal discussion in small groups. ("Let's talk about how that conversation went.")
  - ○ Encourage learners to write about thought-provoking experiences.
  - ○ Dedicate teaching rounds to discussing multiple examples of the same experience, for example, relaying bad news.
  - ○ Relate current experience to future changes in practice. ("What will you do differently next time?")
  - ○ During the teaching session, reflect on your own performance and ask the team, "What went well?" "What could be improved?" Recognize that we as teachers need knowledge and skills to teach effectively in the clinical setting. Learning what is wrong with an approach and adapting appropriately is a good thing, not a failure.
  - ○ As a role model for life-long learning and personal investment in teaching, encourage feedback and be willing to hear constructive criticism.
  - ○ Observe other teachers.

BIBLIOGRAPHY

Armstrong EG, Barsion SJ. Using an outcomes-logic-model approach to evaluate a faculty development program for medical educators. *Acad Med.* 2006 May;81(5):483–488.

Beckman TJ, Lee MC, Rohren CH, et al. Evaluating an instrument for the peer review of inpatient teaching. *Med Teach.* 2003 Mar;25(2):131–135.

Kaufman DM. Applying educational theory in practice. *BMJ.* 2003 May 3;326(7396):986.

Knowles MS. *The Adult Learner: The Definitive Classic in Adult Education and Human Resource Development.* 5th ed. Houston, TX: Butterworth-Heinemann; 1998.

Kripalani S, Pope AC, Rask K, et al. Hospitalists as teachers. *J Gen Intern Med.* 2004 Jan;19(1):8–15.

Mann KV. The role of educational theory in continuing medical education: has it helped us? *J Contin Educ Health Prof.* 2004;24(Suppl 1):S22–S30.

Mann KV. Thinking about learning: implications for principle-based professional education. *J Contin Educ Health Prof.* 2002;22(2):69–76.

McLean M. Qualities attributed to an ideal educator by medical students: should faculty take cognizance? *Med Teach.* 2001 Jul;23(4):367–370.

Prideaux D, Alexander H, Bower A, et al. Clinical teaching: maintaining an educational role for doctors in the new health care environment. *Med Educ.* 2000 Oct;34(10):820–826.

107 TEACHING VENUES FOR THE HOSPITALIST

Bradley A. Sharpe

INTRODUCTION

- • Inpatient teaching (attending) rounds are defined by the Accreditation Council for Graduate Medical Education (ACGME) as "patient-based sessions in which current cases are presented as a basis for discussion of such points as interpretation of clinical data, pathophysiology, differential diagnosis, specific management of the patient, the appropriate use of technology, the incorporation of evidence and patient values in clinical decision making, and disease prevention."
- • Inpatient attending rounds remain a fundamental and crucial component of resident and student education; the inpatient setting provides a unique teaching environment where the patient is a captive "textbook," the learners can be a captive audience, and there is full and easy access to patient information and the medical literature.
- • Hospitalists have the potential to be excellent teaching attendings because of their expertise in general inpatient medicine, their bedside availability throughout the day, and the role modeling of the provision of high-quality and efficient care.
- • There are many challenges to teaching in the inpatient setting including high patient census, billing requirements, short patient lengths of stay, and resident duty hours.
- • In addressing these challenges, there are specific principles and skills that can help the academic hospitalist overcome these challenges and teach effectively in multiple teaching settings.

GENERAL PRINCIPLES

- • Inpatient teaching physicians must participate in faculty development activities that focus on teaching skills. They must make time to prepare for teaching rounds and make themselves available to their inpatient team.
- • Variability and versatility in the location, content, teaching style, and structure of teaching rounds is essential to teaching success. One should avoid getting stuck in a repetitive "rut" in teaching rounds.
- • Under increasing time pressures and potential distractions, establishing clear expectations and ground rules for attending rounds is important (see Chap. 108).

○ Clearly define the start and stop time for each session and then start and stop *on time*.

○ Negotiate with the team how they should handle potential interruptions. Should they answer pages during attending rounds? Are they permitted to complete paperwork or check laboratory values during teaching?

• When possible, separate teaching rounds from "patient management rounds." One way to accomplish this separation is to deliver the teaching rounds in a designated area such as a conference room.

○ Clearly state the distinction to the learners: "Today, for *teaching* rounds, we will be discussing diffuse alveolar hemorrhage."

• Teaching rounds can be in a conference room, at the bedside, or you can employ a "mobile classroom."

CONFERENCE ROOM TEACHING

GENERAL PRINCIPLES

• The typical attending teaching rounds is a regularly scheduled (often daily) meeting of the attending and the learners in a standard location, usually a conference room within the hospital.

• At the beginning of the rotation, the hospitalist attending should make introductions and then assess the learners' (both residents and students) educational needs and *their* goals and expectations for attending rounds.

○ "Are there particular topics or diseases you wanted to learn about this month?"

○ "What have you liked and *disliked* about attending rounds you have had in the past?"

• When teaching in the conference room setting, strive to establish a lively, fun, open, engaging, and yet challenging learning climate (see Chap. 108).

CONTENT OF CONFERENCE ROOM TEACHING

• The content taught in conference room attending rounds should focus on patients currently cared for by the team and not just general medical topics. Previous research supports the value of case-based teaching.

• Variability in content and focus is essential to broaden the educational experience and keep the learners actively engaged. Hospitalist attendings should be versatile and teach on the important knowledge, skills, and attitudes of hospital physicians.

• See Table 107-1 for examples of content to be taught in the conference room setting.

TABLE 107-1 Examples of Content for Conference Room Teaching

1. Examples of knowledge-based topics
   • Treatment of community-acquired pneumonia
   • The evidence for gastrointestinal prophylaxis in the inpatient setting
   • The clinical features and treatment of anti-phospholipid antibody syndrome
2. Examples of skills-based topics
   • Interpretation of electrocardiograms (ECG)
   • Interpretation of chest radiographs
   • How to read an article on a case-control study
3. Examples of attitude-based topics
   • Understanding the impact of socioeconomic status on health
   • Appreciating the role of teamwork and communication in modern healthcare

• In a given teaching rounds, resident and student fatigue and information overload often limit the retention of information. Always finish each teaching session with clear, concise, memorable "take-home points," which highlight the most essential principles.

• Use the conference room setting for reflection and discussions about patients who have died or for whom an end-of-life discussion is anticipated. If there is an unexpected or emotionally difficult death on the team, use the next attending rounds to reflect on the care provided and the experience of the team members.

MEDIA/MATERIALS

• Try to vary the media through which the knowledge, skills, and attitudes are taught.

○ Powerpoint presentations are useful for teaching broad knowledge-based topics.

○ "Chalk talks" using a whiteboard allow for active engagement of the material and questioning of the learners.

○ Reviewing handouts that summarize a clinical issue or topic can provide a visual reinforcement to the auditory teaching.

• Distribute key and pertinent reading materials to the team (or directions on how to access them).

○ Avoid distributing articles or handouts "in a vacuum"—only hand outmaterials if you have actively taught on the material or plan to do so.

TEACHING TECHNIQUES

• Engage learners in substantive discussions about patients to promote student/resident satisfaction with teaching rounds.

• Avoid teacher-dominant, solely didactic teaching rounds.

- Use open-ended, nonthreatening questions of learners to keep them engaged and evaluate their knowledge and understanding.
- Employ a variety of questioning techniques. Not all of the techniques will necessarily be employed during a given teaching session. Some suggestions include:
  ○ *Round-robin*: When asking for the differential diagnosis, go around the room where each learner gets one answer, starting with the medical students.
  ○ *Next step*: Ask "what would you do at this point?" to move the discussion along and focus on diagnostic or therapeutic options.
  ○ *What if?*: Change one variable in the case, keeping all others constant. "What if the creatinine were 3.5 mg/dL instead of 0.7 mg/dL?" This will challenge learners to think beyond the specific case and is particularly useful if the case is straightforward.
  ○ *Assess feelings*: Ask "How do you *feel* about this case/incident?" To senior learners to assess feelings and attitudes. These questions are particularly useful in challenging or complex cases.

LEARNER HETEROGENEITY

- One of the greatest challenges of attending rounds is managing the vast differences in knowledge and experience, ranging from third-year clerks on their first rotation to senior residents in the final months of training, for example, "the one-room schoolhouse effect."
- If teaching rounds do not target learners at all levels, you risk exclusion of individuals, confusion, or boredom.
- There are multiple strategies to cope with learner heterogeneity.
  ○ The resident on the team can act as the *"teaching assistant."* Have him or her answer questions that arise and take advantage of prior experience.
  ○ *"Escalate"* the level of content and questioning in your teaching.
    ▪ Begin with students, focusing on anatomy and physiology, "Can you describe the feedback loop in the hypothalamic-pituitary-adrenal (HPA) axis?"
    ▪ Transition to interns, focusing on clinical skills, "What are the typical signs and symptoms of acute adrenal insufficiency?"
    ▪ Use the resident to discuss complex diagnostics or therapeutics, "How much hydrocortisone should we give this patient with adrenal insufficiency?"
  ○ Consider occasionally conducting teaching rounds for students separately. Separation allows the attending to focus on student-level topics (e.g., basic physical examination skills, patient interviewing skills, etc).

SHARED TEACHING

- The hospitalist attending should not be completely responsible for the education of the team. It is a shared responsibility.
- Have the medical students give 5-minute "mini talks" on specific topics which can fill gaps in knowledge or skills and allow them to begin practicing their teaching skills.
- At one institution, residents wanted to be responsible for one-third of the teaching and to help set the teaching agenda.
- The attending physician can "role model" self-directed learning in researching unanswered questions but should also assign tasks to members of the team and expect them to report back.

BEDSIDE TEACHING

GENERAL PRINCIPLES

- As William Osler stated, there should be "no teaching without the patient for a text, and the best teaching is often that taught by the patient himself."
- Teaching at the bedside should be a fundamental component of resident and student education and yet there has been a gradual decline in the amount of time spent with learners at the bedside.
- Identified barriers to bedside teaching include teacher anxiety about their own examination and teaching skills, difficulty in finding patients, resistance from learners, and fear of patient discomfort.
- Yet, evidence reveals patients favor bedside teaching, feel they are appropriate, and enhance understanding of their disease.
- Bedside teaching also allows the attending to gather additional historical or examination information; directly observe the skills and attitudes of the learners; and role model respect, empathy, and the foundations of the patient-doctor relationship.
- Hospitalist teachers can be experts at initially evaluating and establishing relationships with acutely hospitalized patients and thus are particularly suited for bedside teaching.

APPROACH TO BEDSIDE ROUNDS

- *Preparation*: Take time to plan the bedside teaching encounter and it will improve the experience for both learner and teacher.
  ○ Select appropriate patients for bedside teaching and make sure they are willing and will be available.

○ Decide on a particular focus for each encounter.
  ▪ Examples
    • Taking a better history
    • Eliciting a particular examination finding
    • Observing a learner giving bad news
○ Remain limited in your scope: Each bedside encounter should be no more than 10–15 minutes.
• *Expectations/ground rules*: Meet with the group before you see the patient to orient the learners to the session.
  ○ Outline the time you will spend with the patient and the goals of the session, remaining relatively focused.
  ○ Assign roles to different team members to engage all the learners (one person to take a history, one to do the chest examination, one the cardiovascular examination, etc).
  ○ Remind the team that sensitive issues should not be discussed in front of the entire group.
• *Introductions*: When entering the room, clearly introduce yourself, all of the members of the team, and explicitly state the teaching purpose of the exercise.
• *Case presentation*: Ask the primary care giver (student or resident) to present the case or provide a brief clinical summary. Ideally this is less than 5 minutes and focuses on the key components.
• *Teaching*: Focus teaching on details concerning that patient.
  ○ Role model Physician behavior by sitting down, avoiding medical jargon, and showing respect and empathy.
  ○ Engage all of the learners and team members including the patient's primary nurse if possible; have them answer the patient's questions or perform different aspects of the physical examination.
• *Closure*: In leaving, allow the patient to ask any final questions or clarifications and thank them for their cooperation.
• *Review*: Outside the room or in a conference room, meet again as a group, recap the key teaching points, and answer any final questions.

THE MOBILE CLASSROOM

GENERAL PRINCIPLES

• Add variability and versatility to attending rounds by changing the teaching location, employing the "mobile classroom."
• Hospitalists must have a sophisticated understanding of the hospital and processes of care and are well-situated to teach in different settings.
• When changing the location of attending rounds, you still must clearly outline the expectations and goals

for the session with the team, maintain an appropriate learning climate, and keep control of session.
  ○ Prepare ahead of time and decide on the key teaching and take-home points for the teaching session.
  ○ Coordinate the time and place with the appropriate representative for each destination.
• Take the team to examine the primary data on your patients.
  ○ Examples
    ▪ Visit radiology or the echocardiography lab to review studies.
    ▪ Review pathology or hematology slides if pertinent.
• Observe and evaluate different aspects of the process of care in the hospital with your team.
  ○ Go to the microbiology lab and learn how blood cultures are processed and evaluated by the lab, improving understanding of diagnostic testing.
  ○ Visit the pharmacy to learn about how orders for medications are filled and dispensed to patients, identifying potential sources of error.
• Provide "hands-on" experiences for your residents and students.
  ○ Meet with a respiratory therapist and learn about the mechanical ventilator to enhance management of patients who are intubated.
  ○ Visit the treadmill lab when a team patient is exercising and then interpret the results prior to the final reading by the cardiologist.
• If time permits, take field trips out of the hospital to see other aspects of modern healthcare.
  ○ Tour a skilled nursing facility (SNF) to improve the understanding of the patient experience after discharge.
  ○ Coordinate a tour of an inpatient hospice facility.
  ○ Perform a home visit and reconcile medications post discharge.

SELF-REFLECTION ON TEACHING

GENERAL PRINCIPLES

• Successful teaching in different venues requires self-reflection on performance.
• Regardless of location, after each teaching session, take 3 minutes to reflect on the session.
  ○ Which aspects went well?
  ○ What did not work?
  ○ Which are the teaching techniques I will use in the future?
• Solicit direct feedback from your learners.
  ○ Periodically during your time on service, take the last 5 minutes of a teaching session to get their group feedback on prior sessions.

○ During your midrotation feedback session in a private, nonthreatening setting, provide individual feedback and, solicit feedback about your approach to teaching. Ask specifically about your teaching rounds.
* For more details on feedback, see Chap. 109.
* Hospitalists may play a leadership role in promoting peer review of teaching.
* Hospitalists can master the knowledge, skills, and attitudes necessary to teach effectively in the inpatient clinical setting.
* Consequently, hospitalists are well-positioned to initiate faculty development programs for clinician educators. Further, hospitalists can develop and implement objective, structured tools for peer review and assessment of clinical teaching.

BIBLIOGRAPHY

ACGME Program Requirement for Education in Internal Medicine. *http://www.acgme.org/acWebsite/downloads/ RRC_progReq/140pr703_u704.pdf* Revised July 1, 2004.

Guarino CM, Ko CY, Baker LC, et al. Impact of instructional practices on student satisfaction with attendings' teaching in the inpatient component of internal medicine clerkships. *J Gen Intern Med.* 2006;21(1):7–12.

Hauer KE, Wachter RM. Implications of the hospitalist model for medical students' education. *Acad Med.* 2001;76(4): 324–330.

Irby DM. What clinical teachers in medicine need to know. *Acad Med.* 1994;69(5):333–342.

Janicik RW, Fletcher KE. Teaching at the bedside: a new model. *Med Teach.* 2003;25(2):127–130.

Kroenke K. Attending rounds: Guidelines for teaching on the wards. *J Gen Intern Med.* 1992;7:68–75.3.

Kroenke K, Simmons JO, Copley JB, Smith C. Attending rounds: a survey of physician attitudes. *J Gen Intern Med.* 1990;5(3):229–233.

LaCombe MA. On bedside teaching. *Ann Intern Med.* 1997;126:217–220.

Lehmann LS, Brancati FL, Chen M, et al. The effect of bedside case presentations on patients' perceptions of their medical care. *N Engl J Med.* 1997;336:1150–1155.

Pinsky LE, Monson D, Irby DM. How excellent teachers are made: reflecting on success to improve teaching. *Adv Health Sci Educ Theory Pract.* 1998;3(3):207–215.

Pistoria MJ, Amin AN, Dressler DD, et al. The core competencies in hospital medicine. *J Hosp Med.* 2006;1(supplement 1): 2–95.7.

Ramani S. Twelve tips to improve bedside teaching. *Med Teach.* 2003;25(2):112–115.

Wang-Cheng RM, Barnas GP, Sigmann P, et al. Bedside case presentations: why patients like them but learners don't. *J Gen Intern Med.* 1989;4(4):284–287.

108 TEACHING ON A TEAM
Cindy Lai

INTRODUCTION

Hospitalist clinician-educators currently work in both academic and community teaching hospitals to teach residents and students.
* Most of this instruction takes place at the bedside as hospitalists work alongside trainees on teams. These hospitalists often serve as both the attending of record and teaching attending.
* There is a defined set of principles and skills that the hospitalist attending can use to help students and residents take an active role in their education.
* Hospitalists can play a central role in teaching, observing, and measuring teamwork and communication competency on the micro level, the medical team.
* Incorporating important lessons learned from other industries such as aviation, hospitalists can model effective teamwork and decision-making as a way of reducing error.

GUIDING PRINCIPLES OF TEACHING ON A TEAM

* Effective teaching attendings have the ability to focus group energy on a shared vision, excellent patient care and team learning. They create enthusiasm and inspire others to strive for excellence.
* For hospitalist attendings, preparation is the key to effective leadership of the team and rounds. The following three points are ingredients that will help the hospitalist achieve success on the wards:
  ○ Set explicit expectations for team members:
    ▪ The attending, residents, and students must mutually understand goals and needs and state these explicitly at beginning of the rotation; they should then be revisited throughout the rotation.
    ▪ The attending should familiarize himself with students' formal clerkship or rotation objectives.
  ○ Table 108-1 contains a summary of training-level-specific teaching needs. The following is a guide to what each team member appreciates from the attending:
  ○ Structure teaching rounds to maximize learning
    ▪ The attending should develop a practical plan on how to structure each type of teaching opportunity (e.g., bedside rounds, conferences).
  ○ Create a "safe" learning climate

TABLE 108-1   Training-Level-Specific Teaching Preferences

- Resident: autonomy and responsibility
- Intern: primary responsibility of patient care and communication with families; seeing how a more experienced physician interacts with patients
- Fourth year medical students: responsibility with support and help when needed
- Third-year students: being an integral member of team, one-on-one teaching sessions

TABLE 108-2   Summary: Five Common Characteristics that Facilitate Teaching in Clinical Settings

1. Anchor instruction in cases
2. Actively involve learners
3. Model professional thinking and action in clinical decision-making
4. Provide direction and feedback
5. Create a collaborative learning environment

SOURCE: Irby DM. Clinical teacher effectiveness in medicine. *J Med Edu.* 1978:53:808–815.

- The attending should foster dialogue between all team members, and create an environment in which all opinions are valued.
- The attending should also encourage critical thinking and asking questions about specific management issues.

CLINICAL TEACHING SKILLS

- Overall teaching effectiveness occurs when the attending is enthusiastic and stimulating, establishes rapport, actively involves learners, and provides direction and feedback.
- Given their bedside presence, hospitalists are well-positioned to practice their clinical teaching skills and involve learners in clinical care.
- Several strategies have been noted in the literature to enhance student satisfaction with quality of teaching. These all require conscious attempts to integrate learners into patient-centered learning. Effective attendings incorporate the following practices:
  - Engage students in discussions.
  - Take advantage of teaching moments.
  - Demonstrate enthusiasm and interest in teaching.
  - Deliver both spontaneous and prepared talks.
  - Evaluate new patients with team.
  - Be "available" to team.
  - Treat team members with trust and respect.
  - Encourage acceptance of increasing responsibility.
  - Explain approaches to problems and reasons for decisions.
  - Align teaching with clerkship expectations and goals.
- The hallmark of teaching on the wards is case-based teaching. Case-based teaching allows students and residents to understand the relevance of their reading and learning. They will be motivated to learn and more likely to remember general concepts when given a clinical context.
- Regardless of teaching styles, there are five common characteristics that facilitate teaching in clinical settings (Table 108-2).
  - Anchor instruction in cases.

- Teaching through actual cases allows students and residents to understand the information's clinical relevance.
- They will be able to make connections to their prior knowledge, interpret current case facts, and finally develop general principles from the case.
- Actively involve learners.
  - Teach through questions, problem-solving exercises, reflection.
  - The Socratic method—"guided questioning" through a series of probing questions and answers—allows the attending to assess learners' knowledge base and to guide learners' thinking process by focusing on relevant issues.
  - Model professional thinking and action in clinical decision-making. Bedside and conference teaching are venues for role modeling.
  - Bedside teaching is an excellent venue to model professionalism, including empathy and communication with patients. Going to the bedside is especially helpful if there are any unanswered questions in a case presentation.
  - Teaching in a conference room is an ideal setting in which to articulate and model clinical synthesis skills. Select a few teaching points from a case, and communicate these points through questions and discussion.
  - Draw from learner's prior knowledge. When limits of learners' knowledge is reached, provide clinical cues (e.g., essential features of an illness, what is relevant, what should be prioritized, what can be ignored) and explain how to investigate further.
- Provide direction and feedback.
  - Establish team member interests and expectations at beginning of rotation. Ongoing two-way feedback will allow the hospitalist attending to better understand team needs.
  - Observe students and residents in action—for example, case presentations, physical examination—to be able to identify and correct misconceptions, and to reinforce teaching points.

- Be aware of group dynamics, which can affect team members' ability to achieve their goals.
  ○ Create a collaborative learning environment.
    - Model how to encourage questions and share ideas: offer to look up answers and report back to team.
    - Be comfortable with saying "I don't know"—a model for self-disclosure and self-assessment.
    - Be respectful of students' and residents' time; be flexible depending on their clinical load.
    - Debrief and reflect after stressful situations, such as unexpected outcome, code, or difficult patient or family interaction.
    - Model how to effectively work within a team by encouraging everyone to participate and share information.

MICROSKILLS MODEL OF CLINICAL TEACHING

- In a busy inpatient setting, hospitalists need to teach in a time-efficient manner. Microskills teaching (also known as "one minute preceptor" in the ambulatory setting) is a learner-centered "teaching script" that a teacher uses to probe and evaluate students' understanding of a case.
- This is a sequence of five open-ended "what" questions that permits the teacher to simultaneously diagnose the patient, evaluate students' understanding, and instruct. You do not need to use all the steps in each encounter. See Table 108-3.
- Evidence supports the efficiency and effectiveness of the five-step microskills model. A microskills model has been shown to

TABLE 108-3   Five-Step Microskills Teaching Script

MICROSKILL	RATIONALE	APPLICATION
First microskill: Get a commitment Cue: After presenting the facts of a case, the learner asks you a specific question or remains silent—in effect, waiting for your interpretation Attending: Instead of interpreting the facts, benignly ask an open-ended question about what the learner thinks about the data just presented. The learner will then process the information he or she has just gathered	Getting a commitment requires that the learner processes the information gathered (problem generation and solving). This is not to be confused with further data collection. This microskill helps the teacher assess more efficiently the learner's needs	"What do you think is going on with this patient?" "What do you want to do to workup the patient's wheezes?" If complex case, "How are you going to chip away at this situation?"
Second microskill: Probe for supporting evidence Cue: After committing to a particular stance, the learner looks to the teacher for confirmation Attending: Instead of passing judgment, ask the learner what evidence supports this commitment, or ask what other choices were considered and what evidence supports or refutes these alternatives	"Thinking out loud" allows attending to evaluate learner's knowledge and clinical reasoning underlying the commitment. This is also a good springboard for teacher to identify future key teaching points	"What factors did you consider in making that management decision?" "What else did you consider? How did you rule those things out?" "How did you choose this particular antibiotic for the patient's pneumonia?"
Third microskill: Teach general rules Cue: A teaching point should be apparent after the first two microskills Attending: Goal is to target your teaching to the learner. Give a few teaching points related to symptoms, physical findings, treatment, missed connections, or resources	Teaching a general principle from a specific case will help learners retain information so that they can apply it to future cases	"The point to take away from this case is…" "When this (x) happens, do this (x)…" "This is the first time I've seen a patient with this syndrome. The best genetics website is this xxx. I would also consult with our specialist, Dr. xxx."
Fourth microskill: Reinforce what was done right Cue: The learner has handled a situation in a way that has benefited the patient or colleagues Attending: Comment on a specific behavior that was done right	Verbally reinforcing behavior that led to desired outcome will encourage learner to internalize and repeat	"That was a good assessment of the patient's new wheezes. It shows that you've taken a thorough history and examination, considered her age and studies, and have considered alternative reasons for wheezes such as CHF and COPD. I agree that her wheezes are due to an asthma flare."
Fifth microskill: "Correct mistakes" Cue: Mistake or omission is made in data gathering or problem solving Attending: Allow learner to critique own performance first. Discuss specifically what went wrong and how to correct the error in the future. Suggest new behaviors that may be helpful in future	Mistakes that are not corrected have a good chance of being repeated	"I agree that last week's normal head CT is reassuring in ruling out a brain tumor, but we still need to do a neurologic examination given the change in headache to rule out other life-threatening causes." "It is important to check a daily room air O_2 saturation on every patient requiring supplemental oxygen."

SOURCE: Adapted from Neher JO, Gordon KC, Meyer B, et al. A five-step "microskills" model of clinical teaching. *J Am Board Fam Pract*. 1992;5:419–424; Neher JO, Stevens NG. The one-minute preceptor: shaping the teaching conversation. *Fam Med*. 2003;35(6):391–393; Gordon K, Meyer B, Irby D. The one minute preceptor: five microskills for clinical teaching. Handout, Teaching Scholars Lecture. 2006.

○ Enable the learner to correctly diagnose the clinical problem more often

○ Improve attending's confidence in evaluating the learner on presentation skills, clinical reasoning skills, and fund of knowledge

○ Improve attending's ability to facilitate self-directed learning (SDL)

○ Improve specificity and overall quality of feedback

EMPOWERING RESIDENTS TO BECOME TEAM LEADERS

- Although the hospitalist attending has ultimate responsibility for patient care and for the team, the resident leader has the most impact on a daily basis, and he/she is the true driver of the daily activities, team morale, and overall function.

- It is the hospitalist's responsibility to make sure that the resident leader feels well-supported and has the framework to become an effective leader. To best provide the framework for the resident, the attending should consider the following issues with their residents:

- *Setting explicit expectations with the resident about team management*
  ○ Residents need to understand your clear direction, and vice versa.
  ○ Residents want autonomy and responsibility, but appreciate the attending who is readily available for guidance.
  ○ Sit with the resident at the beginning of the rotation and clarify roles of each team member and the resident's goals for the rotation. This will also help you assess your resident's management of the team.
  ○ What are the residents' expectations for him/herself as team leader, and for the attending? Find out how you, the attending, can help your resident succeed. When do you want to touch base regarding patient admissions? Do you want to be called when patients' clinical status changes? How are they going to give/get feedback from interns and students?

- *Teaching strategies for the resident*
  ○ How is the resident planning to fit teaching into a busy schedule? Team teaching strategies include
    ▪ Providing case-based, relevant five-minute prepared discussion on a patient-related issue (e.g., a question that arose the day before)
    ▪ Delegating time to answer questions to medical students, with clear expectations specified for reporting back to team
    ▪ Teaching pearls during clinical care
    ▪ Demonstrating important physical examination findings

▪ Taking field trips to view peripheral blood smears of patients, pathology, urine microscopy

- *Team morale*
  ○ The resident's enthusiasm will set the stage for the entire team's energy and commitment. The team will work hardest when they feel that they are well-supported and their opinions valued, and when there is an enjoyable, respectful working dynamic.
  ○ How will the resident keep morale up during a busy inpatient month? How will they "build" the team? Strategies may include eating together on-call, frequent "check-ins" with team members, daily teaching, and pitching in with work when interns are busy.

USING "SELF-DIRECTED LEARNING"

- Strategies employing SDL can be used to engage learners to take charge of their own learning. SDL is an adult learning principle in which the learner is involved in formulating questions and finding and organizing the answers (Kroenke). Potential strategies (Jennett, Kroenke) include
  ○ *Set up a learning agenda that the attending and learner mutually agree on*
    ▪ This helps learners to adopt a learning style that works best for them, and engages them in own learning. Also decompresses teaching load on attending—shares responsibility of teaching
    ▪ Open discussion with, "What bothers you most about this case?" or "What would you most like to talk about, given our limited time?"
  ○ *Select one or two issues to teach on the spot*
  ○ *Convert some of learners' questions into SDL assignments.*
    ▪ Assign the learner to look up one to two relevant issues that involve searching the literature, critiquing, and applying it to learner's case
  ○ *Role model*
    ▪ Voice confusion with challenging topics: "Let's both look this up"
    ▪ Demonstrate use of SDL in "real-time": access online resources together: "Let's look this up now"
  ○ *Close the loop*
    ▪ Set time and method for report back to team: "Can you report back to us tomorrow at the beginning of rounds? A 2-minute discussion would be fine."
  ○ *Ensure retention*
    ▪ Apply newly gained knowledge to another patient soon

BIBLIOGRAPHY

Aaggard E, Teherani A, Irby DM. Effectiveness of the one-minute preceptor model for diagnosing the patient and the learner: proof of concept. *Acad Med.* 2004;79:42–49.

Bellet PS. Teaching by hospitalist physicians: a practical approach. *Med Teach.* 2002;24(4):434–436.

Elnicki DM, Cooper A. Medical students' perceptions of the elements of effective inpatient teaching by attending physicians and housestaff. *J Gen Intern Med.* 2005;20:635–639.

Ferrante J. Learner contracts. *Fam Med.* 1998;30(10):703–704.

Frankel A., Leonard MW, Denham CR. Fair and just culture, team behavior, and leadership engagement: the tools to achieve high reliability. Health Research and Educational Trust. 2006 August;41(4 Part II):1690–1709.

Gordon K, Meyer B, Irby D. The one minute preceptor: five microskills for clinical teaching. Handout, Teaching Scholars Lecture. 2006.

Guarino CM, Ko CY, Baker LC, et al. Impact of instructional practices on student satisfaction with attendings' teaching in the inpatient component of internal medicine clerkships. *J Gen Intern Med.* 2006;21:7–12.

Irby DM. Three exemplary models of case-based teaching. *Acad Med.* 1994;69:947–953.

Irby DM. Clinical teacher effectiveness in medicine. *J Med Edu.* 1978:53:808–815.

Jennett PA, Swanson RW. Lifelong, self-directed learning: why physicians and educators should be interested. *J Contin Educ Health Prof.* 1994;14:69–74.

Kroenke K. Practical tips for self-directed learning. http://www.im.org/facdev/7meeting/cycle3/material/kroenke.htm. Accessed June 1, 2006.

Neher JO, Gordon KC, Meyer B, et al. A five-step "microskills" model of clinical teaching. *J Am Board Fam Pract.* 1992;5:419–424.

Neher JO, Stevens NG. The one-minute preceptor: shaping the teaching conversation. *Fam Med.* 2003;35(6):391–393.

Parrott S, Dobbie A, Chumley H, et al. Evidence-based office teaching—the five-step microskills model of clinical teaching. *Fam Med.* 2006;38(3):164–167.

109 FEEDBACK AND THE HOSPITALIST

Anjala Tess

INTRODUCTION

Feedback has been defined by J. Ende as "information that a system uses to make adjustments in reaching a goal."

- In all levels of medical education, this has been interpreted as a description of students' or residents' performance that can be used to improve their behavior.
  - Beyond training, feedback from senior clinicians can help less experienced clinicians improve attitudes or practice and vice versa. Feedback among hospitalists is an emerging area of practice and inquiry and is important for hospitalists in a variety of academic and community settings.
  - Despite the fact that clinical education requires mistakes to be corrected and superior performance to be recognized, this feedback is often not given or, when given, is not conveyed in the most constructive ways.
  - Reasons for the reported dearth of feedback could include lack of time, lack of faculty training or role models, reduced direct observation, and faculty members' discomfort with giving constructive feedback in a relationship that may be longitudinal. In addition, the absence of explicit attention to feedback may lead students to not recognize feedback as it is given and thus underreport when asked.

KEY DEFINITIONS

- There is a difference between feedback and evaluation. Feedback is considered *formative*, that is, intended to guide or change behavior midstream. Evaluation is considered *summative*, that is, a final assessment of whether the learner has reached intended goals and bears the connotation of a grade, comparison, or judgment.
- Feedback can be divided into *brief, formal,* and *major feedback.*
  - *Brief feedback* is delivered while observing and teaching, for example, while teaching a procedure or correcting a presentation on rounds.
  - *Formal feedback* is usually delivered after a specific teaching or clinical encounter to deliver useful feedback to the learners; for example, debrief with the team after a code, or after a family meeting led by the learner. The goal is to discover what went well and what could have been done better.
  - *Major feedback* includes a session that is prescheduled to deliver overall and specific feedback. These sessions are also sometimes used to address significant issues that relate to performance such as professionalism or communication problems. These should be done in private and can take place at midpoint of the teaching relationship, allowing for opportunity to improve before the final evaluation is made.
- Positive feedback is often known as *reinforcing feedback*. Negative feedback is known as *constructive* or *corrective feedback*.
- Knowles has written, "Good feedback is an informed, nonevaluative, objective appraisal of performance intended to improve clinical skills."

GENERAL PRINCIPLES

- Educators have established key central principles to be followed when delivering feedback (see Table 109-1).
- The teacher and learner should meet together as allies with a common goal and not as adversaries. The feedback session should
  - Promote bidirectional feedback sessions including both the learner's input in addition to the faculty member's observations.
  - Aim to be kind, supportive, open-minded, and nonjudgmental.
- Individuals conveying feedback should
  - Deliver feedback that relates to a specific event close to the event so that both you and the learner can remember the details.
  - Establish expectations early including a timeline for both formal and major feedback.
- Components of the feedback delivered should consist of
  - Direct observation whenever possible.
  - Specific examples of positive performance and areas for improvement rather then general statements so that the learner understands exactly which behaviors are desired and which need correction.
    - "Great job today!" becomes "Your presentation was well organized and concise."
  - Proposed specific corrective actions so that comments are deflected away from judgments against the learner as a person.
    - "You were disorganized on rounds today" becomes "I noticed you switched between the history of present illness and the examination four times in your presentation today."
- Feedback should be aimed at behaviors that are remediable and delivered in appropriate quantity and should not consist of
  - Asking a learner to change something about their physical appearance or another feature beyond their control.
  - Overwhelming the learner with a long list of things to improve in a limited time.

TABLE 109-1 Key Points in Feedback

Establish expectation for bidirectional feedback early in the relationship

Choose a safe environment for the learner or peer to receive comments

Select an appropriate time and place for exchange

Allow learner or peer to self-assess

When providing feedback, be specific, timely, and base comments on observable and correctable behavior

Include both positive and corrective feedback

Recap the discussion and review plan for improvement at end of session

GENERAL APPROACH

- Allow the learner to do some self-assessment before the teacher begins commenting.
  - This self-reflection gives the teacher an indication of how to proceed with feedback and how to reinforce desirable behaviors.
- At the time of the first feedback session, orient the learner and set a safe environment.
  - Set the expectation of a feedback and schedule a session early on in your relationship.
  - Establishing a comfortable, safe environment for the discussion is as important as setting a safe learning environment.
  - Meet with the learner in private, that is, separate from his peers where no one can overhear.
  - Make sure the time is appropriate for the learner (not post-call or when overly busy) and that you will both have time to complete the conversation.
- Deliver the feedback
  - Begin by summarizing what the learner has said to reinforce mutual understanding.
  - Include both reinforcing and corrective comments along with examples of desired behaviors.
  - Be specific and avoid general comments about the learner.
    - Focus on actions and behaviors.
    - Do not overwhelm: Choose one or two areas or specific behaviors to address.
  - Allow learner to react to and reflect on your comments as well.
- Plan for improvement
  - Try to arrive at suggestions that you agree on together based on common goals.
  - Focus on specific behaviors that are achievable.
  - Establish a specific timeline.
  - For worrisome behavior, let the learner know if things don't improve, you have a responsibility to let the program leadership know.
- Review and summarize
  - Ask learner to review for you what was discussed and the plan for improvement.

THE ROLE OF THE HOSPITALIST

- Hospitalists can facilitate learning models that promote feedback by working together with the learner or peer to prepare a learning context.
- In the academic setting, hospitalists are in a prime position to establish the expectation of feedback and deliver constructive, ongoing feedback to learners. This opportunity is primarily mediated through the following factors
  - They have already been recognized by both students and residents as highly rated educators.

- ○ As they see patients alongside students and residents on the wards, they can deliver specific feedback in real time based on direct observation.
- ○ They spend more months per year on the wards and so may have a better sense of the progression and appropriate milestones that learners usually make over their training period. This allows hospitalists to not only effectively evaluate learners but also play a role in developing appropriate evaluation tools.
- Beyond teaching settings, hospitalists are in a position to help peers standardize clinical practice and continue to learn.
  - ○ Hospitalists can develop common communication and practice standards that set the service apart from other groups. Through feedback to peers these standards can be established.
  - ○ Hospitalist leaders can sit down with newly hired hospitalists and work together to understand the work environment, expectations of service, and other duties. Hospitalist leaders should periodically give feedback on performance and expect feedback as well.

BIBLIOGRAPHY

Branch W, Paranjape A. Feedback and reflection: teaching methods for clinical settings. *Acad Med.* 2002;77:1185–1188.

Ende J. Feedback in clinical medical education. *JAMA.* 1983;250:777–781.

Hunter A, Desai S, Harrison R, et al. Medical student evaluation of the quality of hospitalist and nonhospitalist teaching faculty on inpatient medicine rotations. *Acad Med.* 2004;79:78–82.

Knowles MS, Holton EF, Swanson RA. *The Adult Learner.* Houston, TX: Gulf; 1998:12–13.

Kulaga M, Charney P, O'Mahony S, et al. The positive impact of hospitalist clinician educators. *J Gen Int Med.* 2004;19:293–301.

110 SCHOLARSHIP AND CAREER DEVELOPMENT FOR THE HOSPITALIST CLINICIAN EDUCATOR

Preetha Basaviah and Subha Ramani

INTRODUCTION

At academic medical centers and community teaching hospitals, hospitalists are increasingly visible as clinician educators,[1] with professional goals to excel as clinicians,

teachers, and scholars. For clinician educators to advance academically and become educational leaders, scholarship is an essential component of their professional growth. It is also important for institutional leadership and promotion committees to recognize that faculty, whose educational activities fulfill established criteria, are scholars and must be recognized and rewarded. Educational scholarship can be demonstrated in the following areas:[2]

- Teaching: innovative teaching should be coupled with demonstration of effectiveness and impact.
- Curriculum development: In residency education, this would refer to any curricula that would fulfill the ACGME requirements.[3] The six steps outlined by Kern and colleagues[4] provide a scholarly framework that curriculum educators can apply to their own educational programs and curricula (Table 110-1).
- Assessment: An essential element of any educational program or innovation is rigorous assessment so that achievement of program outcomes can be demonstrated.
- Mentoring and advising: A scholarly approach to mentoring with appropriate documentation will add value to any teacher's portfolio.
- Educational administration: The impact and success of educational leadership and administration can also be measured and disseminated within or outside the institution.

TYPES OF SCHOLARSHIP

In 1990, Boyer from the Carnegie Foundation for the Advancement of Teaching proposed that the term "scholarship" can be applied to four major academic areas.[5] They include:

1. The scholarship of *discovery* includes traditional research and refers to new knowledge which contributes to the existing knowledge in the field. Educational research fits into this category.
2. The scholarship of *integration* builds links across disciplines and provides a context for understanding that goes beyond the original discipline.

TABLE 110-1 A Six-Step Approach to Curriculum Development

Step 1	Identification of the problem and general needs assessment
Step 2	Needs assessment of target learners
Step 3	Defining curricular goals and objectives
Step 4	Developing educational strategies
Step 5	Implementation of curriculum
Step 6	Evaluation of curriculum and/or learners and curricular changes based on feedback

SOURCE: Adapted from Kern DE, Thomas PA, Howard DM, et al. *Curriculum Development for Medical Education: A Six-Step Approach.* Baltimore, MD: The Johns Hopkins University Press; 1998.

3. The scholarship of *application* refers to application of research findings to practice.
4. The scholarship of *teaching* (educational scholarship) emphasizes the creation of new knowledge about teaching and learning in the presence of the learners.

APPLYING SCHOLARSHIP TO EDUCATION

Education becomes *scholarship* when it demonstrates current knowledge of the field, invites peer review, and involves exploration of students' learning. Building on Boyer's work, Glassick et al. distilled six essential criteria of scholarship that can be applied to traditional research as well as education. These six criteria include:
- Clear goals
  - The purpose of the work is clearly stated.
  - The goals and objectives are realistic and achievable.
  - The work addresses an important question or need.
- Adequate preparation
  - Mastery and understanding of current knowledge in the field and acquisition of skills to carry out the work.
  - Identifying and obtaining the resources needed to complete the work.
- Appropriate methods
  - Using and applying appropriate methods to achieve the stated goals.
  - Modification of methods to deal with changing circumstances.
- Significant results
  - Achievement of the stated goals and objectives.
  - Noteworthy addition to the field and open up additional areas for further exploration.
- Effective presentation
  - Using suitable style and organization to present the work at appropriate venues.
  - Presentation of results with clarity and integrity.
- Reflective critique
  - The scholar critically evaluates his or her own work.
  - The scholar uses evaluations to improve the quality of future work.

Teaching becomes scholarship when:[6]
- Work is made public.
- Work is available for peer review.
- Work is reproduced and built on by others.

PROGRESSION OF SCHOLARSHIP

The following three steps can help transform an educator into an educational scholar:[2]

STEP 1:
- Select one or two of the following educational areas to focus on scholarship: teaching, curriculum development, assessment, mentoring and advising, and educational administration.
- Document all activities with details of the activity, number of learners impacted, and so on.

STEP 2:
- Adopt a scholarly approach to the activity by reviewing available literature, attending faculty development workshops.
- Outline clear goals and plan assessment of educational activities to study intended outcomes.

STEP 3:
- Demonstrate scholarship in the activity by inviting peer review.
- Disseminate work within and outside the institution, publish, and present.

FACULTY DEVELOPMENT

- Faculty development can improve the educational vitality of our institutions through attention to the competencies needed by individual teachers and to the institutional policies required to promote academic excellence.[7,8]
- Faculty development should enhance educational knowledge and skill of faculty members so that their educational contributions can extend to advancing the educational program rather than just teaching within it.
- Specific goals of faculty development include
  - Enhancing knowledge and skills of teaching
  - Increasing understanding of new curriculum and academic program development
  - Developing knowledge and skills in educational research
  - Strengthening academic leadership and career development skills
- The number of faculty development programs for medical educators is growing, and it is essential that clinician educators be encouraged to participate. See Table 110-2.

MENTORSHIP

Mentoring as a scholarly activity includes both the ability to *serve as a mentor* and *to identify appropriate mentors* for oneself to advise on different roles. The ultimate goal in mentoring relationships is that all participants produce a legacy, that is, influence extends to the next generation of scholars.[9]

TABLE 110-2 Applying Glassick's Criteria to Compare Research and Educational Scholarship

GLASSICK'S CRITERIA	RESEARCH	EDUCATIONAL SCHOLARSHIP
Clear goals	Clear hypothesis, experimental design	Teaching strategy, clear, measurable objectives
Adequate preparation	Background literature review	Knowledge of subject; organization of material based on educational objectives
Appropriate methods	Study design; statistical analysis	Appropriate teaching methods; selection of appropriate assessment measures to evaluate outcomes
Significant results	Results of the experiment: hypothesis tested and proved or disproved	Quality and effectiveness of educational presentation; demonstration of learners' accomplishment of objectives
Effective presentation	Publication and presentations at local, regional, national venues	Publication and presentations at local, regional, national venues
Reflective critique	Critical reflection on results to guide the direction of future research	Critical analysis of educational activity and appropriate changes in future educational strategies

SOURCE: Adapted from Fincher RM, Simpson DE, Mennin SP, et al. Scholarship in teaching: an imperative for the 21st century. *Acad Med.* 2000;75:887–894.

Table 110-3 from the SGIM Education Committee presentation, "A Map of the Clinician Educator World", outlines clearly the different stages of career development of a clinician educator and how mentoring is useful in this progression.[10]

NETWORKING AND COLLABORATING

- To network is to interact or engage in informal communication with others for mutual assistance or support.
- A hospitalist clinician educator can establish contacts through several venues.
  - Expand curricular projects: Survey other schools while planning, collaborate outside your department.
  - Participate on committees/task forces relevant to your areas of interest within your institution, regionally, or nationally.
  - Attend local/national meetings in your field, bring your card and obtain information from others with similar interests.
  - Submit a workshop proposal and invite collaborators from outside your institution.
  - Present work at poster/abstract sessions at meetings, promoting discussion about your work, and potential connections with others.
  - Start focus groups with hospitalists in your local area to strategize on how to address common challenges facing hospitalists as teachers.
  - A hospitalist clinician educator can facilitate promotion through the development of innovative

TABLE 110-3 Examples of Faculty Development Opportunities

TYPE OF PROGRAM	EXAMPLES
Workshops and meetings within an institution	• Workshop series on preparing oral presentations, small group teaching, giving feedback, writing test questions • Introduction to clinical research (e.g., ORACLE) • Seminars reviewing faculty promotion process • "Works in progress" meetings, medical education journal clubs • Teaching observation and feedback programs
Faculty development programs within an institution	• Teaching/medical education fellowships, teaching scholars programs or faculty development programs at Harvard, UCSF, Johns Hopkins, University of Washington, UCLA, Medical College of Wisconsin, University of North Carolina Family Medicine Faculty Development Fellowship Program, Michigan State University Primary Care Faculty Development Fellowship, among others
Regional meetings	• Western Group on Educational Affairs (of the AAMC)
Faculty development nationally	• Stanford Faculty Development Center (SFDC), Harvard Macy Program for Health Science Educators, AAMC sponsored Fellowship in Medical Education Research, AAMC Early and Mid-Career Faculty Development for women, American College of Physician Executives course, Society of Hospital Medicine Leadership Retreat, among others
Advanced degrees	• Masters in medical education or public health

educational activities for members of the multidisciplinary care team. Examples include "hospitalist's rounds" for trainees, "hospitalist" educational updates (with CME obtained from your local medical school) for members of the hospitalist service, a hospitalist track within a residency program, or a hospitalist fellowship.
- ○ Hospital medicine is a new, emerging specialty and there are many opportunities to change how we educate ourselves and our trainees based on the core competencies in hospital management.

DISSEMINATION OF WORK

- The scholarship of teaching builds on the process of scholarly teaching. Essential elements of all forms of scholarship are peer review and public dissemination.[11]
- Peer review and public dissemination can be achieved and sustained through four key mechanisms:
  (1) Publications
  (2) Presentations
  (3) Educational products
  (4) Documentation through an educator's portfolio

(1) PUBLICATIONS
- Publishing curricular work is facilitated when one studies what one sees.
  - ○ For example, a hospitalist clinician educator who plays a role in residency program leadership may evaluate the effectiveness of a new hospital medicine and quality improvement longitudinal elective designed for internal medicine residents.
  - ○ Begin planning for publishing at the beginning of the curriculum development process. This process will likely lead to a better product and experience for the trainee. See Table 110-4.
- Consider journals specific to medical education (e.g., *Academic Medicine, Medical Teacher, Medical Education, Teaching and Learning in Medicine*) or specialty journals that publish articles about education (e.g., *Advance in Physiology Education, Journal of General Internal Medicine*).
- Consider technology peer-reviewed venues to disseminate work such as MedEdPORTAL.[12]

TABLE 110-4 How to Make Your Curricular Work Publishable

PHASES OF CURRICULUM DEVELOPMENT	IMPLICATIONS
Problem identification and general needs assessment	• Review existing curricula and related medical education literature • You will likely identify a healthcare problem, document deficiencies in current training approaches, and justify the need for a new approach: "problem identification"
Needs assessment of targeted learners and other contextual variables	• A local needs analysis of trainees at a particular program or institution may be accomplished by a combination of several methods • These include surveys, focus groups, faculty interviews, or formal objective assessments of the learners • Other needs analysis is needed to identify and catalogue local resources, including faculty time, faculty expertise, space, administrative support, equipment, and nonfaculty human resources (like standardized patients) • This needs analysis will help constrain the curriculum within the limitations or seek institutional or external funding
Goals and specific measurable learning objectives	• Explicitly declaring learning objectives should be partnered with development of instructional and evaluation strategies to meet them
Instructional strategies	• Decision-making about objectives, content, structure and instructional strategies represents the culmination of the development process
Implementation	• Consider feasibility and sustainability of the implementation experience

Evaluation and feedback	• Collect information that will help continuously refine one's curriculum
	• Collect information that will help justify activities and aid in seeking support from chair or administrative leadership
	• Ensure outcome measures are linked to learning objectives, have established validity and reliability, and can be feasibly collected
	• Decide on level of evaluation
	• Learner satisfaction is helpful to document for local purposes, but this will not be appealing to editors and reviewers
	• Consider demonstrating *effectiveness* of your curriculum with such outcome measures as
	  ○ Knowledge (examinations)
	  ○ Skills or competence (observation through mini-CEX or OSCE)
	  ○ Attitudes (questionnaires, interviews)
	  ○ Behaviors or performance (vignettes, record audits)
	  ○ Patient-level outcomes (record audits)

SOURCE: Adapted from Irby DM, Cooke M, Lowenstein D, et al. The academy movement: a structural approach to reinvigorating the educational mission. *Acad Med.* 2004;79:729–736.

(2) PRESENTATIONS

- Presentations of your curricula or area of expertise may take the form of workshop proposals, abstract and poster submissions at regional/national meetings, local presentations (grand rounds, noon conference), or CME presentations.

(3) EDUCATIONAL PRODUCTS

- The creation of enduring educational materials is a form of scholarship, and sharing products with other institutions should be documented (see portfolio below). Products include course syllabi, instructional video clips, Web site tutorials, and CD-ROMs.

(4) DOCUMENTATION: EDUCATOR'S PORTFOLIO

- An educator's portfolio is an effective way to document a faculty member's peer-reviewed activities in education and allow for formal assessment for promotion or advancement in education. The structured format may include such categories as educational philosophy, professional development, direct teaching, curriculum development, advising and mentorship, educational administration and leadership, and educational scholarship.

- Learn about the specifics of your medical school promotion process for clinician educators so that you can tailor your portfolio accordingly. See Table 110-5 for the UCSF format. More details of an educational portfolio are described in the following section.

MORE ON EDUCATOR'S PORTFOLIOS[10]

WHAT IS IT?

- It is not a CV.
- It is an evidence and analysis of one's effectiveness as a teacher.
- It is a factual description of a teachers strengths and accomplishments.

WHY AN EDUCATIONAL PORTFOLIO?

- To complement your CV
  - When applying for academic positions, promotion, or a teaching grant or award
  - Preparing for a performance appraisal
- To document the skills you can transfer into another environment
- For the medical school to review, to ensure the standard of teaching is satisfactory

TABLE 110-5   Potential Categories in an Educator's Portfolio: Evidence of Success in Medical Education

CATEGORY	EXAMPLES
Philosophy on teaching	• Brief reflective paragraph on one's personal goals and philosophy on teaching
Direct teaching	• Systematic student reviews (e.g., include tabular summary of teaching evaluations in past 5 years, comparison with mean of course)
	• Systematic peer review
	• Teaching awards, honors, nominations
Curriculum development, instructional design, and assessment of learner performance	• Reports by education consultants
	• Measures of learning including end of course examinations, national board examination scores, OSCEs
	• Peer reviews
	• Systematic student reviews, follow-up surveys
	• For residency, number of positions filled
	• For an elective, number of students enrolled
Advising and mentorship	• Number of students advised, time spent with each, and their current status
	• Example of work of student while under your guidance
	• Impact statements
Educational administration and leadership	• Reports by education consultants
	• Measures of learning including End-of-Course examinations, national board examination scores
	• Program evaluations, external reviews
	• Authorship of administrative reports
	• Impact statements
Educational scholarship and the creation of enduring educational materials	• Regional/national presentations and publications
	• Peer reviewer for education, education-related conferences or journals
	• Education-related grants or contract including title, source dates, and amount
	• Membership and service in education-related professional organizations
Personal/faculty development	• CME courses
	• Institutional faculty development programs
	• National faculty development programs (AAMC Professional Development Seminar for Women Faculty)
	• Fellowships (AAMC Fellowship in Medical Education Research)
	• Degree-granting programs (e.g., master's degree in education)
	• Participation in medical education journal clubs and research meetings

SOURCE: Adapted from *http://www.medschool.ucsf.edu/academy/programs*

KEY CONTENT

- Material from the teacher
  - Reflective statement: philosophy, strategies, objectives, methods
    - What you are trying to achieve
    - What you are doing to try and make this happen
    - To what extent you have been successful
    - What remains the challenge for you
  - Teaching responsibilities (with details of the scope of activity, demographics, etc)
    - Past experience
    - Where: size of class, course
    - How and what: format, role in teaching, learning, assessment
  - Representative learning materials and syllabi
  - Instructions/innovations developed and their effectiveness
  - Service to the institution, for example, leading and participating in important committees
  - Institutional program leadership: if you organize all the conferences for the hospital medicine unit, consider asking for the title of curriculum coordinator, hospital medicine unit.
  - Regional teaching output and evaluations
    - Grand rounds at other institutions
  - National teaching output and evaluations
    - Invited presentations
    - Conference presentations
  - Awards
  - Publications
  - Teaching goals for the next 5 years
  - Professional development
    - Research on teaching and learning
    - Courses undertaken, conferences attended
    - Involvement in educational professional societies
  - Evidence to support claims of effectiveness
- Material from others
  - Student evaluations
  - Statements from colleagues who have observed your teaching or reviewed your teaching materials
  - Honors (internal and external)
  - Evidence of regard from outside sources (invitations to teach elsewhere)
- Products of teaching
  - Syllabi
  - Articles
  - Workshop handouts
  - Multimedia productions (CD-ROMS, videotapes)

SELF-REFLECTION

- To promote life-long, self-directed learning for learners and teachers, one should reflect on one's teaching, activities, and career path.

- To evaluate one's overall career path and potential opportunities that arise, the hospitalist clinician educator can ask herself
  1. Where am I in my career, in terms of current roles and activities?
  2. What are my 5-year career goals, 10-year career goals? What academic niche would I like to establish within my hospitalist service?
  3. Is this new opportunity one that involves an area about which I am passionate? Does it advance my career goals? Does it build on developing areas of expertise, or introduce new areas of expertise in which I want to advance?
- Scholars should ask reflective questions of their own work and their colleagues' work as educators. To what extent does the individual do the following:[13,14]
  - Enhance teaching skills through reading, discussion with colleagues, or participation in workshops.
  - Seek and respond to feedback regarding their teaching.
  - Translate insights from reflective critique to teaching practices.
  - Engage in continuing professional development to hone relevant administrative skills.
  - Use results to develop and implement strategies for ongoing assessment (continuous quality improvement).

SUMMARY

- Develop area of expertise or focus in an area you are passionate about.
- Think of scholarship from the beginning.
- Set aside time for scholarly activities.
- Document all activities, collect evaluations.
- Publish/present all scholarly activity.
- Set and meet goals and objectives with your mentor.
- Network and collaborate with educators within and outside your institution.
- Be active in getting yourself promoted.
- Develop curricula or other educational projects.
- Disseminate your educational products and document whether other educators are using your resources.
- Maintain and update your educational portfolio regularly, do not wait until promotion time.

REFERENCES

1. Kripalani S, Pope AC, Rask K, et al. Hospitalists as teachers. *J Gen Intern Med.* 2004;19:8–15.
2. Hafler JP, Blanco MA, Fincher RM, et al. Educational scholarship. In: *Guidebook for Clerkship Directors.* 3rd ed. Alliance for Clinical Education; 2005.

3. ACGME. Outcome Project. *http://www.acgme.org/outcome/assess/toolbox.asp*
   A brief description of 13 assessment methods and references to articles where more complete and in-depth information about each method can be found.
4. Kern DE, Thomas PA, Howard DM, et al. *Curriculum Development for Medical Education: A Six-Step Approach.* Baltimore, MD: The Johns Hopkins University Press; 1998.
5. Boyer EL. *Scholarship Reconsidered: Priorities of the Professoriate.* Princeton, NJ: Carnegie Foundation for the Advancement of Teaching; 1990.
6. Hutchings P, Shulman LS. The scholarship of teaching new elaborations and developments. *Change.* 1999 Sept/Oct:11–15.
7. Rubeck RF, Witzke DB. Faculty development: a field of dreams. *Acad Med.* 1998;73(supplement September):S32–S37.
8. Wilkerson L, Irby DM. Strategies for improving teaching practices: a comprehensive approach to faculty development. *Acad Med.* 1998;73:387–396.

9. Berk RA, Berg J, Mortimer R, et al. Measuring the effectiveness of faculty mentoring relationships. *Acad Med.* 2005;80:66–71.
10. A Map of the (Clinician Educator) World. Achieving Success While Doing What You Love: A workshop for clinician educators at the Annual SGIM meeting, 2003. *http://sgim.org/am03Handouts/WD02.pdf*
11. Fincher RM, Work JA. Perspectives on the scholarship of teaching. *Med Educ.* 2006;40:293–295.
12. *http://www.aamc.org/meded/mededportal*
    A peer-reviewed technology venue providing opportunities to disseminate education work, also known as MedEdPORTAL.
13. Fincher RM, Simpson DE, Mennin SP, et al. Scholarship in teaching: an imperative for the 21st century. *Acad Med.* 2000;75:887–894.
14. Glassick CE, Huber MT, Maaeroff GI. *Scholarship Assessed: Evaluation of the Professoriate.* San Francisco, CA: Jossey-Bass; 1997.

INDEX

Entries denoted by an italic *t*, *f*, or *n* indicate figures, tables, or notes, respectively.

A

AAFP. *See* American Association of Family Practitioners
abbreviations, unapproved, 23
ABCs (Airway, Breathing, and Circulation), 388
abdominal pain
  acute, 212*t*
  clinical presentation, 211–212
  colitis and, 227
  Crohn's disease and, 232
  diagnosis, 211–212
  disease management strategies, 212–216
  diverticulitis and, 240–241
  epidemiology, 211
  nonsurgical disorders causing, 213*t*
  SCD and, 264
  UC and, 236
ABG. *See* arterial blood gases
ABI. *See* absolute benefit increase
ABIM. *See* American Board of Internal Medicine
abnormal automaticity, 137
abscesses
  intrarenal, 293
  lung, 431
  perinephric, 293
absolute benefit increase (ABI), 88
absolute risk reduction (ARR), 87
  calculating, 88*t*
abstraction, 318*t*
A/C. *See* assist-control
academic detailing, 99
ACC. *See* American College of Cardiology
ACC/AHA guidelines. *See* American College of Cardiology/American Heart Association guidelines
accelerated idioventricular rhythm (AIVR), 153
accessory pathway, 139

ACCP. *See* American College of Chest Physicians
Accreditation Council for Graduate Medical Education (ACGME), 8
  adult learning and, 615
  handoffs and, 62, 68
  Inpatient Teaching Rounds, 617
  quality improvement and, 41
ACE inhibitors
  ARF and, 446
  ARF caused by, 447*t*
  proteinuria reduction and, 462*t*
ACE. *See* angiotensin-converting enzyme
ACEI/ARB, 594
acetaminophen
  overdose, 362–365
  plasma nomogram, 365*f*
ACGME. *See* Accreditation Council for Graduate Medical Education
acid suppression therapy, 254
acid-base disorders
  care transitions, 476
  clinical presentation, 470–472
  diagnosis, 470–472
  diagnostic approach to, 471*t*
  disease management strategies, 476
  epidemiology, 469
  initial management, 472
  pathophysiology, 469–470
  potassium and, 485
  triage, 472
  types, 473–476*t*
acidemia, 470
acidosis
  in ARF triage, 456
  dilutional, 475*t*
  metabolic, 470
  respiratory, 476*t*
  reversing, 193
Acinetobacter baumannii, 314

ACLS algorithms. *See* advanced cardiac life support algorithms
ACOVE. *Se* Assessing Care of Vulnerable Elders
ACP Journal Club (ACPJC), 89
ACPJC. See ACP Journal Club
acquired immunodeficiency syndrome (AIDS). *See also* human immunodeficiency virus
  CAP triage and, 417
  FUO and, 281
ACS conditions. *See* ambulatory care sensitive conditions
ACS. *See* acute chest syndrome; acute coronary syndromes; American College of Surgeons
activated protein C (APC), 436–437
active failures, 17
activities of daily living (ADL)
  confusion and, 321
  deconditioning management and, 519
acute chest syndrome (ACS), 264, 265–266
acute coronary syndromes (ACS), 105, 120
  care transitions and, 124–126
  communication and, 126
  discharge and, 126
  management strategies, 124
  medications for, 125*t*
  risk stratification and, 124–126
  stress testing for, 126*t*
  triage of, 120–124
Acute Decompensated Heart Failure National Registry (ADHERE), 164
acute lung injury (ALI), 442, 443–444*t*
acute management, 110
acute myocardial infarction (AMI), 106
  diagnosing, 108
  JCAHO core measures, 121*t*

acute nonthyroidal illness, 206
acute pancreatitis (AP), 242–243. *See also* pancreatitis
acute phosphate nephropathy, 455–456
acute renal failure (ARF)
  care transitions, 457
  caused by ACE inhibitors, 447*t*
  clinical presentation, 454–456
  diagnosis, 454–456
  disease management strategies, 457
  epidemiology, 446, 452–453
  exogenous causes of, 446*t*
  heme pigment-induced, 447
  initial management, 456–457
  major causes of, 453*t*
  pathophysiology, 446–447, 453–454
  post-renal, 457
  preventive strategies, 447–448
  triage, 456–457
  urinalysis findings, 454*t*
acute respiratory failure (ARF)
  arterial blood gases in, 410*t*
  care transitions, 412
  classification of, 408*t*
  clinical presentation, 408–411
  diagnosis, 408–411
  disease management strategies, 411–412
  epidemiology, 407
  hypercapnic, 408*t*
  hypoxemic, 408*t*
  pathophysiology, 408
  potential causes of, 409*t*
  triage, 411
ADA. *See* American Diabetes Association
addiction
  opioids and, 532
  service consultation, 379
adenosine, 139
ADEs. *See* adverse drug events
ADH. *See* antidiuretic hormone
ADHERE. *See* Acute Decompensated Heart Failure National Registry
adherence. *See* patient adherence
adjunctive therapies, for skin and soft tissue infections, 303–304
ADL. *See* activities of daily living
administrative policies, personality dysfunction and, 358–359
administrative structure, 50
administrators, 100
admission
  assessment for CAP, 422*t*
  bradycardia and, 149–150
  medication discrepancies and, 24–25
  medication list, 26–28
  medication reconciliation at, 27*f*, 28
  preventing polypharmacy at, 33*t*
adrenal axis, in sepsis management, 436
adrenal function, measuring, 436

adrenal incidentalomas, 186
adrenal insufficiency
  noncardiac surgery and, 590
  postoperative fever and, 606*t*
adrenalectomy, 187
adult learning, 615
  practical approaches to, 615–617
  questions, 616*t*
adult respiratory distress syndrome (ARDS), 297
  PEEP in, 444*t*
  ventilation management for, 442, 443–444*t*
advanced cardiac life support (ACLS)
  algorithms, 127
  bradycardia triage and, 150
  VT and, 155
advanced care planning, 552–553
  SNF and, 580–582
advanced directives, 354, 552–553
adverse drug events (ADEs)
  contributing factors, 22
  cost of, 21
  definition of, 21
  epidemiology of, 21
  hospitalists and, 23
  identifying, 22
  injuries and, 22*f*
  IT and, 23
  medication discrepancies and, 24
  patient safety and, 13
  pharmacists and, 26
  reducing, 19, 22–23
  risk factors, 25
adverse drug reaction (ADR), 21
adynamic ileus, 248
AEDs *See* antiepileptic drugs
AF. *See* atrial fibrillation
AFl. *See* atrial flutter
aflutter, 137
AGA. *See* American Gastroenterological Association
Agency for Healthcare Policy and Research, 59
Agency for Healthcare Research and Quality (AHRQ), 10, 14, 21
  ADE costs and, 21
  NGC and, 90
  test results follow-ups and, 76
  vulnerable populations and, 557
agitation management, 326–327
AHA. *See* American Heart Association
AHRQ. *See* Agency for Healthcare Research and Quality
AIDS. *See* acquired immunodeficiency syndrome
aim statements, 43
  examples of, 43*t*
aims, 19

air hunger, 412
airway, in sepsis triage, 434
AIVR. *See* accelerated idioventricular rhythm
alcohol
  behavioral disturbances and, 356–357
  clinical effects of, 374*t*
  intravenous, 378
  toxic ingestion of, 367*t*
  withdrawal, 366–367
  withdrawal syndromes, 374–376
alcohol abuse. *See also* substance abuse
  acute, 373–374
  bedside evaluation, 376
  care transitions, 379
  epidemiology, 373
  pathogenesis, 373
  secondary HTN and, 182–183
  syndromes, treatment, 377*t*
  triage, 377
  withdrawal prophylaxis, 376–377
  withdrawal risks, 374
  withdrawal treatment, 377–379
alcoholic hallucinosis, 375
aldosterone
  antagonists, 165
  deficiency, 492
  hyperkalemia and, 490
aldosteronism. *See* primary aldosteronism
alfa-2 agonists, 537
ALI. *See* acute lung injury
alkalemia, 470
alkalosis
  chloride-responsive metabolic, 487
  metabolic, 475*t*
  respiratory, 476*t*
allergies
  asthma and, 396
  medication, 28*t*
allocation concealment, 83–84
allodynia, 528
alloimmunization, 275
alpha-2-agonists
  noncardiac surgery and, 588
  perioperative medication management and, 592–593
alpha-agonists, alcohol withdrawal treatment and, 378
alpha-beta blockers, 593–594
alpha-blockers, 593–594
alternative medicine, overdoses, 371*t*
Alzheimer's disease (AD)
  confusion and, 321
  in frail older adults, 565–567
ambulatory care sensitive (ACS) conditions, 557
American Academy of Family Physicians, 83
American Academy of Neurology, 317

American Association of Family Practitioners (AAFP), 72
American Board of Internal Medicine (ABIM), 4
American College of Cardiology (ACC), 117
  pacemakers and, 150–151
American College of Cardiology/ American Heart Association (ACC/AHA) guidelines
  AMI and, 121
  CK-MB and, 115
  ETT and, 117
  for Perioperative Cardiac Evaluation, 586, 586f
  systolic HF and, 160
American College of Chest Physicians (ACCP), 498
American College of Clinical Endocrinologists (ACCE), 194
American College of Endocrinology (ACE), 198
American College of Graduate Medical Education (ACGME), 14
American College of Physicians Clinical Guideline, 608
American College of Surgeons (ACS), Statement on Principles Underlying Perioperative Responsibility, 612, 613t
American Diabetes Association (ADA), 194
  hyperglycemia and, 198
American Gastroenterological Association (AGA), 246
American Heart Association (AHA)
  CPR and, 127
  endocarditis and, 283
  pacemakers and, 150–151
American Hospital Association
  2005 Survey, 1
  vulnerable populations and, 560
American Medical Association (AMA), on SCM ethics, 612t
American Society of Gastrointestinal Endoscopy, 253t
American Thoracic Society, 421t
AMI. *See* acute myocardial infarction
amino acids, 521
amiodarone, 208
  AF management and, 134
  postoperative AF and, 133
amphetamines, abuse management, 381
analgesics. *See also* PCA
  adjuvant, 537, 538t
  history, 529
  for mechanical ventilation, 442
  modalities, 531–534
  non-opioid, 532, 532t

opioids, 532–537
  pain management guidelines and, 528–529
  urinary, 291
anaphylaxis, 129t
  dyspnea triage and, 394
  transfusion risks and, 273
anemia
  care transitions, 263
  chronic blood loss, 276
  CKD management and, 463, 463t
  clinical presentation, 261–262
  diagnosis, 261–262
  disease management strategies, 263
  epidemiology, 260
  initial management, 262–263
  pathophysiology, 260–261
  perioperative, 590
  physiologic response to, 272t
  preoperative testing and, 600
  RBC morphology and, 262t
  transfusion and, 277
  triage, 262–263
  UC and, 238
  workup, 261f
anesthesia
  local, 537
  SCD and, 267
anger, communication and, 551
angina
  CP and, 108t
  systolic HF care transition and, 166
  unstable, 108–109
angina pectoris
  approach to, 113–114
  characteristics of, 113t
  clinical presentation of, 113–115
  diagnosis of, 113–115
  differential, 113–115
  pathophysiology of, 113
  suspected, 112
  triage of, 115–116
angiodysplasias, 256
angiography
  coronary, 166
  ICH diagnosis and, 336
  LGI bleeding and, 259
  therapeutic, 255
angiotensin receptor blockers (ARBs), 119–120
  proteinuria reduction and, 462t
  systolic HF management and, 165
angiotensin-converting enzyme (ACE), 119–120
  inhibitors, 164
anion gap, 190t
anorexia, appendicitis and, 214
antiarrhythmic therapy
  AF management and, 135

perioperative medication management and, 594
  SVT and, 144
  SVT management and, 145
antibacterial agents, encephalitis and, 343
antibiotic resistance, 310
  care transitions, 315
  infection control issues, 314
  mechanisms of, 311t
  pathogens, 311–314
  pathophysiology, 310–311
  prevention, 315
  risk factors, 311
antibiotics. *See also* antibiotic resistance
  acute cholecystitis, 216
  bacterial endocarditis and, 286–287
  for bacterial meningitis, 341t
  CAP management and, 420
  CAP triage and, 417
  colitis induced by, 226–227
  cystitis and, 290–291
  diabetic foot infections and, 305
  diverticulitis and, 241–242
  for drug-resistant bacteria, 313t
  empiric, 302–303, 303f
  for endocarditis with enterococci, 287t
  initial empiric for HAP, 425t
  initial empiric for HCAP, 425t
  initial empiric for VAP, 425t
  initial empiric selection, 421t
  for native valve endocarditis, 286t
  neutropenic fever and, 576f
  pancreatic necrosis and, 245–246
  prophylaxis, for endocarditis, 289
  prostatitis and, 292
  for prosthetic valve endocarditis, 287t
  pyelonephritis and, 291
  SBO triage and, 250
  SCD and, 267
  in sepsis management, 435–436
  SSIs and, 605–607, 607t
  UTI prevention and, 293
anticholinergics
  for asthma relievers, 401
  for asthma triage, 398
anticoagulant therapy
  adverse effects of, 507t
  epidemiology, 506
  pathophysiology, 506–507
  summary of, 514t
  for VTE, 505t
anticoagulants, 508–513
  AF and, 133
  AF management and, 135
  dosing, 510t
  perioperative medication management and, 595–596
  systolic HF management and, 165
anticytokines, 598

antidepressants
  palliative care and, 547
  perioperative medication management
    and, 597–598
  tricyclic, 537
antidiuretic hormone (ADH), 477
antidotes, 364*t*
antiemetics, 543
antiepileptic drugs (AEDs), 537
  perioperative medication management
    and, 597
  regimens for seizures, 349*t*
  seizure management and, 348–349
  seizure triage and, 347
  side effects, 349*t*
antifungal therapy, 575*t*
antigenic drift, 297
antigravity muscles, deconditioning and,
  515–516
antihypertensive agents, 332–333
  HTN emergencies and, 178
  perioperative medication management
    and, 592–594
anti-IgE treatment, 401
anti-Parkinson medication, 597
antiplatelet therapy, 508
  ischemic stroke management and, 333
  perioperative medication management
    and, 594–595
  VT management and, 155
antipsychotics
  anxiety treatment and, 547*t*
  perioperative medication management
    and, 597–598
antiretroviral therapy, thrombocytopenia
  and, 271
anti-saccharomyces cerevisiae antibodies
  (ASCA), 233
antispasmodics, 537
antithrombotic therapy, 333
antiviral agents, 298*t*
  encephalitis and, 343
anxiety
  palliative care and, 546–547
  treatment, 546
  treatment approaches, 547*t*
anxiolytics, 598
aorta, coarctation of, 187
AP. *See* acute pancreatitis (AP)
apathetic thyrotoxicosis, 206
APC. *See* activated protein C (APC)
aplastic crisis, 264
  treatment, 265
apologies, patient safety and, 38–39
appendicitis
  acute, 214–215
  atypical, 214–215
  colitis and, 224*t*
  in elderly, 215
  imaging and, 215*t*

application, scholarship of, 628
applied Bayesian analysis, 92–95
ARBs. *See* angiotensin receptor blockers
ARDS. *See* adult respiratory distress
  syndrome
ARF. *See* acute renal failure
ARF. *See* acute respiratory failure
argatroban, 513
ARR. *See* absolute risk reduction
arrhythmias. *See also* ventricular
  arrhythmias
  causes of, 152
  noncardiac surgery and, 588
ARTEMIS trial, 497
arterial blood gases (ABG), 388
  acid-base disorder diagnosis and, 470
  in ARF, 410, 410*t*
  for COPD management, 406
arterial oxygenation. *See* FiO_2
arterial perfusion, 304
arterial puncture, 389
ASCA. *See* anti-saccharomyces cerevisiae
  antibodies
ascites, 222
  cirrhotic, 222*t*
ascorbic acid, CIN prevention and, 451
ask-tell-ask approach, 551
aspiration
  postoperative events, 608
  tube feeds and, 524
  UG bleeding and, 251–252
aspirin
  angina pectoral and, 115
  as anticoagulant, 508
  MI and, 106
  perioperative medication management
    and, 594
  STEMI and, 122
Assessing Care of Vulnerable Elders
  (ACOVE), 559
assessment, 627
assist-control (A/C), 439
  modes, 441
asthma
  acute exacerbations of, 399
  care transitions, 401
  chronic, 399
  clinical presentation, 396
  controllers, 399–401
  diagnosis, 396
  differential diagnosis, 397*t*
  discharge, 401*t*
  disease management strategies, 399–401
  epidemiology, 395
  exacerbation, 397*t*
  hospitalization considerations, 398*t*
  ICU considerations, 399*t*
  initial management, 397–398
  levels of control, 400*t*
  management approach, 400*f*

  pathophysiology, 395–396
  perioperative medication management
    and, 596
  postoperative, 609
  relievers, 399–401
  risk factors, 395*t*
  severity classifications, 399*t*
  triage, 397–398
  triggers, 396*t*
  ventilation management for, 443–444*t*
asymptomatic bacteriuria, 290
asystole, 129*t*
AT. *See* atrial tachycardia
atelectasis, 589
  postoperative, 607
atherosclerotic dysplasia, 183
atherosclerotic renal artery stenosis, 185
atrial fibrillation (AF), 128*t*
  care transitions, 135–136
  causes of, 130*t*
  CHADS2 score and, 136*t*
  chemical cardioversion medications,
    133*t*
  clinical presentation of, 130–131
  diagnosis of, 130–131
  diastolic HF and, 156
  disease management strategies, 134–135
  ECG of, 131*f*
  epidemiology of, 129–130
  ischemic stroke management and, 333
  management of, 131–133
  mechanisms of, 130*t*
  pathophysiology of, 130
  postoperative, 132–133
  rate control medications, 132*t*
  symptoms of, 130*t*
  triage of, 131–133
atrial flutter (AFl)
  care transitions, 135–136
  disease management strategies, 135
  epidemiology of, 129–130
  pathophysiology of, 130
  SVT and, 137
atrial tachycardia (AT), 137
atrioventricular (AV) blocks
  diagnosis, 147–150
  pathophysiology, 147
  QRS complex and, 149
  types of, 149, 149*f*, 150*t*
atrioventricular (AV) nodal blocking
  drugs, 135
  SVT management and, 145
atrioventricular nodal reciprocating
  tachycardia (AVNRT), 137–138
atrioventricular reciprocating tachycardia
  (AVRT), 137–138
atropine, 150
attending rounds. *See* inpatient attending
  rounds
attention, confusion and, 318*t*

audit systems, for discharge, 71
auras, 345, 345t. *See also* seizure
automaticity disorder, 152
autonomy
    adult learning, 616
    pathways and, 60
    patient, 562
AV blocks. *See* atrioventricular blocks
avian influenza A (H5N1), 297
aviation industry, 17, 18t
AVNRT. *See* atrioventricular nodal
    reciprocating tachycardia
AVP V$_2$-receptor agonists, 482
AVRT. *See* atrioventricular reciprocating
    tachycardia
azathioprine, 234

B
bacteremia, 432. *See also* bloodstream
        infections
    catheter-associated UTI and, 292
    clinical presentation, 295
    diagnosis, 295
    disease management strategies, 295
    epidemiology, 294
    initial management, 295
    triage, 295
bacteria. *See also* gram-negative
        bacteria
    antibiotic resistance and, 311
    colon infections, 226t
    drug-resistant, antibiotics for, 313t
    gram-positive, 283
    skin infections and, 301
bacterial endocarditis
    antibiotics for enterococci, 287t
    care transitions, 288–289
    clinical presentation, 284–286
    diagnosis, 284–286
    epidemiology, 282
    initial management, 286–287
    microbiology of, 284t
    prevention, 289
    triage, 286–287
bactrim, 312
bad news, 552, 552t
Balthazar-Ranson grading system, 244t
barbiturates
    abuse management, 381
    overdose, 369–370
basal energy expenditure (BEE), 521–522
bed position, 516f
bedside teaching, 619–620
BEE. *See* basal energy expenditure
behavior
    deconditioning and, 518
    diagnosing confusion and, 317
    disorders, 582–583
behavioral disturbances, 355–356
    medical causes of, 356–357

behavioral sciences, 17
benzodiazepines, 321, 537
    abuse management, 381
    alcohol withdrawal treatment and,
        377–379
    anxiety treatment and, 547t
    delirium and, 327
    GCSE and, 348
    overdose, 369
beta-2-adrenergic agonists, 493
beta-2-agonists
    ARF triage and, 411
    for asthma triage, 397–398
    long-acting, 401
beta-blockers (BBs)
    AF management and, 134
    alcohol withdrawal treatment and, 378
    noncardiac surgery and, 586–588
    overdose, 369
    perioperative medication management
        and, 593
    postoperative AF and, 133
    SVT and, 140–144
    SVT care transitions and, 146
    syncope management and, 174
    systolic HF management and, 165
    VT management and, 155
beta-lactamases, 310
bicarbonate, 193
bifascicular blocks, 149
billing, 50
biopsies
    ARF diagnosis, 455
    FUO management and, 282
bioresorbable membranes, 250
bisphosphonates, 571–572
bites, animal, 306
bladder stones, 293
bleeding
    acute, 276
    drotrecogin alpha and, 437
    intraparenchymal, 335
blood gas analysis, 389
blood loss
    chronic, 276
    transfusion and, 272
blood pH, 469–470
blood pressure (BP)
    between arms, 110
    cerebral hemorrhage triage and,
        337
    CKD management and, 461
    classification, 174–175
    control, 175
    diastolic HF and, 157
    HTN emergencies and, 177
    ischemic stroke triage and, 331
blood tests
    CAP triage and, 415
    for endocarditis, 285

blood urea nitrogen (BUN)
    ARF diagnosis and, 454
    delirium and, 324
    systolic function triage
        and, 162
bloodstream infections, 294t. *See also*
        bacteremia
    catheters and, 295t
    definition of, 295t
    nosocomial, 294, 295t
BMI. *See* body mass index
BMJ Updates, 89
BNP. *See* brain natriuretic peptide
body mass index (BMI)
    hyperglycemia and, 197
    secondary HTN and, 183
body temperature, cerebral hemorrhage
    triage and, 338
body weight, ideal, 441t
bones
    deconditioning and, 516
    resorption, 570
bonuses, 47
bowel rest
    diverticulitis and, 241
    UC and, 238
bowels
    abdominal pain and, 212
    closed loop obstructions, 248
    of frail older adults, 565
    irrigation, 363t
    malignant obstruction, 542–543
    strangulated, 248
bradycardia. *See also* sinus
        bradycardia
    admission and, 149–150
    causes of, 148t
    hemodynamically stable, 149
    unstable, 129t, 150
brain
    arterial territories of, 330f
    biopsy, 341
    herniation, 339
brain natriuretic peptide (BNP)
    diastolic HF and, 157
    differentiating CHF, 391f
    dyspnea diagnosis and, 390–391
    systolic HF triage and, 163
breakthrough dose, 540t
breathing, 548, 548t. *See also* shortness
        of breath
British National Health Service, 98
bronchitis, 403
bronchodilators, 406
    ARF triage and, 411
bronchospasms, postoperative,
        607–608
Buckman, Robert, 552
BUN. *See* blood urea nitrogen
Byock, Ira, 555

C
CAD. *See* coronary artery disease
calciphylaxis, 468
calcitonin, 572
Calcitriol, 570
calcium
  CKD management and, 463*t*
  ischemic stroke and, 329
calcium channel blockers (CCBs)
  non-dihydropyridine, 134
  overdose, 369
  perioperative medication management
    and, 594
  SVT and, 140–144
  syncope management and, 174
calculation, confusion and, 318*t*
calories, 521
CAM. *See* Confusion Assessment Method
Campylobacter, 223
CA-MRSA. *See* methicillin-resistant
    Staphylococcal aureus
cancer
  hypercalcemia of malignancy and, 571
  WHO ladder and, 540
Cannibis sativa, 382
CAP. *See* community-acquired pneumonia
carbohydrates, 522
  consistent, 200
carcinoma, hepatocellular, 223
cardiac arrest
  pulseless, 128*t*
  sudden, 127
  syncop *v.,* 168
Cardiac Arrhythmia Suppression Trial
    (CAST), 82
cardiac catheterization, 97
  without preliminary noninvasive testing,
    117
cardiac murmurs, 284–285
cardiac remodeling, 159–160
cardiac resynchronization therapy, 167
cardiogenic edema, dyspnea triage and,
    392–393
cardiomyopathy, syncope management
    and, 174
cardiopulmonary resuscitation (CPR), 127
cardiothoracic surgery, 110
cardiovascular collapse, 154
cardiovascular disease (CVD)
  ESRD and, 467
  influenza management and, 299
  risk factors in CKD, 459*t*
  smoking cessation counseling and, 158
cardiovascular evaluation, 585–588
cardiovascular medications, 592–594
cardiovascular system, deconditioning
    and, 517
cardioversion, 132
  AF management and, 135

care transitions, 6
  ACS and, 124–126
  CAD and, 120
  chest pain and, 112
  discharge, 68–69
  efficiency of, 60–61
  hospitalist programs and, 50
  polypharmacy and, 35
  SNF and, 579
  teamwork and, 56
Care Transitions Project, 569
career satisfaction, 2–3
Carnegie Foundation for the Advancement
    of Teaching, 627–628
carotid massage, 171
case managers, 61
case mix index (CMI), 68
case-controlled studies, 84
CASS. *See* coronary artery surgery study
cathartics, 363*t*
catheters. *See also* Foley catheters
  ablation, 146
  antibiotic resistance prevention and, 315
  bacteremia and, 294
  bloodstream infections and, 295*t*
  hemodialysis, 465
  impregnated urinary, 294
  parenteral nutrition and, 525
  removal, 295–296
  site insertion, 296
cauda equina syndrome, 575
causation, determining, 84
CBC. *See* complete blood count
CBF. *See* cerebral blood flow
CCBs. *See* calcium channel blockers
CCU. *See* critical care unit
CDC. *See* Centers for Disease Control
CDI. *See* central diabetes insipidus
cellulitis, 300
  facial, 307
  orbital, 307
Centers for Disease Control (CDC)
  Campylobacter and, 223
  influenza infection control and, 298
  on norovirus, 309
  SSIs and, 605
Centers for Medicare and Medicaid
    Services (CMS)
  AMI and, 106
  pneumonia core measures, 413*t*
  quality improvement and, 41
central diabetes inisipidus (CDI), 482
central pontine myelinolysis, 481
cerebral blood flow (CBF), 329
cerebral hemorrhage. *See also*
    intracerebral hemorrhage
  clinical presentation, 335–336
  diagnosis, 335–336
  epidemiology, 335

initial management, 336–338
  pathophysiology, 335
  triage, 336–338
  warfarin algorithm, 338*f*
cerebral hypoperfusion, 168
cerebral infarction, 328
cerebrospinal fluid (CSF) profiles,
    meningitis and, 340*t*, 341
CHADS2 score, 136*t*
charcoal therapy, 363*t*
chart reviews, 22
checklist
  discharge, 70, 70*t*
  handoff, 67, 67*f*
chemotherapy
  neutropenic fever and, 573
  systemic, 578
chest pain (CP), 105
  acute pericarditis and, 110–111
  angina and, 108*t*
  angina pectoris diagnosis and, 113
  assessment of, 109*f*
  cardiac etiologies of, 109
  care transitions and, 112
  causes of, 107*t*
  clinical presentation of, 106–112, 132
  cocaine-associated, 106
  diagnosis of, 106–112
  in dialysis patients, 467–468
  etiology of, 106
  initial management of, 105–106
  ischemic cardiac, 109
  pretest probability and, 107
  risk stratification and, 114*t*
  triage, 105–106
chest pain centers (CPCs), 106
chest radiography (CXR)
  acute PE and, 110
  ARF diagnosis and, 410
  CAP diagnosis and, 413
  CAP management and, 420
  cardiogenic edema and, 392
  empyema and, 431
  for hemodialysis patients, 466
  nonresolving pneumonia and, 427
  pleural effusion and, 427–430
  preoperative testing and, 603
  pulmonary edema, 393*f*
  systolic function triage and, 162
chest tube, 431
Child-Pugh criteria, 222*t*
  decompensated cirrhosis and, 221
  LFTs and, 602
chlamydia, 290
chloridiazepoxide, 377–378
chlorpromazine, 544
cholecystitis, 215–216
cholecystitis, acute. *See* gallbladder
    disease

chronic illness, 73–74
  patient education and, 72
chronic kidney disease (CKD)
  anemia therapy for, 463*t*
  cardiovascular risk factors, 462
  care transitions, 463–464
  clinical presentation, 459–461
  complications of, 462–463
  CVD risk factors in, 459*t*
  diagnosis, 459–461
  disease management strategies, 461–463
  epidemiology, 458
  pathophysiology, 458–459
  precautions in managing, 461*t*
  remission targets, 461*t*
  risk factors, 459*t*
  stages of, 459*t*
  uremic symptoms of, 460*t*
chronic obstructive pulmonary disease
    (COPD), 378
  acute exacerbations of, 404, 404*t*
  care transitions, 407
  clinical presentation, 403–405
  diagnosis, 403–405
  differential diagnosis, 404*t*
  discharge indications, 407*t*
  disease management strategies, 405–407
  dyspnea and, 389
  epidemiology, 402
  indications for hospitalization, 405*t*
  indications for ICU, 405*t*
  initial management, 404–405
  pathophysiology, 402–403
  postoperative, 609
  postoperative exacerbation of, 607
  risk factors, 402*t*
  severity, 403*t*
  stable, 403–404, 404*t*
  therapy stages, 406*f*
  triage, 404–405
  ventilation management for, 443–444*t*
CI. *See* confidence intervals
cilostazol, 595
CIN. *See* contrast-induced nephropathy
cirrhosis, 220
  care transitions, 223
  common etiologies, 221*t*
  compensated, 220–221
  decompensated, 221–222
  disease management strategies, 220–223
  gastrointestinal bleeding and, 222*t*
  noncardiac surgery and, 591
  physiological changes in, 220*t*
  pleural effusion and, 429
  testing, 221*t*
CIWA. *See* Clinical Institute Withdrawal
    Assessment
CKD. *See* chronic kidney disease (CKD)
CK-MB, 115

clinical condition competencies, 4
clinical decision support, 23
clinical evidence, 89
  errors in interpreting, 91
Clinical Institute Withdrawal Assessment
    (CIWA), 376
clinical pulmonary infection score (CPIS),
    424*t*
clinical research, process improvement *v.*,
    18–19
clinical significance, statistical
    significance *v.*, 85
clinical testing. *See* testing
clopidogrel, 122, 508
Clostridium difficile
  clinical features, 230*t*
  Crohn's disease and, 233
  diagnosis, 230*t*
  diarrhea and, 226–227
  management, 229
  neutropenic fever and, 573
  SNF and, 582
  testing, 227–228
  treatment, 230*t*
  VRE and, 312–313
clot formation, 506–507
CMI. *See* case mix index
CMS. *See* Centers for Medicare and
    Medicaid Services
CMV. *See* controlled mechanical
    ventilation
coagulation, preoperative testing of, 601
coagulopathy, 258
cocaine
  abuse management, 380–381
  chest pain and, 106
  overdose, 370
Cochrane Library, 89–90
Cockcroft-Gault equation, 460, 512*t*
codeine, 534
cognition
  competency assessment and, 352
  diagnosing confusion and, 317
cognitive impairment, 353
cohort studies, 84
colitis. *See also* ulcerative colitis
  antibiotic-induced, 226–227
  care transitions, 231
  clinical presentation, 227
  diagnosis, 227–228
  differential diagnosis, 224–225*t*
  disease management strategies, 229–231
  epidemiology, 223–227
  infectious, 229
  infectious agents causing, 238*t*
  initial management, 227–228
  ischemic, 229–231, 256–257
  medical history and, 227*t*
  medication-induced, 226

  triage, 227–228
  types, 224–225*t*
collaboration, 629–630
  care transition efficiency and, 61
colon infections, 226*t*
colonoscopy
  Crohn's disease and, 234
  LGI bleeding and, 259
  UC diagnosis and, 237
colorectal cancer (CRC)
  Crohn's disease and, 235
  UC and, 237
coma, encephalitis and, 343
comanagement, with other services, 9*t*
Combined Cardiac Pulmonary Risk Index
    (CPRI), 608
comfort, 553
comments, empathic, 551*t*
communication, 10
  ACS and, 126
  after death, 555
  ask-tell-ask approach, 551
  bad news and, 552
  barriers to, 550–551, 550*t*
  care transition efficiency and, 61
  closed loop, 55
  competency and, 352
  death and, 554–555
  discharge and, 69, 71
  drug abuse triage and, 380
  error reduction and, 20, 39
  good, 550*t*
  handoffs and, 62, 63*t*
  hospitalist programs and, 50
  IT and, 54
  pain management guidelines and, 529
  palliative care and, 549–556
  patient safety and, 36
  physician-nurse, 50
  polypharmacy and, 35
  post-discharge test results and, 79
  SCM and, 613
  spirituality and, 551–552
  teamwork and, 53
  vulnerable populations and, 561–562
  word choice and, 554
community-acquired pneumonia (CAP)
  admission assessment, 422*t*
  care transitions, 421–422
  clinical presentation, 413
  diagnosis, 413
  disease management strategies, 417–421
  epidemiology, 412–413
  guideline/order set, 414–415*t*
  initial management, 413–417
  pathogens, 418–420*t*
  pathophysiology, 413
  prevention strategies, 415*t*
  triage, 413–417

competency
  advanced directives and, 354
  assessment, 351–353
  construct, 350–351
  informed consent and, 351
complete blood count (CBC)
  anemia and, 261
  CAP triage and, 416
  for hemodialysis patients, 466
  systolic function triage and, 162
compliance, 72. *See also* patient adherence
compression ultrasonography, 502
computed tomography (CT)
  abdominal, 213
  ARF diagnosis and, 410
  colitis and, 228
  diverticulitis diagnosis and, 241
  helical, 213–214
  HTN emergencies and, 178
  ICH and, 335
  meningitis diagnosis and, 340
  non-contrast head, 347
  pancreatitis diagnosis and, 244
  of pulmonary edema, 393*f*
  SBO triage and, 250
  severity index, 244*t*
computerized physician order entry
    (CPOE), 23
  CAP management and, 417
  medication reconciliation and, 29
  polypharmacy and, 32
  post-discharge test results and, 79
conduction abnormalities, 152
conference room teaching, 618–619
  examples, 618*t*
confidence intervals (CI), 86, 87*f*
conflicts, 354–355
confusion
  care transitions, 321
  categories of, 319*t*
  clinical presentation, 317
  diagnosis, 317
  disease management strategies, 321
  epidemiology, 316
  initial evaluation, 317–321
  neurological examination of, 318*t*
  pathophysiology, 316
Confusion Assessment Method (CAM), 324*t*
congestive heart failure (CHF), 111
  BNP and, 390
  noncardiac surgery and, 588
consensus statements, 58
consent, 350. *See also* informed consent
constipation
  opioid side effects and, 536
  opioid-related, 541–542, 542*t*
construction, confusion and, 318*t*
consultation, SCM *v.*, 611–612
contraception, oral, 596–597

contractures
  common, 517*t*
  deconditioning and, 516
  preventing, 519
contrast osmolarity, 450–451
contrast volume, 450
contrast-induced nephropathy (CIN), 117
  clinical presentation, 448–449
  differential diagnosis, 448–449
  epidemiology, 448
  pathophysiology, 448
  preventive strategies, 449–451
  prophylactic strategies, 450*t*
  risk factors, 449*t*
control groups, 84
controlled mechanical ventilation (CMV),
    439
COPD. *See* chronic obstructive pulmonary
    disease
coping mechanisms, 358, 358*t*
core competencies, 4, 5*t*, 10
*The Core Competencies: A Framework for
    Curriculum Development* (SHM), 72
*The Core Competencies in Hospital
    Medicine* (TCC), 4, 6, 10
core measure performance, 49
coronary artery disease (CAD), 112
  care transitions and, 120
  LV dysfunction and, 159
  management strategies, 116–120
  noncardiac surgery and, 585
  prevalence of, 112–113
  risk factors, 113*t*
  systolic HF care transition and, 166
coronary artery surgery study (CASS), 108
coronary revascularization
  noncardiac surgery and, 588
  VT and, 155
corticosteroids
  ARF triage and, 411
  Crohn's disease and, 234
  epidural spinal cord compression
      and, 578
  perioperative medication management
      and, 596
  in sepsis management, 436
  septic shock guidelines for, 436*t*
  UC and, 239
Corynebacterium urealyticum, 293
cost-effectiveness analysis, 96–98
  ethical considerations of, 98
  evidence-based outreach and, 99
costs, 2
  of ARF, 453
  of CKD, 458
CP. *See* chest pain
CPCs. *See* chest pain centers
CPOE. *See* computerized physician
    order entry

CPR. *See* cardiopulmonary resuscitation
CPRI. *See* Combined Cardiac Pulmonary
    Risk Index
cranberry juice, 293
CRC. *See* colorectal cancer
creatinine
  ARF diagnosis and, 454
  clearance, 512*t*
  clearance, of frail older adults, 568
crew resource management (CRM), 53
critical care medicine, 3
critical care unit (CCU), 194–195
CRM. *See* crew resource management
Crohn's and Colitis Foundation of
    America, 235, 240
Crohn's disease
  care transitions, 235
  diagnosis, 233
  disease management strategies,
      234–235
  epidemiology, 231
  initial management, 233–234
  medication dosages, 234*t*
  pathophysiology, 231–232
  SBO and, 247
  treatment options, 234*t*
  triage, 233–234
  UC *v.,* 233, 236
Crossing the Quality Chasm, 36
cross-sectional studies, 84
CRUSADE, 558
CSF profiles. *See* cerebrospinal fluid
    profiles
CT pulmonary angiography (CTA), 391
CT. *See* computed tomography
cultural competence, 562
culture, 15
  ADEs and, 23
  changing, 16
  improving, 19
curriculum development, 627
  publishing, 630*t*
  six-step approach, 627*t*
Cushing's syndrome, 187
CXR. *See* chest radiography
cystitis, 290–291
  UTI and, 289
cytology, 430
cytotoxins, 229

D

daily assessment tool, 568*t*
Dana Farber Cancer Institute, 14
daptomycin, 312
DARE. *See* Database of Abstracts of
    Review of Effects
data collection
  for hospitalist report card, 49
  for quality improvement, 43–44

Database of Abstracts of Review of Effects (DARE), 90
D-dimer, 110
death
  communication after, 555
  communication and, 554–555
  hastened, 554
  SNF and, 582
debriefing, 55–56
decision-making
  assessing capacity for medical, 350
  autonomy in, 54
  capacity for, 353
  care transition efficiency and, 60
  clinical, 91
  competent, 352
  diverticulitis, 241t
  impaired, 354–355
  for incompetent patients, 353–354
  spheres of influence, 354f
deconditioning
  care transitions, 519
  clinical presentation, 515–518
  epidemiology, 515
  factors of, 516t
  management strategies, 518–519
  pathophysiology, 515–518
  prevention of, 518t
  sepsis care transitions and, 437
decontamination, from drug overdose, 363t
decreased renal profusion, 446
deep venous thrombosis (DVT)
  diagnostic approach to, 503f
  management, 505t
  PE and, 494
  prevention initiatives, 500t
  prophylaxis, 498
  VTE and, 501
defect rate, 16
defibrillation, 127
dehydration. See hydration
delay days, 58
delirium, 7
  care transitions, 327
  causes of, 326t
  clinical presentation, 323–325
  confusion and, 316
  dementia and, 567
  dementia v., 325t
  depression v., 325t
  diagnosis, 323–325
  differential of, 318t
  disease management strategies, 325–326
  epidemiology, 323
  initial management, 325
  management of, 325f
  opioid-induced, 543–544
  pathophysiology, 323

perioperative medication management and, 597
prevention, 327
suicide and, 384
treatment, 326–327
triage, 325
delirium tremens (DTs), 373, 375
dementia
  behavioral disturbances and, 356
  delirium and, 567
  delirium v., 325t
  depression v., 325t
  differential of, 318t
  in frail older adults, 565
  medications for slowing, 322t
  Mini-Cog and, 566f
denial, 352–353
dental work, endocarditis and, 283
Department of Health and Human Services (DHHS), 557
depolarization abnormalities, 152
depressed ejection fraction, 174
depression
  behavioral disturbances and, 357
  confusion and, 316
  deconditioning management and, 519
  delirium v., 325t
  diagnosing, 384t
  differential of, 318t
  dying patients and, 547t
  in frail older adults, 567
  GDS and, 567t
  palliative care and, 546–547
  suicide and, 384
  treatment, 546
designer drugs, overdose, 365t
detoxification therapy, 372
  alcohol abuse and, 379
device design, 36
dexamethasone therapy, 341–342
DHHS. See Department of Health and Human Services
diabetes
  acid-base disorder management and, 476
  CKD and, 459
  CKD management and, 461–462
  discharge considerations, 204t
  foot infections, 304–305, 305f
  inpatient certification, 199t
  ischemic stroke management and, 333
  mellitus, 198
  MI and, 122 and
  nephrotoxic precautions in, 197t
  noncardiac surgery and, 590
  in noncritically-ill patients, 198t
  perioperative medication management and, 596

pregnancy and, 203–204
preoperative testing and, 601
ulcers and, 304
diabetic ketoacidosis (DKA), 188
  care transitions, 193
  clinical presentation, 189
  diagnosis, 189
  disease management strategies, 190–193
  HHS v., 190t
  initial management, 189–190
  pathophysiology, 188–189
  protocol for managing, 191f
  triage, 189–190
diagnosis related groups (DRGs), 57
Diagnostic and Statistical Manual of Mental Disorders, Fourth Edition (DSM-IV)
  CAM v., 324t
  defense levels and, 360t
  personality dysfunction and, 357
diagnostic decision-making, 5–6
diagnostic testing. See lab tests
dialysis patients
  care transitions, 468–469
  chest pain in, 467–468
  disease management strategies, 464–468
  emergent dialysis in, 467
  epidemiology, 464–465
dialysis. See hemodialysis
diarrhea
  care transitions, 231
  Clostridium difficile and, 226–227
  Crohn's disease and, 233
  disease management strategies, 229–231
  epidemiology, 223–227
  gastroenteritis and, 308–309
  noninfectious, 224t, 229
  rotavirus and, 309
  SNF and, 582
  tube feeds and, 525
  UC and, 236
diastolic dysfunction
  care transitions, 158
  clinical presentation, 157
  diagnosis, 157, 157t
  disease management strategies, 157–158
  epidemiology, 156
  heart failure due to, 156–158
  initial management, 157
  pathophysiology, 156–157
  triage, 157
diazepam, 377–378
diet(s). See also nutrition
  acid-base disorders and, 469
  elemental, 524
  hyperglycemia management and, 200
  polymeric, 524
dietary supplements, overdose, 371–372
dietitians, SNF and, 580

digitalis, 165
digoxin, 134
dilution, 363*t*
dipyridamole, 595
discharge
    ACS and, 126
    asthma and, 401*t*
    CAP and, 421
    care transition efficiency and, 60–61
    checklist, 70, 70*t*
    communication at, 69, 71
    COPD indications for, 407*t*
    deconditioning care transitions and, 519
    diabetes and, 204*t*
    diastolic HF and, 158
    drug overdose and, 372
    effective, 68–69
    epidural spinal cord compression and, 578
    to extended care facilities, 68
    of frail older adults, 569
    HF and, 164
    HTN management and, 181
    hypoglycemia and, 204
    instructions, 74
    insulin and, 204
    medication discrepancies and, 24–25
    medication reconciliation at, 27*f,* 28–29
    medications at, 71
    planning, 69*f*
    preventing polypharmacy at, 33*t*
    SCD and, 267
    skin infections and, 307
    summary, 69, 69*t,* 70–71
    syncope and, 174
    systems improvement, 71
    test results at, 76
    test results management system, 77–80, 78*f*
    vulnerable populations and, 562
disclosure, 38–39
discovery, 627
disease-modifying antirheumatic drugs (DMARDs), 598
disseminated intravascular coagulopathy, 270–271
dissemination, of work, 630
distal nephrons, 485*f*
distributive shock, 433, 434*t*
diuretics. *See also* loop diuretics
    in ARF triage, 456
    perioperative medication management and, 594
diverticular bleeding, 241
diverticulitis, 256
    acute, 241
    care transitions, 242
    clinical presentation, 240–241
    colitis and, 224*t*

decision-making, 241*t*
diagnosis, 240–241
disease management strategies, 241–242
initial management, 241
pathophysiology, 240
triage, 241
DKA. *See* diabetic ketoacidosis
DMARDs. *See* disease-modifying antirheumatic drugs
DNR order. *See* do not resuscitate order
do not resuscitate (DNR) order
    competency and, 354
    SNF and, 581
documentation, 50, 631
    tools, 56
donepezil, 322*t*
dopamine, 150
DRGs. *See* diagnosis related groups
drivers, 42–43
drotrecogin alpha, 436–437, 437*t*
drug abuse. *See also* substance abuse
    clinical presentation, 379–380
    diagnosis, 379–380
    disease management strategies, 380–382
    epidemiology, 379
    initial management, 380
    triage, 380
drug equivalency, 376*t*, 378*t*
drug overdose
    care transitions, 372
    decontamination, 363*t*
    of designer drugs, 365*t*
    epidemiology, 361
    ingestion algorithm, 361*f*
    initial management, 361–362
    lab testing, 362
    management, 362–372, 364*t*
    pathophysiology, 362
    triage, 361–362
drug-disease interactions, 34*t*
drug-drug interactions, 34*t*
dry weight, assessing, 467*t*
drying agents, for breathing, 548*t*
DSM-IV. See Diagnostic and Statistical Manual of Mental Disorders, Fourth Edition
DTs. *See* delirium tremens
Duke criteria, 285*t*
duodenum, rotavirus and, 309
DVT. *See* deep venous thrombosis
DVT-FREE, 497
dyspnea. *See* shortness of breath

E
early withdrawal syndrome, 374–375
EBM. *See* evidence-based medicine
ECG. *See* electrocardiogram
echocardiography
    acute pericarditis and, 111

ARF diagnosis and, 410
stress, 118
two-dimensional, with Doppler, 163
ecstasy. *See* methylenedioxymethamphetamine
ED. *See* emergency departments
education, 8
educational objectives, 4–5
educational portfolio, 631–632, 631*t*
educational products, 631
EEG. *See* electroencephalogram
efficiency, 1
    of care transitions, 60–61
    LOS and, 58
efflux pumps, 311
elderly. *See also* frail older adults
    appendicitis in, 215
    CAP diagnosis in, 413
    medication reconciliation and, 25
    polypharmacy and, 30–31
    protocol for, 323*f*
    purple urine bag syndrome and, 293
    vulnerable populations and, 557
electrocardiogram (ECG), 105
    acute PE and, 110
    acute pericarditis and, 111
    of AF, 131*f*
    AF diagnosis and, 131
    angina pectoris and, 115
    ARF diagnosis and, 410
    criteria favoring VT, 154*f*
    electrolyte repletion and, 192
    HTN emergencies and, 177
    hyperkalemia and, 492*f*
    hyperkalemia triage and, 492
    hypokalemia and, 489*f*
    hypokalemia triage and, 487
    narrow complex tachycardia analysis, 141*f*
    preoperative testing and, 602–603
    of pulmonary embolism, 392*f*
    sinus bradycardia diagnosis and, 147
    SVT and, 139
    SVT care transitions and, 146
    syncopal etiologies and, 172*t*
    syncope and, 172
    systolic function triage and, 162
    tracing in SVT, 141–143*f*
electroencephalogram (EEG)
    confusion and, 321
    seizure diagnosis and, 346
    seizure triage and, 347
electrolytes, 522
    Crohn's disease and, 233
    preoperative testing of, 601
    repletion, 192
    SBO triage and, 250
elements, trace, 522
ELISAs. *See* enzyme-linked immunosorbent assays

emergency departments (ED), 7
    abdominal pain and, 211
    ACS and, 124
    acute ischemic stroke and, 330
    hospitalists and, 10–11
    HTN emergencies and, 176
    HTN management in, 181
    LGI bleeding and, 257–258
    patient education and, 72
    secondary HTN and, 182
    SVT and, 137
    syncope and, 168
    triage surgical patients, 11*f*
emergency medical services (EMS), 127
emergency medicine, 3
emergent vascular surgery, 110
emotion, palliative care and, 551
empathy, 551*t*
emphysematous pyelonephritis, 292
empyema, 430–431
EMS. *See* emergency medical services
encephalitis
    care transitions, 343
    clinical presentation, 339–341
    diagnosis, 339–341
    disease management strategies, 343
    epidemiology, 339
    pathophysiology, 339
    treatment, 343
    triage, 341–343
encephalopathy
    hepatic, 222–223
    stages of, 223*t*
    Wernicke's, 375–376
Ende, J., 625
endocarditis. *See also* bacterial
        endocarditis
    antibiotic prophylaxis, 289
    antibiotics for native valve, 286*t*
    antibiotics for prosthetic valve,
        287*t*
    complications, 285
    culture-negative, 288
    modified Duke criteria for, 285*t*
    testing, 285
endocrine system, deconditioning
        and, 518
endocrinologic evaluation, for noncardiac
        surgery, 590
endoscopic homeostasis, 254
endoscopic retrograde
        cholangiopancreatography
        (ERCP), 246
endoscopic sphincterotomy (ES), 246
endoscopic surgery, 363*t*
endoscopic therapy
    failure of, 255
    UGI risk stratification, 252–253
endothelial dysfunction, 176

end-stage renal disease (ESRD),
        464–465
    CVD and, 467
    drug dosing in, 466*t*, 468
    hyperkalemia and, 467
    PICC lines and, 469
    skin disorders associated with, 468
engineering, 15
    patient safety and, 15–16
enteral access, 524
enterococci, 287*t*. *See also* vancomycin-
        resistant enterococci
enterotoxins, 309
environment
    behavioral disturbances and, 356
    learning, 616
    work, 8*t*, 47
enzyme-linked immunosorbent assays
        (ELISAs), 309
EPCs. *See* evidence-based practice centers
Epidemiology, Practice, Outcomes, and
        Cost of Heart Failure (EPOCH), 559
epidural spinal cord compression,
        575–576
    back pain and, 577*t*
    clinical presentation, 576–577
    diagnosis, 576–577
    disease management strategies, 578
    initial management, 577–578
    symptoms, 576
    triage, 577–578
epilepsy, 344. *See also* seizure
epileptogenesis, 344
epinephrine
    for asthma triage, 398
    unstable bradycardia and, 150
EPOCH. *See* Epidemiology, Practice,
        Outcomes, and Cost of Heart Failure
equinalgesics
    conversion, to methadone, 533*t*
    dosing, 535–537
ERCP. *See* endoscopic retrograde
        cholangiopancreatography
Eron classification system, 302
error(s). *See also* active failures
    in ACS management, 105
    ADEs and, 21, 22
    alpha, 85
    anatomy of, 15
    beta, 85
    communication and, 39
    deaths due to, 36
    disclosure of, 39
    human, 16–18
    interpreting clinical evidence, 91
    measuring, 19
    in medication reconciliation, 25
    of omission, 53
    patient expectations and, 38–39

reduction strategies, 20
    reporting requirements, 38
    risk management and, 39
erythropoietic agents, 262–263
Erythroxylum coca, 370
ES. *See* endoscopic sphincterotomy
Escherichia coli
    catheter-associated UTI and, 292
    UTI and, 289
ESRD. *See* end-stage renal disease
ethanol testing, 362
ethics
    of cost-effectiveness analysis, 98
    patient safety and, 38
    of research, 13
    of SCM, 612, 612*t*
ethics committees, 355
ethyl alcohol. *See* alcohol
ethylene glycol, 367–368
    acid-base disorders and, 473*t*
    toxic ingestion of, 367*t*
ETT. *See* exercise treadmill testing
euthanasia, 554
evaluation, feedback *v.,* 625
evidence, levels of, 82–83
evidence-based medicine (EBM),
        7, 81
    5S model and, 88–89
    conceptual model, 82*f*
    evidence levels, 82–83
    experimental studies, 83–84
    observational studies of, 84–85
    outcome measures, 81–82
    resources, 89–90
    statistical significance and, 85–86
    study design, 83–85
    testing, 91–92
*Evidence-Based Medicine: How to
        Practice and Teach EBM* (Straus,
        Richard, Glaziou, et al), 89
evidence-based outreach, 99
evidence-based practice centers
        (EPCs), 90
exercise
    COPD care transitions and, 407
    deconditioning management and,
        518–519
    systolic dysfunction and, 161
    tolerance testing, 108
exercise treadmill testing (ETT),
        117
exitotoxicity, 329
experimental studies, of EBM,
        83–84
extended care facilities, 68
extended spectrum beta-lactamase
        (ESBL), 313–314
extubation, 444–445
eye contact, 551

F

faces pain scale, 529–530, 529f
faculty development, 628
    opportunities, 629t
failure mode and effect analysis
        (FMEA), 23
    patient safety and, 37
falls, 583
false negatives, 94
false positives, 94
families
    advanced care planning and, 552–553
    after death, 555
    care transition efficiency and, 60
    communication in palliative care,
        550–551
    confronting fears, 553–554
    death and, 554–555
    personality dysfunction and, 358–359
    post-discharge test results and, 79–80
    structured meeting, 555–556, 556t
fatigue, 17
fears, confronting, 553–554
fecoliths, 240
feedback, 616, 625
    constructive, 625
    definition of, 625
    general approach, 626
    key points of, 626t
    principles of, 626
    reinforcing, 625
feeding intolerance, 524
FE_{Na}, 454
fentanyl
    pain management and, 540
    transdermal, 535t
fever
    appendicitis and, 214
    aseptic meningitis and, 342
    drug, 279
    endocarditis and, 288
    factitious, 279
    in hemodialysis patients, 465f
    hyperthyroidism and, 208
    postoperative, 604–607, 606t
fever of unknown origin (FUO)
    care transitions, 282
    clinical presentation, 279–281
    diagnosis, 279–281
    disease management strategies, 281–282
    epidemiology, 278–279
    initial management, 281
    nosocomial, 281
    triage, 281
FFP. See fresh frozen plasma
FHF. See fulminant hepatic failure
fibromuscular dysplasia, 183
FiO_2, 442
    in ARDS, 444t

First Multicenter Intrapleural Sepsis Trial
        (MIST1), 431
fistula, 242
5-aminosalicylate acid (5-ASA), 238–239
    common, 239t
5S model, 88–89, 89f
flecainide, 144
flow cycling, 440–441
fluid management, 336–337
fluid restriction, 163
FMEA. See failure mode and effect
        analysis
Foley catheters
    SNF and, 582
    UTI and, 291–292
    VRE and, 313
fondaparinux, 512
Food and Drug Administration (FDA)
    pregnancy risk categories of, 509t
    VTE therapy and, 504
foot hygiene, 307
forced acid diuresis, 363t
formula, 19
formulary control, 23
fosfomycin, 291
The Four Things that Matter Most
        (Byock), 555
frail older adults
    care transitions, 569
    epidemiology, 563
    improving care for, 569
    initial management, 563–565
    management strategies, 565–569
    triage, 563–565
fresh frozen plasma (FFP), 275
    for elevated INR, 337t
fulminant hepatic failure (FHF), 218–219
functional status tool, 564t
funduscopic examinations, 177
FUO. See fever of unknown origin

G

galantamine, 322t
gallbladder disease, 266
gallstones, 215
    pancreatitis, 246
gamma-hydroxybutyrate (GHB)
    abuse management, 381
    testing, 362
gas gangrene, 306
gastric lavage, 363t
gastroduodenal ulcer disease, 253
gastroesophageal reflux disease
        (GERD), 112
gastrointestinal bleeding
    cirrhosis and, 222t
    portal hypotension-related, 222
gastrointestinal system, deconditioning
        and, 517

gastroparesis, 527
GCS. See graduated compression stockings
GCSE. See generalized convulsive status
        epilepticus
gender
    hospitalization and, 557, 558–559
    readmissions and, 559
    suicide and, 383
generalized convulsive status epilepticus
        (GCSE), 347–348
    treatment protocol, 348f
generalized tonic-clonic (GTC), 345
genetics, 236
genitourinary system, 517
GERD. See gastroesophageal reflux
        disease
geriatric depression scale (GDS), 567t
geriatric pharmacology, 32
geriatricians, 568–569
GFR. See glomerular filtration rate
GHB. See gamma-hydroxybutyrate
Glasgow Coma Scale, 245t
    cerebral hemorrhage triage and, 336
    drug overdose and, 362
Glassick's Criteria, 629t
Global Initiative for Asthma, 399t
glomerular filtration rate (GFR), 460
glomerulonephritis (GN), 454–455
glucagon, 369
glucocorticoids, 537
glucocorticosteroids. *See also* inhaled
        glucocorticosteroids
    for asthma triage, 398
    dosage, 398t
gluconeogenesis, 373
glucose
    control, 195
    hyperkalemia triage and, 493
    pleural effusion and, 430
    preoperative testing of, 601–602
glycemic control, 7
    diabetic foot infections and, 305
glycolic acid, 367
GN. See glomerulonephritis
goal setting, 55
gobbledygook, 74
goiter, 205
gonorrhea
    cystitis and, 290
    prostatitis and, 292
gout, 598
Grading Recommendation, Assessment,
        Development, and Evaluation
        (GRADE), 83
graduated compression stockings
        (GCS), 496
gram-negative bacteria, 301
    antibiotic resistance prevention and, 315
    ESBL-producing, 313–314

grants, 102
Graves' ophthalmopathy, 207
group dynamics, 42
GTC. *See* generalized tonic-clonic
guidelines, 59–60
  for chest pain, 60
Guillain-Barré syndrome, 300
Guyatt, Gordon, 89
gylcohemoglobin, 333

H
H2 blockers, 598
H5N1. *See* avian influenza A
HAART. *See* highly active antiretroviral
  therapy
Haldol, 543
hallucinations, alcohol withdrawal and,
  374–375
hallucinogens, abuse management,
  381–382
haloperidol, 378
handoffs
  checklist, 67, 67*f*
  communication and, 63*t*
  coordination, 63*t*
  increasing number of, 68
  in-hospital physician, 65–66*t*
  patient safety and, 63*t*
  problem of, 62
  process map, 66–67, 66*t*
  protocol, 65–67
  strategies for, 63–65
  systems improvement, 65–67
handover, 62
HAP. *See* hospital-acquired pneumonia
Harris-Benedict equation, 521–522
Harrison Narcotic Act of 1914, 370
The Harvard Medical Practice Study,
  13–14
HBV. *See* hepatitis B virus
HCAP. *See* healthcare-acquired
  pneumonia
HCUP. *See* Health Care Utilization
  Project
HCV. *See* hepatitis C virus
head-up tilt table (HUTT) testing, 172
Health Care Utilization Project (HCUP),
  557–558
Health Insurance Portability and
  Accountability Act (HIPAA), 380
health outcome, EBM and, 82
healthcare
  costs, 97
  teamwork in, 53–54
healthcare systems
  aviation industry *v.*, 18*t*
  chapters, 5–6, 5*t*
  competencies, 5–6
healthcare value, 41

healthcare-acquired pneumonia (HCAP)
  care transitions, 426
  clinical presentation, 423
  common pathogens, 424*t*
  diagnosis, 423
  disease management strategies, 424–426
  epidemiology, 422–423
  initial empiric antibiotics for, 425*t*
  initial management, 423–424
  pathophysiology, 423
  triage, 423–424
Healthy People 2000, 32
heart disease
  AF and, 130*t*
  cost of, 113
  endocarditis and, 283
  occult coronary, 157
  syncope and, 172*t*
heart failure (HF). *See also* congestive
  heart failure; diastolic dysfunction;
  systolic dysfunction
  acute, 161
  acute decompensated, 160
  ancillary testing for, 57
  core measures, 159
  discharge instructions and, 164
  due to diastolic dysfunction, 156–158
  due to systolic dysfunction, 159–167
  perioperative, 609
  postoperative, 609–610
  refractory, 167
  smoking cessation counseling and, 164
  stages, 160*f*
  therapy, 160*f*
  treatment, 158*t*
  two dimensional echocardiography and,
    163
Helicobacter pylori, 254
heliox, 411
HELLP syndrome, 180
HELP. *See* Hospital Elder Live Program
hemagglutinin, 297
hematemesis, 251
hematochezia, 236
hematologic abnormalities
  for noncardiac surgery, 590–591
  SCD and, 263–264
hematologic system, deconditioning
  and, 517
hemochromatosis, 163
hemodialysis. *See also* dialysis patients
  alcohol abuse and, 374
  ARF care transitions and, 457
  in ARF triage, 456
  catheter, 465
  CIN prevention and, 451
  emergent, 467
  fever in, 465*f*
  hypercalcemia of malignancy and, 571

indications from salicylates, 366*t*
  vascular access, 465
hemodynamics, 251*t*
hemofiltration
  CIN prevention and, 451
  systolic HF triage and, 163
hemoglobin
  anemia and, 260
  LGI bleeding and, 258
  preoperative testing of, 600
hemorrhages, palliative care and, 549
hemorrhoids, 257
hemostasis, 594–596
Henderson equation, 470
heparin. *See also* low molecular weight
  heparin; unfractionated heparin
  overdose, 510
  perioperative medication management
    and, 595–596
  STEMI and, 122
heparin-induced thrombocytopenia (HIT),
  269, 511–512
  platelet transfusion and, 274–275
  treatment, 271
hepatic alcohol dehydrogenase, 368
hepatic systems, 591
hepatitis
  acute, 217–219
  acute, clinical presentation, 217–218
  acute, diagnosis, 217–218
  initial management, acute, 218–219
  triage, acute, 218–219
hepatitis B virus (HBV), 273
hepatitis C virus (HCV), 273
hepatobiliary complications, 527
herbal supplements
  overdose, 371–372, 371*t*
  perioperative medication management
    and, 599
hernias, 247
HF. *See* heart failure
HHS. *See* hyperosmolar hyperglycemic
  state
HICPAC. *See* Hospital Infection
  Control Practices Advisory
  Committee
hierarchical relationships, 54
highly active antiretroviral therapy
  (HAART), 271
HIPAA. *See* Health Insurance Portability
  and Accountability Act
HIT. *See* heparin-induced
  thrombocytopenia
HIV. *See* human immunodeficiency
  virus
homeless
  hospitalization of, 558
  respite care for, 561
homeostenosis, 30–31

hormone replacement therapy (HRT)
epidural spinal cord compression and, 578
perioperative medication management and, 596–597
hospice care, 555. *See also* palliative care
benefits of, 555*t*
dyspnea and, 545
Medicare and, 25
SNF and, 579, 582
hospital admission. *See* admission
hospital discharge. *See* discharge
Hospital Elder Live Program (HELP), 569
hospital employment models, 48
Hospital Infection Control Practices Advisory Committee (HICPAC), 605–607
hospital medicine. *See also* hospitalist movement
alignment of priorities, 8*t*
challenges facing, 2–3
core values, 8*t*
goals, 8*t*
growth of, 3
improving, 3
mortality benefit to, 2*t*
multidisciplinary approach of, 6
threats to, 3*t*
hospital-acquired pneumonia (HAP)
care transitions, 425*t*
clinical presentation, 423
common pathogens, 424*t*
diagnosis, 423
disease management strategies, 424–426
epidemiology, 422–423
initial empiric antibiotics for, 425*t*
initial management, 423–424
pathophysiology, 423
risk factors, 423*t*
triage, 423–424
hospitalist(s)
ADEs and, 23
antibiotic resistance prevention and, 315
care transition efficiency and, 61
career satisfaction, 2–3
companies, 47–48
definition of, 1, 4
ED and, 10–11
feedback and, 12–13
focus of, 15
goals, 632
group models, 47–48
hiring, 47–48
key attributes of, 2
as leader, 7–8
in patient safety, 13
as physician advisor, 9
private practice, 48
report card, 49

research dimensions, 100*t*
as researcher, 99–102
role of, 6, 42
SCM and, 613
as teacher, 8, 615
hospitalist movement, 1–2. *See also* hospital medicine
hospitalist programs
financial viability of, 49
starting, 48–49
successful, 49–50
hospitalization. *See also* psychiatric hospitalization
considerations for asthma, 398*t*
COPD indications, 405*t*
deconditioning and, 515
hazards of, 57*t*
medication reconciliation process, 27*f*
nutrition and, 520–527
preventing polypharmacy at, 33*t*
tracking, 557–558
VTE prophylaxis in, 499*t*
How to Break Bad News: A Guide for Health Care Professions (Buckman), 552
HRT. *See* hormone replacement therapy
HTN. *See* hypertension
human immunodeficiency virus (HIV)
CAP triage and, 417
FUO and, 281
skin infection and, 307
systolic HF triage and, 163
thrombocytopenia and, 271
transfusion risk, 273
HUTT testing. *See* head-up tilt table testing
hyberbilirubinemia, 522
hydration
aseptic meningitis and, 342
colitis and, 231
cystitis and, 291
parenteral, 549
rotavirus and, 309
SNF and, 582, 583
hydrocephalus, 337
hydrocodone, 534
hyperaldosteronism. *See* primary hyperaldosteronism
hyperalgesia, 528
hypercalcemia
differential diagnosis, 570*t*
leukemia and, 570
of malignancy, 569–572
medications, 572*t*
types of, 570
hypercoagulable workup, 231
hyperglycemia, 526
care transitions, 197
in CCU, 194–195
clinical presentation, 199–200

critical illness-induced, 194*t*
diagnosis, 199–200
initial management, 195–196
in noncritically-ill patients, 198–204
oral agents, 200, 200*t*
pathophysiology of, 199
perioperative management of, 197
postoperative management of, 197
treatment goals, 195*t*
triage, 195–196
hyperkalemia, 193
in ARF triage, 456
care transitions, 493–494
CKD management and, 462–463
clinical presentation, 490
diagnosis, 490–492
diagnostic approach to, 491*f*
disease management strategies, 493
ECG changes and, 492*f*
epidemiology, 484
ESRD and, 467
initial management, 492–493
pathophysiology, 484–485
reduced renal potassium excretion and, 490*t*
triage, 492–493
hypernatremia
care transitions, 484
causes of, 483*f*
clinical presentation, 477–478
diagnosis, 477–478, 482–483
disease management strategies, 483
epidemiology, 477
initial management, 483
triage, 483
hyperosmolar hyperglycemic state (HHS), 188
care transitions, 193
clinical presentation, 189
diagnosis, 189
disease management strategies, 190–193
DKA *v.,* 190*t*
initial management, 189–190
pathophysiology, 188–189
protocol for managing, 192*f*
triage, 189–190
hyperparathyroidism, 187, 464*t*
hyperphosphatemia, 464*t*
hypertension (HTN). *See also* portal hypertension
cerebral hemorrhage and, 335
classifications, in pregnancy, 180*t*
diastolic HF and, 156
emergencies, causes of, 176*t*
emergencies, clinical presentation, 177–178
emergencies, diagnosis, 177–178
emergencies, initial management, 178–181

emergencies, triage, 178–181
emergency, care transitions, 181
emergency, disease management
    strategies, 181
epidemiology, 174–176
identifiable causes of, 178t
ischemic stroke management and, 332
management in ICH, 336t
managing, 115–116
noncardiac surgery and, 588
parenteral drugs and, 178, 179t
pathophysiology, 176
pharmacologic strategies, 175t
pheochromocytoma and, 187
in preeclampsia, 181t
primary aldosteronism and, 186–187
pulmonary, 111
renal parenchymal disease and,
    185–186
renovascular, 183–185
resistant, 176
secondary, causes, 183t
secondary, clinical features, 184t
secondary, epidemiology, 182
secondary, etiologies, 182–187
severe asymptomatic, 177
substances associated with, 185t
therapy, in CKD, 462t
UGI bleeding and, 255
urgencies/emergencies, 174–181
hyperthyroidism
    amiodarone-induced, 208
    care transitions, 208
    clinical presentation, 205–206
    diagnosis, 205–206
    disease management strategies, 207–208
    hypercalcemia and, 570
    initial treatment, 208t
    pathophysiology, 205
    perioperative medication management
        and, 596
    subclinical, 206
    symptoms, 206t
hypertriglyceridemia, 527
hypnosis, 531
hypnotics, overdose, 369–371
hypoalbuminemia, 526
hypoglycemia, 526
    care transitions, 204
    perioperative medication management
        and, 596
    risk factors, 203t
hypokalemia
    clinical presentation, 485–486
    diagnostic approach to, 488f
    disease management strategies, 489–490
    ECG and, 489f
    epidemiology, 484
    initial management, 487–489

pathophysiology, 484–485
    renal potassium excretion and, 486f
    triage, 487–489
hyponatremia
    clinical presentation, 477–478
    diagnosis, 477–481
    disease management strategies, 482
    epidemiology, 477
    euvolemic, 479–480, 482
    hypervolemic, 480, 482
    hypovolemic, 479, 481
    initial management, 481–482
    triage, 481–482
hypophosphatemia, 571
hyporeninemic hypoaldosteronism, 492
hypotension
    algorithm, 162f
    ARF management and, 457
hypothyroidism
    care transitions, 210
    clinical presentation, 209
    diagnosis, 209
    disease management strategies, 209–210
    pathophysiology, 208–209
    subclinical, 209
    symptoms, 206t
    therapy, 209t
hypoventilation, 408
hypovolemia, 433
hypoxemia, 438
hypoxia
    COPD and, 403
    postoperative, 608

I

IBD. *See* inflammatory bowel disease
ibuprofen, overdose, 366
ibutilide, 144
ICD. *See* implantable cardioverter
    defibrillator
ICH. *See* intracerebral hemorrhage
ICOPER. *See* International Cooperative
    Pulmonary Embolism Registry
ICU. *See* intensive care unit
IDSA. *See* Infectious Disease Society of
    America
IHI. *See* Institute for Healthcare
    Improvement
ILAE. *See* International League Against
    Epilepsy
imaging
    abdominal pain and, 212
    appendicitis and, 215t
    ARF diagnosis and, 455
    CIN prevention and, 449
immigration, FUO and, 281
immobilization, deconditioning and,
    515–516
immune system, UC and, 236

immune thrombocytopenia purpura
    (ITP), 271
immunizations
    frail older adults and, 564
    systolic HF management and, 164
immunosuppression
    FUO and, 281
    skin infections and, 307
implantable cardioverter defibrillator
    (ICD), 154
    systolic HF care transition and, 166, 167
    VT management and, 156
IMV. *See* intermittent mandatory
    ventilation
incident reports, 22
infection(s). *See also* bloodstream
    infections; skin infections; soft tissue
    infections; surgical site infections
    catheter removal and, 295–296
    colitis and, 238t
    colon, 226t
    control issues, 314
    Crohn's disease and, 233
    diabetic foot, 304–305, 305f
    FUO and, 278–279
    influenza and, 297–298
    influenza control, 298t
    LGI bleeding and, 256–257
    with multidrug resistant pathogens, 423t
    neutropenic fever and, 573t
    postoperative fever and, 605–607
    proctitis and, 238t
    SIRS and, 433
    SNF and, 580–582
    surgical consultation and, 302
    water-related, 306
Infectious Disease Society of America
    (IDSA), 295, 421t, 573
inferior vena caval (IVC) filter, 496
inflammation, FUO and, 279
inflammatory bowel disease (IBD), 231
    colitis and, 224t
    extraintestinal manifestations of, 232t
    LGI bleeding and, 257
    management, 233
infliximab, 235
influenza. *See also* avian influenza A
    antiviral agents, 298t
    chemoprophylaxis, 300
    clinical presentation, 297
    diagnosis, 297
    disease management strategies, 298–300
    epidemiology, 296–297
    infection control, 298t
    initial management, 297–298
    pathophysiology, 297
    prevention, 299–300
    triage, 297–298
    vaccination, 299–300, 299t

information technology (IT)
    ADEs and, 23
    communication and, 54
    hospitalist programs and, 50
    medication reconciliation and, 29
informed consent, 351
inhaled glucocorticosteroids (ICS), 401
inotropes, 435
Inouye, Sharon, 569
inpatient attending rounds, 617
    bedside, 619–620
    mobile classroom and, 620
    principles, 617–618
    teaching on a team and, 621–624
inpatient care delivery, 56
inpatient procedures, 5
Inpatient Teaching Rounds, 617
INR. *See* international normalization ratio
Institute for Healthcare Improvement (IHI), 10, 14–15
    rapid cycle improvement, 18–19
Institute of Medicine (IOM), 14
    on care transition efficiency, 60
    LOS and, 57
    patient education and, 72
    patient safety and, 36
    Preventing Medication Errors 2006, 21
insulin
    deficiency, 199*t*
    discharge and, 204
    DKA and, 191–192
    dose adjustment, 203
    duration of action, 201*t*
    effective regimens, 201, 202*t*
    hyperkalemia triage and, 493
    inhibition, 521
    inpatient regimen, 203
    intravenous, 200, 201*t*
    intravenous *v.* subcutaneous, 196*t*
    management issues, 195*t*
    nutrition and, 202*t*
    nutrition monitoring and, 527
    perioperative, 203
    perioperative medication management and, 596
    postoperative, 203
    resistance, 199
    sliding scale, 201, 202*t*
    subcutaneous, 196*t*, 201
    therapy, 195–196
    titration, 203*t*
insurance, 97
integration, 627
integument, 516–517
intensive care unit (ICU)
    bacterial meningitis in, 342*t*
    cerebral hemorrhage triage and, 336
    considerations for asthma, 399*t*

COPD indications, 405*t*
    delirium and, 323
    HTN emergencies and, 178
    sepsis care transitions and, 437
interdisciplinary care, 579–580
intermediate outcome, 81–82
intermittent mandatory ventilation (IMV), 440
    modes, 441
International Classification of Diseases, Ninth Edition, Clinical Modification (ICD-9-CM), 176
International Cooperative Pulmonary Embolism Registry (ICOPER), 504
International League Against Epilepsy (ILAE), 344*t*
international normalization ratio (INR)
    anticoagulants and, 508–509
    medications to reverse, 337*t*
interpersonal styles, 357–359
InterQual, 58
intestinal ischemia, 226
intestinal pseudo-obstruction, 248
intoxication, 366–367
    acute, 373–374
    behavioral disturbances and, 356
intracerebral hemorrhage (ICH), 335. *See also* cerebral hemorrhage
    hypertension management, 336*t*
intracranial arterial circulation, 330*f*
intrahepatic crisis, 266
intra-hospital transfer, 28
intravenous (IV) drug use, 283
intravenous fluids, 479*t*
intravenous inotropic agents, 163
intrinsic PEEP (iPEEP), 442–444
intubation, considerations for, 439
IOM. *See* Institute of Medicine
ipecac, syrup of, 363*t*
iPEEP. *See* intrinsic PEEP
iron treatment, 262
ischemia, 329
    diastolic HF and, 157
    systolic HF care transition and, 166
ischemic cardiomyopathy, 166*f*
ischemic stroke
    algorithm, 332*f*
    care transitions, 333
    clinical presentation, 329–331
    diagnosis, 329–331
    differential diagnosis, 330*t*
    disease management strategies, 331–333
    epidemiology, 328–329
    initial management, 331
    pathophysiology, 328–329
    risk factors, 332*t*
    triage, 331
    vascular symptoms, 330*t*
isopropanol

overdose, 368
    toxic ingestion of, 367*t*
IT. *See* information technology
ITP. *See* immune thrombocytopenia purpura
IV. *See* intravenous drug use
IVC filter. *See* inferior vena caval filter

J
JC. *See* Joint Commission
JCAHO. *See* Joint Commission of Accreditation of Healthcare Organizations
jejunum, 308–309
job fit, 47
Joint Commission of Accreditation of Healthcare Organizations (JCAHO), 14
    acute MI core measures, 121, 121*t*
    AMI and, 106
    handoffs and, 62, 63*t*
    HF and, 159
    inpatient diabetes certification, 199*t*
    medication reconciliation and, 25
    pain assessment, 528*t*
    pain management, 527
    patient education and, 72
    patient safety and, 38
    pneumonia core measures, 413*t*
    quality improvement and, 41
    test results follow-ups and, 76
joints
    common contractures of, 517*t*
    deconditioning and, 516
jugular venous pressure (JVP), 390
junctional tachycardia, 137
JVP. *See* jugular venous pressure

K
kava, 599
ketoacidosis, 473*t*
    alcohol, 367
ketogenesis, 189
ketosis, 368
kidney stones, 213
kidneys, 458
kidneys, ureter, bladder (KUB), 213–214
King's College Criteria, 219
Klebsiella pneumoniae, 313–314
Knowles, Malcolm, 615, 625
Korsakoff's syndrome, 376
kyphoscoliosis, 389

L
lab tests. *See also* testing
    ARF diagnosis and, 410, 454–455
    CAP triage and, 415–417
    dyspnea diagnosis and, 390–391
    for hyponatremia, 481

MRSA and, 302
  neutropenic fever and, 573
  pleural effusion and, 427–430
  redundant, 69
lactulose, 223
lamotrigine, 349
language, 318*t*
laparoscopy, 250
laparotomy, 247
late withdrawal syndrome, 375
latent conditions, 17
latex agglutination, 309
laws
  patient safety and, 38
  suicide and, 386–387
leadership, 7–8
  academies, 50
  by example, 55
  teaching and, 621
  teamwork and, 624
Leapfrog Group, 14
learner heterogeneity, 619
learning
  environment, 616
  self-directed, 624
  systems, 18
Lee Revised Cardiac Risk Index, 586
left ventricular ejection fraction (LVEF),
    119, 156. *See also* systolic
    dysfunction
  diagnosis, 157, 157*t*
  evaluation, 124–126
  HF and, 156
  treatment, 158*t*
Lehman, Betsy, 14
length of stay (LOS)
  ADE costs and, 21
  care transition efficiency and, 61
  data, 49
  definition of, 57–58
  efficiency and, 58
  history of, 57
  hyperglycemia and, 198
  increasing factors, 58
  optimizing, 59*t*
  QI and, 59–60
lepirudin, 512–513
leukemia, 570
leukotriene modifiers, 401
levothryoxine (LT4), 209
LFTs. *See* liver function tests
LGI bleeding. *See* lower gastrointestinal
    bleeding
ligaments, deconditioning and, 516
likelihood ratio (LR), 93–94
  nomogram, 95*f*
  physical examinations and, 95–96
linezolid, 312
lipase, 243

lipid lowering agents, 594
lipids, 522
  in TPN, 526
listening, 561
literacy
  assessing for, 74–75
  health, 73, 558
lithium, 597
liver disease
  end-stage, 220*t*
  noncardiac surgery and, 591
liver enzymes, abnormal, 217*t*
liver failure
  acetaminophen overdose and, 362
  acute, 218–219, 219*f*
  King's College Criteria, 219
liver function tests (LFTs), 602
liver injury, hepatocellular, 218*t*
liver transplantation, 221
LMWH. *See* low molecular weight
    heparin
loop diuretics
  ARF prevention strategies and, 448
  in ARF triage, 457
  hypercalcemia of malignancy and, 571
  intravenous, 163
lorazepam, 543
LOS. *See* length of stay
low molecular weight heparin (LMWH),
    496–497, 499
  drug action, 510–511
  outpatient therapy, 506*t*
  in prophylaxis, 511
  in treatment, 511
  VTE therapy and, 504
lower gastrointestinal (LGI) bleeding
  care transitions, 259
  clinical presentation, 256–257
  diagnostic evaluation, 259
  ED triage, 257–258
  epidemiology, 256
  initial management, 258
  management algorithm, 258*t*
LR. *See* likelihood ratio
LT4. *See* levothryoxine
lumbar puncture (LP)
  ICH diagnosis and, 336
  meningitis diagnosis and, 339
  seizure triage and, 347
LVEF. *See* left ventricular ejection fraction

M
magnesium, 193
magnetic resonance imaging (MRI)
  abdominal pain and, 214
  cardiac, 118
  cost-effectiveness analysis of, 97
  epidural spinal cord compression and, 577
  FUO management and, 282

ICH diagnosis and, 336
  pancreatitis diagnosis and, 244
malignancy
  hypercalcemia of, 569–572
  hypercalcemia of, medications, 572*t*
malnutrition. *See also* nutrition
  algorithm, 523*f*
  care transitions, 527
  disease management strategies, 526–527
  epidemiology, 520
  initial management, 521–522
  pathophysiology, 521
  triage, 521–522
malpractice, 39
management, 47
manuscript format, 102
marijuana, abuse management, 382
MAT. *See* multifocal atrial tachycardia
measure, 19
measurement, 19–20
  for quality improvement, 43–44
mechanical ventilation
  initiating, 439
  management, 442–444
  modes, 441
  physiologic goals, 441–442
  sedation and, 442
  types, 439–441
  weaning from, 444–445
Meckel's diverticulum, 257
MedEdPORTAL, 630
MEDENOX trial, 496–497
Medicaid, 14
medical conditions, categorization of, 13
medical history
  ARF diagnosis and, 408
  colitis and, 227*t*
  concomitant, 530
  drug abuse and, 380
  dyspnea diagnosis and, 389
  pain management, 530
  pancreatitis diagnosis and, 243
  seizure triage and, 346–347
  syncope and, 170
  UC and, 237–238
Medicare
  Cooperative Cardiovascular Project, 559
  HF and, 159
  hospice care and, 25
  patient safety and, 14
  SNF and, 581*t*
medication discrepancies, 24
  causes of, 24–25
  risk factors, 25
medication history
  medication discrepancies and, 24
  pharmacists and, 29
  preadmission, 26
  tips, 28*t*

medication list
    preadmission, 26–28
    pre-discharge, 26
medication reconciliation, 19
    at admission, 28
    CPOE and, 29
    at discharge, 28–29
    elderly and, 25
    errors, 25
    evidence of, 25–26
    at intra-hospital transfer, 28
    process, 26–29, 27f
    sinus bradycardia care transitions
        and, 151
    staffing and, 29
medications. *See also* polypharmacy
    for ACS, 125t
    adherence, 24
    for AF chemical cardioversion, 133t
    for AF rate control, 132t
    allergies, 28t
    ARF and, 446
    behavioral disturbances and, 356
    common stroke, 334t
    for confusion, 321
    cost-effectiveness analysis of, 97
    de-marketing, 99
    at discharge, 71
    dosage, for Crohn's disease, 234t
    drug fevers and, 280t
    ESRD, 466
    frail older adults and, 564, 567–569
    increasing, 68
    overuse of prophylactic, 31
    parenteral, 178, 179t
    perioperative medication management
        and, 592
    postoperative fever and, 606t
    processes, 22–23
    to reduce INR, 337t
    for slowing dementia, 322t
    unnecessary, 581t
medicolegal issues, suicide and, 386–387
medullary renal ischemia, 448
meetings, family, 555–556, 556t
megacolon, 213
MELD score, LFTs and, 602
melena, 251
memantine, 322t
memory, confusion and, 318t
meningitis. *See also* primary amebic
        meningitis
    antibiotics for bacterial, 341t
    aseptic, 342, 343
    bacterial, 341
    bacterial, in ICU, 342t
    care transitions, 343
    clinical presentation, 339–341
    CSF profiles and, 340t, 341

diagnosis, 339–341
disease management strategies, 343
epidemiology, 339
pathogens, 340t
pathophysiology, 339
triage, 343
viral, 342
Meningitis Foundation of America, Inc., 343
mental status, of frail older adults, 565
mentorship, 100, 627, 628–629
meta-analysis, 85
    plot, 87f
metabolic cart, 522
metabolic system, deconditioning and, 518
methadone
    equinalgesic conversion to, 533t
    pain management and, 540
methanol
    acid-base disorders and, 473t
    overdose, 368–369
    toxic ingestion of, 367t
    toxicity, 368t
methenamine hippurate, 293
methenamine mandelate, 293
methicillin-resistant *Staphylococcal
        aureus* (MRSA), 284
    antibiotic-resistant pathogens and,
        311–312
    carrier state, 312
    community acquired, 304, 312
    control issues, 314
    in sepsis management, 436
    skin infections and, 301
methimazole, 207
methotrexate, 234
methylenedioxymethamphetamine
        (ecstasy), 382
metronidazole, 229
MI. *See* myocardial infarction
MIC. *See* minimum inhibitory
        concentration
microskills model
    five-step, 623t
    of teaching, 623–624
migraines, seizures and, 346
Mini-Cog dementia screen, 566f
minimum inhibitory concentration
        (MIC), 286
MIST1. *See* First Multicenter Intrapleural
        Sepsis Trial
mitral valve prolapse, 111–112
mobility
    barriers to, 519
    of frail older adults, 565
Modification of Diet in Renal Disease
        equation, 460
monitoring, 18
mood disorders, suicide and, 384
morphine, 163

mortality
    benefit, 2t
    LOS and, 58
Motorola, 18
MPI. *See* myocardial perfusion imaging
MRI. *See* magnetic resonance imaging
MRSA. *See* methicillin-resistant
        Staphylococcal aureus
multidisciplinary collaboration, 7
    ED and, 10
    teamwork and, 54
multidisciplinary team, 41–43
    ground rules, 42t
Multifactorial Risk Index, 608
multifocal atrial tachycardia (MAT), 137
Murphy's sign, 215
muscle relaxants, 537
myasthenia gravis, 597
mycobacterium tuberculosis (MB), 430
myelopathy, 576
myelosuppressive chemotherapeutic
        agents, 573
myocardial infarction (MI)
    aspirin and, 106
    AV blocks and, 148
    CCU hyperglycemia and, 196
    CIN and, 448
    CK-MB and, 115
    cost-effectiveness analysis of, 97
    diabetes and, 122 and
    missed diagnosis of, 105
    noncardiac surgery and, 585
    sinus bradycardia and, 148
myocardial perfusion imaging (MPI), 118
myochosis, 240
myoclonus, opioid-induced, 544
myxedema coma, 209

N

NAC. *See* N-acetylcysteine
N-acetylcysteine (NAC), 451
NAO inhibitors, 597
narrative reviews, 85
narrow complex tachycardia
    diagnosis of, 140t
    ECG analysis of, 141f
    management of, 144f
nasogastric suctioning, 589–590
nasogastric (NG) tubes
    SBO triage and, 249–250
    UGI bleeding and, 251
NASPE. *See* North American Society for
        Pacing and Electrophysiology
National Adult Literacy Survey, 73
National Coordinating Council Medication
        Error Reporting Program
        (NCCMERP), 21
National Council on Alcoholism and Drug
        Dependence, 372

National Guideline Clearinghouse (NGC), 90, 412
National Healthcare Disparities Report (NHDR), 559, 560–561
National In-patient Survey (NIS), 558
National Institute for Health and Clinical Excellence (NICE), 90
National Institute of Health Stroke Scale (NIHSS), 336
National Institute on Drug Abuse, 372
National Institutes of Health (NIH)
    endoscopy and, 253
    grants, 102
    hypertension and, 115–116
National Nosocomial Infections Surveillance (NNIS), 295, 605
    definition of bloodstream infection, 295t
national performance targets, 11
National Quality Forum (NQF), 14
National Vital Statistics Report, 383
nausea
    appendicitis and, 214
    opioid side effects and, 536
    opioid-related, 542–543
    treatment, 543t
NCCMERP. See National Coordinating Council Medication Error Reporting Program
NDI. See nephrogenic diabetes inisipidus
necrotizing fasciitis (NF), 304, 306
needs assessment, 616
negative predictive value (NPV), 92f, 93
negligence, 39
Neisseria meningitidis, 339
neoplasms, 279
    LGI bleeding and, 257
nephrogenic diabetes inisipidus (NDI), 482
nephrogenic systemic fibrosis (NSF), 468
nephrons, 458
nephrotoxicity, 446
    aminoglycoside-induced, 447
    diabetes and, 197t
    direct, 448
nephrotoxins, 446–447
    ARF management and, 457
    CIN prevention and, 449
networking, 629–630
neuraminidase, 297
    inhibitors, 298–299
neurodegenerative disease, 316
neuroimaging, 317
neuroleptics
    opioid-induced nausea and, 542
    for terminal restlessness, 549t
neurologic systems
    deconditioning and, 518
    noncardiac surgery and, 591
neurological disorders, 319–320t

neurological sequelae, 343
    methanol overdose and, 369
neuromuscular disease, 388
neuropathy, 304
    neutropenic fever, 572–575
    antifungal therapy and, 575t
    febrile, 574f
    infection and, 573t
    management, 574f
New York Heart Association (NYHA), 161
NF. See necrotizing fasciitis
NG tubes. See nasogastric tubes
NGC. See National Guideline Clearinghouse
NHDR. See National Healthcare Disparities Report
NICE. See National Institute for Health and Clinical Excellence
NICHE. See Nurses Improving Care for Health System Elders
nicotine cessation, 116
night coverage, 47
NIH. See National Institutes of Health
NIHSS. See National Institute of Health Stroke Scale
NIPPV. See noninvasive positive pressure ventilation
nitrates, perioperative medication management and, 594
nitric oxide, inhaled, 411
nitrofurantoin, 291
NIV. See noninvasive mechanical ventilation
NMDA antagonists, 537
NNIS. See National Nosocomial Infections Surveillance
NNT. See number-needed-to-treat
Nolan, Tom, 42f
nomogram, 94
    LR, 95f
    plasma, 365f
noncardiac surgery, 585
    ACC/AHA guidelines, 588f
    cardiovascular evaluation and, 585–588
    endocrinologic evaluation for, 590
    hematologic for, 590–591
    pulmonary evaluation for, 588–590
non-compete clauses, 48
noninvasive mechanical ventilation (NIV), 405
noninvasive positive pressure ventilation (NIPPV)
    ARF triage and, 412
    contraindications for, 438, 439t
    definition, 438
    goals, 438
    indications for, 438
    initiation of, 439

non-ST-elevation myocardial infarction (NSTEMI), 120, 122–124
    TMI risk score for, 124f
nonsteroidal anti-inflammatory drugs (NSAIDs)
    ARF and, 446
    colitis induced by, 226
    overdose management, 365–366
    UGI bleeding and, 251
    ulcer disease and, 254
normal sinus rhythm (NSR), 133
    AF management and, 135
norovirus, 308
    diagnosis, 308–309
North American Society for Pacing and Electrophysiology (NASPE), 150–151
Norwalk gastroenteritis, 582
NPV. See negative predictive value
NSAIDs. See nonsteroidal anti-inflammatory drugs
NSF. See nephrogenic systemic fibrosis
NSR. See normal sinus rhythm
nuclear medicine, 281
null hypothesis, 85
number-needed-to-treat (NNT), 86–88, 88t
Nurses Improving Care for Health System Elders (NICHE), 569
nursing home. See skilled nursing facility
nutrition. See also diet; malnutrition
    care plans, 520–521
    CKD management and, 462, 463
    daily assessment tool, 568t
    deconditioning management and, 519
    enternal, 522–523
    of frail older adults, 567
    hospitalization and, 520–527
    insulin and, 202t
    monitoring, 526–527
    pancreatitis triage and, 245
    parenteral, 525
    screening, 521
    SNF and, 582
    support, initiating, 522–526
NYHA. See New York Heart Association

O
OACs. See oral anticoagulants
obesity, 522
    secondary HTN and, 182–183
observational studies, of EBM, 84–85
obsession, 353
obstructive sleep apnea (OSA)
    secondary HTN and, 183
    sinus bradycardia and, 148
odds ratio, 87f
OG. See osmolar gap
olanzapine, 543–544
ondansetron, 543

opioid(s)
  abuse management, 381
  addiction and, 532
  administration, 534
  breakthrough dose, 540t
  characteristics, 533t
  choices, 534
  classification, 532t
  conversion, 535t
  dosing, 534
  dyspnea and, 545–546
  overdose, 370
  palliative care and, 548
  perioperative medication management
    and, 598
  respiratory depression induced by, 537t
  rotation, 540t
  side effects, 536, 537, 541–544
  starting doses, 534t
  sustained-release, 535
  terminology, 532
  therapy, 532–534
  tolerance, 537, 541–544
  weaning, 536
oral anticoagulants (OACs), 504
organ dysfunction criteria, 433t
orthostatic hypotension, 173
OSA. *See* obstructive sleep apnea
Osler, William, 619
osmolar gap (OG), 472
osteomyelitis, 304–305
outcome measures, 43
  EBM, 81–82
oxalate crystals, 367
oxcarbazepine, 349
Oxford Centre for Evidence-Based
  Medicine, 83
oxygen therapy
  for acute exacerbations of COPD,
    404–405
  for asthma triage, 397–398
  CAP triage and, 417
  delivery *v.* demand, 434t

P
P value, 85–86
PA. *See* physician advisor; plasma
  aldosterone
pacemakers, 150–151
packed red blood cells (pRBCs), 274
PaCO$_2$, 470
Paget-Schroetter Syndrome, 502
pain, 527. *See also* abdominal pain
  acute, 527
  acute, in opioid tolerant, 537
  aseptic meningitis and, 342
  assessment, 528t, 529
  back, 577, 577t
  chronic, 528

consequences, 528t
consultation, 538
determine mechanism of, 530, 530t
epidural spinal cord compression
  and, 576
evaluation, 539–541
intensity, 529–530
numerical rating scale, 529
palliative care and, 548
referred, 211t
scales, 529–530, 529f
suicide and, 384–385
pain management, 527
  definitions, 527–528
  guidelines, 528–531
  non-pharmacologic measures, 531–532
  palliative care and, 539–541
  SCD and, 266
  suggested, 531t
pain/palliative care, 539–541
palliative care. *See also* hospice care
  advanced care planning and, 552–553
  anxiety and, 546–547
  comfort and, 553
  communication and, 549–556
  depression and, 546–547
  dying patients and, 545
  of imminently dying patient, 548–549
  overview, 25
  pain management and, 539–541
  psychiatric consultation and, 547t
  psychosocial issues and, 551–552
  spiritual distress and, 547–548
palpitations, 138t
PAM. *See* primary amebic meningitis
p-ANCA. *See* perinuclear antineutrophil
  cytoplasmic antibodies
pancreatic necrosis, 245–246
pancreatitis
  care transitions, 246
  clinical presentation, 243–244
  diagnosis, 243–244
  disease management strategies, 246
  epidemiology, 242
  gallstone, 246
  initial management, 244–246
  pathophysiology, 242–243
  triage, 244–246
papillary necrosis, 266
PA/PRA ratio, 186
paraldehyde, 474t
paranoia, 353
  personality dysfunction and, 358
parapneumonic effusion, 430–431
parasites, of colon, 226t
parathyroid hormone (PTH), 463t
partial thromboplastin time (PTT), 601
  UH and, 509
Partners Healthcare, Inc., 29

PAS. *See* physician-assisted suicide
pathophysiology, 62
pathways, 59–60
patient(s). *See also* dialysis patients; frail
    older adults; suicidal patients
  advanced care planning and, 552–553
  angina pectoral and, 115
  autonomy, 562
  communication in palliative care,
    550–551
  confronting fears, 553–554
  death and, 554–555
  depression and, 547t
  dying, 545
  expectations, 38–39
  functional decline in, 516t
  handoffs, 7
  imminently dying, 548–549
  incompetent, 353–354
  instructions, 69
  portals, 80
  postoperative, 132–133
  preferences, 560
  questions of, 73t
  refusing transfusion, 277t
  satisfaction, 2
  triage surgical, 11f
patient adherence
  to medication, 24
  to prescribed therapies, 72–73
patient bill of rights, 13
patient education, 72
  for AF, 135
  CAP management and, 417
  chronic illness and, 73–74
  competency and, 352
  deconditioning management and, 518
  on discharge, 69
  ischemic stroke and, 333
  literacy and, 74–75
  for LMWH therapy, 506t
  polypharmacy and, 35
  UC and, 240
patient outcomes research team (PORT)
    study, 417
patient safety, 13
  apologies and, 38–39
  background of, 36
  defect rate and, 16
  disclosure and, 38–39
  engineering and, 15–16
  examples, 37t
  handoffs and, 63t
  history of, 13–15
  hospital-specific interventions, 37–38
  improvement, 18–20
  improvement cycle, 19
  improvement model, 19f
  key principles, 38t

laws, 38
patient education and, 72
principles, 36–37
regulations, 38
teamwork and, 56
terms, 37*t*
patient-centered care, 72
patient-controlled analgesia. *See* PCA
pay-for-performance incentives, 11
patient safety and, 15
PBPs. *See* penicillin-binding proteins
PCA (patient-controlled analgesia),
536, 536*t*
PCI. *See* percutaneous coronary
intervention
PCPs. *See* primary care physicians
PCV. *See* pressure control ventilation
PDSA cycle. *See* plan, do, study, act cycle
PE. *See* pulmonary embolism
PEA. *See* pulseless electrical activity
peak expiratory flow (PEF) assessment,
396
peak pressures, 441, 441*t*
PEEP. *See* positive-end expiratory pressure
peer review, 38
PEF assessment. *See* peak expiratory flow
assessment
penicillin-binding proteins (PBPs), 310
percutaneous coronary intervention
(PCI), 121
complications, 123*t*
urgent, 124
percutaneous transluminal renal
angioplasty (PTRA), 185
perfusion, in sepsis triage, 434–435
pericarditis, 110–111
uremic, 468
perinuclear antineutrophil cytoplasmic
antibodies (p-ANCA), 233
perioperative cardiac events, 585–586
perioperative medication management,
592
by drug type, 592–598
summary of, 593*t*
peritonitis, 214
permanent pacing, 151*t*
personal leverage, 359
personality
defense levels, 360*t*
dysfunction, 357–359
issues, 353
suicide and, 384
perspective, in cost-effectiveness
analysis, 98
PET imaging, 118
pharmacists
ADEs and, 26
medication history and, 29
phenobarbital, overdose, 369

phenytoin, 348
pheochromocytoma
noncardiac surgery and, 590
secondary HTN and, 187
phosphorus, 463*t*
phyncyclidine (PCP), abuse management,
382
physical examination
abdominal, 211–212
acute hepatitis and, 217
ARF diagnosis and, 408–410
for asthma, 396
for dialysis patients, 466
dyspnea diagnosis and, 389–390
of frail older adults, 565
HTN emergencies and, 177
LR and, 95–96
pain management and, 530–531
pancreatitis diagnosis and, 243
SBO diagnosis and, 248
syncope and, 170–171
physician advisor (PA), 9
physician override functions, 9
Physician Payment Review Commission, 59
physician-assisted suicide (PAS), 554
physicians
biases, 560
in SNF, 580*t*
test results awareness of, 77
PICC lines, 469
PICO format, 81
questions, 82*f*
"pill-in-the-pocket" approach, 145–146
PIOPED. *See* prospective investigation of
pulmonary embolism diagnosis
placebos, 528
plan, do, study, act (PDSA) cycle, 43
planning and prioritization process, 8*f*, 9*t*
planning, research and, 100
plasma aldosterone (PA), 186
plasma osmolality, 190*t*, 477
plasma renin activity (PRA), 186
plateau pressures, 441, 441*t*
platelets
aggregation, 176
bleeding risk and, 268
clot formation and, 507
decreased production, 268*t*
peripheral destruction, 269*t*
preoperative testing of, 600–601
transfusion, 274–275
transfusion triggers, 275*t*
UGI bleeding and, 252
pleural effusion, 427–430
algorithm, 429*t*
CAP triage and, 415
differential diagnosis, 430*t*
postoperative, 608
pleural fluid, 428–429

pneumonia. *See also* community-acquired
pneumonia
aspiration, 393–394
bacterial, 299
complications from, 426–427
core measures, 413*t*
criteria for hospitalization, 582*t*
nonresolving, 427, 428*f*
postoperative, 607
severe, 420*t*
SNF and, 582
viral, 298
pneumothorax
acute, 111
dyspnea triage and, 394
point estimate, 86
poison, antidotes, 364*t*
polypharmacy
care transitions and, 35
communication and, 35
conditions caused by, 32–33*t*
contributors, 35*t*
definition, 30
epidemiology of, 30–31
etiology, 31–32
management strategies, 32–35, 35*t*
prevention, 31*t*, 33*t*, 34*f*
rational, 30
risk factors, 33
PORT study. *See* patient outcomes
research team study
portal hypertension
physiological changes in, 220*t*
testing, 221*t*
upper gastrointestinal bleeding, 222
positional orthostatic tachycardia
syndrome (POTS), 138
positive predictive value (PPV), 92*f*, 93
positive-end expiratory pressure (PEEP)
in ARDS, 444*t*
goals, for mechanical ventilation, 441
modes, for mechanical ventilation, 441
positron electron tomography (PET)
imaging. *See* PET imaging
post-endoscopic intervention, 257
post-ischemic ATN, 446
postoperative complications, 604
HF and, 609–610
pulmonary, 607–610
postoperative pulmonary complications
(PPCs), 588–589
odds ratio, 589*t*
potassium. *See also* hyperkalemia;
hypokalemia
acid-base disorders and, 485
disorders of, 484
DKA and, 192
endogenous, 492
exogenous, 491–492

potassium (*Cont.*):
   handling, 485*f*
   hypokalemia triage and, 487–489
   in intravenous fluids, 479*t*
   redistribution, in cells, 486*t*
   redistribution, out of cells, 489*t*
   reduced renal excretion of, 490*t*
   removal, 493
   renal excretion of, 486*f*
   replacement, 489
   salts, 487–489
potassium chloride, 489
   preparations, 490*t*
POTS. *See* positional orthostatic
   tachycardia syndrome
power, 85
PPCs. *See* postoperative pulmonary
   complications
PPIs. *See* proton pump inhibitors
PPS. *See* prospective payment system
PPV. *See* positive predictive value
PRA. *See* plasma renin activity
practice guidelines. *See* guidelines
pRBCs. *See* packed red blood cells
predictive values, 93
preeclampsia, 180
   acute HTN in, 181*t*
   secondary HTN and, 187
pregnancy
   asymptomatic bacteriuria and, 290
   diabetes and, 203–204
   HTN emergencies and, 179
   hypertension classifications, 180*t*
   risk definitions, 509*t*
   seizures and, 349
   SVT management and, 146
   transfusion indications, 274
preoperative screening tests, 599–600
   common, 600–603
   for elective surgery, 600*t*
prescription cascade, 31–32
prescriptions
   patient adherence to, 72–73
   perioperative medication management
      and, 592
   polypharmacy prevention and, 34–35
presentation, 631
pressure control ventilation (PCV), 440
pressure cycling, 440
pressure support ventilation (PSV), 441
pressure ulcers
   preventing, 519
   SNF and, 583
pretest probability, 107
pretibial myxedema, 207
prevalence, 93
PREVENT trial, 497
priapism, 266
primary aldosteronism, 186

primary amebic meningitis (PAM), 341
primary care physicians (PCPs), 50
   abdominal pain and, 211
   care transition efficiency and, 61
   post-discharge test results and, 79
   pressures on, 1
   vulnerable populations and, 562
primary hyperaldosteronism, 186
private hospitalist practice, 48
probability, 86
   LR and, 94
   predictive values and, 93
procainamide, 144
procedure competencies, 5
procedure services, 10
process, 19
   improvement, 18–19
   targets, 11
process measures, 43
   for EBM, 81
prochlorperazine, 542
proctitis, 238*t*
proctocolectomy, 239
projects
   choosing, 42–43
   research, 100
propafenone, 144
propofol, 378
propylthiouracil, 207
prospective investigation of pulmonary
   embolism diagnosis (PIOPED), 110
prospective payment system (PPS), 57
prostatitis, 292
prosthetic heart values, 283
protein, 522
proteinuria
   CKD management and, 462
   reduction, 462*t*
   SCD and, 266
   screening, 460
prothrombin complex concentrate (PCC),
   337*t*
prothrombin time (PT), 252
prothrombin time/international normalized
   ratio (PT/INR), 601
proton pump inhibitors (PPIs), 254
   perioperative medication management
      and, 598
pruritus
   opioid side effects and, 537
   opioid-induced, 544
pseudohyperkalemia, 491
pseudohyponatremia, 480–481
pseudoseizures. *See* psychogenic
   non-epileptic spells
pseudothrombocytopenia, 269
PSV. *See* pressure support ventilation
psychiatric consultation, palliative care
   and, 547*t*

psychiatric disorders
   behavioral disturbances and, 357
   confusion and, 319–320*t*
psychiatric hospitalization, 372
   suicidal patients and, 387
psychiatric illness, 353
psychogenic non-epileptic spells, 346
psychosocial issues, 551–552, 551*t*
psychotic disorders, 384
psychotropic medications, 358
PT. *See* prothrombin time
PTH. *See* parathyroid hormone
PT/INR. *See* prothrombin
   time/international normalized ratio
PTRA. *See* percutaneous transluminal
   renal angioplasty
PTT. *See* partial thromboplastin time
public agency initiatives, 495*t*
public awareness, 16
public health, 231
publications, 630
pulmonary abnormalities, 411*t*
pulmonary artery catheterization, 411
pulmonary complications, 607–610
pulmonary edema
   algorithm, 162*f*
   CT of, 393*f*
   CXR of, 393*f*
pulmonary embolism (PE)
   acute, 110, 391–392, 502
   chest, 110
   diagnostic approach to, 503*f*
   DVT and, 494
   EKG of, 392*f*
   postoperative, 608
   risk stratification, 505*t*
   symptoms, 502
   VTE and, 501
pulmonary evaluation, 588–590
pulmonary function testing, 410–411
pulse oximetry, 389
pulseless electrical activity (PEA), 129*t*
pulsus paradoxus, 389
purple urine bag syndrome, 293
purpura, 276. *See also* immune
   thrombocytopenia purpura
pyelonephritis, 291
   UTI and, 289
pyuria, 291

Q
QALY. *See* quality-adjusted life-year
QI. *See* quality improvement
QRS complex, 149
quality improvement (QI), 41
   choosing projects for, 42–43
   common tools, 44, 44*t*
   effecting change in, 44
   initiatives, 6, 7

LOS and, 59–60
model, 42f, 43
model for, 41–44
monitoring, 44
planning, 43–44
rapid cycle improvement and, 44
quality of care, 2
quality-adjusted life-year (QALY),
97–98
questions
5S model and, 88–89
adult learning, 616t
in conference room teaching, 619
for diagnosing confusion, 317
EBM and, 81
open-ended, 551t
of patients, 73t
psychosocial issues and, 551t
self-directed learning and, 624
using PICO format, 82f
quetiapine, 544
quinupristin-dalfopristin, 313

R
race
Crohn's disease and, 231
hospitalization and, 557, 558–559
NHDR and, 560–561
readmissions and, 559
radiation proctitis, 257
radiation therapy (RT), 578
radioactive iodine uptake (RAIU), 206
radiography. See also x-rays
colitis and, 228
dyspnea diagnosis and, 390–391
HF diagnosis and, 161
renovascular HTN and, 185
SBO diagnosis and, 249
UC diagnosis and, 237
radionuclide imaging, 259
RAIU. See radioactive iodine uptake
randomized controlled trials (RCTs),
499
of EBM, 83
Ranson criteria, 245t
rapid cycle improvement, 18–19
quality improvement and, 44
rapid response teams (RRTs), 7, 9–10
IHI and, 15
rapid ventricular response (RVR),
130–131
rate control, 134, 135
RBCs. See red blood cells
RBI. See relative benefit increase
RCA. See root cause analysis
RCTs. See randomized controlled trials
RDW. See red cell distribution
read-backs, 64
reading level, 74

readmission
LOS and, 58
race/gender, 559
rates, 49
receiver operating characteristic (ROC)
curves, 94–95
graph, 95f
red blood cells (RBCs). See also packed
red blood cells
anemia and, 261
morphology, 262t
red cell distribution (RDW), 260
REE. See resting energy expenditure
reentrant circuits, 137
reentry, 152
regressive behavior, 358–359
regulations
LOS and, 58
patient safety, 38
rehabilitation therapy, 372
for ischemic stroke, 333
relative benefit increase (RBI), 88
relative risk (RR), 86–87
calculating, 88t
relative risk reduction (RRR), 87
calculating, 88t
reliability, 15–16
religion. See spirituality
renal disease
atheroembolic, 455–456
CCU hyperglycemia and, 196–197
HHS and, 193
renal failure. See also acute renal failure
acid-base disorders and, 474t
CIN and, 448–449
renal function, preoperative testing
of, 602
renal parenchymal disease, 185–186
renal profusion, 447
renal replacement therapy, 456
renal systems, 591
renal tube acidosis (RTA), 474–475t
renal-angiotensin activity, 186
Rennie, Drummond, 89
reperfusion strategies, 122
repetition, 74
repolarization abnormalities, 152
report card, 8t
research
assistants, 101
coordinators, 101
dimensions for hospitalists, 100t
disseminating, 102
ethics of, 13
funding, 101–102
manuscript format, 102
necessary steps, 100t
necessary steps in, 100–102
researchers, hospitalists as, 99–102

resident(s)
as team leaders, 624
work hours, 2
work-hour restrictions, 10
respiration, in sepsis triage, 434
respiratory depression
dyspnea and, 388
opioid-induced, 537t
opioid-related, 541
respiratory failure. See also acute
respiratory failure
dyspnea and, 388
mechanical ventilation initiation and,
439
respiratory rate, for mechanical
ventilation, 441
respiratory system, deconditioning and, 517
respiratory therapy, 439
respite care, for homeless, 561
resting energy expenditure (REE), 522
resting pulmonary congestion, 161
resuscitation
algorithm for septic shock, 435f
in sepsis triage, 434–435
reticulocyte production index (RPI), 260
revascularization
in ischemic cardiomyopathy, 166f
NSTEMI and, 124
systolic HF care transition and, 166
rhabdomyolysis, 455–456
rhythm control, 134
rifampin, 288
RIFLE criteria, 452, 453t
right ventricular (RV) dysfunction, 503
risk
baseline, 88t
definition of, 86
denial and, 352–353
management, 39
reduction, 86–88
risk stratification
ACS and, 124–126
AMI and, 121
chest pain and, 114t
polypharmacy and, 32–33
systolic HF triage and, 164
rivastigmine, 322t
Rockall scoring system, 253t
role models, 624
root cause analysis (RCA), 37
rotavirus, 308
RPI. See reticulocyte production index
RR. See relative risk
RRR. See relative risk reduction
RRTs. See rapid response teams
rules, breaking, 17
RV dysfunction. See right ventricular
dysfunction
RVR. See rapid ventricular response

S

SAH. *See* subarachnoid hemorrhage
salaries, 47
salicylates
  acid-base disorders and, 474*t*
  indications for hemodialysis from, 366*t*
  overdose management, 366
sample size, 86
SBAR, 55
  handoffs and, 64–65, 64*t*
SBO. *See* small bowel obstruction
SBT. *See* spontaneous breathing trials
SCD. *See* sickle cell disease
schizophrenia
  behavioral disturbances and, 357
  confusion and, 316
scholarship
  education and, 628
  progression of, 628
  research *v.* educational, 629*t*
  types of, 627–632
SCM. *See* surgical comanagement
Scottish Intercollegiate Guidelines
    Network (SIGN), 90
sedatives
  mechanical ventilation and, 442
  opioid-related, 541
  overdose, 369–371
seizure(s)
  absence, 345
  AED regimens, 349*t*
  alcohol withdrawal, 375
  care transitions, 349
  cerebral hemorrhage triage and, 338
  clinical presentation, 344–346
  diagnosis, 344–346
  differential diagnosis, 346
  disease management strategies,
    348–349
  encephalitis and, 343
  epidemiology, 344
  generalized, 345
  ILAE classification of, 344*t*
  initial management, 346–348
  partial, 344–345
  partial, temporal lobe, 345*t*
  pathophysiology, 344
  post-ictal symptoms, 345*t*
  syncope and, 170
  triage, 346–348
selective estrogen receptor modulators
    (SERMs), 596–597
selective serotonin reuptake inhibitors
    (SSRIs)
  anxiety treatment and, 547*t*
  palliative care and, 547
  perioperative medication management
    and, 597
self-management strategies, 73–74

self-reflection
  educational portfolio and, 632
  on teaching, 620–621
  vulnerable populations and, 561
self-reporting
  adult learning and, 617
  palliative care and, 540
sensitivity, 92–93, 92*f*
  of cardiac stress testing, 118*t*
  false negatives and, 94
sepsis
  CAP triage and, 413–415
  care transitions, 437
  catheter-related, 525
  clinical presentation, 433
  diagnosis, 433
  disease management strategies, 435–437
  epidemiology, 432–433
  focus control, 435–436
  initial management, 434–435
  pathophysiology, 433
  resuscitation algorithm, 435*f*
  sources of, 434*t*
  stages of, 432*t*
  triage, 434–435
septic shock, 433
  CAP triage and, 415
  corticosteroid guidelines for, 436*t*
  resuscitation algorithm, 435*f*
SERMs. *See* selective estrogen receptor
    modulators
Seroquel. *See* quetiapine
serum creatinine, 186
serum leukocytosis, 291
1700 rule, 196*t*
SHEA. *See* Society for Healthcare
    Epidemiology of America
SHM. *See* Society of Hospital Medicine
shock algorithm, 162*f*
shortness of breath (dyspnea), 545–546,
    549
  clinical presentation, 389–391
  diagnosis, 389–391
  differential diagnosis, 388*t*
  epidemiology, 388
  initial management, 391–394
  pathophysiology, 388–389
  postoperative, 608
  triage, 391–394
shunt, 408
SIADH. *See* syndrome of inappropriate
    antidiuretic hormone
sick sinus syndrome, 147–148
sickle cell disease (SCD)
  clinical features, 263–264
  discharge planning, 267
  epidemiology, 263
  painful episode management, 266
  surgical considerations, 267

  treatment, 265–267
  triage, 264–265
sigmoidoscopy
  Crohn's disease and, 234
  UC diagnosis and, 237
SIGN. *See* Scottish Intercollegiate
    Guidelines Network
sign-out, 62
  quality, 65*t*
sign-over, 62
simulations, 17
SIMV. *See* synchronized intermittent
    mandatory ventilation
sinus abnormalities, 148*f*
sinus bradycardia
  care transitions, 151
  clinical presentation, 147–150
  diagnosis, 147–150
  epidemiology, 147
  initial management, 150
  pathophysiology, 147
  triage, 150
sinus tachycardia (ST), 138
SIRS. *See* systemic inflammatory response
    syndrome
situation debriefing model, 64*t*
Six Sigma, 18
skilled nursing facility (SNF), 579
  advanced care planning, 580–582
  common clinical issues, 582
  deconditioning care transitions and, 519
  infection control, 582
  interdisciplinary care, 579–580
  Medicare and, 581*t*
  physician responsibilities in, 580*t*
  transitional care, 579
skin disorders
  associated with ESRD, 468
  of frail older adults, 565
skin infections
  adjunctive therapies and, 303–304
  anatomical correlations, 300*t*
  care transitions, 307
  clinical presentation, 301–304
  diagnosis, 301–304
  disease management strategies,
    304–307
  empiric antibiotic selection and, 303*t*
  epidemiology, 300–301
  microbiology, 301
  pathophysiology, 301
  predisposing factors, 301*t*
sleep apnea. *See* obstructive sleep apnea
small bowel obstruction (SBO)
  causes, 248*t*
  clinical presentation, 248–249
  diagnosis, 248–249
  disease management strategies, 250
  epidemiology, 247

initial management, 249–250
pathophysiology, 247–248
triage, 249–250
SMOG, 74, 75*t*
smoking
   COPD and, 402
   pharmacotherapy for cessation of, 406*t*
   PPCs and, 589
smoking cessation counseling
   asthma management and, 401
   cardiovascular disease and, 158
   HF and, 164
   homosexuality and, 561
   ischemic stroke management and, 333
   postoperative, 608
SNF. *See* skilled nursing facility
social history, of frail older adults, 564
social workers, 580
Society for Healthcare Epidemiology of
   America (SHEA), 295
Society of Hospital Medicine (SHM), 15
   discharge checklist of, 70
   formation of, 1
   management and, 47
   patient education and, 72
   research and, 100
   support, 49
   TCC and, 10
   Wachter and, 4
Society of Thoracic Surgeons (STS), 197
sodium. *See also* hypernatremia;
   hyponatremia
   acid-base disorder diagnosis and,
      470–472
   in intravenous fluids, 479*t*
   water balance, 478*f*
sodium bicarbonate, 493
soft tissue infections
   adjunctive therapies and, 303–304
   anatomical correlations, 300*t*
   care transitions, 307
   clinical presentation, 301–304
   diagnosis, 301–304
   disease management strategies,
      304–307
   empiric antibiotic selection and, 303*t*
   epidemiology, 300–301
   microbiology, 301
   pathophysiology, 301
solitary rectal ulcers, 257
SORT. *See* Strength of Recommendation
   Taxonomy
SPARCS database. *See* Statewide Planning
   and Research Cooperative Systems
   database
specificity, 92–93, 92*f*
   of cardiac stress testing, 118*t*
   false positives and, 94
spheres of influence, 354*f*

spinal cord compression. *See* epidural
   spinal cord compression
spirituality
   communication and, 551–552
   distress, 547–548
   role of, 552*t*
spirometry, 396
   classifications in, 411*t*
   stable COPD and, 403
splenectomy, 263
splenic sequestration
   crisis, 264
   treatment, 265
spontaneous breathing trials (SBT),
   444–445
sputum for Gram culture, 416
SSIs. *See* surgical site infections
SSRIs. *See* selective serotonin reuptake
   inhibitors
ST. *See* sinus tachycardia
staffing
   medication reconciliation and, 29
   splitting of, 359
standardization
   care transition efficiency and, 61
   of discharge, 71
   of discharge summaries, 69
   of handoffs, 65–66
   lack of, 22
Staphylococcal aureus, 282. *See also*
   methicillin-resistant *Staphylococcal*
   aureus
   catheter removal and, 296
   methicillin and, 284
Statewide Planning and Research
   Cooperative Systems (SPARCS)
   database, 559
statins
   noncardiac surgery and, 588
   VT management and, 155
statistical significance, 85–86
statisticians, 101
ST-elevation myocardial infarction
   (STEMI), 121–122
   complications, 123*t*
   therapies, 122*t*
stent placement, 97
stool cultures
   colitis and, 227–228
   hemoccult positive, 232
Strength of Recommendation Taxonomy
   (SORT), 83
Streptococcus milleri, 430
Streptococcus pneumoniae, 339
stress testing
   for ACS, 126*t*
   alternatives to, 119*t*
   cardiac, 117
   cardiac, with imaging, 118

   contraindications to, 119*t*
   limitations to, 119*t*
   practice guideline on, 117*t*
stress tests, 108
stroke. *See also* ischemic stroke
   CCU hyperglycemia and, 196
   common medications, 334*t*
   definition, 328
   noncardiac surgery and, 591
   SCD and, 264, 266–267
structure measures, 43
STS. *See* Society of Thoracic Surgeons
studies, 88
   of EBM, 83–85
subarachnoid hemorrhage (SAH), 335
substance abuse. *See also* alcohol abuse;
   drug abuse
   behavioral disturbances and, 356
   at discharge, 71
   suicide and, 384
suffering, intractable, 549
suicidal patients
   care transitions, 387
   characteristics, 383*t*
   clinical presentation, 383–386
   diagnosis, 383–386
   epidemiology, 383
   management strategies, 386–387
   risk factors, 383*t*
suicide
   assessment, 385*t*
   attempts, 385
   medicolegal issues and, 386–387
   prevention, 386
   risk factors, 384–385
summaries, 88
support groups, 372
supraventricular tachycardia (SVT)
   acute treatment of, 144*t*
   care transitions, 146
   clinical presentation, 138–139
   diagnosis, 138–139
   ECG tracing in, 141–143*f*
   epidemiology, 137
   initial management, 139–144
   long-term management, 145*f*
   management strategies, 145–146
   mechanism of, 138*f*
   pathophysiology, 137–138
   syncope management and, 174
   triage, 139–144
   VT *v.,* 154
   wide complex, 139
surgery. *See also* noncardiac surgery
   improving, 19
   postoperative complications, 604
   preoperative screening tests,
      elective, 600*t*
   SCD and, 267

surgery (*Cont.*):
  SCM and, 612
  VTE prophylaxis in, 497–498
  VTE risk factors, 499*t*
surgical comanagement (SCM), 611
  agreement for, 613
  building, 612–614
  consultation *v.*, 611–612
  ethical pitfalls, 612
  outcome measures, 614*t*
  protocol considerations, 613*t*
  value of, 612
surgical consultation, infection and, 302
surgical site infections (SSIs), 306, 605–607
  antibiotics for, 607*t*
  postoperative fever and, 606*t*
  risk factors, 607*t*
SVT. *See* supraventricular tachycardia
swimming, meningitis and, 341
symptom management, palliative care
    and, 539
synchronized intermittent mandatory
    ventilation (SIMV), 440
syncope
  care transitions, 174
  causes of, 169*t*
  clinical presentation, 168–170
  diagnosis, 168–170
  diagnosis algorithm, 171*f*
  disease management strategies, 173–174
  ECG findings and, 172*t*
  epidemiology, 168
  indications for hospitalization, 170*t*
  initial management, 170–173
  neurocardiogenic, 170
  neurological causes of, 173
  pathophysiology, 168
  seizures and, 346
  survival, 169*f*
  triage, 170–173
syndrome of inappropriate antidiuretic
    hormone (SIADH), 479
  causes of, 479*t*
  hyponatremia management and, 482
systematic reviews, 84–85
systemic inflammatory response syndrome
    (SIRS)
  CAP triage and, 413–415
  infection and, 433
  sepsis and, 432
systemic thromboembolism, 135
systems, 88
  organization and improvement, 6
  specialists, 13
systems improvement
  discharge, 71
  for handoffs, 65–67
  medication reconciliation process and,
      26–29

systolic dysfunction
  care transitions, 165–167
  clinical presentation, 160–161
  diagnosis, 160–161
  disease management strategies, 164–165
  epidemiology, 159
  heart failure due to, 159–167
  initial management, 57–60
  pathophysiology, 159–160
  triage, 57–60

T
T3. *See* triiodothyronine
T4. *See* thyroxine
tachycardia, 128–129*t*. *See also specific types*
  diagnosis of, 140*t*
  diastolic HF and, 157
tamponade physiology, 111
TB. *See* tuberculosis
TBW. *See* total body water
TCC. *See The Core Competencies in
    Hospital Medicine*
teachers
  attributes of, 616*t*
  hospitalist as, 8, 615
teaching
  bedside, 619–620
  in clinical settings, 622*t*
  clinical skills, 622–623
  conference room, 618–619, 619*t*
  educational portfolio and, 632
  feedback, 626
  five-step microskills, 623*t*
  goals, 632
  leadership and, 621
  learner heterogeneity and, 619
  materials, 618
  microskills model of, 623–624
  mobile classroom and, 620
  scholarship and, 627–628
  self-directed learning and, 624
  self-reflection on, 620–621
  styles, 622
  teamwork and, 620, 621–624
  techniques, 618–619
  training-level-specific, 622*t*
  venues, 617–621
team-based care models, 55–56
teamwork, 53. *See also* multidisciplinary
    team
  care transitions and, 56
  effective *v.* ineffective, 55*t*
  error reduction and, 20
  in healthcare, 53–54
  leadership and, 624
  model, 55*f*
  patient safety and, 56
  promoting, 54
  teaching and, 620, 621–624

technology, diffusion of, 560
TEE. *See* transesophageal
    echocardiography
telemetry monitoring, 131
temporal lobe, simple partial seizures,
    345*t*
temporary mechanical circulatory
    assistance, 163
tendons, deconditioning and, 516
tenesmus, 236
TENS. *See* transcutaneous electrical nerve
    stimulation
terminal restlessness, 548, 549*t*
test results
  abnormal, 78–79, 599
  centralized, 78
  continuous, 599
  at discharge, 76
  follow-ups, 76
  high-risk, 78–79
  information systems-based, 79
  physician awareness of, 77
  post-discharge cases, 79*t*, 80*t*
  post-discharge management system,
      77–80, 78*f*
  responsibility for, 77–78
  summary points, 79*t*
testing. *See also* lab tests; preoperative
    screening tests
  of cirrhosis, 221*t*
  cycles, 20
  for endocarditis, 285
  HTN emergencies and, 177
  measurements for evaluating, 92–95
  pancreatitis diagnosis and, 243
  of portal hypertension, 221*t*
  rational use of, 95–96
  shotgun approach to, 92
THC, abuse management, 382
thecal sac, 575
theophylline, 401
  perioperative medication management
      and, 596
therapeutic debridement, 33
therapists, SNF and, 580
thoracic aortic dissection, 110
Thorazine. *See* chlorpromazine
three-tier design, 16
  human error and, 17–18
thrombocytopenia
  care transitions, 271
  clinical evaluation, 270*f*
  clinical presentation, 269
  diagnosis, 269
  disease management strategies, 270–271
  epidemiology, 268
  initial management, 269–270
  LGI bleeding and, 258
  noncardiac surgery and, 591

pathophysiology, 268–269
primary HIV-associated, 271
triage, 269–270
thromboembolism
AF care transitions and, 135–136
CHADS2 score and, 136t
FUO and, 279
thrombolysis, 504
in STEMI, 123t
thrombolysis in myocardial infarction
(TIMI)
in-hospital mortality and, 122t
risk score, 121, 124f
thrombolytic agents, 507
thrombolytic therapy, 331
thromboplastin reagents, 509
thrombosis, 507
thrombotic thrombocytopenic purpura-
hemolytic uremic syndrome
(TTP-HUS), 270
thyroid disease, 187
thyroid gland, 205
thyroid nodular disease, 210
thyroid peroxidase antibody (TPO
antibody), 209
thyroid storm, 205–206, 207
thyroidectomy, 207
thyroid-stimulating hormone (TSH), 205
thyroid nodular disease and, 210
thyrotoxicosis, 207
thyrotropin, 147
thyroxine (T4), 205
TIA. See transient ischemic attack
tidal volumes, 441
time
constraints, 54
frail older adults and, 563
TIMI. See thrombolysis in myocardial
infarction
tissue-type plasminogen activator (tPA),
331
TLS. See tumor lysis syndrome (TLS)
To Err Is Human: Building a Safer
System, 21
LOS and, 57
patient safety and, 36
toluene, 474t
tolvaptan, 482
torsades de pointes, 153
drugs that cause, 153t
therapy, 155
total body water (TBW), 477
total parenteral nutrition (TPN), 521
calculation of, 525t
pancreatitis triage and, 245
prescription, 525–526
toxic inhalants, 382
toxic shock syndrome, 306–307
influenza management and, 299

toxicology testing
drug abuse diagnosis and, 380
drug overdose and, 362
Toyota Lean, 18
tPA. See tissue-type plasminogen activator
TPN. See total parenteral nutrition
TPO antibody. See thyroid peroxidase
antibody
TPR. See true positive rate
training, 53
discharge, 71
transaminases, 218t
transcutaneous electrical nerve stimulation
(TENS), 531
transesophageal echocardiography (TEE),
285
catheter removal and, 296
transfusion
acute hemolytic, 276
adverse effects of, 273t
anemia and, 263, 272, 277
care transitions, 277
clinical presentation, 275–276
diagnosis, 275–276
disease management strategies, 276–277
epidemiology, 272
indications for, 274–275
initial management, 276
pathophysiology, 272–273
patients refusing, 277t
platelet, 274–275
platelet, triggers, 275t
postoperative fever and, 606t
risks of, 273–274
SCD guidelines, 267
triage, 276
trigger, 274
transient ischemic attack (TIA), 328–329.
See also ischemic stroke
care transitions, 333
disease management strategies, 332–333
seizures and, 346
transitional care, 579
transmural inflammation, 232
transtentorial herniation, 337
transthoracic echocardiography (TTE),
285–286
transtubular potassium gradient (TTKG),
485
travel
FUO and, 281
meningitis and, 341
treatment refusal
algorithm, 351f
competency assessment and, 352
tricyclics
overdose, 370–371
perioperative medication management
and, 597–598

trifascicular blocks, 149
triggers, identifying ADEs and, 22
triiodothyronine (T3), 205
troponin, 115
elevated, 116t
true positive rate (TPR), 92
TSH. See thyroid-stimulating
hormone
TTE. See transthoracic echocardiography
TTKG. See transtubular potassium
gradient
TTP-HUS. See thrombotic
thrombocytopenic purpura-hemolytic
uremic syndrome
tube feeds
aspiration and, 524
diarrhea and, 525
enteral access, 524
initiating and advancing, 524–525
intolerance, 523
tuberculosis (TB), 292
tumor lysis syndrome (TLS), 447–448
tumors
epidural spinal cord compression and,
575–576
SBO and, 247
12-step groups, 372
typhlitis, 224t

U
UAG. See urine anion gap
UC. See ulcerative colitis
UGI bleeding. See upper gastrointestinal
bleeding
UH. See unfractionated heparin
UHC. See University HealthSystem
Consortium
ulcer disease, 254
ulcerative colitis (UC), 231
care transitions, 239–240
clinical presentation, 236–237
conditions that mimic, 237t
Crohn's disease v., 233
diagnosis, 236–237
disease management strategies,
238–239
epidemiology, 235–236
initial management, 237–238
pathophysiology, 236
triage, 237–238
ulcers. See also pressure ulcers
diabetic foot infections and, 304
perforated peptic, 215
ultrasound
abdominal pain and, 214
acalculous cholecystitis
ARF diagnosis and, 455
pancreatitis diagnosis and, 244
pleural effusion and, 427–430

unfractionated heparin (UH), 496–497
  drug action, 509
  nomogram, 510t
  in prophylaxis, 509
  in treatment, 509–510
University HealthSystem Consortium
    (UHC), 10
  wRVU and, 49
unnecessary days, 58
unstable angina (UA), 120, 122–124
upper gastrointestinal (UGI) bleeding, 251
  bleeding survey, 253t
  causes of, 253–254
  criteria, 252t
  initial evaluation, 251–252
  predictors for, 252t
  recurrent, 253t, 254–255
  risk stratification, 252–253
  Rockall scoring system for, 253t
  treatment of, 254–255
upper GI evaluation, 259
urinalysis
  acid-base disorder diagnosis and,
    470–472
  CKD diagnosis and, 460–461
  findings in ARF, 454t
  preoperative testing and, 602
  secondary HTN and, 186
urinary retention, opioid-induced, 544
urinary tract infections (UTIs)
  antibiotic-resistant pathogens and, 311
  clinical presentation, 290–293
  complications, 293
  diagnosis, 290–293
  epidemiology, 289
  infection control, 293
  management, 290–293
  nosocomial catheter-associated,
    291–292
  pathophysiology, 289–290
  prevention, 293–294
  upper, 291
urine alkalization, 363t
urine anion gap (UAG), 472
uropathogens, 293
U.S. Prevention Services Task Force
    (USPSTF), 82–83, 90
*User's Guide to the Medical Literature:
    Essential of Evidence-Based Clinical
    Practice* (Guyatt & Rennie), 89
USPSTF. *See* U.S. Prevention Services
    Task Force
utilization management, 9
UTIs. *See* urinary tract infections

V
vaccination
  contraindications to, 300
  influenza, 299t

  NHDR and, 560–561
  SNF and, 582
vagal maneuvers, 139
vaginal estrogens, 293–294
vaginal irritation, 290
vancomycin
  antibiotic resistance and, 312
  colitis management and, 229
  for endocarditis, 288
  indications for, 574t
  neutropenic fever and, 574
vancomycin-resistant enterococci (VRE),
    312–313
  control issues, 314
VAP. *See* ventilator-associated pneumonia
vasodilation, sepsis and, 433
vaso-occlusive conditions, 264
vasopressors, 127
  in sepsis triage, 435
venous thromboembolism (VTE)
  anticoagulant therapy, 505t
  clinical presentation, 502–503
  diagnosis, 502–503
  discharge follow-up, 504–506
  epidemiology, 494, 501
  implement gap, 497–500
  initial management, 503–506
  initial therapy, 504t
  pathophysiology, 501–502
  pretest probability, 502t
  prevention, in surgical patients, 495t
  prophylaxis, in hospitalized patients,
    499t
  prophylaxis modalities, 496–497
  prophylaxis of, 7, 10, 507
  public agency initiatives related to, 495t
  risk assessment tools, 495–496
  risk factors for developing, 495
  risk factors, in surgical patients, 499t
  risk stratification, 503
  scope of, in hospital patients, 494–496
  systems improvement, 500
  therapy, 503–504
  triage, 503–506
ventilator-associated pneumonia (VAP)
  care transitions, 425t
  clinical presentation, 423
  common pathogens, 424t
  diagnosis, 423
  disease management strategies, 424–426
  epidemiology, 422–423
  initial empiric antibiotics for, 425t
  initial management, 423–424
  pathophysiology, 423
  triage, 423–424
ventilators, 440t
ventilatory support, 438
ventricular arrhythmias
  clinical presentation, 152–154

  diagnosis, 152–154
  epidemiology, 152
  pathophysiology, 152
ventricular dyssynchrony, 167
ventricular ectopy, 155
ventricular fibrillation (VF), 152, 154. *See
    also* ventricular
    tachycardia/ventricular fibrillation
ventricular premature complexes
    (VPCs), 152
  initial management, 155
ventricular tachycardia (VT)
  disease management strategies, 155–156
  ECG favoring, 154f
  initial management, 155
  non-sustained, 153t
  non-sustained *v.* sustained, 153
  polymorphic, 155
  stable monomorphic, 155
  SVT *v.*, 154
  syncope management and, 173
  triage, 155
ventricular tachycardia/ventricular
    fibrillation (VT/VF), 127, 128t
verification bias, 119t
VF. *See* ventricular fibrillation
video-assisted thorascopic surgery
    (VATS), 431
viral gastroenteritis, 308
Virchow's Triad, 495t
viruses
  colon infections, 226t
  FUO and, 279
vision, of frail older adults, 565
vitamin K, 337t
vitamins, 522
  perioperative medication management
    and, 599
volume cycling, 439–440
volume repletion, 449–450
vomiting
  appendicitis and, 214
  ICH and, 336
  opioid-related, 542–543
  treatment, 543t
VPCs. *See* ventricular premature
    complexes
V/Q scanning, 391
VRE. *See* vancomycin-resistant
    enterococci
VT. *See* ventricular tachycardia
VTE. *See* venous thromboembolism
VT/VF (ventricular fibrillation), 124
VT/VF. *See* ventricular tachycardia/
    ventricular fibrillation
vulnerable populations, 557
  attitudes for, 561–562, 561t
  disparities among, 559–560
  in hospital settings, 560t

outcomes, 558–559
process of care of, 558
skills and practices, 560–561, 561t

W

Wachter, Robert, 4
warfarin
  cerebral hemorrhage algorithm, 338f
  cerebral hemorrhage triage and, 338
  drug action, 508
  fresh frozen plasma and, 275
  ischemic stroke management and, 333
  in prophylaxis, 508
  systolic HF management and, 165
  in treatment, 508–509
water, 522. *See also* hydration;
    hypernatremia; hyponatremia
  sodium balance, 478f
WBC count. *See* white blood cell count
WCT. *See* wide complex tachycardia
weight loss, SNF and, 583

Wernicke-Korsakoff syndrome, 357
Wernicke's encephalopathy, 375–376
white blood cell (WBC) count
  diverticulitis diagnosis and, 241
  endocarditis and, 286
  preoperative testing of, 600
white papers, 102
WHO. *See* World Health Organization
wide complex tachycardia (WCT),
    154, 154f
withdrawal
  alcohol abuse and, 374
  behavioral disturbances and, 357
  dyspnea diagnosis and, 389
  prophylaxis, 376–377
  syndromes, 374–376
  treatment, 377–379
Wolf-Parkinson-White (WPW)
    syndrome, 132t
work relative value unites (wRVU), 49
workflow structures, 56

work-hour restrictions, 8
  residents, 10
workup bias. *See* verification bias
World Health Organization (WHO)
  herbal supplements and, 371
  ladder, 540
WPW syndrome. *See* Wolf-Parkinson-
    White syndrome
written research protocol, 101t
wRVU. *See* work relative value unites

X

xanthogranulomatous pyelonephritis
    (XGP), 292
XGP. *See* xanthogranulomatous
    pyelonephritis
x-rays. *See also* chest radiography;
    radiography
  abdominal pain and, 212
  epidural spinal cord compression
    and, 577